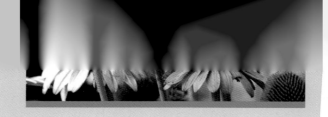

BOTANICAL MEDICINE FOR WOMEN'S HEALTH

SECOND EDITION

AVIVA ROMM, MD

Forewords by:

MARY L. HARDY, MD
Simms/Mann-UCLA Center for Integrative Oncology
University of California
Los Angeles, California

SIMON MILLS, MCPP, FNIMH, MA
Peninsula School of Medicine
Plymouth University
Plymouth, Devon, United Kingdom

ELSEVIER

ELSEVIER

3251 Riverport Lane
St. Louis, Missouri 63043

BOTANICAL MEDICINE FOR WOMEN'S HEALTH, SECOND EDITION ISBN: 978-0-7020-6193-6

Notices

Library of Congress Cataloging-in-Publication Data
Names: Romm, Aviva Jill, author.
Title: Botanical medicine for women's health / Aviva Romm ; forewords by Mary
    L. Hardy, Simon Mills.
Description: Second edition. | St. Louis, Missouri : Elsevier, [2017] |
    Includes bibliographical references.
Identifiers: LCCN 2016029888 | ISBN 978-0-7020-6193-6 (pbk. : alk. paper)
Subjects: | MESH: Genital Diseases, Female--drug therapy | Phytotherapy |
    Women's Health | Pregnancy
Classification: LCC RC48.6 | NLM WP 140 | DDC 615/.321082--dc23 LC record
available at https://lccn.loc.gov/2016029888

Senior Content Strategist: Linda Woodard
Content Development Manager: Luke Held
Content Development Specialist: Kathleen Nahm
Publishing Services Manager: Hemamalini Rajendrababu
Project Manager: Janish Ashwin Paul
Design Direction: Renee Duenow

Printed in India

Last digit is the print number: 18   17   16   15   14   13   12

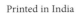

This book is dedicated to all those who have given their lives
to health freedom, to all women ready for a change in health care,
and to all practitioners willing to make those changes.
And to the plants, and the people who have trusted me
with them - you have been my primary teachers.

FOREWORD

Botanical Medicine for Women's Health is being published at an interesting time and speaks simultaneously to a number of converging constituencies. It is a time of growing stress on both the medical system and the patient. Medical care is in crisis with large numbers of underinsured or uninsured patients needing care. Costs are rising from the practice of increasingly technical medicine while patients are unhappy with of the decreasing time and attention they are receiving from their medical providers. Further, the burden of chronic disease is growing in an aging population. In one response to these stressors, patient interest is forcing inclusion of alternative medicines and philosophies into mainstream practice. However, in the case of herbal medicine, incorporation into conventional medicine would represent the return to (pardon the pun) the deepest roots of our own medical tradition.

The lineage of herbal medicine is long, distinguished, and of great importance to Western medical tradition. Herbal medicine has been a significant component of an array of healing systems beginning early on with those of Egypt, Mesopotamia, Greece, and Islam and continuing through the development of medical practice in medieval and modern Europe. Traditional medical practices from Asia and India, as well as Aboriginal traditions on every continent, have also used extensive herbal pharmacopeias. Many of our modern pharmaceutical drugs owe their origins to herbal medicine, with more than one hundred of the most commonly used drugs derived directly or indirectly from plants.

It is particularly appropriate that this book focuses on the herbal treatment of women's conditions. Historically, women, when given the opportunity to train in medical professions or to operate as lay practitioners, often focused their care on women and their children—either by choice or necessity. Often the transmission of this tradition was suppressed or marginalized and women had to use the products of the natural world around them rather than the often more toxic products favored by their conventional counterparts. Thus women's medicine, overseen by female goddesses like Isis or practiced by female practitioners such as Hildegard of Bingen, was largely based on herbal therapies. In fact, rarely were the contributions of these female herbalists recognized by conventional medical history. So, for example, the "discovery" of foxglove as a treatment for cardiac conditions is attributed to Sir William Withering and his source, the old lady of Shropshire, is largely forgotten. Thus I am particularly satisfied that this important herbal textbook is giving serious and scholarly consideration to this traditional practice.

But herbal medicine is not a dead or esoteric art. The World Health Organization estimates that 80% of people in developing countries depend on herbal medicine and traditional practitioners for their primary care. As people migrate from their countries of origin to more industrialized areas, they often bring their traditional practices with them. In modern industrial countries, at least 20% to 30% of people regularly use herbal medicines. For certain conditions, such as HIV, cancer, or other chronic diseases, the numbers have reportedly been much higher. Underinsured patients often substitute herbs or dietary supplements for drugs because of poor access to care or cost of therapy.

These statistics and examples reflect the trend of incorporating traditional healing systems into modern life, moving from self-treatment of self-limiting illness to the care of chronic and more serious medical conditions. Despite the fact that these users are also active consumers of conventional medical services, they often do not disclose their use of herbal medications to their medical practitioners. This withholding arises from a number of causes. Often cited by patients is the belief that most physicians will react negatively to the use of natural products, or worse, that physicians are not knowledgeable about the natural products patients are interested in.

Ironically, despite the fact that herbalists have been advising patients on the use of phytomedicines for millennia and patients are increasing their use of herbal products, herbal practitioners in North America have not generally been incorporated into conventional medical practice. These practitioners and their practices have been largely invisible to the conventional system for a variety of reasons. Patients may self-prescribe from an exploding array of natural health products without the benefit of consultation with an herbalist. In traditional medical systems, other components may be more recognized than the herbal therapy. For example, considering Traditional Chinese Medicine as practiced in the West, acupuncture is better known and more broadly used than Chinese herbal medicine. Most importantly, in the United States the practice of herbal medicine is variable, eclectic, and without standardization or licensure. Whether or not the development of standard herbal practice would represent a desirable outcome, it is a fact that much of the public and most conventional medical practitioners are largely uninformed about what constitutes appropriate training for herbalists and what their appropriate scope of practice should be.

Thus the clash of cultures and lack of understanding inherent in the crisis of our current medical system offer our greatest opportunity. We will need our traditional knowledge to care for our aging population. Our traditional practitioners will have the opportunity to become more closely integrated into the conventional medical model and thus reach a broader array of patients. Better communication between paradigms and practitioners is crucial if we are going to meet the needs of our patients and address the growing problems in our medical system. This book, and hopefully others like it, will aid this process by contributing to our mutual understanding. The careful explication of the practice of traditional herbal medicine will be valuable to conventional practitioners attempting to fill their knowledge gaps and advise their patients appropriately. On the other hand, the inclusion of information from the Western conventional paradigm, especially involving physiology or conventional treatment, will help orient the traditional practitioner to more conventional medical concerns.

It is my hope that in the crisis of modern medicine, we all take the opportunity this book offers to learn from other systems and perhaps reclaim some of the values that have always been at the heart of the practice of the art of medicine.

Mary L. Hardy, MD
Simms/Mann-UCLA Center for Integrative Oncology,
University of California, Los Angeles, California

FOREWORD

There is a significant gap in modern health care and *Botanical Medicine for Women's Health* goes a long way to fill it. There are many illnesses that women may suffer from that are inadequately addressed by modern medical advances. These deficiencies are both specific to the types of health problems involved and also to a wider shift in the direction of health care since the Industrial Revolution.

For most of history, medicine was overwhelmingly women's work. People in traditional hunter-gatherer and pastoral societies, the background to the vast majority of human experience, consistently associated child-rearing, food preparation, and health care as a continuum of services most ably performed by women. Women shared their experiences of menstruation, pregnancy, and child care almost exclusively; men very rarely understood how to handle cases when problems arose. Women understood the plants in their environment and appreciated their roles as foods and remedies. Whereas men were visible as shamans or priests, anecdotal accounts often suggested that the "wise woman" performed a popular service.

Medicine in those far-off times may now seem primitive and ineffective. There is much in *Botanical Medicine for Women's Health* that should cause us to rethink this impression. On the other hand, there are many women who could say that modern medicine is primitive and ineffective. If you have painful or erratic periods, disabling premenstrual symptoms, endometriosis, chronic pelvic inflammation, or cystic ovaries and are only offered the dictative regime of hormones, the sad prescription of antidepressants or tranquillizers, or the erratic and intrusive prospects of surgery, you may think those options need modernizing. If in pregnancy you are one of many for whom a rich life change is encroached upon by the demands of hospitalized obstetrics rather than nurtured in a relationship with an autonomous midwife, you may really feel the loss of something fundamental in health care. If in the upheavals immediately after birth you find yourself alone to cope, you could be forgiven for wondering how sophisticated modern medicine really is. The days when male doctors routinely diagnosed hysteria for any woman's problem they could not understand may now happily be past, but there are still occasional gynecologists who recommend precautionary hysterectomies on the basis that "you will not miss it." Fortunately, there is a refreshing feminizing of medicine today. There are many more women's wellness centers. In some countries, most medical students are now women. However, the techniques available for women doctors to use in women's health care are still blunt.

Perhaps there is still value in reviewing approaches to women's ill health that were developed by women and among women. We can be sure that, over the centuries, many of these approaches emerged because they appeared to work and were reinforced by other women's experiences. Lack of fertility, for example, was such a dire prospect for women that it is not surprising that genuinely interesting remedies emerged: To discover that it is possible with some plants to facilitate long-term regulation of the menstrual cycle is truly exciting. The relief of pain and suffering in pelvic conditions that stubbornly resist other medical treatments is immensely rewarding. To find alternatives for emotional and mental anguish can bring transformation. Women's empirical discoveries included plants that we now know contain potentially modulatory steroidal molecules and other components with prehormonal activity. Some appear to reduce pain and spasm in the womb and other organs. Most old remedies worked softly, apparently in rhythm with the woman's body, mind, and spirit, rather than imposing change. Early women's medicine emphasized remedies that were interactive with functions that we now understand are wonderfully complex and interactive. Most importantly, the techniques were embedded in a world where women themselves created the language of care.

In a modern Western context, it is only recently that those who understand the old remedies have found the voice they deserve. This book has brought together the voices of those practitioners who have worked for years with women in real need. They have learned the hard way what does and does not work. Yes, there are midwife herbalists here, too. That they can bring their years of experience into engagement with modern standards is wonderful. That women at last have an opportunity to rediscover their legacies and well-trodden paths to improved wellness is a cause for celebration.

Simon Mills, MCPP, FNIMH, MA
Peninsula School of Medicine, Plymouth University,
Plymouth, Devon, United Kingdom

Judgments about which phenomena are worth studying, which kinds of data are significant, as well as which descriptions (or theories) of those phenomena are most adequate, satisfying, useful, even reliable, depend critically upon the social, linguistic, and scientific practices of those making the judgment in question.

Evelyn Fox Keller, PhD

Intuition without knowledge is only so valuable. Knowledge without intuition is just a bunch of facts. Knowledge with intuition starts us on our way to wisdom.

Tieraona Low Dog, MD

Women, even those in western nations with access to the best modern medicine has to offer, are drawn to using herbal medicines for a variety of reasons that are important to comprehend if we are both to understand our clients/patients, and if we are to understand some of the deficits of modern medicine that perhaps could be fortified into a more cohesive system that truly meets women's needs physically, emotionally, and spiritually; as we now know, healing encompasses all levels.

One key reason women choose botanical medicines is a desire for a greater level of personal empowerment than is typically engendered by conventional medical care. Botanicals represent a path that is outside of conventional medicine, using self-selected remedies or those recommended by a practitioner who has usually taken the time to investigate the whole of the woman's experience—this is a hallmark of the more "holistic" model of the type of practitioner more apt to be knowledgeable of botanicals. Though conventional medical education has begun to place a greater emphasis on patient-centered care and a collaborative model, in reality, most doctors are too busy to engage personally, inquisitively, and for any length of time with their patients, leading women who visit the doctor's office to feel unheard. Further, most doctors just do not have enough knowledge of natural medicines, nor time to discuss them, leaving patients to seek this information on their own, either through visits to more naturally oriented health care providers such as naturopathic doctors and acupuncturists, who provide an important role in the greater health care system, or to the Internet, which is not always a reliable source.

Another reason women are interested in using herbal medicines as part of their health care plan is the very reasonable desire to avoid potentially harmful or overly aggressive medical interventions whenever possible. Research is revealing reason for concern, as emerging data highlights the potentially serious risks of using common medications like NSAIDs and statins, the latter particularly problematic in women, even at normally recommended doses and durations. Overuse of surgical interventions from hysterectomies to cesarean sections is also a concern.

Many want a deeper sense of connection to the natural world as part of their healing process, and want an eco-friendlier health choice. Natural foods and botanical medicines as therapies leave a much lower carbon footprint than conventional therapies.

Statistics demonstrate that women are the greatest consumers of complementary and alternative (CAM) therapies, including herbal medicines, and that they are willing to pay out-of-pocket for both practitioners and products that they believe will provide what they are seeking. Herb sales in the US alone are currently estimated at approximately $5 billion per year.

THE NEED FOR THIS BOOK

It is my belief that one goal of health care providers should be to serve as a resource for our patients, easing the onus that so typically falls to the patient to not only be sick, but to become an expert in their own care regarding any number of conditions and treatments available to them on the vast menu of medical or alternative choices. Although medical curricula and practices are rapidly expanding to accommodate consumer demand for a more expansive menu therapies, it is challenging for the primary care provider to sort through the surfeit of books, magazines, and medical journal articles available on botanical medicines to determine what is safe and efficacious for patients. Yet the responsibility of learning about these therapies is accepted by the committed practitioner to help patients (many of whom are already using botanical products) make the best choices for effectiveness, safety, product quality, and affordability. A practitioner who is a constant, active learner and critical thinker is able to relieve a tremendous pressure from their patients, allowing them to focus instead on the work of being ill and healing, to whatever capacity possible.

Botanical Medicine for Women's Health strives to offer a realistic appraisal of the therapeutic possibilities of botanical medicines for women in a comprehensive and easily accessible format. Herbal medicines are not universally effective nor are they always the appropriate primary treatment, but they can be an important part of an integrative approach to patient care, and for certain common, mild to moderate, self-limiting, or chronic conditions may be an appropriate initial approach.

Every patient has the right to accurate information about her options. There is a tremendous amount that remains unknown about botanical medicines, as well as women's reproductive conditions. We know very little, for example, about the interactions between plants and the endocrine system. We also know very little about common gynecologic conditions, for example, what causes endometriosis, chronic pelvic pain, or uterine fibroids. We do know that many conventional treatments currently being utilized are not supported by evidence of long-term efficacy or safety—for example, the treatment of chronic pelvic pain with hysterectomy—and that the search for safe and effective alternatives to many gynecologic treatments is necessary and justified. This book compiles information on traditional and contemporary herbal practices associated with many of the most common gynecologic and obstetric problems women face—perhaps as treatments, perhaps as possibilities for further research.

As an author, I faced innumerable challenges in presenting topics that often have very little scientific substantiation, yet are widely used by herbalists, and conversely, making meaning of data for which there is in vitro evidence or evidence in animal models, but which lacks human clinical evidence or the precedence of historical use. It is my hope that readers provide comments on the usability, value, and omissions that need to be addressed to make subsequent editions increasingly helpful and clinically relevant. The importance of elucidating, to the greatest possible extent, herbal practices that are currently being prescribed by practitioners or taken by patients via self-medication, is significant for practitioners and patients, as is the value of admitting there are unanswered questions. It is only by asking the right questions that we can begin to expect meaningful answers. This book seeks to suspend judgment and posits that separate biomedical care and botanical care find the common denominator that patients seek from their practitioner, which is simply—care. It seeks to conceptually combine the rigor of biomedical thinking, reductionism, and skepticism with the holistic, nature-trusting, biophilic orientation of the modern herbalist.

THE STRUCTURE OF BOTANICAL MEDICINE FOR WOMEN'S HEALTH

Botanical Medicine for Women's Health begins with Part I: Foundations of Botanical Medicine, which presents introductory chapters on the recent evolution of integrative care in the United States, the role of botanical medicines in this evolution and in clinical practice, the history of botanical medicines for women, and the principles of botanical medicine including safety, formulation and dosing, identification of quality products, and forms of preparation and administration. Understanding the principles and philosophies underlying herbal medicine practice and product quality optimizes clinical success and safety with herbs; therefore it is suggested that readers review Part 1 before using this book as a quick reference text.

Part II reflects the common conditions women might face or are at risk of developing; Parts III to V describe common conditions in order of their chronology in women's reproductive life cycles from menarche through general gynecology, into childbearing, and finally onto perimenopause/menopause. Each section reviews both the relevant medical background of the condition, and commonly available traditional and evidence-based botanical treatments. Although the review of the literature for this textbook was exhaustive, and has been updated through 2015 in this current edition, obscure and difficult-to-obtain botanicals, and those with promising yet extremely scant research, were omitted for practical reasons for the user.

Chapters follow a standard format, facilitating the book's use as a clinical reference or classroom text. It was tempting to rank each herb for its "level of evidence," or to present them in some hierarchical scheme; however, the current ranking schemes, although quite useful for those seeking to practice within a narrow range of what is considered "acceptable evidence," lend a bias against the use of herbs at all for some conditions, and limit the use of herbs severely for other conditions, simply because of lack of certain forms of evidence, when in many cases, the research has simply not been done. Therefore it was ultimately decided to present the herbs alphabetically, and allow the reader to make her/his determination of what to use based on the reader's own values in ranking of evidence. Readers will be informed when use of an herb is predicated on traditional or historical use alone and when there is scientific evidence.

At the end of the book the reader will find useful dosing information consolidated into a table.

CONTRIBUTING AUTHORS

This book was, in part, made possible by the generous help of the authors whose names appear at the footer on the first page of the chapter to which they contributed in the first edition. Each is a well-respected member of the herbal, naturopathic, midwifery, or integrative medicine community. These authors freely donated their time to research and write as part of their overarching commitment that there be a greater understanding not only of botanical medicines, but of integrative healing for women. The authors of this textbook faced unique challenges in finding buried evidence to support what they know so well from the clinic. Creating language to describe an emerging paradigm is no small feat, nor is taking one paradigm and translating it into a language that others will understand and to which they can relate.

While chapters have now been substantially rewritten by the primary author of this text for the purpose of consistency, style, format, and at times to include a more comprehensive or current literature search than individual authors were able to accomplish, every attempt was made to reflect the original intention and tone of the contributors. It is with tremendous gratitude to each of these originally contributing authors that second edition was written.

IN CONCLUSION

It is my hope this text provides readers with the confidence to begin safely integrating botanical therapies for women's health into their practices, playing a small part in turning an already changing tide of medicine in a direction that includes a patient-centered, integrative approach and that respects the healing power of nature and most importantly, patient choice. The possibility that this book may bring intelligent botanical medicine guidelines into the consulting room, and a small alleviation of suffering for those women who use botanical therapies as part of their medicine, is my fondest expectation.

Aviva Romm, MD
June 18, 2016

PREFACE REFERENCES

1. Keller EF: *Refiguring life: metaphors of twentieth-century biology*, New York, 1995, Columbia University Press, pp 99–118.
2. Rabin, RC. A New women's issue: statins May 5, 2014. http://well.blogs.nytimes.com/2014/05/05/a-new-womens-issue-statins/?_r=0.
3. Mansi I, et al.: Statins and new-onset diabetes mellitus and diabetic complications: a retrospective cohort study of US healthy adults, *J Gen Intern Med*, 2015. http://dx.doi.org/10.1007/s11606-015-3335-1.
4. Shah RV, Goldfine AB. Statins and risk of new-onset diabetes mellitus. Circulation. 126:e282-e284, 2012. doi: 10.1161/CIRCULATIONAHA.112.122135.

ACKNOWLEDGMENTS

This first edition of this book took 8 years to write. The updates for the second edition another year.

Over this time a great number of people provided immeasurable support in numerous ways. My husband Tracy Romm held down the fort at home while I wrote, thought, researched, and wrote some more; my four children Iyah, Yemima, Forest, and Naomi reminded me to remember to play-often; my brainiac herbalist friend Jonathan, treasure helped to "develop my gray matter," as he'd call our conversations in which he'd challenge my ideas; and Roy Upton was a constant cheerleader on this project, fleshing out concepts, research and listening to me talk things out ad infinitum, generously sharing resources, and telling me there was nobody more qualified to write this book. Deep gratitdue to Kerry Bone and Simon Mills who helped me to get this book into the right hands for publication, and Mark Blumenthal, James Duke, and The American Botanical Council for their generous recognition of this book as the James A. Duke Best Botanical Book of 2010. Finally, Renee Davis' deep dive into the botanical literature allowed me to bring this second edition to you. *Each of you helped bring this book to the world and the tens of thousands of women who have been – and will continue to be – helped by its contents.*

This second edition of *Botanical Medicine for Women's Health* saw a consolidation of materials, a lightening of the chapter contents, and research updates to allow this version to be as clinically user friendly as possible. I extend a deep bow to the authors and co-authors of the chapters in the first edition of the book, including Kathy Abascal, Lise Alschuler, Bhaswati Bhattacharya, Mary Bove, Isla M. Burgess, Bevin Clare, Mitch Coven, Robin Dipasquale, Margi Flint, Lisa Ganora, Paula Gardiner, Wendy D. Grube, Christopher Hobbs, David Hoffmann, Sheila Humphrey, Angela J. Hywood, Laurel Lee, Roberta Anne Lee, Clara A. Lennox, Elizabeth Mazanec, Amanda McQuade Crawford, Linda Ryan, Jillian E. Stansbury, Ruth Trickey, Roy Upton, Susun S. Weed, David Winston, Eric Yarnell, and Suzanna M. Zick.

Over the past 35 years of working in women's health, a number of very special women helped me to cultivate my women's wisdom and my skills as a midwife. I particularly want to thank Sarahn Henderson, Ina May Gaskin, and Jeannine Parvati Baker (who passed away before this book was born) for inspiring and guiding me in work that has never grown old.

I also have a beautiful extended community of colleagues in the herbal and integrative medicine worlds who have added to my knowledge, my wisdom, and my success including David Winston, Mary Bove, Chanchal Cabrera, Amanda McQuade Crawford, Steven Dentali, Tieraona Low Dog, Lesley Tierra, Michael Tierra, Susun Weed, Donnie Yance, Mark Blumenthal, Robin DiPasquale, Christopher Hobbs, David Hoffmann, Jeff Jump, Ed Smith, Jill Stansbury, and Joe Betz.

In gratitude.

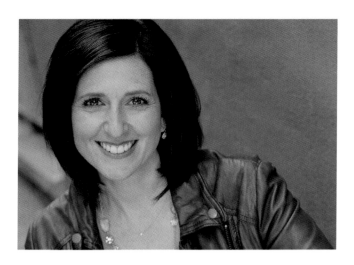

Dr. Aviva Romm, *The Women's Natural Doctor*, has bridged her training in traditional medicine and midwifery with her knowledge of hard science for over 3 decades. A midwife and herbalist for 25 years, as well as a Yale trained MD, Board Certified in Family Medicine with Obstetrics, she completed the Integrative Medicine Residency through the University of Arizona, and practiced Functional Medicine for 2 years at The UltraWellness Center with Dr. Mark Hyman.

In additional to her expertise in botanical medicine, Dr. Romm focuses on the impact of stress physiology on women's health, energy, immunity, willpower, food cravings, weight, chronic disease, and hormone imbalance. She is an avid environmental health advocate, focusing on the impact of toxins on fertility, pregnancy, women's hormones, chronic illness, and children's health.

Dr. Romm is one nation's leaders in the field of botanical medicine and is the author of seven books on natural medicine for women and children, including the first edition of *Botanical Medicine for Women's Health* which received the American Botanical Council's James Duke Award for Excellence in Botanical Writing. She is the integrative medicine curriculum author for the Yale Internal Medicine and Pediatric Residencies, is co-author of the Botanical Safety Handbook, and is the Medical Director for the American Herbal Pharmacopoeia.

She lives and practices medicine in Massachusetts and New York City, and is a nationally sought speaker, author, and consultant.

Aviva Romm, MD is a Board Certified Family Physician, certified professional midwife, herbalist, and the creator of Herbal Medicine for Women, a distance course with over 800 students around the world. An internationally respected authority on botanical and functional medicine for women and children, with 30 years of clinical experience, she is the author of seven books on natural medicine, including *Botanical Medicine for Women's Health*, winner of the American Botanical Council's James Duke Award. A graduate of Yale School of Medicine where she received the Internal Medicine Award for "outstanding academic achievement and community service," Aviva completed her internship in Internal Medicine at Yale where she was instrumental in creating the school's first integrative medicine curriculum. She completed her residency in Family Medicine at Tufts University School of Medicine. She is a member of the Advisory Board of the Yale Integrative Medicine Program, is Medical Director of the American Herbal Pharmacopoeia and Therapeutic Compendium, and sits on the expert panel of the American Herbal Products Association's Botanical Safety Handbook, Prevention Magazine, and serves on the Advisory Committee of the American Botanical Council. Dr. Romm is a leader in the revolution to transform the current medical system into one that respects the intrinsic healing capacities of the body and nature, while helping women take their health into their own hands. Dr. Romm's focus is on women's and children's health, with an emphasis on the impact of stress on health, willpower, food cravings, weight, chronic disease, and hormone imbalance. She is also an avid environmental health advocate, focusing on the impact of toxins on fertility, pregnancy, women's hormones, chronic illness, and children's health. Dr. Romm is a national leader in the field of botanical medicine and is the author of seven books on natural medicine for women and children, including the textbook *Botanical Medicine for Women's Health*, and she is the integrative medicine curriculum author for the Yale Internal Medicine and Pediatric Residencies. She lives and practices medicine in Massachusetts and NYC and is a nationally sought speaker, author, and consultant. She is a gardener, artist, and visionary physician.

TABLE OF CONTENTS

Appendices

From Complementary and Alternative Medicine to Functional Medicine
Health Care's Emerging Evolution

Aviva Romm

The U.S. medical care system is self-validating. Biomedicine is rarely viewed as a historical and cultural byproduct, but rather is considered to be entirely factual, scientific, and universal. Furthermore, many powerful groups have an interest in the maintenance of existing approaches. Nonetheless, several problems have been identified with this medical care delivery system, including issues of access, quality of care, quality of life, technology use, and costs. The conservative, self-validating nature of biomedicine places severe limits on our ability to rethink our approach to medicine and deepen innovative and viable solutions to these problems. Alternative health care systems exist as a rich readily accessible resource for testable ideas about the practice and organization of medical and health care. By virtue of their popular nature, they seem generally to be well-received, low technology, and low-cost approaches to health problems. The potential contribution of these systems to solutions for the medical care problems we face would seem to be great.

–Carol Sakala[1]

FROM ALTERNATIVE TO FUNCTIONAL MEDICINE: WHAT ARE WE TALKING ABOUT?

When I began the first edition of this textbook, the notion of using natural medicines was still quite fringe. At that time, it was described as "alternative" and relegated to the realms of those practicing—legally or not—outside of the hallowed confines of what constituted conventional medical practice.

In the decade and a half since, the landscape has changed. Though I would not say it is common for physicians to prescribe natural therapies to their patients, most now incorporate *some* substances that were previously considered alternative, but which now, as a result of research demonstrating safety, efficacy, or both, have been incorporated into standard medical practice. These include the use of probiotics, fish oil, and flax seeds, to name a few natural products. We have also seen the incorporation of an array of mind-body practices, such as mindfulness meditation and relaxation techniques, as well as physical manipulation and other therapies, such as massage, acupuncture, and reiki, which also has a spiritual component[2,3] (Fig. 1-1).

The evolution of what is now more commonly referred to as "integrative medicine" is perhaps nowhere more evident than in the evolution of the name of the branch of the National Institutes of Health (NIH) assigned to investigate practices that fall into this broad category. Established initially by the Federal Government as the Office of Alternative Medicine (OAM) in 1991, the OAM was given $2 million in funding and was charged with investigating and evaluating promising unconventional medical practices. By 1998, with a rapidly growing national interest in these therapies, knowledge that almost half of Americans were using them, and a growing economic sector of natural products in the national market, the NIH National Center for Complementary and Alternative Medicine (NCCAM) was established by Congress. This name acknowledged that some of the therapies being used and under investigation were alternative to the medical standard of care, but also recognized that some may have a complementary – or supportive adjunct — role in patient health.

The most recent evolution in the name of this center is significant. In December 2014, NCCAM's name was changed to the National Center for Complementary and Integrative Health (NCCIH). The change was made to more accurately reflect the Center's research commitment to studying promising health approaches already in use by the American public and being integrated into conventional medical care settings by physicians and other health care providers. As one patient recently

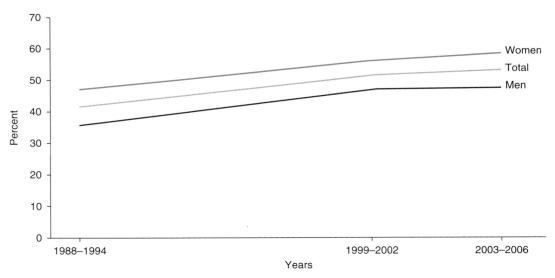

Notes: Significant linear trend from 1988 to 1994 through 2003 to 2006. Statistically significant difference for men compared with women for all time periods, $p < 0.05$ for comparison between genders within survey periods. Age adjusted by direct method to the year 2000 projected U.S. population.

FIGURE 1-1 Dietary supplement use in the United States has increased since the National Health and Nutrition Examination Survey (NHANES) III (1988–2006). From Centers for Disease Control and Prevention, National Center for Health Statistics: *National Health and Nutrition Examination Surveys.*

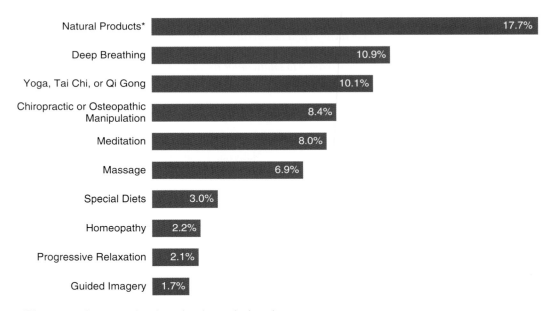

*Dietary supplements other than vitamins and minerals.

FIGURE 1-2 The ten most common complementary health approaches among adults (in 2012). From Clark TC, Black LI, Stussman BJ, et al: Trends in the use of complementary health approaches among adults, United States, 2002-2012. *National Health Statistics Reports;* no 79. Hyattsville, MD: National Center for Health Statistics, 2015.

expressed to me, "Now when I get a cold, if I think it's serious I call my doctor for an antibiotic, then I see my naturopath for herbs, and then go get a treatment from my acupuncturist." This is an increasingly common approach by many individuals, particularly women. Indeed, more than 80% of the US public uses nonconventional practices and complementary medicines adjunctive to conventional medical care.[4]

The term *alternative medicine* created a sharp distinction between the worlds of nonconventional therapies and conventional medicine in an either/or dichotomy, whereas the term complementary medicine brought these worlds closer "describing what many people in reality really do; they combine the two worlds."[5] The term "integrative" now most closely reflects the growing integration of a broader variety

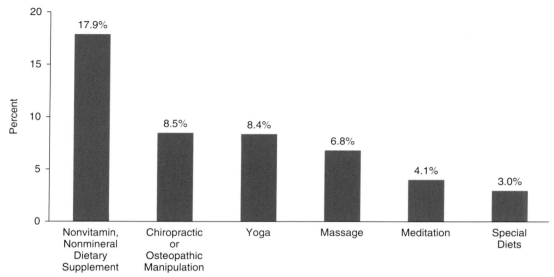

FIGURE 1-3 Percentage of adults who used complementary health approaches in the past 12 months, by type of approach: United States, 2012. From Centers for Disease Control and Prevention, National Center for Health Statistics: *National Health Interview Survey,* 2012.

of previously unconventional therapies into the medical toolbox.

Fig. 1-2 is a graph showing the most commonly utilized complementary and alternative medicine (CAM) therapies by US adults, courtesy of the NCCIH.

Unifying themes among CAM practices include individualized treatment plans; belief in the healing power of nature; union of mind, body, and spirit; and often, more time spent with patients."[5]

The NCCIH defines CAM as "a group of diverse medical and health care systems, practices, and products that are not presently considered to be part of conventional medicine."[6] Complementary medicine is considered to be those therapies used in conjunction with conventional medicines, whereas alternative medicine is considered to be those therapies used in lieu of conventional medicine; for example, the use of a specific herb to reduce perimenopausal symptoms in lieu of hormone replacement therapy (HRT).[6] The term "integrative," according to the NCCIH, involves bringing conventional and complementary approaches together in a coordinated way.

WHERE DO BOTANICAL MEDICINES FIT IN?

According to the NCCIH, herbal, or botanical, medicines fall under the classification "biologically based therapies," which refers to substances found in nature, including herbs, foods, and vitamins. These substances are broadly classified as dietary supplements. The term *dietary supplement* is specifically defined by the 1994 Dietary Supplement Health and Education Act (DSHEA) as a product other than tobacco taken by mouth and intended to supplement the diet, including vitamins, minerals, herbs, and a number of other nutritional supplement products. Forms in which dietary supplements may be sold include extracts and concentrates, tablets, capsules, gel caps, liquids, and powders. Herbal medicines continue to

be the most popular and frequently used CAM/integrative therapies; the use of nonvitamin, nonmineral dietary supplements (17.9%) is greater than any other complementary health approach used by US adults in 2012[7-10](Fig. 1-3).

HOW WIDESPREAD *IS* CAM USE?

Globally, it is estimated that 70% of all health care is provided by traditional, nonconventional medicine.[11] The World Health Organization (WHO) *Traditional Medicine Fact Sheet* states "countries in Africa, Asia, and Latin America use traditional medicine to help meet some of their primary health care needs. In Africa, up to 80% of the population still relies on traditional medicine for primary health care."[12] One of the most commonly used forms of traditional medicine worldwide is botanical medicine.

Surveys indicate that 50% to 80% of all Americans acknowledge having used CAM therapies.[4,13-16] The actual rate of use is likely higher than reported in the United States, suggested by the fact that as many as 50% of patients do not report CAM use to their conventional doctors.[11,17] Surveys typically exclude non–English-speaking respondents, thereby eliminating from the statistical pool those demographic pockets of Americans whose use may be even higher than in the average population; for example, large numbers of Hispanic Americans in certain locales regularly use herbs and spiritual healing practices.[9]

David Eisenberg's seminal surveys on CAM use by Americans conducted between 1990 and 1997 revealed a 45% increase in the use of CAM therapies during that period with estimated out-of-pocket expenses of up to $27 billion in 1997—up from $14 billion in 1990.[9] American patients' visits to CAM practitioners have been estimated at $600 million per year, exceeding the sum of all visits to primary care physicians.[5,7-9,11,17,18] Because these visits are mostly out of pocket, fewer individuals might currently use CAM therapies than if they were fully reimbursed by insurance or deductibles were lower. It is likely that there will be a significant increase in CAM use as more coverage is available from insurance companies, and as greater numbers of conventional practitioners integrate their practices to include a broader range of therapies or increase their number of referrals to a wider range of complementary therapists, such as acupuncturists, naturopathic physicians, and herbalists.

WHO USES CAM?

The average US CAM user is a well-educated health consumer, generally with at least a college education and an annual income of $50,000 or greater. Most are women between 30 and 59 years of age.[8,11,17] Individuals whose personal values include a holistic approach to health, environmentalism, feminism, or a desire for personal spiritual growth are more than twice as likely to use CAM therapies.[8,9,17] Additionally, members of numerous ethnic communities, such as Hispanics, African Americans, Asian Americans, and Native Americans incorporate traditional cultural practices, including the use of herbal medicines, into their healing practices. Having a chronic disease is also an independent predictor of CAM use.[17-19]

WHY ARE PATIENTS TURNING TO CAM?

According to Wayne Jonas, MD, former director of NCCAM, "CAM is a health phenomenon that is largely driven by the public, and this is rather unique in medicine."[7] What is it, in this age of life-saving antibiotics, surgeries, and other seemingly miraculous medical therapies that causes so many individuals to seek therapies outside of conventional medicine? Ostensibly, there are many answers to this question.

CAM therapies are generally seen by Americans as desirable for the prevention of common chronic illnesses, including heart disease, obesity, cancer, and numerous other widespread conditions. In the past 10 years, there has been a dramatic rise in awareness of the benefits of preventative health measures, both by health practitioners and the general public. This awareness is summarized in the following statement: "Preventive health measures, including education, good nutrition, and appropriate use of safe nutritional supplements will limit the incidence of chronic diseases, and reduce long-term health care expenditures...healthful diets may even mitigate the need for expensive medical procedures."[20] This message has been reinforced by cancer and heart disease prevention societies, and the multibillion-dollar-a-year nutritional supplements industry. In response, Americans have turned to the health food store as their pharmacy, self-medicating with dietary supplements—which categorically include herbal products. Too often, individuals are getting health information from the Internet, friends and family, magazines and other popular media, and product manufacturers, rather than from well-trained CAM professionals.

A desire for safer products also leads patients to turn to CAM. Consumers place a strong belief in the high margin of safety of dietary supplements, with 53% of 1027 US adults in a survey commissioned by the Dietary Supplement Education

Alliance (DSEA) stating they feel that some dietary supplements offer benefits that are not matched by conventional drugs. Fifty-six percent of respondents stated that some dietary supplements offered benefits comparable with those of drugs but with fewer side effects.[16] According to Jonas and Linde, concern about the adverse effects of conventional medicines is the third most commonly stated reason for turning to CAM.[7] Many individuals maintain the sometimes erroneous belief that "natural" means safer and gentler.

Numerous patients hold a simple pragmatic reason for using CAM therapies—they have seen many doctors and tried many medications, and they are still sick. Jonas states, "In such circumstances, it is logical that patients search for something else that works. So they seek out other alternatives without necessarily abandoning conventional care."[7] Conventional medicine may be at its best when treating acute crises, but for the treatment of chronic problems it may fall short of offering either cure or healing, leading patients to seek out systems of treatment that they perceive as addressing the causes of their problem, not just the symptoms. Many prefer palliative solutions that seem safer and less invasive than the medical options with which they may be presented.

High costs of conventional medical care are also a factor. "Studies indicate that consumers are placing increased reliance on the use of nontraditional health care providers to avoid excessive costs of traditional medical services and to obtain more holistic consideration of their needs."[20] Although high-quality professional herbal products are not inexpensive, there may be hidden costs to conventional therapies, including more side effects than many herbal medicines. In one study comparing St. John's wort with a typical tricyclic antidepressant drug, both proved close to equally effective in treating depression, although the St. John's wort cost one-fourth the price of the drug and caused one-tenth the side effects of the conventional medication.[7] Cost-effectiveness studies comparing medical interventions with CAM interventions are scarce, and should be conducted more widely.

The desire for a holistic approach and for increased participation in their own care may be one of the most significant forces driving the desire for complementary medicine. "Patients increasingly do not want to be treated simply as a body with a kidney, blood pressure, or blood sugar problem. Rather they want the accompanying social and psychological aspects of their ailments addressed as well."[7] Many patients simply feel that using alternative and complementary therapies more accurately reflects their personal belief systems.[11,21,22]

Interestingly, dissatisfaction with conventional medicine is not an independent predictor of CAM use, with greater than 95% of Americans still regularly relying on conventional medical doctors.[17,23] It appears that most Americans seek to supplement rather than supplant traditional medical care.[11] According to Brokaw and colleagues, "Clearly, CAM is offering something that many patients want but are not getting from conventional medical services."[22]

Some see the use of CAM therapies as an act of self-empowerment and an opportunity to take their health more into their own hands; perhaps a response to the days when "doctors made the decisions; patients did what they were told."[8,24] Dr. Atul Gawande, in his compelling and best-selling book, *Complications: A Surgeon's Notes on an Imperfect Science,* states that "little more than a decade ago…doctors did not consult their patients about their desires and priorities, and routinely withheld information—sometimes crucial information, such as what drugs they were on, treatments they were being given, and what their diagnosis was. Patients were even forbidden to look at their own medical records: it wasn't their property. They were regarded as children, too fragile and simpleminded to handle the truth, let alone make decisions…and they suffered for it. And they missed out on treatments they might have preferred."[25]

Chambliss observes, "Poor physician–patient communication may increase the chance that a patient will turn to alternative medicine. Conventional physicians sometimes alienate patients by minimizing the connection between the mind and the body."[11] Snyderman and Weil, in *Integrative Medicine: Bringing Medicine Back to Its Roots,* observe that the marked improvements in medical understanding that have been the hallmark of the scientific model have been accompanied by "an unexpected and unintended erosion of the patient–physician relationship…Burgeoning medical knowledge has created specialties and subspecialties, all of which are necessary; however it has created a dizzying array of practitioners, who generally focus their attention on small pieces of the patient's problem.… Managed care, capitation, increased need for documentation and productivity, and major constraints in health care funding have further eroded the patient–physician relationship and, at times, have forced physicians into positions of conflict with patients' needs…Physicians simply do not have the time to be what patients want them to be: open-minded, knowledgeable teachers and caregivers who can hear and understand their needs."[13] Table 1-1 compares a conventional medical consultation and a CAM consultation.

TABLE 1-1 CAM Consultations versus Conventional Medicine Consultations

	CAM	Conventional Medicine
Time	More	Less
Touch	More	Less
History taking	Holistic	Specific
Language used	Healing	Cure
	Holistic	Dualistic
	Subjective	Objective
	Wellness	Illness
Patient's role	Consumer	Sick role
Decision making	Shared	Doctor in paternalistic role
Bedside manner	Empathetic	Professional
Consulting room	Counseling	Clinical

Adrian Furnham, PhD, of the Department of Psychology at University College, London, researches the difference between CAM consultations and conventional consultations. His observations suggested these differences.
Can alternative medicine be integrated into mainstream care? From the NCCAM-Royal College of Physicians Symposium, January 23–24, 2001, London.

Linda Hughes, MD, of the University of California, San Francisco, suggests that "Complementary and alternative medicine is attractive to many people because of its emphasis on treating the whole person, its promotion of good health and well-being, the value it places on prevention, and its often more personalized approach to patient concerns."[17] Many CAM practitioners and researchers corroborate this view.*

David Spiegel, MD, professor of medicine and biochemistry at Stanford University School of Medicine, described the current state of health care delivery in the United States as having turned doctors into "biomechanics" and "providers." "They are drowning in paperwork," he said, "especially when it comes to reimbursement for CAM modalities…They haven't been good in helping people reconstitute a relationship with their body and deal with the emotional effects of their disease."[27]

In summary, CAM has increased because in many aspects, it "fills patients' needs."[26]

HOW OFTEN DO WOMEN SEEK CAM THERAPIES AND WHY?

Women seek medical care overall more frequently than men, and also follow more preventative health measures.[28] Therefore it is no surprise that one of the largest subgroups of CAM users is women. Specifically, they are college-educated, employed women of reproductive age, between 30 and 59 years old.[8,11,14] Women are up to 40% more likely to use CAM therapies compared to men.[8]

Although not all women who use CAM define themselves as feminist, in a study by Astin, feminism was cited as one of the three most common personal values contributing to CAM use, with twice as much CAM use likely by women who identified themselves as feminist.[8] This may be a reflection of CAM use as a tool of self-empowerment. The Consumer Healthcare Products/Roper 2001 survey reported that 60% of women, versus 46% of men, were regular dietary supplement users.[28] This pattern of increased use by women is likely to continue. In 1998 the US Surgeon General predicted that gender would be the greatest contributing factor to people's health over the next century, with women predicted to experience significant increases in health-related problems, particularly as baby boomers move into their menopausal years.[28]

The need for personal connection and relationship with health care providers may be a motivating factor for women seeking care from integrative or alternative practitioners. According to feminist theory on gender, communication, and models of learning, women thrive better in environments emphasizing connection.[29] The rampant perception of the depersonalization of medicine and disregard for subjective experience leaves many women feeling alienated. Noted childbirth educator and author Sheila Kitzinger states: "There remains a deep-seated suspicion of women's own accounts, which are often dismissed as mere anecdote…female experience, [particularly in relation to childbearing] is often

---

*References 5, 8, 11, 13, 22, 26.

ignored or trivialized because it does not match with 'observable facts' or because it does not match with ['expert'] perceptions of the same event or process."[30] This phenomenon is recognizable in the cases of premenstrual syndrome (PMS) and postnatal depression; though they are now acknowledged medical syndromes, historically women experiencing these syndromes were dismissed or pathologized. Models of objectivity and distrust of the experiential in favor of the evidence-based may be contrary and counterintuitive to women, who may place more value on intuition and personal experience as valid means of "knowing."[29] CAM therapies, typically patient-centered in their philosophies, are inherently more inclusive of the subjective voice—of the "intuitive and personalized."[29]

Doctor–patient interactions are frequently hurried, with little time for the patient to ask questions and have concerns addressed. Women often feel uncomfortable questioning or disagreeing with their physician, particularly if the physician is male, and especially if they already feel vulnerable as a result of a challenging health condition. Many women, by social convention, do not exercise their assertive voice (i.e., "speak up"), and thus do not experience satisfaction at their medical appointments. Seeing themselves as the passive recipients of health care services rather than consumers with the right to expect certain services for the fees they have paid, women often leave medical appointments feeling vaguely dissatisfied and marginalized.[31]

Because personal interaction with the patient is typically lengthier, and establishment of a partnership rather than hierarchical relationship between client and provider is an important aspect of most CAM therapies, women are more likely to feel that their questions and concerns have been acknowledged and addressed in the course of a CAM appointment and are less likely to feel marginalized. CAM therapies, inherently personalized and individualized, incorporate the client's subjective experience into the development of the protocol. Thus CAM therapies may be more compatible with women's emotional and psychological needs in the health care relationship.

The absence of the feminine voice in our health institutions may also be a primary contributing factor to women seeking health care outside of these institutions and returning to traditional healing methods, such as the use of herbal therapies. There is a need for inclusion of the emerging feminist perspective, known in academic circles as "women's ways of knowing," into the discussion of potential new paradigms for women's medicine. Jeanne Achterberg, in *Woman as Healer: A Panoramic Survey of the Healing Activities of Women from Prehistoric Times to the Present*, states insightfully that

> *The dissonance between women's talents and women's fate bears close attention as it reflects the evolution of institutions that lack the feminine voice. The absence of balance in these institutions has perpetuated a crisis that now extends alarmingly through all levels of health—from the health of tissues, mind, and relationships, to the health of the environment upon which life itself is dependent.[32]*

Women also have significant concerns over the safety of some of the therapies specifically prescribed for women's health. For example, recent backpedaling by the medical and pharmaceutical establishments on the actual safety and efficacy of HRT has led many women to lose confidence in a range of pharmaceutical interventions. Turning to herbs and nutritional supplements for the symptomatic relief of menopausal complaints, and even the prevention of cardiovascular disease, seems to many a practical and relatively safe response to the HRT confusion. Erosion of confidence in conventional care makes women increasingly vulnerable to "natural product" marketing schemes by pharmaceutical and nutraceutical companies.

With the number of women in the 40 and above age range increasing by 10 million in the next decade, it is expected that women are likely to be targets for massive dietary supplement, functional food, and over-the-counter (OTC) product advertising campaigns; this represents multimillions of dollars of profit to the dietary supplements industry. It is essential that health professionals give direct attention to the safety and efficacy of dietary supplements and CAM therapies aimed toward women to sort the reality from the hype, lest marketing at the expense of their health and pocketbooks victimize women.

WHAT PATIENTS DO NOT TELL THEIR DOCTORS AND HOW THAT MAY NEGATIVELY AFFECT PATIENTS' HEALTH

"Most patients who are using CAM are, unfortunately, not talking with their practitioners about it," states Ellen Hughes, MD, in *Integrating Complementary and Alternative Medicine into Clinical Practice*.[23] Statistics vary, but research indicates that 20% to 72% of all patients do not inform their physicians of their use of herbs, nutritional supplements, and other CAM therapies.*

In one significant example, almost 50% of patients undergoing surgery at a University of Colorado hospital never informed their doctors about using an alternative therapy within the 2 weeks before the surgery.[11]

Among patients older than 50 years of age, who are the most likely to be on multiple medications when taking dietary supplements, fewer than 30% are likely to report their supplement use to their doctors.[34]

Wendy Kohatsu, MD, in *Complementary and Alternative Medicine Secrets*, emphasized that it is "of great concern that two-thirds of patients do not tell their doctors about the use of CAM. Because of growing data about interactions between conventional and CAM therapies, open communication is imperative for all concerned."[5]

There are several probable reasons for such nondisclosure. Two commonly cited reasons are "Doctors don't ask because they don't want to know and/or don't feel they have the time; and patients feel reluctant to volunteer such information because they are afraid doctors will think less of them and/or don't feel it's relevant."[8] According to Hughes, 61% of patients

---

*References 8,9,11,23,26,33.

in one survey simply felt it was not important to reveal CAM use to their doctors; 60% stated that their practitioner "didn't ask"; 31% asserted that it was none of their care provider's business; 20% felt their provider was not knowledgeable enough about CAM to make it worth mentioning; and 13% felt their physician would disapprove and discourage their use of CAM.[17] In an article in *U.S. Pharmacist,* Michael Montagne, PhD, a professor at Massachusetts College of Pharmacy, confirms the possibility that care providers might make derogatory remarks: "words used by conventional health professionals to describe…why people choose alternative therapies tend to be pejorative, paternalistic, sarcastic, ethnocentric, or negatively biased in some way."[35] The perception that derogatory attitudes toward CAM users exist, or that physicians are just not interested in taking time to serve as advocates and educators for patients, may play a dramatic role in keeping patients from talking to their doctors about CAM use.

Patients may pay the price. Recent surveys indicate that 18% (15 million) of US adults take prescription drugs concurrently with herbs or vitamins, and most are unaware of the potential risks and contraindications of the herbal remedies they use.[34,35] Nondisclosure of CAM use to physicians could result in unfavorable consequences for the patient.[11] For example:

- A patient might be using a less effective CAM treatment in place of a more effective standard therapy.
- A patient might be using an ineffective CAM therapy, wasting the patient's time and money.
- Combining dietary supplements (e.g., herbs, vitamins, minerals) with pharmaceutical drugs can lead to unknown or known adverse reactions.
- A patient could be using a potentially dangerous CAM therapy.

Fortunately, and as a general testament to the overall safety of botanical medicines, "despite this widespread concurrent use of conventional and alternative medicines, documented drug–herb interactions are sparse."[35]

Approximately 25% of Americans end up substituting herbs for prescription drugs.[17] Lack of knowledge of the use of a complementary therapy may lead the practitioner to misinterpret the effects, including the benefits, of a conventional therapy.[4,33] If health care providers are going to provide safe and effective therapies to their patients, they must be open-minded and knowledgeable enough about CAM therapies to have honest, meaningful, and respectful discussions with their patients, and be able to at least advise their patients about the safety and efficacy of the most common therapies, or be able to provide appropriate resources for information and referrals for competent care.

WHY DOCTORS ARE TURNING TO INTEGRATIVE MEDICINE

It is really no secret why doctors are turning to integrative medicine. Medical practitioners, especially those in primary care fields, are increasingly dissatisfied with their profession. Low reimbursement rates from insurers require doctors to see a high volume of patients to pay the bills. Additionally the medical-legal environment and insurers require an ever-increasing amount of documentation in the form of electronic medical records, transforming what was once considered the satisfying experience of seeing patients into a mountain of unanswered calls and e-mails, unfinished patient charts at the end of the day, and disgruntled patients who got only about 10 minutes of real time with their physician, who often seems hurried and harried.

Further, many medical doctors are increasingly aware of the limits of conventional medicine to truly prevent—and even treat—many diseases. Some have themselves experienced being a patient who recovered from a complex, chronic, or even debilitating set of symptoms only after a change in diet, lifestyle, and the addition of meditation and supplements to their daily health care plan, and realize they want to offer the same options to their patients.

CAM/INTEGRATIVE MEDICINE EDUCATION IN CONVENTIONAL MEDICINE

Health professionals are aware of the growing need for a minimum understanding of CAM and integrative medicine, even if only to be prepared to have meaningful safety discussions with patients using such therapies. Further, many physicians and medical students express a direct interest in learning to incorporate CAM/integrative practices. As many as 60% of doctors have recommended an alternative therapy to their patients at least once, and half have used them themselves.[5] Yet presently, few medical professionals are fully comfortable with or knowledgeable enough about CAM/integrative therapies to actually integrate them as a part of the clinical repertoire, or to be able to thoroughly or accurately educate their patients about the benefits and risks of CAM therapies.[14,17] This lack of comfort with and knowledge about CAM/integrative therapies extends to pharmacists and dieticians.[37] They may be particularly concerned about the safety of herbs because they contain pharmacologically active constituents, as opposed to other therapies that may not contain measurable active constituents (i.e., homeopathy) or that are not ingested (i.e., massage therapy, aromatherapy, Reiki).[14] Then again, the known potential for pharmacologic activity is exactly what makes botanical medicines of special interest.

Many medical students, aware of the growing trend for patients to use nonconventional therapies, admit that they would like to receive training in CAM therapies—particularly botanical medicine.[13,14] Currently, most receive little training, if any, in the use of phytotherapy during the course of their medical education.[13] There is little consensus in the conventional medical world as to what extent and how to integrate such therapies into medical training and practice.

As of a 1997 to 1998 survey of 125 medical schools in the United States, 64% of the 117 schools that responded were offering courses in CAM either as required courses or electives, with only one third of schools requiring CAM study as part of the formal curriculum.[17,22] This number doubled from 34% in 1995 and has increased steadily since, though in most medical curricula such training is a small part. Most of the courses are brief, with fewer than 20 contact hours, and in a lecture series on multiple modalities, students typically receive no more than 2 hours of lecture on any single modality; thus such classes are more likely to be introductory survey courses than in depth presentations of clinically applicable information and techniques.[22,33] Additionally the majority of physicians currently practicing received no training in CAM modalities.[23]

David Eisenberg states, "Unless medical students or physicians in practice or in training are exposed to these therapies … unless they actually see a demonstration on a patient, a volunteer, a medical colleague, or themselves, they are simply unable to prescribe it. And they are unable to appreciate the conversation that they may need to have with a patient who wants a referral."[38]

Presently only one fourth of CAM courses surveyed by Wetzel and Kaptchuk use a case-based teaching approach.[39] Further, it is not realistic to expect physicians to be fully fluent in a wide range of alternative medicines and treatments while under pressure to remain current on all the developments in their own fields.[39] Although Hughes suggests that the number of "bilingual" physicians – those who understand both conventional and CAM models of care, will be in great demand, she points to the need for a cooperative environment between physicians and alternative practitioners—in this case, skilled herbalists and naturopathic doctors—for the purpose of referrals and mutual support of the patient.[23,26]

There is an unmistakable demand for increasing the number of CAM courses in medical schools, botanical medicine conferences for health professionals, and even postgraduate courses in botanical medicine for doctors and pharmacists. However, if these courses provide only superficial information, most of which is based on the limited number of herbs for which there is comprehensive scientific evidence, and taught in a way that presents herbs as substitutes for pharmaceutical drugs, then patients are not necessarily going to get what they are asking for—an increased sense of individuality, personal care, and attention to their holistic needs in the course of seeking to improve or restore health. This results in what is called green allopathic medicine - herbs substituted for pharmaceuticals, but using the same value system used by conventional medicine. A shift is required not just in the medicines we use, but in the thinking that leads to prescribing. *Functional Medicine* may provide that bridge for conventional practitioners.

FUNCTIONAL MEDICINE

Functional Medicine, which defines itself as a system addressing the underlying causes of disease using a systems-oriented approach and engaging both patient and practitioner in a therapeutic partnership, has emerged as what some think of as the next evolution of integrative medicine. It is on the cutting edge of integrating the latest in genomics and epigenetics, environmental and personalized medicine, the gut microbiome, and the root causes of inflammation and other chronic conditions in combination with what have been classically CAM and integrative types of therapies, particularly dietary, botanical, and nutritional supplement strategies, to develop individualized protocol for patients. As it is a more recent arrival on the integrative medicine scene, Functional Medicine is not recognized as a separate therapy by NCCIH, and it is taught in only a couple of medical schools in the United States. However, and substantially, as of 2015 the Cleveland Clinic collaborated with the Institute for Functional Medicine (i.e., the leading national organization certifying health care practitioners in Functional Medicine) to establish a Center for Functional Medicine as one of its research centers under the guidance of Dr. Mark Hyman.

Much of the philosophy underlying Functional Medicine is built on the foundations of classic naturopathic medicine. Although this book has not been revised to fully reflect the Functional Medicine approach that I now incorporate into my medical practice, the concepts on Functional Medicine are very consistent with the botanical approach of looking to the root causes of disorders. Both attempt to restore and support the patient's body in its natural inclination toward health rather than merely suppressing and controlling symptoms as is typically done with a conventional medical approach.

TOWARD AN INTEGRATED FUTURE OF HEALTH CARE

There is a crisis in our current health care system. As health professionals, we have the opportunity to remake the health care system into a model that includes compassion, mutual patient and practitioner satisfaction, intelligent scientific rationale, the best technology, and the best natural therapies. In fact, these qualities together may be considered characteristic of what is being referred to as *integrative medicine*. Integrative medicine embodies characteristics that are inherent in the foundational principles of botanical medicine and naturopathic medical care, and is emerging as a discrete model and speciality training in the halls of conventional medicine.

Ben Kligler, MD, and Roberta Lee, MD, leaders in this field, define integrative medicine as

> *a practice that is oriented toward prevention of illness and toward the active pursuit of an optimum state of health. It is the marriage of conventional biomedicine, other healing modalities, and traditional medical systems (Chinese medicine, Ayurveda, homeopathy, and Western herbalism, among others).*[40] *This involves an understanding of the influences of mind, spirit, and community, as well as the body. It entails developing insight into the patient's culture, beliefs, and lifestyle that will help the provider understand how best to trigger the necessary changes in behavior that will result in improved health. This cannot be done without a sound commitment to the doctor–patient relationship.*[41]

Medical residencies and postdoctoral fellowships in integrative medicine have arisen to meet the educational needs of physicians interested in such training, and a national organization, the Consortium of Academic Health Centers for Integrative Medicine, arose and for many years supported the development of undergraduate integrative medical education for emerging physicians. Harvard Medical School, Yale School of Medicine, Stanford University, and Johns Hopkins University are among the many schools now a part of this group. The Consortium defines integrative medicine as follows:

Integrative Medicine is the practice of medicine that reaffirms the importance of the relationship between practitioner and patient, focuses on the whole person, is informed by evidence, and makes use of all appropriate therapeutic approaches, healthcare professionals and disciplines to achieve optimal health and healing.

—Developed and adopted by The Consortium, May 2004, edited May 2005

Integrative practitioners embrace both conventional and alternative practices critically, prioritizing therapeutic options according to the level of benefit, risk, potential toxicity, and cost to the patient. Although integrative practitioners have a wide range of modalities at their disposal, they often are not specialists in any specific modality, having gained only brief exposure to a variety of modalities in their medical training. Some integrative physicians have specialized in a specific modality outside of medical school, for example, obtaining a license in acupuncture or specific training in botanical medicine. Many work in integrative clinics that employ a variety of types of practitioners, or work in conjunction with CAM practitioners in their communities. Integrative medicine practitioners can serve as a bridge for patients seeking both conventional and alternative modalities, with the integrative physician serving as a central figure assisting the patient in orchestrating his or her health care options.

Natural therapies incorporating herbs tend to acknowledge the multifaceted nature of a client. Finally, there is a growing trust in herbal medicine and a belief in its ability to heal. These factors combine to form a foundation for transforming illness into wellness. How this renewal is achieved by herbal medicine is not through mimicking a medical model of pathology or substituting "natural" drugs. One alternative objective in herbal medicine is to assess and address functional disturbances rather than pathology. We look for simple causes that affect our normal function rather than suspecting disease first.

—Amanda McQuade Crawford, MNIMH, RH (AHG)

History of Herbal Medicines for Women

Such "fathers of herbal medicine" as Dioscorides did not simply pull their therapeutic theories out of the air. His herbal was the human, largely female heritage finally recorded by a man interested enough in the subject and literate enough to be able to write it down. Ironically, the early records of women's knowledge could be read by very few women.[1]

Jennifer Bennett, Lilies of the Hearth: The Historical Relationship Between Women and Plants

WOMEN, HERBS, AND HEALTH REFORM: A HISTORICAL SUMMARY

Women's history has always been woven with plants and the healing arts, particularly botanical medicine and midwifery.[1-4] In virtually every culture, without exception, women maintained knowledge of herbal healing for the prevention and treatment of common maladies that afflicted their communities, including herbal treatments for women's complaints. A textbook on botanical medicine for women would not be complete without recognition of the historical role of women healers.

Few records exist to tell us the stories of ancient women healers: their training, their successes, the clinical challenges they faced, or their experiences as women with medical careers.[2] The limited historical records that do exist, however, give us a glimpse of some of the remarkable women healers in ancient times. Given the pharmacy of their day, it is clear that many of these women were highly skilled herbalists.[3,5] Modern history leaves no doubt as to the important role women have played in the resurgence of herbal medicine and traditional healing practices in present-day medicine.

WOMEN HEALERS THROUGHOUT HISTORY

There is a remarkable absence of women healers in the archives of medicine. Information on the practices of women healers must be "carefully teased out of a few surviving works written by women healers, from relics and artifacts, from myth and song, and from what was written about women."[2] Although women have long handed herbal knowledge down to their daughters, both orally and in the form of "stillroom" books—the herbal equivalent of family recipe books—only a minority of women from the most privileged, educated backgrounds managed to keep comprehensive records or documentation of herbal "recipes." Negligibly few women published serious medical works. On the rare occasion one did, it was frequently under a male pseudonym. Jeanne Achterberg states:

> *The experience of women healers, like the experience of women in general, is a shadow throughout the record of the world that must be sought at the interface of many disciplines: history, anthropology, botany, archaeology, and the behavioral sciences. . . . The available information on woman as healer in the western tradition spans several thousand years, stretching far back into prehistory when conditions were likely to support women as independent and honored healers. During and following those very early years, the role of women healers has been inexorably married to shifts in the ecology, the economy, and the politics in the area in which they lived.[2]*

Women Healers of Ancient Egypt and Ancient Greece

The oldest report of a woman physician dates to circa 3000 BCE. Records from this time indicate that a well-known practicing female physician lived in the city of Sais, where later there was a medical school. One of the earliest known medical documents, the Kahun papyrus (circa 1900 BCE) from Egypt, addresses the diseases of women and children. It has been suggested that this papyrus was written for women practitioners, as in ancient Egypt only women treated women's diseases.[3] Egyptian queens, including Queen Hatshepsut (who reigned from 1503 to 1482 BCE), encouraged women to become physicians. Hatshepsut herself set up three medical schools, as well as botanical gardens. Women healers were responsible for planting medicinal herb gardens and maintaining pharmacies.

Egyptian belief in the afterlife led to the practice of burying with the dead those things that were important to them in life and that would be needed in their next existence. At least one Egyptian queen, Mentuhotep, is purported to have been found buried with alabaster ointment jars, vessels for tinctured herbs, dried herbs, and spoons for measurement.

Polydamna, also a queen and physician of Egypt, was reputed to have given knowledge of the healing properties of the opium poppy, one of the possible ingredients in the famous sedative nepenthe. She was also alleged to have trained Helen of Troy (circa 2000 BCE), who is thought to have brought herbal knowledge from ancient Egypt to ancient Greece.[3]

The role of women healers was well established in ancient Greece, whereas in Egypt, priestesses were often physicians and keepers of healing traditions. Their practices represented a synthesis of the physical and spiritual aspects of healing. One of the most revered deities of healing in ancient Egypt was the goddess Isis, to whom supplicants directed their prayers for healing. The medical practices of ancient Greece led to the development of later Western medical healing practices, including surgery. It has been suggested by scholars that women may have been largely responsible for the initial development of surgical techniques and therapeutics. Leto was the goddess of surgery.

Hygiea, an important goddess in the Greek pantheon and daughter of Asclepias, the legendary father of medicine (circa 900 BCE), is still a part of medicine today. Her statue is found on the fronts of hospitals and her name is invoked daily in our word hygiene, as is her sister's—Panacea—often mentioned in medicine. Both sisters were invoked for the restoration of good health—the practice of hygiene now considered central to preventive medicine. Hundreds of shrines dedicated to this family were erected in ancient Greece. Each woman in the family of Asclepias had her own staff, much like Asclepias', with a snake winding around it—a symbol that has persisted for thousands of years as emblematic of healers, and that is still used today as the symbol of Western medicine.

By the time of Hippocrates (400 BCE), women's role in society had been minimized to that of servants; their role in the healing arts was likewise marginalized. Nonetheless, the contributions of several women healers were recorded. Aristotle's wife Pythias was known to "assist" Aristotle in his work; together they wrote a text of their observations of the flora and fauna of one of the Greek islands. She was also involved in the study of anatomy and left detailed illustrations of chick and human embryologic studies. Queen Artemisia of Caria (350 BCE) has been praised by Pliny the Elder and Theophrastus for her healing abilities, and is credited by them for introducing wormwood (*Artemisia* spp.) as a cure for numerous ailments, although there is some debate over the attribution of the botanical name for the *Artemisia* species to Queen Artemisia as opposed to the goddess Artemis. Pliny (c. 50 CE) wrote of several women who authored medical books, including Elephantis and Lais.[3]

A famed ancient Athenian woman healer, Agnodice, left an extraordinary legacy. At the time of her birth in Greece, women were forbidden to study medicine; the penalty for doing so was death. Women throughout the entire Greek empire recognized her as having started a female medical revolution in Athens, which eventually influenced the practice of medicine. It is said that Agnodice felt so called to practice medicine as a response to the number of women dying as a result of refusal by medical doctors to treat them that she dressed as a man and enrolled at the medical school in Alexandria. Upon graduating, she established her practice, still disguised as a man, but upon being discovered to be a woman, local women flooded to her practice. When authorities discovered her proper identity, she was arrested and put on trial. It is purported that when her patients discovered her plight they threatened to rebuke their husbands by withholding "marital favors" if they did not support Agnodice's liberation. Congregating at the courthouse, they threatened to commit suicide en masse if she was not released. Successful in their efforts, Agnodice was freed and permitted to practice—in any manner of clothing she pleased. More significantly, women, with the exception of slaves, were permitted to openly study and practice medicine, treating only the diseases of women and children. This led to a new avenue of social and economic freedom for women in Greece. Numerous famed female physicians followed in Agnodice's footsteps: Theano, Aspsasia, Antiochis, and Cleopatra, a physician practicing at the time of Galen (second century CE). These women specialized in gynecologic and obstetric complaints, wrote extensively, and were renowned for their work.

At the University of Athens there is a fresco of the famed woman physician Aspasia in the company of such leaders as Socrates, Plato, and Sophocles. Her writings remained the standard textbook of gynecology until the time of Trotula. Aspasia employed treatments for problems as diverse as difficult labor, retained placenta, uterine tumors, and peritonitis, for which she performed successful surgeries. Cleopatra also wrote an extensive gynecology text that was distributed throughout Greece and Rome, and used as a standard treatise by doctors and midwives well into the sixteenth century. However, her work had been falsely attributed to a male writer of the sixth century CE. Soranus is later thought to have plagiarized her work extensively in his famed text, *Gynaecology*. This was not uncommon: What is believed to be the oldest medical treatise, written by a woman named Metrodora, was attributed to a man named Metrodorus. The original manuscript written by Metrodora still survives in Italy.

Women Healers in Ancient Rome

Before Greek influence in Rome, physicians were disparaged. Families were expected to tend to their own health needs. The spiritual attributions of health and disease received more recognition than the physical, with goddesses such as Diana, Minerva, and Mater Matuta presiding over women's reproductive concerns. Women had better social status in ancient Rome than in ancient Greece, and Roman women met the arrival of female physicians from Greece with great receptivity. It may be that Roman male rulers were less pleased. Pliny the Elder is quoted as having said that women healers should practice inconspicuously "so that after they were dead, no one would know that they have lived."[2] Nonetheless, women healers, mostly from aristocratic families, were busily practicing by the first century CE, being greatly sought after and handsomely paid for their work.

Two successful practitioners were Leoporda and Victoria, both of whom are mentioned in medical writings of the day, with Victoria receiving the dedication to a medical book. In the preface of the book *Rerum medicarum,* she is recognized as being a knowledgeable and experienced physician. Inscriptions of tombstones of women physicians from Rome include such accolades as "mistress of medical sciences" and "excellent physician."[3] Several celebrated women physicians include Olympias, Octavia, Origenia, Margareta (an army surgeon), and Fabiola. The former two wrote books of prescriptions, and the latter was considered to possess remarkable intellectual ability as well as unusual charity. Fabiola opened a hospital for the poor in Rome—the first civil hospital ever founded and thought to be one of the best in Europe at the time. It is said that when she died, thousands attended her funeral procession.

Western Europe: The Middle Ages

The Middle Ages were an ambivalent time for women healers. Emerging from the early Middle Ages, during which women healers were considered to be diabolic, little respect was left for ancient traditions deifying women, their bodies, and their connection to nature. St. Jerome, ironically a dear friend and supporter of the healer Fabiola, is quoted as having said that "woman is the gate of the devil, the path of wickedness, the sting of the serpent, in a word, a perilous object."[2]

Although midwives were well respected as skilled practitioners within their communities, many so-called cunning women, who were often poor and illiterate, were accused of and tried for witchcraft. Cunning women were thought to be dabbling in sorcery and bewitchment; midwives were often called as witnesses to testify against them at witchcraft trials.[6] Midwives were seen as protectors of the expectant mother; a midwife was "the key figure in preventing harm. . . who guaranteed and subtended the order threatened by the witch."[7]

Midwives were not impervious to accusations of witchcraft. There are notable cases, such as Walpurga Haussmann of Dillenge, who was tried as a witch and executed.[6] However, they are mainly notable because they are anomalous cases; some prosecutions were a result of political positioning, whereas others were of previously respectable midwives who slipped into "irregular healing methods."[6]

Overall, midwives tended to be well respected in their communities; however, their skills and expertise varied tremendously. Because there were neither formal education programs for midwives nor standards of practice, the quality of care and skill a midwife possessed was largely individual. Nonetheless, there are impressive, if few, records of women from the Middle Ages who dedicated themselves to healing and medicine. Empress Eudoxia (420 CE) is attributed with the founding of two medical schools and a hospital in Syria, Jerusalem, and the land that eventually became Mesopotamia. Princess Radegonde of Burgundy studied medicine and opened a hospital for lepers, and Hilda of Whitley was an Anglo-Saxon princess who became a physician and in 657 CE built an abbey where she practiced medicine and taught many classical academic subjects.

Jacoba Felicie is an example of one tried for the practicing medicine without a license. Brought to trial in 1322 by the Faculty of Medicine at the University of Paris, she was a literate woman from an affluent family. Jacoba, with unspecified medical training, had successfully treated numerous patients who testified at her trial. Yet the testimonies were used against her as proof that she had committed the cardinal crime, not of healing, but of attempting to cure. In fourteenth-century England, educated women practitioners were likewise the target of campaigns by English physicians seeking to rid themselves of "worthless and presumptuous women who usurped the profession," seeking fines and long imprisonment for women who attempted the "practyse of Fisyk."[4] Women practitioners whose lives were spared had enough fear instilled in them to practice their crafts extremely covertly, if at all.

Although volumes of women's herbal healing traditions were lost during this time, Europeans still depended on plants for medicine, so common household cures persisted. Numerous lay books on herbal medicinal cures were sold for the "gentlewoman" to use for keeping her family well, and ironically these books offered much of the same materia medica in use by physicians during that time. However, the revered place of women healers in their communities had been dramatically altered. Attitudes about nature, women, and their bodies also changed considerably, with the Baconian belief that all three were conquerable by medicine and technology.[8]

When the Moors conquered Spain, Spanish women trained in the healing arts of midwifery and alchemy alongside men, with an emphasis on the treatment of gynecologic and obstetric conditions. The renowned Arabic physician Rhazes is said to have learned many new remedies from women, and to have admitted jealousy of women healers, whom he said were often able to find cures where he had failed to successfully treat a patient.

Trotula of Salerno is a legendary female healer of the Middle Ages. It is alleged that Trotula was considered the most distinguished teacher at the medical college in Salerno, Italy, a gathering place for men and women of Greek, Arab, Latin, and Jewish backgrounds studying medicine. She is said to have been the first female professional of medicine at Salerno, in the eleventh or twelfth century, and was called to medicine because she saw women suffering from obstetric and gynecologic complaints that they were too embarrassed to discuss with male doctors. Trotula was an early advocate of healthy diet, regular exercise, hygiene, and reduced stress. Although her history is not known with certainty, one of the most significant historical discourses on obstetrics and gynecology, referred to as *The Trotula,* actually a compendium of three texts, was either written in part by her, named after her, or is based on her teachings.[9] *The Trotula* remained an authoritative text for several centuries. It is predicated on religious and philosophic notions of the period (i.e., the curse of Eve and women's fall from grace), but the author(s) do not pathologize the normal processes of a woman's body and assert that women have particular needs that should only be evaluated and treated by other women. The clinical portions of the book refer to the menses as "flowers," describing menstruation as a process necessary for fertility, much as trees need flowers to produce fruits. Diagnoses are based on keen observation and include assessment of physical findings from pulse and urine, as well as the patient's features and speech patterns. The text advanced theories and procedures, and was the first to define the diagnosis of syphilis based on its dermatologic manifestations. Trotula appears to have treated all manner of conditions with a variety of practices ranging from medicated oils to cesarean section, with awareness of the need for antisepsis in surgery, prescribing topical and internal herbal treatments that may have been efficacious, based on what is known today about their actions. Sensitivity to the intimate needs of women is expressed, for example, by publishing the prescription of a procedure that will allow a woman who has previously lost her virginity to appear a virgin upon first intercourse after marriage, lest she face difficult political, legal, and social consequences. Jeanne Achterberg in *Woman as Healer* describes Trotula of Salerno:

> She personified the balance that is so critical to the advancement of woman as a health care professional; a knowledge of science, attention to the magic that is embedded in the mind, a mission of service, awareness of suffering and the gift of compassion. She also had the courage to speak, write, and teach with conviction.[2]

The place of women healers continued to decline dramatically, but another woman healer of the Middle Ages, Hildegard of Bingen, achieved such significant fame that her story bears telling. Hildegard, like many of the other famed women healers, was born of a noble family. She lived between 1098 and 1179 CE in Germany. At 3 years of age, she began receiving visions* and she began religious education at age 8. Her gift of prophecy gave her the uncanny ability to understand religious scriptures immediately, and from an early age she drew the attention of nobles and religious leaders. She also received visions of how life at her abbey was to be lived, ranging from ornate clothing to the development of a language used in the convent—of which nearly a thousand words survive today. Hildegard was known as a gifted intellectual, skilled in both academia and the arts—the latter as a musician and composer. One of her many books, *Cause et Curae,* a collection of five tomes, is a comprehensive medical work in which she describes diagnosis based on four humoral types (i.e., sanguine, phlegmatic, melancholic, and choleric), reminiscent of ancient Greek medical descriptions; appropriate behaviors for lifestyle, including recommendations for diet, stress reduction, and moral behaviors; and astrological predictions, for example, for conception. She provides an extensive discourse on gynecology, with recipes for external and internal preparations, as well as applications for over 200 medicinal plants. Her recommendations also included the use of gemstones, incantations, and hydrotherapy.[3]

Another of her collections, *Physica,* is comprised of nine books containing treatises on plants and trees, minerals and metals, and animals, including their medicinal and "energetic" qualities, and again drawing upon Greek medical descriptions. As is the case with most healers, Hildegard of Bingen's medical protocol reflected the cultural and religious context in which she lived; thus Christian mysticism pervades her writing. Yet her role as a woman healer also ran contrary to the common trends of the society in which she lived. Unlike some of the healers already mentioned who made deliberate political choices to develop their arts contrary to popular opinion on the role of women in medicine, Hildegard's calling came to her unbidden, as did her dedication to monastic life. Nonetheless, she represents a high level of intellectual achievement, forwardness in her discussion of women's gynecologic and sexual concerns, and an exemplary level of dedication to social service.

Women Herbalists in the Eighteenth and Nineteenth Centuries

"In the year 1775 my opinion was asked concerning a family recipe for the cure of dropsy. I was told that it had long been kept a secret by an old woman in Shropshire who had sometimes made cures after the more regular practitioners had failed."[10] This statement was made by the illustrious Dr. William Withering, discussing his discovery of the use of foxglove. He is purported to have paid the woman, a Mrs. Hutton, an undisclosed sum of gold coins for sharing the family "recipe," consisting of 20 herbs for the treatment of what was then considered a virtually incurable condition. Little mention of Mrs. Hutton or her herbal practice, if indeed that is what it was, is otherwise made, but the story of the development of the still-used drug digitalis for the treatment of congestive heart failure is medical legend.

Samuel Thomson, the founder of Thomsonian Herbalism, which for a time was a rival to the "regular" doctors, wrote in 1834, "We cannot deny that women possess superior capacities for the science of medicine."[4] Thomson, like Withering, learned herbal medicine from a countrywoman well versed in the subject, although Thomson studied botanical medicines extensively, whereas Withering learned the secret of only one formula. Yet in the Victorian era, women interested in the healing arts and plants were relegated to the study of botany, which was considered to provide good gentle exercise for the mind and body. Women were discouraged and prevented from the practice of medicine, and eventually even midwifery; the latter was taken over, initially by an untrained class of physicians referred to as barber surgeons—an accurate name as they were both barbers and surgeons.

Women, considered the weaker gender, were seen to be in need of protection from the rigors of intellectual exercise, which might "damage their delicate constitutions." In the Victorian era, a sharp distinction was made between science and superstition. A line was drawn between the intuitive, folkloric, and nonacademic approaches of traditional healers and the linear, academic approaches of medical doctors and scientists. It is ironic, however, that the cures of early doctors were largely unsuccessful; with the use of heroic treatments such as

---

*The description of the physical symptoms by which Hildegard's visions were accompanied is remarkably consistent with the characteristics of migraine headaches, including the prodromal or "aural" phase, through to the blinding lights and pain, and finally with the euphoric postmigraine phase. Thus she may have been a lifelong sufferer of migraine headaches.

purges, bleedings, and mercury-based drugs, they often led to more harm than good. In direct contrast, although herbal cures were not always successful, they often were, and they rarely caused anything near the magnitude of adverse physical problems caused by the cures of the regular doctors.

By necessity, women resumed their roles as active community healers during the settlement of the United States, delivering babies and tending to the health care needs of families from the east to the west coasts during westward expansion. Some women brought healing remedies with them from Europe, eventually planting gardens with herbs that have now become naturalized throughout much of the United States. Many learned to replace their traditional remedies with indigenous plant species, not infrequently learned from their native neighbors.

As in Europe, the politics of medicine, which in the United States ultimately gave rise to the American Medical Association (AMA), once again eventually usurped the role of the community-wise woman. From witchcraft accusations of seventeenth-century New England to the systematic discrediting of midwives and women doctors through the early 1900s, the history of medicine in the United States tells a story of competing political interests, smear campaigns against "irregular" doctors and women, and the development of a medical monopoly by regular physicians.

Until the early 1900s, medical schools for women, blacks, and Native Americans coexisted with medical schools that allowed only males. In 1912 the Flexner report, commissioned by the Carnegie Foundation, effectively led to the closure of the former schools, and only those schools sanctioned by the report remained operational.*

Although many of the criticisms made in the Flexner report may have accurately portrayed the dismal state of numerous medical programs, there appears to have been no effort made after the report to ensure access to medical education for those whom these schools served.

WOMEN'S HEALTH MOVEMENTS

In spite of numerous imposed limitations—or perhaps because of them—women in the United States have been active in health care reform for the better part of the last two centuries. Waves of activism have tended to occur periodically and coincidentally with other social reform movements, such as abolition, suffrage, and the women's rights movement. Women's involvement in health care has transformed medicine in this country, from changing medical practices to humanizing health care institutions, consequently enhancing the status of women socially, economically, and politically.

The Popular Health Movement

The Popular Health Movement is one of the underacknowledged examples of a major women's health reform movement in the United States.[11] Taking place between the 1830s and 1840s, it was a broad-based social movement focused on educating individuals about their bodies, their health, and disease prevention. It was a strategic reaction against the status of the elitist, formally trained physicians who promoted heroic, dangerous treatments that were frequently as incapacitating or deadly as they might have been life-saving.[11] Popular health movement educators instead emphasized healthy lifestyles, proper diet, exercise, eliminating corsets, and advocated the use of birth control and abstinence in marriage to limit family size.

An emphasis was placed on lay practitioners, including midwives, as it was perceived that gentler treatments were to be found in the hands of women and domestic healers.[11] Alternative health establishments, such as water cure centers, were popularly frequented; physiologic societies were founded that provided women opportunities to learn about and discuss their health concerns. Women were strongly encouraged to go to medical school and liberate information for others. It was firmly believed that medical information should be accessible to all and that the specialized language of doctors, medical journals, and textbooks prevented nonmedical practitioners from understanding what should rightfully be common knowledge.[11]

Although this movement eventually ceded to the times, the post–Civil War period marked the beginning of widening opportunities for women to access greater education. There was a significant increase in the number of women attending medical schools, with women comprising up to 6% of all physicians in the United States. This is a remarkable statistic, since as recently as 1973 in the United States, only 9% of all physicians were female.†

The Women's Medical Movement

Women physicians, continuing the philosophic tradition of the Popular Health Movement, established the women's medical movement as a way to publicly challenge the popular medical philosophies regarding women's health championed by conventional physicians. These theories included the belief that women were fragile and that education damaged the female reproductive organs. Limited by constraints that prevented them from working in male-run hospitals, they founded exemplary and successful women's hospitals, employing doctors and nurses of both genders. Boston Women's Medical College became the first contemporary medical school established for the training of female physicians. Eventually merging with Boston University because of financial troubles, the school still exists as the prestigious Boston University College of Medicine.

The Progressive Era

In the early 1900s, referred to as the Progressive Era, the women's health movement wrestled with the issue of legalization of contraception, led by activist Margaret Sanger,

---

*Many of the medical programs, for example, Johns Hopkins University and Harvard Medical College, are among those medical colleges that continue to thrive today.

†Currently, the number of female and male medical students is approximately equal, with there often being slightly more female students than male entering medical school classes; however, specialties such as surgery are more common to men than women.

which eventually led to the legalization of birth control and the maternal and child health movement, which was trying to increase the safety of motherhood through the establishment of prenatal care and maternal health clinics.[12] New York City was the center of activity for both efforts.

The Women's Health/Self-Help Movement

The 1960s and 1970s saw the rebirth of the women's health movement, once again arising to challenge a male-dominated medical system. The women's self-help movement has continued to tackle such difficult issues as abortion rights, rape, women's cancers, childbirth reform, and the excessive use of surgeries such as hysterectomies, mastectomies, and cesarean sections.

The return to natural medicines and lay healers that occurred in the post–Civil War era resurfaced in the mid-1960s along with the women's self-help movement. Herbalists—both women and men—began to reclaim the use of herbal medicines in response to perceptions of overcontrol by the medical system, as well as overuse of medications and invasive treatments. Back-to-nature philosophies consistent with using gentler and more natural remedies and the desire to be independent of conventional institutions (i.e., the medical establishment) created the modern-day role of herbalists who began to quietly practice their art. These herbalists trained by studying the plants themselves, apprenticing themselves to indigenous healers, and studying old texts such as the eclectic medical books. Similarly, women found themselves training as midwives to meet the needs of increasing numbers of women seeking home births to give birth without intervention and outside the confines of medical establishments and protocol. Some women learned the arts of midwifery and herbal medicine simultaneously, serving their communities much as the wise women of more ancient times. Many of the most well-known and respected herbalists and midwives of today's herbal movement are those who began in the 1960s and 1970s.

Rebirth of Alternative and Traditional Healing in the Contemporary United States

In recent decades, increasing numbers of women have become disenchanted with the interventionist and impersonal nature of obstetrics, gynecology, and other specialties, such as oncology, and have turned to alternative healers for care. Articles on the large number of iatrogenic diseases caused by mismedication and unnecessary use of procedures in hospitals and doctors' offices has fueled the desire of many to seek more natural medical approaches. This strong public interest in herbal medicine has fed a large economic boom in the natural products industry. Scientific evaluation of herbal medicines has begun, frequently looking to the traditional use of the herbs to direct researchers toward possible medical applications.

Both midwifery and herbal medicine are experiencing resurgence, largely as a result of demand by women patients. Women are making connections between their health and their environments—whether their personal lives, work lives, or physical, ecologic environment. Stress, past abuses, and environmental health risks are increasingly recognized as important factors influencing health. It is fascinating to appreciate that the transformations currently taking place in health care are not sudden or new, but the result of centuries of effort for health care reform by women healers and those unique men practicing alongside these remarkable women, who together continue to shape the history of health care.

ANCIENT TO MODERN HERBAL PRESCRIBING

Detailed records of the herbs used as medicines for women's health concerns have survived the centuries, primarily through ancient treatises and the works of leading herbalists and physicians of their day; included are Soranus, Galen, Dioscorides, Rhazes, Avicenna, Trotula, Hildegard, and Gerard, among many others who published on gynecologic and obstetric herbal medicine. By the seventeenth century in England, primary health care was most commonly provided by lay people, including family members, "housewyfs," local wise women, midwives, and clergy. This led to a flood of "self-help" medical books, which included information on diagnosis and treatment; the latter was often largely based on herbal prescriptions and the practice of what has been called "empirical medicine."[13] The herbal prescriptions in these books drew from the works of earlier authorities, for example, Gerard and Dioscorides, and were consistent with the standard conventional medical practices of the day, in contrast with today's self-help or alternative health movement, whose practices often differ vastly from conventional therapies.[13]

Although Western herbal medicine has not enjoyed the unbroken lineage of other traditional medicine systems, for example, traditional Chinese medicine or Ayurveda, it is remarkable to observe that many of the herbs used today for gynecologic and obstetric complaints are the same as those used hundreds or thousands of years ago. There are also many obscure, even bizarre, treatments that fortunately are no longer implemented. The materia medica of Western herbal medicine has been augmented and improved by the addition of herbs that were used by the indigenous inhabitants of North America, and that have been learned by European immigrants in the 400 years since their arrival in North America.

COMMON WOMEN'S HEALTH CONCERNS DISCUSSED IN ANCIENT TEXTS, TREATISES, AND TABLETS

The problems that have arisen historically in gynecologic and obstetric care are not entirely different from those women face today, and some conditions, such as recto-vaginal fistula, which were devastating for women 5000 years ago, remain so today for women in developing nations who lack access to proper preventative and reparative care. Box 2-1 gives a partial list representative of the types of topics that were discussed in herbals for women, although the names of conditions may have differed (e.g., amenorrhea was typically referred to as retention of menses).

BOX 2-1   Topics Commonly Addressed in Ancient Herbals for Women

Afterbirth retention
Ano-vaginal fistula
Breast lesions
Breast pain
Childbirth difficulties
Coagulation problems; excessive bleeding
Conception
Constipation
Contraceptives
Depilatories
Diarrhea
Diuresis
Excessive heat
Excessive menstruation
Fetal death/expulsion
Hair care
Heart conditions
Hemorrhoids
Infertility
Lochial flow
Menopause
Miscarriage
Nausea
Prolapsed uterus
Pudendal itching
Tumors
Uterine problems
Vaginal hygiene
Vaginal problems

TABLE 2-1   Herbs Used as Aphrodisiacs

Location	Herbs
Ancient Assyria	Five aphrodisiacs were described in *The Assyrian herbal*, a monograph published in 1942 on Assyrian herbal medications based on fragments of cuneiform script on approximately 660 medical tablets:
	• Asafoetida *(Ferula foetida)*
	• Stinging nettle seed *(Urtica dioica)* (Fig. 2-1)
	• Red poppy *(Papaver rhoeas)*
	• Berberis spp.
	• Camphor *(Cinnamomum camphora)*
Arabia	• Cubeb *(Piper cubeba)*
	• Galanga *(Alpinia galanga)*

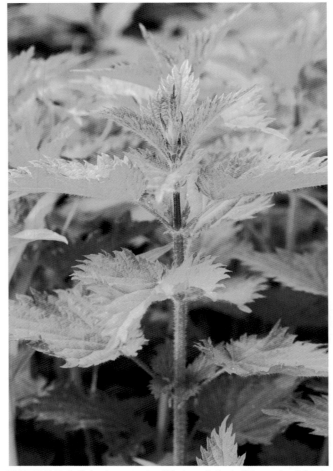

FIGURE 2-1 Stinging nettle *(Urtica dioica)*. (Photo by Martin Wall.)

COMMON HERBAL PRESCRIPTIONS FOR SELECTED WOMEN'S HEALTH CONCERNS

This chapter is not meant to be an exhaustive accounting of all of the herbal remedies used for women's health since time immemorial. It is meant to illustrate some of the more important remedies that were used historically, occasionally highlighting the unique or strange, and to provide a demonstration of the long historical use of herbs for women's health. The ways in which these herbs may have been used medicinally is highly variable, and included oral administration, topical applications (usually to the affected area), fumigation, douching, as amulets and charms, or with incantations or prayers, in ancient times to one of the many goddesses or gods who presided over the health of women. Although the information presented in the following is strictly botanical, the materia medica of ancient peoples included a variety of nonherbal medicaments, for example, castoreum (i.e., musk from the perianal sacs of beavers), which was used by ancient Egyptian midwives to expedite labor, or stones such as malachite and copper salts. The primary resource for this information is *The History of Medications for Women* by Michael J. O'Dowd, a gem of a book for those interested in the history of medicines for women from ancient to modern times.[5]

The information is presented by highlighting selected common gynecologic or obstetric conditions or herbal actions (e.g., lactation, aphrodisiacs), further subdivided by time or culture, and the medicines used. Botanical names are provided when these were identified in the source materials.

Aphrodisiacs

The use of aphrodisiacs to increase libido is documented in most cultures throughout history, even as far back as ancient Assyria (Table 2-1).[5] Herbal sexual stimulants remain popular products and are commonly available over the counter. Women today are most likely to seek aphrodisiac herbs for the treatment of sexual debility, such as in the perimenopausal years, rather than simply to increase an otherwise healthy sex drive.

Breast Abscesses/Breast Disease

Breast disease is commonly mentioned in ancient texts and treatises (Table 2-2). Although the type of breast disease is often not differentiated, it is believed that breast abscesses and breast cancer are usually the subjects. Many herbs, often in the form of poultices and washes, were used topically to treat breast disease.

Labor

A safe, expedient, and minimally painful labor was no less a goal of women living in ancient times than it is today. Herbs were used for all manner of problems that might have arisen during the childbearing process, from the need for pain relief to the need to augment a delayed or stopped labor. Categorically, herbs for childbearing can neatly be split into analgesics and oxytocics (Table 2-3).

Lactation

Concerns about insufficient breast milk have long plagued lactating mothers, and a number of herbs have been described for improving the quantity and quality of milk (Table 2-4).

TABLE 2-2	Herbs Used for Breast Disease
Location	**Herbs**
Ancient Assyria	• Chaste berry *(Vitex agnus-castus)* extract was applied, either alone or in rose water, as a poultice for breast disorders.
	• Fenugreek *(Trigonella foenum-graecum)* was applied as a paste, mixed with flour. It was still listed in the 1983 *British Herbal Pharmacopoeia (BHP)* as a treatment for suppurating wounds.
	• Pine (similar to oil of turpentine)
Ancient Greece and Rome	• Cabbage *(Brassica oleracea var. capitata)*
	• Celery *(Apium graveolens)*
	• Cumin *(Cuminum cyminum)*
	• Fenugreek
	• Linseed *(Linum usitatissimum)*
	• Mallow *(Althea* spp.)
	• Olive oil
Europe: Late Middle Ages	• Celandine juice *(Chelidonium majus)*
	• Linseed

TABLE 2-3	Herbs Used for Childbearing
Location	**Herbs**
Analgesics	
Ancient Assyria	Many of the ancient Assyrian pain-relieving herbs contained hyoscine (i.e., scopolamine) and are herbs that are not considered gentle or safe for use today, with gentler choices preferred by midwives, and controlled pharmaceutical drugs being preferred when there is the need for strong action.
	• Fox grape *(Vitis labrusca)*
	• Henbane *(Hyoscyamus niger)*
	• Mandrake *(Mandragora officinarum)*
Oxytocics	
	Many oxytocic herbs were strong purgatives, and did not exert a direct action on the uterus, whereas others may have had a true oxytocic effect. These are mostly out of use in favor of gentler herbs or controlled pharmaceuticals.
Ancient Assyria	• Galbanum *(Ferula galbaniflua):* used as a fumigant to facilitate childbirth
	• Castor oil *(Ricinus communis)* was mixed with beer and applied topically to the abdomen overlying the uterus to stimulate contractions, a practice still used today, though without the beer.
	• Juniper *(Juniperus communis):* taken alone or with psyllium *(Plantago ovata)* to speed delivery (Fig. 2-2)
Ancient Egypt	• Birthwort *(Aristolochia clematis)* to induce labor
	• Basil *(Ocimum basilicum)*
	• Fir *(Abies* spp.)
	• Frankincense *(Boswellia* spp.)
Ancient Greece and Rome	• Anise seed *(Pimpinella anisum)*
	• Cedar resin
	• Dittany *(Origanum dictamnus)*
	• Southernwood *(Artemisia abrotanum)*
	• Sweet bay *(Laurus nobilis)*
Europe: Late Middle Ages	• Hyssop *(Hyssopus officinalis)*
	• Madder roots in honey as a suppository *(Rubia tinctoria)*
	• Roses in wine *(Rosa* spp.)

TABLE 2-4	**Herbs Used for Lactation**
Location	Herbs
Ancient Egypt Europe: Late Middle Ages	• Wild lettuce (*Lactuca virosa*) • Vervain (*Verbena* spp.) in lukewarm white wine

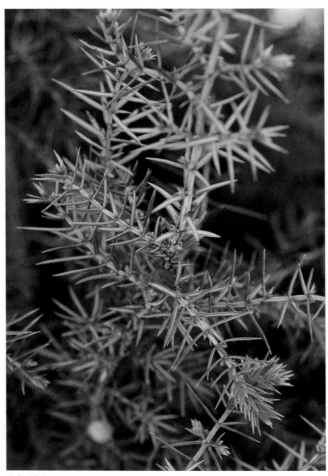

FIGURE 2-2 Juniper (*Juniperus communis*). (Photo by Martin Wall.)

Wild lettuce (*Lactuca virosa*), for example, known to have grown wild in ancient Egypt, was given to women after childbirth to promote the increased flow of breast milk. It was described in 1652 by Culpepper in his herbal and in 1735 by John K'Eogh in *Botanologia Universalis Hibernica* as such.[5] It is not used today for this purpose; it is used instead mostly as an anodyne and sedative, for which it also has been used traditionally.

Menstruation

Common menstrual problems included failure to menstruate (possibly because of pregnancy, but also primary or secondary amenorrhea), dysmenorrhea, or excessive menstruation. Remedies for these conditions were widely discussed in ancient and historical texts.

BOX 2-2	**On Paucity of the Menses**

From *The Trotula*[9]

If women have scant menses and emit them with pain, take some betony or some of its powder. Some pennyroyal, sea wormwood, mugwort, of each one handful. Let them be cooked in water or wine until two parts have been consumed. Then strain through a cloth and let her drink it with the juice of fumitory.

From Green M: The Trotula: An English Translation of the Medieval Compendium of Women's Medicine, Philadelphia, University of Pennsylvania Press, 2002.

TABLE 2-5	**Herbs Used for Amenorrhea**
Location	Herbs
Ancient Assyria	• Sweet bay (*Laurus nobilis*) • Caper (*Capparis spinosa*) • Cypress (*Cupressus* spp.) • Calendula (*Calendula officinalis*) (Fig. 2-3) • Papyrus (*Cyperus papyrus*) • Saffron (*Crocus sativus*)
Ancient Egypt	• Caper (*Capparis spinosa*) • Cumin (*Cuminum cyminum*) • Dates (*Phoenix dactylifera*) • Juniper (*Juniperus communis*) • Pine oil (*Pinus* spp.) • Rue (*Ruta graveolens*) • Sesame (*Sesamum indicum*)
Ancient Greece and Rome Europe: Late Middle Ages	• Cucumber (*Cucumis sativus*) • Hellebore (*Veratrum* spp.) • Anise seed (*Pimpinella anisum*) • Clove (*Syzygium aromaticum*) • Fennel (*Foeniculum vulgare*) • Fern roots • Feverfew (*Tanacetum parthenium*) • Horehound (*Marrubium vulgare*) • Hyssop (*Hyssopus officinalis*) • Lilies • Mugwort (*Artemisia vulgaris*) • Rue (*Ruta graveolens*) • Shepherd's purse (*Capsella bursa-pastoris*) • Southernwood (*Artemisia abrotanum*) • White pepper (*Piper nigrum*) • Wormwood (*Artemisia absinthium*) (Fig. 2-4) • Yarrow (*Achillea millefolium*)

Amenorrhea

Amenorrhea is the absence of one or more menstrual periods in a woman of reproductive age. The treatment for amenorrhea (Box 2-2), for which there were many different attributed causes, was generally in the form of emmenagogues administered orally and topically (Table 2-5). Many emmenagogues are also abortifacients, and may have been used as such. A number of these herbs may have also been used to induce uterine contractions to dispel a dead fetus (i.e., from miscarriage or intrauterine fetal death).

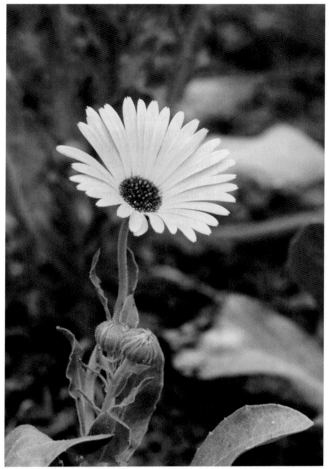

FIGURE 2-3 Calendula *(Calendula officinalis).* (Photo by Martin Wall.)

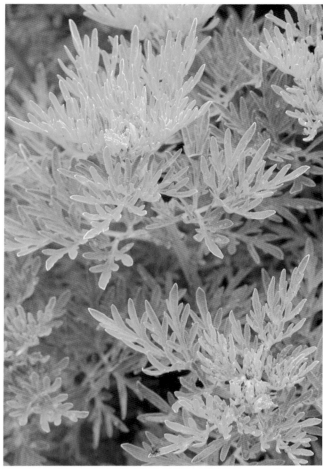

FIGURE 2-4 Wormwood *(Artemisia absinthium).* (Photo by Martin Wall.)

Dysmenorrhea

Painful menstruation commonly mentioned in ancient texts remains a common problem addressed in modern herbals for women today (Table 2-6).

Excessive Menstrual Bleeding

Box 2-3 includes an excerpted, translated section from an extensive protocol on uterine prolapse taken from *The Trotula.* Table 2-7 lists some herbs used for excessive menstrual bleeding.

HISTORY OF AMERICAN BOTANICAL MEDICINE: FROM THOMSON TO THE ECLECTICS

In the early part of the nineteenth century, medical practice in the United States was in a dismal state. General lack of medical knowledge, poor hygiene, and allopathic medicine's adherence to dangerous treatments made going to a physician both a frightening and hazardous experience. The overuse of bleeding, mercury, arsenic, opium, emetics, and purgatives weakened patients almost as much as the diseases did.[14] In response to the common practice of excessive bleeding and purging, physician William Cobbett said, "It was one of those

TABLE 2-6	**Herbs Used for Dysmenorrhea**
Location	**Herbs**
Ancient Assyria	• Asafoetida • Calendula *(Calendula officinalis)* • Hemp seeds *(Cannabis sativa):* taken in beer as an analgesic and for heavy menstruation • Dried rose *(Rosa* spp.) cooked in wine • Poppy *(Papaver somniferum)* • Mandrake *(Mandragora officinarum)*
Ancient Egypt	• Frankincense *(Boswellia* spp.) • Cannabis sativa
Ancient Greece and Rome	• Artemesia absinthium • Bayberry *(Myrica* spp.) • Cumin *(Cuminum cyminum)* • Dill *(Anethum graveolens)* • Linseed *(Linum usitatissimum)*

great discoveries which are made from time to time for the depopulation of the earth."[15]

Many of the botanicals used in contemporary herbal practice in both the US and Europe derive from the knowledge

BOX 2-3   On Descent of the Womb

From *The Trotula*[9]

If it happens that after birth the womb descends too far down from its places, let oats, have first been moistened and put into a sack, be heating and applied.

Sometimes the womb is moved from its place, and sometimes it descends, and sometimes it goes all the way out through the vagina. And this happens on account of a weakening of the ligaments and an abundance of cold humors inside.

Treatment

If it descends and does not come all the way out, aromatic substances ought to be applied to the nose, such as balsam, musk, ambergris, spikenard, storax, and similar things. Let her be fumigated from below...

But if the womb has come out, let aromatic substances be mixed with juice of wormwood, and from these things let the belly be anointed with a feather. Then take rue, castoreum, and mugwort, and let them be cooked in wine until two parts have been consumed, then give it in a potion.

From Green M: The Trotula: An English Translation of the Medieval Compendium of Women's Medicine, Philadelphia, University of Pennsylvania Press, 2002.

TABLE 2-7   Herbs Used for Excessive Menstrual Bleeding

Location	Herbs
Ancient Assyria	• Cassia (a form of cinnamon); cinnamon is still used by herbalists and midwives for heavy uterine bleeding • Calendula *(Calendula officinalis)* • Stinging nettle leaf *(Urtica dioica)* • Windflower *(Anemone pulsatilla)*; pulsatilla is still used by herbalists and midwives today, mostly as an analgesic and antispasmodic for the treatment of dysmenorrhea
Ancient Egypt	• Aloe vera • Date juice *(Phoenix dactylifera)* • Flax tampons
Ancient Greece and Rome	• Grape seed *(Vitis vinifera)* • Lotus *(Nelumbo nucifera)* • Myrtle *(Myrtus communis)* • Pine *(Pinus* spp.) • Pomegranate peel *(Punica granatum)* • Quinces *(Cydonia oblonga)* • Tart wine
Arabia	• Raspberry *(Rubus* spp.)
Europe: Late Middle Ages	• Betony *(Stachys betonica)*

of two sects of medical practitioners prominent in the US in the eighteenth through the very early twentieth centuries: the Physiomedicalists and the Eclectics. Also included is a maverick individual named Samuel Thomson (1769-1843), a poorly educated New Hampshire farmer, who was severely disenchanted with the "regular" doctors of his day and who was impelled to create an herbal alternative—Thomsonian Medicine. This system borrowed heavily from Native American herbal traditions, native sweat baths, and New England folk remedies.

The most successful sect of botanic physicians—the Eclectic physicians—was founded in the 1820s and was responsible for popularizing many now well-known herbs including echinacea *(E. angustifolia)*, goldenseal *(Hydrastis canadensis)*, black cohosh root/macrotys *(Actaea racemosa)*, cactus *(Selenicereus grandiflorus)*, wild indigo *(Baptisia)*, blue cohosh root *(Caulophyllum thalictroides)*, cascara sagrada *(Rhamnus purshiana)*, and kava kava *(Piper methysticum)*. The Eclectic philosophy allowed physicians to select therapies from other medical sects such as allopathy, homeopathy, and hydrotherapy that would benefit individual patients; botanical products were considered to be and were produced as pharmaceuticals. In the golden era of Eclectic medical practice (1875 to 1895) there were over 8000 Eclectic physicians practicing throughout the United States and eight legitimate Eclectic medical schools.

The change in centuries brought new ideas that the Eclectics were reluctant to embrace, such as bacteriology, vaccination, and pharmacology. The onslaught of the AMA and the Carnegie Foundation monies, which fueled the AMA's growth and increasing dominance, changes in medical education, and the Flexner report, which damned most sectarian medical schools, all led to a steady decline in status of and enrollment Eclectic schools. The Eclectics, who were always most popular in rural America, were increasingly seen as a relic of older days. They were considered unscientific, clinging to plant medicines rather than the new miracle drugs created in laboratories (e.g., aspirin, sulfa drugs). No longer was orthodox medicine bleeding or poisoning patients, and improved hygiene had reduced the dangers of many terrible diseases that were once common. In this changing social, political, and cultural climate, the Eclectics could only be seen to belong to the past, not the bright industrial future of the twentieth century. The Eclectic Medical College, the last school of Eclectic medicine, closed its doors in 1939.

 SPECIFIC INDICATIONS FOR BOTANICALS FOR WOMEN: ECLECTIC MEDICAL TRADITION

Tables 2-8 and 2-9 contain a summary and comparison of remedies acting on the reproductive organs of women that were popular among the selected medical physicians.

A note concerning eclectic medicines and doses

Although many Eclectic physicians made their own tinctures, the most popular medicines were Specific Medicines made by Lloyd Brothers of Cincinnati and "normals" made by W.S. Merrill, also of Cincinnati. These products were highly concentrated extracts, thus the dosage levels were quite low, especially compared with tinctures.

TABLE 2-8   Eclectic Remedies Acting on the Reproductive Organs of Women

Botanical	Black haw (*Viburnum prunifolium*)	Pulsatilla (*Anemone spp.*)	Blue cohosh (*Caulophyllum thalictroides*)	Black cohosh (Macrotys; *Actaea racemosa*)	Chaste tree (*Vitex agnus-castus*)
Action	Acts mildly as a nervine and antispasmodic. Produces muscular relaxation and reduction of reflex irritation during pregnancy. Has a tonic and soothing influence on the entire uterine structures.	Strong-acting nervine and anxiolytic, especially for menstrual, premenstrual, or menopausal problems with intense emotional symptomology.	Has a wide influence on the reproductive organs, increasing activity and reducing pain; widely used for uterine and ovarian pain with fullness, ovarian neuralgia, endometritis, endometriosis pain, and mittelschmerz.	Exercises a wide influence on the nerve centers and their blood supply. Is a mild motor depressant and nerve sedative. Positively relieves muscular soreness or aching, induced or idiopathic, from whatever cause. Relieves erratic nervous conditions; acts directly upon the reproductive functions.	Corpus luteum insufficiency with elevated estrogen and/or deficient progesterone. Highly effective remedy for premenstrual and menopausal anxiety, hot flashes, and uterine fibroids.
General Influence on the Menstrual Function	Indicated in dysmenorrhea, with cramplike or spasmodic pains. Corrects nervous irritation and sympathetic disturbances.	Usually for delayed or scanty menses caused by anxiety; fear; shock; or in weak, depleted anemic girls.	A direct emmenagogue and antispasmodic, it is indicated in amenorrhea, dysmenorrhea, irregular menstruation, and premenstrual syndrome (PMS) anxiety.	In menstrual disorders, accompanied with aching or muscular soreness, and cool skin. Relieves amenorrhea with these symptoms; will control congestive dysmenorrhea. Its influence here is enhanced by aconite or belladonna. Is beneficial in menorrhagia and metrorrhagia; is given in menstrual irregularities of young girls.	Hyper- or polymenorrhea, amenorrhea caused by hormonal imbalance. Helps to reestablish normal cycle *after* use of birth control pills. Useful for treating a wide range of PMS symptoms.
Prevent Miscarriage or Abortion	The best of remedies for this purpose, reliable in emergencies if given in full doses, frequently repeated. Reliable in habitual abortion; will prevent induced abortion if membranes are not ruptured. Should be given in advance in habitual cases, and continued past the time.		In atonic conditions during pregnancy, it will restore tonus to the uterus and promote a normal labor. In small quantities mixed with viburnum it has a reputation for preventing premature labor. NOT RECOMMENDED FOR SELF-MEDICATION DURING PREGNANCY. PROFESSIONAL USE ONLY.	Cannot be depended upon. Acts more like ergot; is given only in small doses, for its specific indications.	May be used up to third month of pregnancy to prevent miscarriage and to remedy morning sickness.

Continued

TABLE 2-8 Eclectic Remedies Acting on the Reproductive Organs of Women—cont'd

As a Partus-preparator	Abates nerve irritation, restlessness, hysterical symptoms, and erratic pains; contributes to a normal condition; prevents morning sickness and premature contractions; induces cheerfulness and hopefulness and prevents accidents.	In atonic conditions during pregnancy, it will restore tonus to the uterus and promote a normal labor.	The most frequently used remedy for this purpose; less reliable than mitchella; removes erratic pains and irregular conditions; overcomes hysteria; soothes general muscular irritation; conducive to a normal, easy, short labor.	Frequently used in combination (e.g., mother's cordial), it prevents false labor pains, anxiety, and promotes a healthy, easy labor. May cause fetal congestive heart failure. Best to avoid during pregnancy.	Has no direct influence.
In Labor	Promotes normal conditions, with regular normal contractions; soothes undue muscular irritation. Prevents hemorrhage.	It is beneficial in labors with sluggish, ineffectual, and weak contractions.	Stimulates strong, productive contractions. Useful in pokey labor (i.e., rigid os, 4-5 cm)	A most reliable oxytocic; produces normal regular intermittent pain; does away with erratic and irregular pains, especially of rheumatic or neuralgic origin. Prevents postpartum hemorrhage; relieves nervous irritation.	Has no direct influence.
After Labor	Restores normal tone and normal capillary circulation; prevents subinvolution, prolapse, and malposition.	Can be of benefit with *Cimicifuga* for postpartum depression.	Helps to expel placenta; reduces postpartum pain; prevents uterine subinvolution.	Relieves severe aching and muscular soreness; controls postpartum hemorrhage; promotes normal involution; prevents the recurrence of uterine misplacement; cures persistent leukorrhea, especially if accompanied with relaxation and hypertrophy.	As a galactagogue to stimulate and maintain milk production (most effective first 10 days after birth).
For other Conditions, Including Menopause	Valuable during protracted or eruptive fevers, where there is irregular menstruation, with impending uterine inflammation and sepsis. May reduce cyclical outbreaks of herpes.	Excellent remedy for PMS and menopausal anxiety or depression and nervous headaches. Avoid use in acute inflammatory conditions.	Effective for menopausal pain; low back pain with pain radiating down the legs; arthritic pain in small joints; spasmodic coughing.	It is of value in fevers with its specific symptomology and in inflammation of the kidneys and bladder. Aching and muscular soreness are its specific indications; helps with menopausal symptoms, including depression and hot flashes.	Teenage acne—boys and girls; premenstrual oral and genital herpes; carminative. Hormonally related constipation. Menopausal symptoms, including hot flashes, excessive sweating, formication, and anxiety.

Adapted from Ellingwood F: New American Materia Medica.

TABLE 2-9 Additional Female Reproductive Remedies Used by the Eclectics

Herb, Part Used	Used for
American mistletoe, herb (Phoradendron serotinum)	Uterine hemorrhage, including postpartum bleeding. Used as an oxytocic to stimulate labor; considered more effective than ergot.
Canada fleabane, herb (Conyza canadensis)	Profuse vaginal discharge or menorrhagia.
Cottonroot, bark (Gossypium herbaceum)	Clotty, scanty menses with lower backache, a feeling of fullness, and weight in the pelvis and bladder.
Cramp bark (Viburnum opulus)	Spasmodic uterine pain; dysmenorrhea, perineal pain.
Helonias (Chamaelirium luteum)	Female reproductive system amphoteric; increases fertility, regulates hormonal levels. Useful for pelvic congestion.
Licorice (Glycyrrhiza glabra)	Contains isoflavones (i.e., phytoestrogens)—use with white peony and saw palmetto for polycystic ovary syndrome.
Motherwort (Leonurus cardiaca)	Anxiolytic; antispasmodic; premenstrual syndrome; and menopausal anxiety.
Partridge berry (Mitchella repens)	Uterine astringent, menorrhagia, uterine prolapse, feeling of heaviness in abdomen, tender with pressure.
Peach tree, bark (Prunus persica)	Irritation of the stomach and upper gastrointestinal tract; severe morning sickness.
Raspberry, leaf (Rubus spp.)	Uterine tonic; useful throughout pregnancy and postpartum, uterine prolapse, and menorrhagia.
Saw palmetto (Serenoa repens)	Uterine tonic; useful for polycystic ovary syndrome, infertility, and pelvic fullness syndrome.
Shepherd's purse, herb (Capsella bursa-pastoris)	Heavy bleeding caused by fibroids.
Thuja (Thuja occidentalis)	Used topically and orally for venereal warts resulting from human papillomavirus. Also indicated for leukorrhea and urinary dribbling.
Tiger lily (Lilium lancifolium)	Used for pelvic congestion and stagnation; ovarian neuralgia.
True unicorn, root (Aletris farinosa)	Polymenorrhagia with laborlike pain and a sense of debility in the pelvis.
Water eryngo (Eryngium aquifolium)	Urinary irritation experienced as a constant sexual urge.
White ash, bark (Fraxinus americana)	Fibroids, especially with heavy bleeding. Uterine hypertrophy with profuse leukorrhea and menstrual bleeding.
White baneberry, root (Actaea alba)	Ovarian cysts with pronounced tenderness upon palpation.
Yarrow, herb and flower (Achillea millefolium)	Atonic menorrhagia, vaginal leukorrhea, postpartum bleeding, and heavy bleeding from fibroids.

Fundamental Principles
of Herbal Medicine

Not everything that can be counted counts, and not everything that counts can be counted.
Albert Einstein

THE EVIDENCE BASE FOR BOTANICAL MEDICINE

In the past decade, herbal medicine has been undergoing a resurgence in popularity, as well as a rapid evolution, as divergent streams of thought meet to redefine and apply it in a modern clinical context. Many Western herbalists and naturopathic physicians share the concern that the mainstreaming of herbal medicine threatens to uproot it from its classical foundations. However, a growing number of medical doctors are eager to add potentially helpful botanical medicines to the repertoire in integrative therapies; yet they are fearful of herb-drug interactions, product quality, and side effects. Consequently they prefer a very limited evidence-based approach in their selection process. Most clinical practitioners desire a high level of reassurance, via scientific validation methods, that the products they recommend or which their patients might already be using meet basic standards of safety, quality, and efficacy.[1-4]

Interestingly, patients may be more interested in anecdotal evidence of safety and risk in comparison with practitioners, who are more likely to want detailed objective evidence of benefit, safety, and risk.[5] There is a tremendous need for a consistent and comprehensive way to evaluate herbal medicine efficacy and safety and integrate the concerns and experiences of all of the partners in health care: medical doctors and scientists, traditional practitioners, and those taking herbal medicines both for self-care and as patients.

This chapter proposes an integrative model of evidence-based herbal medicine that allows an intelligent synthesis of the various possible forms of data in the evaluation of botanical medicines, including traditional wisdom (its own form of evidence), scientific findings, and expert consensus based on clinical observation. This chapter also discusses the evidence upon which this text is based.

In its broadest and most liberal interpretation, evidence-based medicine (EBM) can embody an ideal fusion of "clinical and laboratory research data with human experience," as suggested by herbalist Simon Mills, rather than the

reductionist, prepackaged mind-set that it has been accused of engendering.[6] An integrative model of presenting evidence can be seen in the monograph collections of the European Scientific Cooperative on Phytotherapy (ESCOP), the World Health Organization (WHO), and the *American Herbal Pharmacopoeia (AHP),* all of which acknowledge multiple levels of evidence including traditional use, clinical applications, and relevant science.

WHAT IS EVIDENCE-BASED MEDICINE?

The concept of EBM was first articulated in mid-nineteenth-century Paris, and perhaps even earlier.[7] Described more recently as "the conscientious, explicit, and judicious use of current best evidence in making decisions about the care of individual patients,"[7] EBM has been widely adopted in conventional medical circles as a hierarchic methodological model of evaluating and ranking evidence for the determination of what is considered the best and most objective clinical practice. EBM as a packageable product concept has become big business in medicine—a profitable host of commodities that include national conferences; hand-held computers that can be taken into patient consultations and programmed to generate EBM protocols for patients on the spot; books and journals; undergraduate and postgraduate training programs; and Web-based courses.[7] Centers for the study of EBM have been established, as have extensive databases.[7]

Yet responses to EBM as a medical paradigm based solely on external, objective evidence to the exclusion of the practitioner's clinical judgment and experience have been highly equivocal, with criticisms ranging from "evidence-based medicine being old hat" to it being a "dangerous innovation, perpetrated by the arrogant to serve cost-cutters and suppress clinical freedom." EBM has been "criticized for the inappropriateness of much evidence and its application to clinical practice, for logical inconsistencies, for potentially reducing the role of clinical judgment, for difficulties integrating into everyday professional practice, and for cultural bias."[8] EBM has been critically called "cookie-cutter" medicine, systematizing patient treatments according to specified protocol.[9] Ironically, this appears to be a backward step in light of patients' increasing demands for greater individual attention

The editor wishes to thank *Botanical Medicine for Women's Health,* Edition 1 contributors to this chapter: Lisa Ganora, David Hoffmann, Eric Yarnell, Kathy Abascal, and Mitch Coven.

in medical care. Accusations of EBM being a cost-cutting measure are based upon the belief that streamlining diagnoses and treatments will represent cost savings to managed care organizations.[7-9]

Practitioners naturally want to provide their patients with the best options. Many believe that relying solely on external, quantified evidence will relieve them of the burden of responsibility (or culpability) inherent in exercising individual clinical judgment. However, removing subjective observation and judgment entirely from clinical decision making requires objectifying and homogenizing patients. John Astin, PhD, writing in *Academic Medicine*, states:

> *Decisions in medicine, irrespective of how much objective evidence we gather, always involves the weighing of probabilities . . . To suggest that randomized controlled trials, meta-analyses and clinical practice guidelines will eliminate the need for clinical judgment is to misrepresent the realities of clinical medicine (both CAM [complementary and alternative medicine] and conventional). If medicine could be purely evidence-based (which is highly debatable both practically and financially), then in theory medical care . . . could essentially be administered by computers and computer algorithms.*[2]

EBM proponents such as David Sackett argue that the concepts of EBM have been misinterpreted to be a one-dimensional orthodoxy based solely on objective, quantitative research methodologies, and that it is actually a much broader model than has been typically conveyed, with external evidence being only one of three important aspects of EBM.[7] The other arms of EBM are the patient's preferences, needs, and circumstances, and the practitioner's clinical experience (Fig. 3-1).

Sackett's description of EBM demonstrates its potential to serve as an integrative model:

> *The practice of evidence-based medicine means integrating individual clinical expertise with the best available external clinical evidence from systematic research. By individual clinical expertise we mean the proficiency and judgment that individual clinicians acquire through clinical experience and clinical practice. Increased expertise is reflected in many ways, but especially in more effective and efficient diagnosis and in the more thoughtful identification and compassionate use of individual patients' predicaments, rights, and preferences in making clinical decisions about their care. By best available clinical evidence we mean clinically relevant research, often from the basic sciences of medicine, but especially from patient centered clinical research . . . Without clinical expertise, practice risks becoming tyrannized by evidence, for even excellent external evidence may be inapplicable to or inappropriate for an individual patient. Without current best evidence, practice risks becoming rapidly out of date, to the detriment of patients . . . External clinical evidence can inform, but can never replace, individual clinical expertise, and it is this expertise that decides whether the external evidence applies to the individual patient at all and, if so, how it should be integrated into a clinical decision.*[7]

According to this, EBM need not be restricted to reductionist forms such as randomized controlled trials (RCTs) and meta-analyses as some suggest (Box 3-1, Fig. 3-2). At its best, it is a "triangulation of knowledge from education, clinical practice, and the best research available for a given condition or therapy."[9]

SUPPORTING EVIDENCE FOR BOTANICALS DISCUSSED IN THIS TEXT

The WHO and numerous individual nations, in recognition of the widespread use and significance of traditional medicines as accessible, safe, and cost effective forms of medicine in their countries and the value of varying levels of evidence in informing botanical use, have adopted standards for evaluating and approving the efficacy and safety of traditional herbal medicines. Acceptable forms of evidence include:

- Scientific evidence
- Expert opinion, including those based on contemporary clinical use by practitioners
- Historical and traditional data
- Ethnobotanical information

It is upon these forms of evidence that this book relies for its supporting data. Readers can determine for themselves whether the supporting evidence accompanying each herb, along with the safety data, adequately substantiates the use of that herb in the context of the practitioner's own practice and expectations of evidence.

Scientific Evidence

Scientific data included in this book may fall into any of the following categories:

- Meta-analyses of randomized controlled trials (RCTs)
- Systematic reviews
- Individual RCTs
- At least one well-designed controlled study with expert recommendations
- Other types of well-designed experimental studies
- Other studies: open, comparative, correlation, case control; expert opinion of a committee

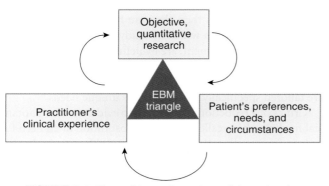

FIGURE 3-1 The evidence-based medicine triangle.

BOX 3-1 Research Methods for Beginners

For those unfamiliar with research jargon, here is a brief overview of research methodologies and terminology. Research methods are categorized hierarchically in order of highest to lowest value of objectivity and reliability of the levels of evidence. The "evidence pyramid" is one such scheme for classifying research methods (Fig. 3-2).

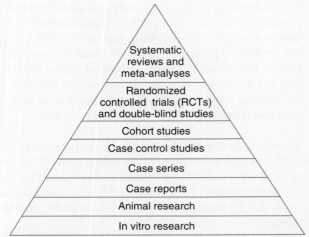

FIGURE 3-2 The evidence pyramid. (Courtesy of SUNY Downstate Medical Center.)

Definitions

A *systematic review* is a method of reviewing multiple clinical trials using a system that minimizes study biases. It consists of a comprehensive survey of all of the primary studies of the highest level of evidence on a topic that have been systematically identified, ranked, and summarized according to explicit methodologies.

A *meta-analysis* is a survey in which the results of the studies included in the review are statistically similar and are combined and analyzed as if they were one study. Meta-analyses have several limitations: Studies rarely agree precisely and often sample sizes of single studies limit the conclusions that can be drawn; biases may be built in if authors selectively include studies that support their own conclusions; studies that demonstrate positive outcomes tend to be selectively published over those that do not; if several weak studies are combined, they may cumulatively give the impression of a strong study.

A *randomized controlled trial* (RCT) is comprised of two groups: a treatment group and a control group. The former receives the treatment being evaluated; the latter receives either no treatment or a default treatment. Participants are then randomly assigned to all groups.

A *double-blind study* is one in which neither the participant nor practitioner knows whether the participant is receiving the treatment being studied or the control treatment. This type of study is thought to be the most effective at eliminating confounding variables such as a placebo effect and bias.

In a *cohort study*, participants with a specific condition or those receiving a particular treatment are followed over time and are compared with another group not affected by the condition or receiving the treatment. Cohort studies have a number of limitations, including possible variability between the two groups and length of time for the studies; the latter could lead to changes in participant condition, as well as participants dropping out of the study.

Case control studies are those in which patients with a certain condition are compared with those who do not have the condition. Advantages are that they can be done quickly and do not require researchers to have special methods; rather, they depend more upon questionnaires. Case control studies are considered less reliable than RCTs and cohort studies.

Case series and *case reports* are either collections of reports on a series of patients, or a report on the treatment of a single patient. Case reports are considered to lack statistical validity because there are no control groups with which to compare study outcomes.

- Toxicology studies; in vivo and in vitro studies
- Animal studies*

Problems with Conventional Research Methodologies for Botanical Therapies

Not all complementary and alternative medicine (CAM) therapies (e.g., prayer, homeopathy) are expected to stand up to classic methods of safety and efficacy testing and yet are considered safe for use, even if some question their therapeutic efficacy. However, because herbs contain pharmacologically active substances, there is an implicit expectation that if herbs "really work" they should be able to measure up to the standards established for conventional drugs.

Although this is theoretically sound, it is not reasonable in practice. Whole herbs are not the same as isolated drugs, nor are they applied as such by botanical medicine practitioners. A distinction can be made for single isolated active ingredients derived from botanicals, which are much more like pharmaceutical drugs than they are herbal products. RCTs for herbal products, in which all study group participants all receive the same treatment, are by definition given in a model that is different than the way herbs are applied clinically by herbalists, wherein choice of herbs, formulation, and dosage are tailored specifically to the patient's unique needs.[6,9]

Critics of a reductionist approach to evidence-based botanical medicine have called the mere substitution of an herb for a drug "green allopathy," asserting that although herbs can work effectively this way, there is more to take into account, including differing "root" or underlying causes leading to similar external manifestations or symptoms. The belief of herbal

---

*Note that the author is philosophically opposed to the mistreatment of animals for the benefit of science, strongly favoring instead the development of harmless animal studies and ethical human study models. However, given the value of certain information derived from animal studies, for example, teratogenicity and mutagenicity studies, animal studies are regrettably included.

"energetics," the traditional notion of herbs being hot or cold, for example, can be found almost ubiquitously in traditional cultures across the globe; though apparently based in cosmology and spiritual attributes, this belief may eventually bear out in plant pharmacology, personalized medicine, and genomics.

There is frequently a discrepancy between the dose or form of an herb used in a clinical trial from that used in actual clinical practice by herbalists and other practitioners; further, clinical trials typically use single plants or even isolated plant constituents, whereas traditional and modern herbal practice tends to rely on combinations of herbs, which may create a unique gestalt with benefits that exceed those of single plants.[10]

According to the WHO:

Experience has shown that there are real benefits in the long-term use of whole medicinal plants and their extracts, since the constituents in them work in conjunction with each other. However, there is very little research on whole plants because the drug approval process does not accommodate undifferentiated mixtures of natural chemicals, the collective function of which is uncertain. To isolate each active ingredient from each herb would be immensely time-consuming at unsupportable cost, and is almost impossible in the case of preparations.[11]

Although RCTs may show positive effect, lack of positive RCTs does not indicate inefficacy; it may simply denote a lack of studies, or an inappropriately or ineffectively applied protocol. RCTs can only answer specific questions about general populations: Does this herb given in this group, at this time, in this form, and at this dose treat this condition? They do not answer specific questions about individual patients, and individual patient care is the crux of botanical medicine practice.

Additionally, botanical medicines are rarely prescribed in isolation—nutritional, lifestyle, and mind–body practices used in conjunction with botanical products add yet unknown elements to the gestalt of what creates a therapeutic protocol for any individual.

Limits of Research and Research Biases

Implicit in relying upon the results of RCTs and other classic trials is the belief that they represent unbiased analyses. This may be a mistaken assumption. Even the RCT, the gold standard of research methodologies and one of the most reliable methodologies for limiting study biases, is not impervious to bias and is not without limitations.[12] Methodological features of RCTs, including trial quality, have been shown to influence effect sizes; and some researchers believe that eliminating the psychological component of clinical care from trials and minimizing placebo effect may cause studies to bear little resemblance to clinical practice.[13,14]

Politics also influences the choice of which studies get funded; what questions are asked; and whether, where, and how outcomes are published.[15] Limited financial incentive on the part of pharmaceutical companies and researchers to investigate herbal products, particularly whole herbs, is due in part to the limited patentability of botanicals, and leads to fewer funding

opportunities.[16,17] Publication bias on the part of medical journals also has recently been raised as a significant concern. Additionally, there may be negative biases in the publication of case reports, with emphasis placed on the negative side effects of botanicals.[3] John Astin, MD, writing on CAM, states that the "approach of selectively citing one negative article while failing to cite any of the positive systematic reviews or meta-analyses is the antithesis of evidence-based medicine. It is, in short, opinion based medicine."[2] He states further that "The failure to cite such evidence contributes to a very misleading picture of the state of the scientific evidence base underlying CAM."[2]

Frequently, herbal medicine as a whole is indicted on the basis of a small number of published negative case reports that are typically followed by a cascade of negative popular media. Although adverse effects and potential harm are rightfully brought to the attention of professionals and the public, there appear to be double standards in the reporting of the potential harmfulness of herbs compared with the volume and severity of reports on the risks of pharmaceutical medications.

Nonetheless, in spite of the billions of dollars of herbal products sold in the United States alone, there are negligible reports of adverse herbal events compared with the volume of reported adverse drug events. In Europe, where millions of units of herbal products are sold and market surveillance and adverse events reporting systems are well established, there too are an amazingly small number of adverse reports.[8] This is in stark contrast to the gross number of adverse events, and even adverse event–related deaths, in the US alone from properly prescribed and properly taken medications. Acetaminophen is a major contributor to liver damage; statin drugs have been found to increase diabetes and heart disease incidence in large numbers of otherwise healthy adults, especially women, and the combination of nonsteroidal antiinflammatory drugs (NSAIDs) and selective serotonin reuptake inhibitors (SSRIs) has been found to cause intracranial bleeding.[18,19]

A major concern expressed about herbal medicine is the questionable safety of botanical medicines in pregnancy. Although indeed many are not to be used in pregnancy because of uncertainty about their safety, more than 90% of medications approved since 1980 have not been properly tested for mutagenicity or teratogenicity.[20] Further, a growing body of evidence suggests that only 20% to 37% of conventional medical practices that are commonly accepted and used across a broad range of medical specialties are predicated on evidence from RCTs. Coronary bypass surgery was used for more than 20 years before it was subjected to clinical trials.[16,21,22] Although these statistics do not justify lack of evidence for nonconventional therapies and do not negate the necessity for reliable clinical evidence, they do illustrate that there are sometimes double standards influencing attitudes about nonconventional therapies, and that there may at times be a suspension of common sense in pursuit of the holy grail of evidence (Box 3-2).

Expert Opinion

Well into the early twentieth century, observational studies were considered an important source of medical evidence, declining in perceived value only over the past 20 years.[12]

BOX 3-2   A Satirical View of Evidence-Based Medicine

Parachute Use to Prevent Death and Major Trauma Related to Gravitational Challenge: Systematic Review of Randomized Controlled Trials*

Abstract objectives: To determine whether parachutes are effective in preventing major trauma related to gravitational challenge.

Design: Systematic review of randomized controlled trials (RCTs).

Data sources: Medline, Web of Science, Embase, and the Cochrane Library databases; appropriate Internet sites and citation lists.

Study selection: Studies showing the effects of using a parachute during free fall.

Main outcome measure: Death or major trauma, defined as an injury severity score > 15.

Results: We were unable to identify any RCTs of parachute intervention.

Conclusions: As with many interventions intended to prevent ill health, the effectiveness of parachutes has not been subjected to rigorous evaluation by using RCTs. Advocates of evidence-based medicine (EBM) have criticized the adoption of interventions evaluated by using only observational data. We think that everyone might benefit if the most radical protagonists of EBM organized and participated in a double-blind, randomized, placebo-controlled, crossover trial of the parachute.

*Data from Smith GCS and Pell JP: *BMJ* 327:1459–1461, 2003, www.bmj.com.

Clinical decision making in medicine was based on observation, personal experience, and intuition.[12] Even the RCT is only 50 years old and has been established as the definitive method of testing new drugs only since the 1980s.[23]

Although herbal medicine is frequently "dismissed by the orthodoxy as a fringe activity,"[6] there are actually thousands of well-trained, highly knowledgeable, and experienced clinical Western herbalists in numerous countries—England, Scotland, Germany, Australia, New Zealand, Canada, and the United States, to name a few. In Europe, particularly in Germany, phytotherapy is an accepted part of medical practice. Botanical experts are either trained as part of medical education if they are physicians, or in recognized botanical medicine educational programs with consistent curricula. In the United States, 17 states currently recognize naturopathic physicians who have graduated from accredited 4-year naturopathic colleges and passed their medical boards as legitimate physicians whose scope of practice includes botanical medicine. Over the past decade, a number of physicians have also gained significant experience in the clinical use of herbs. Although anecdotal evidence has largely been dismissed as invalid, the consensus of a large body of experts is entirely valid.

A large collective body of knowledge from contemporary clinical practitioners provides compelling evidence for the use of herbal medicines. Case studies (*n* = 1 study), case series, uncontrolled trials, observational reports, and outcome-based studies all contribute important information to the dialogue on botanicals, ranging from establishing clinical effects that merit further study to providing clinical insights that corroborate traditional uses with modern pharmacologic effects.[24,25] "Case study research provides a useful tool for investigation of unusual cases or therapies for which effectiveness data are lacking and for preliminary investigation of any factor that may influence patient outcome." Qualitative research methods need to be developed further to fully evaluate the efficacy and safety of nonconventional therapies.[23] Collaboration between conventionally trained researchers and traditional and medical herbalists to systematically document herbalists' clinical use of botanical medicines is a rich and yet untapped area for botanical medicine research.

This textbook draws extensively upon the valuable resource of "contemporary clinical consensus" (expert opinion) derived from communication with practitioners, surveys, published and unpublished reports, texts, training materials, and symposia.

Historical and Traditional Evidence

Historical information referred to in this text is largely derived from classical botanical medicine texts, treatises and herbals, pharmacopoeias, monographs, and academic books on the history of botanical medicines. These appear in the references corresponding to individual chapters. Herbalist Kerry Bone best explains traditional use:

> *Traditional use occurs in the context of a traditional medicine system. This healing system may have evolved over thousands of years and be part of a great culture, or it may be part of a smaller or more primitive system. The important point is that traditional use is the refined knowledge of many generations, carefully evaluated and re-evaluated by many practitioners of the craft. It is not just the anecdotal accounts of a few practitioners.[26]*

Bone defines folk use "as small-scale use; often in an isolated context . . . Folk use should therefore not be confused with traditional use. That is not to say that folk use is without value. More that it should be placed in the context of the hypothetical rather than the definite."[26]

Traditional sources for this text include pharmacopoeias, classic texts on traditional Western herbal practices, and classic texts and materia medica from recognized traditional systems, for example Traditional Chinese Medicine (TCM) and Ayurveda. Additionally, herbs that are regulated as traditional medicines in nations with established traditional medicine categories are included as traditional medicines.

Ethnobotanical Information

Ethnobotanical evidence can be a useful source of information on the historic and cultural uses of herbs—especially when illustrating the length of time for which an herb has been used or the diversity of cultures in disparate locations that have independently arrived at a similar use for a specific plant. However, unless how the herb was prepared for use is stated in

---

BOX 3-3   Integrative Medicine Texts, Herbal Texts, and Herbal Monographs Referenced in the Book

Barrett M: *Handbook of Clinically Tested Herbal Remedies,* New York, 2004, Haworth Press.

Barton S: *Clinical Evidence,* London, 2001, BMJ Publishing Group.

Blumenthal M: *The ABC Clinical Guide to Herbs,* Austin, 2003, American Botanical Council.

Blumenthal M, Busse W, Goldberg A, et al: *The Complete German Commission E Monographs Therapeutic Guide to Herbal Medicines,* Austin, 1998, American Botanical Council.

Blumenthal M, Goldberg A, Brinckmann J: *Herbal Medicine: Expanded Commission E Monographs,* Newton, 2000, Integrative Medicine Communications.

Bone K: *A Clinical Guide to Blending Liquid Herbs,* St. Louis, 2003, Churchill Livingstone.

Bone K: *Clinical Applications of Ayurvedic and Chinese Herbs,* Queensland, 2000, Phytotherapy Press.

Bruneton J: *Pharmacognosy,* Paris, 1999, Technique and Documentation.

Bruneton J: *Toxic Plants Dangerous to Humans and Animals,* Paris, 1999, Technique and Documentation.

European Scientific Cooperative on Phytotherapy (ESCOP): *ESCOP Monographs: The Scientific Foundation for Herbal Medicinal Products,* ed 2, New York, 2003, Thieme.

Evans WC: *Trease and Evans' Pharmacognosy,* London, 1998, Saunders.

Felter HW, Lloyd JU : *King's American Dispensatory, 1898,* vols 1 and 2, ed 18, Sandy, 1983, Eclectic Medical Publications.

Hoffmann D: *Medical Herbalism: The Science and Practice of Herbal Medicine,* Rochester, 2003, Healing Arts Press.

Kligler B, Lee R: *Integrative Medicine: Principles for Practice,* New York, 2004, McGraw-Hill.

Kohatsu W: *Complementary and Alternative Medicine Secrets,* Philadelphia, 2002, Hanley & Belfus.

Kraft K, Hobbs C: *Pocket Guide to Herbal Medicine,* New York, 2004, Thieme.

Low Dog T, Micozzi M: *Women's Health in Complementary and Integrative Medicine: A Clinical Guide,* St. Louis, 2004, Elsevier.

McGuffin M, et al: *American Herbal Products Association botanical safety handbook,* Boca Raton, 1997, CRC Press.

McKenna DJ, Jones K, Hughes K, et al: *Botanical Medicines: The Desk Reference for Major Herbal Supplements,* New York, 2002, Haworth Press.

Mills S, Bone K: *Principles and Practice of Phytotherapy,* Edinburgh, 2000, Churchill Livingstone.

Moerman D: *Native American Ethnobotany,* Portland, 2000, Timber Press.

O'Dowd MJ: *The History of Medications for Women: Materia medica Woman,* New York, 2001, Parthenon Publishing Group.

Rakel D: *Integrative Medicine,* Philadelphia, 2003, Saunders.

Rotblatt M, Ziment I: *Evidence-based Herbal Medicine,* Philadelphia, 2002, Hanley & Belfus.

Upton R: *American Herbal Pharmacopoeia and Therapeutic Compendium Series,* Santa Cruz, 2004, American Herbal Pharmacopoeia.

Weiss R, Fintelmann V: *Herbal Medicine,* ed 2, New York, 2000, Thieme.

Wichtl M: *Herbal Drugs and Phytopharmaceuticals: A Handbook for Practice on a Scientific Basis,* Stuttgart, 2004, Medpharm.

World Health Organization: *The World Health Organization Monographs,* Geneva, 1999, WHO.

---

the ethnobotanical reference, it is often difficult to extrapolate a practical, clinical application. Indigenous peoples commonly use plant medicines externally, ceremonially, and symbolically without the patient ingesting or medicinally applying the herb. Blowing the smoke of an herb over a patient or having the patient wear a piece of a root in a pouch as an amulet is drastically different than having the patient take a concentrated decoction of many grams of the roots. Ethnobotanical uses cited in this book imply ingestion or topical medicinal application of the herb unless otherwise specified.

REFERENCES USED IN THE DEVELOPMENT OF THIS TEXT

The following were considered acceptable forms of references for inclusion in this text:

- Academic articles from peer-reviewed medical and CAM journals
- Classic botanical medicine texts and recognized pharmacopoeia
- Definitive evidence-based botanical medicine texts and reference books

- Recognized monographs (e.g., those published by *AHP,* ESCOP, and WHO)
- Ethnobotanical and historic references

Box 3-3 give a complete list of botanical medicine texts, monographs, and databases consulted for this book.

IS THERE ADEQUATE EVIDENCE FOR BOTANICAL MEDICINES?

Although it is frequently stated that botanical medicines are poorly studied, a quick examination of a comprehensive database (e.g., Ovid, Cochrane) should dispel that myth. In addition to an exponentially growing body of clinical studies, there are numerous in vitro and in vivo human tissue, cell, and animal studies on herbal products and isolated constituents.[8] In Europe, clinical research into herbal medicine has been established for decades.[17] With the establishment of National Center for Complementary and Alternative Medicine (NCCAM) (now National Center for Complementary and Integrative Health [NCCIH]), the priority for herbal research has continued to grow in the United States. Although there are a limited number of RCTs for most herbs, those that have been conducted should establish a compelling argument for the efficacy of herbal medicines. Efficacy studies and meta-analyses are growing in number and include positive reports in the Cochrane Collaboration on ginkgo for cognitive impairment and dementia, echinacea for cold treatment, St. John's wort for treatment of mild to moderate depression, and feverfew for the treatment of migraines; and RCTs for St. John's wort for treatment of mild to moderate depression, kava kava for anxiety, chaste tree berry for premenstrual syndrome (PMS), and horse chestnut for venous insufficiency, among others.[8,26]

It is also important to remember that few botanical approaches have been disproved or proved dangerous.[2] As conventional medicine moves toward a more integrated model of health care that incorporates herbal medicines, and as botanical medicine practitioners increasingly work with medical professionals, there will be an inherent need to blend languages and approaches to create a useful and mutually respectful paradigm. Change will have to be reflected not only in clinical and educational settings but also in research models. An inclusive, holistic interpretation of EBM allows the possibility of it being used as an ideal model incorporating the best available objective evidence (e.g., scientific, traditional, ethnobotanical) with practitioner experience and patient preferences and circumstances.

THE ACTIONS OF HERBS

The therapeutic information in this textbook is presented using the traditional vocabulary of botanical medicine alongside that of contemporary science and medicine. One of the defining characteristics of herbal medicines are what are classically referred to as their "actions," or their observed effect on the body; for example, increased urination after using a diuretic, or a dry feeling in the mouth as a result of ingesting an astringent herb as a tea.

Barring a few modern terms such as *adaptogen* and *phytoestrogen,* the terms describing the actions of herbal medicines have been in constant use for centuries. Some terms, such as *astringent, diuretic,* or *analgesic* will be familiar to the reader and remain a part of the modern pharmacist's and physician's lexicon. Others, such as *bitters,* are terms used by lay folk and practitioners alike, in this case describing the herbs' taste, but also associated with the physiologic action of facilitated digestion caused by stimulation of gastric juices and bile release.

Some terms, and the concepts that belie them, may seem both unfamiliar and archaic; for example, using the term *alterative* to describe "blood detoxification." Although scientific research has not specifically, to my knowledge, explored this action category as a whole, many of traditional actions do interact with commonly known physiologic and biochemical pathways, including the detoxification pathways, which are supported by botanical chemical constituents such as flavonoids found abundantly in fruits, especially berries, vegetables, and herbal medicines.

Many of the actions described in this section are identical to those used in conventional medicine; for example,

diaphoretic, analgesic, diuretic, or *antimicrobial,* although the mechanisms of action of herbs may or may not correspond to those of conventional medications. An understanding of these terms is essential to understanding numerous botanical texts, both old and modern, which employ them.

This section is not an exhaustive presentation of herbal actions nor are all of the herbs associated with each action listed. Rather, it is an overview, focusing on terms and herbs that are relevant to the conditions presented in this book. This section is divided into "General Actions" and "Gynecologic and Obstetric Actions." General botanical textbooks such as *Principles and Practice of Herbal Medicine* and *Medical Herbalism* offer in-depth discussions of herbal actions and their relationships to botanical science.

GENERAL ACTIONS

Adaptogens

Soviet scientists coined the term *adaptogen* in 1964 to describe herbs that increase the body's nonspecific resistance and vitality, helping the individual adapt to and defend against the effect of allostatic load on the body—the wear and tear of acute and chronic exposure to stressors. These herbs are used to increase work capacity, efficiency, and cognitive function, including memory, decision making, and concentration; to regulate the stress response hormones and neurotransmitters, including cortisol; and to improve nonspecific immunity and blood sugar regulation. Chapter 5 offers a comprehensive discussion of adaptogens.

For an herb to be classified as an adaptogen it must:
- Show nonspecific activity
- Have a normalizing influence independent of the nature of the pathologic state
- Be innocuous and not influence normal body functions more than required

Herbs are classified as adaptogens based upon both clinical and in vitro research (Box 3-4 and Fig. 3-3).

Alteratives

Alteratives are so called because they are thought to "alter" the body's metabolic processes, improving a range of functions from nutrition to elimination (Box 3-5 and Fig. 3-4). Folk healing traditions sometimes invoke the concept of "blood cleansing," which, although hinting at much, is technically inaccurate, as blood does not require "cleansing." Traditionally these herbs may have been used, along with bitters (see later discussion) for "spring cleansing" (what are now thought of as *detoxes*), or when there was infection or skin disease. Herbs in this category help the body eliminate waste through the kidneys, liver, digestive system, lungs, or skin, whereas others work through unknown mechanisms of action. Immunologic research on certain secondary plant products, especially saponins, has led to some interesting suggestions for the basis of alterative action; however, the specifics of plant activity are the result of the way the whole plant works upon the human body,

BOX 3-4 Adaptogenic Herbs

American ginseng *(Panax quinquefolius)*
Ashwagandha *(Withania somnifera)*
Eleuthero *(Eleutherococcus senticosus)*
Holy basil *(Ocimum sanctum)*
Korean ginseng *(Ginseng)*
Licorice *(Glycyrrhiza glabra)* (see Fig. 3-3)
Nettle *(Urtica dioica)*
Reishi *(Ganoderma lucidum)*
Rhaponticum *(Rhaponticum carthamoides)*
Rose stonecrop *(Rhodiola rosea)*
Schisandra *(Schisandra chinensis)*

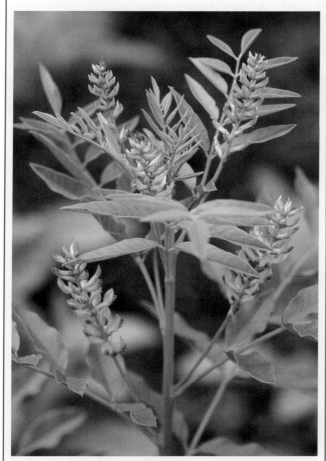

FIGURE 3-3 Licorice *(Glycyrrhiza glabra)*. (Photo by Martin Wall.)

BOX 3-5 Alterative Herbs

Blood root *(Sanguinaria canadensis)*
Blue flag *(Iris versicolor)* (see Fig. 3-4)
Burdock *(Arctium lappa)*
Calendula *(Calendula officinalis)*
Cleavers *(Galium aparine)*
Dandelion *(Taraxacum officinale)*
Echinacea *(Echinacea* spp.)
Figwort *(Scrophularia nodosa)*
Garlic *(Allium sativum)*
Goldenseal *(Hydrastis canadensis)*
Oregon grape *(Mahonia aquifolium)*
Red clover *(Trifolium pratense)*
Sarsaparilla *(Smilax* spp.)
Wild indigo *(Baptisia tinctoria)*
Yellow dock *(Rumex crispus)*

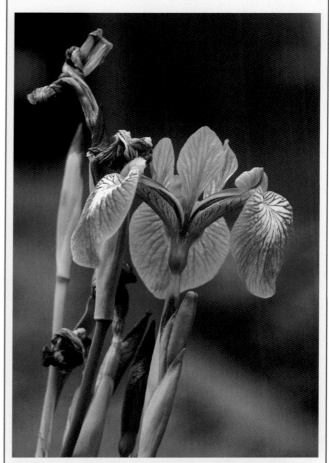

FIGURE 3-4 Blue flag *(Iris versicolor)*. (Photo by Martin Wall.)

not simply specific active ingredients. Alteratives can be used as supportive therapy in many diverse conditions, including inflammatory skin diseases, arthritis, and a wide range of autoimmune problems. Alteratives are considered "cooling" from a traditional energetic perspective.

Analgesics

Analgesics (Box 3-6 and Fig. 3-5) relieve pain. They can range from mild (i.e., anodynes) to strong effects (i.e., sedatives) and may owe their activity to antiinflammatory action (e.g., *Dioscorea villosa*) or central effects (e.g., *Piscidia piscipula, Piper methysticum*). Many of the strongest herbal analgesics are not available legally without a prescription (e.g., opium products such as morphine, cannabis products). Analgesics are generally considered "cooling" from a traditional energetic perspective.

Antiemetics/Antinauseants

Antiemetics are the herbs that alleviate nausea and prevent or reduce vomiting (Box 3-7 and Fig. 3-6); this is a property generally attributed to the presence of volatile oils in the plant, many of which have antispasmodic effects in the stomach. Some may also have a direct action on the medulla (i.e., vomiting center) of the brain. They are useful in the treatment of nausea and vomiting in pregnancy, *Hyperemesis gravidarum*, motion sickness, chemotherapy-induced nausea, and nausea related to colds and general stomach upset.

Antiinflammatories

Antiinflammatory herbs (Box 3-8 and Fig. 3-7) relieve inflammation without the potentially hazardous side effects of steroidal and nonsteroidal antiinflammatory drugs. They are beneficial for relieving pain and discomfort, and also the underlying inflammation associated with numerous health conditions. Antiinflammatory herbs can be classified in relationship to the body system (Table 3-1) or tissue for which they are most appropriate, or by their pharmacologic mode of action. The four primary categories of antiinflammatory herbs are salicylate-containing, steroid precursors, essential oil–rich, and resin-containing.

BOX 3-6   Herbal Analgesics

Ashwagandha *(Withania somnifera)*
Black cohosh *(Actaea racemosa)*
Black haw *(Viburnum opulus)*
Birch *(Betula* spp.)
California poppy *(Eschscholzia californica)*
Cramp bark *(Viburnum prunifolium)*
Corydalis *(Corydalis* spp.)
Dong quai *(Angelica sinensis)*
Jamaican dogwood *(Piscidia piscipula)*
Kava kava *(Piper methysticum)*
Marijuana *(Cannabis sativa)*
Pulsatilla *(Anemone pulsatilla)*
Rupturewort *(Herniaria glabra)*
Wild yam *(Dioscorea villosa)*
Willow *(Salix* spp.) (see Fig. 3-5)

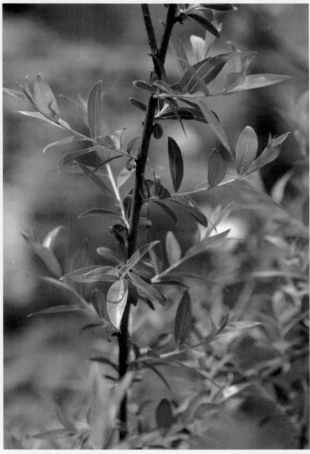

FIGURE 3-5 Willow *(Salix* spp). (Photo by Martin Wall.)

BOX 3-7   Herbal Antiemetics/Antinauseants

Chamomile *(Matricaria recutita)*
Cinnamon *(Cinnamomum zeylanicum)*
Ginger *(Zingiber officinalis)*
Marijuana *(Cannabis sativa)*
Peppermint *(Mentha piperita)* (see Fig. 3-6)

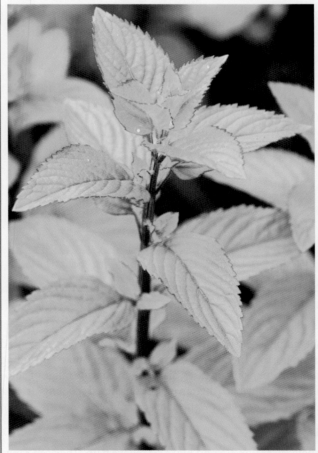

FIGURE 3-6 Peppermint *(Mentha piperita)*. (Photo by Martin Wall.)

Salicylate-Containing

These herbs are most useful for musculoskeletal inflammatory conditions. They do not pose the dangers to the stomach associated with aspirin. In fact, *Filipendula ulmaria*, rich in salicylates, has been used to staunch mild stomach bleeding. *Viburnum prunifolium* and *Actaea racemosa* are other examples of herbs in this category, commonly recommended in this book.

Steroid Precursors

Steroids were first isolated from plant material, and some herbs contain molecules that may be metabolized by the body into inflammation-fighting steroidal molecules. Herbs rich in these steroids are effective antiinflammatories, and are especially useful in the treatment of inflammation of autoimmune origin. Examples are *Glycyrrhiza glabra* and *Dioscorea villosa*, which contain diosgenin.

Essential Oil–Rich

Many aromatic herbs rich in essential oils have antiinflammatory actions. One of the best of these remedies is *Matricaria recutita*, which is rich in terpenes such as bisabolol and chamazulene. These herbs are especially useful internally for irritable bowel syndrome (IBS) and inflammatory bowel disease (IBD), and topically for skin inflammation. *Calendula officinalis* and *Hypericum perforatum* are other well-known plants containing oils that soothe and reduce inflammation.

Resin-Containing

A number of resin-containing plants reduce inflammation, but may cause gastric inflammation, limiting their usefulness. Many, nonetheless, are invaluable in the treatment of arthritic conditions. Examples are *Menyanthes trifoliata*,

---

BOX 3-8 Antiinflammatory Herbs

Angelica *(Angelica archangelica)*
Birch *(Betula* spp.)
Black cohosh *(Actaea racemosa)*
Black haw *(Viburnum prunifolium)*
Borage *(Borago officinalis)*
Butterbur *(Petasites hybridus)*
Calendula *(Calendula officinalis)*
Chamomile *(Matricaria recutita)*
Chickweed *(Stellaria media)*
Chinese skullcap *(Scutellaria baicalensis)*
Cleavers *(Galium aparine)*
Comfrey *(Symphytum officinale)*
Corn silk *(Zea mays)*
Cramp bark *(Viburnum opulus)*
Devil's claw *(Harpagophytum procumbens)*
Dong quai *(Angelica sinensis)*
Echinacea *(Echinacea* spp.)
Feverfew *(Tanacetum parthenium)*
Ginger *(Zingiber officinale)*
Goldenrod *(Solidago canadensis)*
Green tea *(Camellia sinensis)* (see Fig. 3-7)
Horse chestnut *(Aesculus hippocastanum)*
Lady's mantle *(Alchemilla vulgaris)*
Lavender *(Lavandula officinalis)*
Licorice *(Glycyrrhiza glabra)*
Marshmallow *(Althaea officinalis)*
Meadowsweet *(Filipendula ulmaria)*
Peppermint *(Mentha piperata)*
Plantain *(Plantago major)*
Quaking aspen *(Populus tremuloides)*
Rehmannia *(Rehmannia glutinosa)*
Sage *(Salvia officinalis)*
St. John's wort *(Hypericum perforatum)*
Turmeric *(Curcuma longa)*
White peony *(Paeonia lactiflora)*
Wild yam *(Dioscorea villosa)*
Willow *(Salix* spp.)
Witch hazel *(Hamamelis virginiana)*
Yarrow *(Achillea millefolium)*

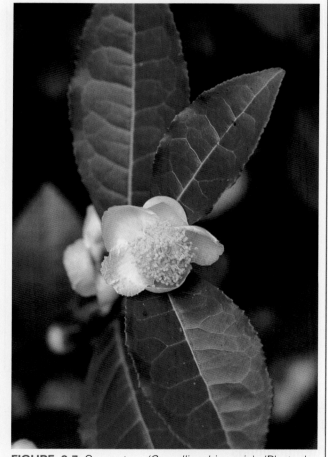

FIGURE 3-7 Green tea *(Camellia chinensis)*. (Photo by Martin Wall.)

TABLE 3-1	Body System Affinities of Antiinflammatory Herbs
Body System	**Examples of Herbs**
Circulatory	Achillea millefolium, Aesculus hippocastanum, Crataegus spp., Tilia platyphyllos
Digestive	Althaea officinalis, Calendula spp., Dioscorea villosa, Glycyrrhiza glabra, Hydrastis canadensis, Matricaria recutita, and Mentha piperita.
Urinary	Solidago virgaurea, Zea mays
Reproductive	Alchemilla vulgaris, Caulophyllum thalictroides
Musculoskeletal	Actaea racemosa, Betula spp., Dioscorea villosa, Filipendula ulmaria, Harpagophytum procumbens, Populus tremuloides, Salix spp., Tanacetum parthenium
Nervous	Hypericum perforatum
Skin	Arnica montana, Calendula officinalis, Commiphora molmol, Hydrastis canadensis, Hypericum perforatum, Plantago major, Stellaria media

---

BOX 3-9 Herbal Antimicrobials

Aniseed (Pimpinella anisum)
Bearberry (Arctostaphylos uva-ursi)
Blood root (Sanguinaria canadensis)
Calendula (Calendula officinalis)
Cranberry (Vaccinium macrocarpon)
Echinacea (Echinacea spp.)
Eucalyptus (Eucalyptus spp.)
Garlic (Allium sativum)
Goldenseal (Hydrastis canadensis)
Goldthread (Coptis chinensis)
Lavender (Lavandula officinalis)
Lemon balm (Melissa officinalis)
Licorice (Glycyrrhiza glabra)
Myrrh (Commiphora molmol)
Olive (Olea europaea)
Oregano (Origanum vulgare)
Oregon grape (Mahonia aquifolium)
Peppermint (Mentha piperata)
Plantain (Plantago major)
Reishi (Ganoderma lucidum)
Rosemary (Rosmarinus officinalis)
Sage (Salvia officinalis)
St. John's wort (Hypericum perforatum)
Tea tree (Melaleuca alternifolia)
Thuja (Thuja occidentalis)
Thyme (Thymus vulgaris)
Usnea (Usnea barbata)
Wild indigo (Baptisia tinctoria)
Wormwood (Artemisia absinthium)
Yarrow (Achillea millefolium)

TABLE 3-2	Body System Affinities for Antimicrobials	
Body System	**Examples of Herbs**	
Urinary	Arctostaphylos uva-ursi, Achillea millefolium	
Reproductive	Calendula officinalis, Echinacea spp., Allium sativum, Thymus vulgaris	
Nervous	Hypericum perforatum, Melissa officinalis	

interactions with pathogens or indirectly mediated via the herb's interaction with the immune system. As examples of the diversity of mechanisms involved (Table 3-2), consider the following: *Melaleuca alternifolia* (tea tree) contains an oil rich in terpinene-4-ol that directly interferes with a pathogen's metabolism, thus killing it. Other herbs rich in volatile oils also work directly to kill microorganisms. Examples include *Allium sativum, Thymus vulgaris,* and *Eucalyptus* spp. *Echinacea* spp. directly stimulate the body's own immune response, and thus are often effective antimicrobial agents. *Vaccinium macrocarpon* (cranberry) blocks the adhesion of uropathogenic *Escherichia coli* to the walls of the bladder, thus offering a useful treatment for cystitis.

Antispasmodics/Spasmolytics

Antispasmodic herbs (Box 3-10 and Fig. 3-8) relieve muscle tension and spasm, both in the musculoskeletal system and the smooth muscle of the hollow organs (i.e., bladder, uterus, stomach, intestine, gallbladder) (Table 3-3). *Spasmolytic* is a synonymous term. Uterine antispasmodics, which typically ease spasms in the bladder as well, are listed separately under gynecologic and obstetric actions. Antispasmodics usually have peripheral action and generally are not sedating.

Astringents

The basic action of astringents (Box 3-11 and Fig. 3-9) is to tonify or tighten tissue. They are sometimes called *styptics* when applied externally to stop bleeding, and *antihemorrhagics*

Harpagophytum procumbens, and *Guaiacum officinale.* These herbs are not discussed further in this textbook.

Antimicrobials

Antimicrobial herbs (Box 3-9) inhibit or destroy pathogenic microorganisms, including bacteria, fungi, and viruses. It would be a mistake to attempt an overarching generalization about mechanisms of action for herbal antimicrobials. Antimicrobial effects may be related to direct

BOX 3-10   Antispasmodic Herbs

Angelica *(Angelica archangelica)*
Aniseed *(Pimpinella anisum)*
Black cohosh *(Actaea racemosa)*
Black haw *(Viburnum prunifolium)*
California poppy *(Eschscholzia californica)*
Catnip *(Nepeta cataria)*
Chamomile *(Matricaria recutita)*
Cramp bark *(Viburnum opulus)*
Damiana *(Turnera diffusa)*

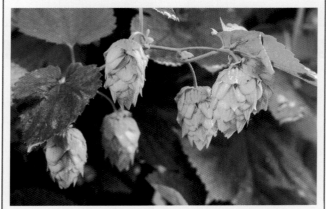

FIGURE 3-8 Hops *(Humulus lupulus)*. (Photo by Martin Wall.)

Fennel *(Foeniculum vulgare)*
Feverfew *(Tanacetum parthenium)*
Ginger *(Zingiber officinale)*
Hops *(Humulus lupulus)* (see Fig. 3-8)
Jamaican dogwood *(Piscidia piscipula)*
Kava kava *(Piper methysticum)*
Lavender *(Lavandula* spp.)
Licorice *(Glycyrrhiza glabra)*
Linden *(Tilia platyphyllos)*
Lobelia *(Lobelia inflata)*
Motherwort *(Leonurus cardiaca)*
Mugwort *(Artemisia vulgaris)*
Peppermint *(Mentha piperita)*
Skullcap *(Scutellaria lateriflora)*
Skunk cabbage *(Symplocarpus foetidus)*
St. John's wort *(Hypericum perforatum)*
Sundew *(Drosera rotundifolia)*
Thyme *(Thymus vulgaris)*
Wild lettuce *(Lactuca virosa)*
Wild yam *(Dioscorea villosa)*

TABLE 3-3   Body System Affinities with Antispasmodics/Spasmolytics

Body System	Examples of Herbs
Cardiovascular	*Leonurus cardiaca, Viburnum opulus, Actaea racemosa*
Digestive	*Matricaria recutita, Viburnum opulus, Viburnum prunifolium, Valeriana officinalis, Humulus lupulus, Mentha piperita, Salvia officinalis, Foeniculum vulgare, Dioscorea villosa*
Urinary	*Viburnum opulus, Viburnum prunifolium, Dioscorea villosa, Piper methysticum*
Reproductive	*Viburnum opulus, Viburnum prunifolium, Dioscorea villosa, Actaea racemosa*
Musculoskeletal	*Piper methysticum, Viburnum opulus, Viburnum prunifolium, Lobelia inflate, Valeriana officinalis, Scutellaria lateriflora, Actaea racemosa*

that astringent, tannin-rich remedies create precipitates with herbs high in alkaloids. This alteration of protein is how animal skin is turned into leather. In other words, astringents produce a kind of temporary leather coat on the surface of tissue. Because of this activity, tannins have a number of therapeutic benefits. They:

- Reduce irritation on the surface of tissues through a sort of numbing action
- Reduce surface inflammation
- Create a barrier against infection, which is of great help for wounds and burns

Astringents have a role in a wide range of problems in many parts of the body (Table 3-4) but are of great importance in wound healing and conditions affecting the digestive system. In the gut, they reduce inflammation, improve symptoms of diarrhea, and are widely used in various diseases of digestion. However, long-term use as medicine or too much tea in the diet can be deleterious to health, as this will eventually inhibit proper food absorption across the gut wall.

Bitters

Bitters are remedies (Box 3-12 and Fig. 3-10) that have a bitter taste ranging from mildly bitter-tasting (e.g., *Achillea millefolium, Taraxacum officinale* leaf) to profoundly distasteful (e.g., *Ruta graveolens, Artemisia absinthium*). Absinthin, found in plants of the genus *Artemisia*, such as *A. absinthium*, is so bitter it can be tasted at dilutions of 1:30,000.

The constituents that contribute bitterness to an herb are described as *bitter principles*. Taste is a phenomenon of chemoreception; a range of molecular structures share the bitter property. Great diversity and complexity are found among these bitter principles, but it appears that they all work in a similar way by triggering a lingual sensory response. A reflex

when used for internal bleeding. Astringent action results from a diverse group of complex chemicals called tannins or gallotannins that share chemical and physical properties. The name *tannin* comes from the use of these constituents in the tanning industry. They have the effect of precipitating, or denaturing, protein molecules. They also precipitate starch, gelatin, alkaloids, and salts of heavy metals. One of the few incompatibilities found when making herbal medicines is

BOX 3-11   Herbal Astringents

Bayberry *(Myrica cerifera)*
Bearberry *(Arctostaphylos uva-ursi)*
Blackberry *(Rubus villosus)*
Cranesbill *(Geranium maculatum)*
Green tea *(Camellia sinensis)*
Goldenrod *(Solidago virgaurea)*
Horse chestnut *(Aesculus hippocastanum)*
Horsetail *(Equisetum arvense)*
Oak *(Quercus* spp.) (see Fig. 3-9)
Plantain *(Plantago major)*
Raspberry *(Rubus* spp.)

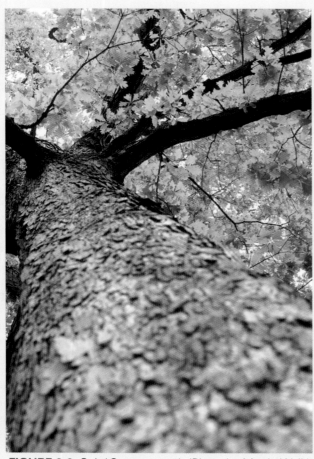

FIGURE 3-9 Oak *(Quercus* spp.). (Photo by Martin Wall.)

Sage *(Salvia officinalis)*
Shepherd's purse *(Capsella bursa-pastoris)*
Witch hazel *(Hamamelis virginiana)*
Yarrow *(Achillea millefolium)*

TABLE 3-4   Body System Affinities with Astringents

Body System	Examples of Herbs
Digestive	*Quercus* spp., *Hamamelis virginiana, Geranium maculatum, Hydrastis canadensis, Salvia officinalis*
Urinary system	*Equisetum arvense, Achillea millefolium*
Reproductive	*Alchemilla arvensis, Hydrastis canadensis, capsella bursa-pastoris, Achillea millefolium*
Skin	*Achillea millefolium, Hamamelis virginiana, Plantago major, Quercus* spp.

BOX 3-12   Herbal Bitters

Barberry *(Berberis vulgaris)*
Boneset *(Eupatorium perfoliatum)*
Centaury *(Centaurium erythraea)*
Chamomile *(Matricaria recutita)*
Dandelion *(Taraxacum officinale)*
Gentian *(Gentiana lutea)*
Goldenseal *(Hydrastis canadensis)*
Horehound *(Marrubium vulgare)*
Mugwort *(Artemisia vulgaris)*
Rue *(Ruta graveolens)*
Tansy *(Tanacetum vulgare)* (see Fig. 3-10)
Wormwood *(Artemisia absinthium)*
Yarrow *(Achillea millefolium)*

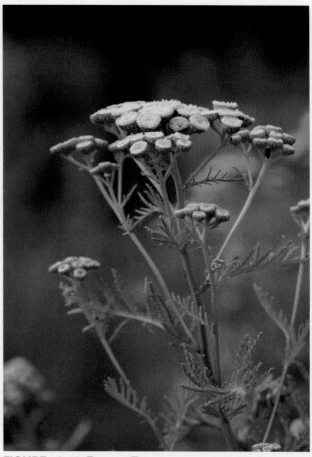

FIGURE 3-10 Tansy *(Tanacetum vulgare)*. (Photo by Martin Wall.)

is stimulated by bitter taste, directed by the nerves to the central nervous system. From there, a message goes to the gut, giving rise to the release of the digestive hormone gastrin. This in turn leads to a whole range of effects, all of value to the digestive process. Among the many actions of bitters, they:
- Stimulate appetite
- Stimulate release of digestive juices from the pancreas, duodenum, and liver

TABLE 3-5	**Body System Affinities for Bitters**
Body System	**Examples of Herbs**
Cardiovascular	*Leonurus cardiaca*
Digestive	*Artemisia vulgaris, Berberis vulgaris, Centaurium erythraea, Chelidonium majus, Gentiana lutea, Hydrastis canadensis*
Reproductive	*Achillea millefolium*
Nervous	*Humulus lupulus, Valeriana officinalis*
Skin	*Taraxacum officinale, Arctium lappa*

- Aid the liver in detoxification work and increase the flow of bile
- Help regulate secretion of pancreatic hormones that regulate blood sugar, insulin, and glucagon
- Help the gut wall repair damage

The tonic effects of these remedies go beyond specific digestive hormone activity. As digestion and assimilation of food is basic to health, bitter stimulation can often fundamentally affect health far beyond the simple mechanics of digestion (Table 3-5). It is not necessary to taste the bitter taste to receive the benefits because the gut has bitter receptors downstream from the oral cavity.

There are a number of contraindications to the use of bitters including use with the following conditions:

- Pregnancy
- Kidney stones
- Gallbladder disease
- Gastroesophageal reflux
- Hiatal hernia
- Gastritis
- Peptic ulcer disease

Cardiac Herbs

Some of the remedies in the cardiac group (Box 3-13 and Fig. 3-11) are powerful cardioactive agents, such as *Digitalis* (foxglove), whereas others are gentle and generally safe cardiotonics, like *Crataegus* (hawthorn) and *Tilia* (linden).

- *Cardiotonics* have an observable beneficial action on the heart and blood vessels but do not contain cardiac glycosides. Flavones appear to be major contributors to their beneficial actions. Examples include *Crataegus, Tilia platyphyllos, Allium sativum,* and *Leonurus cardiaca.*
- *Cardioactive* plants owe their effects on the heart to their content of cardiac glycosides, and thus have both the benefits and drawbacks of these constituents. The main danger is that glycosides will accumulate in the body, as their elimination rates tend to be low. *Convallaria majalis* is an example of a botanical used by medical herbalists to augment cardiac function. Care must be taken with these herbs, particularly when patients are on cardiac medications or have cardiac conditions.

BOX 3-13   Cardiovascular Herbs

Bugleweed (*Lycopus* spp.)
Cayenne *(Capsicum annuum)*
Coleus *(Coleus forskohlii)*
Garlic *(Allium sativum)*
Ginkgo *(Ginkgo biloba)*
Hawthorn *(Crataegus* spp.)

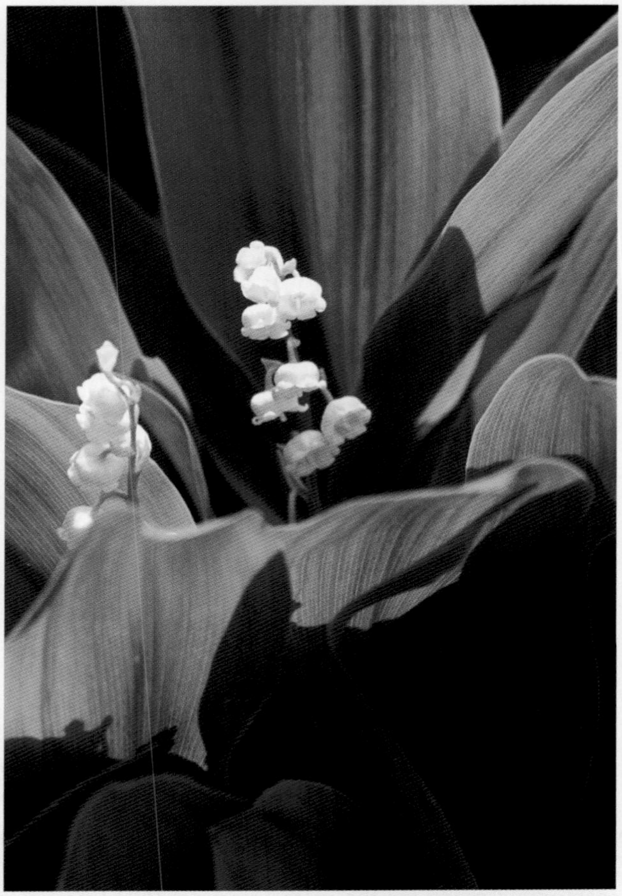

FIGURE 3-11 Lily of the valley *(Convallaria majalis).* (Photo by Martin Wall.)

Horse chestnut *(Aesculus hippocastanum)*
Lemon balm *(Melissa officinalis)*
Lily of the valley *(Convallaria majalis)* (see Fig. 3-11)
Linden *(Tilia platyphyllos)*
Motherwort *(Leonurus cardiaca)*
Rosemary *(Rosmarinus officinalis)*
Yarrow *(Achillea millefolium)*

Carminatives

Carminatives (Box 3-14 and Fig. 3-12) are specifically antispasmodic to the bowel, easing cramping, griping, and discomfort caused by flatulence. Their mode of action is attributed to volatile oils. These terpene oils have local anti-inflammatory and antispasmodic effects upon the mucosal and muscular layers of the alimentary canal. An example is farnesene, a constituent of many complex plant volatile

BOX 3-14 Herbal Carminatives

Angelica *(Angelica archangelica)*
Aniseed *(Pimpinella anisum)* (see Fig. 3-12)
Caraway *(Carum carvi)*
Cardamon *(Elettaria cardamomum)*
Chamomile *(Matricaria recutita)*
Cinnamon *(Cinnamomum* spp.)
Dill *(Anethum graveolens)*
Fennel *(Foeniculum vulgare)*
Ginger *(Zingiber officinale)*
Hops *(Humulus lupulus)*
Lemon balm *(Melissa officinalis)*

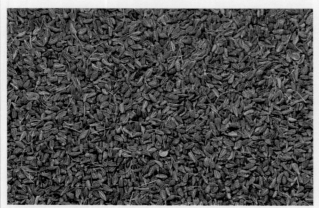

FIGURE 3-12 Aniseed *(Pimpinella anisum)*. (Photo by Martin Wall.)

Peppermint *(Mentha piperita)*
Sage *(Salvia officinalis)*
Thyme *(Thymus* spp.)
Valerian *(Valeriana officinalis)*

BOX 3-15 Herbal Cholagogues

Artichoke *(Cynara scolymus)*
Balmony *(Chelone glabra)*
Barberry *(Berberis vulgaris)*
Black root *(Leptandra virginica)*
Blue flag *(Iris versicolor)*
Boldo *(Peumus boldus)*
Boneset *(Eupatorium perfoliatum)*
Butternut *(Juglans cinerea)*
Celandine *(Chelidonium majus)*
Dandelion *(Taraxacum officinale)*
Fringe tree bark *(Chionanthus virginicus)*
Fumitory *(Fumaria officinalis)*
Gentian *(Gentiana lutea)*
Goldenseal *(Hydrastis canadensis)*
Lemon balm *(Melissa officinalis)*
Oregon grape *(Mahonia aquifolium)*
Rosemary *(Rosmarinus officinalis)*
Sage *(Salvia officinalis)*
Wild indigo *(Baptisia tinctoria)*
Wild yam *(Dioscorea villosa)*
Yellow dock *(Rumex crispus)*

- Acute cholecystitis, unless gallstones have been ruled out
- Acute viral hepatitis
- Liver disorders

Demulcents

Demulcent herbs (Box 3-16 and Fig. 3-13) soothe and protect irritated or inflamed tissue. Used topically, they are called emollients. Demulcents are rich in carbohydrate mucilage made up of complex polysaccharide molecules. They become slimy and gummy when they come in contact with water. This physical property has a clear and direct action on the lining of the intestines, where it soothes and reduces irritation by direct contact. However, some demulcents have similar actions far from the site of their absorption into the body, for example, the urinary tract or lungs (Table 3-6), which is less easily explainable and likely caused by reflex action or as yet unclear systemic action. In general, mucilage-containing demulcents share the following properties:

- Reduce irritation down the whole length of the enteric system
- Lessen the sensitivity of the digestive system to gastric acids and to digestive bitters
- Help prevent diarrhea secondary to inflammation/ irritation
- Reduce digestive muscle spasms that cause colic
- Ease coughing by soothing bronchial tension
- Relax painful spasms in the bladder and urinary system, and sometimes even in the uterus

Diuretics

Strictly speaking, a diuretic (Box 3-17) is a remedy that increases urination. In traditional herbal medicine, the term *diuretic* tends to be applied more broadly to herbs that

oils with carminative actions, such as *Matricaria recutita*. *Origanum compactum* is a species of oregano used as an antispasmodic remedy for the gastrointestinal (GI) tract, especially in Morocco. Belgian researchers have found that the infusion of flowers and leaves inhibits contractions triggered in guinea pig ileum by acetylcholine, histamine, serotonin, nicotine, 1,1-dimethyl-4-phenylpiperazine iodide, and even electrical stimulation. The main active components in the essential oil were identified as thymol and carvacrol. This example may help explain the well-known actions of all of the carminative remedies.

Cholagogues

Cholagogues (Box 3-15) stimulate the flow of bile from the liver. Most bitters and hepatics are also cholagogues. These herbs are of great help to digestion, assimilation, and elimination.

Cholagogues are contraindicated in the presence of the following conditions:
- Painful gallstones
- Acute bilious colic
- Obstructive jaundice

BOX 3-16   Herbal Demulcents

Coltsfoot *(Tussilago farfara)*
Comfrey *(Symphytum officinale)* (see Fig. 3-13)
Cornsilk *(Zea mays)*
Flax *(Linum usitatissimum)*
Iceland moss *(Cetraria islandica)*
Irish moss *(Chondrus crispus)*
Licorice *(Glycyrrhiza glabra)*

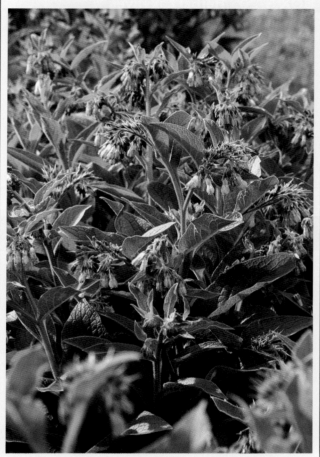

FIGURE 3-13 Comfrey *(Symphytum officinale)*. (Photo by Martin Wall.)

Oat *(Avena sativa)*
Marshmallow *(Althaea officinalis)*
Mullein *(Verbascum thapsus)*
Slippery elm *(Ulmus rubra)*

TABLE 3-6   Body System Affinities for Demulcents

Body System	Examples of Herbs
Digestive	*Symphytum officinale, Althaea officinalis, Cetraria islandica, Chondrus crispus, Glycyrrhiza glabra, Linum usitatissimum, Ulmus rubra*
Urinary	*Althea officinalis*
Skin	*Symphytum officinale, Althaea officinalis, Plantago major, Stellaria media, Ulmus rubra*

BOX 3-17   Herbal Diuretics

Boldo *(Peumus boldus)*
Buchu *(Agathosma betulina)*
Celery seed *(Apium graveolens)*
Corn silk *(Zea mays)*
Dandelion leaf *(Taraxacum officinale)*
Juniper *(Juniperus communis)*
Linden *(Tilia platyphyllos)*
Parsley *(Petroselinum crispum)*
Pellitory of the wall *(Parietaria judaica)*
Saw palmetto *(Serenoa repens)*

TABLE 3-7   Types of Urinary Tract Herbs

Action	Herbs
Antiinflammatory	*Arctostaphylos uva-ursi, Galium aparine, Zea mays, Althea officinalis*
Antilithic	*Collinsonia canadensis, Eupatorium purpureum*
Antimicrobial	*Achillea millefolium, Arctostaphylos uva-ursi, Vaccinium macrocarpon*
Astringent	*Achillea millefolium, Arctostaphylos uva-ursi, Equisetum arvense*
Demulcent	*Arctostaphylos uva-ursi, Zea mays*

TABLE 3-8   Body System Affinities for Diuretics

Body System	Examples of Herbs
Bladder	*Vaccinium macrocarpon, Achillea millefolium, Zea mays, Arctostaphylos uva-ursi*
Cardiovascular	*Convallaria majalis, Taraxacum officinale, Achillea millefolium*
Skin	*Galium aparine, Taraxacum officinale*

have some sort of beneficial action on the urinary system (Table 3-7); for example, urinary demulcents and antiinflammatory remedies (Table 3-8). I rarely ever use *diuretic* herbs for the true purpose of diuresis; however, urinary antispasmodics and demulcents are used in this book, and in such cases, these terms are specified. Many diaphoretic herbs act as diuretics when taken cold.

Hepatics

Hepatic herbs (Box 3-18) are used to stimulate or support liver function in a range of ways. Traditionally, they were used to tone and strengthen liver function, and, in some cases, increase the flow of bile (also see Bitters). They are classically included as primary components of treatments for skin conditions. They are also widely used by herbalists in protocol for the treatment of gynecological conditions in which there is hormonal dysregulation; this use is based on the premise that improved liver function will improve hormonal conjugation and elimination. Western herbs such as *Leonurus cardiaca* and *Taraxacum officinale* are commonly used this way, as is the TCM herb

BOX 3-18 Hepatic Herbs

Agrimony (*Agrimonia eupatoria*)
Artichoke (*Cynara scolymus*)
Balmony (*Chelone glabra*)
Barberry (*Berberis vulgaris*)
Centaury (*Centaurium erythraea*)
Dandelion (*Taraxacum officinale*)
Fringe tree (*Chionanthus virginicus*)
Gentian (*Gentiana lutea*)
Goldenseal (*Hydrastis canadensis*)
Milk thistle (*Silybum marianum*)
Motherwort (*Leonurus cardiaca*)
Oregon grape (*Mahonia aquifolium*)
Tumeric (*Curcuma longa*)
Yarrow (*Achillea millefolium*)
Yellow dock (*Rumex crispus*)

BOX 3-19 Hepatoprotective Herbs

Calendula (*Calendula officinalis*)
Milk thistle (*Silybum marianum*)
Rosemary (*Rosmarinus officinalis*)
Schizandra (*Schisandra chinensis*)
Tumeric (*Curcuma longa*)

BOX 3-20 Herbal Laxatives

Aperient herbs
Licorice (*Glycyrrhiza glabra*)
Yellow dock (*Rumex crispus*)

Bulk laxatives
Flax seed (*Linum usitatissimum*)
Psyllium seed (*Plantago ovata*)

Demulcent laxatives
Irish moss (*Chondrus crispus*)
Licorice (*Glycyrrhiza glabra*)
Slippery elm bark (*Ulmus rubra*)

TABLE 3-9 Body System Affinities for Hepatic Herbs

Body System	Examples of Herbs
Digestive	*Agrimonia eupatoria, Berberis vulgaris, Juglans cinerea, Taraxacum officinale* root, *Chionanthus virginicus* bark, *Gentiana lutea*
Reproductive	*Hydrastis canadensis, Berberis vulgaris*
Skin	*Iris versicolor, Taraxacum officinale, Hydrastis canadensis, Mahonia aquifolium, Rumex crispus*

TABLE 3-10 Body System Affinities for Nervines

Body System	Examples of Herbs
Cardiovascular	*Melissa officinalis, Tilia platyphyllos, Leonurus cardiaca*
Digestive	*Melissa officinalis, Matricaria recutita, Lavandula* spp., *Humulus lupulus, Valeriana officinalis*
Reproductive	*Actaea racemosa, Caulophyllum thalictroides, Viburnum* spp., *Leonurus cardiaca*
Musculoskeletal	*Actaea racemosa, Viburnum prunifolium*
Skin	All nervines may help the skin in an indirect way, but the following have a good reputation for skin conditions: *Scutellaria lateriflora, Hypericum perforatum, Actaea racemosa*

Bupleurum falcatum, in combination with other TCM or Western herbs. The hepatic herbs listed in Box 3-18 are otherwise not largely used this way gynecologically but are used to improve digestion and phase 1 and 2 detoxification (Table 3-9).

Hepatoprotective herbs (Box 3-19), which are given their own separate category, specifically serve as antioxidants, and support phase 1 and phase 2 detoxification. Some—for example, *Silybum marianum*—protect the hepatocytes from oxidative and other damage. Vegetables in the *Brassicaceae* family (e.g., broccoli, kale, collard greens, cabbage) are also hepatoprotective.

Laxatives

Herbal laxatives (Box 3-20) stimulate the bowel as a result of anthraquinones and other constituents that stimulate bowel peristalsis—some quite aggressively (i.e., purgatives) whereas others are more gentle (i.e., aperients)—or via mechanical action, either by lubrication or by providing bulk.

Nervines

A nervine is an herb with a restorative or relaxing effect upon the nervous system. Nervines are commonly included in many herbal protocols because many illnesses are caused by stress; illness, especially when chronic, is almost universally accompanied by a stress component, affecting sleep and ability to relax (Table 3-10). Nervines are divided into categories based on their effects, some of which are elaborated on in Table 3-11 (Fig. 3-14).

Nervine Tonics

Nervine tonic herbs are commonly prescribed in cases of acute or chronic emotional or mental stress or nervous debility, often in conjunction with adaptogens. This invaluable group of tonic remedies is best exemplified by *Avena sativa*. Nervine tonics that also have a relaxing effect include *Scutellaria lateriflora* and *Hypericum perforatum*. Some nervines may also be stimulating to the nervous system, imparting a sense of energy; Mate (*Ilex paraguariensis*) is an example; see Table 3-11 for additional examples.

Nervine Relaxants

Nervine relaxants (Box 3-21) are most important in times of stress, anxiety, and feeling overwhelmed. They are used in a broad holistic way to bring calm and emotional ease at lower doses and gently promote sleep at higher doses. Many can be

TABLE 3-11	Nervine Categories
Nervine Action	**Herbal Examples**
Antispasmodic	*Piper methysticum, Valeriana officinalis* (see Fig. 3-14), *Viburnum opulus, Actaea racemosa, Passiflora incarnata*
Antidepressant	*Hypericum perforatum, Melissa officinalis*
Adaptogen	*Withania somnifera*
Analgesic	*Piscidia piscipula, Gelsemium sempervirens*
Anxiolytic	*Piper methysticum, Passiflora incarnata*
Relaxant	*Passiflora incarnata, Scutellaria lateriflora, Valeriana officinalis, Verbena officinalis*
Sedative	*Humulus lupulus, Passiflora incarnata, Valeriana officinalis*
Stimulant	*Coffea arabica, Camellia sinensis, Cola vera, Paullinia cupana,* Mate (*Ilex paraguayiensis*)
Tonic	*Avena sativa, Hypericum perforatum, Scutellaria lateriflora,* (see Adaptogens)

BOX 3-21   Nervine Relaxants

Ashwagandha (*Withania somnifera*)
Black cohosh (*Actaea racemosa*)
Black haw (*Viburnum prunifolium*)
California poppy (*Eschscholzia californica*)
Chamomile (*Matricaria recutita*)
Cramp bark (*Viburnum opulus*)
Damiana (*Turnera diffusa*)
Hops (*Humulus lupulus*)
Jamaican dogwood (*Piscidia piscipula*)
Kava kava (*Piper methysticum*)
Lavender (*Lavandula* spp.)
Lemon balm (*Melissa officinalis*)
Linden (*Tilia platyphyllos*)
Lobelia (*Lobelia inflata*)
Milky oats (*Avena sativa*)
Motherwort (*Leonurus cardiaca*)
Passionflower (*Passiflora incarnata*)
Pulsatilla (*Anemone pulsatilla*)
Pulsatilla (*Pulsatilla vulgaris*)
Skullcap (*Scutellaria lateriflora*)
St. John's wort (*Hypericum perforatum*)
Valerian (*Valeriana officinalis*)
Vervain (*Verbena officinalis*)
Wood betony (*Stachys betonica*)
Ziziphus (*Ziziphus spinosa*)

BOX 3-22   Sedative Herbs

Ashwagandha (*Withania somnifera*)
California poppy (*Eschscholzia californica*)
Corydalis (*Corydalis ambigua*)
Hops (*Humulus lupulus*)
Jamaican dogwood (*Piscidia piscipula*)
Pulsatilla (*Anemone pulsatilla*)
Valerian (*Valeriana officinalis*)

BOX 3-23   Anxiolytic Herbs

Ashwagandha (*Withania somnifera*)
Blue vervain (*Verbena officinalis*)
California poppy (*Eschscholzia californica*)
Chamomile (*Matricaria recutita*)
Kava kava (*Piper methysticum*)
Lavender (*Lavandula officinalis*)
Motherwort (*Leonurus cardiaca*)
Passionflower (*Passiflora incarnata*)
Skullcap (*Scutellaria lateriflora*)
Valerian (*Valeriana officinalis*)

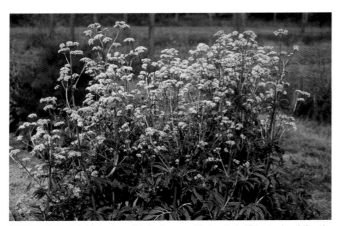

FIGURE 3-14 Valerian (*Valeriana officinalis*). (Photo by Martin Wall.)

selected on the basis of their secondary actions to treat additional problems. This is one of the great benefits of using herbal remedies to help with stress and anxiety. In addition to the herbs that work directly on the nervous system, antispasmodic herbs—those that affect the peripheral nerves and the muscles—may have an indirect relaxing action on the whole system. Putting the physical body at ease promotes ease in the psyche. Many nervine relaxants have this antispasmodic action. Sedating herbs (Box 3-22), or hypnotics, can be used to induce deeper relaxation when there is extreme tension, inability to sleep, or pain.

Anxiolytics

Herbs in the anxiolytic category (Box 3-23) are used to relieve the mental and physical symptoms of anxiety. They are generally not sedating or consciousness-impairing at lower doses, at which they can be used regularly to relieve chronic anxiety.

They can be applied at higher doses or higher dose frequencies for relief of acute anxiety. *Lavandula officinalis, Leonurus cardiaca,* and the nervine *Rhodiola rosea* are examples of anxiolytics.

Antidepressants

Much media attention and scientific research has gone into the herb St. John's wort, which is the most widely used antidepressant agent in Europe for the treatment of mild

BOX 3-24 **Herbal Antidepressants**

Ashwagandha *(Withania somnifera)*
Kava kava *(Piper methysticum)*
Lavender *(Lavandula officinalis)*
Lemon balm *(Melissa officinalis)*
Motherwort *(Leonurus cardiaca)*
Passionflower *(Passiflora incarnata)* (see Fig. 3-15)
St. John's wort *(Hypericum perforatum)*

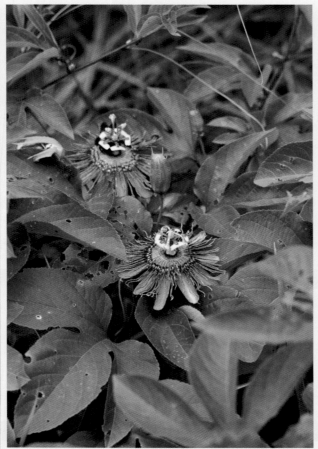

FIGURE 3-15 Passionflower *(Passiflora incarnata).* (Photo by Martin Wall.)

BOX 3-25 **Herbal Aphrodisiacs**

Cardamom *(Elettaria cardamomum)*
Cinnamon *(Cinnamomum* spp.)
Damiana *(Turnera aphrodisiaca, T. diffusa)*
Dong quai *(Angelica sinensis)*
Epimedium *(Epimedium aceranthus)*
Garlic *(Allium sativum)*
Ginseng *(Panax ginseng)*
Ho shou wu *(Polygonum multiflorum)*
Licorice *(Glycyrrhiza glabra)*
Longan *(Euphoria longan)*
Marijuana *(Cannabis* spp.)
Milky oats *(Avena sativa)*
Rehmannia *(Rehmannia glutinosa)*
Saw palmetto *(Serenoa repens)*
Schisandra *(Schisandra chinensis)*
Shatavari *(Asparagus racemosus)*
Tribulus *(Tribulus terrestris)*
Wolf berry *(Lycium chinense)*
Yohimbe *(Pausinystalia yohimbe)*

GYNECOLOGICAL AND OBSTETRIC ACTIONS

Aphrodisiacs

Herbal aphrodisiacs (Box 3-25) have a long history of use both as sexual stimulants for pleasure's sake and for the treatment of sexual debility. The ability to improve sexual function is ascribed to numerous herbs from many cultures. Their activity is variously attributed to stimulating action, especially the warming, spicy, and fragrant herbs; kidney tonic function; improved strength of the reproductive/sexual activities; nervine relaxation activity; improved vaginal tissue tone and lubrication; and increased pelvic circulation. A few of these have research or clinical trials behind them, including *Centella asiatica, Humulus lupulus, Panax ginseng,* and *Avena sativa.*

Emmenagogues

Strictly speaking, emmenagogues (Box 3-26 and Fig. 3-16) are herbs that stimulate menstrual flow, and are typically used to treat amenorrhea. Several are abortifacient; thus emmenagogues are contraindicated in pregnancy. In TCM, the concept of an emmenagogue is applied to those herbs that increase general blood flow—for example, *Salvia miltiorrhiza*—and may be used for gynecologic purposes, but are also used to improve cardiovascular function. Today, many herbals use the term *emmenagogue* broadly to denote remedies that tone and normalize the function of the female reproductive system; however, this is inaccurate. Of the many plants that stimulate menstruation, some also have a tonic effect. Some appear to work through hormonal activity, others through local irritation, and some may have effects on coagulation or uterine circulation. They should be used with great care.

Galactagogues

Galactagogues (Box 3-27) stimulate the production or flow of breast milk in lactating women. They may act hormonally, or

to moderate depression. The actions of most herbs used as antidepressants continue to be elucidated, and new herbs are added to the treatment panoply as our understanding of depression evolves. St. John's wort contains active ingredients that appear, among other actions, to act as monoamine oxidase inhibitors (MAOIs). The historical use of this herb as an antidepressant is ancient, long preceding the existence of psychiatry as a medical field. More recently, *Curcuma long* extracts have been found effective in the treatment of depression, most likely because of the inflammation that can cause this condition. Depression, as with other conditions in the herbal clinic, is treated comprehensively, with attention to the whole patient, not just his or her neurotransmitters. Herbs can play an important role in the botanical clinical treatment of depression (Box 3-24 and Fig. 3-15).

BOX 3-26   Herbal Emmenagogues

Blue cohosh (*Caulophyllum thalictroides*)
Cotton root (*Gossypium herbaceum*)

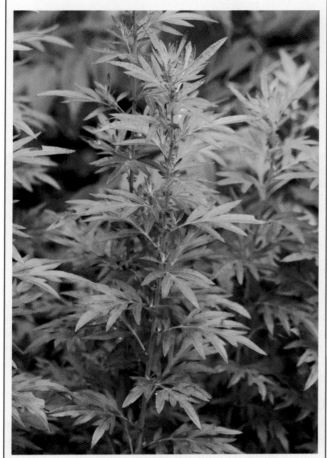

Dong quai (*Angelica sinensis*)
Feverfew (*Tanacetum parthenium*)
Ginger (*Zingiber officinale*)
Motherwort (*Leonurus cardiaca*)
Mugwort (*Artemisia vulgaris*) (see Fig. 3-16)
Pennyroyal (*Mentha pulegium*)
Rue (*Ruta graveolens*)
Sage (*Salvia officinalis*)
Tansy (*Tanacetum vulgare*)

FIGURE 3-16 Mugwort (*Artemisia vulgaris*). (Photo by Martin Wall.)

BOX 3-27   Galactogogue Herbs

Anise seed (*Pimpinella anisum*)
Chamomile (*Matricaria recutita*)
Chaste berry (*Vitex agnus-castus*)
Fennel (*Foeniculum vulgare*)
Fenugreek (*Trigonella foenum-graecum*)
Marshmallow (*Althea officinalis*)
Milky oats (*Avena sativa*)

BOX 3-28   Hormone-Regulating Herbs

Black cohosh (*Actaea racemosa*)
Blue cohosh (*Caulophyllum thalictroides*)
Blue vervain (*Verbena officinalis*)
Chaste berry (*Vitex agnus-castus*)
Dong quai (*Angelica sinensis*)
False unicorn (*Chamaelirium luteum*)
Fennel (*Foeniculum vulgare*)
Licorice (*Glycyrrhiza glabra*)
Motherwort (*Leonurus cardiaca*)
Red clover (*Trifolium pratense*)
Sarsaparilla (*Smilax ornata*)
Soy (*Glycine max*)
Tribulus (*Tribulus terrestris*)
White peony (*Paeonia lactiflora*)
Wild yam (*Dioscorea villosa*)

BOX 3-29   Ovarian Tonic Herbs

Blue cohosh (*Caulophyllum thalictroides*)
Chaste berry (*Vitex agnus-castus*)
False unicorn (*Chamaelirium luteum*)
White peony (*Paeonia lactiflora*)

may include herbs that are nutritive to improve milk quality and quantity. Nervines are commonly combined with galactagogues to encourage relaxation and thereby facilitate the letdown reflex.

Hormonal Modulators

Many claims are being made about plants that affect hormonal balance (Box 3-28), but we will limit our discussion here to those that have a measurable influence. The most important of these herbs in the European tradition is *Vitex agnus-castus*.

Other herbs such as *Humulus lupulus* and *Salvia officinalis* have measurable estrogenic effects.

Ovarian Tonics

Herbs in the ovarian tonic category (Box 3-29) have demonstrated or alleged direct or indirect stimulating effects on the ovaries and are thus used when there is hormonal dysregulation at the level of the ovary; infertility; when there is poor ovarian circulation suspected; and when there are ovarian cysts or endometriosis of the ovary.

Oxytocic or Partus Preparator

Oxytocic or partus preparators are herbs (Box 3-30) that have been used to promote or increase uterine activity, facilitating labor or expulsion of the placenta. (See Chapters 15 and 20 for a complete discussion of this category of herbs.)

Phytoestrogen

Phytoestrogen is a relatively new term in the herbal nomenclature, referring to herbs that contain isoflavones with estrogen-like activity. Many herbs in this category are legumes, such as soy and red clover. Several volatile oil–rich herbs may also

---

BOX 3-30 Oxytocic (Partus Preparator) Herbs

Blue cohosh (*Caulophyllum thalictroides*)
Cotton root (*Gossypium herbaceum*)
Partridge berry (*Mitchella repens*)
Schisandra (*Schisandra chinensis*)
Spikenard (*Aralia racemosa*)

BOX 3-31 Uterine Astringent/Antihemorrhagic Herbs

Bayberry (*Myrica cerifera*)
Bethroot (*Trillium erectum*) (see Fig. 3-17)
Cinnamon (*Cinnamomum* spp.)
Cranesbill (*Geranium maculatum*)
Erigeron (*Canada fleabane*)
Lady's mantle (*Alchemilla vulgaris*)
Shepherd's purse (*Capsella bursa-pastoris*)
Panax notoginseng
Raspberry (*Rubus idaeus*)
Witch hazel (*Hamamelis virginiana*)
Yarrow (*Achillea millefolium*)

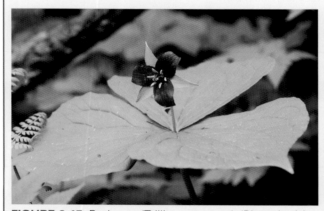

FIGURE 3-17 Bethroot (*Trillium erectum*). (Photo by Martin Wall.)

BOX 3-32 Uterine Antispasmodic Herbs

Black cohosh (*Actaea racemosa*)
Black haw (*Viburnum prunifolium*)
Chamomile (*Matricaria recutita*)
Corydalis (*Corydalis ambigua*)
Cramp bark (*Viburnum opulus*)
Dong quai (*Angelica sinensis*)
Jamaican dogwood (*Piscidia piscipula*)
Motherwort (*Leonurus cardiaca*)
Pulsatilla (*Anemone pulsatilla*)
White peony (*Paeonia lactiflora*)
Wild yam (*Dioscorea villosa*)

BOX 3-33 Uterine Circulatory Stimulant Herbs

Cinnamon (*Cinnamomum cassia*)
Dong quai (*Angelica sinensis*)
Ginger (*Zingiber officinalis*)
Motherwort (*Leonurus cardiaca*)
Peony (*Paeonia* spp.)

---

have estrogen activity, such as anise seed and fennel, and herbs such as hops and sage have also been found to have estrogenic potential. A great deal of attention has been directed toward research on the potential health benefits of phytoestrogens for the prevention of a variety of conditions and diseases, especially menopausal complaints, cancer, and osteoporosis, as well as their risks. Other herbs that have been proposed to have hormonal activity, for example, black cohosh and dong quai, do not and work through other mechanisms of action; for example, black cohosh most likely works via serotonin pathways that help with the neurovegetative symptoms of perimenopause.

Uterine Astringents/Antihemorrhagics

A number of herbs (Box 3-31 and Fig. 3-17) are used to reduce uterine blood loss whether related to menorrhagia, metrorrhagia, or organic disease, such as fibroids. How these herbs work is an important but unanswered question. No astringent tannin can reach uterine tissue from the gut. It is possible that some, but not all, of these herbs have some kind of hormonal effect. Of the many valuable remedies listed as astringents earlier in this chapter, perhaps the most valued is *Achillea millefolium*.

Uterine Antispasmodics

There are a number of valuable remedies (Box 3-32) that affect the complex autonomic innervation and smooth musculature of the reproductive system. These are used for the treatment of dysmenorrhea, endometriosis, chronic pelvic pain, irritable uterus of pregnancy, painful labor contractions, and other painful or spasmodic conditions of the uterus.

Uterine Circulatory Stimulant

Uterine circulatory stimulant herbs (Box 3-33) are a subset of uterine tonics, and are used to improve circulation to the uterus when there is ischemic pain, for example, with dysmenorrhea. They are also used to improve circulation to reduce uterine/pelvic congestion, such as with uterine fibromyomas. They are mostly contraindicated during pregnancy unless otherwise specified (e.g., *Zingiber officinalis* for nausea and vomiting of pregnancy [NVP]).

Uterine Tonic

The term *emmenagogue* is sometimes used to describe herbs that are actually uterine tonics (Box 3-34) but that do not necessarily stimulate menstrual flow. These are plants that have a toning, strengthening, and nourishing effect upon both the tissue and function of the female reproductive system. We do not have a good understanding of how and why they work, but this should not invalidate their observed

> ### BOX 3-34   Uterine Tonic Herbs
>
> Black cohosh (*Actaea racemosa*)
> Black haw (*Viburnum opulus*)
> Bethroot (*Trillium erectum*)
> Blue cohosh (*Caulophyllum thalictroides*)
> Cramp bark (*Viburnum prunifolium*)
> Dong quai (*Angelica sinensis*)
> False unicorn (*Chamaelirium luteum**)
> Goldenseal (*Hydrastis canadensis*)
> Lady's mantle (*Alchemilla vulgaris*)
> Motherwort (*Leonurus cardiaca*)
> Partridge berry (*Mitchella repens*)
> Raspberry leaf (*Rubus idaeus*)
> Yarrow (*Achillea millefolium*)

*False unicorn is an endangered botanical; therefore use only cultivated herbal products.

therapeutic value. They are commonly applied for conditions such as endometriosis, uterine fibromyomas, dysmenorrhea, metrorrhagia, dysfunctional uterine bleeding, and other conditions in which the uterus is "boggy," there is regularly excessive bleeding, or there is pain and spasmodic activity. For the latter, they are often combined with uterine antispasmodics.

SELECTION CRITERIA, FORMULATION, AND PRESCRIBING

> *Herbal medicine encourages the physician to treat the patient as an individual and, hence, to switch from a fixed therapy regimen to a more individualized type of therapy.*
> *Rudolph Weiss*[27]

The herbal products market offers consumers and practitioners an overwhelming array of individual products and formulae from which to choose for virtually every conceivable symptom and condition. This creates both convenience and potential confusion: Which herbs and formulations are effective? Safe? Some products are based on traditional formulation principles and herbal indications, and others seemingly contain a kitchen sink of herbs based on marketing trends and, sometimes, misinformation.

Understanding the principles of herbal formulation allows the practitioner to effectively understand and evaluate formulae—both their individual ingredients and how they work as a whole—and to select those that might offer benefit to their patients and reject those that are ineffective at best, and potentially harmful at worst.

Building a successful herbal formula—determining the correct herbs, their correct proportions, and the dosing strategy—is a central skill in herbal medicine practice. It is in custom formulation that herbal medicine is most tailored to patients' unique needs, and most greatly departs from conventional medical care with its standardized prescriptions. It is also where much of the science with which we struggle to validate herbal medicine efficacy becomes

limited and we are forced to rely on practitioner experience and tradition.[27,28]

There are numerous factors to consider when choosing which herbs to include in a formula, the exact proportions of all of the herbs, and the prescribing schedule. Dosing is discussed separately in this chapter.

SELECTION CRITERIA

Multiple factors influence the selection of herbs for the individual patient, including the patient's condition; the system of herbal medicine used by the practitioner; the actions of specific herbs and the systems they affect; herbs' availability, environmental sustainability, and cost; and likelihood of patient commitment* (Table 3-12).

Prescribing for the Individual Patient's Condition

The most important factor determining the selection of herbs is the patient's condition, both currently and constitutionally. This is determined by differential diagnosis and physical assessment, the patient's overall health status (i.e., current and past medical history), and an understanding of underlying factors associated with the disease or disorder process, including but not limited to health of the major body systems (e.g., whether there are chronic digestive or circulatory problems) and social, emotional, and psychological stressors and factors affecting the patient.

The Herbal Medicine System

The system of herbal medicine to which the practitioner subscribes determines the language of the diagnosis, which in turn influences the selection of herbs and the rationale for their use. For example, a Western biomedical herbal practitioner diagnosing a patient with symptoms of vaginal itching, yellowish-white discharge, and frequent urination might diagnose *vaginal candidiasis*, whereas a TCM practitioner might diagnose the same patient with damp heat and blood deficiency. Although there is some crossover in the herbs that are selected by each practitioner (e.g., both may end up with a berberine-containing herb in the final formula, perhaps *Coptis chinensis* [goldthread] or *Hydrastis canadensis* [goldenseal]), the language to describe their inclusion differs.

The Western practitioner would include one of these herbs for their antimicrobial, antiinflammatory constituents; the TCM

---

*In the first edition of this book I used the word "compliance" here, where it is now changed to commitment. *Compliance* is a word that I have eliminated from my own doctor–patient lexicon. This shift is more than semantic; it reflects a change in the patient–doctor relationship to one of mutual understanding and practitioner efficacy in determining and working with the patient to overcome obstacles to what is ideally a commitment to adhering to a protocol, compared with the outdated model in which a patient "complies" with the "doctor's orders." It is also an evolution beyond "adherence" and "concordance," which the reader can learn more about here: Aronson JK: Compliance, concordance, adherence, *Br J Clin Pharmacol* 63(4):383–384, 2007.

TABLE 3-12	**Summary of Factors Affecting Herb Selection Criteria**
Factor	**Description**
Individual patient's condition	Accurate diagnosis, understanding of underlying or concomitant factors, history
Herbal medicine system	Assessment of patient and understanding and prescribing of herbs is consistent with an herbal medicine system or context (e.g., Western herbal medicine, Traditional Chinese Medicine, Ayurveda)
Herbal actions	Understanding the pharmacologic, biological, traditional, and synergistic actions of herbal medicines
Availability	Patients' ability to obtain ingredients in herbal formulae
Financial considerations	Patients' ability to afford herbal formulae in adequate amounts and for adequate durations for efficacy
Ecological considerations	Use of herbs that are not endangered or rare; recognizing the intrinsic relationship between planetary and individual health in medical health choices
Patient commitment and esthetics	Patients' ability to commit to protocol, based on ease of obtaining and preparing herbs, and palatability

practitioner would describe these same effects as "heat clearing" and "cooling." The TCM practitioner might also include herbs that nourish the blood, such as a combination of *Angelica sinensis* and *Rehmannia glutinosa* as part of a larger formula for treating the perceived underlying blood deficiency. The Western practitioner may also separately provide tonics for the patient who has recurrent problems with vaginal candidiasis.

Practitioners must define for themselves the system of herbal medicine they are using, and from this they can define the language that will shape their system of herb selection. This book focuses primarily on a Western system of herbal medicine, using both Western biomedical knowledge of herbs, as well as traditional Western herbal philosophies. Additionally, representing the synthesis of herbal traditions that now compose Western herbal medicine, herbs from the Chinese and Indian materia medica are included, based on both their traditional uses and actions and modern pharmacologic understanding of these herbs.

The Herbs and Their Actions

Integral to the ability to create an herbal formula is knowledge of the properties, actions, appropriate indications, and contraindications of each herb. The American Herbalists Guild, the oldest and largest professional organization for herbal practitioners in the United States, requires their professional members to have a working knowledge of at least 150 different herbs. The British medical herbalist regularly uses more than 250 herbs in practice, and a TCM practitioner might select from among 2000 different medicines in the Chinese pharmacopoeia.[29] This breadth of knowledge is something that comes with time and experience, as well as a great deal of study. Practitioners must also have on hand a selection of reliable reference books, including materia medica, monographs, and pharmacopoeias. At first, the practitioner frequently refers to these books, but over time gains intimate knowledge of a wide variety of herbs that allow more spontaneity in formula development. However, even experienced practitioners regularly turn to their reference books—or most reliable Internet sources.

Practitioners can learn a great deal about the actions and energetics of herbs from their own clinical observations and those of their colleagues. For example, the herb *Angelica sinensis* (Dong quai), classified as a warming herb in TCM, is traditionally used as a postnatal tonic. Yet, as a midwife, I observed three distinct cases in my practice in which a breastfeeding newborn

developed the appearance of a heat rash in conjunction with the mother's consumption of the herb as part of a tea. In each case the rash disappeared with cessation of tea intake, and in one case, with retrial, reappeared. Such observations should not be discounted but gathered and collated to add to the growing body of knowledge of modern herbal medicine. This side effect of *A. sinensis* case is now documented in the *Angelica sinensis* monograph of the *AHP* and the *A. Sinensis Survey of the American Herbalists Guild*.[30,31] Herbal practitioners generally develop a repertory of herbs they most frequently use and that they find most effective. The selection varies with the practitioner's specialty; in other words, a gynecologic specialist draws from a slightly different materia medica than a practitioner who specializes in immune disorders. Of course, practitioners must be cautious about overvaluing their own or their colleagues' observations—there can be a tremendous amount of bias in the accuracy, interpretation, and reporting of individual clinical observations.

Availability of Herbs

Patients must be able to readily obtain the herbs and products in their prescriptions. Many herbal practitioners prefer to fill the prescription themselves to retain quality control and guarantee that the patient leaves an appointment with the intended formulae. If the practitioner plans to fill the prescription from his or her own dispensary, the herbs must be in stock, or a similar and adequate substitute must be available.[28] Not all health professionals want to run a complete dispensary through their practice because of time involved, costs, space availability, or even perceived conflicts of interest. There are several high-quality and reliable herb companies that provide formulation services, filling prescriptions and shipping products directly to patients. They allow practitioners to choose the discount available to patients, ranging from no mark-up, allowing patients to receive wholesale costs, to a full-retail price, creating a profit for the practitioner.

Financial Considerations

In the United States, herbal prescriptions, even when made by a licensed practitioner, are not usually reimbursable by insurance companies.[32] Although Americans have demonstrated that they are willing to pay out-of-pocket for herbal medicines, cost is a major concern for many. It is important to discuss financial ability with patients to provide a protocol that will allow them to take enough of the herbs for a sufficient duration of time to have the desired effect, and not add high herbal costs to their burden of health care costs.[28]

Herbal prescriptions may need to be tailored to meet the needs of the patient's budget, such as prescribing teas as a less expensive option to tinctures, and teaching patients to make their products whenever possible, rather than purchasing them premade at health food retailers.[28] Expensive, exotic, "designer" herbs and herbal products are not necessarily more effective than simple herbs, and in fact, many trendy products may be less safe and effective than time-tested home remedies.

Herbal formulae often need to be changed or modified as patients start to experience results; also, sometimes the correct formula is not achieved immediately, requiring a new prescription (and thus the patient must purchase a different formula) after trying an initial protocol for only a short time. In TCM, it is not uncommon for the Chinese doctor to alter an herbal prescription every few days. Careful attention to formulating and prescribing the minimum effective dose can reduce product waste and loss of money to the patient; however, it is not possible to entirely eliminate this factor from herbal practice, and this should be clearly explained to patients before initiating an herbal protocol.

Herbal practitioners may choose to maintain a dispensary as a way to offer a cost saving to their patients, making herbal products available to their patients nearly at cost, marking the products up only enough to cover the cost of stocking and maintaining the inventory and filling prescriptions. Keep in mind that a busy practice might require the help of a full- or part-time employee solely for that purpose. This service allows the practitioner to provide high-quality products at a fraction of their cost in retail institutions. Practitioners choosing to do this will want to investigate the good manufacturing practices (GMPs) of their jurisdiction to comply with all manufacturing and labeling laws that might pertain to them. Additionally, practitioners might want to consider carrying product liability insurance.

Environmental Sustainability

Widespread use of herbal medicines can lead to overharvesting of frequently used or rare plant populations. This is exacerbated by the vagaries of fashion, whereby a certain herb will be promoted excessively (and often inappropriately). This problem has a historical precedent; consider the destruction of large stands of the American ginseng population by Daniel Boone and other pioneers who profited from its harvest and export to China, or the depopulation of the American lady's slipper (*Cypripedium pubescens*) owing to its popularity in the nineteenth and early twentieth centuries as a sedative. Modern examples of this are *Hydrastis canadensis* (goldenseal) and *Chamaelirium luteum* (false unicorn), an American woodland plant endangered in the wild and difficult to cultivate. In a broader philosophic sense, one cannot ultimately separate the health of the environment from the health of the individual; thus attention to ecological herbalism is part of the responsibility the practitioner assumes in assuring the long-term health of patients. Thus a responsible herbalist avoids the use of endangered plants and seeks appropriate substitutes wherever possible (Box 3-35).[28,29]

> ### BOX 3-35 The United Plant Savers' Plants at Risk and to Watch Lists for Herbs Discussed in this Textbook
>
> Plants on these lists should only be used when obtained from manufacturers observing sustainable growing and harvesting practices.
>
> **"At Risk" List**
> - American ginseng (*Panax quinquefolius*)
> - Black cohosh (*Actaea racemosa*)
> - Blue cohosh (*Caulophyllum thalictroides*)
> - Echinacea (*Echinacea* spp.)
> - False unicorn root (*Chamaelirium luteum*)
> - Goldenseal (*Hydrastis canadensis*)
> - Lady's slipper orchid (*Cypripedium* spp.)
> - Slippery elm (*Ulmus rubra*)
> - Sundew (*Drosera* spp.)
> - Trillium, Bethroot (*Trillium* spp.)
> - Wild yam (*Dioscorea* spp.)
>
> **"To Watch" List**
> - Arnica (*Arnica* spp.)
> - Cascara sagrada (*Frangula purshiana*)
> - Gentian (*Gentiana* spp.)
> - Goldthread (*Coptis* spp.)
> - Kava kava (*Piper methysticum*) (Hawaii only)
> - Lobelia (*Lobelia* spp.)
> - Mayapple (*Podophyllum peltatum*)
> - Oregon grape (*Mahonia* spp.)
> - Partridge berry (*Mitchella repens*)
> - Pipsissewa (*Chimaphila umbellata*)
> - Spikenard (*Aralia racemosa, A. californica*)
> - Stone root (*Collinsonia canadensis*)
> - Wild indigo (*Baptisia tinctoria*)

Adherence and Obstacles to Commitment

Herbal preparations can be time consuming for patients to make and are not always pleasant tasting, factors that can reduce a patient's commitment to an otherwise good herbal protocol. If the herbs are not taken, they will not work. An in-office dispensary reduces the need for the patient to seek out herbs on his or her own, minimizing time and expense, and maximizing the likelihood that the herbs will actually be obtained. Selecting the form of the herb that will most likely encourage its use is also important. For example, a single working mother may be more likely to take a tincture, tablets, or capsules that she does not have to prepare, and which can easily fit into her purse, than a tea that she has to prepare at home and carry along on her busy day. These considerations can be discussed with patients before writing their prescriptions.

Taste is not always possible to fully mask with herbs, particularly with bitters, in which the bitter taste is partly necessary for the effects of the medicine. However, much can be done to improve the taste of many herbs. In teas, infusions, and decoctions a corrigent (i.e., a flavoring agent) such as licorice, anise seed, spearmint, or peppermint may be used; in tinctures, glycerine, elderberry syrup, the aforementioned herbs, or one or two drops of a pleasant-flavored essential oil, such as anise seed, cinnamon, peppermint, or spearmint may be used. Tinctures may be taken heavily diluted in water, or taken in a small amount of juice to mask the taste. With experience, practitioners can learn to combine herbs to maximally enhance their taste; however, it is inevitable that some herbs have a very strong taste. This should be explained to patients in advance, and if necessary a very small amount (e.g., ½ ounce of tincture) of the herbal product mixed and sent home with the patient to see if the product is tolerable before assembling a full prescription. For patients who find the taste of liquid and alcohol extracts intolerable, capsules and tablets may be substituted for some herbs.

FORMULATING

An effective formula will lead to the desired health outcome with maximal benefits, patient commitment, and minimal, if any, side effects. It will be cost-effective and ecologically sustainable. Most herbalists have a single technique they prefer for formula development, and create all formulae based on a skeleton model of their preferred method. There is no right or wrong way to design an herbal formula—herbal formulation is as much an art as it is a science. General formulation strategies follow.

Establishing Therapeutic Goals and Priorities

Before developing protocol and formulae for an individual patient, clear therapeutic goals and priorities must be established. These should be based on the patient's needs and personal treatment goals, an understanding of the condition from a Western biomedical perspective, and an understanding of the condition based on the traditional concepts of the system of herbal medicine being practiced.[33]

Therapeutic priorities are based on the immediate needs of the patient and a ranking of the urgency of various presenting symptoms and conditions. Optimally, a therapeutic plan is devised that addresses the most urgent and challenging symptoms for the patient, and begins to address underlying conditions in a systematic manner. Kerry Bone, in his book *A Clinical Guide to Blending Liquid Herbs,* defines the following as goals for Western herbal prescriptions for the individual patient. These key concepts can be considered guiding principles for identifying the overall therapeutic goals for the formula[33]:

- Raise the vitality to enhance the patient's ability to resist disease.
- Relieve the underlying causes that either predispose the patient to illness or provoke the disease process.
- Reduce the effect of the sustaining causes of the disease process; for example, inflammation.
- Promote and nourish healthy functioning of tissues, organs, and systems related to the condition being treated.
- Control counterproductive symptoms that interfere with healing.

The Structure of an Herbal Formula

Herbal formulae follow many styles, from single-drug ingredients (*monotherapy* or *simples*) to the 15-to-20-ingredient formulae typical of TCM. All herbs in a formula should support the therapeutic goals either directly or by supporting the actions of the primary herbs in the formula. An herbal formula should not contain so many ingredients that the patient is receiving inadequate amounts of the individual herbs.

Key formula ingredients are as follows:

- The *primary* or *main* ingredient(s)
- The *adjuvant*(s), *supporting,* or *secondary* ingredient(s) that enhance or complement the effects of the primary ingredients in a specific manner
- A *corrigent,* an ingredient to enhance the flavor or tolerance of the preparation

Additionally, herbalists may add one or more of the following to a formula:

- *Warming, carminative* herbs such as ginger or cinnamon to prevent digestive discomfort from an herbal formula and to enhance the metabolism of the formula. This practice is now being validated by research demonstrating that the addition of a spice (e.g., black pepper or its constituent piperine) to an herbal, or even a pharmaceutical protocol such as antibiotic therapy, enhances the uptake of the drug and reduces the amount of drug required for therapeutic efficacy.
- *Trophorestorative* or *tonic herbs* that support specifically stressed body systems.
- *Nervines;* stress is a common component of health problems, either as an underlying factor or as a result of the presence of illness.
- *Antiirritants* are herbs that reduce the irritating effects of other herbs in the formula; for example, a mucilaginous herb.

Generally, one to three main ingredients are used, one to two adjuvants, one corrigent, and one "warming" herb.[27] Commonly a single herb in the formula will serve multiple purposes; an herb such as ginger or cinnamon may act as both a corrigent and a carminative.

The German Commission E further specifies that herbs should be included in herbal combination products if:

- The use of the various components with identical or different effects leads to additive or synergistic effects;
- The combination leads to a superadditive effect of the fixed combination compared with that of the individual components;
- The combination leads to reduction or elimination of undesirable effects of individual components;
- The combination leads to a simplification of therapy or improvement in therapy safety, patient commitment, or absorption.[27]

Exquisite formulating; that is, using the minimal number of the most exact herbs in a formula, should be every practitioner's goal. For some patients a single formula with only a few herbs may be effective for treatment. For many patients, it will be necessary to provide more than one formula at a time;

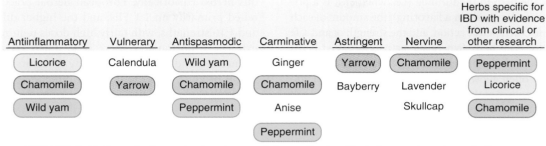

Therapeutic Goals:
• Heal damaged intestinal lining (antiinflammatory, vulnerary)
• Address intestinal spasms (antispasmodic), gas and bloating (carminative), and diarrhea (astringent)
• Consider underlying stress (nervine)

Antiinflammatory	Vulnerary	Antispasmodic	Carminative	Astringent	Nervine	Herbs specific for IBD with evidence from clinical or other research
Licorice	Calendula	Wild yam	Ginger	Yarrow	Chamomile	Peppermint
Chamomile	Yarrow	Chamomile	Chamomile	Bayberry	Lavender	Licorice
Wild yam		Peppermint	Anise		Skullcap	Chamomile
			Peppermint			

FIGURE 3-18 Sample formula development for patient with inflammatory bowel disease (IBD). Note: see page 50 for formula.

for example, the use of one formula to address underlying causes with another for acute symptoms, the use of a tincture and a topical application in the case of a skin condition or vaginal infection, or the prescription of a formula for acute use and another for chronic use. For example, a patient with chronic anxiety during the day and insomnia at night may be prescribed a general nervine tonic with adaptogens for regular daily use, with a separate formula consisting of sedative herbs for acute insomnia to be taken only before bed or as needed.

TCM bases the structure of the formula on the ancient Chinese structure of government. There is an emperor who determines the overall approach (i.e., the primary herb), various ministers who support and carry out the wishes of the emperor (i.e., adjuvants), assistants who create the agenda for government and set the political climate and tone, and servants who carry out the work (i.e., warming stimulants). In the context of the herbal formula, this means that the herbs are layered or each considered in juxtaposition to the other parts of the formula, as well as for their own merit. The Chinese art of compounding, or making herbal formulae, is impressive and their energetic principles may be successfully applied to Western herbal formulations as well.[28]

Steps to Developing a Formula

Mills and Bone best elucidate key formulation concepts in their textbook, *Principles and Practice of Phytotherapy: Modern Herbal Medicine*. To develop a formula[6]:

1. Determine the treatment goals based on traditional herbal concepts, the conventional medical understanding, and the patient's case.
2. Make sure the goals are individualized to the needs of the specific case.
3. Decide upon the immediate treatment priorities.
4. Determine what actions are required based on the treatment goals.
5. Choose reliable herbs that have the desired actions, with as much overlap as possible to minimize the number of herbs in the overall formula.

6. If a particular action needs to be emphasized, select more than one herb with this action, or include a single very effective herb with the desired action.
7. Combine the herbs in appropriate proportions and doses.

Selecting the Herbs

Once the therapeutic goals and necessary herbal actions have been determined, the specific herbs must be selected. The simplest method, especially when one is a beginner, is to take a fresh piece of paper and create columns of the various therapeutic actions needed for the formula. Under each column, select herbs from your references and knowledge base that fit the category and the specifics of the patient's condition.

Because many herbs have multiple actions, you will find that herbs appear more than once on the page, under different columns. Narrow your selection by first choosing those herbs that address more than one need (Fig. 3-18). For example, if there is upper respiratory infection and you are seeking an herb that is antiviral, antiinflammatory, and expectorant, licorice might be an excellent choice, as it possesses all of these actions. It is also a corrigent, thus minimizing the need for an additional flavoring agent for an infusion or tincture.

Next, select herbs that most specifically address any remaining symptoms or conditions that are intended to be addressed by this formula, keeping an eye to the key components of a formula outlined in the preceding. Finally, make sure that there are no contraindications to any of the herbs you have selected for the patient, including potential herb–drug interactions, herb–herb interactions within the formula, or herb–herb interactions between formulae if more than one prescription has been given.

Note that the form of preparation you are giving will also affect your selection of herbs; therefore you must select the preparation form that will allow you to effectively deliver the medication to the patient. For example, if you are prescribing highly bitter or unpleasant tasting herbs, you will want to use a form that is most palatable, probably a tincture or possibly a capsule; if you are prescribing demulcent, mucilaginous herbs, you will want to use a tea or infusion, as many mucilaginous herbs are not highly soluble in alcohol.

Determining the Correct Proportions of Herbs in a Formula

The amount of each herb in a formula depends on the relative importance of the herb in the formula (i.e., whether it is a primary herb, a secondary herb, or a flavoring), the amount of each herb required for therapeutic action, and the strength of and safe dosing range for each herb. Synergistic activity between herbs should be considered; the presence of more than one herb with a similar action often allows the formulator to reduce the volume of one or another of the herbs. Tincture formulae are built around a final product volume of 100 mL. Infusions can be prepared by the cup, typically 1 to 3 tsp of herb per cup of water, and decoctions are typically based on a ratio of 28 g (1 ounce) of herbs to 1 L (1 quart) of water.

The herbs in infusions and decoctions are measured in "parts," or the proportion of individual herbs compared with the whole. If you consider a formula to be composed of 100 parts as a total amount, then each herb would be assigned a certain number of parts, similar to the percentage of the herb in the formula. The word *parts* can then be translated into ounces, grams, or teaspoons based on the measurement you are using and the total volume you need to prepare. In this book, rather than assuming 100 parts for a whole formula, the formulae assume 10 parts to make the numbers more manageable. Here is a sample formula as an example of the parts system:

🌿 SAMPLE COLD INFUSION (MACERATE)

Bowel Antiinflammatory Blend

Marshmallow root	(Althaea officinalis)	4 parts
Chamomile	(Matricaria recutita)	4 parts
Ginger	(Zingiber officinalis)	1 part
Peppermint	(Mentha piperita)	1 part
	Total:	**10 parts**

To prepare: Mix the herbs. Steep 1 tbsp herb:250 mL cold water for 1 hour, stirring a couple of times. Strain; bring to a boil for 1 minute; serve warm or at room temperature.

Dose: 1 to 3 cups per day as needed.

Indications: Irritable bowel syndrome (IBS); bowel inflammation; stomach upset; dyspepsia (heartburn).

In this example, you can see that there are 10 parts total. The parts are written in descending order of volume. In this case, marshmallow and chamomile happen to also be the primary herbs in the recipe. Ginger and peppermint are important bowel antiinflammatory herbs, but in this recipe also serve as secondary and adjunct herbs; the ginger warms the digestion and improves the taste, and the peppermint acts as a carminative and also improves the taste.

Selecting Herb Strength When Using Tinctures

Tincture strength based on the weight to volume (w:v) ratio is discussed in Botanical Preparations. When preparing a formula, the practitioner must determine what strength of each herb in the formula to use. The relationship between extract strength and clinical efficacy is a matter of debate, and has been poorly evaluated. The preparations available, even to professionals, are highly variable, ranging from 1:1 fluid extracts (FEs) through 1:5 extracts for commonly used herbs and 1:10 for highly potent, restricted, or potentially dangerous herbs. Historically, European herbal practitioners have relied primarily on 1:1 FEs, and the higher dilutions of 1:5 and 1:10 strengths, with fairly high doses required for the 1:5 extracts. Unfortunately, there is so much variability in the US market, and such a wide variety of factors that determine actual product potency, that it is difficult to determine the resulting clinical difference in the various strengths available, the difference becoming theoretical and somewhat arbitrary.

The potency of the final product is determined by numerous factors, including the quality of the starting material, the plant parts used (e.g., one herb manufacturer may prepare a *Hypericum* tincture using the entire 2 to 4 feet of the plant, whereas another company may use only the active, medicinal top 4 to 8 inches of the flowering plant, resulting in a potentially very different product), the solubility of the individual herb(s), use of the proper solvent, solvent percentage, and w:v ratio. Because of this variability, it becomes almost impossible to recommend specific w:v ratios and alcohol percentages in the sample formulae in this text. It is assumed that tinctures are being purchased from manufacturers who prepare their products according to proper standards and specifications, using high-quality starting materials.

Practitioners should not be concerned if the suggested strength is not available, requiring the practitioner to rely on a slightly higher or lower w:v ratio, as long as one stays within the 1:2 to 1:4 strength range. Going from a tincture to an FE (1:1) can significantly increase the potency of a product and is not recommended as a substitute in the suggested formulae. When a 1:5 or 1:10 is recommended, this indicates that an herb is potentially toxic in higher amounts and this strength should not be exceeded unless the formula is properly modified to include a reduction in the overall volume of that herb.

Putting It All Together

The following sample formula is based upon the herb selection strategy presented earlier in this section; this formula represents a standard herbal prescription, including common and botanical names for the herbs, herbs' strengths and volumes, and recommended dose. The vegetable glycerin is optional for taste, and may be replaced with 10 mL of *Pimpinella anisum* (anise seed).

🌿 SAMPLE FORMULA FOR INFLAMMATORY BOWEL DISEASE

Mix the following tinctures:

Chamomile	(Matricaria recutita)	30 mL
Wild yam	(Dioscorea villosa)	25 mL
Licorice	(Glycyrrhiza glabra)	15 mL
Yarrow	(Achillea millefolium)	10 mL
Peppermint	(Mentha piperita)	10 mL
Vegetable glycerin		10 mL
	Total:	**100 mL**

Dose: 5 mL of tincture in a small amount of warm water, two to three times daily.

The Prescribing Schedule

How often a patient should take the prescribed formula(e) depends on the severity and urgency of the condition, the strength and safety of the herbs, and the likelihood of the patient's adherence. The following is a general summary of the prescribing range for various herbal products:

- Tinctures: 2 to 7 mL, 1 to 3 times daily
- Decoctions: ¼ to 2 cups daily
- Infusions: 1 to 6 cups daily
- Capsules and tablets: 1 to 3 capsules, 1 to 3 times daily

TABLE 3-13 Plant Parts

English and Latin Names, and Abbreviations

Plant Part	Latin Name Singular (Plural)	Abbreviation
Leaf	folium (folia)	fol.
Flower	flos (flores)	Flor.
Fruit	fructus (fructus)	fruct.
Herb	herba (herbae)	herb.
Root	radix (radices)	rad.
Rhizome	rhizoma (rhizomae)	rhiz.
Bark	cortex (cortices)	cort.

From Kraft K, Hobbs C: *Pocket guide to herbal medicine,* Stuttgart, 2004, Thieme. (Reprinted with permission.)

Occasionally, products are prescribed with special instructions, for example, *Vitex agnus-castus* is often prescribed in a single 5 mL dose in the morning, or other herbs may be prescribed for taking before bed, with meals, or only during a specific phase of the menstrual cycle.[34]

In acute conditions the prescribing schedule may be more aggressive. For example, a woman experiencing uterine contractions with a threatened miscarriage may take a uterine antispasmodic formula every 15 minutes for a set period of time (e.g., 2 hours) in a reduced dose until relief is achieved.

Where adherence is a concern, the practitioner may ask the patient how often she will realistically take the prescribed formula, and adjust the individual dose to accommodate a daily therapeutic dose in that intake frequency. For example, if a woman tells you she will not take her formula at the office, prescribing a formula to be taken 2.5 mL four times daily will be ineffectual. Better to prescribe a dose of 5 mL twice daily, if the herbs in the compound are safe in that individual dose.

PRESCRIPTION WRITING

In Europe, where herbal medicine is part of the norm in the health care system, herbal prescription writing follows traditional prescription nomenclature (Tables 3-13 and 3-14), allowing herbal formulae written by the practitioner to be

TABLE 3-14 Prescription Writing

Terms and Abbreviations

English Instruction	Latin Equivalent	Precription Nomenclature/Abbreviation
Equal parts of each ingredient	ana partes aequales	Aa. (aa.)
Water	aqua	aqu.
Add	adde	add.
Or similar	aut similia	aut. simil.
With	cum	c.
Cut	consisus	cc., conc.
Crushed	contusus	cont.
Give the patient	da	d.
Give and label as follows	detur signetur	d.s.
Make, prepare	fiat	Ft.
Drops	gutta, guttae	Gtt. (gtt.)
Make an infusion	infunde	Inf
Mix	misce	m.
Mix and make	misce, fiat	M. f.
Mix and make a tea	misce fiat species	M. ft. spec.
Mix and make an ointment	misce fiat unguentum	M. ft. ungt.
Mix, give, label as	misce, da, signe	M.D.S.
After meals	post cibum	p.c.
Pills	Pilliulae	pill.
Powder, pulverize	pulvus, pulveratus	pulv.
Take	recipe	Rx
Label	signa	S.
Tea	species	spec.
Suppository	suppositorium	supp.
Divide into X doses	tales doses	Tal. dosis No. X
Tincture	tinctura	tct., tr.
Ointment	unguentum	ungt.

easily read and prepared in the pharmacy. Although most practitioners in the United States will not likely be sending their patients to the "herbal pharmacy" to have their prescriptions filled, it is worthwhile to understand the formal language of the prescription, especially when using European herbals and pharmacopoeia. Latin binomials should be given for all plants in a prescription to guarantee use of the proper plant genus and species in the product. Practitioners should at all times create an accurate record of exactly what was prescribed in each patient's chart.

BOTANICAL PREPARATION FORMS*

Herbal products range from simple, crude herbs in raw and tea forms to sophisticated standardized extracts with fixed concentrations of specific constituents. Using the most appropriate forms of administration can maximize efficacy and patient commitment. Patient-determined factors, such as time limitations, financial considerations, taste aversions, and extenuating factors (e.g., history of alcohol abuse leading to current alcohol avoidance), help to narrow preparation choices to further the likelihood of patient implementation. This section reviews the various types of commonly used herbal preparations, their advantages and disadvantages, and preparation methods (Table 3-15).

Gynecologic conditions sometimes require the use of special botanical preparations for direct application of herbal medicines to affected tissue. The most common of these preparations are vaginal rinses, douches, sitz baths, suppositories, and pessaries. This section also provides instructions for preparing the special herbal applications used in this book and not described fully in Botanical Preparations. Specific herbs for various conditions are presented under their respective conditions and may be incorporated into these general instructions. Most of these preparations are easy to prepare, inexpensive, and require minimal supplies.

PREPARATION FORMS

Powdered Herbs, Capsules, Tablets, and Pills

Powdered herbs—the finely ground form of the crude herb—are a simple and cost-effective way for patients to take herbal medicines. Generally, the powder is pressed into tablets or pills, or may be encapsulated (Fig. 3-19), but occasionally palatable herbs are taken with hot water or even sprinkled onto foods.

Advantages. Tablets, pills, and capsules are inexpensive and are a widely recognized form of medicine to patients accustomed to Western medicine, thus are easily accepted by most. Powdered herbs present the whole herb to the patient's digestive system and thus may be a preferred choice when the therapeutic goal requires direct contact between the herb and

the GI tract, as is the case with mucilaginous and vulnerary herbs used to treat IBS.

Disadvantages. The grinding of the herb into powder generates heat that may degrade valuable medicinal constituents. Once ground, powdered herbs oxidize more readily than whole herbs, given the vast increase in exposed surface area. The time from harvest to purchase is an unknown factor that may significantly affect the medicinal qualities of the preparation. Thus the medicinal activity and quality of powders is highly variable and can be unreliable; practitioners must evaluate individual companies and products for quality.

Liquid Extracts

The most common forms of liquid extracts are:
- Aqueous extracts (e.g., teas, infusions, decoctions)
- Hydroethanolic extracts (e.g., tinctures, fluid extracts)
- Glycerin extracts (e.g., glycerites)

Any of these forms may be further manufactured into additional product forms, such as by concentrating liquid extracts and adding binders to form tablets or transforming a decoction into syrup. Plant constituents may be water soluble, soluble only in alcohol, or have extractability somewhere in between. For instance, alkaloids are typically soluble in 45% alcohol, but hydrastine, an alkaloid found in *Hydrastis canadensis* (goldenseal) root (Fig. 3-20), may require a 70+% alcohol menstruum for full extraction. On the other hand, berberine, another alkaloid found in goldenseal, is poorly soluble in alcohol. A high-percentage alcohol tincture will have a different hydrastine to berberine ratio than a tincture made with a lower-percentage alcohol; an aqueous extraction may have berberine but no hydrastine. The situation is complicated by the fact that multiple constituents within the herb interact in solution and affect each other's solubility.

The choice of solvent, or menstruum, changes the chemical profile and thus the medicinal qualities of the product (Table 3-16). This is an area where comparative outcome research is lacking, although a few basic studies do exist. For example, one French study found that a 30% ethanol tincture of *Viburnum opulus* (cramp bark) was five times more potent as a spasmolytic in vitro than a 60% ethanol tincture.[35] Herbalists will commonly report that one form of an herb over another is consistently more effective in the clinic; for example, many find licorice decoction more effective than tincture for controlling inflammation. Herbal manufacturers and practitioners rely largely on pharmacopeial values for determining extraction methods and standards.

Advantages. The advantages of liquid extracts over solid forms vary with the specific form of liquid extract and the herb. In general, liquid extracts are easy to swallow, absorb, and assimilate. Water-based preparations are typically inexpensive to prepare and often have a wide margin of safety because they are relatively diluted, although this is not a reliable safety guideline; hydroethanolic extracts are characteristically concentrated and thus easy to store, transport, and take in small but high-potency doses.

*The editor wishes to thank *Botanical Medicine for Women's Health,* Edition 1 contributors Eric Yarnell; Kathy Abascal; Mitch Coven; Ed Smith, RH (AHG); and David Bunting.

TABLE 3-15 Summary of Internal Botanical Preparations

Preparation Type	Solvent(S)	Shelf-Life*	Benefits	Problems	Other Notes
Crude powdered herb	None	12 months for above-ground parts and up to 3 years for roots, if properly stored	Whole herb (all constituents present), pills readily accepted, relatively inexpensive, easy to dispense and formulate	Damaged by processing, mold contamination; batch-to-batch variability high; may be difficult to swallow and hard to digest	Freeze-dried powders may have longer shelf-life
Granule	Water, sometimes wine or oil	12-24 months	Decreased dose needed, palatable, easy to dispense and formulate, relatively inexpensive	Little research, short history of use, batch-to-batch variability high	Starch may be added
Standardized extracts	Variable	Variable (12-24 months presumably)	Well researched (sometimes), dosing objectively determined, easy to dispense, less batch-to-batch variability	Relatively expensive, may have solvent residues, little history of use, cannot formulate, potential loss of beneficial constituents not assayed, capsules possibly difficult to swallow	Higher environmental effect if solvents used
Hot infusion or decoction	Water	Hours to days (if refrigerated)	Inexpensive, easy to formulate, benefits of water†	Time consuming to prepare, complex to dispense, bad taste	Will not extract hydrophobic constituents
Cold infusion	Water	Hours to days (if refrigerated)	Inexpensive, easy to formulate, benefits of water†	Time consuming to prepare, complex to dispense	Will not extract hydrophobic constituents
Tincture	Ethanol, water, sometimes glycerin	Years to decades	Easy to formulate and dispense, relatively broad extract, easy to swallow and absorb, fast acting	Moderately expensive, contain ethanol, flavor often unpalatable	Differing ethanol and ratio concentrations; extracts different ranges of constituents
Fluid extract	As tincture	As tincture	As tincture but more concentrated, thus lower doses required	As tincture, increased processing may damage some constituents, only works with dry raw material	As tincture
Glycerite	Glycerin, water	2-5 years	Easy to formulate and dispense, easy to swallow, palatable	Moderately expensive	Only extracts hydrophilic constituents
Syrup	Simple carbohydrate, water	1-2 years	As glycerite	Moderately expensive, relatively poor preservative	As glycerite
Acetract	Vinegar, water, sometimes ethanol and/or glycerin	1 year or more depending on formula	Easy to formulate and dispense, easy to swallow, effectively extracts alkaloids	Moderately expensive, poor preservative, does not extract other constituents well	Used exclusively with alkaloid-rich herbs
Volatile oil, steam distilled	None	1-3 years	Easy to formulate and dispense, multiple modes of application, very low doses needed (concentrated), some objective doses established	Expensive, narrow therapeutic window (concentrated)	
Volatile oil, supercritical carbon dioxide	Carbon dioxide	Unknown (presumably 1-3 years)	As volatile oil, steam distilled	As volatile oil, steam distilled	New technology with little clinical research or use
Hydrosol	Water	Weeks to months	Inexpensive, dilute tinctures for topical use	Questionable if medicinally useful, extremely dilute, spoils quickly	

*Assuming optimal storage conditions.
†The patient takes in the water simultaneously with the herb, which brings additional benefits, such as increased diuresis.

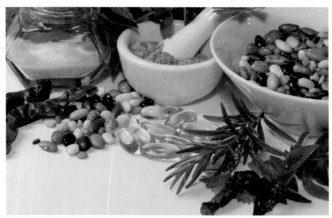

FIGURE 3-19 Herbs in various forms. (Photo © istock.com)

TABLE 3-16 General Solubility of Botanical Compounds

Phytochemical Category	MOST SOLUBLE IN...	
	(Ethanol %)	Water Solubility
Proteins, lectins	25%	Very high
Tannins	25%-30%	High (in hot water)
Saponins	25%-30%	High
Carbohydrates	25%-30%	High (in cold water)
Glycosides	25%-30%	High
Alkaloids	45%	Marginal
Alkaloid salts	25%-30%	High
Monoterpenoids, sesquiterpenoids, diterpenoids	60%	Low
Phenylpropanoids	60%	Low
Lignans	80%-90%	Very low
Resins	90%	Very low
Lipids	90%	Very low

Note: There are exceptions in every category.
From Yarnell E: *Phytochemistry and pharmacy for practitioners of botanical medicine,* Wenatchee, 2003, Healing Mountain Publishing.

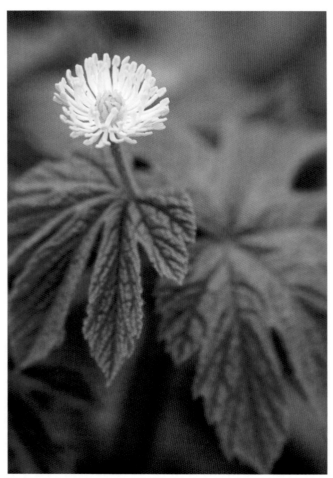

FIGURE 3-20 Goldenseal *(Hydrastis canadensis).* (Photo by Martin Wall.)

Disadvantages. Water-based products such as teas, infusions, and decoctions require patient preparation, may be cumbersome to transport, have a short shelf-life, and often present palatability issues. Aqueous extracts make only the water-soluble constituents available to the patient, which may be undesirable or desirable, depending on the therapeutic goal and required constituents. Hydroethanolic products require

alcohol consumption, present a more concentrated product with thus a potentially smaller margin of safety for many herbs, and can be costly. Products prepared with solvents other than ethanol may contain undesirable solvent residues.

Aqueous Extracts (Teas, Infusions, and Decoctions)

Historically, herbs were most commonly prescribed as simple aqueous extracts to be consumed orally or used in baths, douches, rinses, compresses, and other applications. There are four basic aqueous extracts:

- Teas
- Hot infusions, made by steeping the herbs in hot water for varying lengths of time
- Cold infusions (i.e., macerates), made by steeping the herb in cold water for a prolonged period (4 to 8+ hours)
- Decoctions, made by simmering or boiling the herb in water generally from 20 minutes to 1 hour

Tea is considered a culinary preparation; however, many teas, such as green tea, can provide significant medicinal benefit when consumed in adequate amounts over a prolonged period of time.

Infusions are principally made from the above-ground parts of dried herbs, including leaves, stems, flowers, aromatic seeds (e.g., anise and fennel seeds), and fruits. The water is boiled, the heat turned off, the water poured over the herbs in a vessel (e.g., cup, tea pot, glass canning jar), and the steeping carried out in the closed vessel. When prepared this way, fragile plant parts are extracted with minimal damage to constituents. To some extent, even volatile oils contained in aromatic plants are preserved, as they condense on the lid and fall back into the water. Dried or fresh plant material can be used. Infusions are a poor choice where hydrophobic constituents are sought for their medicinal effect, including alkaloids, resins, and lipids, although it is a misconception that alkaloids are not extracted well in water because many are. Typically 1 tablespoon of dried herb per cup (250 mL) of boiling water is used. Steeping time is generally as follows:

- Aromatic plants/plant parts: 10 to 15 minutes
- Nonaromatic leaves and flowers: 30 minutes to 1 hour
- Woody plant parts and soft roots: 1 to 4 hours

Cold infusions, also called *macerates,* are prepared by steeping the dried herb in an appropriate volume of cold water, typically from 2 to 8 hours, depending on the herb and its extractability. Cold infusions are well suited to extracting mucilaginous compounds in a palatable manner and are also often preferred when one wants to minimize tannin extraction from tannin-rich herbs, such as uva ursi (*Arctostaphylos uva ursi*) or red raspberry leaf (*Rubus idaeus*). Because no boiling water or alcohol is used to prepare cold infusions, microorganisms that would otherwise be killed might remain in the final cold infusion product. Caution may be warranted in using cold infusions with immuno-compromised patients. A solution is to prepare the cold infusion, and then bring it to a quick boil before consuming.

Decoctions are prepared by simmering or boiling aqueous extracts. Decoctions use the seeds, roots, and barks of dried plants, with the exclusion of aromatic seeds. The additional heat provided through simmering or boiling enables water to penetrate into the dense tissue and release constituents. As with infusions, the quality of the herb is paramount. Root decoctions are often quite bitter and unpalatable to the general public, and as a result, patient willingness to drink decoctions may be poor. This is certainly a disadvantage when compliance is desired. Typically 7 to 28 grams (¼ to 1 ounce) of herb is used per liter of boiling water, and simmered 20 minutes or longer depending on the desired strength and concentration.

Vaginal rinses are commonly recommended for the treatment of vulvovaginitis to reduce pain and inflammation, and when there is dysuria associated with urinary tract infection (UTI), or to reduce perianal microbial contamination that can lead to UTI, such as from *E. coli*. They may also be used postnatally for the repair of episiotomy damage or perineal tears from birth.

To prepare a vaginal rinse: Fill a "peri" bottle or a clean, plastic squeeze bottle with a well-strained, strong infusion or decoction. Squeeze the warm or room temperature liquid over the affected area either during or after urination. This significantly reduces inflammation and stinging, and promotes tissue healing. One to two teaspoons of sea salt may be added to each 8-ounce bottle.

Douches are prepared the same way as vaginal rinses, except that the infusion or decoction is placed in a douche bottle or bag apparatus. Vulnerary, antimicrobial, and astringent herbs are commonly used, and may include *Calendula officinalis, Thymus vulgaris, Usnea barbata, Achillea millefolium, Myrica cerifera,* and many others. The addition of several drops of antimicrobial essential oil is common when douching is intended for the treatment of vaginal infection,

however, regular douching is not recommended and can be counterproductive.

Herbal baths can be a rejuvenating ritual, an opportunity for relaxation, or a healing external application. They are useful for a variety of complaints: sore muscles, exhaustion, stress, irritability, insomnia, headache, and respiratory congestion. Sitz baths can be used to facilitate tissue repair (e.g., to heal an episiotomy wound), to reduce inflammation (e.g., hemorrhoids, postnatal perineal trauma), and to treat genitourinary infection (e.g., vaginal candidiasis). Care must be taken with baths to avoid burns from overly hot water.

A full herbal bath can be made two ways. One is to fill a cotton cloth, clean sack, or large cotton tea sack with at least 1 ounce of aromatic or mucilaginous herbs. Fasten the closed cloth to the faucet and let hot bath water run through the sack while filling the tub. Squeeze the sack now and then to wring out the "tea." This will make a mild but pleasant herb bath. The second method is to prepare 2 quarts of a strong herbal infusion or decoction, strain out the herbs, and pour the liquid into the tub of water. Additionally, a few drops of essential oil may be added to the bath after it is filled to add to the aromatic or antimicrobial effects of the bath.

If using aromatic herbs, keeping the door to the bathroom closed while filling the tub will allow the aroma of the herbs to fill the air. This adds to the relaxing effect of the bath.

A sitz bath is prepared as the second method of the full herbal bath. One quart of strong decoction, or 2 quarts of strong infusion, are placed in a sitz bath, or alternatively, in a shallow tub filled with just enough water to reach hip level. Sea salt and antimicrobial essential oils such as lavender, thyme, rosemary, or oregano are commonly added to the water for additional antiseptic effects.

Syrups

Syrups are concentrated, sweet preparations made from a water infusion or decoction base that has been simmered down to a significantly reduced volume, usually one quarter of the original volume. Sucrose and honey are the most commonly used sweeteners. A sweet alcohol such as brandy, or glycerin or another preservative may be added to extend the shelf-life of syrup from several days to several weeks or even months. Refrigeration is typically required to keep homemade syrups. The concentration of simple sugars needed to prevent microbial growth is fairly high, often between 25% and 50% of the total volume. Syrups are very palatable medicines but expose the patient to the regular consumption of sugar, and thus may not be optimal for regular, long-term use. Syrups can be used for short-term delivery when the unpalatability of the herbs would otherwise prevent commitment.

Hydroethanolic Extracts (Tinctures and Fluid Extracts)

Tinctures are hydroethanolic extracts. The combination of water and alcohol optimizes the solubility of plant constituents when both water- and alcohol-soluble constituents are desired in the final product. Alcohol content ranges from 30% to 95% ethanol depending on the amount of alcohol required for optimal extraction and preservation of the desired constituents. Tinctures have a long shelf-life (frequently many years), preserving the tincture from bacteria and fermentation, even when left at room temperature; however, they should ideally be kept in a cool location away from direct heat and light.[36] Some research shows substantial degradation of individual constituents at room temperature after 3 to 6 months; thus studies are needed to determine optimal storage conditions and shelf-life for various plants. This could play a significant role in cost-savings to patients and industry, as well as play a substantial role in plant preservation by eliminating waste that occurs as a result of unnecessarily short expiration dates. Also, by determining which plants have a short shelf-life, such studies could help to maximize medicinal plant efficacy by ensuring that patients receive fresh product. Indeed, some constituent may degrade over time, making certain medicines less effective for specific conditions requiring the presence of those constituents, but other constituents may remain intact, preserving the usefulness of the plant for other conditions. Table 3-16 illustrates the effectiveness of alcohol at extracting many constituents.

Hydroethanolic extract potency is expressed as a ratio: w:v. A 1:1 extract or a FE signifies that 1 g of the herb material by weight was extracted with 1 mL of liquid solvent; a 1:2 extract uses 1 g of herb to 2 mL of liquid solvent, and so on. The weight of the fresh plant macerations includes the water weight of the raw material. An average fresh herb is 67% water by weight, so 3 pounds dry down to 1 pound. The amount of actual plant tissue in 1:2 fresh plant maceration is equivalent to 1:4 dry plant maceration. This can be confusing because the 1:2 fresh plant maceration seems more potent by three-fold, yet they use the same amount of plant tissue and can be viewed as equivalent. The significance of w:v ratios in terms of clinical potency and formulation is discussed in Selection Criteria, Formulation, and Prescribing and Dosing.

There are four main types of hydroethanolic extracts:
- Fresh plant tinctures prepared by maceration
- Dried plant tinctures prepared by maceration
- Dried plant tinctures prepared by percolation
- Dried plant FEs prepared by percolation

Fresh Plant Macerations. Fresh plant macerations are prepared by soaking the freshly cut herb in a hydroethanolic menstruum for 14 to 30 days, after which the mixture is pressed under high pressure then filtered to obtain a final extract. Most fresh plant concentrations have a 1:2 or 1:3 w:v ratio; however, sometimes herbs that are potentially toxic are intentionally made more dilute (e.g., 1:10). Fresh plant tinctures capture constituents close to harvest without exposing plants to the drying process, which for many plants can reduce their potency. Thus certain herbs with temperature-sensitive constituents are prepared only as fresh tinctures. The actions of herbs may be different depending on whether they are prepared fresh or dried. *Lobelia inflata,* for example, is parasympathomimetic when fresh and primarily emetic when dried; fresh pulsatilla is significantly more toxic than dried; and *Frangula purshiana* (cascara sagrada) bark must be dried before preparing to eliminate the plant's cathartic qualities.

Dried Plant Macerations. Dried plant macerations are prepared in the same way as fresh, but the starting material is first dried. Owing to the reduced water volume in the dried starting material, these tinctures are generally prepared in 1:4 w:v concentrations. It is difficult to make these more concentrated. Except in very resinous plants such as *Commiphora molmol* (myrrh), the menstruum seldom exceeds 60% to 70% ethanol. Tinctures with a lower w:v ratio have often been concentrated by evaporation techniques.

Dried Plant Tinctures Prepared by Percolation. Percolation is a distinctly different process than maceration (Fig. 3-21). In percolation, the powder is first macerated in a small amount of alcohol for 24 hours. The moistened herb is next packed into a percolation cone and the menstruum poured over the top of the herb. The menstruum is allowed to "percolate" through the herb in a continuous flow, with an extraction rate of one to three drops per second. Menstruum is moved through the herb until the desired amount of tincture has been produced. The w:v ratio is predetermined, and historically was done to a 1:4 concentration. Percolations are being produced at much higher concentrations of 1:2 and 1:3 ratios, although these have not been shown to represent more thorough extractions.

It is undetermined whether percolation provides a superior tincture compared with maceration. Maceration allows

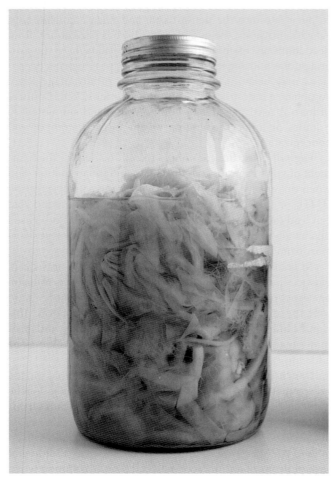

FIGURE 3-21 Maceration setup.

the use of fresh or dry starting material and requires less equipment, whereas percolations can only be performed with dried, powdered starting material and percolation cones. Percolations can be produced at much higher concentrations and in a shorter period of time, typically 2 to 3 days.

Dried Plant Fluid Extracts Prepared by Percolation. Percolation can yield an FE; by definition, an FE is a 1:1 w:v extract. FEs are concentrated and thus are particularly suitable for herbs that require high dosing for efficacy. FEs cannot be prepared by maceration without the application of additional heat or vacuum to remove excess liquid, processing steps that may damage important plant compounds. A straight FE is also not a true 1:1 unless repercolation is used to fully exhaust the plant material. There is no consensus on the potency of fluid extracts compared with other tinctures. Most manufacturers and practitioners agree that fluid extracts are not proportionally more potent than other concentrations; for example, a 1:1 percolate is *not* necessarily five times more potent than a 1:5 percolate or macerate, owing to the fact that phytochemicals remain in the marc (the solid plant material remaining after extraction) after a 1:1 extract. Clinical trials have not compared fluid extracts to tinctures of the same plant, so exact differences in potency are not known. Many plants are unsuitable as fluid extracts. At 1:1 concentrations, the solvent can become supersaturated, and with certain herbs, the resulting product may become an unusable, gelatinous mass.

Care must be taken in combining tannin- and resin-containing tinctures in formulae to avoid precipitating out the tannins and possibly the resins, as well. Tannins will also form insoluble complexes with alkaloids and thus tannin- and alkaloid-rich tinctures are generally considered incompatible. It is unknown to what extent mixing other tinctures precipitates out desired compounds. In many cases, mixing will only result in minor precipitates that are invisible to the naked eye and likely remain bioavailable when ingested.

Glycerin Extracts (Glycerites)

Glycerin, technically an alcohol, has solubility very similar to water, a sweet taste, and a viscous consistency. It is used to prepare "alcohol-free" tinctures, and to preserve and sweeten the taste of liquid extracts. Glycerin has very different biological properties than ethanol. It is suitable for preparing extracts of plants that contain primarily water-soluble compounds, and is not generally able to dissolve alkaloids, resins, lipids, lignins, phenylpropanoids, or terpenoids. Glycerin can be obtained from plants, animals, or petroleum. Most tincture manufacturers use vegetable glycerin, but it is advisable to inquire to make sure that this is the case. Today, there are many glycerites of plants containing constituents that are not soluble in water, such as some of goldenseal's alkaloids. Typically, an alcohol tincture is prepared, the alcohol is evaporated off, and glycerin is added, although this process removes volatile constituents.

Advantages. Glycerin tastes sweet. This makes glycerites relatively palatable to many consumers compared with ethanol tinctures. Glycerin can be used to make macerations from fresh or dry starting material, using a procedure otherwise identical to tincturing by maceration. However, this is only efficacious if water-soluble compounds are desired.

Disadvantages. Unlike ethanol, which actually slightly increases absorption of many constituents, glycerin slightly interferes. Glycerites have a shorter shelf-life than tinctures. A minimum of 50% glycerin is necessary to prevent microbial growth in glycerites. Glycerin's viscosity and stickiness make it unsuitable for percolation. That said, glycerin is sometimes added in small percentages to hold constituents in solution even in percolations, as in the case with *Cinnamomum verum* (cinnamon). Typically, 5% glycerin is added to the menstruum in such instances.

Standardized Extracts

Standardization (Box 3-36) refers to the manufacture of botanical extracts with consistent methods and materials to ensure that products contain the desired ingredients and consistent, reliable quality. Optimal standardization practices begin with the starting materials: guaranteeing correct plant species, quality of the materials to be used, and sometimes the identification of marker compounds to ensure identity, quality, and strength. Marker compounds are then reassessed in the final product to confirm that the contents and quality of the final products match that of the starting materials. This is particularly common for hydroethanolic extract. Unfortunately, the concept of standardization has been misconstrued by manufacturers and consumers, and sometimes misrepresented as a marketing tool by the former, to mean "active constituents."

There is insufficient research detailing the exact role of chemical markers in clinical efficacy. In some cases, markers play a critical role in plant efficacy, for example, as with the flavonolignan complex known as silymarin from *Silybum marianum* (milk thistle). In other instances, the markers chosen have been clearly shown to be only one among many important compounds, such as hypericin from *Hypericum perforatum*.[37] In still other cases, the markers chosen have not yet been definitively shown to even be associated with quality raw materials, such as echinacoside from *Echinacea* spp.[38]

Advantages. Standardization of manufacturing procedures and material quality provides a measure of control over batch-to-batch variability and adds greater certainty to dosing. When using extracts that were used in clinical trials, it increases the likelihood of similar efficacy.

Disadvantages. There are no fixed requirements for standardization in the United States; there is a near total absence of published research showing that any particular standardization scheme is clinically superior to any other type of product; and there is some evidence that concentrating plants to specific constituents may actually have detrimental effects clinically. For example, recent evidence suggests that the practice of concentrating *Hypericum* products to higher hyperforin concentrations than found in nature may lead to the highly publicized effects of the herb interfering with cytochrome P450 (CYP), leading to herb–drug interactions with this plant.

Blending poor-quality batches of raw product with higher-quality batches to obtain desired standardization of certain constituents, or "spiking" batches with the marker compound, are known practices among less reputable manufacturers. This practice reduces overall batch quality, and potentially product

BOX 3-36   The American Herbal Products Association: Standardization of Botanical Products White Paper

In recent years, the US marketplace has seen an increasing appreciation of the health-promoting benefits of herbal preparations. Both consumers and health care practitioners are becoming more receptive to their use. Many people, however, have reservations about the use of herbal products because of the chemical complexity of such products and the perceived difficulty in ensuring batch-to-batch product reproducibility. To address this concern, there has been a trend in the marketplace toward the use of "standardized" preparations; and in most cases, the word *standardized* is associated with a quantitative claim for the content of a particular constituent or constituents. The constituent or constituents that are the subject of such a quantitative claim are commonly known in the United States as *marker compounds* or *markers*.

Based on the attention such a specification focuses on the marker compound(s), the layperson often naturally assumes that the marker content is of paramount importance in guaranteeing the reproducibility or even the efficacy of the extract. Furthermore, it is often assumed that the marker is the only factor of such importance. Neither of these assumptions is correct. Marker compounds often bear little or no relationship to the efficacy of the preparation, and reproducible marker content is indicative of a reproducible product only if used in the context of a complete body of raw material and manufacturing controls. Standardization is a complex process requiring attention to a

wide variety of parameters, with the ultimate goal of enhancing the batch-to-batch reproducibility of the entire spectrum of constituents, not just one or a few.

In broad terms, standardization is the complete body of information and controls that serves to optimize the batch-to-batch consistency of a botanical product. Standardization is achieved by reducing the inherent variation of natural product composition through quality assurance practices applied to agricultural and manufacturing processes. Standardization seeks to enhance the reproducibility of a product's safety and efficacy by providing the product with a more consistent composition. In any botanical, there are many compounds and types of compounds that work together once the product is ingested. Some compounds in the plant may enhance or diminish the physiologic effects of others. Other compounds, although having no direct physiologic effect, may nevertheless influence the stability, solubility, and bioavailability of the physiologically relevant compounds. Therefore by directly or indirectly enhancing the reproducibility of the complete composition of the product, standardization serves to enhance the batch-to-batch consistency of the product's effect.

American Herbal Products Association: Excerpts from *Standardization of botanical products: white paper*, Silver Spring, June 2003, AHPA.

safety, with aggressively concentrated "actives." It has proved to be relatively easy to fool standardization testing methods with inferior products.

The potential also exists for crowding out yet unmeasured but beneficial constituents with aggressive standardization. Standardization may also leave undesirable solvent residue in the final product. It is not required that solvents be listed on the label, thus such products may mislead the practitioner or consumer expecting a "natural" product free of chemical contamination.

Careful label reading is essential to ensure that the patient actually gets a product that contains the desired amount of the standardized constituent. For example, some manufacturers sell 300-mg milk thistle seed capsules containing 80-mg silymarin, whereas others offer 300-mg milk thistle seed capsules standardized to 80% silymarin. The latter contains 240 mg silymarin; significantly more than the former product, although on a quick read the products seem identical.

Concentrated Powdered Extracts (Granules)

Granules originated in traditional Chinese and Ayurvedic herbalism. Crude herbs are first decocted, usually in water, but traditionally may have been decocted in wine or stir-fried in honey. The liquid extract is then concentrated and vacuum dried onto small particles of herb or starch. The final granules usually have a 5:1 w:v concentration (5 g of crude herb concentrated into 1 g of granule extracted). The granules can then be taken as is, chased by water or another beverage, or reconstituted into a tea by dissolving in hot water. They can also be pressed into pills or encapsulated. Some companies

capture the essential oils during processing and add them back in before vacuum drying.

Advantages. Granules allow practitioners to dispense relatively high doses of plant material in a small volume. They also reduce palatability problems, particularly when taken as a pill. They are easy to dispense and formulate. They are fairly stable and last at least 2 years if stored in a dark, cool place.

Disadvantages. Damage may occur to some constituents during the extraction process, and thus not all herbs may be optimally effective in this dose form. Also, herbs high in low water–soluble phytochemicals are not optimally extracted into 5:1 decocted powder extracts either. The appropriate traditional decoction method (e.g., water, alcohol) must be chosen to extract the intended constituents before granulation, or efficacy may be decreased. Practitioners should question manufacturers about production processes to ensure that proper preparation procedures are in effect.

Fluid Acetracts

A fluid acetract is technically an extract of a plant in 100% acetic acid; however, 100% acetic acid is dangerous to handle and ingest. Practically it refers to an extract using 3% to 6% acetic acid (i.e., vinegar). At this concentration, microbial growth will occur, so ethanol is often included in the menstruum, changing the solvent nature of the menstruum. Acetracts are prepared by maceration in the same way as tinctures, have a shelf-life of no longer than a year, and must be kept refrigerated.

Vinegar extracts are uncommon for medicinal use today, but have a long history of use in botanical medicine. Alkaloids from alkaloidal salts become water soluble in acidic solvents. As a result, vinegar is a good extraction medium for alkaloid-containing plants like goldenseal, lobelia, and *Sanguinaria canadensis* (bloodroot). Vinegar extracts will have a longer shelf-life when water is not added in the preparation process. It has been suggested that macerations of dried plants may produce better results than extracts from fresh plants, where the water contained in the plant may excessively dilute the vinegar.

Essential Oils

Essential oils are traditionally prepared by steam distillation. The phenylpropanoids and/or terpenoids in the starting material boil and are condensed along with water into a capture vessel. The resulting oil can then easily be decanted from the water, with which it will not mix. Note that the heat involved in this process changes many of the constituents, and thus distilled volatile oils do not exactly match the compounds found in the plant. Research on a volatile oil cannot thus be directly extrapolated back to use of the crude herb. For example, *Matricaria recutita* (chamomile) leaf and flower contains matricin, which is converted to chamazulene by steam distillation. Chamazulene is not found in unheated, crude chamomile. Many medicinal properties of chamazulene have been discovered that do not necessarily apply to crude chamomile.

Volatile oils of all types are highly concentrated, potent extracts. Most plants contain at most 1% to 2% terpenoids and/or phenylpropanoids, which are therefore being concentrated 50 to 100 times to produce a volatile oil. They are always used in extremely low doses and with great care. These complex mixtures are lipophilic and thus have serious potential, in case of overdose, to cause harm to the highly fatty tissues of the nervous system in particular. With oral dosing, there is also concern about potential harm to the liver. A typical oral dose for an average-sized adult is three drops three times daily, although this will vary with the oil. Essential oils are thus generally administered only by inhalation or topically. Note that transcutaneous absorption of significant amounts of essential oil can also lead to toxicity; topical use can also lead to contact dermatitis. They are generally not applied undiluted (i.e., neat) to the skin. Instead, they are mixed into a carrier oil, usually almond, coconut, avocado, or other high quality oil, allowing greater distribution of the essential oil over a larger surface area, while protecting the skin from the potentially caustic nature of many essential oils. A sample of the oil should be patch-tested before extensive application, and a highly diluted product should be used.

Processes other than steam distillation can also produce essential oils. Some plants will yield oil by simple expression, whereas others are extracted using organic solvents. Petroleum ether is one of the most common solvents in current use, having replaced the highly toxic benzene.

Supercritical Carbon Dioxide Extracts

In recent years, supercritical carbon dioxide (CO_2) technology has been applied to extraction of botanical medicines. When carbon dioxide is placed under enormous pressure, it changes into a state between a liquid and a gas known as the supercritical state. When the pressure is removed from a supercritical system, the carbon dioxide returns to a gaseous state and leaves the final extract free of solvent. Supercritical carbon dioxide is a fairly broad spectrum solvent of many constituents of interest in plants, particularly low molecular weight terpenoids and phenylpropanoids; however, according to Steven Dentali, PhD, a natural products chemist, other solvents are often added to supercritical CO_2 because its solvent range is limited. Fatty acids and their glycerides are slightly soluble. Simple organic acids, carbohydrates, amino acids, proteins, and most inorganic salts are virtually insoluble. Thus supercritical carbon dioxide extracts are usually most like volatile oils, although they are chemically distinct because there are none of the heat-generated byproducts unique to steam-distilled volatile oils. There is no historical data, and little research, to support the use of supercritical extracts as an alternative to a tincture or a tea. Owing to the potential toxicity of essential oils when used internally, caution is advised in evaluating the use of these extracts as medicines although they appear highly useful as a method for concentrating specific constituents.

Freeze-Dried Botanicals

Freeze-drying (i.e., lyophilizing) is a dehydration process that removes the water from a substance by exposure to dry, freezing air. It is variously described as a process in which no heat or chemicals are involved and as a process in which chemical solvents are used, after which the extract is flash-evaporated at low temperature in a partial vacuum to remove the solvents. The solid residue is then packed into capsules.

Opinions vary, with some claiming that freeze-dried herbs are superior to other types of dried herbs and others arguing that freeze-dried herbs are unstable owing to their hygroscopic nature, which leads to rapid degradation upon exposure to air once a product bottle is opened by the consumer. Studies may support this concern. One study showed that air-dried oregano had a lower rehydration rate than freeze dried.[39] Another study found that freeze-drying of spearmint resulted in substantial losses in oxygenated terpenes and sesquiterpenes compared with oven or air drying.[40] In a study of basil, freeze-dried leaf had a lower content of volatile oils than oven-dried.[41] Freeze-dried aloe had a lower content of organic and fatty acids compared with oven-dried aloe.[42] On the other hand, freeze-dried seaweed had a higher content of total amino acids, lipids, and vitamin C compared with sun- and oven-dried seaweed, although the oven-dried variety had the highest mineral content.[42] A pilot clinical trial found that 600 mg of freeze-dried, powdered *Urtica dioica* (stinging nettle) leaf one or more times a day was significantly more effective than placebo at reducing symptoms of allergic rhinitis.[43] In addition, many studies, especially pharmacologic studies, use lyophilized herbs. Whether freeze-drying is beneficial may depend on the plant in question. Research comparing the activity of freeze-dried versus herbs preserved by other means has not been conducted in any systematic fashion.

Injectable Botanicals

Injection of botanical extracts by various routes has been practiced since at least the end of the nineteenth century, when intradermal or intramuscular injection of extracts of *Lobelia inflata* (lobelia), among other herbs, was popular among the Eclectic physicians in North America. Since that time, more sophisticated extracts suitable for intravenous injection have appeared in Europe and Asia, where herbal products are largely regulated as pharmaceutical drugs; but these are rarely encountered in North America.

Crude herbs and extracts of herbs are generally unsafe for injection, particularly intravenous injection. Saponins are often hemolytic and tannins can damage the liver, kidneys, and nervous system.[6] Many modern injectables, such as silymarin, glycyrrhizin, and schisandra represent single compounds or a limited number of compounds. Others, for example, extracts of *Viscum album* (European mistletoe) or *Echinacea* spp., are complex extracts. All preparations intended for injection must be sterile.

There are a number of older studies of injectables in the European, and particularly German, literature. For example, intramuscular injectable extracts of *Echinacea* spp. have been shown to be helpful for treatment of pertussis.[44] One of the best-studied injectable botanicals is an extract of European mistletoe used subcutaneously to induce immune responses for treatment of cancer and acquired immunodeficiency syndrome (AIDS) patients.[45] Intravenous glycyrrhizin combined with cysteine and glycine (2:1:20 ratio) has been effective in clinical trials for patients with hepatitis B, hepatitis C, and human immunodeficiency virus (HIV) infection.[46-48] Intravenous silymarin has been used in German and other European hospitals to treat poisoning by *Amanita phalloides* (death cap mushroom).[49] Use of injectable botanical extracts and botanical compounds is common in China. Extracts for intravenous and/or intramuscular injection from *Angelica sinensis* (dong quai) root, *Rabdosia rubescens* (dong ling cao) herb, *Salvia miltiorrhiza* (Chinese sage, danshen) root, *Allium sativum* (garlic) bulb, *Corydalis yanhusuo* (yan hu suo) root, *Artemisia annua* (sweet Annie, qing hao) herb, and many others have been the subject of numerous Chinese clinical trials showing efficacy.[50]

Few generalizations can be made about injectable botanicals. Each individual agent must meet unique standards specific to that herb. Anyone purchasing injectable botanical extracts should be certain about the safety of the product. Various professional licensing laws do not specifically mention injectable botanicals in almost all cases. Some licensed health professionals use them quietly or under more general provisions of medical licenses with unknown potential for legal problems. Ultimately, it is anticipated that as research evidence supporting efficacy of these agents mounts, injectable botanicals will become more available and officially recognized.

Topical Applications

Numerous dose forms are available to deliver herbs to the skin or for transcutaneous absorption (Table 3-17). Each will be reviewed in turn later.

There is surprisingly little information on the extent to which plant constituents are absorbed cutaneously. Most botanicals used topically have a long history of use and have

TABLE 3-17 Summary Chart of External Preparations and Bases

Preparation Type	Typical Base
Bath, sitz bath, hand-and-foot bath	Aqueous
Compress	Aqueous
Cream	Oil/aqueous to which has been added or in which has been extracted one or a combination of the following: whole herb, powder, tincture, essential oil
Douche	Aqueous
Enema	Aqueous
Gel	Aqueous
Oil	Oil
Pessary	Whole herb/tincture/essential oil
Plaster	Whole herb
Poultice	Whole herb
Powder	Whole herb
Salve/ointment	Oil and wax to which has been added one or a combination of the following: whole herb, powder, tincture, essential oil
Steam inhalation	Aqueous
Suppository/bolus	Oil to which has been added or in which has been extracted one or a combination of the following: whole herb, powder, tincture, essential oil
Wash	Aqueous or dilute hydroethanolic

good safety profiles. However, certain compounds such as toxic pyrrolizidine alkaloids and methyl salicylate reportedly are absorbed to some extent through the skin—enough to potentially warrant concern with significant or long-term use, or use on open skin or inflamed skin and wounds that will absorb compounds more readily and extensively.

Creams

A cream is an oil-in-water emulsion and is essentially the same as a lotion (although lotions tend to be thinner). Creams and water-based extracts, including tinctures, mix together well. Fixed oils such as safflower and sunflower seed oils are typically used as a base.

Creams are thin, easily applied, and are generally well absorbed. Because they tend to be moistening or only mildly drying, they are preferred in cold, dry climates. They are not appropriate for application to open wounds. Both short-term and chronic uses are appropriate. Creams have long shelf-lives, particularly if natural antioxidants and antimicrobials are included to reduce oxidation and microbial growth. Synthetic preservatives are not recommended.

Salves and Ointments

Salves are oil-based preparations used for healing skin trauma and irritated or dry tissue. They are relatively easy to prepare; stored in a cool, dark environment, they have a long shelf-life—often up to a year or more. Salve can be made from premade infused oil or by simmering herbs in oil to extract

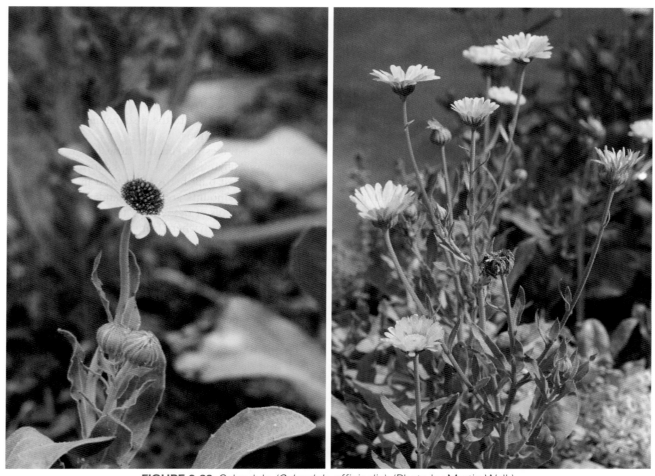

FIGURE 3-22 Calendula *(Calendula officinalis).* (Photo by Martin Wall.)

their constituents. Additionally, dried powdered herbs, essential oils, and tinctures can be added to a salve. Herbs commonly used in salves include *Calendula officinalis, Plantago lanceolata, Stellaria media, Hamamelis virga urea, Hypericum perforatum, Commiphora molmol, Hydrastis canadensis,* and *Symphytum officinale* (radix or folia).

(Note: If making salve from premade oil, begin with step 3. See the following for directions on making herbal oil.) To prepare herbal salve:

1. Place 1 ounce of dried herbs and ½ cup of good-quality olive oil in a small saucepan. Simmer for 1 hour on a very low flame with the pot covered. Add additional oil if necessary to keep the herbs immersed, and watch carefully to avoid scorching.
2. Strain the herbs well through a cotton cloth or cheesecloth, squeezing as much of the oil as possible out of the plant material. You may need to let the oil cool before this can be done.
3. Pour the extracted oil into a clean, dry saucepan, adding ½ ounce of grated beeswax per every 4 ounces of oil. Melt over a low flame, stirring constantly until the beeswax is fully dissolved.
4. Check for readiness by pouring 1 teaspoon of the product into a small, clean glass jar and placing in the freezer

for 3 to 5 minutes. The salve should be firm and solid without being so hard that it cannot melt onto your skin. If the consistency is correct, then pour the salve into small jars, cool to room temperature, cover, label, and store. If your salve is too soft, add more beeswax; if it is too hard, add more oil.

Preparing herbal oil for use in salve: Take the finely cut herb(s) of your choice and place in a clean, dry glass jar with a lid. Cover the herb material with olive oil, extending 1 inch above the top of the herbs. Cover and place the container in the sun or a warm location for 2 weeks. Shake the container daily. Strain the liquid into a clean glass jar, discarding the herb material. Store in a cool, dark place. This oil can be used to prepare salve, or alone as a medicated oil. The herbs used must be extractable in oil.

Suppositories and Pessaries

Suppositories allow for the insertion of herbal preparations into a body orifice. They are commonly used for vaginal and rectal complaints. The word suppository is derived from the Latin *suppositorium,* which means, "something placed beneath." *Pessary* is an interchangeable term, but refers specifically to a vaginal suppository. Suppositories, like many of the other preparations discussed in this section, are made from herbs that are antiinflammatory to the mucous membranes, astringent to excessive discharges and damaged tissue, and antimicrobial. They are used extensively for vaginal infections and inflammation, cervical dysplasia, rectal fissures, and hemorrhoids.

Suppository molds can easily be prepared at home by patients, using aluminum foil that has been folded several times lengthwise, and then widthwise, to form a trough approximately 8 inches in length and ½ inch in width. Alternatively, suppository molds can be purchased from apothecary supply shops. The base of the suppository is a combination of coconut oil and cocoa butter, to which is added the desired combination of medicated oils, powdered herbs, and tinctures. This is then poured into the mold, refrigerated to harden, cut into pieces the size of the patient's pinky finger, and inserted as needed. It is recommended that women wear a sanitary napkin when the suppository is in place, lest the melting oil stain the undergarments.

To prepare a suppository:
1. Melt ¼ cup each of cocoa butter and coconut oil.
2. Add 2 tablespoons of powdered herbs, for example, a combination of *Hydrastis canadensis*, *Ulmus rubra*, and *Althea officinalis* powders.
3. Add 15 drops of essential oil, for example, *Lavandula officinalis* and *Thymus vulgaris* and/or 1 tablespoon of appropriate herbal tincture.
4. Add 1 tablespoon of infused oil of *Calendula officinalis* (Fig. 3-22).
5. Stir well and pour into the suppository mold. Refrigerate until firm. Insert vaginally or rectally as needed.

Suppositories will keep in the refrigerator or freezer for many weeks.

Poultices and Compresses

A poultice is the direct application of the crude, fresh herb to the skin. A compress or fomentation is the application of a cloth that has been soaked in a plant extract. Usually, the extract (i.e., tea, dilute tincture) is an infusion or decoction, although diluted tinctures are also applied this way. Poultices, compresses, and powders are primarily used short term for wounds, bruises, sprains, or strains. They can be messy and generally require the patient to sit or lie still during use for 30 minutes or longer several times a day for optimal results. Poultices and compresses have extremely short shelf-lives, and must be prepared for each application.

Great care is warranted to make sure that contaminated herbal material is not put into or on any wound. In early stages of wound healing, moist herbal compresses will generally work best, provided they are changed many times a day. Ointments applied too early can delay healing, and should never be applied to puncture wounds, as this can create an anaerobic environment.

Powder

Powdered herbs can be applied directly to the skin or mixed with water or other extracts to form a paste. They are typically applied dry to weeping skin conditions to absorb discharge and impart antimicrobial or vulnerary action.

BOTANICAL MEDICINE DOSING

The goal of the practitioner is to provide an effective dose of a medication—enough to elicit a therapeutic response, yet not so much as to cause undesirable side effects or toxicity. Finding a *minimum effective dose* is ideal because it maximizes efficacy and safety; is also the most economical for the patient; and contributes to the sustainability of wild and cultivated plant populations.

What constitutes an effective dose is a matter of some debate among phytotherapists. For solid forms of herbal medicines (e.g., dried bulk herbs to be used in teas and decoctions), dosing amounts are fairly standard. However, there are varying schools of thought for tincture prescribing, with practices ranging anywhere from giving single drops ("drop dosing") of a botanical medicine to using large doses (as much as 5 to 10 mL of tincture three times daily), the latter common in European herbal medicine and among medical herbalists.

The drop dose strategy is not consistent with traditional prescribing practices, nor do most herbalists feel it bears out clinically, but seems to be based on homeopathic prescribing patterns and interpretations of the apparently low doses used in Eclectic medicine. The homeopathic dose application is not conducive to the use of herbs for their phytochemical constituents, but reflects an *energetic* model of herbal medicine. Although Eclectic medicines may have been used in low doses, they were actually highly concentrated pharmaceutical-like preparations requiring a low dose. Looking to traditional systems of herbal medicine such as TCM and Ayurvedic medicine, one finds that high doses of botanical prescriptions are the norm, with patients instructed to take as many as 30 g per day of an herb in tea or decoction form. Tinctures were not typically used other than in the form of medicated wines.

Western herbal practitioners worldwide most commonly subscribe to what is referred to as a "physiologic" dosing strategy, giving only enough of the botanical medicine to have a therapeutic effect; others may prefer a "pharmacologic" dosing strategy, prescribing larger doses to elicit a marked response.[51] Physiologic dosing is most appropriate for herbal products that are intended for long-term, regular use, as in the treatment of chronic conditions, or for the treatment of mild conditions. Pharmacologic dosing is more commonly used for acute or serious conditions requiring a quick response.

The complexity of dosing with tinctures is because of the fact that tinctures do not come in a single standard strength. They are available in a variety of strengths and concentrations; are made from both fresh and dried material; are made from material harvested at various times, leading to natural chemical variation in the product; and are made from starting materials of varying quality. As described in Herbal Preparations, tinctures are prepared in varying strengths, with ratios of herb to extraction menstruum (e.g., 1:2, 1:3, 1:4) affecting the strength of the final product.

Further, even if two different tinctures of the same herb are 1:5, that does not mean they are the same strength. Take a 1:5 feverfew *(Tanacetum parthenium)* tincture, for example. One may be made from whole feverfew plants (i.e., woody stem and all), and another from only leaves and flowers that have been stripped clean of stems, greatly affecting the composition and strength of the final product. Some companies use the whole St. John's wort *(Hypericum perfoliatum)* plant (2 to 4 feet tall), stems and all; others use only the medicinal flowering tops and an additional 2 to 6 inches, depending on the height of the plants. The latter will yield a more potent medicine. One calendula *(Calendula officinalis)* tincture may be made from old, faded, odorless, fumigated calendula flowers, and another from recently and properly dried, organically cultivated calendula that is still rich in color, aroma, flavor, and activity. Two different tinctures could be 1:5 from the same herb material, but can still be different strengths because different menstruum or extraction methods were used, or the same extraction methods may have been used, but with different extraction efficiencies.

Fresh herb tinctures can appear stronger than they actually are, but that is because of the math. For example, 1:2 fresh tinctures, when calculated according to equivalent dry herb tinctures, are often only around 1:8 or 1:10, depending on the amount of water weight of the fresh herb. Some herbs require curing to extract their full therapeutic potential. For example, it is necessary to activate endogenous enzymes in wild cherry bark *(Prunus serotina)* during extraction to enable hydrolysis of the bark's cyanogenic glycosides. Thus two 1:4 wild cherry tinctures—one hydrolyzed, and one not—are by no means equal in potential therapeutic activity (or potential toxicity). Simply put, there is no universal menstruum, herb/menstruum ratio, or extraction technique for all herbs. Each herb needs to be extracted according to its own unique physical and chemical characteristics and the strength and activity of the medication desired.

It is important to note that the ratio of herb to menstruum in a tincture is not always reflective of tincture strength. Although a 1:2 tincture is a stronger tincture than a 1:3, 1:4, or even 1:10 of the same herb, a 1:10 is not always a weak tincture. Many herbs that would be toxic in more concentrated strengths are standardly prepared as 1:10 tinctures according to the Brussels Protocol of the early twentieth century. Arnica *(Arnica montana),* for example, is prepared as such based on pharmacopeial standards, and given its potential toxicity, a 1:10 may still provide quite a strong medicine.

Although it may seem most reasonable to rely on the results of botanical clinical trials, using only those doses that were found to be successful, most herbs have not been subject to clinical trials and therefore there are only a limited number of herbs that have scientifically established doses. The preparations used in clinical trials do not necessarily have phytoequivalence to herbs sold on the common market, often making clinical trial doses irrelevant to the consumer and the practitioner. Further, the success of doses in clinical trials is relevant to those patients in the clinical trial, and does not necessarily apply to others who may not match the characteristics of trial subjects, for example, weight, age, metabolism, and health status. In fact, age, weight, and clinical status (e.g., pregnancy, immune status) will all affect what is an appropriate dose for an individual patient. Finally, clinical trials most often do not reflect traditional or modern clinical herbal practice strategies, and thus dosing information derived from clinical trials may be irrelevant to how the herb is used by the herbalist, which will most likely be in combination with other herbs.

Dosages for the individual patient can be derived from a standard dosage range, as presented in Appendix I. These were derived from a composite of what are considered some of the most authoritative information sources currently available in botanical medicine, with the traditional dose referring to the doses expected to be used by herbalists in clinical practice, and the clinical trial dose being based on the ranges determined effective in positive clinical trials, when available. Doses are provided for the form in which each herb is typically used.

The dosage range for tinctures assumes that a 1:4 tincture is being used unless otherwise indicated. Should practitioners be using more or less concentrated products, such as 1:3 or 1:5 strengths, doses can easily be adjusted mathematically, or the given dose can simply be used at the lower or higher range, respectively. Although extrapolation from a 1:4 to a 1:2 or 1:1 extract cannot be directly made by simply proportional adjustment, one can get a relatively good approximation of a safe and effective dose by dividing the dose of a 1:4 tincture by 4.

Doses are based on the assumption that the patient is a nonpregnant adult with an average weight of approximately 140 pounds. Adjustments for substantial weight variations, particularly for women who are more slight, can be made by using herbs in the lower range for women significantly (>20 lb) below the average. Lower doses are also generally appropriate for chronic conditions, whereas higher doses may be required in acute conditions; however, lower doses can also be given with greater frequency for acute conditions.

Dosing of herbal medicines, unlike pharmaceutical drugs, is not an exact science. Traditional doses are based on experience, trial and error, and historical use. Individual patients may benefit with lower doses or may require slightly higher doses. A complete list of doses for all herbs included in this text is found in Appendix I.

Guidelines for Herbal Medicine Use

BOTANICAL MEDICINE SAFETY: GUIDELINES FOR PRACTITIONERS

Estimates suggest that as many as 50% of Americans use some type of herbal supplement, as many as 18% use a supplement in conjunction with a pharmaceutical drug, and most do not inform their health care providers of herbal medicine use (see Chapter 1).[1-9]

Botanical medicine safety has therefore become a critical issue for practitioners, whether they themselves are prescribing herbal medicines in practice, or are caring for patients who are self-medicating with herbs.

One central role of the practitioner must be to maximize patient safety and treatment efficacy, minimize the likelihood of risk, and help patients to make the most appropriate decisions regarding both conventional and natural therapies.

Assessing the safety of individual botanical medicines can be challenging because of lack of a rigorous scientific evidence base for many herbs. Practitioners must rely on either a relatively small selection of herbal medicines for which evidence has been solidly established, or on a composite of information from the medical literature, historical literature, adverse events reports, safety reviews, books, herb–drug interaction charts, and botanical monographs to assemble a clear picture of whether an herb is not only generally safe, but safe for an individual patient. This takes time and requires quick access to the information, as well as knowledge of which sources are reliable, and can still leave the practitioner with a sense of uncertainty.

Numerous and complex factors influence botanical medicine safety and risk, including:

- The safety profile of individual plants
- Potential allergic or idiosyncratic reactions
- Potential or known interactions with other substances (e.g., herb–drug interactions)
- Product adulteration or contamination (e.g., heavy metals, pharmaceuticals, other contaminants)
- Substitutions (i.e., the accidental or deliberate use of the wrong herb)
- Timing of use (e.g., before surgery, during pregnancy/lactation)
- Dosage

- Duration of use (e.g., potential for accumulate toxicity)
- Lack of appropriate therapy for a medical condition

Botanical medicine safety is a broad and complex subject, far larger than can be adequately addressed in a single chapter. Nonetheless, a text on botanical medicine would be incomplete without addressing this critical topic. This chapter provides an overview of the most pertinent botanical medicine safety concerns relevant to clinical practice.

The author highly recommends the *Botanical Safety Handbook (BSH)*, second edition, as a resource. The *BSH* is available in hardback and online and is the most definitive source of safety information on individual botanical medicines. Additional recommended references appear in Table 4-1.

The *BSH* has classified herbs according to the following safety scale:

Class 1. Herbs that can be safely consumed when used appropriately.

- No significant adverse events in clinical trials
- No case reports with significant adverse events and high probability of causality
- No identified concerns for use during pregnancy or lactation
- No innately toxic constituents
- History of safe traditional use
- Toxicity associated with excessive use is not a basis for exclusion from this class
- Idiosyncratic, minor, or self-limiting side effects are not bases for exclusion from this class

Class 2. Herbs for which the following use restrictions apply, unless otherwise directed by an expert qualified in the use of the described substance:

2a: For external use only

- Toxicity demonstrated with crude preparation taken at traditional dose
- Adverse event data in humans with probability of causality of toxicity (e.g., hepatotoxicity, nephrotoxicity, neurotoxicity)

2b: Not to be used during pregnancy

- Adverse event data in humans and probability of causality
- Data in animals suggest teratogenicity or fetal wastage
- Traditional use contraindicates (e.g., abortifacient, uterine stimulant)

2c: Not to be used while nursing

- Potential hepatotoxicity or neurotoxicity

The editor wishes to thank *Botanical Medicine for Women's Health*, Edition 1 contributor Roy Upton for his significant contributions to this chapter.

TABLE 4-1   Resources for Assessing Botanical Medicine Safety

Botanical	Author/Editor	Publisher
Texts		
Adverse Effects of Herbal Drugs (three volumes)	DeSmet P	Springer Verlag
Botanical Dietary Supplements: Quality, Safety, and Efficacy	Mahady G, Fong H, Farnsworth N	Swets and Zeilinger
Botanical Safety Handbook	Gardner Z, McGuffin M, Upton R, et al	CRC Press
Commission E (translated)	Blumenthal M (ed.)	American Botanical Council
Expanded Commission E	Blumenthal M (ed.)	American Botanical Council
Herb-Drug Interaction Handbook	Herr SM	Church St. Books
Herb, Nutrient, and Drug Interactions	Stargrove M, Treasure J	Mosby
The Essential Guide to Herbal Safety	Bone K, Mills S	Churchill Livingstone
Toxicology and Clinical Pharmacology of Herbal Products	Cupp M	Humana Press
Monographs		
American Herbal Pharmacopoeia (AHP)	Upton R (ed.)	AHP
European Scientific Cooperative of Phytotherapy (ESCOP)	ESCOP	ESCOP
World Health Organization (WHO)	WHO	WHO
Web sites		
The Cochrane Library	www.cochrane.org	
Health Canada	www.hc-sc.gc.ca	
The National Center for Complementary and Integrative Health (NCCIH)	https://nccih.nih.gov	National Institutes of Health
Natural Medicines Comprehensive Database	www.naturaldatabase.com	
Examine	www.examine.com*	
Natural Standard Herb and Supplemental Handbook: The Clinical Bottom Line	Basch E, Ulbricht C	Mosby
Natural Standard Herb and Supplement Reference: Evidence-Based Clinical Reviews	Ulbricht C, Basch E	Mosby
Office of Dietary Supplements (ODS)	www.ods.od.nih.gov	National Institutes of Health
TOXNET	http://toxnet.nlm.nih.gov	National Library of Medicine

*Requires subscription.

- Bioavailability in breast milk has been demonstrated
- Traditional use contraindicates
- Adverse event data in humans and probability of causality

2d: Other specific use restrictions as noted
- Information exists for unsafe use by specific populations

Class 3. Herbs for which significant data exist to recommend the following labeling:

"To be used only under the supervision of an expert qualified in the appropriate use of this substance." Labeling must include proper use information: dosage, contradictions, potential adverse effects and drug interactions, and any other relevant information related to the safe use of the substance.
- Narrow therapeutic range
- Identified safety concerns in many populations

Class 4. Herbs for which insufficient data are available for classification.
- No significant history of traditional use

Applying this framework, along with the ethical guidelines and Kemper-Cohen algorithm (Fig 4-1) discussed later one can assess whether to use a botanical therapy for a specific patient.

ADVERSE DRUG REACTIONS, HERBAL ADVERSE EVENT REPORTS, AND ADVERSE EVENTS REPORTING SYSTEMS

According to the World Health Organization (WHO), an adverse drug reaction (ADR) is defined as "Any response to a drug which is noxious and unintended, and which occurs at doses normally used in man for prophylaxis, diagnosis, or therapy of disease, or for the modification of physiologic function."[10] For reporting purposes, the Food and Drug Administration (FDA) categorizes a serious adverse event as one in which "the patient outcome is death, life-threatening (real risk of dying), hospitalization (initial or prolonged), disability (significant, persistent, or permanent), congenital anomaly, or required intervention to prevent permanent impairment or damage."[11] The American Society of Health-System Pharmacists (ASHP) defines a significant ADR as any unexpected, unintended, undesired, or excessive response to a drug that:

- Requires discontinuing the drug
- Requires changing the drug therapy
- Requires modifying the dose (except for minor dosage adjustments)
- Necessitates admission to a hospital
- Prolongs stay in a health care facility
- Necessitates supportive treatment
- Significantly complicates diagnosis
- Negatively affects prognosis
- Results in temporary or permanent harm, disability, or death

Consistent with this definition, allergic and idiosyncratic reactions are also considered ADRs.[12]

In contrast, and not technically defined as ADRs, are side effects, which are defined by the ASHP as "an expected, well-known reaction resulting in little or no change in patient management (e.g., drowsiness or dry mouth caused by administration of certain antihistamines, nausea associated with the use of antineoplastics)" with "a predictable frequency and an effect whose intensity and occurrence are related to the size of the dose." Also not categorized as ADRs are "drug withdrawal, drug-abuse syndromes, accidental poisoning, and drug-overdose complications."[12]

After the thalidomide disaster of the 1950s, which led to over 10,000 cases of a severe limb deformity called phocomelia and a 50% mortality rate in infants whose mothers had been exposed in pregnancy, WHO established and has maintained an international adverse drug events reporting system. Since 1978, the WHO International Drug Monitoring Program (IDMP) has collected ADR reports from 60 participating nations, and now includes both pharmaceutical and botanical medicine information. Of the more than 2.5 million reports in their International Drug Information System (INTDIS) database, approximately 10,000 relate to herbal medicines, primarily involving multiple ingredients.[13] This demonstrates a remarkably low incidence of serious ADRs resulting from herbal products, especially compared with that of pharmaceutical drugs and the much larger worldwide consumption of botanicals compared with conventional medications. Many of the reports were associated with negative interactions with conventional medications and most side effects were reported for people 60 to 69 years of age.

Between 1983 and 1989 a total of 1070 inquiries were made. Not all inquiries represented adverse effects. Twenty-five percent of reports ($n = 267$) were of subjects with acute symptoms.[14] This is suggestive of a very low incidence of reporting of adverse effects caused by herbal preparations. Ernst conducted a survey of complementary and alternative medicine users in the United Kingdom. Of those who had reported use of herbal medicines, 8% reported having observed adverse effects, none of which were considered serious,[14] similarly suggesting a low incidence of adverse effects

with herbal products; though, as with ADRs for pharmaceutical medications, these are likely underreported.[15,16]

In the US, the Dietary Supplement and Nonprescription Drug Consumer Protection Act mandates for manufacturers and marketers of dietary supplement products to report "serious adverse events" to the FDA within 15 days of the report. Additionally, the product marketer is required to document and assess every allegation of an adverse event associated with a dietary supplement to determine whether or not it meets the "serious" criteria for reporting to the FDA. All records related to any adverse event report (AER) must be kept for no less than 6 years, regardless of whether the adverse event was reported to FDA. These records must be readily available for inspection by FDA compliance officers upon request.

The main AER systems for dietary supplements are the same as for pharmaceutical medications, represented by local and national poison control centers and the FDA's MedWatch program, all of which have serious limitations. Most reporting systems, including these, are passive systems with no criteria for submission, no verification of the authenticity or accuracy of reports, and no effective follow-up or investigation. To be meaningful, AERs must be critically reviewed and products analyzed. Yet when a report is made through Poison Control Centers or MedWatch, neither a systematic review of the patient or event is conducted, nor is the product involved in an event typically analyzed, making it impossible to establish a causal relationship between an event and an herb/herbal product. Further, recording practices are highly variable between systems and between centers within the same reporting system, and there is often selection bias.[17]

The US poison control centers evaluated the incidence of AERs for all dietary supplements.[17] In a 10-month period, 1466 reports of potential events caused by ingestion of supplements were made. More than one third of these (534) were unintentional ingestions; 471 reported no symptoms. Half (741) of the total reports produced symptoms. The reviewers reported that 66% (489) of symptoms were associated with dietary supplement exposure with varying degrees of confidence and 27% (132) were considered to be either definitely or probably related, whereas 34% (166) were reported as definitely or probably unrelated. The balance of reports (39%; 190) represented a 50% chance for the event to be correlated to supplement use. Ninety of the subjects used supplements in an attempted suicide, whereas the others used supplements for various reasons, ranging from the treatment of specific conditions (35%) to enhanced athletic performance (10%) and dieting (14%), among others.

From 2008 through 2011, the FDA received 6307 reports of adverse effects through the newly mandated Dietary Supplement and Nonprescription Drug Consumer Protection Act. Of these, 71% were considered to be serious, as defined in the Act. Most adverse effects were associated with combination versus single-ingredient products.[18] The following findings were reported:

53% (3370) resulted in unspecified important medical events of a serious nature
29% (1836) resulted in hospitalization

20% (1272) resulted in serious injuries or illnesses

8% (512) resulted in a life-threatening condition

2% (92) resulted in death

In previous decades, botanicals most frequently associated with adverse events included ma huang *(Ephedra sinensis),* which was removed from general commerce in the US in 2004, St. John's wort *(Hypericum perforatum),* the caffeine-containing guarana *(Paullinia cupana),* and ginseng (species not identified). Of a total of 401 calls to poison control centers specifically related to adverse events of dietary supplements, 286 events were classified as mild, 89 as moderate, and 22 as severe, with a total of four deaths. Subjects experiencing symptoms were taking as many as 44 ingredients concurrently and had more serious adverse events than did those taking fewer supplements long-term.

In comparison, a total of 61,229 calls regarding adverse events caused by other consumed substances, mostly pharmaceuticals, were made in the same time period. These data again show a relative paucity of adverse effects reported for herbal supplements despite widespread use of herbal products; this is consistent with pharmacovigilance findings internationally (see later discussion). Nevertheless, as also reflected in the data, herbal products should not be regarded as benign and should be used and prescribed responsibly and with full knowledge of the potential for therapeutic efficacy, positive and negative interactions with conventional medications, and adverse effects.

CATEGORIES OF COMMON HERBAL ADVERSE EFFECTS

The Toxicologic Medical Unit of Guy's and St. Thomas Hospital in London conducted a 5-year toxicologic review of adverse events caused by herbal drugs based on reports made to the National Poison Control Center.[19] Drowsiness and dizziness, as well as vomiting, diarrhea, abdominal pain, and nausea were the most commonly reported side effects. Other events of note included agitation and irritability, cardiac arrhythmias, psychological disturbances, and facial flushing. Interaction of botanical and conventional anticoagulants has resulted in reports of abnormal bleeding, and effects of interactions with herbs that rely on the cytochrome P450 (CYP) enzyme system have resulted in elevations or decreases in serum drug concentrations, affecting clearance times, efficacy, and toxicity. Reports of liver abnormalities were most commonly associated with Chinese herbal medicines.

Allergic and Idiosyncratic Reactions

An allergic reaction is defined as an immunologic hypersensitivity, occurring as the result of unusual sensitivity to a drug.[12] Allergic reactions occur via immune-mediated mechanisms; for example, the development of drug-specific antibodies, reactions to drug–antibody complexes, or release of inflammatory compounds. They are largely unpredictable and can range from minor complaints, such as itchy eyes, runny nose, and minor skin reactions, to fatal anaphylactic shock. Allergic reactions to herbal medicines are uncommon, but may result

from a compound inherent to the plant, or from contamination of the plant with molds, fungi, or other agents.

Patients with known sensitivity to specific allergens, for example, members of the *Asteraceae* family, should use herbs in this family with caution or avoid them altogether. Plants in this family are rich in sesquiterpene lactones, a constituent with known allergenicity primarily responsible for allergic reactions; however, any plant may cause a reaction in any individual.[20]

An idiosyncratic reaction is defined as an abnormal susceptibility to a drug peculiar to the individual.[12] Idiosyncratic drug reactions (IDRs) are also immune mediated, and may result in severe skin reactions, anaphylaxis, blood dyscrasias, hepatotoxicity, and internal organ involvement. Symptoms such as fever and joint pain may accompany an IDR. The immune involvement appears to be a result of the interaction of cellular proteins with reactive drug metabolites, and thus differs slightly from the etiology of allergic reactions. These types of reactions occur very infrequently, are independent of dose, and are highly unpredictable.

Risk factors for idiosyncratic reactions include increasing age, concurrent use of multiple medications (i.e., polypharmacy), hepatic disease, renal disease, malnutrition or decreased body weight, chronic alcohol consumption, and gender (i.e., women are more susceptible to IDRs). Specific enzyme deficiencies may be involved in some IDRs. Hepatotoxicity reactions reported with use of kava kava *(Piper methysticum)* are most likely a result of idiosyncratic reaction to this herb.[20]

Skin reactions such as contact dermatitis, irritation, and burns are the most common types of allergic reaction to herbs, and are associated with the topical application of irritating herbs or repeated exposure through handling of herbs, such as among employees in the herbal manufacturing industry. Asthma is also known to occur as a result of repeated exposure in this latter population. Care must therefore be taken when applying external therapies and also with repeated exposure to herbs and dust from herbs. Reports of contact dermatitis, allergic reaction, or other skin irritation are especially common with garlic *(Allium sativum),* mustard powder, cayenne pepper *(Capsicum annum),* and members of the *Asteraceae* family. Oral administration of the following herbs has also been associated with general skin reaction: echinacea *(Echinacea* spp.), goldenrod *(Solidago virgaurea),* and kava.[20]

Adverse Reactions Caused by Overdose

There are a number of reported incidences of overdose with herbal products, including unintentional overdose, as well as suicide attempts, most of which have failed likely because of the overall low toxicity of even those plants that would be considered potentially fatal enough to attempt overdose.[21] There is little information regarding the treatment of overdose of herbal products. As with all pharmacologic agents, treatment should be based on the herb's mechanisms of action and the reaction.

Reactions Caused by Specific Herbs and Toxic Compounds in Plants Discussed in This Textbook
Kava Kava *(Piper methysticum)*

Since 2000, the traditionally used South Pacific anxiolytic herb kava kava has been reported to be associated with approximately 60 reports of hepatotoxicity. About 26 reports were generated between Germany and Switzerland, several in the United Kingdom, and the FDA collected another 26. A large number of the subjects were concomitantly taking potentially hepatotoxic drugs; some had been diagnosed with elevated liver enzymes before kava use, and in at least one case, elevated liver enzymes returned to normal when the subject discontinued combined kava use and chemotherapy. In the majority of these cases and based on formal toxicologic reviews of the available data, causal relationship could not be established.

Of these cases, it appears that in 4 of the original 26 European reports, hepatotoxicity may have been exacerbated by kava, and from the available information, there appears to have been one person whose hepatotoxicity was directly related to kava consumption. The majority of other cases could not be linked directly to kava.

Nevertheless, based on these reports, several countries adopted restrictions on kava sales. In Australia, kava products must be prepared as aqueous (nonalcohol) solutions of whole or peeled rhizome, and must not contain a recommended daily dose of more than 250 mg of kava lactones; tablets or capsules must not exceed 125 mg/tablet; tea bags must not exceed 3 g/tea bag. If a product contains more than 25 mg/dose, then appropriate warning labels must accompany the product. In the United Kingdom, legislation was enacted as of 2002 to prohibit the sale of foods containing kava, and herbal products were limited to 625 mg/dose.

In June 2002, Germany banned the therapeutic use of kava completely.[20] A review was conducted by the FDA. Because of the lack of compelling data about a causal relationship, no ban was imposed in the United States. However, fear of potential litigation has caused product liability insurance carriers to deny coverage for kava products, ostensibly eliminating widespread availability of kava. Such events have to be juxtaposed against prevalence of use. In Europe alone, more than 100 million daily doses are used.

The Swiss regulatory agency in charge of the control of medicines reported the following: "It is estimated that eight cases of hepatotoxicity have occurred in a total of 40 million daily doses or one case per 170,000 courses of treatments of 30-days duration."[22] The normal incidence of hepatotoxicity in the population at large is 10 in 10,000. This suggests that hepatotoxic events of kava are much less than what is normally observed in the population at large.

Toxic Plants Not Typically Used

Some plants contain known toxins so potent that the plants are not typically used medicinally nor sold on the common market. If they are prescribed, they are generally done so by licensed care providers (e.g., ND, MD, LAc) and under strict controls. Therefore these herbs pose little threat to the average patient, with the exception of accidental substitutions (e.g., that of digitalis leaf in a plantain product in the late 1990s), use of toxic herbs by medical herbalists, or as a result of prescription by a licensed care provider.

BOX 4-1   Botanicals Containing Toxic Pyrrolizidine Alkaloids

Borage leaf *(Borago officinalis)* (not borage seed oil)
Butterbur leaf and root *(Petasites hybridus)* (PA-free material available)
Coltsfoot leaf *(Tussilago farfara)*
Comfrey leaf and root *(Symphytum officinalis, S. asperum, S. uplandicum)*
Ragwort *(Packera aurea)*

Many plants—including commonly consumed foods—contain compounds that might be toxic if consumed in large doses or for prolonged periods of time. If used properly, these too pose little risk to the average patient. However, several compounds found in herbs that have recently been or continue to be sold on the market should signal a red flag to practitioners because they are known or suspected to cause significant damage when taken in medicinal doses or for a sustained time. These are discussed briefly in the following.

Pyrrolizidine Alkaloids

The unsaturated form of pyrrolizidine alkaloids (PAs) found in a number of commonly used medicinal plants, for example, comfrey *(Symphytum officinale)*, coltsfoot *(Tussilago farfara)*, or plants in the genus *Senecio*, can directly cause veno-occlusive disease (VOD) and have resulted in fatalities, usually when consumed as a survival food during times of drought or famine or when used medicinally over a prolonged period of time or in susceptible individuals.

Because a number of botanicals used medicinally contain toxic PAs, and because some herb references continue to recommend such botanicals, caution is warranted (Box 4-1). Not all forms of PAs, such as the saturated PAs found in *Echinacea* species, are converted to toxic pyrroles, and therefore plants containing nontoxic saturated PAs should be distinguished from those that are toxic.[20]

Aristolochic Acids

Aristolochic acid (AA), even in small amounts, can cause both stomach and kidney cancer.[23] Although no AA-rich plants are discussed in this textbook, this discussion is included because of risk of adulteration in imported botanical products. A ban on AA-containing plants (Table 4-2) has been implemented in many countries, and the FDA issued a consumer advisory and import alert in 2001 warning the public and regulatory agencies about this problem. However, many products that may contain AA remain on the market in Asia. Domestically, plants that may be confused with AA-containing plants have been subjected to systematic analysis at the point of importation before they are allowed in commerce. Herbal practitioners must be vigilant about herbal and supplement products that may be mixed with AA-containing plants and ensure that manufactured products prescribed have the necessary controls to avoid adulterants.

TABLE 4-2 Botanicals Containing Aristolochic Acids or Those that May Be Mixed with Aristolochic Acid–Containing Plants

AA-Containing Plants	Possible Substitutions*
Aristolochia (*Aristolochia fangchi*)	Stephania (*Stephania tetrandra*)
Aristolochia manshuriensis	Akebia (*Akebia* spp.)
	Clematis (*Clematis* spp.)
Wild ginger (*Asarum* spp.)	Used intentionally

*These botanicals do not contain aristolochic acid (AA). It is recommended that these botanicals be subjected to AA testing to prevent adulteration. For a more complete listing see: http://www.fda.gov/Food/RecallsOutbreaksEmergencies/SafetyAlertsAdvisories/ucm095272.htm

Botanical Quality Standards and Reactions Caused by Contamination and Adulteration of Herbs

The safety of any medicinal product is partly dependent on the manner in which the product is produced. In the US, dietary supplements must be made according to federally mandated good manufacturing practices (GMPs) that were implemented by FDA; all manufacturers are subject to FDA inspection; and the FDA maintains the authority to remove from the market any unsafe ingredient or product that was not made in conformity with GMPs. Although individuals, organizations, industry, and government are actively working to ensure compliance with national quality GMP standards, noncompliance remains an issue, both for products made in the US and abroad.

European herbal product standards are generally stricter than most other countries, including the US; thus European-made herbal products have a greater likelihood of safety, quality, and efficacy. The most important aspects of quality control (QC) include the accurate identification, relative purity, and relative quality of raw material used in herbal products (Tables 4-3 and 4-4).

The safety of plants may also be affected by the presence of contaminants not naturally occurring in the plants, including heavy metals (e.g., taken up from the soil naturally, resulting from pollution, or their addition as part of traditional formulation or processing, as may be the case with Traditional Chinese Medicine [TCM] or Ayurvedic preparations and prescriptions), microbial contamination (e.g., owing to animal feces or poor handling under unhygienic conditions), or processes that are applied to the plant (e.g., sterilization with ethylene oxide gas, pesticides, fungicide, or gamma irradiation). By law, herbal products that enter the market must be safe for consumption as a food and be free of toxic microbial contamination. Similarly, certain treatments, such as with pesticides and irradiation, are not permitted on herbal products unless expressly approved. Nonetheless, because herbs are obtained from a variety of sources worldwide, many of which routinely use such treatments, herbal products may contain one or more of these contaminants. However, the General Accounting Office (GAO) analyzed 40 different supplement

TABLE 4-3 Potential Toxic Plant Adulterations Causing Safety Concerns

Botanical Nomenclature	Potential Adulterant	Potential Adverse Event
Black cohosh (*Actaea racemosa*)	Other species of cohosh	Some species of cohosh are toxic
Echinacea purpurea and other species	Missouri snakeroot	Allergic reaction in sensitive individuals
Eleutherococcus senticosus	Chinese silk vine	Birth defects if used in pregnancy
Skullcap (*Scutellaria lateriflora*)	Germander	Hepatotoxicity
Chinese star anise (*Illicium verum*)	Japanese star anise	Convulsions
Stephania tetranda	Aristolochia (*Aristolochia fangchi*)	Nephrotoxicity, cancer

TABLE 4-4 Potential Contaminants of Herbal Products

Adulterating Agent	Examples
Botanicals	Aristolochic acid-containing plants, belladonna, Chinese silk vine, digitalis, germander, Japanese star anise, nonmedicinal plant parts
Filth	Dirt, insect fragments
Microorganisms*	Toxic strains of *Escherichia coli*, *Staphylococcus aureus*, salmonella, shigella, *Pseudomonas aeruginosa*
Microbial toxins	Aflatoxins, bacterial endotoxins
Pesticides†	Chlorinated pesticides (e.g., dichlorodiphenyltrichloroethane [DDT], dichlorodiphenyldichloroethylene [DDE], aldrin, dieldrin), fungicides, herbicides
Sterilization agents‡	Ethylene oxide, methyl bromide, phosphine, gamma irradiation
Heavy metals§	Arsenic, cadmium, lead, mercury
Conventional drugs¶	Analgesics, anticoagulants, antiinflammatories, benzodiazepines corticosteroids, hormones

*Current law prohibits the presence of toxic microorganisms in herbal products. Contaminated products can be removed from the market. To date, there have been no published reports of herbal products toxicity from such microorganisms.
†Although some of these pesticides have been banned in the United States for decades, they may still be in use in other countries. Conversely, some pesticides may be approved for use in common foods but lack approval for use on herbal products.
‡These sterilization processes, although approved for use in certain foods, are not approved for use on herbal products.
§Heavy metals in food and water is a problem worldwide but have been specifically noted to occur in numerous herbal medicine products manufactured in China.
¶It is prohibited to combine conventional drugs in products marketed as dietary supplements.

products and ingredients for pesticide and metal contamination.[24] According to the report, "The levels of contaminants found do not exceed any FDA or Environmental Protection Agency (EPA) regulations governing dietary supplements or their raw ingredients, and FDA and EPA officials did not express concern regarding any immediate negative health consequences from consuming these 40 supplements."

The best way for practitioners to avoid potentially contaminated or adulterated products is to become knowledgeable of the practices of suppliers and manufacturers, and identify those with high quality standards (see Selecting and Identifying Quality Herbal Products). Companies that are run by or employ qualified herbalists on their staff and that serve the needs of health professionals are often the most reliable, but this in itself is not a guarantee of quality.[25]

Traditional Chinese Herbal Medicines Mixed with Conventional Pharmaceutical Drugs

It is not uncommon for Chinese herbal products made in Asia, including those sold in the United States, to be adulterated with conventional pharmaceutical drugs.[26] Adulterants have included caffeine, paracetamol, indomethacin, hydrochlorothiazide, prednisolone, barbiturates, and corticosteroids.[27] The purpose for the inclusion of pharmaceutical drugs in botanical products is presumed increased efficacy. However, inclusion of such substances is not consistent with the principles of TCM. In a survey evaluating herbal products used in hospitals in Taiwan, approximately 24% of 2406 herbal drugs tested contained pharmaceuticals.[26-28]

Significantly, in most cases the pharmaceutical adulterants are not disclosed on the product label or packaging. Herbal products adulterated with conventional medications have been found to be manufactured in mainland China, Hong Kong, and Taiwan.[29] In the United States, under dietary supplement regulations, such products are considered to be adulterated and are subject to removal from the market. Thus far, there have been no reports of the addition of pharmaceuticals in domestically made Chinese herbal products. Although there are undoubtedly high-quality herbal products manufactured in Asia, it is currently almost impossible for consumers and most health professionals (even trained TCM practitioners) to differentiate between adulterated and nonadulterated products. Thus patients using some traditional Chinese herbal medicine products in combination with conventional medications may also be unknowingly subjected to unexpected drug–drug interactions via a pharmaceutical adulterant.

Ayurvedic Herbs and Heavy Metal Contamination

In traditional Ayurvedic medicine, the addition of metals is common in selected herbal preparations. These are considered to contribute specific desired activities and are processed in a manner in which it is believed reduces their toxicity, although this latter assertion has not been critically documented. Additionally, if indeed processing does reduce the toxicity of heavy metals, there is no guarantee that all manufacturers apply these techniques appropriately. The prevalence of heavy metals in Ayurvedic preparations has been reported.

In a study conducted by Saper and colleagues, it was found that one in five Ayurvedic herbal products produced in South Asia and sold in Boston-area South Asian grocery stores contained potentially harmful levels of lead, mercury, and/or arsenic. If taken as recommended by the manufacturers, 20% of products could result in heavy metal intakes above published regulatory standards.[26] The Indian government made testing for heavy metals compulsory and labeling for heavy metals within permissible limits mandatory for Ayurvedic medicine products produced in India and destined for export beginning in January 1, 2006, as part of an attempt to address this problem; however, permissible limits may not meet optimal health and safety standards for patients concerned about any unnecessary exposure to toxic metals.[28]

HERB–DRUG INTERACTIONS

Herb–drug interactions are the most prevalent source of reported adverse effects worldwide and warrant serious concern, particularly given the frequency of polypharmacy in most US adults. According to a 1998 report by Eisenberg and coworkers, 61.5% of patients who used nonconventional therapies did not disclose this to their physicians.[30] In another survey, conducted among patients at the Mayo Clinic, even though patients were asked about supplement use in a written intake form, approximately half did not disclose this until engaged in a structured interview.[31] The same subjects similarly did not report on their prevalence of over-the-counter (OTC) medication use. A more recent report found that among individuals older than 50, many of whom are on at least one if not multiple medications, only as many as 30% report their use of dietary supplements to their doctors.[9]

These findings suggest that health professionals *must* be proactive in garnering information about both supplement and OTC drug use. Herbs and pharmaceutical drugs can interact either predictably or unpredictably with both positive and negative results (Table 4-5). Such modulation may be caused by direct pharmacologic activity or may lead to changes in the CYP enzyme system that affects drug metabolism.

For orally consumed medications, hydrophilic fibers and demulcents can interfere with absorption of conventional drugs, thereby decreasing their efficacy, whereas certain spices (e.g., black pepper, ginger) may increase drug absorption. Many botanicals that contain tannin (e.g., white oak bark, witch hazel) are capable of binding to both alkaloid and mineral drugs, resulting in decreased absorption of these. (See Appendix III for a comprehensive table of potential herb–drug interactions for common herbs.) The *BSH* provides a list of botanicals known to interact with conventional medications.

Combining any substances (e.g., herbs–drugs, drugs–drugs, herbs–herbs) can lead to additive, synergistic (i.e., potentiating) or antagonistic (i.e., negating) effects. Only synergistic effects truly constitute herb–drug interactions in that a new substance is formed in the interaction. In additive effects, the substances are not actually interacting with each other; they are simply both having simultaneous effects on the body. This is not widely explained in the herbal literature, but is an important distinction.

TABLE 4-5   Potential Interactions of Commonly Used Herbs with Conventional Pharmaceuticals

Botanical	Conventional Medication	Interaction	Evidence
Aloe *(Aloe vera)*	Glyburide	Potentiates activity	Human studies
Ashwagandha *(Withania somnifera)*	Barbiturates; diazepam, clonazepam	Additive effect; prolongs barbiturate-induced sleeping times; potentiates the effects of diazepam and clonazepam	Case report; animal studies
Astragalus *(Astragalus* spp.)	Acyclovir, interleukin, interferon; immunosuppressive agents	Enhances effectiveness of each; may antagonize the effects of immunosuppressives	Pharmacologic mechanisms
Chaste tree *(Vitex agnus-castus)*	Dopaminergic agents	May potentiate the effects	Animal studies
Chinese sage *(Salvia miltiorrhiza)*	Anticoagulants	Potentiates effects	Case report
Dong quai *(Angelica sinensis)*	Anticoagulants	Increased risk of bleeding	Case report
Eleuthero *(Eleutherococcus senticosus)*	Digoxin	Increased plasma level	Case report validated by rechallenge
Ephedra *(Ephedra sinensis)*	Stimulants	Potentiates the effects of stimulants	Case reports; pharmacologic mechanisms
Garlic *(Allium sativum)*	Anticoagulants; ritonavir, saquinavir	Potentiates anticoagulant activity; gastrointestinal discomfort; 51% decrease in plasma levels of saquinavir	Case reports; pharmacologic mechanisms
Ginkgo *(Ginkgo biloba)*	Anticoagulants	Potentiates anticoagulant activity	Case reports, in vitro assays; clinical studies fail to show a potentiation
Ginseng *(Panax ginseng)*	Phenelzine; warfarin; hypoglycemic medications; corticosteroids; digoxin; furosemide; ERT	Mania; increased cAMP; increased anticoagulant effects; increased hypoglycemic effects; increased side effects of corticosteroids; increased serum digoxin levels; decreased efficacy of furosemide; postmenopausal bleeding or mastalgia when taken with ERT	Case reports
Goldenseal *(Hydrastis canadensis)*	Drugs metabolized by CYP system	Inhibits CYP 3A4	Pharmacologic mechanisms
Gymnema *(Gymnema sylvestris)*	Insulin	May increase insulin-producing islet cells; enhances the effects of glyburide and tolbutamide	Animal studies; human clinical trials
Hawthorn *(Crataegus* spp.)	Digoxin, cardiac glycosides in general; theophylline, caffeine, papaverine, adrenaline, sodium nitrate, adenosine; barbiturates	Additive effect on cardiac glycosides; increases coronary artery-dilating effects of a number of drugs; increases barbiturate-induced sleeping times	Clinical experience, pharmacologic mechanisms
Hydrophilic fibers (flax seed, guar gum, psyllium seeds)	Digoxin, paracetamol, bumetanide, metformin, phenoxymethylpenicillin, glibenclamide	Slows gastric absorption	Case reports
Kava Kava *(Piper methysticum)*	Alprazolam, anesthetics, anxiolytics and barbiturates in general, cimetidine, levodopa, terazosin	Potentiation or additive effects resulting in CNS depression; dopamine antagonism	Case reports; pharmacologic screening

Continued

TABLE 4-5   Potential Interactions of Commonly Used Herbs with Conventional Pharmaceuticals—cont'd

Botanical	Conventional Medication	Interaction	Evidence
Licorice (*Glycyrrhiza* spp.)	Corticosteroids; potassium sparing diuretics; MAOIs; oral contraceptives	Potassium loss; increased corticosteroid plasma levels; increased salt and water retention; increased side effects of MAOIs; glycyrrhizin decreases plasma clearance, increases AUC plasma concentrations of prednisone; potentiates cutaneous vasoconstrictor response	Case reports of hypokalemia; may cause preterm birth; most reports caused by excessive consumption of licorice candy, which is most often made with anise (*Pimpinella* spp.); case reports
Papaya (*Carica paw paw*)	Warfarin	Increased INR	Case reports
Pepper (*Piper nigrum*)	Phenytoin	Increased absorption of conventional drugs	Clinical trials; pharmacologic mechanisms
Psyllium (*Psyllium ovata*)	Lithium	Decreased lithium concentrations	Case reports
Reishi mushroom (*Ganoderma lucidum*)	Chlorpromazine, reserpine, barbitals; amphetamines; anticoagulants; statin drugs; immunosuppressive agents	Increases sedative effects of conventional drugs; antagonizes amphetamines; may potentiate the effects of anticoagulants and statin drugs; may antagonize the effect of immunosuppressant agents	Pharmacologic mechanisms
Schisandra (*Schisandra chinensis*)	Chlorpromazine, reserpine, pentobarbital; amphetamines; caffeine; Adriamycin, acetaminophen; vasoconstrictors; sympathomimetics	Prolongs barbital-induced sleeping times; enhances CNS-inhibitory effects of chlorpromazine, reserpine, and pentobarbital; antagonizes CNS-stimulatory effects of amphetamines and caffeine; reduces cardiotoxicity of Adriamycin and hepatotoxicity of acetaminophen; may increase risk of hypertension if taken with vasoconstrictors and sympathomimetics	Pharmacologic mechanisms
Stinging nettle (*Urtica dioica*)	NSAIDs	Increased therapeutic effect	Controlled trial
St. John's wort (*Hypericum perforatum*)	5-Aminolevulinic acid, amitriptyline, cyclosporine, digoxin, indinavir, midazolam, nefazodone, nevirapine, paroxetine, phenprocoumon, saquinavir, sertraline, simvastatin, tacrolimus, trazodone, theophylline, warfarin, photosensitizing agents, oral contraceptives	Increases metabolic capacity of cytochrome P enzymes (reduces plasma levels of medications metabolized via these pathways); increases activity of P-glycoprotein; synergistic serotonin uptake inhibition; may potentiate photosensitization, mild serotonin syndrome, and decreased theophylline concentrations; reduces efficacy of oral contraceptives	Case reports/case series
Valerian (*Valeriana officinalis*)	GABAergic agents; barbiturates	Additive effects; prolongs barbiturate-induced sleeping times	Clinical findings
Yohimbe (*Pausinystalia yohimbe*)	Centrally acting antihypertensives, tricyclic antidepressants	May antagonize guanabenz and methyldopa; clinically observed CNS effects and hypertension when given with tricyclic antidepressants	In vitro assays; clinical findings

ERT, Estrogen replacement therapy; *cAMP,* cyclic adenosine monophosphate; *CYP,* cytochrome P450; *CNS,* central nervous system; *MAOIs,* monoamine oxidase inhibitors; *AUC,*; *INR,* international normalized ratio; *NSAID,* nonsteroidal antiinflammatory drug; *GABA,* gamma-aminobutyric acid.

Reports of Interactions

The literature consists mainly of case reports and in vitro pharmacologic data that have not been assessed for clinical relevance.[32] Patients or physicians make most individual case reports, usually after having experienced or observed an unexpected adverse reaction. Case reports, which typically are not subjected to critical review, are among the most unreliable body of information from an evidence-based perspective.

There have been a few critical reviews that provide some meaningful guidance regarding herb–drug interactions (Box 4-2). Researchers Izzo and Ernst conducted a systematic review of herb–drug interactions of seven of the most popularly used botanicals: garlic, ginkgo, St. John's wort, saw palmetto, kava kava, Asian ginseng, and echinacea.[33] Clinical data were collected from standard databases, recent articles and books, and interviews with herbal product manufacturers,[11] herbal experts,[8] and organizations related to medical herbalism.[28] In a 21-year period (1979 to 2000), a total of 41 case reports or case series in 23 publications and 17 clinical trials were obtained. Of these, only 12 interactions could be considered life threatening; these were mostly associated with a dangerous reduction in blood plasma levels of cyclosporine in organ transplant patients using St. John's wort, owing to a putative effect on CYP systems.[33]

The paucity of incidences of herb–drug interactions for these seven botanicals should also be viewed within the context of their total use. Definitive data regarding actual herb use are lacking, but available published marketing reports for ginkgo, kava, and St. John's wort provide some guidance. The available scientific literature is discussed further later.

BOX 4-2 Herb–Drug Interactions Literature: Case Reports Evaluation

The following 10-point evaluation scheme was established by medical herbalist Jonathan Treasure as a means to determine the validity and reliability of herb–drug interactions as presented in case reports in the medical literature. Many botanical researchers/authors have postulated that without a complete report, including the information described in the following, it is not possible to make an accurate evaluation of the significance of an herb–drug interaction case report.

1 to 5: Necessary
1. Positive identification (ID) of herb (i.e., form, brand, ingredients, dose, duration)
2. Adequate description of case (i.e., full details of the adverse drug reaction [ADR] and patient history)
3. Plausible pharmacologic timing
4. Other possible explanations ruled out
5. Concomitant medications noted (including dosage or none stated)

6 to 10: Substantiating
6. Confirmation by objective measures (e.g., serum levels of drug)
7. Plausible or established pharmacologic mechanism
8. ADR ceases on withdrawal of herb
9. ADR event reproduced by rechallenge
10. Previous exposure linked to same ADR

Categories of Herb–Drug (and Purported) Interactions

Anticoagulants

One of the most significant areas of concern regarding herb–drug interactions relates to coagulation. A number of plants have been reported to interact with anticoagulant agents, most specifically with warfarin and aspirin. The most common interaction reported has been enhancement or potentiation of anticoagulant effects. However, inhibition of anticoagulant effects is also possible through vitamin K pathways. Many foods and herbs contain high amounts of vitamin K and may decrease the efficacy of warfarin, thereby increasing the risk of thrombosis or myocardial infarction. Most available reports are from individual cases and may represent isolated events. Other researchers and reviewers have raised concerns over theorized mechanisms of action or the presence of specific compounds that may affect coagulation. Some of these may present real concerns, whereas others have not resulted in adverse events in actual clinical use. Regardless, caution is advised when using any medication with purported anticoagulation activity in conjunction with other anticoagulants, before surgery, and in those with bleeding problems.

Ginkgo. Ginkgo extract is by far the most widely used and prescribed medicinal herb in the world. According to a review of DeFeudis, from 1979 to 1998, approximately 110 million daily doses of ginkgo leaf extract were sold in France alone. According to market data of Dr. Willmar Schwabe GmbH, the maker and world's leading marketer of the most clinically tested ginkgo extract (EGb 761), in the period from 1979 to 1997, it was estimated that more than 2 billion daily doses of ginkgo extract were distributed worldwide. A more recent report estimates that from 1997 to 2002, 1.375 billion daily treatments of ginkgo single preparations have been administered in Germany alone. Until 2003, a total of only four case reports of potential interactions between ginkgo and conventional medications had been published.[34] Two of these were associated with bleeding events. This has led to significant concerns regarding its potential to increase the effects of anticoagulants. However, such events, if causal, are rare. More than 40 clinical trials with several thousand subjects have been conducted using the EGb 761 ginkgo extract with no reports of increased bleeding. A number of studies have specifically looked at its potential for increasing the anticoagulant effects (i.e., international normalized ratio [INR]) of aspirin and warfarin with negative results; it has been included in pharmacovigilance reviews throughout Europe for decades and few reports of adverse effects exist.[34]

Garlic. Garlic has been reported to thin the blood by at least three different mechanisms; fibrinolytic activity, inhibition of platelet aggregation, and decreased fibrinogen activity. Most of these findings were from human studies with very small patient populations.[35] Consumption of garlic as a food has not been implicated in bleeding events, suggesting that cooked garlic, which is most commonly consumed, does not contain the compounds responsible for the anticoagulant effects. This is likely as numerous studies suggest that allicin, which is lost in cooking, is associated with its putative anticoagulant activity. Thus varying preparations may elicit different actions, depending on the constituents present in the preparation. Primarily, supplemental forms of garlic preparations, especially those delivering allicin, should not be used, or should be used very cautiously in those with bleeding problems, using anticoagulants, or before surgery.

Herbs that contain salicin, such as willow (*Salix* spp.), meadowsweet (*Filipendula ulmaria),* and birch (*Betula* spp.), have been noted as potential substances that may enhance the effects of anticoagulants. This is based on the fact that salicin was a precursor of acetyl salicylic acid (i.e., aspirin). However, with few exceptions clinical trials with salicin-containing herbs have yet to demonstrate any blood-thinning activity of these substances. Salicin does not appear to affect platelet aggregation in the same manner as does aspirin. There have been two case reports regarding anticoagulant activity of the oils of birch and wintergreen, both of which contain methylsalicylates.

Herbs that contain coumarin or closely related compounds have also been suspected of causing bleeding events or enhancing the effects of anticoagulants. Coumarin itself is not active in humans; for it to have activity it must undergo a transformation caused by different types of molds. Reports of bleeding caused by coumarin-containing herbs, most notably sweet melilot (*Melilotus officinalis),* have been made owing to consumption of fermented leaves by cattle. Reports regarding an anticoagulant effect of coumarin-containing herbs in humans have only rarely been made.

Other Botanicals. Other botanicals that have been reported to potentiate the effects of anticoagulants include those that inhibit platelet aggregation through an inhibition of thromboxane synthetase (e.g., ginger), arachidonic acid (e.g., those rich in essential fatty acids), or epinephrine (e.g., garlic). A number of Chinese herbs have been implicated in bleeding problems. Most notably these include Chinese salvia (*Salvia miltiorrhiza),* dong quai (*Angelica sinensis),* and corydalis (*Corydalis yanhusuo).* These botanicals are classified as possessing blood-thinning properties from a traditional Chinese medical perspective and so such an effect is predictable. In the case of dong quai, which is commonly used in the treatment of gynecologic conditions and anemia, a 46-year-old woman experienced a greater than twofold elevation in prothrombin time (from 16.2 to 27 seconds) and INR (from 2.3 to 4.9) after consumption of a commercial dong quai product. No other cause for the increase could be determined and coagulation values returned to acceptable levels within 1 month after discontinuing dong quai.[36] Similar increases in INR have been reported for Chinese salvia, one of the most commonly used botanicals in Chinese medicine for increasing blood circulation. Conversely, high doses of green tea (*Camellia* spp.), as well as ginseng, have been reported to decrease the effects of warfarin.[37,38]

A relatively large number of medicinal plants can potentially interact with conventional anticoagulant medications. Therefore monitoring of bleeding signs and INR is warranted when using botanicals with known effects on bleeding mechanisms in conjunction with anticoagulant therapy or those with a history of use in altering circulation. These same botanicals should also be avoided immediately before surgery (Table 4-6).

Anesthetics, Anticonvulsants, Barbiturates, Benzodiazepines, Opioids, and Sedatives

Hundreds of plants have been used historically for their sedative, pain-killing, and anticonvulsant activity. Used in combination with similarly acting medications, enhancement of activity resulting in loss of muscular coordination or a prolongation of anesthesia- or barbiturate-induced sleeping times has been observed. Compounds in valerian root, for example, display an affinity for barbiturate, gamma-aminobutyric acid-A (GABA-A), peripheral benzodiazepine, serotonin, and opioid receptors, whereas California poppy (*Eschscholzia californica*) contains the alkaloid chelerythrine, which is a protein kinase inhibitor (Table 4-7).

Cardiovascular Medications

A number of botanicals directly or indirectly affect the cardiovascular system and may interact with cardiovascular medications. A variety of mechanisms of action may be included in these effects: direct antihypertensive activity through diuresis (e.g., juniper berry), vasodilatation (e.g., hawthorn leaf with flower), and muscular relaxation (e.g., cramp bark). A number of other botanicals can affect blood pressure indirectly through a number of functions, including: cholesterol-lowering effects (e.g., garlic [*Allium sativum];* guggul [*Commiphora mukul]),* adaptogens (e.g., eleuthero), nervines (e.g., skullcap [*Scutellaria lateriflora];* zizyphus [*Zizyphus spinosa]),* and weight loss aids (guggul [*Commiphora mukul]).* The most widely studied botanical in Western herbal medicine for the treatment of cardiovascular disease is hawthorn (*Crataegus* spp.). It possesses a number of pharmacologic activities that make it ideal for the treatment of stage I and II cardiac insufficiency. Most importantly it primarily exhibits positive inotropic activity, thereby slowing the heart and making for a stronger, more efficient heartbeat, much like beta-blockers. Because of this it can potentiate the effects of other positively inotropic agents such as digitalis. In the 1980s in Germany, it was a relatively common practice for physicians to prescribe hawthorn alternately with digitalis preparations to reduce the prevalence of accumulated toxicity often associated with digoxin glycosides. However, taken together without modifying the dose of digitalis can result in additive and potentially dangerous effects.

Cholesterolemic drugs, such as the statins, inhibit cholesterol biosynthesis through an inhibition of hydroxymethylglutaryl-CoA-coenzyme reductase. Any botanical that has a cholesterol-lowering effect through the same pathway (e.g., guggul) may result in potentiation. The primary botanicals used by American consumers for reducing cholesterol levels include red yeast (contains lovastatin, which acts similarly to statin drugs), garlic, and gum guggul resin. Although this potential interaction is not life threatening, it may require modifying the dose of conventional medications. Other classes of botanicals, such as laxatives, may indirectly negatively interact with cardiovascular medications by causing potassium loss (Table 4-8).

Drugs Metabolized via the Cytochrome P450 System

In recent years, a number of botanicals have been shown to affect the metabolizing of numerous conventional medications through a modulation of the CYP enzyme system.

TABLE 4-6 Botanicals Best Avoided Before Surgery or with Anticoagulant Use

Botanical	Action
Alfalfa leaf *(Medicago sativa)*	Potential anticoagulant effect if the material was subjected to fermentation; potential coagulant activity caused by vitamin K content
Angelica *(Angelica* spp.)	Possible anticoagulant effects
Asafoetida root *(Ferula foetida)*	In vivo anticoagulation
Black currant seed oil *(Ribes nigrum)*	Possible anticoagulant effects of gamma linolenic acid (GLA)
Borage seed oil *(Borago officinalis)*	Possible anticoagulant effects of GLA
Cayenne pepper *(Capsicum annum)*	Antiplatelet aggregation caused by capsaicin
Chamomile flowers *(Matricaria chamomilla)*	Potential anticoagulant effect
Chinese salvia root *(Salvia miltiorrhiza)*	Anticoagulant effect
Chinese skullcap *(Scutellaria baicalensis)*	Inhibits vitamin K reductase
Cornsilk *(Zea mays)*	Contains vitamin K
Devil's claw *(Harpagophytum procumbens)*	Possible anticoagulant effects
Evening primrose seed oil *(Oenothera biennis)*	Possible anticoagulant effects of GLA
Fenugreek seed *(Trigonella foenum-graecum)*	Anticoagulant effect
Feverfew leaf *(Tanacetum parthenium)*	Inhibits platelet aggregation
Garlic bulb *(Allium sativum)*	Anticoagulant effect; can interact with warfarin
Ginger root *(Zingiber officinale)*	Inhibits platelet aggregation
Ginkgo leaf *(Ginkgo biloba)*	Potential anticoagulant effect
Ginseng root *(Panax ginseng)*	May exacerbate hypertension; inhibits platelet aggregation
Horse chestnut seed *(Aesculus hippocastanum)*	Potential anticoagulant effect caused by saponin compounds (e.g., esculetin, osthole)
Licorice root *(Glycyrrhiza* spp.)	Potential anticoagulant effect
Papaya *(Carica papaya)*	Potential for increased bleeding caused by papain
Parsley leaf *(Petroselinum crispum)*	Contains vitamin K
Pau d'Arco bark *(Tabebuia* spp.)	Potential anticoagulant effect caused by lapachol, which works similarly to warfarin
Red clover blossoms *(Trifolium pratense)*	Potential anticoagulant effect
Shepherd's purse herb *(Capsella bursa-pastoris)*	Contains vitamin K
St. John's wort herb *(Hypericum perforatum)*	Prolongs effects of anesthesia
Stinging nettle leaf *(Urtica dioica)*	Contains vitamin K
Turmeric root *(Curcuma longa)*	Potential anticoagulant effect

TABLE 4-7 Botanicals That May Interact with Sedatives

Botanical	Interacting Medications	Possible Effect
Ashwagandha *(Withania somnifera)*	Barbiturates	Potentiation
Black currant seed oil *(Ribes nigrum)*	Anticonvulsants	May decrease seizure threshold
Borage seed oil *(Borago officinalis)*	Anticonvulsants	May decrease seizure threshold
California poppy *(Eschscholzia californica)*	Analgesics, sedatives	Potentiation
Catnip *(Nepeta cataria)*	Barbiturates	Potentiation
Chamomile *(Matricaria recutita)*	Barbiturates	Potentiation
Cramp bark *(Viburnum opulus)*	Anticonvulsants	Contains salicylates; may increase effect
Eleuthero *(Eleutherococcus senticosus)*	Barbiturates	Potentiation
Evening primrose *(Oenothera biennis)*	Anticonvulsants	May decrease seizure threshold
Hops *(Humulus lupulus)*	Sedatives	Potentiation
Kava kava *(Piper methysticum)*	Anesthetics, barbiturates	Prolonged sedation times
Passionflower *(Passiflora incarnata)*	Barbiturates	Potentiation
Schisandra *(Schisandra chinensis)*	Barbiturates	Potentiation
St. John's wort *(Hypericum perforatum)*	Anesthetics, benzodiazepines	Prolonged anesthesia times; decreased efficacy in some cases, increased effects in others; binds to gamma-aminobutyric acid (GABA) receptor
Valerian *(Valeriana officinalis)*	Anesthetics, barbiturates, benzodiazepines	Prolonged sedation times; binds to multiple neurologic receptors
Willow *(Salix* spp.)	Anticonvulsants	Contains salicylates; may increase effect
Wintergreen *(Gaultheria procumbens)*	Anticonvulsants	Contains salicylates; may increase effect

Approximately 80% of drugs are metabolized by this system and include calcium channel blockers, cyclosporine, loxapine, oral antihistamines, and oral penicillin, to name just a few. Taking a botanical that affects this system can elicit an inhibitory or stimulatory activity, resulting in either too slow or too rapid drug clearance, with either negative or positive effects. Stimulation of this system can cause substances to be metabolized rapidly, compromising the clinical efficacy of the drug if effective concentrations are not maintained. If this system is inhibited, drugs can accumulate in the blood too fast or for extended periods of time, thus increasing their toxicity. No formal human investigations to date regarding the potentially positive interaction between botanical and conventional medications have been conducted.

Several botanicals have demonstrated a relatively strong in vitro effect on CYP450 3A4 (CYP3A4), including St. John's wort *(Hypericum perforatum),* goldenseal *(Hydrastis canadensis),* cat's claw *(Uncaria tomentosa),* echinacea *(Echinacea angustifolia),* chamomile *(Matricaria chamomilla),* and licorice *(Glycyrrhiza glabra).*[39] However, in vitro data may not accurately reflect what occurs in humans. Most CYP effects that are reported are caused by negative observations derived from case reports or from in vitro data showing changes in drug pharmacokinetic values AUC (i.e., area under curve) that may have no clinical relevance.

St. John's Wort. As of 2001, St. John's wort was the primary antidepressant used throughout Europe with approximately 66 million daily doses in Germany, outselling most conventional antidepressants. Up until the 2000 review of Izzo and Ernst, a total of 29 potential interactions were reported. Most of those were associated with decreased blood cyclosporine levels caused by enhanced hepatic enzyme induction (CYP). Others were associated with an additive effect of St. John's wort with selective serotonin reuptake inhibitors (SSRIs). Interaction with oral contraceptives (OCPs) has also been noted. In one study of 12 women, concomitant use of St. John's wort was associated with a significant ($p < 0.05$) increase in the oral clearance of norethindrone and a significant reduction in the half-life of ethinyl estradiol. The oral clearance of midazolam was significantly increased during St. John's wort

administration, but the systemic clearance of midazolam was unchanged. Serum concentrations of follicle-stimulating hormone, luteinizing hormone, and progesterone were not significantly affected by St. John's wort dosing ($p > 0.05$). Breakthrough bleeding occurred in 2 of 12 women in the control phase compared with 7 of 12 women in the St. John's wort phase. The oral clearance of midazolam after St. John's wort dosing was greater in women who had breakthrough bleeding.[40]

No pregnancies have been reported in the literature as a result of OCP–St. John's wort interactions. Again, considering the prevalence of St. John's wort use, such incidences of adverse effects are rare. With increased understanding that St. John's wort does affect CYP enzyme systems, such interactions can be more readily predicted and therefore minimized (see Drugs Metabolized via the Cytochrome P450 System).[33]

In a few of the most noted cases, St. John's wort was shown to inhibit CYP3A4 in vitro and stimulate it in vivo. According to case reports, two transplant patients were medicated with cyclosporine to prevent organ rejection. After self-medicating with St. John's wort, cyclosporine plasma levels were found to be 25% to 50% lower than expected, resulting in acute organ rejection in one of the subjects. Upon discontinuation of the botanical, drug plasma levels returned to expected levels. Other such case reports have been made, suggesting strongly that St. John's wort and other botanicals that upregulate the CYP system must not be used in conjunction with immunosuppressant drugs in organ transplant patients (see http://medicine.iupui.edu/clinpharm/ddis/main-table for a regularly updated resource on substances that interact with the cytochrome system).[41]

Hypoglycemic Agents

There are definitive data on the appropriate use of antidiabetic botanicals in the treatment of diabetes specifically for their effects on blood sugar regulation and reduction in insulin resistance. Use of such herbs in conjunction with hypoglycemic therapies can potentially result in decreased glucose absorption that can alter insulin needs. Among the most widely used botanicals with putative blood sugar lowering

TABLE 4-8 Botanicals That May Interact with Cardiovascular Medications		
Botanical	**Therapeutic Category**	**Effect**
Digitalis,* lily of the valley, squill See Table 4-5	Antiarrhythmics Anticoagulants	All contain cardiac glycosides
Digitalis, garlic, hawthorn, lily of the valley, squill	Antihypertensives	
Coltsfoot	Calcium channel blockers	
Digitalis, figwort, lily of the valley, squill; eleuthero; hawthorn	Cardiac glycosides	Some contain cardiac glycosides; eleuthero can increase plasma digoxin levels; hawthorn is positively inotropic
Artichoke, fenugreek, garlic, ginger, guggul, red rice yeast	Cholesterolemic agents	Increased therapeutic effect; red rice yeast contains lovastatin
Agrimony, arjuna, birch leaves, celery seed, corn silk tassels, couch grass, goldenrod, horsetail, juniper berry, phyllanthus, rehmannia	Diuretics	Increased potassium loss

*Digitalis is not available as a botanical dietary supplement and is rarely prescribed by medical herbalists.

effects include: cinnamon (*Cinnamomum* spp.), bitter melon (*Momordica charantia*), fenugreek (*Trigonella foenum-graecum*), and prickly pear (*Opuntia* spp.), this latter species being widely used in Hispanic communities. High fiber intake can also inhibit glucose absorption, as can consumption of mucilaginous herbs (Box 4-3).

Immune Suppressants and Immune-Enhancing Therapies

Many botanicals possess immunomodulatory activity. Some of these, such as echinacea, are used for the prevention or reduction of severity of colds and flu. Others, such as astragalus and reishi mushroom, are used for general immune enhancement or specifically in conjunction with conventional cancer therapies. Prudence dictates that such herbs should not be used in conjunction with immunosuppressant therapies such as those used in organ transplant patients or in those with autoimmune disease. There are case reports of echinacea exacerbating symptoms of lupus and rheumatoid arthritis. There are very little data regarding the use of botanicals with immunosuppressive therapies (Box 4-4). No well-designed trials regarding such combined therapies are available. There are limited data suggesting a positive effect of immunomodulating botanicals when used in conjunction with conventional therapies, showing enhanced efficacy of chemotherapeutic therapies.[42-45] The use of immune-modulating botanicals must be weighed against the cytotoxic therapies of Western medicine.

Diuretics

Pharmacologic evidence regarding definite diuretic activity of many botanicals is lacking, yet they are very commonly used. In general, use of diuretics can lead to potassium loss, which can potentially lead to fatal arrhythmias. This does not appear to have been reported with use of herbal diuretics. There are, however, some reports of potassium loss through the excessive use of purging cathartics as part of weight loss programs; some also contained diuretics. Part of the reason may be that many herbal diuretics, for example dandelion leaf (*Taraxacum officinale*), also contain high amounts of potassium, which may actually result in increased serum potassium levels (Box 4-5). Nonetheless, care should be taken when using diuretics with patients on medications that have narrow therapeutic windows, or when potassium depletion may place the patient at risk.

Tannins and Iron Availability

Botanicals rich in tannins, a common constituent of many barks and leaves, can decrease the absorption of certain classes of drugs, most notably alkaloidal and mineral drugs such as colchicine, ephedrine, copper, iron, and zinc; thus individuals with specific deficiencies (e.g., iron, zinc) may be advised to avoid tannin-rich botanicals for the duration of supplementation (Box 4-6).

LACK OF APPROPRIATE THERAPY OR DISCONTINUATION OF CONVENTIONAL CARE

Many conventional medical practitioners are legitimately concerned that a patient may defer "proper" treatment of

---

BOX 4-3 Botanicals That May Interact with Hypoglycemic Agents

Agrimony (*Agrimonia eupatoria*)
Alfalfa (*Medicago sativa*)
Aloe juice (*Aloe* spp.)
American ginseng (*Panax quinquefolius*)
Bilberry leaves (*Vaccinium myrtillus*)
Bitter melon (*Momordica charantia*)
Dandelion root (*Taraxacum officinale*)
Devil's club (*Oplopanax horridus*)
Fenugreek (*Trigonella foenum-graecum*)
Garlic (*Allium sativa*)
Ginseng (*Panax ginseng*)
Guar gum (*Cyamopsis tetragonoloba*)
Gymnema (*Gymnema sylvestre*)
Jambul seeds (*Syzygium cumini*)
Madagascar periwinkle (*Vinca rosea*)
Maitake mushroom (*Grifola frondosa*)
Marshmallow root (*Althaea officinalis*)
Prickly pear cactus (*Opuntia* spp.)

BOX 4-4 Botanicals Generally Contraindicated with Immunosuppressive Therapies

Astragalus (*Astragalus membranaceus*)
Atractylodes (*Atractylodes* spp.)
Echinacea (*Echinacea* spp.)
Eleuthero (*Eleutherococcus senticosus*)
Ginseng (*Panax ginseng*)
Grifola mushroom (*Grifola umbellata*)
Licorice root (*Glycyrrhiza glabra*)
Maitake mushroom (*Grifola frondosa*)
Poria (*Poria cocos*)
Reishi mushroom (*Ganoderma lucidum*)
Schisandra (*Schisandra chinensis*)

BOX 4-5 Herbal Diuretics

Agrimony (*Agrimonia eupatoria*)
Arjuna (*Terminalia arjuna*)
Birch leaves (*Betula* spp.)
Boldo (*Peumus boldus*)
Celery seed (*Apium graveolens*)
Corn silk (*Zea mays*)
Couch grass (*Agropyron repens*)
Dandelion leaf (*Taraxacum officinalis*)
Elder flowers (*Sambucus* spp.)
Goldenrod (*Solidago* spp.)
Horsetail (*Equisetum arvense*)
Juniper berry (*Juniperus communis*)
Parsley leaf (*Petroselinum crispum*)
Phyllanthus (*Phyllanthus niruri*)
Rehmannia (*Rehmannia glutinosa*)
Shepherd's purse (*Capsella bursa-pastoris*)
Stinging nettle (*Urtica dioica*)
Yarrow (*Achillea millefolium*)

a condition in hope that a natural therapy can resolve their problem; that a natural therapy may interfere with the safety or efficacy of a conventional treatment being followed; or that a patient may discontinue an effective treatment in hopes of benefit from a potentially ineffective natural treatment. Unfortunately, there are few clear guidelines for determining the relative efficacy of an herbal versus conventional drug therapy. As noted, a number of studies have compared herbal with conventional medications, with some studies either showing equal or greater efficacy. Some have also demonstrated a better safety profile than the conventional medicine and conventional nosotropics (St. John's wort versus imipramine). However, these are few and far between and more research in this area is needed. Where the literature is clear, one role of the practitioner can be to help the patient choose the therapy that has the greatest level of efficacy and safety. Health professionals must additionally balance the right of patients to choose the therapy they feel is best for them with the best medical opinion that can be offered. Additionally, most surveys show that the majority of patients using complementary and alternative medicine (CAM) therapies are also under the care of their primary physician or other health professional.[30]

TIMING OF HERB USE

Use of Herbs Before Surgery

A number of botanicals should be avoided, or used with care, before or when undergoing surgery; largely this is because of theoretical or known risks of interactions with coagulation therapies or anesthesia. Patients must also be queried regarding their use of botanicals at this time. As noted, there are a number of botanicals with blood-thinning potential, such as ginkgo, garlic, dong quai, and red clover, whose use is so common that patients might not report these in a standard medical history intake. There are also botanicals that have been reported to interact with general anesthesia, most notably, St. John's wort, which may intensify or prolong the effects

---

BOX 4-6   Tannin-Rich Botanicals

Agrimony (*Agrimonia eupatoria*)
Bahera (*Terminalia belerica*)
Bayberry (*Myrica cerifera*)
Blackberry leaf (*Rubus villosa*)
Black walnut (*Juglans nigra*)
Green tea (*Camellia* spp.)
Guarana (*Paullinia cupana*)
Horse chestnut (*Aesculus hippocastanum*)
Maté (*Ilex paraguariensis*)
Raspberry leaf (*Rubus idaeus*)
Rhubarb (*Rheum palmatum*)
Sheep sorrel (*Rumex* spp.)
Uva ursi (*Arctostaphylos uva-ursi*)
White oak (*Quercus* spp.)
Willow (*Salix* spp.)
Witch hazel (*Hamamelis virginiana*)
Yellow dock (*Rumex crispus*)

---

of anesthesia. The American Society of Anesthesiologists (http://www.asahq.org/.../patient-brochures/asa_supplements-anesthesia_final/en/2) recommends that patients stop taking herbal supplements 2 weeks before surgery because they may affect anesthesia and bleeding times and cause dangerous fluctuations in blood pressure. If there is not enough time before surgery to stop, patients are recommended to bring the products to their primary care physician so an assessment of any danger can be made.

Use of Herbs in Pregnancy and Lactation

There are many conditions associated with pregnancy for which expectant mothers seek natural therapies, sometimes in the hopes of avoiding what they perceive to be more toxic conventional medications. Such conditions include morning sickness, threatened miscarriage, vaginal infections, anemia, varicose veins, hemorrhoids, depression, anxiety, and sleeplessness. One survey of emergency room visits reported that 14.5% of women used herbal remedies during pregnancy.[46] In addition to unsupervised herb use by consumers, approximately 50% of midwives and naturopathic physicians routinely prescribe herbal medicines during pregnancy, including a prominent use of botanicals such as black and blue cohosh (*Actaea racemosa, Caulophyllum thalictroides*), castor oil (*Ricinus communis*), and evening primrose oil (*Oenothera biennis*) for inducing labor. Considering whether to use an herbal medicine during pregnancy requires skill and sound judgment on the part of the practitioner, or in the case of self-medication, careful consideration on the part of the consuming woman. Minimally, the relative health of the expectant mother, the indication, and the appropriateness or inappropriateness of other medications or therapies must be considered. Ultimately, with herbal medicines, the choice of medications should be made by the expectant mother with full knowledge of the potential consequences. There are also significant legal liabilities that are incurred when using herbs in pregnancy. A list of botanicals that should not be used in pregnancy except under the care of a qualified health care professional is provided in Chapter 15, where the special considerations of herb safety during pregnancy are extensively addressed.

THE RELATIVE SAFETY OF CONVENTIONAL DRUGS AND HERBAL MEDICINES: KEEPING IT ALL IN PERSPECTIVE

When assessing the safety of herbal medicines, it is important to remain cognizant of the relative risks associated with approved medications, used singly and in combination with other agents. It is a common misconception that because a medication is FDA approved it is safe when used as indicated. In 1990 the United States GAO reviewed 198 FDA–approved drugs and reported that of these, approximately 102 (51.5%) had serious postapproval side effects. These included anaphylaxis, cardiac failure, hepatic and renal failure, birth defects, blindness, and death.[47] At the time of the report, all but two of the medications remained on the market. One study reported that among 1000 older adult patients admitted to the hospital from the emergency room, 538 were exposed to 1087 drug–drug interactions.[48] In a review of hospital surveillance reports of adverse events associated with approved medications, Lazarou and colleagues reported that 2,216,000 patients experienced serious adverse effects resulting in 60,000 to 140,000 fatalities annually as a result of the correct use of conventional drugs.[49] Not included in this figure were deaths caused by misuse of medications (e.g., improper prescribing, dosing, combining), which accounts for another 200,000 patients annually.

These figures make adverse events caused by approved conventional medications one of the leading causes of death in the United States—almost as many as are associated with smoking, and more than those related to alcohol, recreational drugs, and firearms. Additionally, adverse events associated with conventional drugs have been reported to be the number one cause of hospital admissions (at a cost of $116 million annually), and once in the hospital, approximately 35% of patients are likely to experience an additional ADR. In total, this represents estimated extra health care costs of $77 billion annually (2010 numbers).[50-51] reported 4.3 million adverse drug events in 2001, showing an upward trend from 1995 to 2001. A 2008 memo of the European Commission shows that dangers associated with pharmaceutical medications are not isolated to the US. In acknowledging the need for legislative changes to improve drug safety, the European Commission estimated that 5% of all hospital admissions in the EU are caused by an ADR, that ADRs are the fifth most common cause of hospital death, and that ADRs are responsible for approximately 197,000 deaths annually. In reporting on the prevalence of adverse effects caused by conventional medications, the US Department of Health and Human Services (CDC), which oversees the FDA, stated: "The United States is in the midst of an unprecedented drug overdose epidemic. Drug overdose death rates have increased five-fold since 1980." a phenomenon that has been widely observed and discussed in medical journals worldwide.

With this perspective in mind, it may be advantageous for practitioners to counsel patients about the potential benefits of herbal medicines as a means of reducing the high propensity for adverse events caused by conventional medications.

Such a belief is reflected in the experience of numerous integrative medical practitioners, conventionally trained physicians who gain further training in various aspects of natural medicine. According to David Rakel, one leading CAM practitioner, "Although it's important to be aware of drug–herb interactions, we need to be less concerned about them than about interactions between prescribed drugs. Drug–herb interactions are generally much less severe than drug–drug interactions."[53] Samuel D. Benjamin, Director of the Center for Complementary and Alternative Medicine and Associate Professor of Pediatrics and Family Medicine at the State University of New York, Stony Brook, stated that "The overwhelming majority of interactions are not related to the use of herbals. Drug–herb interactions don't compare to drug–drug interactions. Herbals are less toxic than pharmaceuticals."[53] According to medical researcher

Adriane Fugh-Berman, Assistant Clinical Professor of Health Care Sciences at George Washington University School of Medicine and Health Sciences, drug–drug "interactions kill people every day. What I have been really trying to convey to people . . . is that drug interactions are much more common and severe than drug–herb interactions. As clinicians we should be alert to both types but take pains to keep drug–herb interactions in context."[53]

GUIDELINES FOR PRACTITIONERS

Emergency Room Personnel

Emergency room attendants should be aware of the conditions they are most likely to encounter in patients who have reported a reaction thought to be correlated with consumption of an herbal product. These include the following:

- *Allergic reactions:* Any therapy can elicit allergic reactions in any individual in an unanticipated manner. Most specifically, anaphylaxis, angioedema, bronchospasm, contact dermatitis, and urticaria may occur. Cross-reactivity may occur with substances known to commonly cause allergic reactions such as ragweed pollen. Although rare, such reports have been made in those consuming plants of the ragweed family.
- *Skin rash:* There are numerous reasons for skin rashes to be caused by herbal products, including allergic reactions (e.g., ragweed family or iodine-containing plants in those sensitive to these agents), photosensitizing agents (e.g., St. John's wort, rue, psoralen-containing herbs such as some angelica species and lomatium *[Lomatium dissectum]*), or topical irritants (e.g., garlic, mustard, and poke root plasters; most essential oils).
- *Elevated liver enzymes:* This is one of the more common adverse effects caused by herbal products. Those most associated with this reaction include: direct hepatotoxins such as PA-containing herbs; botanical preparations with added pharmaceuticals; potentiation of hepatotoxic pharmaceuticals or other product adulterations; and idiosyncratic reactions.
- *Hypertension/hypokalemia:* Herbal stimulants, including cola nut, caffeine, guarana, and most commonly, ephedra (now banned in the US), can exacerbate already existing hypertension. Licorice has been reported to cause severe hypokalemia-induced hypertension at doses of up to 100 g daily. This reaction has only been reported rarely with licorice root and mostly with licorice candy, which is typically prepared with anise. There is, however, one case report of low-dose licorice root intake as part of a laxative tea causing hypokalemia. This may have been a result of the fluid loss owing to the laxative more than the physiologic effect of licorice. Asian ginseng *(Panax ginseng)* may exacerbate already existing hypertension. Yohimbe has been associated with hypertensive effects.
- *Mouth ulcers:* These can be caused by herbs rich in sesquiterpene lactones, such as feverfew *(Tanacetum parthenium)* and Missouri snake root *(Parthenium integrifolium)*.

- *Hemorrhagic events:* A number of botanicals have the potential to contribute to bleeding events, though the literature does not support an association for all of these (e.g., ginkgo). Case reports of subconjunctival hemorrhage, subdural hematomas, potentiation of bleeding effects of aspirin, and postsurgical bleeding complications have been associated with ginkgo *(Ginkgo biloba),* garlic *(Allium sativum),* and dong quai *(Angelica sinensis).* Bleeding abnormalities may occur with members of the legume family such as alfalfa or red clover, which contain coumarins. However, fermentation of these herbs is required to develop active coumarins. Such events have been reported for red clover. Feverfew may interfere with blood coagulation.
- *Exacerbation of gastroesophageal reflux disease (GERD):* There have been rare reports of peppermint *(Mentha piperita)* exacerbating GERD symptoms. It conversely is used to treat digestive upset.
- *Palpitations, cardiac arrhythmias, and tachycardia:* Sympathomimetic agents and central nervous stimulants commonly affect cardiac rhythm. Botanicals associated with such effects include: cola nut *(Cola nictida),* guarana *(Paullinia cupana),* lobelia *(Lobelia inflata),* and ma huang *(Ephedra sinensis).* Excessive intake of licorice candy (typically prepared from anise) may result in pseudoprimary aldosteronism with edema, hypertension, and hypokalemia. One case of near-fatal cardiac arrest has been reported. Excessive use of laxatives, which can cause fluid loss, has resulted in fatalities. Yohimbe has been associated with tachycardia.
- *Threatened miscarriage/abortion:* There have been a number of cases of attempted abortions using botanicals. Those most widely used include: black cohosh *(Actaea racemosa),* blue cohosh *(Caulophyllum thalictroides),* and pennyroyal *(Mentha pulegium)* oil.

Oncologists

Use of herbal medicines is prevalent among cancer patients, including in pediatric care, where up to 84% of children with cancer are using some form of CAM therapy[54] compared with up to 80% of adults with cancer. The seriousness of the disease leads patients to seek a variety of therapies regardless of the level of evidence supporting their use. Unfortunately, there are few well-designed trials examining the usefulness of botanical supplements for the direct treatment of cancer or in conjunction with conventional therapies, and what information exists is conflicting. Most commonly used are herbal therapies to enhance immune function, directly combat cancer, and yet others to provide palliative relief from side effects associated with conventional cancer therapies. There are two primary safety considerations regarding botanical therapies in cancer: (1) ensuring that potentially ineffective therapies are not substituted for potentially effective conventional therapies, and (2) making sure that botanical therapies do not lessen the effects of conventional therapies. Most of the published data, however, show there is no lessening of efficacy of chemotherapeutic drugs and does demonstrate decreased side effects of chemotherapy

and radiation; thus some experts here and abroad suggest that immune-supportive therapies should be standard of care.

Among the most common herbs used to counter the immunosuppressive effects of chemotherapeutic drugs are: reishi mushroom *(Ganoderma lucidum),* turkey tail *(Trametes versicolor),* astragalus *(Astragalus membranaceus),* maitake mushroom *(Grifola frondosa),* evening primrose oil *(Oenothera biennis),* green tea *(Camellia sinensis),* mistletoe *(Viscum album),* shiitake mushroom *(Lentinula edodes),* garlic, turmeric *(Curcuma longa),* and ginseng. There are a plethora of human and preclinical data demonstrating the potential for benefit of these in conjunction with conventional cancer therapies. The immunomodulating mushrooms, for example, contain a broad spectrum of compounds with demonstrable preclinical antitumor activity and some clinical data showing positive effects on preserving or restoring immunocompetency during and after chemotherapy. Actions associated with numerous compounds within botanicals include antiinflammatory, immunomodulating, and cytotoxic effects, tubulin-binding agents, topoisomerase inhibitors, phytoestrogens, and direct anticarcinogenic effects.[55] One meta-analysis of the use of astragalus in conjunction with conventional platinum-based chemotherapy for advanced non–small-cell lung carcinoma suggested increased efficacy over chemotherapy alone. Most notably, in some of the studies reported, the addition of astragalus to the chemotherapy protocol resulted in a significant reduction of death at 12 and 24 months and reduction of chemotherapy toxicity, and enhanced chemotherapy efficacy.[56]

In a phase I clinical trial of women with breast cancer, women treated with turkey tail mushrooms trended toward increased lymphocyte counts, increased natural killer cell function activity, and dose-related increases in CD8+ T cells and CD19+ B cells. According to a review of botanical medicine and cancer, Boon and Wong (2004) state that current evidence suggests that soy, tomatoes, ginseng, garlic, and green tea have cancer preventive properties and that ginger may be effective to allay chemotherapy-induced nausea and vomiting; they further report on the potential of numerous other botanicals to reduce side effects associated with chemotherapy.[57]

In another similar review, Olaku and White (2011) report on a number of clinical cases with botanicals that report lowering of prostate-specific antigen and tumor markers and partial and complete regressions of tumors, as well as documenting adverse effects of some botanicals in cancer care.[58]

Although there are methodological limitations to most of these studies, nevertheless they show significant potential for benefit and a low risk of adverse effects or negative interactions with conventional therapies.

Other herbal therapies believed to help treat cancers directly include the Hoxsey formula and Essiac, both multi-ingredient formulae for which there are little clinical data but are widely used.

Botanicals That Should Only Be Used by Qualified Health Professionals

The majority of botanicals that have remained on the commercial market have persisted because of their relatively high degree of safety when used by consumers without the guidance of a health professional. Most do not present a significant enough health risk to warrant prescription-only status. However, historically, relatively toxic botanicals (e.g., aconite, digitalis, gelsemium) have been used by medical herbalists. Most of these have not remained in the commercial market as dietary supplements. The use of such toxic herbs should be limited to well-trained medical herbalists.[59] Recommendations regarding the use of botanicals that should only be used by skilled individuals can be found in the *BSH*.

CONCLUSION

With the increasing prevalence of the use of herbal products, and the fact that many consumers and patients are using herbal products in conjunction with conventional medications, it is becoming increasingly important for health care providers to be aware of potential adverse effects and interactions. Based on a review of the world's data, adverse effects caused by herbal medicine are relatively rare. A number of botanicals have compared favorably in clinical trials with conventional medications for the same indications, and a critical review of the literature demonstrates a remarkable safety record. For example, ginkgo (*Ginkgo biloba*) has been shown to be similarly effective to conventional nosotropics and better tolerated; whereas contrary to inaccurate media reporting, St. John's wort (*Hypericum perforatum*) has been shown to be equal to or more efficacious than standard antidepressant medications but with approximately half the rate of adverse events.[60-62] Another herb, kava kava (*Piper methysticum*), has demonstrated efficacy equal to many standard anxiolytics, with greater safety than the commonly prescribed benzodiazepines.[63]

Conversely, there are a number of safety concerns about which practitioners must remain aware. These include potentiating or antagonistic effects of herb–drug interactions (especially potential anticoagulant effects), some of which are predictable, although others are not; potential contaminations and adulterations of herbal products; and the potential for patients to forgo effective therapies. A review of the literature clearly shows that adverse effects caused by herb–drug interactions are the most common concern but, according to numerous experts, are far less significant than drug-drug interactions. Understanding the in vivo pharmacologic effects of botanical medicines can help to increase the predictability of potential interactions. There are increasing resources designed for health care providers, including textbooks, online databases, and training programs. Additionally, the majority of medical schools now offer some level of training in CAM therapies, which include some review of herbal product use. As use of herbal medicines grows, practitioners will be forced to obtain some level of education regarding their appropriate use. For many integrative medical practitioners, that time has already arrived, and this will lead to a greater understanding of how botanicals can best be used in conjunction with conventional medications, and therefore, how best to serve the patient.

INTEGRATING BOTANICAL MEDICINES INTO CLINICAL PRACTICE: ETHICAL CONSIDERATIONS AND GUIDELINES

There is a growing recognition by conventional medicine practitioners that botanical medicines possess therapeutic value, often with a high safety profile, and that they may be a reasonable addition to the options available to patients before starting or along with accepted pharmaceuticals. The need for alternatives becomes more acute as we recognize that many of our most trusted remedies—from acetaminophen to statins—carry sometimes as many risks as benefits.

However, many health professionals face the ethical dilemma of whether, and to what extent, to integrate herbal medicines into their practices; how much to support patient use; the challenge of learning which products are efficacious and safe; and when to be concerned about herb-drug interactions. Thus they are reasonably reluctant to integrate herbal medicines into their practices.[64] Most lack adequate training in botanical medicine use unless specifically trained in integrative medicine with an emphasis on botanicals.

Lack of knowledge of how to apply herbal therapies not only prevents practitioners from using valuable medical options; hesitation about or frank disapproval of them has been demonstrated to reduce patient disclosure of use to their primary care practitioners. Thus this behavior prevents practitioners from serving as effective advisors and advocates for their patients regarding safe and effective herb use and the avoidance of potential herb–drug interactions.[9]

ADDRESSING ETHICAL CONSIDERATIONS

Jeremy Sugarman, in the *JAMA* article, Physicians' ethical obligations regarding alternative medicine, suggests that physicians facing ethical dilemmas about integrating CAM into their practices, or at least trying to decide how to address CAM use by patients, consider applying a "set of inherent ethical principles of the medical profession: respect for persons, nonmaleficence, beneficence, and justice" into their decision-making process.[65] These principles, are well known to physicians:

1. *Respect for persons,* also referred to as *autonomy,* implies respecting the patient's personal preferences, including the right to "reject unwanted interventions and to make choices that are consonant with their values."[65] Implicit in respect for autonomy is informed consent and shared decision making—also a cornerstone of integrative medicine and CAM practices.

2. *Nonmaleficence* means not harming patients in the provision of medical care. In relationship to CAM, it becomes incumbent on the practitioner to elicit comprehensive information about the patient's CAM use to prevent harmful interactions between conventional and alternative therapies and to alert the patient to concerns the practitioner might have about a treatment.[4,65]

3. *Beneficence* suggests that patients have the right to effective interventions. Thus if effective CAM therapies exist,

patients have the right to be informed of them and practitioners have some "limited obligation . . . to make patients aware of safe and effective alternative medicine modalities."[65] This is, of course, limited by the availability and dependability of such information, as well as by the realistic time constraints that prevent practitioners from becoming fully knowledgeable about the range of therapies that exists. However, it is the responsibility of practitioners choosing to use CAM therapies to be adequately knowledgeable about those therapies. Further, referral and consultation is appropriate if the patient will benefit and the referral is to a qualified practitioner.

4. *Justice* refers to equity in health care—meaning that patients should have "fair access to alternative therapies that are known to be safe, effective, and appropriate for their conditions."

GUIDELINES

Once practitioners have recognized that their patients have an ethical right to information on the safe and effective use of botanical therapies, or possibly even botanical products, how are they to advise patients about them? Wayne Jonas suggests that health practitioners follow a simple set of practical rules he calls the "four Ps": protect, permit, promote, and partner.[66] He defines these as follows:

- *Protect:* Determine whether the product or procedure is safe, low-cost, and nontoxic.
- *Permit:* Support the use of those therapies that are safe and affordable, even if they have not been definitely proved. Jonas suggests that such therapies may "empower the patient and enhance nonspecific effects" (i.e., placebo effect).
- *Promote:* Encourage the use of proven practices, in some way making them safely available to patients.
- *Partner:* Respect your patient's right to self-determination and work in partnership with the patient and her or his complementary medicine provider. Be actively engaged in gathering and assessing information that will allow you to make professional recommendations to your patient.

Karen Adams, in *Ethical Considerations of Complementary and Alternative Medical Therapies in Conventional Medical Settings*, suggests consideration be given to the following: (1) whether evidence supports both safety and efficacy; (2) whether evidence supports safety but is inconclusive about efficacy; (3) whether evidence supports efficacy but is inconclusive about safety; or (4) whether evidence indicates either serious risk or inefficacy.[64] She advises the following steps as guidelines:

If evidence supports both safety and efficacy, the physician should recommend the therapy but continue to monitor the patients conventionally. If evidence supports safety but is inconclusive about efficacy, the treatment should be tolerated and monitored for effectiveness.

BOX 4-7   Factors in Risk–Benefit Analysis of Complementary and Alternative Treatments versus Conventional Medical Treatment

- Severity and acuteness of illness
- Curability with conventional treatment
- Degree of invasiveness, associated toxicities, and side effects of conventional treatment
- Quality of evidence and efficacy of the desired complementary and alternative medicine (CAM) treatment
- Degree of understanding of the risks and benefits of the CAM treatment
- Knowledge and voluntary acceptance of those risks by the patient
- Persistence of the patient's intention to use the CAM treatment

From Adams K, Cohen M, Eisenberg D, et al: Ethical considerations of complementary and alternative medical therapies in conventional medical settings, *Ann Int Med* 137(8):660–664, 2002.

If evidence supports efficacy but is inconclusive about safety, the therapy still could be tolerated and monitored closely for safety. Finally, therapies for which evidence indicates either serious risk or inefficacy obviously should be avoided and patients actively discouraged from pursuing such a course of treatment.[64]

The risk–benefit analysis shown in Box 4-7 should be considered when there is insufficient evidence for or against a particular treatment.

There are numerous medical practices that were once considered fringe, such as biofeedback, that are now a routine part of conventional medicine. As practitioners gain increased experience and confidence with a modality, and as both clinical and pharmacologic studies are done that continue to demonstrate the safety and efficacy of the modality, the less fringe a practice seems. Botanical medicines have always been part of human and medical history; their use should not seem entirely foreign today.

Another algorithm to follow when considering whether to recommend or endorse the use of botanical medicines or other integrative therapies was established by Kathi Kemper, MD and Michael Cohen, JD. Figure 4-1 reflects the principles set out by Karen Adams to assess safety and efficacy.

SELECTING AND IDENTIFYING QUALITY HERBAL PRODUCTS

The quality, therapeutic efficacy, and safety of botanical products are of concern to practitioners, manufacturers, regulators, and consumers alike. This section is a primer on the standards practitioners may want to look for when selecting

---

The editor wishes to thank Roy Upton for his contributions to the discussion on GMPs in this chapter.

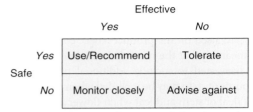

	Effective	
	Yes	*No*
Safe *Yes*	Use/Recommend	Tolerate
No	Monitor closely	Advise against

FIGURE 4-1 Ethical framework for therapies.

botanical medicine products. The section focuses on the characteristics of quality botanical products, the issue of phytoequivalence, and recommendations for selecting products.

REGULATIONS GOVERNING BOTANICAL PRODUCTS

It is frequently asserted in the media and among critics of dietary supplements that botanical dietary supplement products in the United States are not subject to any regulatory standards. This is inaccurate. The Dietary Supplement Health and Education Act (DSHEA) of 1994 defines dietary supplements and dietary ingredients, establishes a framework for product safety, outlines guidelines for literature displayed where supplements are sold, provides for use of claims and nutritional support statements, requires ingredient and nutrition labeling, and grants the FDA the authority to establish GMP regulations beyond those for food, which already apply to this class of goods.[67]

In 2007, the FDA issued GMPs for dietary supplements, a set of requirements and expectations by which dietary supplements must be manufactured, prepared, and stored to ensure quality. Manufacturers are expected to guarantee the identity, purity, strength, and composition of their dietary supplements, as well as set limits on contamination. In addition, all supplement products are required by law to provide certain information about their formulation.[68] Any supplement that does not conform to these basic guidelines is subject to regulatory action by the FDA.[5]

MANUFACTURING QUALITY BOTANICAL PRODUCTS

Ultimately, the quality of the starting materials is essential to the quality of any product, as is the proper preparation/manufacture of each ingredient in a product. A number of manufacturing steps can maximize the quality, safety, and efficacy of botanical products, including:
- Proper identification
- Proper harvest times and collection practices
- Use of proper plant part
- Analysis of purity
- Organoleptic analysis
- Chemical assay when appropriate
- GMPs
- Proper preparation
- Proper drying conditions if using dried herbs

- Proper labeling and marketing
- Appropriate enforcement FDA/Federal Trade Commission (FTC)

Batch-to-batch consistency is an important measure of a product's quality, and perhaps one of the most clinically significant aspects of a product. Thus practitioners will want to purchase from companies that have internal standards that allow them to guarantee a consistent product over time (Box 4-8).

Proper Identification

Proper identification is essential to product safety and efficacy. Identity testing can include organoleptic analysis and chemical assay. With whole plant material, organoleptic analysis can often be adequate for identification; however, with powdered herbs, microscopy can be very useful in plant identification, and chemical assays can be necessary because identification of material can be more difficult when the whole herb form is no longer available.

The plant should be identified in the field by the harvester and checked in the manufacturing facility to ensure there has been no mislabeling of the herb between harvest and delivery to the manufacturer. Misidentification (not to mention substitution, contamination, and adulteration) can lead to hazardous consequences for the consumer should a toxic or contraindicated herb replace the desired herb. The classic case illustrating problems with identification is that of a pregnant woman who was unknowingly consuming an herb called *Periploca sepium* in place of *Eleutherococcus senticosus* throughout her pregnancy because of the misidentification or adulteration of a product; her baby suffered from androgenization.[69]

Regulations require that any named ingredient on dietary supplement packaging be accurately labeled, which means that product marketers must have a scientifically valid means for determining identity. The final rule requires the manufacturer to perform "at least one appropriate test or examination to verify the identity of any component that is a dietary ingredient" and for finished products, "appropriate tests or examinations . . . [on] a subset of finished dietary supplement batches that you identify through a sound statistical sampling plan (or for every finished batch) . . . to determine compliance with . . . one or more established specifications . . . that, if tested or examined on the finished batches of the dietary supplement, would verify that the production and process control system is producing a dietary supplement that meets all product specifications." This basically means that finished products need to be tested to make sure they are in conformity with what is said on the packaging.

In much of the industry, QC personnel rely solely on an affidavit from the ingredient supplier as to the identity of the ingredient. This is conveyed via a document known as a certificate of analysis (COA). Oftentimes, a COA provides no more information than "green powder" to describe the ingredient and "conforms" to describe the test that was performed to determine identity. This is completely insufficient for making a determination of identity. One key component of this regulation is that manufacturers cannot rely on a COA for determining identity, but rather must perform at least one specific identity test.

Harvest Times and Collection Practices

Plant constituent profiles are not static; rather, the concentrations of individual constituents have peaks and nadirs at various times, both seasonally and even daily. Harvesting herbs with an understanding of their optimal harvest times can improve the quality of individual herbs for their optimal medicinal activity. Contemporary agricultural, analytical-chemical, and traditional guidelines may be used to determine proper harvest times and practices for various herbs. Manufacturers producing quality herbal products start with raw materials that were properly harvested to preserve the desired properties and hence the desired chemical profile.

Plant Part

The chemical profile of an herb also varies greatly within the plant itself; the roots, stems, leaves, flowers, fruits, and seeds usually contain different constituents or the same ones in different amounts, which results in different biological activities. The root of dandelion, for example, is a bitter tonic and gentle laxative, whereas the leaf of dandelion is a powerful diuretic. The flowering tops of St. John's wort contain much higher quantities of the constituents believed responsible for the herb's antidepressant activity, whereas the leaves and stems possess much lower amounts; thus a more active medicine is produced by manufacturers harvesting the uppermost flowering parts rather than the entire above-ground portion. Most herb books name the medicinal part of the plant, making it easy for the practitioner to identify whether they should be using root, leaf, or another part.

However, not all manufacturers strictly include just the medicinal plant part (although by law they are required to state the plant part used on the product label); costs of buying often dictates, meaning that the most desired plant part may be haphazardly harvested to include additional parts. For example, large amounts of stem may be included when only leaf is desired, or a great deal of stem and leaf when flower is desired. This can be nearly impossible to detect in powdered or extracted products (although it is often obvious with bulk whole herb); thus it is important to question manufacturers about their practices, which can include strict specifications for the plant part used and acceptable amounts of foreign matter (i.e., undesired other plant parts). They may even be able to specify which pharmacopeial monograph, if any, applies to their product.

Purity

The *purity* of a dietary supplement refers to that portion or percentage of a dietary supplement that represents the intended product.

Strength

The strength of a dietary supplement relates to its concentration (for example, weight/weight, weight/volume, or volume/volume).

Composition

A dietary supplement's *composition* refers to the specified mix of product and product-related substances in a dietary supplement. Under current rules, ingredients must be listed in order of predominance.

Limits on Contaminants

Dietary supplement products, like conventional foods, must be free of pathogenic microbes. AHPA recommends specific maximum-tolerated levels for dried raw agricultural commodities, including cut and powdered commodities, that are used as botanical ingredients in dietary supplements and that are subject to further processing, as follows[68]:

- *Total aerobic plate count:* 10^7 colony-forming units/gram
- *Total yeasts and molds:* 10^5 colony-forming units/gram
- *Total coliforms:* 10^4 colony-forming units/gram
- *Salmonella:* absent in 10 grams
- *Escherichia coli:* not detected in one gram
- *Aflatoxins B_1, B_2, G_1, and G_2:* 20 µg/kg (parts per billion [ppb])
- *Aflatoxin B_1:* 5 µg/kg (ppb)

Practitioners may want to inquire as to whether a manufacturer uses irradiation as a technique to reduce microbial count because this is a common practice that has no federal allowance for most herbs.

Labeling

Supplement labels must provide consumers with nutritional information. Unlike foods, supplements must state the quantity of each of the contained ingredients (except for "proprietary blends") that make up a product. All herbal products are required to identify the parts of each plant ingredient used, and label them with their accepted common names. The FDA specifies exactly what kind of claims are allowed on product labels and prohibits the use of any statement that would brand the product as a drug. Herbal supplements are not allowed to make statements regarding prevention, cure, mitigation, or treatment of diseases. Instead, their claims are limited to statements that are legally defined as "statements of nutritional support" that include "structure/function statements."[68]

To Learn More About Botanical Product Regulations

For those who wish to learn more about the regulations governing dietary supplement in the US, visit the FDA web site at www.fda.gov. The National Institutes of Health Office of Dietary Supplements also provides a wealth of information about specific dietary supplements, as well as more global issues at http://dietary-supplements.info.nih.gov. For those wishing to study herbal products in clinical trials, visit the National Center for Complementary and Integrative Health (NCCIH) at www.nih.gov/about/almanac/organization/NCCIH.htm. The FTC guidelines for claims substantiation can be found at www.ftc.gov.

ETHICAL CONSIDERATIONS

Sustainability

Sustainability is of key importance to the survival of many important botanical medicine species, some of which have been lost historically because of overuse, such as the once relied-upon sedative lady's slipper (Cypripedium pubescens), the gynecologic remedy false unicorn (Chamaelirium luteum), or the antimicrobial herb goldenseal (Hydrastis canadensis). Herbalists should prioritize sustainability in attention to harvesting, cultivation, and choice of plants prescribed in the clinic; regularly inform their patients of the need for sustainability; and be highly knowledgeable about sustainable alternatives to at-risk and endangered species. Thus the sustainability of herbs is also an important factor in selecting herbal products. Practitioners can become informed about which herbs are endangered and make efforts to use only those herbs that are cultivated if on an endangered list, or use alternatives to those herbs.

Efficacy

Product efficacy can be determined by clinical observation, patient reporting, clinical trials, or a combination of these. Practitioner observation and patient reporting are subject to a host of biases; however, the collective clinical knowledge of herbal practitioners is an important and valuable source of information. Though rigorous clinical testing of botanicals remains limited compared with the vast potential pharmacopoeia available to us, quite a number of herbs have now been found to be tremendously efficacious for a range of conditions and symptoms. However, lack of clinical trials does not mean a botanical medicine is inefficacious, and presence of a clinical trial does not mean that the same herb will perform identically when not manufactured to the exact specifications and given in a different dosage.

In countries such as the United Kingdom, Canada, and Australia that have Traditional Medicines categories as part of the governmental regulatory framework for botanical medicines, efficacy is determined by a combination of factors, including historical use, traditional use, contemporary clinical use within a given period of time (e.g., the past 15 to 30 years), and scientific evaluation (e.g., clinical trials). Increasingly, there are companies that offer professional lines of products that are aware of the unique needs and concerns of botanical practitioners.

Helping Patients to Select Quality Products

Perhaps one of the most challenging areas of botanical medicine practice is knowing which companies and products are reliable. Several independent organizations offer quality testing and allow products that pass these tests to display their seals of approval. These seals of approval provide assurance that the product was properly manufactured, contains the ingredients listed on the label, and does not contain harmful levels of contaminants. These seals of approval do not guarantee that a product is safe or effective. Organizations that offer this quality testing include:

U.S. Pharmacopeia
ConsumerLab.com
NSF International

However, this testing can be costly, prohibiting some reputable companies from participating; additionally, questions have been raised as to whether these companies are performing the proper tests to assess product ingredients. For example, consider the use of DNA barcoding by the New York State Attorney General's office in an attempt to discredit herbal products, when this form of analysis is an inappropriate method for proper plant ingredient identification in the herbal products that were investigated.[70]

The Role of the Herbalist in the Botanical Products Industry

Skilled herbalists with combined training in botany, organoleptic and macroscopic plant identification, product formulation, and clinical practice, can offer unique insights regarding product quality, efficacy, and strength to today's herbal industry. Perhaps the most illustrative example of this occurred a number of years ago when a large batch of plantains distributed to United States botanical products manufacturers was contaminated with digitalis. Several consumers were poisoned by this adulterated product. However, because of the identification skills of an herbalist employed by one of the companies that received the bad shipment, this company rejected the batch and therefore did not distribute harmful product.

Programs such as Bastyr University's bachelor of science in botanical medicine are attempting to train herbalists to work in industry. Herbalists and herbalist-manufacturers, those botanical manufacturing companies run by herbalists, approach issues of product quality and efficacy informed by an amalgamation of information drawn from traditional practices, observation of therapeutic response, experiential knowledge of the plants, and contemporary scientific studies. This synthesis of knowledge may represent a significant contribution to the conversation on medicinal plant product standards. Cooperation between scientific researchers and botanical practitioners/small manufacturers may present novel approaches to understanding optimal conditions for growing, harvesting, preparing, storing, and delivering medicinal plant products.

Endocrine Disorders and Adrenal Support

HYPOTHYROIDISM AND HYPERTHYROIDISM

Untreated and undertreated thyroid disorders can exact pronounced consequences on health and quality of life.[1,2] Thyroid dysfunction in women can alter weight, mood, cognition, sleep, and menstrual regularity; it also affects reproduction, leading to infertility and miscarriage. Children born to women with untreated thyroid disorders during pregnancy can experience long-term consequences, including permanent cognitive developmental delays.[3-7]

Long-term, untreated thyroid conditions in adult women significantly increase the risk of cardiovascular disease, osteoporosis, reproductive cancer, and multisystem failure. Approximately 5% of Americans report having thyroid disease or taking thyroid medication, and numerous individuals have undiagnosed thyroid disorders.[2] The most common thyroid disorders are hypothyroidism, both clinical and subclinical, and hyperthyroidism. Detection and treatment of most thyroid disorders is straightforward and can prevent long-term and potentially disastrous sequelae that may occur in the absence of appropriate care.

HYPOTHYROIDISM

Hypothyroidism is persistent insufficiency of either thyroid hormone production or receptor sensitivity to thyroid hormone, leading to a generalized decrease in numerous metabolic functions (Box 5-1). It is the most prevalent of the pathologic hormone deficiencies, and can reduce physical and mental functional ability, quality of life, and long-term health.[2,8] Hypothyroidism is classified on the basis of onset (congenital or acquired), endocrine dysfunction level (primary, secondary, or tertiary), and severity, which is classified as overt (clinical) or mild (subclinical) hypothyroidism.[8] The total frequency of hypothyroidism, including subclinical cases, among adult females from all age groups ranges from 3% to 7.5%, with significantly higher rates in women older

than 60 years old.[1] Hypothyroidism occurs at a rate approximately 10 times higher in women than men, and some consider it to be widely underdiagnosed.[9-12]

Pathophysiology

Hypothyroidism is classified as primary, secondary, or tertiary. Primary hypothyroidism is significantly more common than secondary, occurring at a rate of approximately 1000:1; tertiary hypothyroidism, resulting from disease in the hypothalamus, is rare.[8,13] Myxoedema refers to severe or complicated cases of overt hypothyroidism with cretinism syndrome, and is extremely rare.[8]

Those at increased risk of developing hypothyroidism include[9]:

- Postpartum women
- Women with family history of autoimmune thyroid disorders (AITD)
- Those with previous head, neck, or thyroid surgery or irradiation
- Those with other autoimmune endocrine disorders (e.g., type 1 diabetes mellitus, adrenal insufficiency, ovarian failure)
- Those with nonendocrine autoimmune disorders (e.g., vitiligo, multiple sclerosis)
- Patients with primary pulmonary hypertension
- Those with Down's or Turner's syndromes

The following biological activities are particularly impaired by hypothyroidism[8]:

- Calorigenic modification
- Oxygen consumption throughout most tissues
- Protein, fat, and carbohydrate metabolism
- Augmentation of calcium adenosine triphosphatase (ATPase) activity in cardiac muscle
- Mitochondrial adenosine triphosphate (ATP) production
- G-protein–coupled membrane receptor activity
- Organ-specific effects

The editor wishes to thank *Botanical Medicine for Women's Health,* Edition 1 contributors Mary Bove and Jillian Stansbury for their original contributions to this section.

The editor wishes to thank *Botanical Medicine for Women's Health,* Edition 1 contributor Angela J. Hywood for her original contributions to this chapter.

BOX 5-1   Thyroid Hormone: a Review of Synthesis and Release

Iodide, which is primarily nutritionally derived is concentrated by the thyroid gland, converted to organic iodine by thyroid peroxidase (TPO), and then incorporated into tyrosine in thyroglobulin in the thyroid. Tyrosines are iodinated at one (i.e., monoiodotyrosine) or two (i.e., di-iodotyrosine) sites and then joined to form the hormones thyroxine (T4) and tri-iodothyronine (T3). Another source of T3 within the thyroid gland is the result of the outer ring deiodination of T4 by a selenium-based enzyme. T3 and T4 are cleaved from thyroglobulin by proteolytic lysosomes, resulting in the release of free T3 (FT3) and free T4 (FT4). The iodotyrosines (i.e., monoiodotyrosine and di-iodotyrosine) are also released from thyroglobulin, but little reaches the bloodstream.

The T4 and T3 released from the thyroid reach the bloodstream, where they are bound to thyroid hormone–binding serum proteins (primarily thyroxine-binding globulin [TBG] and transthyretin) for transport. About 0.03% of the total serum T4 and 0.3% of the total serum T3 are free and in equilibrium with the bound hormones, and only FT4 and FT3 are available to the peripheral tissues for thyroid hormone action. T3 is the metabolically active hormone.

Thyroid-stimulating hormone (TSH), or thyrotropin, controls all reactions necessary for the formation of T3 and T4 and is itself controlled by the pituitary gland through a negative feedback mechanism regulated by the circulating level of FT4 and FT3 and by conversion of T4 to T3 in the pituitary. Increased levels of free thyroid hormones inhibit TSH secretion from the pituitary, whereas levels of T4 and T3 result in an increased TSH release from the pituitary. TSH secretion is also influenced by thyrotropin-releasing hormone (TRH) synthesized in the hypothalamus.

The thyroid produces about 20% of the circulating T3. The remaining 80% is produced by peripheral conversion of T4, primarily in the liver. A variation of this process also may produce reverse T3 (rT3), which has minimal metabolic activity. rT3 levels increase in chronic liver and renal disease, acute and chronic illness, starvation, carbohydrate-deficient diets, and possibly during extreme or prolonged stress. These states result in decreased production of the active hormone, T3, and in increased serum rT3 levels because of decreased rT3 clearance. The decreased production of T3 might be an adaptive response to illness, and can be seen in hypothyroidism.

The clinical manifestations of hypothyroidism (see Signs and Symptoms) are the result of effects occurring at the molecular level because of the effect of thyroid hormone insufficiency.[8]

Primary Hypothyroidism

Primary hypothyroidism is the most common form of hypothyroid disorder. It may be either congenital or acquired. Globally, the most common cause of congenital hypothyroidism is endemic iodine deficiency; however, it may also result from thyroid gland agenesis, defective thyroid hormone biosynthesis, or rarely hemangiomas, which also may occur in young children.[8,9] (Congenital hypothyroidism is not discussed in the remainder of this section.)

The most common form of primary hypothyroidism in geographic areas of normal iodine intake is acquired primary hypothyroidism. It is most frequently a result of autoimmunity, in which case it is referred to as autoimmune thyroid disorder (AITD) or autoimmune thyroiditis (Hashimoto's disease).[1,7,8] Antibodies are formed that bind to the thyroid (specifically against the thyroid peroxidase [TPO] enzyme, thyroglobulin, and thyroid-stimulating hormone [TSH] receptors) and prevent the manufacture of sufficient levels of thyroid hormone. In addition to binding to thyroid tissue, these antibodies also may bind to the adrenal glands, pancreas, and parietal cells of the stomach.

Autoimmunity as an etiologic factor is supported by the presence of lymphatic infiltration of the thyroid gland and the presence of circulating thyroid autoantibodies in nearly all affected patients.[8] In fact, the most common risk factor for both hypothyroidism and hyperthyroidism is the presence of TPO autoantibodies.[1] Genetic predisposition (i.e., autosomal dominant inheritance) is a major factor in the etiology of AITD, accounting for as much as 79% of susceptibility to autoimmunity, though there appear to be significant hormonal and environmental factors contributing to manifestation of disease.[1,8] Autoimmune thyroiditis is increased in areas of high iodine intake, for example, in Iceland, suggesting an antigenic response.[1,8]

Recent evidence supports the belief that fluoride, including in normal amounts of exposure through fluoridated water, is involved in the etiology of Hashimoto's thyroiditis.[14,15]

Evidence also points to the role of celiac disease in Hashimoto's thyroiditis.[16,17]

Other causes of hypothyroidism include iatrogenesis secondary to radiation or medications that interfere with thyroid function, genetic defects of the T3 hormone receptors, and excessive consumption of goitrogens (i.e., substances that interfere with thyroid hormone production and release). Postpartum hypothyroidism is a transient form of hypothyroidism that affects 5% to 10% of postpartum women in the United States.[18] Transient hypothyroidism may occur secondary to subacute thyroiditis caused by infection. Primary hypothyroidism is often idiopathic, with no definable cause.[7]

The long-term consequences of untreated overt hypothyroidism are significant, and include elevated cholesterol and atherosclerosis, cardiac, renal, and neurologic diseases, increased susceptibility to infectious diseases, possibly increased rates of reproductive cancers, and ultimately, multiple organ failure if the disease progresses.[7,19,20] Hypothyroidism is readily detectable and treatable; therefore these consequences should be almost entirely avoidable with screening and early treatment.

Subclinical Hypothyroidism

Subclinical hypothyroidism refers to patients with primary hypothyroidism with normal serum free thyroxine (FT4) and elevated TSH.[2] These individuals may or may not be symptomatic. Dr. Low Dog suggests that *symptomatic euthyroid state* is a more appropriate label for these patients.[13]

The prevalence of subclinical hypothyroidism is highest in the United States among white women (5.8%), and is 5.3% and 1.2% among Hispanic American and African American women, respectively. Rates tend to increase significantly with age, reaching as high as 8% to 10% in women ages 45 to 74 years, and 17.4% in women older than 75 years of age.[21]

There is strong evidence from high-quality longitudinal studies that subclinical hypothyroidism places women at significant risk for the later development of overt hypothyroidism, yet it frequently goes undetected and untreated.[2] Untreated subclinical hypothyroidism can lead to daily interference with optimal physical, neurologic, psychological, and emotional functioning, and can cause a diminished quality of life. Controversy exists regarding the routine screening and treatment of subclinical hypothyroidism for all women, a practice that has not been well studied or determined to be conclusively beneficial.[7-9]

Its proponents argue that preventative treatment with T4 is relatively safe, effective, and inexpensive, and can prevent the development of overt hypothyroidism and its consequences.[7,8] Further, women who have been treated for subclinical hypothyroidism have retrospectively reported improvements in their physical and mental wellness.[7] Patients with subclinical hypothyroidism and abnormal lipid profiles may experience improvement within 1 month of T4 treatment.[7] Subtle and reversible changes in myocardial performance also have been reported in women with mild hypothyroidism.[8] Careful follow-up is essential, with periodic reevaluation of relevant laboratory markers and symptoms. Because of the frequency of hypothyroidism in older women, routine screening and treatment may be justified in this population. Routine screening also may be prudent during pregnancy because of the serious consequences of long-term cognitive dysfunction and decreased intelligence in the offspring of women with untreated prenatal hypothyroidism.[6]

Secondary Hypothyroidism

Secondary hypothyroidism can result from diseases that interfere with thyrotropin-releasing hormone (TRH) production by the hypothalamus, its delivery by the pituitary stalk, or with problems of pituitary thyrotropin production (e.g., pituitary adenomas, hypothalamic tumors, or their treatments such as surgery or radiation therapy). Head trauma, metastatic disease, and infection can also lead to secondary hypothyroidism.[8] Iatrogenic hypothyroidism is the second most common cause and is the result of radioactive iodine therapy or ablation treatment for Graves' disease and other forms of hyperthyroidism.

Signs and Symptoms

Any of the symptoms listed in Box 5-2 may be present in degrees ranging from mild (i.e., requiring careful discernment of the clinical picture) to severe. Hypothyroidism may also be asymptomatic, detectable only by laboratory screening. Hypothyroidism is commonly overlooked clinically because of the presence of these symptoms in any number of other diseases.

Diagnosis

Diagnosis of hypothyroidism should be sought on the basis of family history, clinical signs, age, and pregnancy status (because of risks for the fetus in cases of untreated maternal hypothyroidism). Diagnosis remains somewhat controversial because of variations in acceptable ranges of laboratory values among different labs and institutions. Because of this, thyroid dysfunction

---

BOX 5-2 Signs and Symptoms of Hypothyroidism

Ataxia
Bradycardia
Carpal tunnel syndrome
Cold intolerance
Constipation
Decreased energy
Decreased exercise tolerance
Delayed reflexes
Depression
Diastolic hypertension
Dry or brittle hair
Dry skin
Fatigue
Galactorrhea
Goiter
Hyperlipidemia
Infertility
Loss of libido
Low body temperature
Low-pitched or hoarse voice
Menstrual irregularities
Miscarriage
Muscle cramps
Muscle weakness
Periorbital edema
Poor memory
Psychomotor retardation
Slow speech
Somnolence
Water retention
Weight gain

TABLE 5-1 Biochemical Markers in Thyroid Dysfunction

Thyroid Disorder	TSH Level	Thyroid Hormone Level
Subclinical hypothyroidism	>0.5 - 3.0 mU/L	Low FT4
Overt hypothyroidism	>3 mU/L	Normal FT4
Overt hyperthyroidism	Low or undetectable	Elevated FT4 or FT3
Subclinical hyperthyroidism	Low or undetectable	Normal FT4 or FT3

Data from Wartofsky L, Dickey R A: The evidence for a narrower thyrotropin reference range is compelling. *J Clin Endocrinol Metab*, 90(9), 5483-5488, 2005. doi:10.1210/jc.2005-0455
TSH, Thyroid-stimulating hormone; *L*, liter; *FT4*, free thyroxine; *FT3*, free tri-iodothyronine.

---

in a patient who complains of symptoms but presents with "normal" laboratory values should not be disregarded.

TSH measurement is commonly accepted as the most significant and sensitive measurement for hypothyroidism diagnosis. Elevated TSH identifies patients with primary hypothyroidism regardless of the cause or severity.[8] Primary hypothyroidism presents with a low serum T4 with attendant elevation of serum TSH. Subclinical hypothyroidism is marked by normal serum T4 levels with slight to moderately increased

TSH levels and a normal FTI (Table 5-1). Laboratory tests are considered generally unnecessary to determine the underlying cause of primary hypothyroidism. Factors such as previous neck/thyroid irradiation or surgery, or other exposure to radiation (e.g., pharmaceutical exposure) postpartum status, or other known contributing factors is adequate. Autoimmune causes can be assumed on the basis of ruling out other possible etiologies.[8] An important note is that serum TSH levels may rise in the recovery phase of illness, mimicking values associated with hypothyroidism. Therefore measurement of TSH after complete recovery is appropriate. FT4 is required to give an accurate measurement of thyroid hormone activity, given that only 0.03% of total T4 hormone is unbound and reflects the thyroid hormone activity of T4. The remaining 99.97% of total T4 is bound to carrier proteins and is metabolically inactive. The FT4 or FTI in conjunction with a TSH can be used to categorize most cases of thyroid dysfunction. The exception occurs when FT4 remains normal but free tri-iodothyronine (FT3) is abnormal, as may occur when there is a deficient conversion of T4 to T3.

Measurement of T3 is controversial. The conventional medical belief is that normal serum T3 levels are maintained until severe hypothyroidism occurs. Recently, however, many physicians have begun to evaluate T3 as a part of thyroid screening. Many test T3 levels only when patients are unresponsive to treatment with T4. T3 levels can be decreased in primary and secondary hypothyroidism (serum thyroxine-binding globulin [TBG] is also decreased), by some medications, with low carbohydrate diets, and in euthyroid sick syndrome. Laboratory diagnosis of secondary hypothyroidism is marked by low T4 levels and low or normal TSH levels. Many patients need to have tests repeated several times to achieve an accurate and correct diagnosis.

Basal body temperature (BBT) testing has been suggested as a screening test for subclinical hypothyroidism. However, there are many factors other than thyroid hormones that affect BBT and thus by itself, low BBT is not a pathognomonic indicator of thyroid hormone status, although it does indicate lowered metabolic status.

Conventional Treatment

Treatment of hypothyroidism with thyroid extract has been practiced since 1891, when Murray first reported the use of sheep thyroid extract. Thyroid hormone was first crystallized in 1914, and initial testing with T4 began in 1927.[8] Exogenous thyroid hormone replacement remains the standard treatment, with T4 considered the treatment of choice based on its general efficacy and relatively small risk of adverse effects when given at the proper dose.[7,8] Conventional practice advocates the use of T4 alone over T3 and T4 combinations, the latter of which may provide T3 in excess of normal thyroid secretion.[7] However, many physicians find that the addition of T3 can be beneficial for patients not responding optimally to T4 alone.

Administration of thyroid replacement therapies should be carefully monitored because of the narrow toxic-to-therapeutic ratio of thyroid hormone, with the patient being maintained on the lowest possible effective dose, which will be individually determined. The typical required daily dose is 1.5 μg/lb body weight, with doses for older adults at approximately 70% of that required for younger women.[7] It has been estimated by some researchers that as many as 20% of hypothyroid patients are receiving excessive doses. Adverse reactions to T4 are usually related to excessive doses or increased thyroid hormone activity.[9] T3 supplementation may be implemented for patients unresponsive to T4 treatment alone.

No studies of controlled treatment of subclinical hypothyroidism have been conducted.[2]

Commonly used thyroid medications include:

- Synthetic preparations containing only T4
- Synthetic mixtures of T3 and T4 in similar ratios
- Synthetic T3 preparations
- Desiccated "natural" thyroid preparations (e.g., Armour thyroid): provide T4 and T3, plus amino acids and micronutrients. A popular criticism of natural thyroid preparations is that they lack consistency and reliability, and as stated, may provide T3 in excess.[7]

Botanical Treatment

Traditionally, hypothyroidism would have been recognized and treated by herbal practitioners on the basis of its presenting metabolic deficiency symptoms, rather than as a discrete disease entity. The botanical practitioner recognized the patient picture as one of overall depletion. Herbalists today also view hypothyroidism with the goal of improving overall metabolism and the general integrity of the endocrine system. Many consider primary thyroid dysfunction to be a treatable condition with herbs and specific nutritional supplements (Table 5-2). Symptoms of hypothyroidism (e.g., constipation) may be treated with a symptom-specific protocol.

TABLE 5-2	Botanical Treatment Strategies for Hypothyroidism		
Therapeutic Goal	**Therapeutic Action**	**Botanical Name**	**Common Name**
Stimulate thyroid hormone production/thyroid activity	Thyroid stimulating	*Bauhinia purpurea*	Bauhinia
		Coleus forskohlii	Coleus
		Commiphora mukul	Guggul
		Fucus vesiculosus	Bladderwrack
		Withania somnifera	Ashwagandha
Support metabolic function, reduce damage from oxidative stress, improve energy and vitality	Adaptogens	See Adaptogen section	
Supplement iodine in iodine deficiency-related cases	Iodine-rich	*Fucus vesiculosus*	Bladderwrack

An adequate understanding of the influence of botanical medicines on the thyroid gland, thyroid hormone production, and metabolism is lacking, as are human studies on the use of herbs for hypothyroidism. In fact, there is limited evidence for the botanical treatment of this condition. In contrast, there is a long history of the successful and relatively safe use of thyroid hormone replacement therapy. Thus unless a patient is responding poorly, conventional replacement therapy remains an excellent treatment choice. However, patients with borderline hypothyroidism may prefer and request alternatives to conventional therapy, and symptomatic euthyroid patients, or those with subclinical hypothyroidism, may be good candidates for botanical therapies that might support normalization of thyroid function. Note that botanicals that increase thyroid hormone levels are contraindicated in patients with hyperthyroidism; herbs presented in the discussion of hyperthyroidism for the reduction of thyroid hormone levels are contraindicated for patients with hypothyroidism. Botanical therapies that increase thyroid function should not be combined with thyroid replacement therapies. Patients using botanical therapies to manage thyroid conditions should be monitored regularly (every 6 months) with thyroid testing.

Adaptogens

Adaptogenic herbs play a key role in regulating various metabolic processes through improvement in hypothalamic-pituitary-adrenal (HPA) axis functioning. Both hypothyroidism and hyperthyroidism are associated with enhanced oxidative stress. Adaptogenic herbs counter catabolic processes associated with stress on the body and increase the oxygen consumptive capacity to decrease metabolic markers associated with anaerobic metabolism. Additionally, adaptogens such as *Eleutherococcus senticosus* and many others have been demonstrated to improve fatigue, weakness, and debility.

Ashwagandha (*Withania somnifera)* is the only adaptogen for which a thyroid-related study was identified. In one study, the effects of daily administration of ashwagandha root extract (1.4 g/kg body wt.) and *Bauhinia purpurea* bark extract (2.5 mg/kg body wt.) for 20 days on thyroid function in female mice were investigated. T3 and T4 concentrations were increased significantly by *Bauhinia,* and serum T4 concentration was enhanced by *Withania*. Both the plant extracts showed an increase in hepatic glucose-6-phosphatase (G-6-Pase) activity and antiperoxidative effects as indicated either by a decrease in hepatic lipid peroxidation (LPO) and/or by an increase in the activity of antioxidant enzyme(s). It appears that these plant extracts are capable of stimulating thyroid function in female mice.[22] The importance of *W. somnifera* root extract in the regulation of thyroid function with special reference to type I iodothyronine 5′-monodeiodinase activity in mouse liver was investigated. Although the extract (1.4 g/kg, p.o. [by mouth] for 20 days) increased serum T3 and T4 concentrations and hepatic G-6-Pase activity, hepatic iodothyronine 5′-monodeiodinase activity did not change significantly. Furthermore, the extract significantly reduced hepatic

LPO, whereas the activities of antioxidant enzymes such as superoxide dismutase and catalase were increased. It was concluded that the extract stimulates thyroid activity and also reduces LPO of hepatic tissue.[23]

Bladderwrack

Many herbalists and naturopathic physicians have relied on seaweed species in the treatment of hypothyroidism predicated on their iodine content. *Fucus vesiculosus,* or bladderwrack, for example, contains variable amounts of iodine, up to 600 mg/g. Much of the iodine content is organically bound, a more potent thyroid-stimulating form than mineral-bound iodine.[24] There are case reports of seaweed, especially bladderwrack, causing both hypothyroidism and hyperthyroidism, and evidence suggests thyroid activity. However, there are no studies of efficacy, dosage determination, or safety to support its use, and no standardization of iodine content.[25,26] Using seaweeds with the rationale that its iodine content is what is affecting treatment may be erroneous because most thyroid insufficiency in the United States is not attributable to iodine deficiency. Further, excess iodine, as discussed, can contribute to or worsen hypothyroidism. Bladderwrack may interfere with thyroid replacement therapies such as T4.[24] Bladderwrack also contains organically bound arsenic; although it is rapidly excreted, use caution with large amounts.[26]

Coleus

Coleus spp. have been used for centuries in Ayurvedic medicine.[27] Forskolin stimulates thyroid function with increased thyroid hormone production in the isolated gland. However, in vitro, low forskolin concentrations inhibited thyroid function.[26] No other research on the use of this herb for thyroid conditions was identified.

Guggul

Guggul has shown thyroid-stimulating activity, but not via the pituitary–TSH mechanism. It is thought to have a direct action on the thyroid gland. It acts on the peripheral conversion of T4 to T3, increasing T3 levels without changing T4 levels. By increasing thyroid metabolism and activity, guggul reduces low-density lipoprotein (LDL) cholesterol in individuals with functional hypothyroidism, which may be related to the stimulation of T3 by guggulsterones.[28] The effect of a petroleum ether extract of *Commiphora mukul* was tested on mice thyroid glands grown in organotype of culture using modified Dulbecco's Eagle Medium. There was a significant increase in the structure and function of thyroid cultivated explants using media containing the guggul extract with raised media T3 resin uptake, PBI, and FT4 index. The *C. mukul extract likely* augmented thyroid hormone synthesis and release.[29]

Nutritional Considerations

A variety of food antigens may induce antibodies that cross-react with the thyroid gland. A food elimination diet free of gluten containing grains and casein-containing dairy products may be helpful in the treatment of autoimmune hypothyroidism. The ingestion of goitrogens—foods that block iodine utilization—are best limited in those patients with goiters. Goitrogens include such foods as turnips, cabbage, mustard, cassava root, soybean, peanuts, pine nuts, and millet. A 2011 trial found that women with subclinical hypothyroidism who ingested soy had a threefold risk of developing overt hypothyroidism. (The dose was 30 g soy protein with 16 mg phytoestrogens.)[30] Cooking usually inactivates goitrogens.[31] Rich sources of iodine include ocean fish, sea vegetables (e.g., kelp, dulse, arame, hijiki, nori, wakame, kombu), and iodized salt, and should be included when there is iodine deficiency, but reduced when there is iodine excess.

TINCTURE FOR HYPOTHYROIDISM

Coleus	(Coleus forskohlii)	20 mL
Ashwagandha	(Withania somnifera)	20 mL
Bladderwrack	(Fucus vesiculosus)	15 mL
Licorice	(Glycyrrhiza glabra)	10 mL
Guggul	(Commiphora mukul)	10 mL
Nettles	(Urtica dioica)	10 mL
Reishi mushroom	(Ganoderma lucidum)	10 mL
Ginger	(Zingiber officinalis)	5 mL
		Total: 100 mL

Dose: 5 mL, morning and noon.

Thyroid function may be supported nutritionally, even with the use of thyroid replacement therapy. Nutrients that may be beneficial supplements include selenium; zinc; tyrosine; and vitamins A, D, E, and C.[31] Good sources of zinc include seafood (especially oysters), beef, oatmeal, chicken, liver, spinach, nuts, and seeds. The richest food source of selenium is Brazil nuts, especially those that are unshelled.

Selenium is a cofactor in normal thyroid hormone production. Selenium deficiency decreases conversion of T4 to T3. People with selenium deficiency have elevated T4 and TSH. Patients with normal circulating hormone levels who display clinical hypothyroid symptoms may be selenium deficient; thus selenium levels should be evaluated and supplementation provided if deficiency is present. A double-blind, placebo-controlled trial of selenium supplementation of 100 µg/day for 3 months among older subjects showed an improvement in selenium indexes, a decrease in T4, and a trend toward normalization of the T3:T4 ratio.[13]

Zinc is involved with synthesis of hypothalamic TRH; a zinc deficiency may lower 5′-deiodinase function, thereby contributing to a lower conversion of T4 to T3. Supplementation with zinc acts to normalize the TRH-induced TSH reaction and increase conversion of T4 to T3. The recommended dosage is zinc picolinate, 30 mg/day.[31]

Tyrosine is an amino acid used as a precursor for making thyroid hormone. Tyrosine deficiency can contribute to low thyroid function. Low-protein diets may provide insufficient tyrosine for normal thyroid hormone production. Supplementation of tyrosine at a dose of 500 to 1500 mg daily has therapeutic benefits in hypothyroidism.

TREATMENT SUMMARY

- Improve overall metabolism with diet, exercise, and herbs. Green tea is an excellent herb for gently boosting metabolism, and the adaptogens are a good long-term treatment.
- Remove stressors and improve adrenal and thyroid functioning with the use of adaptogens.
- Use botanicals to directly augment thyroid function.*
- Monitor progress with regular thyroid testing.
- Avoid foods that stimulate antigen cross-reactivity with the thyroid, such as gluten and casein.
- Avoid excessive intake of foods that act as goitrogens.
- Evaluate and ensure adequacy of dietary iodine intake: ocean-caught fish, iodized sea salt, and sea vegetables (e.g., kelp, wakame, nori) are good sources.
- Supplement with zinc; selenium; and vitamins A, C, D, and E.
- Initiate an exercise program to improve metabolism and prevent weight gain; dieting is discouraged because it can reduce metabolic function.

*Do not combine thyroid-stimulating herbal therapies with pharmaceutical thyroid medication. Consult with the patient's physician if the patient wants to make a switch between conventional and botanical therapies. In many cases, conventional treatment is the optimal choice.

Exercise

Regular daily exercise stimulates thyroid gland function and increases tissue sensitivity to thyroid hormones.[31] Exercise is especially important for dieting, overweight, hypothyroid patients; dieting can often put the body into a lower metabolic rate as the body tries to conserve fuel. Adjunctive regular exercise prevents the metabolic rate from dropping with the decrease in caloric intake.

 CASE HISTORY: HYPOTHYROIDISM

Eliza, a 44-year-old woman, reports weight gain without an increase in dietary intake, fatigue, muscle weakness, frequent infections, poor healing skin lesions, and alopecia. Symptoms began about 6 months ago and over the last 5 weeks have increased in severity. She works 30 hours a week as a therapist, lives alone with her two cats, and loves to garden. She takes a daily multivitamin and mineral supplement plus 1000 mg daily of vitamin C.

Her maternal family history is positive for hypothyroidism, allergies, and depression; paternal history is positive for late-onset diabetes, stroke, and allergies. The patient reports a generally healthy diet of whole foods with light meats, eggs, tofu, and fish as her main proteins. She eats mostly organic vegetables and seasonal fruits along with whole-grain breads and cereals. She eats some cheese and butter, but uses rice milk instead of cow milk. She drinks water, herb teas, and one cup of coffee each morning. She often skips breakfast because she has no hunger in the morning.

She experiences sluggish bowels, often skipping a day or two each week, and has frequent gas and bloating. She experiences recurrent sore throat and tonsillitis along with frequent sinus fullness and swollen glands in her neck. She claims to sleep well but wakes too early and often feels tired upon rising. She feels tired often in her day and experiences muscle fatigue. Her menstrual cycle length is every 32 days, with menses lasting 6 to 7 days and accompanied by heavy bleeding and clots for 2 days, and with dysmenorrhea on those first 2 days. Associated complaints include bloating, food cravings, irritability, weepiness, and depression for 5 to 7 days before her menses starts. She reports no children and never having been pregnant. She has no breast complaints and does a monthly self-breast examination. On physical examination, her basal body temperature (BBT) averages 96.4° F over a 5-week period. Her normal blood pressure is 110/66 mmHg, pulse is 68 beats/min, and she has reduced lower extremity reflexes. Her skin is slightly dry to the touch. Laboratory results demonstrate a TSH of 17.04 IU/mL (0.32-5.00), FT4 of 0.8 ng/dL (0.8-1.8), total T3 of 94 ng/dL (60-180), and a T3 uptake of 36% (22-37). Thyroid antibodies, antimicrosomal antibody of 400 (<100), and antithyroglobulin antibodies are normal. She was diagnosed with Hashimoto's disease.

Treatment Protocol

Tincture to be taken internally:

Coleus	(Coleus forskohlii)	20 mL
Ashwagandha	(Withania somnifera)	20 mL
Bladderwrack	(Fucus vesiculosus)	15 mL
Licorice	(Glycyrrhiza glabra)	10 mL
Guggul	(Commiphora mukul)	10 mL
Nettles	(Urtica dioica)	10 mL
Reishi mushroom	(Ganoderma lucidum)	10 mL
Ginger	(Zingiber officinalis)	5 mL
		Total: 100 mL

Dose: 5 mL, morning and noon.

Supplements

Include, along with the balanced diet:
- High-quality multivitamin supplement
- Selenium 100 µg, three times daily with meals
- Zinc 15 mg daily
- Tyrosine 500 mg daily

Patient was evaluated 3 months after starting treatments with the following laboratory values: TSH of 1.27 IU/mL, FT4 1.1 ng/dL, and FT3 4.0. The botanical medicine dose was adjusted to 3 mL, morning and noon. The patient was instructed to continue all else and follow up in 6 months.

HYPERTHYROIDISM

Pathophysiology

Hyperthyroidism, or thyrotoxicosis, is the result of excessive levels of circulating thyroid hormones. It is characterized by elevated total T4, FT4, FT4 index, and/or T3 and T3 resin uptake. Low TSH and normal levels of T3 and T4 characterize subclinical hyperthyroidism, and it has the same causes as overt hyperthyroidism.[2] Graves' disease, an autoimmune disorder in which stimulatory anti-TSH receptor antibodies are formed, makes up the majority of hyperthyroid cases.

In fact, the strongest risk factor for both hypothyroidism and hyperthyroidism is the presence of TPO antibodies.[1] These antibodies are directed toward the receptors in the cell membrane of the thyroid gland, causing the gland to increase growth, size, and function. Graves' disease is characterized by several common features, including thyrotoxicosis, goiter, exophthalmos, and pretibial myxedema. Graves' disease is eight times more common in women than men, typically presents between the ages of 20 and 40 years old, and the most common presentation is a diffuse non-painful goiter. It may be more prevalent in some genetic HLA haplotypes.[32]

There are several types of thyroiditis that can cause hyperthyroidism, including Hashimoto's thyroiditis, subacute thyroiditis, painless thyroiditis, postpartum thyroiditis, and radiation thyroiditis. Other contributing factors include stress, smoking, iodine supplements/excessive iodine intake, drug-induced hypothyroidism, higher pregnancy frequency, being postpartum, and microbial infections. Hyperthyroid patients have a significantly lower exposure to exogenous estrogens than euthyroid patients.[1]

Toxic adenoma is a solitary nodule within the thyroid that produces excessive amounts of thyroid hormones. It typically occurs in the middle-aged and older populations.[13]

Thyroid storm, or thyrotoxic crisis, can occur as a result of a serious stressor, such as surgery, infection, or trauma in a poorly managed case. The mortality rate is approximately 25% even with proper medical treatment.[13]

Hyperthyroidism and subclinical hyperthyroidism affect quality of life, producing symptoms mimicking adrenergic overactivity. Subclinical hyperthyroidism exerts significant effects on the cardiovascular system. It is associated with a higher heart rate and increased risk of supraventricular arrhythmias, and with an increased left ventricular mass, often accompanied by impaired diastolic function and sometimes by reduced systolic performance on effort and decreased exercise tolerance. These changes usually precede the onset of more severe cardiovascular disease, thus potentially contributing to increased cardiovascular morbidity and mortality. Subclinical hyperthyroidism may accelerate the development of osteoporosis and hence increased bone vulnerability to trauma, particularly in postmenopausal women with a preexisting predisposition. Fortunately, subclinical hyperthyroidism and its symptoms are readily preventable and reversible with timely treatment.[33]

Signs and Symptoms

Symptoms of hyperthyroidism are listed in Box 5-3. Menstrual symptoms associated with hyperthyroidism can vary, and may range from amenorrhea to oligomenorrhea, but menstrual cycles also may appear normal. Anxiety, nervousness, and depression rates are higher in hyperthyroid patients than in euthyroid controls.[2] Graves' disease is characterized by a triad of hyperthyroidism, exophthalmos, and pretibial myxedema. Hyperthyroidism symptoms in postmenopausal women present differently than in younger women. Symptoms are usually confined to a single organ system, particularly the cardiovascular or central nervous system (CNS). Goiter is usually absent in 40% of cases, and in older women, a co-occurring disease such as infection of coronary heart disease is usually predominant. The triad of weight loss, constipation, and appetite loss occurs in about 15% of older patients, whereas ophthalmic disease is rare. Practitioners may notice failure to thrive in older patients, with signs of heart disease, unexplained weight loss, and mental or psychological changes signaling possible hyperthyroidism.[7]

Diagnosis

Definitive laboratory diagnosis is based on elevated serum FT4, total T4, FT4 index, and T3 resin uptake. If these are borderline elevated, the T3 should be checked because it is often elevated out of proportion to the T4. TSH is typically decreased. Test for Graves' disease using the serum TSH receptor antibodies (TSH-R-Ab) test. If nodular goiter presents, a thyroid scan to rule out cancer is recommended.[34] As with hypothyroidism, controversy exists as to whether to routinely screen for subclinical hyperthyroidism. Proponents of screening advocate for the potential benefit via prevention of atrial fibrillation, osteoporotic fractures, and other complications of overt hyperthyroidism. Controlled studies of the treatment of subclinical disease have not been conducted.[2]

Conventional Treatment

The primary goal of conventional medicine is to limit the amount of thyroid hormone production by the thyroid gland.[18] Three main treatment methods are available: (1) antithyroid drug therapy, (2) surgery, or (3) radioactive iodine therapy. Although Graves' disease is an autoimmune disorder, conventional treatment of the disorder is aimed at managing the hyperthyroidism.

Antithyroid drug therapy seems to be most useful in young patients with mild disease. The drugs propylthiouracil, carbimazole, and methimazole may be given until spontaneous remission occurs. Twenty to 40% of patients have spontaneous remission within 6 months to 15 years of duration. There is a 50% to 60% relapse rate in patients treated with this method of therapy.[13,32]

Thyroidectomy is the treatment of choice for those patients with large or multinodular goiters. The patient is given antithyroid drugs for 6 weeks to bring the gland to a euthyroid state. The patient is also given potassium iodine for 2 weeks before surgery to diminish the vascularity of the gland and simplify the surgery. Subtotal thyroidectomy is preferred over total thyroidectomy. Patients generally require supplementation with thyroid hormone after surgery.

In radioactive iodine therapy, radioactive iodine is given in one dose, after which the gland shrinks and the patient becomes euthyroid over a period of 6 to 12 weeks. The major complication of this method of therapy is hypothyroidism, which develops in 80% of patients treated.[35]

In mild cases of hyperthyroidism, beta (β)-blockers may be given to provide symptomatic relief of adrenergic symptoms, including arrhythmia, tremor, tachycardia, and anxiety. They also provide minimal prevention of peripheral conversion of T4 to T3. Because β-blockers have no effect on inhibition on the production or release of thyroid hormone, they are an adjunctive therapy alongside of one of the more invasive therapies described in the preceding.[13]

Botanical Treatment

Traditional Western botanical medicine practitioners have found several herbs effective in the treatment of hyperthyroidism, a number of which have demonstrated antithyroid activity, inhibiting the binding of TSH to thyroid tissue (Table 5-3). Additionally, a number of herbs are effective in the treatment of heart palpitations, anxiety, and adrenergic symptoms associated with hyperthyroidism. Note the treatment of mild hyperthyroidism only with botanical medicines is recommended; moderate to severe or persistent cases

---

BOX 5-3 Signs and Symptoms of Hyperthyroidism

Diaphoresis
Diarrhea
Exercise intolerance
Exophthalmia
Goiter
Hair loss
Heart palpitations
Heat intolerance
Increased appetite
Nervousness
Onycholysis (i.e., separation of the nail from the bed)
Personality/psychological changes
Pretibial myxedema
Skin changes
Tachycardia
Thyroid bruit (murmur)
Tremor
Weakness
Weight loss

TABLE 5-3 Botanical Treatment Strategies for Hyperthyroidism

Therapeutic Goal	Therapeutic Action	Botanical Name	Common Name
Inhibit TSH binding	Antithyroid	*Lycopus* spp.	Bugleweed
		Lithospermum officinale	Club moss
		Melissa officinalis	Lemon balm
Relieve palpitations	Antiarrhythmics	*Leonurus cardiaca*	Motherwort
Relieve anxiety	Anxiolytics	*Leonurus cardiaca*	Motherwort
	See Nervines in index	*Melissa officinalis*	Lemon balm

TSH, Thyroid-stimulating hormone.

require medical treatment, and all individuals with hyperthyroidism require medical supervision.[13]

Herbs that increase thyroid activity, as discussed under hypothyroidism, should be avoided in the hyperthyroid patient. Additionally, the use of ephedra is contraindicated in patients with hyperthyroidism, and herbs with high caffeine content should be avoided.[36] Increased consumption of goitrogens (e.g., leafy greens, cabbage, broccoli, Brussels sprouts, soy) can be part of a treatment strategy to reduce thyroid hormone.[13]

Thyroid hormone excess causes an increase in metabolism, and thus an increase in nutritional needs, excessive glucose metabolism, and increased oxidative stress and increased susceptibility to liver damage. Botanical medicines and nutritional supplements to reduce oxidative stress (e.g., adaptogens, antioxidants) and protect the liver (e.g., *Silybum marianum*) also should be included in the protocol (see Additional Therapies).

Bugleweed

Bugleweed (Fig. 5-1) has a long history of use by herbalists for the treatment of palpitations and anxiety.[13] It is widely recommended in medical herbalism texts. Priest and Priest describes it for the treatment of palpations, tachycardia, and dysregulation of the autonomic nervous system. Weiss and

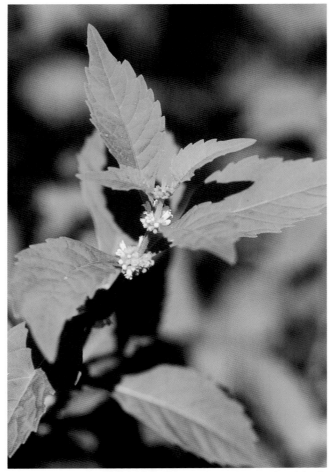

FIGURE 5-1 Bugleweed (*Lycopus* spp.). (Photo by Martin Wall.)

Fintelmann refers to bugleweed as having thyrostatic effects and suggests its use for the treatment of hyperthyroidism, whereas the *British Herbal Pharmacopoeia (BHP)* calls it a T4 antagonist.[37-39] Hoffmann reports it to be indicated for mild forms of hyperthyroidism, especially when symptoms include tightness of breathing, palpitations, and shaking.[40] Priest and Priest recommend combining bugleweed with motherwort for hyperthyroid cardiac reactions, a common practice among herbalists.[39]

In vivo and in vitro evidence has demonstrated that *Lycopus* spp. can be beneficial in the treatment of hyperthyroid symptoms.[13] An open study tested *Lycopus europaeus* in mild hyperthyroidism using measures of urinary T3 and T4 excretion. *Lycopus* administration was associated with increased T4 excretion, possibly involving renal mechanisms.[41] Additionally, an open postmarketing surveillance study aimed to assess the efficacy of *L. europaeus* extract (Thyreogutt). The study consisted of three groups (n = 430)—a prolective assessment in patients receiving product for 4 weeks (n = 146), a retrolective documentation of data from patients who had received at least 4 weeks of product during the previous 2 years (n = 171), and a control cohort receiving no treatment (n = 86). The extract was found to be well tolerated and treatment correlated with statistically significant improvement in mild hyperthyroid symptoms. The dose was not disclosed.[42]

Rosmarinic acid, ellagic acid, chlorogenic acid, and luteolin-7-β-glucoside appear to be the active constituents leading to blocking of TSH receptors and inhibition of peripheral conversion of T4 to T3.[13,43] Aqueous, freeze-dried extracts of *Lycopus* spp., *Lithospermum officinale,* and *Melissa officinalis* have been studied in vivo and in vitro; preliminary results support their use in Graves' disease. This combination was shown to inhibit TSH effects on TSH receptor sites on thyroid cell membranes, block effects of antithyroid immunoglobulins on TSH receptors, and inhibit peripheral deiodination of T4 to T3.[44] No human clinical trials have been conducted using bugleweed.[13] The German Commission E recognizes the use of bugleweed for mild hyperthyroid conditions with neuroanatomic dysfunction based on pharmacologic studies only, and states that in rare cases high doses have resulted in thyroid enlargement, whereas sudden discontinuation of use has increased disease symptoms.[45]

FORMULA FOR HYPERTHYROIDISM

Motherwort	(*Leonurus cardiaca*)	25 mL
Bugleweed	(*Lycopus* spp.)	25 mL
Lemon balm	(*Melissa officinalis*)	25 mL
Nettles	(*Urtica dioica*)	25 mL
		Total: 100 mL

Dose: This is a classic herbal formula for hyperthyroidism.

The late Hein Zeylstra, well-known herbal educator from Tunbridge Wells, United Kingdom, recommended an equal-part mixture of 1:5 tincture of these herbs given in 5 mL doses three times daily.

Club Moss, Gromwell

Like bugleweed, *Lithospermum* has a long history of use for the treatment of hyperthyroid conditions. It was used by the

Eclectic physicians for this purpose, and although less widely used than *Lycopus*, has been equally well studied.[13,46] Animal studies using *Lithospermum officinale* have demonstrated its ability to block TSH activity at the receptor level, block the release of TSH from the thyroid, and suppress the iodide pump. It also inhibits peripheral T4-deiodination and conversion to T3.[44,47] An in vitro study using freeze-dried extract demonstrated the ability to decrease antibody binding to thyroid tissue in Graves' disease.[44] No human clinical trials have evaluated the use of *Lithospermum* for hyperthyroid diseases.[13]

Lemon Balm

Lemon balm (Fig. 5-2), historically referred to as the "gladdening herb," is calming to the nervous system and has been used since ancient times for this purpose. In vitro studies have confirmed this herb's ability to block TSH receptors and inhibit both binding of bovine TSH to human thyroid tissue and binding of autoantibodies in Graves' disease.[44] The herb has a high safety profile and is appropriate for the treatment of mild hyperthyroidism, as well as associated anxiety and depression.[13]

Motherwort

Motherwort (Fig. 5-3) is classically used for the treatment of anxiety, depression, heart palpitations, and tachycardia, making it highly appropriate for symptomatic relief in hyperthyroid disease.[13,37,40] Chemical analytical and animal studies confirm the herb's sedative, anxiolytic, antiarrhythmic, and antispasmodic effects.[13] The German Commission E supports the use of motherwort for the treatment of cardiac disorders associated with anxiety and for the symptomatic relief of hyperthyroidism.[45]

Nutritional Considerations

The risk of oxidative damage is increased in the hyperthyroid patient because of a higher metabolic rate. LPO is increased and activities of antioxidant enzymes are altered. Dietary changes involve an emphasis on goitrogens (i.e., foods that naturally block thyroid hormone synthesis) and the avoidance of certain foods, particularly those high in iodine content (e.g., seaweeds). Dietary goitrogens include broccoli, cauliflower, Brussels sprouts, cabbage, kohlrabi, sweet potatoes, almonds, pine nuts, millet, peaches, and peanuts.[8]

- Include a complex daily antioxidant supplement.
- Flavonoid-containing substances have been shown to decrease serum T4 concentrations and inhibit both conversion of T4 to T3 and 5′-deiodinase activity.[48] Foods and botanical medicines that are high in flavonoid compounds include those fruits and vegetables of yellow-orange, red, and purple colors; such as blueberries,

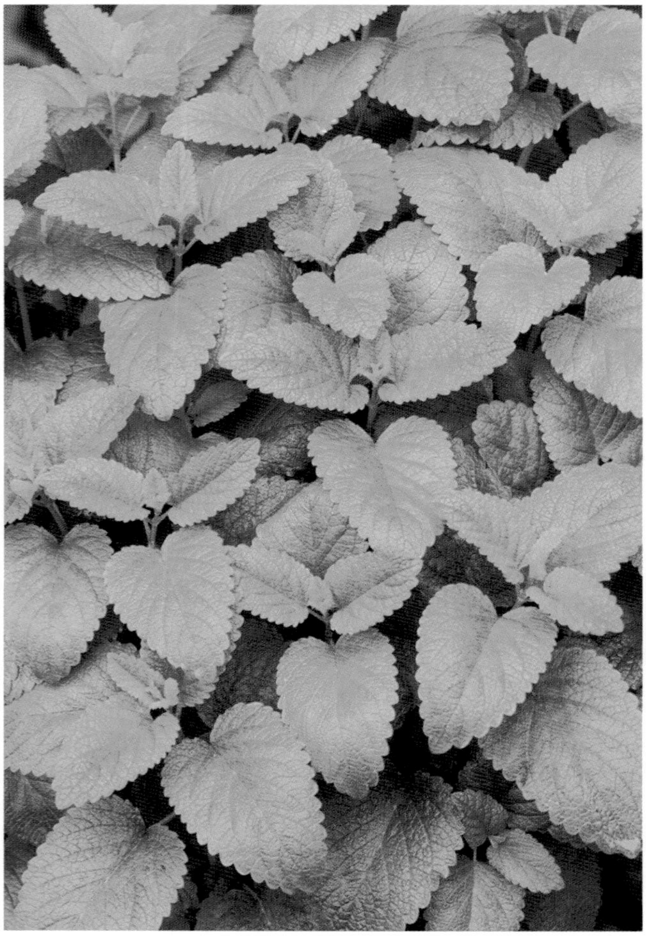

FIGURE 5-2 Lemon balm *(Melissa officinalis).* (Photo by Martin Wall.)

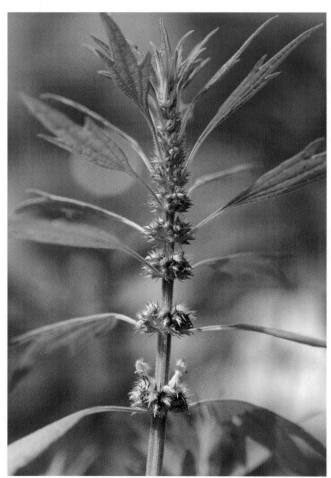

FIGURE 5-3 Motherwort *(Leonurus cardiaca).* (Photo by Martin Wall.)

purple grapes, and cherries. Botanical medicines that provide flavanoid compounds include hawthorne berry, astragalus, ginkgo, licorice, and chamomile.[49]

- Calcium metabolism is altered in hyperthyroidism, making Graves' patients more susceptible to osteoporosis.[7] Adequate prevention of osteoporosis should be an important part of the patient's treatment plan (see Chapter 7).
- Selenium deficiency substantially alters the conversion of T4 to T3 in peripheral tissues such as the liver and kidneys.[43,50] In a randomized, prospective, blinded study, 36 patients with autoimmune thyroiditis were given 200 µg of selenium for 3 months. Thyroid-specific TPOAb concentrations significantly decreased from 100% to 63%; 9 of the 36 had complete normalization of TPOAb concentrations.[51]
- Zinc needs are increased in hyperthyroid patients because of greater urinary zinc excretion.

Additional Therapies

Stress reduction methods include biofeedback, meditation, tai chi, yoga, and prayer therapy, and should be included in a plan for hyperthyroid treatment.

TREATMENT SUMMARY

- Achieve symptomatic relief of heart palpitations and anxiety with herbs.
- Use herbs and antioxidant supplements to protect the liver against the oxidative stress effects of increased metabolism caused by this condition.
- Ensure adequate nutritional intake; metabolism is significantly increased in patients with hyperthyroidism.
- Increase intake of dietary goitrogens to help reduce excessive thyroid function.
- Severe hyperthyroidism requires medical management.

 CASE HISTORY: HYPERTHYROIDISM

A 32-year-old woman presented with a 3-month history of chronic vaginal and nipple candidal infection. She is 8 months postpartum and breastfeeding her daughter, who has also had recurrent thrush for the past 3 months. She reports nearly constant anxiety, heart palpations several times a day, excessive thirst and hunger, irritability, fatigue, and hot flashes. She reports that it is difficult for her to relax and she is bothered by insomnia. She reports a normal first pregnancy and birth and no menstrual cycle since the pregnancy. She experiences frequent colds and sinus infections and is chronically congested in her nasal passages, with postnasal drip and fullness in her left ear. She complains of frequent gas and bloating and reports two or three bowel movements daily, often unformed.

She used Nystatin oral suspension several times for the yeast, as prescribed by her primary care physician, and was taking a prenatal vitamin and eicosapentaenoic acid/docosahexaenoic acid (EPA/DHA) 500 mg two times a day. Her blood pressure is 124/78 mmHg; pulse is 92 beats/min, and respirations are 20 breaths/min. Her physician observed that the woman had extreme nervousness about the well-being

of the baby, how she is caring for the baby, and breastfeeding issues.

Laboratory Values
TSH: <0.01IU/mL (0.4-5.0 IU/mL), T4: 18.8 mcg/dL (4.5-12 mcg/dL), FTI: 7.3 mcg/dL (1.4-3.7 mcg/dL), T3 uptake: 39% (25-36), FT4: 5.1 ng/dL, (8-1.8 ng/dL), total T3: 553 ng/dL (80-180 ng/dL), and TSH-R-Abs positive.

She was diagnosed with hyperthyroidism (Graves' disease).

Treatment Protocol
Tincture to be taken internally:

Bugleweed	(*Lycopus* spp.)	20 mL
Club moss	(*Lithospermum officinale*)	20 mL
Lemon balm	(*Melissa officinalis*)	20 mL
Motherwort	(*Leonurus cardiaca*)	10 mL
Skullcap	(*Scutellaria lateriflora*)	10 mL
Valerian	(*Valeriana officinalis*)	10 mL
Eleuthero	(*Eleutherococcus senticosus*)	10 mL
		Total: 100 mL

Dose: 5 mL, TID (three times per day) with meals.
Also: Astragalus capsules 500 mg twice daily.

Dietary recommendations were to increase dietary goitrogens, including broccoli, cauliflower, Brussels sprouts, cabbage, kohlrabi, sweet potatoes, almonds, pine nuts, millet, peaches, soy, and peanuts.

She was encouraged to practice daily yoga for half an hour, along with aerobic exercise four to five times a week.

Take a 20-minute warm bath at night with essential oils of lemon balm and lavender (five to seven drops each per bath).

The patient was evaluated with labs 2 months later showing TSH: <0.01 IU/mL, T3: 38%, T4: 18.3 mcg/dL, FTI: 5.9 mcg/dL, total T3: 433 ng/dL, and FT4: 3.4 ng/dL . She reports her average pulse as being 84 beats/min and her signs and symptoms are lessening.

Evaluation after 7 months of treatment shows TSH <0.01 IU/mL, T3: 110, FT4: 0.72 ng/dL, and FTI: 2.9 mcg/dL.

STRESS, ADAPTATION, THE HYPOTHALAMIC-PITUITARY-ADRENAL AXIS, AND WOMEN'S HEALTH

Viewed from the perspective of the evolution of the animal kingdom, sustained psychological stress is a recent invention, mostly limited to humans and other social primates.
Robert Sapolsky, author, Why Zebras Don't Get Ulcers

Stress is a fact of life. However, for most of our biological history, stress was a short-term crisis, after which, according to Robert Sapolsky, author of *Why Zebras Don't Get Ulcers*, "It's either over with or you're over with."[52] Modern society, with its 24/7 work requirements, global Internet access, high level of stimulation and demand, and chronic (daily) repeated stresses, has opened us to a whole new realm of chronic, debilitating diseases. Western medicine is beginning to understand what

The editor wishes to thank *Botanical Medicine for Women's Health*, Edition 1 contributor Jillian Stansbury for her original contributions to this chapter.

has long been recognized by traditional medicine systems: that stress, or more traditionally viewed, one's relationship with and response to the world, has an effect on health.

What we now know scientifically is that the challenge of a small amount of stress, whether from positive or negative stressors (i.e., eustress versus distress), can actually increase the overall health and performance of the individual organism; but prolonged or repeated stress leads to wear and tear on the body (i.e., allostatic load), part of a deleterious picture leading to numerous health consequences. These may include reproductive disorders, endocrine dysregulation, insulin resistance (i.e., syndrome X), obesity, chronic fatigue syndrome (CFS), cardiovascular disease, osteoporosis, impaired immunity, autoimmune disorders, cognitive impairment, thyroid disorders, chronic anxiety, postpartum depression, and major depression, to name a few of the big players.[52-57]

It might not surprise readers that women are experiencing these conditions in increasing and significant numbers. Although stress is not the sole cause of these illnesses—as most illnesses have multifactorial etiologies—stress appears to be an underlying factor in many conditions. Unlike exposure to environmental toxins and radiation, traffic patterns, and other factors over which we have little control, stress may be one factor whose effects we have the ability to minimize.

STRESS, HEALTH, AND DISEASE: THE PHYSIOLOGY AND PATHOPHYSIOLOGY OF STRESS AND THE STRESS RESPONSE

The groundwork for the scientific understanding of the physiology of mind–body interactions was first established in the 1930s by the work of Walter Cannon, and was followed in the 1940s by the extensive work of Hans Selye, who first formally elaborated the concept of stress and its effects on physiology.[53,58-62] Selye is also credited with introducing the terms *corticoids, glucocorticoids,* and *mineralocorticoids,* and through his work demonstrated the "triad of stress"—adrenal enlargement, gastrointestinal (GI) ulcers, and thymus gland atrophy—in response to exposure to chronic stressors.[60] George Chrousos summarizes stress and the stress response as follows:

> *Life exists by maintaining a complex dynamic equilibrium, or homeostasis, that is constantly challenged by intrinsic or extrinsic adverse forces or stressors. Stress is, thus, defined as a state of threatened homeostasis, which is reestablished by a complex repertoire of physiologic and behavioral adaptive responses of the organism. The adaptive responses may be inadequate for the reestablishment of homeostasis or excessive and prolonged; in either case a healthy steady state is not attained, and pathology may ensue.[58]*

Stressors are threats to homeostasis and the adaptive responses are the counteracting forces intended to reestablish it.[52,57,61] Selye termed the adaptive stress response *general adaptation syndrome,* and demonstrated that it consisted of a consistent set of physiologic responses that included initial response to the stressor followed by an exhaustion phase and eventually a recovery phase (Fig. 5-4).

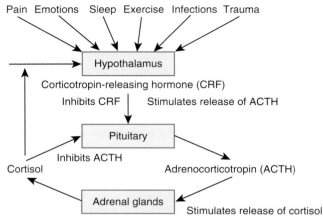

FIGURE 5-4 Stressors, the stress response, and the hypothalamic-pituitary-adrenal (HPA) axis. (Courtesy Robyn Klein.)

More recently the stress response has been renamed *allostasis,* the ability of the organism to maintain stability, or homeostasis, through change.[53,61] McEwen elaborates:

> *The terms, "allostasis" and "allostatic overload," allow for a more accurate definition of the overused word "stress" and provide a view of how the essential protective and adaptive effects of physiological mediators that maintain homeostasis—the body's optimal set points for important factors such as blood pressure, fluid balance, pH, glucose levels, oxygen levels, temperature, etc.—are also involved in the cumulative effects of daily life when they are mismanaged or overused. When mediators of allostasis, like cortisol and adrenaline, are released in response to stressors or to lifestyle factors such as diet, sleep, and exercise, they promote adaptation and are generally beneficial. However, when these mediators are not turned off when the stress is over, or when they are not turned on adequately during stress, or when they are overused by many stressors, there are cumulative changes that lead to a wear-and-tear, called "allostatic load or overload," on the body and brain. The concept of allostasis refers to the network of interacting mediators by which stability, that is, homeostasis, is achieved through change. There are primary mediators of allostasis, such as, but not confined to, hormones of the hypothalamic-pituitary-adrenal (HPA) axis, catecholamines, and cytokines. These mediators interact with each other to create a network of reciprocal effects.[53]*

Our bodies possess complex and elegant mechanisms for responding to and recovering from acute exposure to stressors. The neuroendocrine system has evolved two primary pathways responsible for responding and adapting to potentially harmful or life-threatening encounters: the sympathoadrenal system (SAS) and HPA axis. Both mediate a two-way brain–body communication that sets in motion a series of hormonal and neuroendocrine responses that "switch on" and "switch off" what has been commonly referred to as the "fight or flight" response.[52,61] In response to the alert system being switched on, the body's resources are mobilized for protective action: The heart rate increases and blood is diverted from digestion (who needs to digest when being chased by the proverbial saber tooth tiger?) into the periphery, especially the legs (yup, you want to be able to run away from the tiger!); the respiratory rate increases; blood pressure increases; urinary output decreases; the pupils dilate to increase sight; other senses such as hearing and smell become keener; the mind becomes sharp and alert and vigilance is enhanced; appetite decreases; immunity is suppressed; and large amounts of sugar are delivered to the bloodstream via lipolysis and gluconeogenesis to provide the energy needed for a massive response. Growth, reproduction, and sexual response are inhibited—resources are instead diverted to immediate life-saving needs, rather than toward what Sapolsky refers to as optimistic activities. In the recovery phase, interestingly, the body responds to the need for repair by increasing appetite and storing fat (primarily in the abdomen).[52]

Hormonal and neuroendocrine mediators and messengers from the sympathetic nervous system and HPA axis orchestrate all of these responses. At the first sign of threat, or even a perceived threat, the sympathetic nervous system goes into action. Epinephrine (i.e., adrenaline) and norepinephrine (i.e., noradrenalin) are released from the nerve endings of the adrenal glands and the rest of the body, respectively, and begin to stimulate the body to further reaction in a matter of seconds. The hypothalamus releases a substance called corticotrophin-releasing hormone (CRH), which triggers the release of ACTH (corticotrophin), which within a few minutes reaches the adrenal glands, where it causes the release of glucocorticoids (i.e., cortisol, corticosteroids). The pancreas releases glucagons, which with the glucocorticoids increase the levels of circulating glucose. Glucocorticoids do this via the promotion of protein and lipid degradation from muscle, skin, and fat. Energy is mobilized at the expense of storage. Other hormones are released as well. Prolactin is secreted by the pituitary and plays a role in the suppression of reproduction during stress. Endorphins and enkephalins are released, blunting pain perception. Vasopressin (antidiuretic hormone) is released from the pituitary and maintains blood pressure, forestalling, for example, hypovolemic shock in the event of massive blood loss. Prostaglandins, platelet activating factor, and nitric oxide are all stimulated. The allostatic response also inhibits the release of numerous hormones, for example, estrogen, progesterone, and testosterone, as well as growth hormone and insulin.

Prolonged and repeated exposure to aversive events—as well as anticipation of aversive events (e.g., worry and anxiety about future or impending events such as an interview, an examination, paying the bills)—may lead to a sustained activation and dysregulation of the HPA axis.[52] In time, allostatic states place wear and tear on the regulatory systems of the brain and body, which can lead to the HPA axis hyperfunctioning or hypofunctioning (respectively, the inability to turn off, or turn on the adaptive response): maladaptive responses thought to be causally linked to a number of disorders via glucocorticoid and other effects on the cardiovascular system, mobilization of bone stores of calcium, effects on weight and fat distribution, hormonal effects on the reproductive system, thyroid effects, and so forth.[52,53,56,61]

Women are more likely to experience menstrual irregularities, anovulation, infertility, osteoporosis, chronic fatigue, autoimmunity, cardiovascular disease, syndrome X, and diabetes, for example. Further, there is significant evidence that a history of childhood sexual or psychological abuse predisposes one to HPA dysfunction later in life.[63] Excessive exercise (overtraining) also can lead to HPA dysfunction with increased fatigue and decreased immune response.[64] Irregular and inadequate food intake, regular hypoglycemic episodes, and yo-yo dieting also cause excessive stress and cause blood sugar imbalances that can lead to allostatic overload and eventually HPA dysregulation.

The medical profession does not define a category of illnesses that encompasses the effects of allostatic load. Prevention and treatment of stress and its effects on the HPA axis are not considered a part of preventative care or treatment for the numerous and serious stress-related diseases mentioned earlier, with limited exceptions. Adrenal disease is recognized only in its severest forms: Addison's disease and Shy-Drager syndrome. Yet the symptoms of HPA axis dysregulation are rampant in modern society. Aside from overt dysfunction and disease—reproductive disorders and endocrine dysregulation, insulin resistance (i.e., syndrome X) and obesity, CFS, cardiovascular disease, osteoporosis, impaired immunity and autoimmune disorders, thyroid disorders, cognitive impairment, chronic anxiety, and major depression—Americans are plagued by fatigue and exhaustion, insomnia, emotional frustration, digestive problems, weight problems, menstrual problems, infertility, menopausal problems, headaches, susceptibility to colds, musculoskeletal tension, allergies and asthma, atopic conditions, and numerous other problems that can be related to stress and chronic HPA hyperfunctioning or hypofunctioning.[52-56] The need to address chronic stress as part of the prevention and treatment of chronic illness is more than a lip service to a holistic approach—it is a significant part of a comprehensive medical and public health approach to reducing chronic health problems affecting all populations in the United States. It is also an integral aspect of herbal medicine care, as discussed in the following.

EUSTRESS AND DISTRESS

Interestingly, pleasant and pleasurable activities (e.g., sex, numerous mind-altering and energy-altering substances that are commonly used and abused, heavy exercise) also trigger the stress response. The primary factors distinguishing distress from eustress appear to be the quality and intensity of the stressor, termination of the stress response after a particular stressor has ceased, and the return of homeostasis.[61] Genetic predisposition, life history, and age also seem to play significant roles in the perception of stress and in the stress response.[52,61]

DIFFERENTIAL DIAGNOSIS

HPA dysfunction must be distinguished from specific chronic and acute diseases, as well as from clinical adrenal disease.

Patients complaining of chronic, recurrent symptoms should have serious underlying illness ruled out. HPA dysfunction then becomes a diagnosis based on exclusion of other possible causes.

CONVENTIONAL THERAPIES FOR HYPOTHALAMIC-PITUITARY-ADRENAL AXIS DYSFUNCTION

Although Selye's work was accepted as logical and well supported, and was validated by numerous subsequent researchers, conventional medicine does not recognize generalized HPA dysfunction as a discrete entity, much less propose methods for prevention and treatment. Patients presenting with weakness, fatigue, insomnia, anxiety, susceptibility to colds, stress symptoms, and stress intolerance are typically prescribed antidepressants and anxiolytics. If hypertension and heart palpitations are most prominent, β-blockers or other cardiovascular medications may be prescribed. If low adrenal function has affected progesterone or reproductive function, hormone replacement is typically offered. If dysglycemia and episodic blood sugar difficulties are the presenting symptoms, the case is often misunderstood. Vital signs and routine blood work, including blood glucose, may often be normal, and the individual is typically told all is fine, or perhaps offered psychiatric medications.

BOTANICAL APPROACHES TO STRESS AND HYPOTHALAMIC-PITUITARY-ADRENAL AXIS DYSREGULATION

Adaptogens reduce the cost of homeostasis/allostasis to the organism, preventing or delaying damaging effects caused by stress and aging. By helping to maintain a state of balance throughout the body, adaptogens hold the key to vitality.

Donald Yance

Those using this book may notice the regular inclusion of adaptogens and nervine herbs in the treatment of conditions that on the surface may appear unrelated to the nervous system or HPA axis. By now it is probably evident that the nervous, endocrine, reproductive, and immune systems are immutably interconnected—effects in one have tremendous effects on the regulation of the others. Herbalists recognize the significant effects of stress on physiologic functioning, as well as the role of illness increasing stress response. Therefore many botanical protocols for chronic health problems include herbs that support the ability of the organism to respond to and withstand stress—or allostatic overload.

The primary class of herbs used to support and restore adrenal health and optimal HPA axis functioning is known as the adaptogens. Many are considered "tonics" in traditional medicine systems (e.g., ginseng in Traditional Chinese Medicine [TCM], ashwagandha in Ayurveda). Lazarev, a Russian pharmacologist who researched the resistance of organisms to stress in experimental studies and initially tested pharmacologic drugs, first coined the term *adaptogen*

in 1947. To be considered an adaptogen, the substance had to demonstrate the following[62]:

- Nonspecific effects in that the adaptogen increases resistance to a very broad spectrum of harmful factors (i.e., stressors) of different physical, chemical, and biological natures
- A normalizing effect: it counteracts or prevents disturbances brought about by stressors
- It must be innocuous to have a broad range of therapeutic effects without causing any disturbance (other than very marginally) to the normal functioning of the organism

Lazarev, Brekhman, and other Russian researchers were using the terms *stress* and *stressors* in the classical sense as defined by the work of Selye, and were seeking to develop medications able to mobilize the intrinsic adaptive mechanisms to help individuals cope with and survive in situations of intense or prolonged stress while maintaining physical and mental work capacities. Adaptogens were considered to constitute a new class of metabolic regulators of natural origin that increased the organism's adaptive abilities to environmental factors and prevented damage from these factors. Most studies of adaptogens were originally conducted in Russia and focused on *Eleutherococcus senticosus, Rhodiola rosea, Schisandra chinensis,* and *Bryonia alba.* These herbs were incorporated into official medical practice in the USSR and produced as standardized extracts in various forms. Having been found quite safe, they are still used in Russia in both self-care and physician-prescribed regimens.[57] By 1984, there were over 1500 studies in Russia alone on just three adaptogenic herbs (*Eleutherococcus, Rhodiola,* and *Schisandra*). Interest in adaptogens has also spread worldwide; the term *adaptogen,* for example, is recognized by the Food and Drug Administration (FDA) as a functional term.[62]

A substance that reduces the state and severity of stress and counteracts the effect of stressors is an adaptogen.[65] Adaptogens contain phenolic compounds with a structural resemblance to catecholamines, suggesting an effect on the SAS; tetracyclic triterpenes, similar to the corticosteroids that inactivate the stress system; and oxylipins, unsaturated trihydroxy or epoxy fatty acids resembling leukotrienes and lipoxines.[57] Adaptogens have a range of effects, and appear to act broadly on tissue involved in homeostatic regulatory systems (e.g., immune, endocrine, CNS) rather than having specific targets. There is significant evidence that adaptogens increase exercise capacity, endurance, stamina, cognitive function, and mental alertness, and that they increase nonspecific immunity and stress resistance, relieve fatigue, and improve energy metabolism and tissue repair. Evidence also indicates that administration of adaptogens modulates ACTH and corticosteroid formation and normalizes levels of stress hormones.[62] They may be considered substances that allow the organism to resist stress at higher levels of challenge.

Adaptogens have been used historically as general tonic medicines, thought to gently strengthen the CNS in cases of fatigue, physical exertion, aging, weakness from disease and injury, and prolonged stress. They are considered to induce "states of nonspecifically increased resistance" (SNIR). Many cultures have embraced the widespread use of such herbs in older adults and the infirm: *Panax* in China and Asia,

Eleutherococcus in Russia, and *Withania* in India. They have been historically and clinically reported to improve diabetes, blood pressure, and cardiac action, and relieve mental confusion, headache, and weakness among older adults. These plants are also credited with an affinity for the nervous system and an ability to relieve mental stress in cases of insomnia and anxiety disorders. Muscle fatigue, physical weakness, and immune deficiency were all thought to improve with the use of such herbs. Athletes, for example, sometimes benefit from the use of adaptogens, noting improved stamina and endurance. They also may be used to improve postsurgical healing and convalescence.[57]

It is generally recommended to give a course of adaptogens over a prolonged period of time, a minimum of 3 months generally, or on an ongoing basis for up to several years for severely depleted patients. Adaptogens may be used singly; however, it is preferable to combine them with other herbs to support, direct, and moderate their individual effects. Although adaptogens, by definition, lack serious side effects, their specific qualities may best be tempered by combination with other herbs. For example, *Rhodiola* or *Schisandra* taken alone are both quite drying and astringent, and can be tempered by combining them with herbs that are moistening and sweet, such as licorice. Ginseng, particularly red ginseng, can be heating and stimulating. Looking at TCM, one quickly notices that herbs such as ginseng are only one of several herbs included in a formula for this very reason. Additionally, although adaptogens share many qualities, each individual herb possesses unique characteristics that distinguish it from the others; thus prescribing should still be based on the individual patient. Adaptogens may be used prophylactically before times of physical, emotional, or mental stress, or restoratively, such as after a long illness or prolonged period of debility or stress.

Licorice, which may not be truly classified as an adaptogen, is included because of its marked cortisol-sparing, adrenal-tonic effects. Calmative nervines that act as sympathetic relaxing agents such as *Matricaria recutita*, *Scutellaria lateriflora*, *Avena sativa,* and *Passiflora incarnata,* for example (Table 5-4), are indicated because these may reduce stress-induced CRH stimulation of the adrenal output of cortisol and adrenaline. Parasympathomimetics directly or indirectly increase parasympathetic function, reducing sympathetic dominance. They are indicated for anxiety and stress, and to relieve symptoms that result from adrenergic stress.[66] Evidence for nervines and other herbs listed in Table 5-4 are found elsewhere throughout this text. For insomnia, sedatives may be included; for chronic musculoskeletal problems, antispasmodics may be incorporated into formulae. Adaptogens also may be effectively combined with herbs for individual systems, for example, hawthorn for the cardiovascular system, or chaste berry for the reproductive system.

Ashwagandha

The roots of ashwagandha have long been used as *rasayana* drugs in Ayurvedic medicine to prevent or treat disease through the restoration of a healthy balance of life.[65] Ashwagandha is used in Ayurvedic medicine as a general restorative medicine, and to improve general health,

TABLE 5-4 Botanical Treatments for Improving the Stress Response

Herbal Action	Botanical Name	Common Name
Adaptogens	*Eleutherococcus senticosus*	Eleuthero Ginseng
	Panax ginseng	American
	Panax quinquefolius	ginseng
	Rhaponticum carthamoides	Rhaponticum Rhodiola
	Rhodiola rosea	Schizandra
	Schizandra chinensis	Ashwagandha
	Withania somnifera	
Nervines	*Avena sativa*	Milky oats
	Hypericum perforatum	St. John's wort
	Lavandula officinalis	Lavender
	Leonurus cardiaca	Motherwort
	Matricaria recutita	Chamomile
	Melissa officinalis	Lemon balm
	Passiflora incarnata	Passion flower
	Scutellaria lateriflora	Skullcap
	Valeriana officinalis	Valerian
	Verbena officinals	Blue vervain
Parasympath omimetics	*Anemone pulsatilla*	Pulsatilla
	Lobelia inflata	Lobelia
	Piper methysticum	Kava kava
Anxiolytics	*Avena sativa*	Milky oats
	Eschscholzia californica	California poppy
	Lavandula officinalis	Lavender
	Leonurus cardiaca	Motherwort
	Matricaria recutita	Chamomile
	Passiflora incarnata	Passion flower
	Piper methysticum	Kava kava
	Scutellaria lateriflora	Skullcap
	Valeriana officinalis	Valerian
	Verbena officinalis	Blue vervain
	Withania somnifera	Ashwagandha

longevity, and prevent disease. Ashwagandha is much less stimulating than ginseng, making it preferable for patients with irritability, anxiety, and insomnia, and as a gentle tonic herb for the nervous system.[67] The species name, *somnifera*, indicates the plant's traditional use for sleep induction. Ashwagandha is immunomodulatory and improves energy in patients experiencing stress-induced illness or exhaustion. It is indicated in inflammatory conditions, such as arthritis or other musculoskeletal disorders, and it is combined with other herbs in the treatment of cancer. Ashwagandha is used in Ayurveda and Unani systems of medicine for the treatment of pain, skin diseases, infection, inflammation, gastrointestinal disorders, rheumatism, and epilepsy. It is also used as a general tonic for the improvement of libido, liver health, mental state, cancer, heart disease, and the immune system.[68] In vivo studies support its use for antiinflammatory, immunomodulatory, antioxidant, thyroid-stimulating, anxiolytic, stress-reducing, memory-enhancing, and antineoplastic effects (Table 5-5).[65,68-78] Ashwagandha is also reported to be hematopoietic, making it useful in the treatment of anemia.[79] Ashwagandha is combined with levodopa, tropane alkaloid–containing plants, and other herbs as a therapy for

TABLE 5-5	**Effects and Supposed Mechanisms of Some Actions of Ashwagandha**
Effects	**Supposed Mechanism of Action**
Adaptogenic and immunomodulatory activity	Steroidal lactones 5,20(R)-dihydroxy-6,7 α-epoxy-1-oxo-(5 α)-witha-2,24-dienolide and solasodine are known to possess adaptogenic and immunomodulating activity.[65,68,69,74]
Anticonvulsant activity	May be mediated via a gamma (γ)-aminobutyric acid (GABA)-ergic mechanism, likely through the barbiturate site on the macromolecule ionophore complex.[68,117]
Antiinflammatory effect	May be mediated by decreased glycosaminoglycan synthesis. Ashwagandha extract increased phagocytosis and intracellular killing of peritoneal macrophages but did not increase the number of peripheral leukocytes.[72]
Antistress/antianxiety effects	Ashwagandha has demonstrated inhibition of stress-induced increases in the dopaminergic receptor population in the corpus striatum.[215] Ashwagandha may have a GABA-mimetic action.[76,83,117,216]
Anticancer effects	Withaferin A is the primary antineoplastic agent. Its mechanisms of action are still unclear.[69] It has been found to arrest cellular division at metaphase; has shown inhibition of protein and nucleic acid syntheses in P388 cells in vitro; and has shown inhibition of ribonucleic acid (RNA) synthesis in Sarcoma 180 cells. Withaferin A induces a G2/M block.[68,69] An immunostimulatory effect may be partially responsible for antineoplastic activity but this is uncertain: in animal experiments, Withaferin A has shown both immunostimulatory and immunosuppressive activity.[69] Some studies have focused on the ability to reduce stress-induced oxidative damage.[72] Rat models have been observed for condensation and fragmentation of chromatin as quantitative markers, as well as other observable cellular changes, to assess the cytoprotective properties of *Withania*.[217] Such researchers propose that *Withania* extracts may help prevent free radical–induced cleavage of deoxyribonucleic acid (DNA). *Withania somnifera* has been shown to increase the percentage of cells containing neurites in human neuroblastoma cells, promote the growth of new dendrites, and may aid in the repair of damaged neuronal circuits.[71] Withaferin A is reported to have a radiosensitizing effect that has been noted in animal studies to reduce the toxicity of irradiation therapy and also improve its effects.[69] Antitumor effects of *Withania* have also been investigated.[218,219]
Memory-enhancing effects	*Withania* appears to mediate stress-induced disruption of memory formation and retention. Neuroelectrical, physical stress–induced, and scopolamine-induced disruption of acquisition and retention of memory consolidation all appear to be significantly reduced with the administration of *Withania* extracts.[73] Animal experiments have noted *Withania* to provide protection to neuronal cell bodies when animals are subjected to stressful conditions.[220] Effects may also be caused by increased cholinergic signal transduction cascade in the brain.
Sedative effects	May be caused by the alkaloid somniferum.
Cardiovascular effects	The steroidal lactones have a mild ionotropic and chronotropic effect on the heart.

parkinsonism.[80] Ashwagandha and other herbs may take the place of benzodiazepines and have a calming effect on the nervous system. Applications for ashwagandha based on traditional use, animal studies, and clinical evidence are listed in Box 5-4.

Overall, toxicity studies have demonstrated a high level of safety of ashwagandha and its extracts.[65,79] The American Herbal Products Association has rated it a class 2b herb (i.e., not to be used during pregnancy); however, the evidence contraindicating its use during pregnancy is limited and questionable, and Ayurvedic practitioners have used it traditionally during pregnancy.[79,81] Because ashwagandha reverses cyclophosphamide-induced neutropenia, it may be prudent to avoid its use in patients with leukemia who are being treated with cyclophosphamide.[69]

Eleuthero

Eleuthero, a native of northeast Asia, is used in TCM for general weakness and debility, lassitude, anorexia, insomnia, and dream-disturbed sleep.[82] Its use as an adaptogen originated in the former Soviet Union in the latter half of the twentieth century, when it was researched and promoted by scientists as

BOX 5-4	**Applications for Ashwagandha**

Anxiety
Arthritis
Cancer (animal and in vitro data)
Cardiovascular effects (animal data)
Cyclophosphamide toxicity (animal data)
Debility
Epilepsy (animal data)
Growth and development
Immune system (animal data)
Infection (animal and in vitro data)
Inflammation (animal data)
Insomnia
Liver disease (animal data)
Memory (animal data)
Morphine withdrawal (animal data)
Muscle spasm (animal data)
Oxidation (animal data)
Pain (animal data)
Sedation (animal data)
Stamina (animal data)
Stress (animal data)
Thyroid stimulant (animal data)

a substitute for *Panax ginseng*, which was more expensive and less accessible. Pharmacologic studies have suggested that its effects are at least equal to, and perhaps superior to, those of *P. ginseng*.[82]

Until recently referred to as Siberian ginseng, the herb is now properly referred to as eleuthero; this acknowledges that although the plants are from the same family, their actions arise from very different chemical constituents.[81] Eleuthero's actions much like ginseng in that they are considered immunomodulating, stress reducing, performance and energy enhancing, anabolic, and adaptogenic—hence the original misnomer.[82] The herb has demonstrated the ability to improve adrenal function, stress tolerance, immune function, resistance to infection (including influenza), and selective memory.[25,36,62,83,84] The plant contains phenylpropionates (e.g., syringin, caffeic acid, sinapyl alcohol, coniferyl aldehyde), lignins (e.g., sesamin, syringoresinol and its glucoside), saponins (e.g., daucosterol, β-sitosterol, hederasaponin B), coumarins (e.g., isofraxidin and its glucoside), vitamins (e.g., vitamin E), and provitamins (i.e., provitamin A [β-carotene]). These molecules have demonstrated a wide range of pharmacologic activities and are associated with an extensive literature base.[85] Six secondary compounds found in *Eleutherococcus* have been shown to have various levels of activity, as shown in Table 5-6. Previously, many of these compounds were referred to as *eleutherosides*; however, as these compounds are not unique to this plant, and had been previously identified from other sources, the term eleutherosides is not properly applied to these constituents.[82,85]

Animal experiments have confirmed not only these actions but also the reduction of natural killer (NK) cell activity and the inhibition of corticosterone elevation induced by swimming stress in animal models.[86] Stress-induced gastric ulcers have been prevented in animal models, and positive results have been shown with reduction of serum lipid-peroxide levels and improved lipid metabolism.[82,87] In healthy volunteers, ingestion of fluid extracts led to markedly increased T-lymphocyte counts and studies have demonstrated overall improvements in cellular defense.[45,87] Studies on athletic performance and stress response have shown that eleuthero improves the testosterone to cortisol ratio by over 28%, a marker of reduced stress response in athletes.[88] Clinical findings also have suggested that patients with moderate fatigue in CFS may benefit from use of eleuthero, and that older adults may safely experience improvement in some aspects of mental health and social functioning after 4 weeks of therapy, although these differences attenuate with continued use.[89] Eleuthero also has been shown to cause reductions in cardiovascular stress response in healthy patients. Eleuthero is considered to have a high safety profile. Russian studies have noted a general absence of side effects and adverse reactions, and there are no expected significant herb–drug interactions; however, its use is not recommended for patients with hypertension or during acute phase of infection, although it may be combined with antibiotics for treatment of dysentery.[25,36,45,90] The German Commission E considers it an invigorating tonic to be used in cases of fatigue, decreased work capacity and concentration, and for convalescence.[45,82] It is not

TABLE 5-6	*Eleutherococcus* Constituents and Effects
Effects	**Constituent(s)**
Antioxidant	Syringin, caffeic acid, caffeic acid ethyl aldehyde, coniferyl aldehyde
Anticancer	Sesamin, sitosterol, isofraxidin
Hypocholesterolemic	Sesamin, sitosterol, β-sitosterol, β-sitosterol 3-D-glucoside
Immunostimulatory	Sesamin, syringin
Choleretic	Isofraxidin
Reduce moderate insulin levels	β-Sitosterol and its glucoside
Radioprotectant	Syringin
Antiinflammatory and antipyretic activities	β-Sitosterol
Antibacterial agent	Caffeic acid

Data from Wichtl M: *Herbal drugs and phytopharmaceuticals: a handbook for practice on a scientific basis,* ed 4, Stuttgart, 2004, Medpharm; Davydov M, Krikorian AD: *Eleutherococcus senticosus* (Rupr. & Maxim.) Maxim. (*Araliaceae*) as an adaptogen: a closer look, *J Ethnopharmacol* 72(3):345–393, 2000; Brekhman II, Dardymov IV: New substances of plant origin which increase nonspecific resistance, *Annu Rev Pharmacol* 9:419–430, 1969.

heating or stimulating to the degree of ginseng or *Schisandra*. In fact, herbalists consider it a generally neutral herb that can be used by anyone.[91,92]

Ginseng (*Panax ginseng; Panax quinquefolius*)

Ginseng species include *Panax ginseng* and *Panax quinquefolius*: Asian and American ginseng, respectively (Fig. 5-5). *Panax notoginseng* and *Panax pseudoginseng* are also ginsengs but are not discussed here. *Eleutherococcus senticosus*, formerly referred to as Siberian ginseng, is not, in fact, a ginseng. White and red ginsengs are both forms of *P. ginseng*; white is unprocessed, and red is steam prepared.[93] In TCM, white and red ginseng are considered to have different actions, the former being much less stimulating, and the latter being used for deep deficiencies and to move the qi. Western herbalists consider American ginseng to be less heating and gentler than either type of Asian ginseng, especially compared with red ginseng. The word *Panax* is derived from the word *panacea* in deference to the plant's wide-ranging uses from immune support to energy enhancement to promotion of longevity. Ginsenosides are considered to be the pharmacologically active components of ginseng; however, as stated in Wichtl, "the theory for its use in traditional medicine cannot be explained based on the criteria of western rational medicine."[82,93]

Chinese medicine has included ginseng in its pharmacopoeias for as long as 5000 years. It is not considered a medication for specific conditions; rather, it is a tonic for improving overall energy and sense of well-being. It is, however, included in formulae for specific conditions, especially those associated with debility, fatigue, immunodeficiency, irritability, insomnia, decreased cognitive and memory functions, and impotence or loss of libido; it is also included in

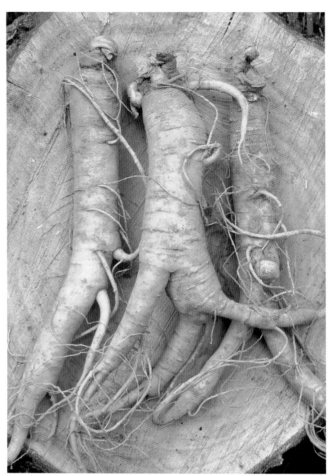

FIGURE 5-5 Ginseng *(Panax ginseng)*. (Photo by Martin Wall.)

BOX 5-5   Summary of Ginseng's Beneficial Effects

Improvement in physical stamina, exercise performance, well-being
Improvement in mental performance, learning, memory
Reduction in fatigue
Improved stress response and functioning under stress
Glucose regulation/blood sugar reduction in non–insulin dependent diabetes (NIDDM)
Improved cardiac function in congestive heart failure
Improved high-density lipoprotein (HDL) levels
Improvement for diminished libido, male fertility problems, erectile dysfunction
Antioxidant activity
Cancer prevention
Improved recovery in infection, especially chronic bronchitis; for the treatment of asthma, chronic obstructive pulmonary disease (COPD), dyspnea
Psychological and physical complaints associated with menopause
Improvement in metabolism; anabolic effects
A tonic for older adults and during convalescence
Reduction in preeclampsia in pregnant women compared with matched controls
Neuralgia, convulsions, neurosis, anxiety, insomnia
Improvement of bifida strains and inhibition of clostridia strains in human intestinal flora

formulae for calming the nerves, promoting the production of moisture in the body, and other conditions. The German Commission E approved its use as a tonic to combat feelings of lassitude and debility, lack of energy and ability to concentrate, and during convalescence.[45] Ginseng is one of the most extensively researched botanical medicines in the world.[93] This review of ginseng is by no means comprehensive, and primarily is intended to convey its overall effects in the context of this section. The actions most ascribed to ginseng are tonic and adaptogenic, demonstrating the ability to enhance nonspecific immunity, inhibit fatigue, and have antiaging effects (Box 5-5).*

Randomized, double-blind, controlled trials have shown that Korean ginseng significantly improves quality of life and well-being measures under stress, including alertness, relaxation, appetite, fatigue levels, sleep quality, recovery from the common cold and bronchitis, and significantly decreases systolic blood pressure compared with controls.[26]

Ginseng's adaptogenic effects are notable in the HPA axis. Ginseng improves recovery from chronic stress by improving corticoid response from the adrenal gland and the corticotropin feedback loops with the HPA.[83,84] Animal

studies have noted ginseng administration to enhance energy metabolism during exercise.[94] *P. ginseng* has been noted to elevate testosterone when low, but not elevate it excessively when within the normal range. *P. ginseng* has been investigated for immune modulating and anticancer activities.[95] Animal and human investigations have shown ginseng to possibly reduce the occurrence of cancer. Mice exposed to carcinogens have fared better when treated with ginseng than untreated controls.[96] In one human trial, *Panax* was shown to be an effective therapy in the treatment of acute infectious bronchitis.[97] Ginseng may improve immune function, as evidenced by increased blood levels of basic immune cells, including natural killer cells, lymphocytes, and macrophages, seen after the administration of ginseng preparations.[98-100]

Enhancing gonadotropin activity may be added to the list of the many uses for *Panax*. Gonadotropin levels have been shown to increase in men with low sperm counts taking ginseng extracts but not in men with normal sperm counts.[101] After 3 months of daily ginseng consumption, testosterone, dihydrotestosterone (DHT), and related sperm counts and sperm motility were noted to improve in the infertile men, whereas normal controls displayed only slight increases, with none of the controls developing abnormally high or excessive levels of hormones. Human clinical studies also observed an increase in libido and erectile function. The Chinese species, Ginseng, is also reported to be a sexual tonic and aphrodisiac useful in maintaining the reproductive organs and sexual desire

*References 26, 82-84, 90, 93-112.

TABLE 5-7   Condition/Botanical Medicine Summary Table

CONDITION/ACTION

Botanical	Adaptogen/Tonic	Antidepressant	Antiinflammatory/Antineuralgia	Antioxidant	Anxiolytic	Cardioprotective/Hypocholesteremic	Chemoprotective	Fatigue/Exhaustion	Antiarrhythmic	Hematopoietic/Erythropoietic	Hepatoprotective	Hyperthyroidism	Hypothyroidism	Immunomodulation	Sedative/Hypnotic	Aphrodisiac	Nootropic	Hypoglycemic	Nervine	Stamina/Energy
Avena sativa					X			X							X	X			X	X
Bauhinia purpurea													X							
Coleus forskohlii													X							
Commiphora mukul													X							
Eleutherococcus senticosus	X	X	X	X	X	X	X	X						X	X		X	X		X
Eschscholzia californica					X														X	
Fucus vesiculosus													X							
Hypericum perforatum		X			X														X	
Lavandula officinalis		X			X														X	
Leonurus cardiaca					X				X			X							X	
Lithospermum officinale												X								
Lobelia inflata					X										X				X	
Lycopus spp.												X								
Matricaria recutita					X														X	
Melissa officinalis		X			X							X							X	
Panax ginseng	X	X		X	X		X	X		X				X	X	X	X	X		X
Panax quinquefolius	X	X			X		X	X									X			X
Passiflora incarnata					X														X	
Piper methysticum		X			X														X	
Rhaponticum carthamoides	X	X		X	X	X	X	X	X						X	X	X		X	X
Rhodiola rosea	X	X		X	X	X	X	X	X					X	X	X	X	X		X
Schisandra chinensis	X		X	X		X	X	X			X			X		X	X			X
Scutellaria lateriflora		X			X														X	
Valeriana officinalis					X														X	
Verbena officinalis					X														X	
Withania somnifera	X	X	X	X	X	X	X			X				X	X	X	X			X

HPA, Hypothalamic-pituitary-adrenal.

into old age. Low sperm counts are a symptom of hypogonadism and hormonal imbalance. There are case reports of acute life-threatening hypopituitarism (i.e., postpartum Sheehan's syndrome) being successfully treated with ginseng and licorice.[102]

Ginseng may improve the stress response by reducing the excessive sympathetic response that promotes a fight or flight cascade. Adrenal cortisol production and activity may be improved, along with corticotropin feedback loops, with the use of adrenal tonic herbs such as *P. ginseng*.[83] Blood sugar reductions have been demonstrated, with potential benefit for patients with type 2 diabetes mellitus.[103,104] Several

human trials have shown clinically useful antianxiety effects with the use of ginseng preparations without any adverse side effects reported.[105] Side effects and drug interactions are not expected with proper use.[35] However, reported side effects in noncontrolled studies in which subjects have been using high doses of caffeine and taking products with additional ingredients have included sleeplessness, anxiety, diarrhea, and skin problems.[35]

Concerns about ginseng abuse syndrome (GAS) occurring with regular use have been entirely debunked, the progenitor of the concept himself retracting his conclusions.[93] Pregnancy use is contraindicated in the *British Herbal*

Compendium to the *BHP;* however, ginseng is traditionally used during pregnancy in China, and studies have shown no teratogenicity, mutagenicity, or other adverse effects, and in fact one study demonstrated a reduction in pre-eclampsia compared with a control group.[93] Neither the American Herbal Products Association nor the German Commission E suggest restricted use during pregnancy; however, given that long-term safety studies are lacking, it is best to avoid except in TCM formulae specifically for pregnancy-related problems and under the supervision of a qualified TCM provider or herbalist skilled in obstetric herbal medicine.[36] Diabetic patients may need to adjust insulin doses; patients taking anticoagulant drugs are recommended to speak with their health care providers before taking ginseng.[36] Herbalists generally discourage the use of stimulants with ginseng, and also may contraindicate ginseng use in patients with hypertension, hyperthyroidism, or other "excess" states (Table 5-7).

Licorice

Although licorice is sometimes categorized as an adaptogen, it does not strictly meet the criteria of one. Its actions are specific rather than nonspecific, and its use in certain patients in high doses or over a prolonged period is not always benign, and in fact can pose serious consequences. However, because of licorice's action on the adrenal glands, as well as on several conditions associated with HPA dysfunction, it raises questions about the potential role of licorice in the prevention and treatment of HPA dysfunction, and merits mention in this section. Peptic ulcer was one of the first conditions ever to be associated with an overactive stress response. Interestingly, licorice extract has demonstrated efficacy against *Helicobacter pylori,* including against clarithromycin-resistant strains.[93,113]

Licorice studies have demonstrated its positive effects in treating viral infection, particularly those caused by herpes simplex virus, an active infection associated with increased stress. A recent study demonstrated that licorice root extract might even interfere with the latency of the herpes virus.[114] Licorice components also have demonstrated the ability to modulate bone disorders in menopausal women because of affinity to 17β-estradiol. This potential exists with or without the presence of vitamin D.[93,115] (Licorice has also demonstrated estrogen-inhibitory effects.[93]) Licorice hydrophobic flavonoids have evidenced abdominal fat-lowering and hypoglycemic effects, possibly mediated via activation of peroxisome proliferator-activated receptor-γ (PPAR-γ).[116]

Researchers examined the effects of licorice on memory and learning in a mouse model and found promise as a memory enhancer in both exteroceptive and interoceptive behavioral models of memory. The antiinflammatory and antioxidant properties of licorice may be contributing favorably to the memory enhancement effect. Because scopolamine-induced amnesia was reversed by licorice, it is possible that the beneficial effect on learning and memory may result from facilitation of cholinergic transmission in the brain.[117] In the treatment of postpartum anterior pituitary insufficiency, 10 patients demonstrated complete recovery with a decoction of licorice and ginseng.[93]

Licorice inhibits corticoid dehydrogenases, prolonging the half-life of cortisol in the body. The *British Herbal Compendium* cites licorice as having adrenocorticotropic activity, indicating it for adrenocorticoid insufficiency.[67] Thus it is sometimes described by herbalists as an adrenal tonic and cortisol sparing.[25,67,118]

Licorice is contraindicated by the German Commission E in patients with cholestatic liver disorders, liver cirrhosis, hypertension, hypokalemia, severe kidney insufficiency, and pregnancy.[45] It is also contraindicated in congestive heart failure and edema.[26] Licorice safety issues are discussed further in discussions of pregnancy and herb safety.

Rhaponticum carthamoides

Rhaponticum carthamoides has been used for centuries in Siberia as a folk medicine for the treatment of fatigue, anemia, and impotence, as well as for convalescence after illness.[119] In 1961, the liquid extract (1:1) was officially recognized and included in the Soviet Pharmacopoeia as a natural agent for overcoming fatigue, improving physical and mental productivity and stamina, and shortening recovery time after illness.[120] The roots and rhizomes are considered the plant's medicinal parts; the active ingredients are primarily phytoecdysteroids (especially ecdysterone), although the plant also contains a number of other biologically active compounds, including flavonoids, sesquiterpene lactones, and polyines.[121,122] *R. carthamoides* extract standardized to 5% ecdysterone is considered the most potent form.[120,123] Several decades of research have demonstrated numerous pharmacologic effects in animal models and human studies.[120,124,125] It is a classic adaptogen with a wide range of activities, including normalizing effect on the CNS and cardiovascular system, sleep, appetite, moods (e.g., neurotic, asthenic, depressive, hypochondriac), mental and physical state, and the ability to function well under stress. It has marked anabolic activities, building lean muscle, reducing body fat, and improving work and athletic capacity and performance; improves mental acuteness; alleviates depression; is a tonic for the vital organ systems; and is erythropoietic and antioxidant, delaying the effects of aging.[120] *R. carthamoides* improves stress response and adaptability to physical and mental challenges, enhances mental and physical capacity for work under stressful conditions, inhibits disorders of energetic metabolism, maintains stable glycogen levels in the skeletal muscles, increases the blood supply to the muscles and brain, and shortens the recovery period after prolonged muscular workloads.[120,126] *R. carthamoides* favorably affects heart rate, improving arterial pressure and hastening recovery after work load.[127,128] In trained athletes, *R. carthamoides* improves endurance, speed, recovery, and physiologic markers, and allows anabolic processes to outpace catabolic processes, leading to greater fitness, endurance, and performance.[120,127,129-132] *R. carthamoides* has also shown some preliminary beneficial outcomes in childbearing women, shortening the duration

BOX 5-6 Therapeutic Actions of *Rhaponticum carthamoides*

Increases protein synthesis, reduces adipose tissue, builds muscle mass

Increases stamina, endurance, athletic performance, work productivity

Improves mental health, learning, memory

Improves additivity to cold climates

Enhances immune activity

Improves insulin sensitivity, stabilizes blood sugar; antidiabetic

Reduces body fat; increases lean muscle

Lowers cholesterol, reduces atherosclerosis; cardiovascular restorative

Antiarrhythmia

Hepatoprotective, hepatoregenerative

Protects against the effects of steroids

Enhances mitochondrial activity

Antioxidant

Stabilizes cell membranes

Anticancer

Antiepileptic

Stimulates erythropoiesis, increasing erythrocytes and hemoglobin

Renal protective

Sexual enhancement

Antidepressant; reduces alcohol cravings

Anti-Giardia; antifungal

of labor and improving postpartum recovery.[120] A comprehensive list of *R. carthamoides'* effects appears in Box 5-6.[119,120,125,132-141]

Rhodiola rosea

Rhodiola rosea, also called golden root, Arctic root, and rose root, grows in arctic and mountain regions throughout Europe, Asia, and America.[142-144] Its use was first recorded by the Greek physician Dioscorides in 77 CE in *De Materia Medica*.[144] It has been used for centuries as a traditional medicine in Russia, Scandinavia, and other countries for the treatment of fatigue, depression, anemia, impotence, GI ailments, infections, and nervous system disorders, and to promote physical endurance, longevity, and work productivity.[144,145] *R. rosea* appeared in the scientific literature of Sweden, Norway, France, Germany, the Soviet Union, and Iceland as early as 1725.[144] Because most of the identified literature on this herb is from foreign language sources, I have relied largely upon secondary sources for this review.[143-145] *R. rosea* has been an accepted medicine in Russia since 1969 for the treatment of fatigue, somatic and infectious illness, psychiatric and neurologic conditions, and as a psychostimulant to increase memory, attention span, and productivity in healthy individuals. It is also officially registered in Sweden and Denmark and is widely used in Scandinavia as a general tonic and to increase mental work ability under stress.[144] *R. rosea* is classified as an adaptogen.[142-145] It contains a range of antioxidant compounds, and its adaptogenic activities are attributed to its unique phenylpropanoids rosavin, rosarin,

and rosidirin, and to phenylethanol derivatives p-tyrosyl and salidroside (also called rhodioloside), as well as to flavonoids, triterpenes, monoterpenes, and phenolic acids. Rosavins are the accepted marker compounds for water and alcohol extracts.[143,144] Research both from animal models and human clinical trials indicates a number of favorable effects associated with its use, including CNS stimulation, pronounced antistress effects, enhanced physical work and exercise performance, increased muscle strength, reduction in mental fatigue, and prevention of high altitude sickness.[142,145-148] Cardioprotective and anticancer effects also have been attributed to its intake.[142,145] Although research on *R. rosea* has been extensive, it has also been described as "fragmentary," with methods, statistics, and controls poorly defined.[142,145] Further, not all studies have yielded positive outcomes for efficacy, although this may be related to product, dose, and duration of administration. *R. rosea* extract exhibited an antiinflammatory effect and protected muscle tissue during exercise.[149] Studies have demonstrated its ability to induce a general sense of well-being and reduce situational anxiety.[144,145] It has demonstrated improvement in depressive syndromes, mental and physical fatigues secondary to medical conditions, sexual dysfunction, thyroid hypofunction (without causing hyperthyroidism), thymus gland functioning, adrenal functioning, and menopause-related conditions.[144,145] Its mechanism of action is partly attributed to the herb's ability to influence levels of monoamines, including serotonin, dopamine, and norepinephrine in the cerebral cortex, brainstem, and hypothalamus through inhibition of degradation enzymes and facilitation of neurotransmitter support in the brain. It also appears to prevent catecholamine release and cyclic adenosine monophosphate (cAMP) elevation in the myocardium, to prevent depletion of adrenal catecholamines by acute stress, and to induce opioid peptide biosynthesis and activation of central and peripheral opioid receptors.[143,150,151] Enhanced antitumor and antimetastatic activity has been demonstrated when *R. rosea* extract is combined with cyclophosphamide (i.e., an antitumor agent).[143,152]

Schisandra

Schisandra, or schizandra, has an ancient history of use in China, where it is called *wu wei zi*, or five-flavored fruit, because of it is said to possess the five flavors of classical Chinese medicine: sour, bitter, sweet, salty, and pungent. Because of this, it is held in high regard in the Chinese materia medica and is still widely used in TCM today.[93,153] In the first century classic herbal compendium, the *Divine Husbandman's Classic of the Materia Medica* (by Shen Nong Ben Cao Jing), schisandra is classified among the superior medicines, purported to "prolong the years of life without aging"; increase energy (qi); treat fatigue, emaciation, and languor; act as a male sexual tonic; and treat asthma.[93,153,154] It was also considered antihepatotoxic, antidiabetic, and antitussive, and is a sedative, tonic, and treatment for cholera. In combination with other herbs, its applications become much broader.[93,154] The fruit is considered highly astringent, and is therefore used for a variety of secretory excesses, including night sweats, chronic diarrhea, and in males, spermator-rhea.[153] Official indications for the fruit include diabetes, frequent urination, night sweats, chronic cough, and dyspnea.[26,93] Schisandra was introduced from eastern Russia into Europe in the 1850s.[93] Since the 1950s, research in the former Soviet Union has focused on its potential uses as an adaptogen, primarily to enhance concentration and increase endurance, and its use is integrated into conventional medical and pharmacy practice in Russia.[62,153] The primary active ingredients are lignans.[93,153,155] It is official in the pharmacopoeias of China, Japan, Korea, and Russia. Current research has focused on its effects in treating diabetes and liver damage related to hepatic disease; for example, hepatitis.[93,153] Hepatoprotective, antioxidant, antiproliferative and chemopreventive, antiinflammatory, cardioprotective, and antimicrobial effects have all been demonstrated in in vivo and in vitro studies.[93,153,156] Hepatoprotective and performance/endurance-enhancing effects have been demonstrated in human clinical studies.[93,157] Research into schisandra's use as an adaptogen was inspired by its TCM use as a tonic for debility. Numerous clinical trials conducted in the 1950s showed improvement in activities requiring concentration, coordination, and endurance, a reduction in fatigue, and an increase in accuracy and work quality.[153] Uncontrolled trials suggest general improvements in mental efficiency in humans, with associated improvement in vision and hearing and skin receptor sensitivity.[158] Animal models have demonstrated adaptogenic effects, including increased renal and gonadal ribonucleic acid (RNA), glycogen, and enzyme levels in older models (rabbits) compared with younger animals.[26] In a double-blind, placebo-controlled randomized controlled trial (RCT) involving race and show-jump horses, treatment with schisandra reduced heart rate, respiratory frequency, and lactate levels, and increased plasma glucose and performance.[26,153] Treated horses also completed the race faster than controls.[153] Similar results demonstrating enhanced performance and recovery after exercise have been found in other studies involving racehorses.[153] In an in vivo study with phenobarbital, ethanol, and ether, intraperitoneal administration of schisandra reduced sleeping time, suggesting antidepressant activity.[26,153] Several other studies have also suggested antidepressant activity, both in animal and human clinical models. One rat study showed a significant increase in dopamine and its metabolites in the rat brain. Stimulating effects on the CNS have been reported, including restlessness, increased aggressiveness, and insomnia at higher doses.[153] Increased resistance to heat and frostbite have both been demonstrated, suggesting the ability of the herb to increase response to environmental stressors.[153] Schisandra is considered to have a high safety profile, and appears to be entirely free of toxicity when used in the recommended dosage range.[153] No clinical reports of overdosage in humans have been identified.[93] According to TCM, schisandra should not be used in cases of excess heat, or in the early stages of a rash or cough.[154] Patients with high gastric acidity or peptic ulcers may experience exacerbation.[153] It is also considered contraindicated in patients with epilepsy, hypertension, and

intracranial pressure.[159] Side effects may include restlessness, insomnia, and dyspnea.[93,154] Schisandra may increase uterine contractility, and is used in TCM to induce or promote prolonged labor; therefore its use is not recommended during pregnancy.[93,153,154]

ADDITIONAL THERAPIES

Dehydroepiandrosterone

Dehydroepiandrosterone (DHEA) and its active metabolite, DHEA sulfate (DHEAS), are endogenous hormones synthesized and excreted primarily by the adrenal cortex in response to ACTH. In women, the synthesis of DHEA and DHEAS occurs almost exclusively in the adrenal cortex. DHEA is classified as an androgen, and may be converted into other hormones, including estrogen and testosterone. DHEA and DHEAS serve as the precursors of approximately 75% of active estrogens in premenopausal women, and 100% of active estrogens after menopause. The levels of DHEA in the blood are typically 10 times those of cortisol.

DHEA is active in the CNS, and is taken up by the amygdala, hippocampus, thalamus, midbrain, and frontal cortex.[160] DHEA and DHEAS also appear to have neurotrophic effects, increasing the number of neurofilament-positive neurons and regulating the motility and growth of corticothalamic projections in cultured mouse embryo brain cells.[161] DHEA and DHEAS output is maximal between the ages of 20 and 30 years and then declines with age at a rate of approximately 2% per year, leaving a residual of 10% to 20% of the peak production by the eighth or ninth decade of life. The exact mechanism of action and clinical role of DHEA and DHEAS remains unclear. Epidemiologic data indicate an inverse relationship between serum DHEA and DHEAS levels and the frequency of cancer, cardiovascular disease (in men only), Alzheimer's disease and other age-related disorders, immune function, and progression of human immunodeficiency virus (HIV) infection.[161]

Beneficial effects of DHEA, based on animal studies, include improved immune function and memory and prevention of atherosclerosis, cancer, diabetes, and obesity. Clinically validated uses of DHEA include replacement therapy in patients with low serum DHEA levels secondary to chronic disease, adrenal exhaustion, or corticosteroid therapy; treating systemic lupus erythematosus (SLE), improving bone density in postmenopausal women; improving symptoms of severe depression; improving depressed mood and fatigue in patients with HIV infection; and increasing the rate of reepithelialization in patients undergoing autologous skin grafting for burns; however, such uses remain controversial.[161] Supporting clinical studies also suggest possible benefit in enhancing immune response and sense of well-being in older adults, and a reduction in some cardiovascular risk factors. Other uses for DHEA, for example, for retarding the aging process, improving cognition, promoting weight loss, increasing lean muscle mass, and slowing the progression of Parkinson's disease and Alzheimer's disease are clinically unsubstantiated.[161]

DHEA supplementation has been found to elevate serum testosterone, estrone, and estriol levels in postmenopausal women. DHEA may lead to an increase in progesterone production indirectly because both DHEA and progesterone require pregnenolone as a precursor. If the body does not have to manufacture DHEA, more pregnenolone may be shunted to progesterone synthesis. Physiologic replacement dosages of oral DHEA in healthy women over 40 range from 5 to 30 mg/day, and are usually given once in the morning. This is generally adequate to raise serum DHEAS to the levels found in adults 20 to 30 years of age and impart the documented benefits of heightened sense of well-being and increased bone mineral density in postmenopausal women.[161] Higher doses may be necessary for increasing suppressed DHEA and DHEAS levels secondary to chronic disease, adrenal exhaustion, and corticosteroid therapy.[161] Pharmacologic dosages of 200 mg/day have been successfully used in patients with SLE. Dosages of 200 to 500 mg/day have been used in HIV-positive patients with depressed mood and fatigue.[161] With physiologic and supraphysiologic doses, the most common side effects include acne and mild hirsutism.[161,162] Rakel suggests that dosages not exceed 50 mg/day of an oral dose regimen in non–adrenal deficient patients.[31] As OTC sources of DHEA are not standardized, inconsistent and insufficient daily administration may be a problem.[31]

The long-term effects of significantly raised androgen levels in women using DHEA are unknown. A case control study of postmenopausal women not taking DHEA or hormone replacement therapy whose levels of endogenous DHEAS were in the highest quartile had a significantly higher risk of breast cancer than women whose levels of endogenous DHEAS were in the lowest quartile. The effects of long-term physiologic or supraphysiologic doses of DHEA on suppression of adrenal cortex are unknown; however, there does not appear to be feedback inhibition of DHEA or DHEAS secretion by the HPA axis.[161] Baseline DHEAS should be checked before initiating therapy and the serum DHEAS level should be checked at least annually to ensure that it is in the normal range.[161] DHEA can affect (raising some, lowering others) serum levels of calcium channel blockers, metformin, corticosteroids, insulin, and triazolam. Diet and exercise also can affect DHEA and DHEAS levels. DHEA supplementation is contraindicated in patients with a history (personal or family) of sex hormone–responsive cancers. DHEA supplementation should be avoided during pregnancy and lactation.[161]

Lifestyle and Reducing the Effects of Stress

Stress is an unavoidable fact of life. Its effects, however, can be mitigated. The effects of lifestyle on preventing and reducing stress and, consequently, stress-related illness, cannot be overstated. The following are simple suggestions for managing stress[52]:

- Avoid emotional eating (overeating and undereating). Teach patients to eat healthy foods, in appropriate amounts for their body and lifestyle, when hungry. This will not only keep the body healthy, but will also lead to weight stabilization. For many women, being overweight is both a result of stress and a cause of stress, leading to a vicious cycle.

- Encourage dietary changes that enrich nutrition and reduce empty calories.
- Take a complex multivitamin and mineral supplement to ensure adequate intake of trace nutrients.
- Drink enough fluids throughout the day.
- Get enough sleep and correct sleep. Sleeping adequate amounts is critical to keeping the neuroendocrine system healthy, reducing stress, and caring well for the body. However, sleeping at optimal hours for the body's hormonal and neurotransmitter systems is also important to health. Cortisol and melatonin, for example, both intrinsic to maintaining proper stress response, have secretory rhythms that are optimized by following diurnal sleep patterns, ideally by going to sleep by 11 PM and rising early in the morning. Although patients with jobs that require night work or women with young children might not be able to achieve this rhythm, lack of this rhythm may be a clue to HPA access disruption and related illnesses such patients are experiencing.
- Get moderate exercise.
- Engage in relaxation techniques, for example, yoga, tai chi, meditation, art "therapy," journaling, and so forth.
- Avoid or minimize caffeine intake.
- Address work–life, relationship, or environmental stressors through making changes, getting counseling, or other means that reduce exposure to life stressors and environmental hazards. Provide patient referral to marriage and family counselors, environmental groups, and so forth as appropriate.
- Social support is one of the most important factors in stress response and life expectancy. Individuals living in isolation respond more poorly to stress and illness, recover more slowly, and have a lower life expectancy than individuals with an established social network and social support.

POLYCYSTIC OVARY SYNDROME

Polycystic ovary syndrome (PCOS) is the most common endocrine disorder in women of reproductive age, spanning adolescence through menopause.[163,164] Previously considered a gynecologic problem diagnosed on the presence of a polycystic ovarian state evidenced by ultrasound, PCOS is now recognized as a complex endocrine disorder with multiple possible etiologies and clinical manifestations, only one of which may be the presence of polycystic ovaries.[165]

PCOS is defined as hyperandrogenism and chronic anovulation in cases in which secondary causes of these signs have been excluded. It is characterized by oligo-ovulation, hyperandrogenism, insulin resistance, an increased luteinizing hormone (LH) to follicle-stimulating hormone (FSH) ratio, decreased sex hormone-binding globulin (SHBG), and hyperlipidemia. Patients may exhibit hirsutism, menstrual irregularities, dysfunctional uterine bleeding (DUB), obesity, anovulatory infertility, miscarriage, acne, alopecia, and affected mood (e.g., irritability, tension, depression).[165-167] PCOS is estimated to affect up to 10% of women of reproductive age in the United States, or 5 million women, although data vary based on the population being studied.[164,167]

PCOS is still considered in the gynecologic realm because patients typically seek gynecologic care for control of abnormal menstrual bleeding, anovulation, and infertility.[164,168] However, it is essential that practitioners expand their view of this condition to recognize the potential long-term and serious health implications associated with PCOS. Available data support significantly increased rates of type 2 diabetes mellitus, dyslipidemia, hypertension, cardiovascular disease, gestational diabetes, gestational hypertension, and endometrial cancer in women with PCOS.[164-166,169-171]

PATHOPHYSIOLOGY

The underlying primary cause of PCOS remains uncertain, and there are numerous proposed etiologies. Several genetic theories have been raised. A genetic predisposition (autosomal dominant) is suggested by familial clustering and increased incidence of female hyperinsulinemia and male pattern baldness in male and female family members of women with anovulation, hyperandrogenism, and polycystic ovaries.[165] Positive findings have been identified in genes that regulate both steroidogenesis and insulin secretion. It is believed that insulin resistance may be caused by aberrations in the insulin receptors. It has also been suggested that PCOS is a result of "thrifty" genes, an adaptive biological response providing advantages (e.g., increased muscle strength, moderate abdominal fatness, and decreased insulin sensitivity, which is an energy-sparing mechanism) to women with this predisposition in times of nutrition shortage. However, a negative response of the mechanism is triggered under conditions of exposure to unlimited food supplies and sedentary lifestyle.[172]

Gestational factors have also been implicated in the development of this condition. In one study, 235 women with PCOS were divided into two groups categorized according to a clinical presentation: obese women with androgenization and elevated LH and testosterone; or under to normal weight women with elevated LH but no androgenization. It was determined that women in the first group had above-average birth weight and were born to obese mothers; women in the second group were born after term (>40 weeks' gestation), reflecting the possibility that events occurring in fetal life may have long-term or irreversible effects on neuroendocrine function.[173,174]

The mechanisms of PCOS are better understood than the causes. In the normal menstrual cycle, gonadotrophin-releasing hormone (GnRH) is secreted from the hypothalamus in a pulsatile manner. GnRH reaches the pituitary gland, where it stimulates the release of FSH and LH. These hormones then act upon the ovaries, where they regulate production of steroid hormones and, as a result, follicular development. LH stimulates production of androgen and progesterone by the theca cells and FSH stimulates the production of aromatase in the granulose cells, which are responsible for the conversion of androgen to estrogen. Local estrogen production nourishes the development of the follicle, whereas nonaromatized androgens inhibit follicular growth. The ovary generally regulates its own environment with feedback mechanisms that cause the decline of FSH secretion as the follicle matures. When estrogen reaches a critical concentration in the general circulation, LH secretion surges, triggering ovulation. After ovulation, progesterone is secreted by the corpus luteum.[163] In PCOS, the GnRH pulsatile frequency is higher than normal, and there is increased circulating LH and decreased FSH. This imbalanced LH:FSH ratio leads to excessive production of androstenedione and testosterone; in the absence of total suppression of FSH, continued follicular growth occurs, but not to the point of maturity, and a resultant atresia of the developing follicles occurs. The classic polycystic ovary results from a state of chronic anovulation. Circulating estrogen levels are elevated owing to increased peripheral conversion of increased amounts of androstenedione to estrogen, primarily in the form of estrone. The chronic absence of progesterone allows an enhanced pulsatile secretion of GnRH, which contributes to the high levels of LH and low levels of FSH in a vicious cycle (Box 5-7).[165]

Elevated Androgens and Hyperactive Cytochrome P450 17 Enzyme

The ovaries and adrenals of women with PCOS are responsible for elevated androgen production. It is postulated that these women have a hyperactive production of cytochrome P450 17 (CYP17) enzyme, responsible for forming androgens from DHEAs at those sites, which is further exacerbated when there is obesity.[165] DHEA is found to be elevated in 50% of women with PCOS. The elevated DHEA is caused by stimulation with ACTH, produced by the pituitary largely in response to stress. The excess DHEA then converts to androgens via adrenal metabolism. This contributes to the typically elevated androgen levels in PCOS. Elevated total and free testosterone levels correlate to the elevated LH levels. The serum total androstenedione is usually elevated to no more than twice the normal range (20 to 80 ng/dL). High androgen levels in the ovary inhibit FSH; hence they inhibit development and maturation of the follicles.[165,175] The skin and adipose tissue add to the complex etiology of PCOS. Women who develop hirsutism have increased sensitivity to androgen activity in the skin; hence they develop abnormal patterns of hair growth. Aromatase and 17-β-hydroxysteroid activities are increased in the fat cells and peripheral

---

> **BOX 5-7**   **Summary of Hormonal Characteristics of Polycystic Ovary Syndrome**
>
> - Elevated luteinizing hormone (LH)
> - Decreased follicle-stimulating hormone (FSH)
> - Overproduction of androstenedione,* testosterone,† dehydroepiandrosterone† (DHA), dehydroepiandrosterone (DHAS), 17-hydroxyprogesterone (17-OHP), and estrone
> - Hyperinsulinemia
> - Inadequate progesterone stimulus owing to anovulatory state
>
> *Almost exclusively adrenal secretion.
> †Mostly ovarian secretion.

aromatization increases with body weight. The metabolism of estrogens by way of 2-hydroxylation and 17-alpha (α)-oxidation is decreased. Estrogen levels increase as a result of peripheral aromatization of androstenedione. This cascade results in chronic hyperproduction of estrogen (i.e., estrogen dominance). Acne is seen in approximately one third of all PCOS patients; also, most women with severe acne have PCOS.[167] Hirsutism occurs in 70% of women with PCOS in the United States, as opposed to only 10% to 20% of Japanese women diagnosed with the syndrome. This may explain the genetically determined differences in 5-α-reductase activity between cultures, or from a holistic standpoint, may reflect differences in endocrine behavior in accordance with local diet and levels of physical fitness.

Estrogen Dominance

Hypothalamic-pituitary-ovarian (HPO) axis imbalance contributes significantly to the etiology of PCOS. The result of increased GnRH output causes an elevation in the pulsatile output of LH and induces an elevated LH:FSH ratio (typically 2:1). Approximately 25% of PCOS patients also exhibit hyperprolactinemia. Hyperprolactinemia results from abnormal estrogen negative feedback from the pituitary gland. Elevated prolactin can contribute to elevated estrogen levels.

Insulin Resistance

In addition to aberrations in HPO axis behavior, insulin resistance and resultant hyperinsulinemia are central to the picture of PCOS.[163,165] Insulin resistance is defined as reduced glucose response to a given amount of insulin, and is commonly referred to as syndrome X. Hyperinsulinemia in hyperandrogenic anovulatory women is accompanied by upper-body obesity characterized by increased abdominal fat.[165,174] Central (android) obesity is associated with significantly increased cardiovascular risk factors including hypertension and poor cholesterol-lipoprotein profiles.[165] A waist to hip ratio of greater than 0.85 indicates android fat distribution.[165] Women with PCOS exhibit substantially increased impaired glucose tolerance (IGT) and a tendency toward non–insulin dependent diabetes (NIDDM) than other women of matched age and weight.[176] The prevalence of IGT is 31.1%, and that of type 2 diabetes is 7.5%, indicating that these women are at significantly increased risk for these conditions and their sequelae.[177] In addition to intrinsic endocrine factors, insulin resistance is caused by poor diet (especially excessive carbohydrate consumption) and stress. Hyperinsulinemia is not always a characteristic of hyperandrogenism but is uniquely associated with PCOS.[175] Thirty percent to 40% of obese women with PCOS have IGT or diabetes. However, women with anovulatory hyperandrogenism can present with normal insulin and glucose tolerance, indicating factors other than IGT involved in the etiology.[175,178]

Acanthosis nigricans—velvety, darkly pigmented skin—is considered a marker of insulin resistance in women with hirsutism. These pigmented lesions can also be found on the nape of the neck, in the axilla, inner thigh, and below the breast. Women with severe insulin resistance can develop

HAIR-AR syndrome, consisting of hyperandrogenism (HA), insulin resistance (IR) and *Acanthosis nigricans* (AR).[167] These women have elevated testosterone (>150 ng/dL) and fasting insulin levels of greater than 25 IU/dL. Insulin alters steroidogenesis secretion (independent of gonadal production) in PCOS because insulin and insulin-like growth factor receptors are located within the ovarian tissue.

Stress

Stress appears to be a factor in the etiology of PCOS. The effects of stress on hormonal dysregulation, cortisol and blood sugar regulation, and adrenal function are well established. One animal study demonstrated that activation of the sympathetic nervous system precedes the induction of polycystic ovaries and that increased sympathetic activity plays a role in the development and maintenance of ovarian cysts. Further research on the role of stress and the development of PCOS is warranted.[179]

SIGNS AND SYMPTOMS OF PCOS

The symptomatology of PCOS is highly variable; therefore close attention should be paid to the presenting clinical picture of the patient.[167] The most common reason for gynecologic evaluation is menstrual irregularity, most commonly oligomenorrhea or amenorrhea.[167,168] Women also commonly seek gynecologic care for infertility and signs of androgen excess.[168]

The following clinical features may be present in PCOS:
- Menstrual irregularity secondary to chronic anovulation or oligo-ovulation
- Dysfunctional uterine bleeding
- Anovulatory infertility
- Hirsutism
- Acne
- Alopecia
- *Acanthosis nigricans*
- Obesity (especially android-type)
- Mood disorders[180]
- Habitual abortion
- Ultrasound evidence of PCOS (not itself indicative of this syndrome)

Menstrual Irregularity

- Eight or fewer menstrual cycles per year
- Unpredictable menstrual cycles
- Amenorrhea for longer than 4 months in the absence of pregnancy or menopause
- Infertility
- History of ovarian cysts
- Irregular bleeding
- DUB (i.e., excessive or heavy bleeding)

Hyperandrogenism

- Acne
- *Acanthosis nigricans*
- Alopecia

- Hirsutism
- Virilization

Obesity

- Seen in approximately 65% of patients with PCOS.[164]
- The body fat is centrally located (truncal, android).[165,174]
- A higher waist to hip ratio (>0.85) indicates an elevated risk of cardiovascular disease and diabetes.[165,167]
- BMI >30[167]
- Presents long-term complications of PCOS

Lipoprotein Profile

An abnormal lipoprotein profile is associated with IGT and is commonly seen in patients with PCOS. The typical PCOS lipoprotein profile includes:

- Elevated total cholesterol
- Elevated triglycerides
- Elevated levels of low density lipoproteins (LDL)
- Low levels of high density lipoproteins (HDL)
- Low apoprotein A-1

The culmination of these factors leads to a marked elevation in cardiovascular risk for the PCOS patient. Another metabolic observation that puts these women at higher cardiovascular risk is the incidence of impaired fibrinolysis, shown by elevated circulating levels of plasminogen activator inhibitor. This is associated with atherosclerosis and hypertension. When these factors are combined, PCOS women are at much higher risk of hypertension, atherosclerosis, and have a sevenfold risk of myocardial infarction.

An ultrasound will reveal ovaries that are enlarged from two up to five times greater than normal, with bilateral microcysts within each ovary, with generally more than five cysts per ovary. The diameter of each cyst is approximately 0.5 to 0.8 cm. As the number of cysts increases and the ovaries become larger, the clinical symptoms become more severe. Polycystic ovaries themselves may be normal and as a single sign are not diagnostic of hyperandrogenism, insulin resistance, or PCOS.

DIAGNOSIS

The major clinical criteria for PCOS include:

- Clinical or biochemical evidence of hyperandrogenism
- Oligo-ovulation or anovulation
- Exclusion of other known disorders (e.g., adrenal hyperplasia, hyperprolactinemia)

Additionally, any of the signs and symptoms presented earlier may be part of the diagnostic picture. Family history of diabetes or menstrual irregularity is significant.

BIOCHEMICAL AND ENDOCRINOLOGY EVALUATION

The following should be evaluated when establishing a definitive diagnosis of PCOS:

- Pituitary and ovarian hormone serum levels:
  - LH
  - FSH

> **BOX 5-8   Risks and Consequences Associated with Polycystic Ovary Syndrome[165]**
>
> - Infertility
> - Menstrual irregularities and dysfunctional uterine bleeding (DUB)
> - Hirsutism, acne, hair loss (i.e., alopecia)
> - Endometrial cancer as a result of unopposed estrogen (and possible increased risk of breast cancer)
> - Cardiovascular disease
> - Diabetes

- Estradiol
- Progesterone
- Prolactin
- β-Human chorionic gonadotropin (HCG) (to rule out pregnancy)
- Circulating androgens and related hormones:
  - Free testosterone and free androgen index (FAI): 17-hydroxyprogesterone (17-OHP)
  - SHBG: 24-hour urinary-free cortisol
  - DHEAS
- Endometrial biopsy
- Glucose tolerance test
- Thyroid panel
- Blood lipid profile

Appropriate diagnosis and treatment are essential to prevention of the sequelae of this condition (Box 5-8).

DIFFERENTIAL DIAGNOSIS

Specific conditions that must be ruled out include[167,174]:
Common:
  Hyperprolactinemia
  Hypothalamic amenorrhea
  Non–PCOS insulin resistance
  Premature ovarian failure
  Obesity from other causes
Rare:
  Cushing's syndrome
  Hyperandrogenism
  Adrenal hyperplasia
Very Rare:
  Androgen-producing tumors

CONVENTIONAL TREATMENT APPROACHES

The overall goals of medical treatment are to:

1. Reduce androgen production and circulation
2. Protect the endometrium against unopposed estrogen
3. Achieve healthy body weight
4. Reduce cardiovascular disease risk
5. Reduce diabetes and hyperinsulinemia risks[165,167]

More specifically, women are currently being treated for their presenting clinical symptoms, including irregular menses, hirsutism, and infertility, as well as according to

TABLE 5-8	Medications Commonly Used for the Treatment of Polycystic Ovary Syndrome
Medication	**Effects/Use**
Oral contraceptives	Combined estrogen and progestin oral contraceptives are known to decrease the adrenal and ovarian production of steroid hormones and reduce hair growth by two-thirds in patients with PCOS and hirsutism. Progestin offers the benefit of lowering elevated LH levels, resulting in reduced ovarian testosterone production. The estrogen increases the liver's production of SHBG, also reducing free circulating testosterone levels. Estrogen inhibits the conversion of testosterone to DHT by inhibiting the enzyme α-5 reductase. The use of oral contraceptives alone is only successful in 10% of cases and insulin resistance can be enhanced by the use of combined oral contraceptives.
Medroxyprogesterone acetate	Oral or intramuscular injection of medroxyprogesterone acetate has been used primarily for contraception and hirsutism. It affects the hypothalamic pituitary axis by decreasing the production of GnRH, hence reducing production of estrogen and testosterone. It also decreases the production of SHBG. If given orally, doses of 20-40 mg daily are suggested; if intramuscular injection is used, 150 mg is administered every 6-12 weeks. It is said to reduce hair production by 95% in responsive patients. Side effects include amenorrhea, headaches, fluid retention, weight gain, liver dysfunction, and depression.
GnRH agonists	These drugs cause ovarian suppression to levels of castration in the patient with PCOS. The drug most commonly used from this class is leuprolide acetate and is given by intramuscular injection every 28 days to suppress ovarian androgens. The oral contraceptive is used concurrently to replace estrogen to prevent bone loss and other menopause-like side effects this drug induces.
Glucocorticoids	Glucocorticoids, such as dexamethasone, are used for patients with adrenal or mixed adrenal and ovarian hyperproduction of androgens. A dose of 25 mg is given daily, which causes suppression of DHEAS production. Excessive doses of this drug can suppress adrenal gland function and cause symptoms of Cushing's syndrome. The drug is used for both hirsutism and acne associated with PCOS.
Ketoconazole	This drug acts by inhibiting key steroid hormone synthesis via inhibition of CYP–dependent enzymes. As a result, when given at a dose of 200 mg per day, it can reduce the production of testosterone, androstenedione, and free testosterone. It also reduces the production of cortisol. Ketoconazole is a strong hepatotoxin.
Spironolactone	Spironolactone specifically inhibits aldosterone-binding sites in the kidney. Originally used as a potassium-sparing diuretic for the treatment of hypertension, spironolactone is used for hirsutism to reduce androgens by inhibiting DHA at the intracellular receptor sites; suppressing testosterone synthesis by decreasing CYP enzymes; increasing androgen catabolism; and inhibiting 5-α-reductase activity in the skin. Moderate improvement in hirsutism can be seen in 70%-80% of PCOS women within 6 months on a dose of at least 100 mg for 6 months. The side effects of this drug include metrorrhagia, which occurs in 50% of women on doses greater than 200 mg per day. Other side effects include urticaria, mastodynia, and scalp hair loss. The patient's potassium and creatinine levels need to be monitored carefully while on this drug. It is essential that a woman uses contraception while on spironolactone because it can cause feminization of a male fetus if she becomes pregnant.
Flutamide	Flutamide is a nonsteroidal antiandrogen first used for prostate cancer. Now used for PCOS, it acts by inhibiting the binding of androgens at target tissue. It also reduces elevated LH and FSH levels typically seen in PCOS and is often combined with the oral contraceptive pill. Side effects include dry skin, reduced libido, hot flashes, increased appetite, liver toxicity, breast tenderness, nausea, and headaches.
Finasteride	This drug is classified as a specific inhibitor of 5-α-reductase activity and reduces the hirsutism associated with PCOS. In clinical trials, most improvement was seen after 6 months on a dose of 7.5 mg per day taken orally. Finasteride is said not to cause menstrual irregularity nor to suppress ovulation. It is often used in combination with an oral contraceptive because it is said to be more effective this way. The oral contraceptive increases circulating SHBG, which further decreases the free testosterone. As with spironolactone, this drug can cause feminization of a male fetus; hence it needs to be used concurrently with contraception.

References 163-165,168,175,178.
PCOS, Polycystic ovary syndrome; *LH*, luteinizing hormone; *SHBG*, sex hormone-binding globulin; *DHT*, dihydrotestosterone; *GnRH*, gonadotrophin-releasing hormone; *DHEAS*, dehydroepiandrosterone sulfate; *DHA*, dehydroepiandrosterone; *CYP*, cytochrome P450; *FSH*, follicle-stimulating hormone.

complaints or desired outcome (e.g., persistent acne, achieving pregnancy).[175,178,181] Table 5-8 provides a comprehensive overview of medications commonly used to treat PCOS.

Irregular Menses

Oral contraceptive pills (OCPs) are commonly used to regulate the menses, and have been the mainstay of long-term PCOS treatment. They suppress pituitary LH, increase SHBG, and decrease androgen secretion. The combined pill often worsens insulin resistance and if the patient falls into the categories of being overweight or obese, this therapy is relatively contraindicated. Also, the long-term safety of OCPs has been questioned. However, recent studies have indicated that a combination of OCPs with metformin improved hyperinsulinemia and hyperandrogenism in nonobese women with PCOS.[163,164,175,178]

Hirsutism

Hirsutism is addressed with the administration of antiandrogens or spirolactone. The action of these drugs is to inhibit binding of DHT to the receptors at the hair follicle site.[163,164]

Infertility

Clomiphene citrate is suggested to women with PCOS with diagnosed fertility challenges. Clomiphene citrate induces ovulation and does increase risk of multiple pregnancies. This drug acts by inhibiting estrogen negative feedback at the hypothalamus, thus enhancing the pituitary's production of FSH.[164]

Oral Hypoglycemic Agents: Metformin

Hyperandrogenism is said to be substantially relieved using metformin therapy, which leads to a decrease in insulin levels and results in improved reproductive function. Metformin is given orally at a dose of 500 mg three times daily. For obese women trying to conceive with PCOS, metformin is combined with clomiphene citrate for best results in restoring ovulation. The most common side effects of metformin are nausea, vomiting, diarrhea, bloating, and flatulence. One study confirmed that diabetics have substantially decreased cardiovascular risks with metformin treatment.[163,164,167,182-184]

Surgical Treatment

Ovarian wedge resections can be performed to reduce androstenedione levels and decrease plasma testosterone levels; however, in patients with hirsutism and PCOS, hair reduction was only noted to a figure of 16%.[165,178]

Weight Management

Numerous clinical studies have demonstrated that in women with obesity, insulin resistance, and PCOS, a weight loss of 5% to 10% of body weight can result in regulation in the menstrual cycle and a dramatic reduction in risk factors, likely through insulin regulation.[166,178,185-189] Richardson describes weight loss as the most successful and globally beneficial therapy for obese women with PCOS but also the most difficult to implement. Weight loss alone has led to achievement of pregnancy in 60% of cases without other medical intervention.[164] Weight loss may improve signs of hyperandrogenism and menstrual irregularity, hyperinsulinemia, restore ovulation and fertility, and improve gonadotrophin pulsatile secretion, and may prevent NIDDM and cardiovascular disease. Weight loss also decreases ovarian P450c17 α-activity and reduces free serum testosterone in obese women with PCOS.[166,178,185-189] Encouragement of lifestyle changes, for example, weight loss and regular exercise, should be part of any treatment plan for overweight women with PCOS. It is interesting to note, however, that short-term caloric restriction does not reduce LH secretion, an apparent paradoxical effect in light of other findings, leaving questions unanswered as to the exact mechanisms

of long-term weight loss, which demonstrates clear improvement of endocrinology markers.[189]

Strategies for weight loss include:
- Moderate weight loss over time (not rapid or drastic)
- Gentle exercise
- Consumption of low glycolic index carbohydrates; reduced intake of fats and simple sugars
- Avoidance of hypoglycemia through frequent meals (4 to 6 times/day)[164]

In addition to the direct health benefits of weight loss, there are the additional and important improvements in body image, self-esteem, and a sense of personal control as a result. These improvements can lead to marked reduction in depression and other affective moods associated with PCOS.[164,180]

BOTANICAL TREATMENT OF PCOS

Little direct research has been done on the use of botanicals for the treatment of PCOS. Nonetheless, many women seek alternatives to reliance on conventional pharmaceutical interventions for this condition. Botanical treatment strategies for PCOS are best directed at stress reduction and management, and improvement of HPA axis response through the use of adaptogens. Adaptogens also play a positive role in glycemic regulation. In fact, the role of adaptogens should be given primary consideration. *Vitex* may play a role in hormonal regulation, particularly hyperprolactinemia and progesterone insufficiency. A small amount of Chinese research has been done on a TCM formula containing *Paeonia lactiflora* and *Glycyrrhiza glabra* for PCOS, and this is or "discussed below".

Adaptogens are discussed generally or "below", and at length elsewhere in this book (see index for "Adaptogens," as well as specific herbs in this category).

The herbs discussed under supporting evidence may have direct benefit in the metabolic or endocrine disruption particular to PCOS. Protocol for the treatment of acne, infertility, amenorrhea, DUB, mood disorders, and other PCOS symptoms should be incorporated into treatment protocol for PCOS as needed. Refer to the relevant sections of this book for these additional treatment strategies. Weight loss should be a primary goal in the care of overweight women with PCOS, and counseling should be recommended as needed, especially when there is poor self-esteem (common with acne, obesity, and hirsutism), or debilitating mood disorders (Table 5-9).

Discussion of Botanicals
Adaptogens and Polycystic Ovary Syndrome
- American ginseng
- Ashwagandha
- Eleuthero
- Ginseng
- Licorice
- Rhaponticum
- Rhodiola
- Schizandra

TABLE 5-9 Summary of Botanical Treatment Strategies for Polycystic Ovary Syndrome

Therapeutic Goal	Therapeutic Action	Botanical Name	Common Name
Improve stress response and HPA function	Adaptogens	*Eleutherococcus senticosus*	Eleuthero
		Glycyrrhiza glabra	Licorice
		Panax ginseng	Ginseng
		Panax quinquefolius	American ginseng
		Rhaponticum carthamoides	Rhaponticum
		Rhodiola rosea	Rhodiola
		Schizandra chinensis	Schizandra
		Withania somnifera	Ashwagandha
Hormonal regulation (increased progesterone secretion; LH:FSH regulation, decreased prolactin)	Hormonal regulators	*Glycyrrhiza glabra/uralensis*	Licorice
		Paeonia lactiflora	White peony
		Tribulus terrestris	Tribulus
		Verbena officinalis	Blue vervain
		Vitex agnus-castus	Chaste berry
Glycemic regulation/improve lipid profile	Antihyperlipidemics	*Gymnema sylvestre*	Gymnema
Treatment of:			
Acne	See Acne		
Amenorrhea	See Amenorrhea		
Dysfunctional Uterine Bleeding	See Dysfunctional Uterine Bleeding		
Depression	See Depression		
Anxiety	See Anxiety		
Infertility	See Chapter 16		

HPA, Hypothalamic-pituitary-adrenal; *LH*, luteinizing hormone; *FSH*, follicle-stimulating hormone.

In response to stress, the adrenals release cortisol, inducing an elevation in prolactin (i.e., the "stress hormone") and increased androgen synthesis, which in turn leads to menstrual cycle dysregulation, especially anovulation, characteristic of PCOS. Physiologically, the HPA axis can be supported with adaptogens.[190] Combining adaptogenic herbs such as ginseng (*P. ginseng* or *P. quinquefolius*), eleuthero, and ashwagandha improve resistance to stress through modulation at the adrenal level. These herbs act to regulate the HPA axis and assist in general adaptation. Many adaptogens (e.g., *Panax* spp.) also have regulatory effects on blood sugar. Licorice is the only adaptogen that has been studied specifically for its effects on PCOS (see Peony; also see Adrenal Support).

Blue Vervain

Blue vervain is a favorite nervine of many herbalists specializing in gynecologic care for its regulating effects on emotional irritability associated with hormonal fluctuations, especially with premenstrual syndrome (PMS). The German Commission E cites its uses for, among other things, irregular menstruation, nervous disorders and exhaustions, and complaints of the lower urinary tract; however, the efficacy for these claims remains unsubstantiated.[191] Many herbalists consider sluggishness of the liver to be at fault, and attribute blue vervain's hormonal action to stimulated liver function and subsequent actions on hormonal metabolism and elimination.

Chaste Berry

Chaste berry should be considered for hyperprolactinemia and low progesterone associated with PCOS. A review of the available literature on *Vitex* indicates evidence of efficacy for hyperprolactinemia, corpus luteum insufficiency, and infertility associated with corpus luteum insufficiency.[192] Hyperprolactinemia and latent hyperprolactinemia are frequent causes for cyclical disorders including corpus luteal insufficiency, which can lead to PMS, secondary amenorrhea, and premenstrual mastalgia. *Vitex* demonstrated the ability to regulate prolactin production through dopamine agonist activity at the hypothalamic-pituitary level.[192-194] The dopaminergic compounds in chaste berry have been identified as the diterpene, including rotundifuran and 6β,7β-diacetoxy-13-hydroxy-labda-8,14-diene. It may be extrapolated from pharmacologic studies that *Vitex* is indirectly progestogenic, and may play a role in conditions where there is unopposed estrogen, an important factor in the association between PCOS and an increased risk of endometrial cancer.[194] Proposed mechanisms of *Vitex* for attenuating hyperprolactinemia include inhibition of estrogen receptor-A expression and an increase of estrogen receptor-B expression in pituitary cells.[195] No studies were identified evaluating the role of *Vitex* in PCOS treatment.

Gymnema

Gymnema is a traditional Indian herb used as an antidiabetic, hypoglycemic, lipid-lowering agent that supports weight reduction. *Gymnema* has a trophorestorative action of the β-cells of the pancreas. The leaf is the plant part used medicinally. The key constituents of *Gymnema* include saponins and gymnemic acids. *Gymnema* is indicated in PCOS for its insulin-modulating activity, with added benefits in reducing elevated triglycerides. Key constituents suppress the perception of the sweet taste on the taste buds, so if taken before

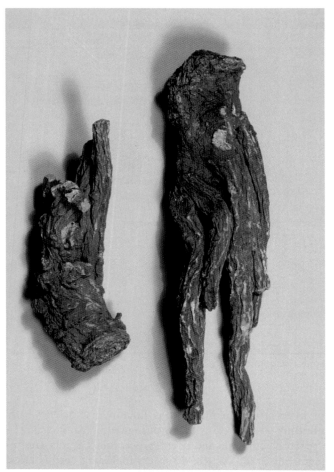

FIGURE 5-6 Peony *(Paeonia lactiflora).* (Photo by Martin Wall.)

food, masks sweet detection and reduces desire for sweet foods and caloric intake for 90 minutes after administration.[196] *Gymnema* has demonstrated hypoglycemic activity in experimental models of diabetes, NIDDM, and hyperglycemia. Its mechanism of action includes the inhibition of glucose absorption in the intestine by the saponin fraction of the herb.[194]

Peony (White)

White peony (Fig. 5-6) is a frequently used gynecologic herb in TCM. Western herbalists use it for PCOS, hyperprolactinemia, endometriosis, ovarian failure, and androgen excess. *Paeonia* has been shown to positively influence low progesterone, reduce elevated androgens (testosterone), and modulate estrogen and prolactin. In vitro, the active constituent paeoniflorin has been shown to affect the ovarian follicle by its action on the aromatase enzyme.[191] Aromatase is necessary for follicle maturation, ovulation, corpus luteum function, steroid hormone synthesis, and the regulation of conversion of androgens to estrogens. The feedback mechanisms of the pituitary and hypothalamus rely on aromatase to regulate prolactin and GnRH. The traditional Chinese formula known as Shakuyaku-Kanzo-To or TJ-68, which

is a decoction of *Glycyrrhiza glabra* and *Paeonia lactiflora,* has been subject to a number of clinical trials, all of which demonstrate activity in hormonal regulation of androgens. In one trial of TJ-68, eight women with hyperandrogenism and oligomenorrhea were given the formula for 2 to 8 weeks. This combination regulated LH:FSH ratios. Over this period of time, serum testosterone levels decreased to less than 50 ng/dL and this resulted in seven of the eight women regularly ovulating.[197] Another trial with TJ-68 involved 20 women diagnosed with PCOS. The formula was successful in lowering testosterone in 90% of the women, of which 25% went on to conceive.[198] It is suggested that TJ-68 acts directly on the ovary, increasing the activity of aromatase, which promotes the synthesis of estradiol from the testosterone, thus lowering serum testosterone levels. It also seems to regulate the LH:FSH ratio. Paeoniflorin has also demonstrated antihyperlipidemic and antihyperglycemic effects in animal models.[199,200] Licorice is contraindicated in patients with hypertension.

Sarei-to

One study reports on the use of the Chinese herbal medicine Sairei-to for the treatment of anovulatory PCOS patients. As a result of treatment, serum LH and the LH:FSH ratio significantly decreased and the ovulatory rate was 70.6%. Serum testosterone levels were within normal limits before the treatment, and did not significantly change during the treatment. The authors concluded that the preparation appears to have a steroidal effect.[201]

Tribulus

As a result of Bulgarian research, *Tribulus* has become a popular herb for the treatment of female and male endocrine disorders.[202] It is considered a general tonic, aphrodisiac, estrogen, and androgenic modulator, and is used to restore vitality and libido, and reduce the physiologic effects of stress. Bulgarian research has identified a steroidal saponin known as a furostanol saponin, calculated to contain no less than 45% protodioscin. The leaf is noted to be higher in the unique saponin rather than the fruit. Other active constituents include phytosterols and spirostanol glycosides. The tonic activities are exacted through intensifying protein synthesis and enhancing the activity of enzymes associated with energy metabolism.[196] Protodioscin, a steroidal saponin in *Tribulus,* has been proven to improve sexual desire via the conversion of protodioscin to DHEA.[203] It has also been observed that *Tribulus* grown in different soils does not consistently produce the important active furosterol, protodioscin. To ensure the desired clinical results, it is recommended to use only the Bulgarian-grown *Tribulus* standardized to 40% furosterol saponins by ultraviolet (UV) analysis. It is not interchangeable with the Chinese or Indian *Tribulus.* It is best used on days 5 to 14 of the menstrual cycle to restore menstrual regularity (Box 5-9).

Black Cohosh

The hormonal aspects of an anovulatory cycle predisposes the ovary to cyst development. One trial (n = 100) assessed

---

BOX 5-9 Sample Botanical Prescriptions for Polycystic Ovary Syndrome

The first two formulae here are recommended by herbalist Amanda McQuade Crawford in her book *Herbal Remedies for Women* as a biphasic treatment for ovarian cysts. They are slightly modified to fit the dosage strategy used in this textbook.

Formula 1: Menstruation through Ovulation (Tincture)

Black cohosh	(*Actaea racemosa*)	30 mL
Blue cohosh	(*Caulophyllum thalictroides*)	25 mL
Milk thistle seed	(*Silybum marianum*)	20 mL
Wild yam	(*Dioscorea villosa*)	10 mL
Black haw	(*Viburnum prunifolium*)	10 mL
Yarrow	(*Achillea millefolium*)	5 mL
		Total: 100 mL

Dose: 5 mL, three times daily.

Formula 2: Ovulation to the Onset of Menstruation (Tincture)

Chaste berry	(*Vitex agnus-castus*)	30 mL
Black cohosh	(*Actaea racemosa*)	30 mL
Dandelion root	(*Taraxacum officinale*)	15 mL
Wild yam	(*Dioscorea villosa*)	15 mL
Black haw	(*Viburnum prunifolium*)	10 mL
		Total: 100 mL

Dose: 5 mL, three times daily.

Hormonal Normalizing Formula for Polycystic Ovary Syndrome (Tincture)

This formula is designed to have a normalizing effect on the hypothalamic-pituitary-ovarian (HPO) axis, and thereby a regulating effect for women with polycystic ovary syndrome (PCOS).

Chaste berry	(*Vitex agnus-castus*)	30 mL
White peony	(*Paeonia lactiflora*)	20 mL
Black cohosh	(*Actaea racemosa*)	20 mL
Dong quai	(*Angelica sinensis*)	20 mL
Hops	(*Humulus lupulus*)	10 mL
		Total: 100 mL

Dose: 5 mL, three times daily.

For women prone to blood sugar dysregulation, also give 2.5 mL each daily of *Gymnema* and fennel tinctures.

---

the effect of a black cohosh preparation in ovulation induction in women with PCOS. Patients were randomized into groups receiving clomiphene citrate (100 mg daily for 5 days) or black cohosh (20 mg daily for 10 days) starting day 2 of the menstrual cycle for three consecutive cycles. Levels of FSH, LH, FSH:LH ratio, progesterone, endometrial thickness, and pregnancy rate were measured throughout the study. The black cohosh group experienced changes in LH and progesterone levels, improved FSH:LH ratio, and increases in endometrial thickness compared with the clomiphene citrate group. (Klimadynon(®) Black cohosh extract).[204]

Cinnamon

Cinnamon may benefit PCOS patients by increasing insulin sensitivity. A 2008 pilot study (n = 15) examined the effects of cinnamon extract in treating PCOS. Participants were assigned to receive cinnamon or a placebo daily over 8 weeks. Using fasting and oral glucose tolerance tests, statistically significant results were seen in the cinnamon group compared with the placebo. (Extract dose not noted.)[205]

CASE HISTORY: POLYCYSTIC OVARY SYNDROME

Sarah, age 34, who is thinking about getting pregnant, presented with irregular menses. She was diagnosed with polycystic ovary syndrome (PCOS) in the past 2 years. Up until 6 months before her naturopathic consultation, she has taken an oral contraceptive in combination with Levoxyl but suffered side effects of heightened emotional lability from these drugs. Her menstrual cycle varied in length from 50 to 70 days and she experienced midabdominal cramping for 24 hours before the onset of her menses. The flow, after starting with brown spotting for 12 to 18 hours, was light to medium, lasted for 4 to 5 days, and was dark red in color. She has had occasional menstrual clots. Her skin was affected badly from the PCOS and she experienced painful, deep cystic acne on her face, chest, and back, which was worse for up to a week before the onset of each menses. She had taken two courses of isotretinoin (Accutane) within the past 5 years and regularly used tetracycline for treatment of her acne. Breast tenderness was an uncomfortable premenstrual feature. She had gained 23 pounds over the past 3 years, which she had difficulty losing despite exercise on a regular basis. She had a high carbohydrate diet and craved sugar intensely. She was a shift worker in a high-stress and high-responsibility occupation; she experienced fatigue daily. She was taking prescription thyroid medication for Hashimoto's thyroiditis, diagnosed 4 years prior, at which time she was also diagnosed as having secondary osteoporosis. Recent evaluation of her spinal density indicated osteopenia; her femoral density indicated osteoporosis; and total hip density indicated severe osteopenia.

Treatment Summary for PCOS
- Achieve a healthy weight.
- Modify the diet and lifestyle for heart protection.
- Control insulin resistance and hyperlipidemia through dietary modification and the use of herbal adaptogens such as eleuthero, licorice, ginseng, *Rhodiola*, and *Schisandra*, among others, and antihyperlipidemics, for example, *Gymnema*.
- Treat hormonal dysregulation with herbs such as licorice, peony, *Tribulus*, blue vervain, and chaste berry.
- Treat symptoms of PCOS such as acne, amenorrhea, dysfunctional uterine bleeding (DUB), depression, and anxiety. See relevant chapters for botanical and additional treatment strategies for these conditions and combine protocol accordingly.
- See Chapter 16 for the treatment of infertility associated with PCOS.

Additional Assessment

Hormonal evaluation showed a typical pattern of a 2:1 luteinizing hormone (LH) to follicle-stimulating hormone (FSH) ratio, with elevated testosterone and hyperlipidemia.

Treatment Protocol

Chaste berry	(Vitex agnus-castus)	20 mL
White peony	(Paeonia lactiflora)	20 mL
Gymnema	(Gymnema sylvestre)	20 mL
Schisandra	(Schisandra chinensis)	20 mL
Echinacea	(Echinacea spp.)	10 mL
Licorice	(Glycyrrhiza glabra)	10 mL
		Total: 100 mL

Dose: 8 mL, twice daily.

Additionally:

Tribulus concentrated extract, equivalent to fucosterol saponins (protodioscin) 300 to 400 mg per day on days 5 to 14 of the cycle to ensure cyclic regularity.

After 5 months on the herbal protocol, the patient's cycle regulated to a 32-day length with a consistent 15-day follicular phase and 17-day luteal phase. Problematic symptoms such as mastalgia, acne, and hirsutism diminished significantly during the 5-month program. The lipid profile has improved to within normal ranges and with the inclusion of a combined regimen of *Gymnema,* and dietary modification (low carbohydrate diet). She lost a total of 12% body weight in the 5 months. The client became pregnant in her second month of actively trying to conceive.

NUTRITIONAL CONSIDERATIONS

An extensive literature review specific to lifestyle factors and PCOS demonstrates that an essential treatment strategy for ameliorating the symptoms of PCOS and aiming to resolve the underlying metabolic derangements is the implementation of a weight loss program. Modulating the diet not only helps reduce hyperinsulinemia and normalizes female endocrine function, but also serves as a preventative against cardiovascular risk factors. Dietary modification is discussed under Weight Management (see earlier discussion).

Supplements

Chromium appears to have a beneficial role in the regulation of insulin action and its effects on carbohydrate, protein, and lipid metabolism, although not all studies have demonstrated favorable effects on blood glucose. Chromium appears well tolerated, with no toxicity even at 1000 μg/day, well above the typically recommended 200 μg/day dose.[206,207] Fish oil may

be protective and beneficial for patients with PCOS and a dyslipidemic profile for its ability to reduce serum triglycerides in diabetics.[207]

N-acetyl-cysteine (NAC) may also be beneficial for PCOS patients. A randomized clinical trial (n = 100) compared the efficacy of NAC with metformin in PCOS treatment. Patients were randomized to receive either metformin (500 mg three times daily) or NAC (600 mg three times daily) for 24 weeks. Outcomes were measured through hirsutism scoring, body mass index (BMI), serum levels of FSH, LH, DHEAS, 17-hydroxyprogesterone, total and free testosterone, androstenedione, TSH, SHBG, prolactin, glucose tolerance tests (i.e., glucose, insulin), TNF-α, and lipids. End point evaluations suggested decrease of LH, total testosterone, and free testosterone and significant increase of SHBG in both groups. Hirsutism also improved in both groups. Nine patients experienced the restoration of menstrual regularity in the metformin group and 11 patients did so in the NAC group (36% vs. 34%). A decrease in LDL was observed in the NAC group but not the metformin group. Both groups exhibited positive differences in HOMA-IR=Homeostatic model assessment for insulin resistance scores.[208]

A combination of 4 g of myo-inositol and 400 mcg of folic acid significantly improved ovulation and conception in women with PCOS, at a rate better than a dose of 1500 mg per day of metformin. D-chiro-inositol, at 1200 mg per day, has been shown to improve insulin sensitivity and reduce serum testosterone levels in women with PCOS. Myo-inositol (up to 4 g per day) may be substituted, or a combination of the two may be used and may even be superior. Legumes are also rich in inositol.

Pinitol, similar to d-chiro-inositol, at 600 mg twice daily for 3 months lowered blood glucose levels by 19%, lowered average glucose levels by 12%, and significantly improved insulin resistance.[209-214]

ADDITIONAL THERAPIES

Stress Management

As discussed throughout this section, stress plays a direct role in HPA hormonal responses that affect the endocrine system and contribute to PCOS. Stress management strategies therefore are an important part of PCOS treatment.

Exercise

Implementing an exercise regime of approximately 30 minutes per day will assist weight loss and improve stress management. Light cardiovascular activity, even just a 30-minute walk daily, can also reduce cardiovascular disease risk.

Sleep, Mood, and Sexual Function

INSOMNIA

Insomnia is defined as dissatisfaction with the quantity, quality, or timing of one's sleep or sleep disturbance occurring at least three times per week for at least 1 month; it is often associated with daytime dysfunction that impairs regular activities at home or work.[1,2] It commonly manifests as the inability to fall asleep (i.e., prolonged sleep latency), sleep interrupted by periods of wakefulness, or early morning waking.

Rest is a critical biological need; individuals with insomnia experience significant consequences caused by lack of restorative sleep, including fatigue, exhaustion, depression, irritability, cognitive disturbances, decreased job performance, weight gain, chronic pain, and even an increased rate of accidents, such as motor vehicle accidents.

Insomnia is divided into two main categories: primary (i.e., extrinsic) insomnia resulting from psychosocial problems, poor sleep hygiene (discussed in the following), situational stresses, or substance misuse or abuse; and secondary (i.e., intrinsic) insomnia, caused by psychophysiologic problems or comorbidities (e.g., sleep apnea, restless leg syndrome [RLS], shift work disorder, and circadian rhythm disorders).[1] It is estimated that between 10% and 50% of Americans report insomnia at any given time.[1,2] It may be transient, short term, or long term.[2]

Common causes of insomnia include sleep rhythm reversals, nightmares, RLS, nocturnal leg cramps, snoring, sleep apnea, pain (e.g., arthritis or other chronic pain), dyspnea (e.g., caused by congestive heart failure), allergies, psychological stress, depression, anxiety, panic disorder, hormonal changes of perimenopause (particularly waning progesterone levels), urinary frequency, gastroesophageal reflux, and hyperthyroidism.[1,3]

Use of substances such as alcohol, caffeine, and nicotine, as well as many prescription and over-the-counter (OTC) medications, is common and can cause or exacerbate insomnia. Some of these agents are also addictive and can cause side effects. Sleep disturbances are more common in women than men, and sleep disorders are more likely to occur at specific times during the female reproductive life cycle; for example, with symptomatic premenstrual periods, physical discomforts associated with pregnancy, nocturnal hypoglycemia in pregnancy, hormonal changes and neurovegetative symptoms

The editor wishes to thank *Botanical Medicine for Women's Health* Edition 1 contributor Clara A. Lennox for her original contributions to this chapter.

(e.g., hot flashes) associated with menopause, and also old age (possibly caused by decreased melatonin production).[4,5]

DIAGNOSIS

The diagnosis of insomnia is typically based on subjective reporting by the patient, and when possible, reporting by the patient's bed partner, who may be able to objectively convey information about the nature of the sleep disturbance.[4] A careful history and routine physical examination are conducted to rule out or determine whether there are associated or underlying problems. The type of insomnia (i.e., difficulty with sleep onset, sleep maintenance, early awakening) can be indicative of associated disorders (Table 6-1).

It is important to query the patient about possible precipitants of sleep problems, such as relationship or work-related problems and other stressors, whether there have been any recent life events that may have led to the sleep disturbance (e.g., recent loss of a loved one, loss of a job, trauma, posttraumatic stress), or any circumstances that might perpetuate sleep disturbances. Examples include working in bed, eating in bed before sleep, watching television in bed, having unrealistic expectations (e.g., that one must have 8 hours of sleep each night to feel rested), trying too hard to sleep and remaining in bed when sleep will not come easily, sleeping with a partner who snores or sleeps restlessly, or having arguments with a spouse or partner in bed.

Patients should be asked about physical problems that may cause them to wake during the night; for example, dyspnea, indigestion, pain, or restless or cramping legs. Sleep studies are rarely necessary for the diagnosis of common sleep disturbances. The phenomenon known as "adrenal fatigue" is associated with hypothalamic-pituitary-adrenal (HPA) axis dysregulation; patients experience a chronic state of hypervigilance associated with being "tired and wired," that is, exhausted but unable to fall asleep or achieve restful sleep. This is attributed to disruption in the diurnal cortisol rhythms and may be demonstrated by elevated evening or nighttime cortisol levels on salivary cortisol testing.

CONVENTIONAL TREATMENT APPROACHES

A range of therapies from nonpharmacologic to drug based are available, and treatments encompass the many possible etiologies of sleep disorders. Nonpharmacologic strategies include promotion of sleep hygiene (Box 6-1), cognitive behavioral

TABLE 6-1   Types of Sleep Disturbance and Associated Conditions

Sleep Disturbance	Possible Causes
Delayed sleep onset	Retiring to bed prematurely
	Poor sleep hygiene
	Anxiety
	Mood disorders, including depression and bipolar disorder
	Restless leg syndrome
Stimulants (e.g., caffeine, medications, drugs)	Pain/neuropathy
	Dyspnea or respiratory disorders
Sleep maintenance	Excessive time in bed
	Mood disorders
	Sleep apnea
	Dyspnea or respiratory disorders
	Pain
	Neurologic disease
Early waking	Major depression
	Learned or conditioned waking
	Required waking for work, school, family responsibilities

Adapted from Becker P: Insomnia: prevalence, impact, pathogenesis, differential diagnosis, and evaluation, *Psychiatr Clin North Am* 29:855–870, 2006.

BOX 6-1   Sleep Hygiene

Sleep hygiene refers to a set of practices that promote restful, effective sleep. These include:

- Wait until you are sleepy to go to bed.
- If you are not asleep after 20 minutes, get out of the bed and do something relaxing; for example, read.
- Use rituals that help you relax each night before bed; for example, take a warm bath.
- Get up at the same time each morning.
- Avoid taking naps if possible.
- Keep a regular schedule for meals, medications, chores, and other activities.
- Do not eat, watch TV, use the computer, or talk on the phone in bed—use bed only for sleep (and sex).
- Do not have caffeine after lunch.
- Do not have a beer, a glass of wine, or any other alcohol within 6 hours of bedtime.
- Do not have a cigarette or any other source of nicotine before bedtime.
- Do not go to bed hungry, but do not eat a big meal near bedtime.
- Avoid rigorous exercise within 6 hours of bedtime.
- Unclutter and clear your bedroom of desks, computers, and other work items.
- Check for potential allergens such as mold, dust, pollen, and mites.
- Ensure that your bed gives proper support. Sagging, lumpy, and overly soft or hard mattresses frequently cause sleep difficulties. Uncomfortable pillows also can be disruptive to sleep.
- Ensure sufficient exercise during the day; adequate exercise helps to promote restful sleep.
- Journal writing at bedtime is a fabulous way to process emotions, feelings, and the day's events, and clears the heart and mind before sleep.
- Use relaxation and stress-reducing techniques before bed, such as yoga, meditation, contemplation and prayer, listening to soothing music, or tuning into the night sky and moon.
- Because irregular sleeping habits lead to sleep problems, create a regular bedtime and stick to it.
- Examine attitudes about not sleeping, especially the emotions and thoughts that arise while not sleeping.
- Make your bedroom quiet, dark, and a little bit cool in temperature.

therapies, stimulus control therapies (e.g., patients are taught to avoid sleep-incompatible behaviors such as watching television in bed and are taught to get out of bed rather than lay there trying to fall asleep if sleep does not come easily), and temporal control therapies (e.g., deliberately waking at the same time each day and getting out of bed regardless of how much sleep was obtained the previous night; avoidance of naps). Pharmacologic interventions include antidepressant and anxiolytic medications, including benzodiazepines, sedatives, narcotics for pain, and the use of dopamine agonists for the control of RLS symptoms.

Nonpharmacologic Treatment Strategies

The nonpharmacologic strategies mentioned earlier have proven effective, safe, and reliable for those with primary and secondary insomnia, whether of psychiatric or medical origin, compared with placebo and pharmacologic interventions, with none of the side effects associated with medications.[1,3,6] Therefore when possible it is preferable to attempt nonpharmacologic methods first, progressing to medications as needed.

THE BOTANICAL PRACTITIONER'S PERSPECTIVE

Many patients prefer a natural approach, related to concerns about dependency and side effects associated with conventional sleep medications.[7] Therefore practitioners may want to consider using botanical therapies in conjunction with nonpharmacologic strategies for the relief of sleep disorders before turning to pharmaceuticals. The herbs presented in this section are those commonly used for general sleep promotion. To be effective, however, it is essential to also treat concurrent or underlying problems that prevent sleep.

Readers are also referred to relevant chapters for the treatment of HPA axis disruption, anxiety, depression, premenstrual tension, pelvic pain, or menopausal symptoms. A number of the herbs herein simultaneously address more than one of these concerns. For example: hops may relieve hot flashes and promote sleep; California poppy may relieve restless legs and promote sleep; and lavender, among others, has been shown to relieve anxiety and also promotes a tranquil state that is conducive to more restful sleep. Adaptogens, principal herbs for the treatment of fatigue, are discussed in Chapter 5, and provide important benefits for patients suffering from the effects of sleep deprivation or HPA axis disturbance.

Herbs for sleep promotion may be taken 30 and 60 minutes before bed. However, herbalists commonly report that

TABLE 6-2	**Herbs for Insomnia**		
Therapeutic Goal	**Therapeutic Activity**	**Botanical Name**	**Common Name**
Sleep promotion	Tranquilizer	*Eschscholzia californica*	California poppy
		Lavandula officinalis	Lavender
		Leonurus cardiaca	Motherwort
		Matricaria recutita	Chamomile
		Melissa officinalis	Lemon balm
		Passiflora incarnata	Passionflower
		Piper methysticum	Kava kava
Sleep promotion	Sedative	*Eschscholzia californica*	California poppy
		Humulus lupulus	Hops
		Lavandula officinalis	Lavender
		Matricaria recutita	Chamomile
		Melissa officinalis	Lemon balm
		Passiflora incarnata	Passionflower
		Piper methysticum	Kava kava
		Scutellaria lateriflora	Skullcap
		Valeriana officinalis	Valerian
Sleep promotion	Hypnotic	*Eschscholzia californica*	California poppy
		Humulus lupulus	Hops
		Piper methysticum	Kava kava
		Valeriana officinalis	Valerian
Sleep promotion	Anxiolytic	*Humulus lupulus*	Hops
		Leonurus cardiaca	Motherwort
		Passiflora incarnata	Passionflower
		Piper methysticum	Kava kava
		Scutellaria lateriflora	Skullcap
		Valeriana officinalis	Valerian

herbs for sleep problems associated with chronic anxiety yield the best results when taken several times throughout the day rather than only before bedtime. It may take several weeks of taking the herbs to notice consistent improvement. The dosage range for most formulae is 2 to 5 mL three to four times daily, with an additional dose of 2 mL taken every half hour two to four times in the few hours before bedtime. Administration may be repeated in the night if the patient wakes and is unable to return to sleep. Herbal teas for relaxation also may be taken before bedtime; however, the need to urinate from drinking tea is apt to lead to waking and thus can be counterproductive. It is not advisable to combine botanical sedatives, tranquilizers, and anxiolytics with conventional pharmaceuticals because of possible interactions and potentiation of sedative action.

A clarification of nomenclature related to sleep promotion is necessary, as the terms sedative, hypnotic, and tranquilizer are not synonymous.[8] Tranquilization refers to an emotional calming that may or may not lead to sleep but that does not promote drowsiness; sedation refers to a reduction in cognitive function that is favorable to sleep promotion; and a hypnotic directly promotes sleep. Readers will note some overlap in the Table 6-2 herbs. Table 6-3 elucidates the strength of each of the herbs in this chapter based on this nomenclature. Readers will note a dose-dependent relationship with herbs and strength of effect.

California Poppy

California poppy, an herb indigenous to California and used by Native Americans as a sedative, hypnotic, and analgesic,

remains widely popular among herbal practitioners today as a reliable treatment for sleep disorders, especially overexcitement and sleeplessness, and also as an antispasmodic when there is muscular tension, restlessness, and pain.[9-11] Of interest is that the liquid extract of this herb was included in the Parke-Davis catalog in 1890, in which it was referred to as an "excellent soporific and analgesic, above all harmless."[11] Its efficacy was compared with morphine but without the side effects associated with that drug (e.g., constipation, addiction).[11]

Animal studies have demonstrated binding of alkaloids in California poppy to gamma (γ)-aminobutyric acid (GABA) receptors. Sedative effects have been demonstrated at higher doses, whereas anxiolytic effects are predominant at lower dose ranges.[12] These effects are may be mediated by interactions of California poppy with benzodiazepine receptors. In vitro and animal studies have demonstrated spasmolytic effects on smooth muscle.[13]

A combination formula containing California poppy (80%) and *Corydalis* (20%) extracts demonstrated in vitro ability to interact with opiate receptors, suggesting an analgesic activity, and in two controlled clinical trials normalized disturbed sleep patterns without carryover effects or dependency.[11]

Hops

Hops, a primary ingredient in beer, has long been used for its sedative effects. Historically, it was taken internally and stuffed into herbal pillows to be slept on for a sedating effect.[9,14] Hops is approved by the German Commission E for

TABLE 6-3 Ranking Levels of Botanicals for Sleep Promotion

Herb	Rank
Lavender	1
Chamomile	1
Lemon balm	1
California poppy	1-3
Motherwort	1-3
Skullcap	1-3
Passionflower	1-4
Valerian	2-4
Hops	2-5
Kava kava	2-5

These herbs are ranked on a scale of 1 to 5. A 1 denotes general relaxation that facilitates sleep rather than sedation (i.e., tranquilization), whereas a 5 is a hypnotic. The range in between denotes sedation. A range suggests that the effects of the herb are dose dependent.

mood disturbances, restlessness, anxiety, and sleep disturbances; it is approved by the European Scientific Cooperative on Phytotherapy (ESCOP) for tenseness, restlessness, and sleep disorders.[14,15]

Hops may have central nervous system (CNS) depressant effects. Animal studies suggest sedative, hypnotic, and spasmolytic effects; however, there is a dearth of good-quality human clinical trials on the use of hops for the treatment of sleep disturbances.[16,17] Recent research has focused more on the phytoestrogenic uses of hops. Hops has a long history of safe use, few anecdotal adverse events reports,[17] and is considered safe when used in recommended doses. It is generally recommended, based on theoretical grounds of drug potentiation, that hops not be combined with herbs that affect the CNS, including barbiturates, antidepressants, sedatives, and antipsychotics.[9,17] Neither ESCOP nor the German Commission E provide contraindication to use nor report on drug interactions.[14,15] For insomnia and sleep disturbances, hops is often combined with other sedative herbs, including passionflower, skullcap, or valerian. Caution is advised when driving or operating heavy machinery. Use of hops is not advised during pregnancy or by women with a history of estrogen-sensitive cancers.

Chamomile

Chamomile is noted both for its effects on the gastrointestinal (GI) system for the treatment of spasms and dyspepsia, and as a tranquilizer and mild sedative. It appears that inhalation of the essential oil–containing vapor when drinking the tea may play an important role in the sedative effects of this herb.[18] Constituents, including flavonoids and apigenins, may bind to benzodiazepine receptors in the CNS.[19] Animal studies demonstrate anticonvulsant and CNS depressant activity.[8] One clinical trial was identified for chamomile in primary insomnia. Participants (n = 34) were randomized to 270 mg of chamomile twice daily or placebo for 28 days. Using sleep diary measures, there were no significant differences observed between experimental or control groups. (Preparation not noted.)[20] Chamomile is a gentle herb considered safe for children, pregnancy, and lactating women, and was immortalized by Beatrix Potter when Peter Rabbit's mother gives it to the naughty Peter to promote sleep. There are no contraindications to use or known interactions.

Kava Kava

Kava kava is used in its native south Pacific islands as a sedative, aphrodisiac, and recreational and religious beverage.[8] It has earned a reputation as a useful botanical for the treatment of anxiety, sleep disorders, restlessness, and as a muscle relaxant.[21] Practitioners might consider it for anxiety-related sleep disorders, muscle twitching, and restless legs that interfere with sleep. Short-term studies suggest that kava kava is effective for insomnia, particularly in improving sleep quality and decreasing the amount of time needed to fall asleep, and that the kava pyrones act centrally as antispasmodics and anticonvulsants.[8,22] The mechanisms of action proposed for kava kava include decreased levels of glutamate (i.e., an excitatory neurotransmitter), activation of dopaminergic neurons, interaction with GABA receptors, direct action on muscles that leads to relaxation, elevation of dopamine and serotonin levels via inhibition of monoamine uptake, and cellular actions similar to mood stabilizers.[23-29] The German Commission E contraindicates kava kava in patients with endogenous depression.[15] Some individuals do not like the feeling they get when taking kava kava, reporting a sensation of numbness that is unpleasant. A lower dose may prevent this feeling, but some patients may just not tolerate kava kava well. There is a possible potentiation of the effects of alcohol, barbiturates, and other substances affecting the CNS when used with kava kava; therefore simultaneous use is inadvisable.[21] Patients with prior or current liver disease, or those taking medications that carry a risk of hepatotoxicity, should not use this herb without the supervision of a medical doctor.

Lemon Balm

A recent multicenter study examined the use of a valerian and lemon balm preparation in children younger than 12 years of age suffering from restlessness and nervous dyssomnia. Out of a total of 918 children, 80.9% who suffered from dyssomnia experienced improvement, and 70.4% of the patients with restlessness reported an improvement of symptoms. (Dose and preparation were not disclosed.)[30] Another randomized controlled clinical trial found lemon balm to be "beneficial in moderating subjective mood in response to mild psychological stress."[31]

ESCOP supports the use of lemon balm as a sedative for tenseness, restlessness, and irritability, as well as the symptomatic relief of minor digestive complaints, for example, spasms.[14] The German Commission E supports its use for nervous sleeping disorders.[15] Like chamomile, lemon balm is considered a gentle herb to be taken as a tea, also rich in volatile oils that calm the mood, and it also may be taken in tincture form.[18] It has been traditionally called "the gladdening herb," which has lent to its modern use as not only a tranquilizer and mild hypnotic but as an anxiolytic and mild antidepressant. The herb is well tolerated and there are no contraindications to use or known interactions.

Lavender

Lavender is a mild sedative used for restlessness, nervous exhaustion, and sleep disorders.[32] It is approved by the German Commission E for the treatment of mood disturbances and functional abdominal complaints (e.g., nervous stomach irritations). It is used as a tranquilizing herb in the form of tea, tinctures, and as an aromatherapy agent.[15] A murine study used inhaled linalool, one of lavender's predominant terpenes, to increase sleep time.[33] Two small human clinical trials have been conducted on lavender inhalation and parameters of sleep quality. A recent controlled pilot study (n = 50) of intermediate care unit patients tested lavender aromatherapy for sleep quality improvement. Control groups received standard care for insomnia and treated patients received 3 mL of 100% lavender oil in a glass jar at the bedside. Sleep quality was monitored through the Richards–Campbell Sleep Questionnaire and vital sign data points taken throughout the night. The treated group exhibited lower blood pressure than the control group ($p = .03$). The mean sleep scores were higher in the intervention than the control groups (48.25 vs. 40.10), but the difference was insignificant.[34] In another study, researchers investigated effect of lavender fragrance on insomnia and depression in 42 female college students. Participants self-reported improvements in sleep latency and sleep satisfaction at lower concentrations, and improvements in depressive moods during treatment weeks at higher concentrations of the lavender fragrance.[35] It is a gentle herb with no reported side effects or expected drug interactions. A relaxing bath can be taken before bed using five to seven drops of lavender essential oil added to a tub of hot water. Alternatively, or additionally, an aromatherapy atomizer containing lavender oil can be sprayed near the sleeping area to promote a sense of calm. The essential oil is not to be taken internally.

Motherwort

Motherwort has been used traditionally as a nervine, tranquilizer, and mild sedative for irritability and tension. Its use is approved by the German Commission E for the treatment of nervous cardiac conditions and thyroid hyperfunction.[15] It is an excellent addition to formulae for sleep disorders in perimenopausal women experiencing anxiety or heart palpitations, and for patients with subclinical hyperthyroid function. Any patients experiencing heart palpitations, other cardiac symptoms, or hyperthyroid symptoms, should seek the care of a qualified medical practitioner before self-medication with motherwort to rule out a serious underlying disorder.

Magnolia

The bark of magnolia has been used traditionally as a nervine, diaphoretic, and antiinflammatory herb in North American and Chinese herbal medicine. In vitro studies suggest sedative activity of several compounds in magnolia, potentially mediated by GABA receptor expression upregulation and activation of adenosine, dopamine, and serotonin receptors.[36,37] A multicenter randomized control trial (n = 89) demonstrated efficacy of a combination containing magnolia extract and magnesium on sleep disturbances in menopause. A formulation containing magnolia bark extract, magnesium, soy isoflavones, lactobacilli, calcium, and vitamin D_3 was administered daily over the course of 24 weeks. Flushing, nocturnal sweating, palpitations, insomnia, asthenia, anxiety, mood depression, irritability, vaginal dryness, dyspareunia, and low libido significantly decreased in severity compared with placebo controls (60 mg magnolia bark extract).[38]

Passionflower

Passionflower is a folk remedy used for anxiety. In Brazil it is called *maracuja* and its juice is used as a popular beverage. Valued by the Eclectic physicians for its use in treating insomnia, passionflower is a useful adjunct in the management of nervous disorders that affect sleep, and is popular among herbalists to include in formulae for general sleep disturbances, perimenopausal sleep disturbances, depression, and anxiety.[32,39] It has not been associated with acute or chronic toxicity. Animal studies have confirmed sleep-inducing effects of the herb.[8,40] A randomized controlled trial (n = 41) evaluated the efficacy of passionflower tea on sleep quality. For 1 week, participants consumed a cup of either placebo or passionflower tea, filled out a sleep diary for 7 days, and completed the Spielberger State-Trait Anxiety Inventory on the final morning. The data suggested significantly improved sleep quality with passionflower tea compared with placebo ($p < 0.01$).[41,42]

The pharmacologic profile of the extracts suggests that large doses may result in CNS depression and bradycardia, prolonged QT interval, and ventricular tachycardia.[43] In a Cochrane Database review, two studies evaluating two distinct passionflower formulations were not able to differentiate *Passiflora* from benzodiazepines for any of the outcome measures. The authors reported that the lack of statistical difference may be interpreted in two ways: (1) the medications were equally effective, or (2) the absence of difference may be caused by type II error (i.e., sample sizes not large enough or insufficient number of studies for inclusion).[44] ESCOP endorses passionflower's use in the treatment of tenseness, restlessness, and irritability, and difficulty in falling asleep.[14] The German Commission E supports its use for the treatment of nervous restlessness.[15] There are no known side effects or contraindications to use, although the theoretic contraindication of sedative herbs with sedative pharmaceuticals is generally applied.

Skullcap

Skullcap has a long historical reputation of use as an anxiolytic, antiseizure, and sedative herb, and is commonly used both for nervous disorders and sleep problems. However, there is surprisingly little clinical research on this herb. Studies with *Scutellaria baicalensis*, a species commonly used in Traditional Chinese Medicine (TCM) as an antiinflammatory, antibacterial, antiviral, and antiatherosclerotic herb, have demonstrated binding of several alleged active flavonoids, including baicalin and its aglycone baicalein, to the benzodiazepine site of the GABA-A receptor.[45] A recent animal study demonstrated significant anxiolytic activity of *Scutellaria lateriflora* crude herb administered as aqueous and hydroethanolic extracts.[45] Extracts were analyzed and compared with valerian and passionflower extract for constituents that might indicate anxiolytic or sedative activity. GABA and glutamine were identified in varying amounts, although it remains uncertain at this time just how much these amino acids contribute to the actions of skullcap.[45] Hepatotoxic reactions have been reported after ingestion of preparations allegedly containing skullcap. Adulteration of skullcap herb by *Teucrium* spp., a known hepatotoxic herb, is recognized, and is most likely the culprit in supposed skullcap-associated hepatotoxicity, rather than skullcap itself. Marketplace standards are (ideally) applied to prevent this from occurring. Nonetheless, it is this possibility of adulteration with *Teucrium* spp. that leads to the contraindication of skullcap during pregnancy. One source reported symptoms of giddiness, stupor, confusion, and seizures associated with overdose of skullcap tincture; similar findings have not been otherwise reported in the herbal literature.[46]

Valerian

Valerian has been used for sleep disorders, nervous conditions, anxiety, musculoskeletal tension, and pain for at least 2000 years.[47] The *ESCOP monographs* indicate valerian for the relief of temporary mild nervous tension and difficulty falling asleep, uses that are corroborated by the German Commission E, the World Health Organization (WHO), and European Medicines Agency.[14,15,48] The WHO further describes valerian as gentler alternative or substitute for stronger sedatives; for example, benzodiazepines and for the treatment of anxiety-related sleep disturbances.[49] A systematic review by Stevinson and Ernst identified nine clinical trials evaluating the efficacy of valerian for sleep promotion. Of these, three found strong evidence of efficacy in reducing sleep latency and improving sleep quality.[50,51] Other recent trial evidence supports the use of valerian for treating sleep disturbances. One trial evaluated the efficacy of valerian for sleep improvement in cancer patients. The patients (n = 227, 119 completed) were assigned to placebo or valerian (450 mg) treatment groups; treatment was administered orally 1 hour before bedtime for 8 weeks. Using the Pittsburgh Sleep Quality Index (PSQI), participants reported fewer sleep disturbances with valerian than a placebo. (Preparation not noted.)[52] Another trial (n = 100) evaluated the efficacy of valerian extract in treating insomnia and sleep disturbances in postmenopausal women. Each group received either 530 mg of concentrated valerian extract or a placebo twice daily for 4 weeks. Using PSQI, participants in the valerian group reported improved sleep quality (30%) compared with the placebo (4%) ($p < 0.001$). (Preparation not noted.)[53] A triple-blinded, randomized, placebo-controlled study compared the valerian with placebo on sleep quality in patients with RLS. Participants (n = 37) were randomly assigned to receive 800 mg of valerian or placebo for 8 weeks. The primary outcome of sleep was sleep quality with secondary outcomes including sleepiness (via PSQI and Epworth Sleepiness Scale) and RLS symptom severity. The patients who consumed valerian reported improved symptoms of RLS and decreased daytime sleepiness. (Preparation not noted.)[54]

Valerian has also been tested in combination products for sleep improvement. One study tested the use of a valerian and lemon balm combination for the treatment of insomnia in 100 menopausal women ranging 50 to 60 years of age, split into treatment and control groups. Using PSQI at the baseline and end point, significant improvements were observed in the valerian group over the controls. (Preparation not noted.)[55]

A double-blind trial investigated a combination product consisting of standardized extracts of valerian, passionflower, and hops in comparison to zolpidem in treating primary insomnia. Subjects were administered one tablet of either the herbal product or zolpidem 10 mg at bedtime for 2 weeks. Using the Insomnia Severity Index and Epworth Sleepiness Scale, subjects in both groups experienced improvement in total sleep time, sleep latency, and number of nightly awakenings. No notable differences were observed between the herbal product and zolpidem groups. Safety assessments were carried out via liver and renal function tests, and no adverse events were recorded except for drowsiness in both groups. (Preparation and dose was one tablet of NSF-3.)[56]

Another double-blind trial was performed to assess the efficacy of a fixed valerian and hops extract combination for insomnia treatment compared with placebo, as well as valerian as a single herb. The treatment period lasted for 4 weeks. The fixed extract combination was significantly superior to the placebo in reducing sleep latency. The single valerian extract was not found be superior to placebo. (The fixed combination consisted of 500 mg valerian extract and 120 mg hops extract [both 45% methanol].)[57] Additionally, a review on the use of valerian and hops in treating insomnia evaluated the relevant literature in the Allied and Complementary Medicine *Database (AMED)* and MEDLINE database. Out of the 16 studies that met the inclusion criteria, 12 concluded that the use of valerian (alone or in combination with hops) is associated with improvements in some sleep parameters.[58,59]

However, valerian as a sleep aid has not demonstrated efficacy in all clinical trials. A phase 2 crossover randomized controlled trial of older women (n = 16) tested efficacy of valerian for insomnia treatment. Participants ingested 300 mg of concentrated valerian extract or placebo 30 minutes before bedtime for 2 weeks. Sleep was assessed in the laboratory and at home by self-report and polysomnography (PSG) at baseline and at the beginning and end of each treatment phase. Using these measures, researchers did not observe statistically significant differences between valerian and placebo. (Preparation not noted.)[60]

Valerian contains sesquiterpenes of the volatile oils (e.g., valeric acid); iridoids (e.g., valepotriates); alkaloids; furofuran lignans; and free amino acids such as GABA, tyrosine, arginine, and glutamine.[47] The valeric acid and valepotriates are commonly cited as the active ingredients in valerian, and although it has been demonstrated that they possess direct sedative effects, it is likely that all of the active constituents of valerian function in a synergistic manner to produce a clinical response.[32,61] Animal studies suggest the inhibition of enzymes that degrade GABA as one possible mechanism of action.

There may be individual variations in valerinic acid metabolism that may affect its physiologic effects. A pharmacokinetic study evaluated valerenic acid in a group of elderly women after receiving a single nightly valerian dose, and after 2 weeks of valerian administration. The researchers found large variability in the pharmacokinetics of valerenic acid and concluded that this may contribute to the inconsistencies with valerian's efficacy as a sleep aid. (Dose was not disclosed.)[62]

Valerian is considered more effective as a sleep aid when used chronically rather than acutely. It is a reasonable mild alternative to benzodiazepines and does not lead to sleepiness or grogginess upon waking. It is well tolerated by most patients, although herbalists have reported paradoxical effects (i.e., stimulation) in as many as 10% of patients. Vivid dreams have been reported as the most common side effect of valerian use.[11] Theoretical dose-related physical impairment may occur within the first few hours after ingestion; thus it is advised that patients do not drive or operate heavy machinery while taking valerian. Chronic use over years may lead to withdrawal symptoms if the herb is discontinued abruptly.[21] Although there are no known contraindications, caution is advised in combining sedative herbs with sedative pharmaceuticals. It is considered safe when used appropriately at a dose of 2 to 3 g of crude herb per cup of tea one to several times daily, 1 to 3 mL tincture one to several times daily, or 10 to 15 mL of tincture 30 to 60 minutes before bed.[9,15] Valerian may be used as a single herb preparation; however, several trials have demonstrated efficacy of multiherb products including valerian, hops, and lemon balm.[21] Valerian root is considered contraindicated in pregnancy because of lack of demonstrated safety and the mutagenic potential of valepotriates, although the actual valepotriate content of commercial products has been found to be extremely low.[21,47]

Ziziphus

Ziziphus spinosa has been widely used in Chinese medicine for GI complaints and as a sedative and anxiolytic herb. Research suggests that the triterpenoid saponins and flavonoid fractions in *Ziziphus spinosa* exert its sedative effects, notably jujubosides and spinosin, respectively.[63] A murine study demonstrated jujubosides increased total sleep and rapid eye movement (REM) sleep, and was potentiated by 5-hydroxytryptophan (5-HTP).[64] Another murine study investigated whether the hypnotic effects of spinosin are mediated via serotonin-1A receptors. The results suggested that spinosin may be an antagonist at postsynaptic 5-HT(1A) receptors.[65] *Ziziphus spinosa* is an ingredient in the traditional Chinese formula Gui Pi Tang (which includes Ginseng and Longan), commonly recommended for women with perimenopausal sleep disturbance.

PROTOCOL FOR SLEEP TROUBLES

For patients with sleep troubles seeking a natural approach, a combination of nonpharmacologic strategies and appropriate botanicals can be effective. The following formulae are examples of how herbs might be combined to address a variety of sleep-related problems. Patients can expect results within a couple of weeks after beginning a therapy, although some may experience rather immediate benefits.

Difficulty Falling Asleep

Tea: Combine equal parts of the following bulk herbs. Prepare by steeping 2 tsp of herbs in 1 cup of boiling water for 10 minutes. It is important to steep the tea in a covered vessel to preserve the medicinal volatile oils.

Lavender	(*Lavandula officinalis*)	1 part
Chamomile	(*Matricaria recutita*)	1 part
Lemon balm	(*Melissa officinalis*)	1 part
	Total: 3 parts	

Dose: Drink 1 to 4 cups daily, but discontinue drinking about 30 minutes before bed to avoid night waking from the need to urinate.

Tincture:

California poppy	(*Eschscholzia californica*)	20 mL
Hops	(*Humulus lupulus*)	20 mL
Passionflower	(*Passiflora incarnata*)	20 mL
Valerian	(*Valeriana officinalis*)	20 mL
Skullcap	(*Scutellaria lateriflora*)	20 mL
	Total: 100 mL	

Dose: Take 2 to 4 mL for four doses starting 2 hours before bedtime. Repeat one to three doses during the night if night waking is a problem. For individuals for whom hops is contraindicated, omit the hops and increase the California poppy and passionflower each by 10 mL. For those who cannot tolerate valerian, omit and increase the passionflower by 10 mL.

Inability to Sleep Associated with Anxiety
Tincture:

Passionflower	(*Passiflora incarnata*)	30 mL
California poppy	(*Eschscholzia californica*)	25 mL
Motherwort	(*Leonurus cardiaca*)	15 mL
Kava kava	(*Piper methysticum*)	15 mL
Skullcap	(*Scutellaria lateriflora*)	15 mL
	Total: 100 mL	

Dose: Take 2 to 4 mL three to four times daily, and two to four doses within the 2 hours before bedtime.

Difficulty Sleeping Caused by Musculoskeletal Pain or Restless Legs
Tincture:

Cramp bark	(*Viburnum opulus*)	30 mL
California poppy	(*Eschscholzia californica*)	25 mL
Corydalis	(*Corydalis ambigua*)	15 mL

Continued

Hops	(Humulus lupulus)	15 mL
Kava kava	(Piper methysticum)	15 mL
		Total: 100 mL

Dose: Take 2 to 4 mL as needed for pain relief, up to six doses daily.

Difficulty Sleeping Associated with Perimenopausal Complaints
Tincture:

Black cohosh	(Actaea racemosa)	30 mL
Hops	(Humulus lupulus)	20 mL
Motherwort	(Leonurus cardiaca)	15 mL
Passionflower	(Passiflora incarnate)	15 mL
Sage	(Salvia officinalis)	10 mL
Lavender	(Lavandula officinalis)	10 mL
		Total: 100 mL

Dose: 3 to 5 mL as needed in the evening and before sleep, up to four doses daily.

NUTRITIONAL CONSIDERATIONS

- L-tryptophan was a popular supplement for sleep promotion. Though its use was banned in 1989 because of association with eosinophilia-myalgia syndrome, it continues to be sold over the counter. Although its use as a supplement is not recommended, L-tryptophan is naturally occurring in milk, traditionally used as a sleep aid taken warmed before bed. Its safety and efficacy in this form has not been evaluated.[1]

- 5-HTP, a form of tryptophan, has been reported in numerous double-blind studies to decrease the time required to get to sleep and to decrease the number of night awakenings. Taking 5-HTP will raise serotonin levels, which helps to initiate sleep. Care should be taken in patients using serotonin-enhancing medications, for example, selective serotonin reuptake inhibitors (SSRIs).

- Melatonin, also an endogenous neurotransmitter involved in sleep regulation, is a popular sleep aid, promoted for treating insomnia caused by circadian rhythm disturbances and preventing jet lag. It is thought that it is the natural decline in melatonin levels as we age that is partially responsible for increasing insomnia in the elderly. A number of substances, including tobacco, alcohol, nonsteroidal antiinflammatory drugs (NSAIDs), calcium channel blockers, benzodiazepines, fluoxetine, and steroids decrease melatonin production. The primary side effect associated with melatonin use is drowsiness. It is typically take in 0.3- to 3-mg doses. It is contraindicated in prepubertal and pregnant women due to potential interference with luteinizing hormone.[1]

- Magnesium supplementation may be effective in promoting high-quality, uninterrupted sleep (225 mg magnesium).[9,66]

- Vitamin B$_6$ supplementation may reduce symptoms of insomnia, depression, and irritability. B$_6$ is involved in the production of the neurotransmitter serotonin, an endogenous chemical responsible for sleep regulation.[9]

- Iron-deficiency anemia has been associated with RLS; women experiencing this discomfort should have their iron and ferritin levels checked to rule out anemia.

- Some women, especially during pregnancy, report that nocturnal leg cramps are improved when they take a calcium and magnesium supplement. A dose of 800 to 1200 mg calcium and 400 to 600 mg magnesium daily is recommended.

DEPRESSION

Depression is a complex state because of its potential multifactorial etiologies ranging from inflammation and hormonal dysregulation to a history of physical or emotional trauma. According to the WHO, depressive disorders are the fourth most important cause of disability worldwide and are expected to become the second most frequent cause of illness by the year 2020.[67,68] Further, mounting evidence suggests a role for depression in the development of coronary heart disease, increasingly a major contributor of morbidity and mortality in women.[69]

Depressed mood, loss of pleasure in activities (or life), or loss of interest in nearly all activities, persisting for at least 2 weeks, constitutes a diagnosis of clinical depression. This state is commonly accompanied by symptoms of sadness, poor self-esteem, anxiety, irritability, anger, social withdrawal, guilt, helplessness, hopelessness, multiple physical complaints or fears, obsessive thoughts, poor concentration, decreased libido, recurrent thoughts of death or suicide, or psychotic symptoms; and there also may be neurovegetative symptoms such as fatigue or loss of energy, sleep disturbance, appetite disturbance, or psychomotor retardation or agitation.[70]

The etiologies of depression are not fully understood but should include an understanding of childhood events, adult traumas, socioeconomic and sociopolitical factors, and the effects of current stressors on the individual.[67,71] Psychosocial causes include domestic violence, bereavement, and personality disorders.[70] There are marked cultural, gender, and age differences in presentation. Many people with depression do not complain of sadness; in fact, they may describe anxiety or somatic symptoms as predominant. A diagnosis of depression should be considered in anyone complaining of fatigue, sleep or appetite problems, or multiple body symptoms.

DIAGNOSIS

Types of depression are classified by the American Psychiatric Association's criteria, set forth in the *Diagnostic and Statistical Manual of Mental Disorders,* ed 4, Text Revision (DSM-IV-TR) as follows[71]:

- *Major depression* manifests as depressed mood and/or loss of interest or pleasure for at least 2 weeks, with at least four other symptoms (appetite disturbance; sleep disturbance; psychomotor retardation or agitation; fatigue or loss of energy; feelings of worthlessness or excessive or inappropriate guilt; diminished ability to think or concentrate, or indecisiveness; recurrent thoughts of death or suicidal ideation).[71] Symptoms should not be caused by the effects of a substance (i.e., alcohol or drugs—illegal or prescription), a medical condition (e.g., hypothyroidism), or bereavement, which are classified separately.

- *Dysthymic disorder* has symptoms similar to major depression, but are persistent for at least 2 years and are less severe.[71]
- *Bipolar disorder* involves the occurrence of one or more manic episodes; often individuals also have had one or more episodes of major depression.
- *Seasonal affective disorder* (SAD) occurs in northern latitudes as light exposure decreases in the fall; symptoms resolve as days lengthen in spring. Overeating (especially carbohydrates) and oversleeping are common.[70] These diagnoses may be applied only after other causes of depression have been eliminated.
- *Prescription drugs* may cause depression as a side effect. Common culprits include beta(β)-blockers, antihypertensives, tranquilizers, antiepileptics, corticosteroids, digoxin, and histamine 2 (H_2)-blockers. Some antidepressants may exacerbate depression.
- *Drugs of abuse* (e.g., alcohol)
- *Toxic-metabolic conditions* such as thyroid disease, diabetes mellitus, Cushing's syndrome, and electrolyte/calcium imbalance.
- *Neurologic conditions* such as stroke, epilepsy, and dementia.
- *Infectious causes* such as viral mononucleosis, hepatitis, human immunodeficiency virus (HIV), syphilis, and Lyme disease.
- *Nutritional deficiency*
- *Other causes* include postsurgery, cancer, chronic fatigue syndrome, fibromyalgia, and rheumatoid disease.[70]

A careful medical, family, and social history, with detailed review of systems must be done; questions about organic causes and depressive symptoms must be covered in detail. If a diagnosis of depression is suspected, an evaluation of suicide risk must be made. Physical examination should address not only possible medical causes of depression but also specific somatic symptoms, providing reassurance about fears of covert illness. Mental status can be assessed during the history and examination, with specific questions about mood and memory. There are no laboratory tests for depression; blood work to rule out organic causes might include a complete blood count (CBC), blood sugar, blood urea nitrogen (BUN), creatinine, electrolytes, liver function tests, albumin, calcium, and thyrotropin (TSH).[70] Some of these would be required before starting psychotropic medications. Diagnostic questionnaires may be used to assess the severity of the depression and monitor clinical response to treatment.

CONVENTIONAL TREATMENT APPROACHES

An immediate referral to a psychiatrist should be made and confirmed by the practitioner in cases involving suicidal ideation, very severe depression, bipolar disease, paranoia, or

psychosis.[68,70] Any underlying cause or contributing factor should be addressed (e.g., alcohol abuse, prescription drug side effects, hypothyroidism, domestic violence). Presuppositions should not be made about who is at risk for suicide based on demographics or educational levels; for example, suicide is a disproportionately high cause of mortality in physicians, particularly in female physicians and domestic violence against women is as common in the most highly educated top socioeconomic tiers as it is in the lowest.[72]

Antidepressant Drugs

Antidepressant drugs are currently the mainstay of standard medical drug treatment of depression in menopause. Noticeable clinical improvement may take 3 to 4 weeks or longer, and may require trying a variety of medications before a "fit" is achieved between medication, patient, and therapeutic response. There is little difference in efficacy among the varied categories of antidepressants; they are all equally effective; they differ in type and severity of side effects.[67]

The most popular category at present is the SSRIs, including fluoxetine (Prozac), sertraline (Zoloft), paroxetine (Paxil), fluvoxamine (Luvox), and citalopram (Celexa).[70] They have energizing or activating effects, which can be useful in patients with low-energy symptoms, but can result in side effects such as anxiety, insomnia, agitation, and restlessness.[70] Paroxetine is effective for treatment of hot flashes, as is venlafaxine.[73]

Concerns have been raised about the safety of SSRIs in the treatment of symptoms other than depression in perimenopausal women, particularly an increased risk of cardiovascular disease and stroke. Further, a combination of NSAIDs and SSRIs identified as a cause of brain bleeding in women using them. So prescribing these medications in these populations should not be taken lightly, and patients on these medications already should be advised of these risks.[74]

A major drawback to successful use of SSRIs is that sexual dysfunction occurs in nearly 60% of patients, is difficult to manage, involves loss of libido and orgasmic dysfunction in both men and women, and is often not discussed unless the practitioner asks about it directly.[75] Serotonin syndrome (includes tremor, agitation, delirium, rigidity, myoclonus, hyperthermia, and obtundation) is a potentially fatal consequence of combining SSRIs with other drugs that also increase serotonin,[75] especially in elders. SSRI inhibition of the liver cytochrome P450 (CYP) isoenzymes causes slowing of hepatic drug metabolism and interactions with other drugs, including phenytoin (Dilantin), warfarin (Coumadin), cimetidine, barbiturates, macrolide antibiotics, antihistamines, benzodiazepines, β-blockers, carbamazepine (Tegretol), cyclosporine, diltiazem, digoxin, *haloperidol* (Haldol), lithium, theophylline, tolbutamide, and many others.[76] Overdose is rarely fatal.[75] These drugs should not be stopped suddenly, or withdrawal symptoms (e.g., flulike symptoms, malaise, dizziness, nausea, paresthesias, depression, sleep problems) may occur.[65,75]

Tricyclic antidepressants (TCAs) such as desipramine (Norpramin), nortriptyline (Pamelor or Aventyl), or doxepin (Adapin or Sinequan) are sedating, making them good choices for women with anxiety, panic, or insomnia symptoms.[70] Side effects are likely to be anticholinergic symptoms (e.g., dry mouth, constipation, sexual dysfunction, urinary retention, blurred vision, increased intraocular pressure, brain fog, sedation, heart block), postural hypotension, and weight gain.[70,75] A full-blown anticholinergic syndrome of agitation, delirium, and fever can occur, especially with antihistamines (including OTC sleep, allergy, and cold medications) and other anticholinergic drugs.[70] Many other severe drug interactions include serotonin syndrome, hypertensive crisis (with clonidine), life-threatening arrhythmia (with quinolone antibiotics); and inhibition of CYP drugs.[76] Tardive dyskinesia may occur, and may be irreversible.[76] Overdoses are fatal with a 10-day supply of 200 mg/day.[75] Withdrawal symptoms may occur; taper slowly.

Trazodone (Oleptro) is sedating and very useful for anxiety, panic, insomnia, alcoholism, and aggressive behavior[76]; patients may respond in 1 week, with good effects in 2 weeks; some patients may take up to 4 weeks.[76] It can be very effective for hot flashes that cause night sweats. It has few common side effects (other than drowsiness and headache) and much less sexual dysfunction, but it can cause serotonin syndrome and CYP drug interactions. Overdose can be fatal, especially in combination with other drugs. Nefazodone (Serzone) is similar, has complex effects on serotonin, and also less sexual dysfunction. There are reports of severe liver failure, all in women; somnolence occurs in 25% and dizziness in 17%; serious interactions occur with CYP drugs.[76]

Bupropion (Wellbutrin) is somewhat activating, so its side effects include anxiety, agitation, and insomnia; it has a fourfold to tenfold increase in risk of seizures, especially in patients with anorexia or bulimia; it can cause hepatocellular injury and increased risk of liver cancer, and interacts with CYP drugs.[76] Overdose can cause death.

Monoamine oxidase inhibitors (MAOIs) are drugs of last choice, when everything else has failed; in addition to more potentially fatal drug interactions than all the other antidepressants, they can interact with a substantial number of common foods (e.g., cheese, pepperoni, beer, red wine, bananas, avocados, coffee, colas, chocolate, and many more); there are cases of dependency and withdrawal; and overdoses can be fatal.[76]

THE BOTANICAL PRACTITIONER'S PERSPECTIVE

In many indigenous medical systems, and for a substantial segment of Western herbal practitioners, beliefs about the causes and meanings or purposes of depression are radically different from those held commonly by orthodox medical practitioners. In addition to consideration of the individual's nutrition, exercise, and relaxation practices, work and family situations, use of drugs and medications, and exposure to toxins (e.g., emotional, spiritual, environmental, endogenously produced byproducts of detoxification), and identification of underlying causes of inflammation and infection (e.g., viruses), the major focus will be on the loss of inner balance

and harmony, and on empowering the client to start to work on restoration.[77]

The illusion of separateness so pervasive in Western cultures is felt by many indigenous traditions to be a major cause of illness. This illusion allows us to ignore the reality that the whole of life is an integrated web, rooted both in earth and in the Divine,[78] one and inseparable; true "interbeing," as Thich Nhat Hanh[79] would describe it.

A sense of lack of connectedness, of lacking a relationship with the entire universe, is for many a cause of emotional disturbance; recognizing this can be the means of its healing. Tibetan Buddhism attributes mental illness, including depression, to leading a life that runs counter to one's deepest spiritual self, especially if that self is resisted, denied, or repressed.[77] On the other hand, a deep sense of connectedness may cause depression in sensitive individuals. Those who have the strongest empathy for the planet and others may suffer emotionally in the face of ongoing worldwide environment, social, and political crises.[80]

The value of connectedness or interrelationship in healing depression includes several major considerations. If interbeing is accepted then healing can take place via developing connections to nature, family, friends, and community.[81] Service to others, especially to the healing of the planet, can be a very powerful path to healing oneself.[81] An interdisciplinary medical literature review showed that "interaction with the natural world positively affects multiple dimensions related to human health: physical, psychological-emotional, social, and spiritual," including less effect of stress on the autonomic nervous system, less pain, shorter surgical recovery time, improvement of deficits in attention, greater satisfaction with life, more positive social interactions, less aggressive behavior, and feelings of "greater interdependence and connectedness."[82] The botanical practitioner views the use of herbs as part of not only healing the body but as part of building a relationship with the natural world.

The following herbs represent only a fraction of those that are used worldwide to treat depression and its related symptoms (Table 6-4). These herbs may be used singly but are more often used in combinations specifically formulated for the unique needs of the patient. In addition to directly treating symptoms of depression, associated complaints such as chronic pain, insomnia, fatigue, and other predisposing health problems should be appropriately addressed through herbal formulae and other strategies.

Albizzia

In TCM, this is considered an herb to "nourish the heart and calm the spirit"; the literal translation of the herb's common Chinese name is "collective happiness bark." It is used for heartbreak, depression, insomnia, poor memory, bad temper, and irritability caused by constrained emotions, giving feelings of calm and peace, and lifting the spirit.[83,84] Studies show sedative properties (increased sleeping time in mice), strong antioxidant activity, improvement in learning and memory, increased levels of serotonin and GABA, and anticonvulsive and antianxiety activities.[85-89] Contemporary use is mainly

TABLE 6-4   Herbs for Depression

Therapeutic Activity	Botanical Name	Common Name
Antidepressant	Hypericum perforatum	St. John's wort
Adaptogen	Asparagus racemosa	Shatavari
	Eleutherococcus senticosus	Eleuthero
	Withania somnifera	Ashwagandha
	Angelica sinensis	Dong quai
Nervine	Anemone pulsatilla	Pulsatilla
	Lavandula officinalis	Lavender
	Leonurus cardiaca	Motherwort
Stimulant	Camellia sinensis	Green tea
	Rosmarinus officinalis	Rosemary

by practitioners of TCM, but it is an herb that can be easily incorporated into Western botanical protocol in tincture and other forms.

Ashwagandha

A classic herb in Ayurvedic medicine and now regarded as one of the best adaptogenic tonics, ashwagandha has been used for over 3000 years to restore, enhance, and preserve energy, strength, memory, and vitality, counteracting the effects of stress on the mind and body, calming a turbulent mind, and promoting inner peace and clarity.[90,91] A review article describes the findings from 58 articles found in a search of four medical databases, concluding that ashwagandha has antiinflammatory, antitumor, antistress, antioxidant, immunomodulatory, hematopoietic, and nutritive properties, and may be of benefit also to the endocrine, cardiopulmonary, and CNS systems; it has little or no toxicity.[92] The review also pointed out that ashwagandha may be even more effective when given in combination with other herbs (as is usually the case in its traditional use). In addition to this extensive review, there are articles supporting the anxiolytic and antidepressant activities of ashwagandha (found to be comparable to that of lorazepam and imipramine); reversal of chemotherapy-induced neutropenia; anticonvulsant activity; improvement or protection of memory from known disruptors; and adaptogenic effects.[88-91,93-102] Mild GI side effects may occur. It is an excellent choice in depression with anxiety and panic, a racing mind, insomnia, exhaustion, heavy bleeding, stress, and low libido.[91] It is also used for helping memory and learning, for malnutrition and anemia, arthritis, inflammation, bronchospasm, immune enhancement, alcoholism, and reproductive system disorders; improvement in libido occurs gradually after at least a month of use.[90] Ashwagandha may be taken in tincture, decoction, or powdered in capsules. Traditionally, the powder is prepared by boiling in milk with a small amount of sugar or honey.

Bacopa

Bacopa is one of the most important Ayurvedic herbs for depression, emotional stress, mental exhaustion, forgetfulness,

and anxiety.[103-106] Its effects on cognitive function (i.e., improvement in learning and memory) have been documented in numerous studies, as has its antioxidant activity in the brain and its ability to regulate brainwave activity and serotonin.[107-110] One study shows significant antidepressant effects comparable to imipramine in a rodent model.[111] Three review articles summarize its documented effectiveness in enhancing learning and memory.[94,112,113] Two studies show protection of brain function from the adverse effects of morphine and phenytoin.[114,115] Two studies found adaptogenic effects protective against stress-induced physical and biochemical changes.[116,117] In view of the growing body of research, its use is increasing among Western herbalists, who combine it in tincture form with other herbs for memory and mood enhancement.

Black Cohosh

Black cohosh was a favorite remedy of the Eclectics, who used it for nervous irritation, hysteria, melancholia, and epilepsy related to menstrual cycles, and for obstetric purposes.[118] The therapeutic efficacy of black cohosh for menopausal symptoms, including hot flashes and mood disorders, has been demonstrated in a number of trials.[119] A double-blind, randomized, multicenter study showed black cohosh to be equipotent to estrogen and superior to placebo in reducing climacteric symptoms, with beneficial effects on serum markers of bone metabolism, no effect on endometrial thickness, and increased vaginal superficial cells.[120]

A 2007 6-month clinical trial evaluated the efficacy of fluoxetine and black cohosh in the treatment of postmenopausal symptoms. Women (n = 120) were randomized into groups either taking fluoxetine and black cohosh or placebo. Alterations in menopausal symptoms were tracked through diaries and questionnaires consisting of a modified Kupperman Index, Beck Depression Inventory, and a RAND-36 Measure of Health-Related Quality of Life. The different depressions indexes yielded varying results over the length of the study (Black cohosh dose and preparation were not disclosed.).[123] Compared with fluoxetine, black cohosh demonstrated greater efficacy in the treatment of hot flushes and night sweats. However, fluoxetine was more effective in improvements shown on Beck's Depression Scale.

It has also been studied in conjunction with standard antidepressants. A 2013 randomized controlled trial (RCT) combined treatment of Remifemin (a black cohosh supplement) and paroxetine for perimenopausal depression. A group of 120 patients were divided into control (paroxetine 20 mg daily for 2 months) and treatment groups (1 Remifemin tablet twice daily *and* paroxetine 20 mg daily for 2 months). Side effects were monitored using blood and urine analysis, electrocardiography, liver function, kidney function, and blood pressure before and after treatment. After 8 weeks, therapeutic efficacy of the treatment group was significantly higher than that of the control group, according to Hamilton (HAMD) and Kupperman scores. No physiologic detections of side effects were seen in either group.[122] An excellent review monograph by McKenna et al reviews the history and clinical studies, concluding that black cohosh is safe (i.e., low toxicity, few and mild side effects), well tolerated, and effective for menopausal symptoms, including anxiety and depression.[123] A recent review reiterated that adverse effects are extremely uncommon, and that there are no known significant adverse drug interactions.[124] Possible dopaminergic activity is being investigated, with early evidence supporting this.[125] Safety concerns have been studied extensively, with findings of no estrogenic effect, no increased growth of human breast cancer cells, and even actual inhibition of some breast cancer cell lines, with enhancement of the effect of tamoxifen.[126-132] Two comprehensive reviews reported that adverse events were rare, mild, and reversible; few reports of severe events were not sufficiently substantiated.[133,134] Contemporary use involves taking preparations of the black cohosh root or rhizome orally, often in tablet form, but also as a tincture.[135] It may be combined in a formula with other herbs to address individual needs.

Crocus

Crocus sativus is well known as the plant that provides the spice saffron from its flower structure. Historically it was used in the Middle East for depression, anxiety, and high blood pressure. It contains crocin-1, which may confer antidepressant effects.[136] An increasing body of literature supports its use as an antidepressant. Moshiri et al (2006) conducted a 6-week outpatient randomized clinical trial (n = 40) comparing 30 mg daily of crocus petal to placebo in treating depression. As measured with the HAMD, the crocus group experienced a reduction in depressive symptoms compared with placebo.[137] The next year (2007), the same research team tested the efficacy of crocus (30 mg daily) against fluoxetine (20 mg) in an 8-week outpatient randomized clinical trial (n = 40). The two groups performed equally in measures of depressive symptoms as rated by the HAMD.[138]

Dong Quai

Dong quai is classified as a "blood tonic" in TCM, and as such is listed in TCM formulae for depression.[84] Lesley Tierra describes current TCM use of dong quai as one ingredient in formulae for stagnant liver qi, which is considered to be the root cause of depression.[139] However, TCM texts describe it as contraindicated for yin deficiency with heat signs, a classic TCM description of menopause.[139] When there is yin deficiency heat, it should be avoided or combined with appropriate herbs to mitigate its warming qualities.

Eleuthero

Eleuthero has been used in TCM for longer than 2000 years as an important adaptogen and to treat depression, anxiety, insomnia, mental strain, stress, and energy depletion.[140,141] Eleuthero has demonstrated adaptogenic and endurance-enhancing effects,[142] immunomodulatory and immunostimulatory effects, radiation protection, improvement in cognitive function and well-being, and stress reduction.[92,143-149] Many herbalists add eleuthero to their treatment protocols for depression with mental exhaustion, for rejuvenating the nervous system, and for restoring energy levels, in keeping with its traditional use.[150]

Ginkgo

Ginkgo may be beneficial in addressing a number of factors that can contribute to the experience of depression in women, particularly during the perimenopausal and menopausal years, including cognitive function changes, anxiety, and decreased sexual function, as addressed in the following.

Ginkgo's efficacy in preserving and improving cognitive function in elders or the cognitively impaired has been systematically demonstrated, especially for increasing accuracy and speed (i.e., working memory), improving complex attention, and significantly increasing speed of performance and mental fluency. Demonstrations include a number of critical reviews; meta-analyses; and well-designed randomized, double-blind, placebo-controlled clinical trials.[150-158] Clinical studies and electroencephalogram (EEG) data have shown cognitive-activating ability and significant efficacy similar to that of conventional nootropic drugs (e.g., tacrine, nimodipine) and probably similar to donepezil (Aricept), but at a tenth of the cost.[159-162] In addition, the frequency of adverse effects was lowest with ginkgo.[162] Please note that almost all of the research has involved one specific type of ginkgo extract (EGB-761) or its equivalent; one study concluded that EEG data showed that other products did not result in similar homogeneous CNS effects.[160] Recent studies have also shown significant improvement in cognitively intact older adults,[163] and dose-dependent improvement in memory and attention in healthy young adults, particularly when combined with *Panax ginseng* or *Bacopa monniera*.[164-167] The critical review by Kleijnen and Knipschild found that ginkgo led to clinically significant improvement in fatigue, depressed mood, and anxiety in patients with chronic cerebral insufficiency.[152] A study by Vorberg in similar patients also concluded that ginkgo improved symptoms of depression.[168] A trial by Lesser and colleagues showed that many people older than age 50 whose depression is unresponsive to antidepressants may have cerebrovascular insufficiency.[169] A randomized, double-blind placebo-controlled study demonstrated impressive improvement in depression resistance by adding ginkgo to the patients' conventional antidepressant; effectiveness was determined by a highly significant drop in scores on the HAMD from 14 to 7 after 4 weeks of treatment, and then down to 4.5 at 9 weeks, whereas the placebo group decreased by only 1 point in 8 weeks.[170] The study by Huguet and coworkers showed the decrease in serotonin receptor sites associated with aging, and the restoration of binding sites by treatment with ginkgo.[171]

A review article on alternative therapies for menopause quotes data that ginkgo helps relieve anxiety and depression among postmenopausal women.[172] A more recent study (randomized, placebo-controlled, double-blind, crossover) described improvement in self-rated mood in healthy young adults taking ginkgo versus placebo.[173] Using PSG (i.e., sleep EEG) to monitor sleep patterns, a pilot study was able to demonstrate that ginkgo significantly improved several sleep parameters in patients with major depression on a TCA.[174] The addition of ginkgo to Haldol also resulted in improvement in patients with treatment-resistant chronic schizophrenia.[175]

There are now several studies showing that ginkgo can ameliorate sexual dysfunction, but this topic remains controversial. One open study also describes improvement in symptoms of antidepressant-induced sexual dysfunction by using adjuvant ginkgo, with particularly good results in women.[176,177] In support of this theory, a case report was published describing one patient with a rare side effect of SSRI treatment, genital anesthesia; her symptoms failed to improve on conventional therapy or yohimbine but did resolve promptly with ginkgo.[178] Another case report tells of a woman who developed decreased libido and complete inability to achieve orgasm on Luvox; after 2 months on 240 mg of ginkgo per day, her symptoms resolved, and have remained under control for over a year, unless she tries to cut back the dose.[179]

A 2002 Cochrane Database Systematic Review done in 2002 concluded that data from the massive number of studies showed no significant difference between ginkgo and placebo in the proportion of participants experiencing adverse effects.[180] The biggest safety issue with ginkgo is the persistent question of whether or not it increases the risk of bleeding, particularly with warfarin (Coumadin) or aspirin. One study (1 year, 309 patients) reported one stroke and one subdural hematoma, both in the placebo group.[158] Considering that ginkgo is highly popular in Europe as an antiasthmatic and circulatory agent, and that in 1988 German physicians wrote 5.4 million prescriptions for it,[181] one might expect that if it caused serious bleeding it would be obvious by now. The question may have been answered by a new study (randomized, double-blind, placebo-controlled, crossover) of outpatients on stable, long-term warfarin, who were given ginkgo or placebo; there was no change in international normalized ratio (INR) or geometric mean dosage of warfarin during all treatment periods.[182] Another study showed no electrocardiogram (ECG) changes with short-term ginkgo in healthy volunteers.[183]

One safety issue, which is seldom raised, is that of the presence of a neurotoxin, ginkgo toxin, in the leaves and other plant parts; heating inactivates it during the extraction process.[159] Perhaps this is an indication that this is one of the few herbs that is safest when taken in standardized extract form.

Ginkgo is used by herbalists all over the planet for many indications, including asthma, vascular disorders, memory problems, sexual dysfunction, macular degeneration, and tinnitus; it is often added to therapeutic protocols for depression, especially in people over the age of 45 with attention and memory symptoms, and is considered to be an important tonic herb for the brain.[150,184,185]

Gotu Kola

Gotu kola is used by Ayurvedic, TCM, and Western herbal practitioners for the treatment of depression, anxiety, stress, memory, and mental fatigue.[105,186] A summary of the research documenting effectiveness as an adaptogen and for improving learning and memory was published in 1997.[94,187-190] Other studies show sedative and antidepressant activity comparable to imipramine and attenuation of the acoustic startle response (supporting anxiolytic claims).[191-193] It is used for memory enhancement, as a sedative nervine, and as an antispasmodic. It is considered to be a "balancing tonic" that both increases energy and relaxes the body; especially useful for insomnia.[194]

Holy Basil

Holy basil (also known as Tulsi) is a sweet, warming herb that has a long record of use in Ayurvedic medicine, where it is revered as a holy and sacred herb. It is classified a rasayana, an herb that improves overall health and well-being. The contemporary use of this herb involves mood improvement, anxiety reduction, adrenal support, and mental focus. Human studies are lacking, but one rodent study found holy basil (200 mg/kg) to confer antidepressant and anxiolytic effects (Holy basil ethanol leaf extract).[195] Holy basil can be taken as tea, tincture, or in capsules for long periods of time for the gradual improvement of mood and the stress response.

Lavender

Used in ancient Greek, Persian, Arab, and Roman medicine as a bath additive for the purification of body and spirit, lavender was also prized in Tibetan and Ayurvedic medicine.[196] Called "the broom of the brain," it was mentioned in an eighth century BCE Indian/Tibetan medical text as an ingredient in psychiatric formulae (as an edible butter; still in use in Tibetan medicine) for insanity and psychoses.[196] Lavender is listed in the *Ayurvedic Pharmacopoeia of India* for depressive states with digestive dysfunction; it is also used as an antispasmodic, sedative, and antirheumatic.[196] European use of lavender as a soothing treatment for emotional overload is well described in Gerard's herbal of 1597, in which he said that lavender "doth help the passion and panting of the heart."[197] Felter stated that it was used by the Eclectics for colic, headache, hysteria, "nervous individuals who faint easily and have hysterical seizures," and also for nervous irritability in children.[198] EEG studies demonstrate that lavender has a relaxing effect (increased alpha [α] and frontal β), with decreased anxiety and tension, and significant decreases in State-Trait Anxiety scores; it promotes drowsiness and induces sleep.[199-203] Cardiac response patterns have also been used to demonstrate the relaxing properties of lavender.[204] In one study of hospitalized children with HIV, all the children reported relief of pain, some completely; their use of analgesic drugs was decreased; muscle spasms caused by encephalopathy and chronic chest pain that had been previously unresponsive to conventional analgesia were eased; and painful neuropathy was alleviated almost completely.[205,206] A study of foot massage with or without lavender essential oil included 100 patients in a coronary care unit, 50% of whom were intubated; a control group rested in a curtained-off area; 90% of those in the massage-with-lavender group showed a significant reduction in heart rate, compared with 58% of those in the massage-only group and 41% in the control group.[205,207] One RCT on a small number of hospitalized patients with rheumatoid arthritis used a 10-minute upper neck and shoulder massage, with or without lavender, on two consecutive nights: analgesia use was decreased; patients reported better sleep or ability to roll over.[205,208] A RCT of 122 CCU patients showed that the aromatherapy group felt "less anxious and more positive" after massage with lavender, compared with massage only or with the control group; conscious patients who were able to respond also felt more able to cope; a modified assessment tool developed specifically for intensive care unit (ICU) patients who are unable to respond verbally was also used.[205,209] Other studies demonstrate lavender's sedative and mood-enhancing properties.[159,210] In contemporary botanical medicine, lavender is felt to have an amphoteric or balancing capacity, cooling and sedating (analgesic, antipyretic, sedating, antiinflammatory), or warming and stimulating (diaphoretic, antiinfective, antidepressant) as needed.[211] Consequently, it is especially useful for depression with mood swings.[212] Varieties with different balances of chemical constituents (i.e., chemovars) have slightly different effects.[159] It is also used to treat anxiety, stress, spasms, cramps, pain, insomnia, and headache, and to enhance meditation and spiritual practices.[194] Lavender is another good friend to have on the windowsill or in the garden.[213]

Motherwort

Motherwort, native to Europe and Asia, was used throughout its original range to treat female reproductive disorders and heart symptoms.[196] The ancient Greeks gave motherwort to pregnant women suffering from anxiety.[194] The English herbalist Gerard (late sixteenth century) noted its effectiveness in treating cardiac weakness. His successor, Culpepper, emphasized motherwort's ability to make the mind cheerful.[196] Ellingwood describes its use by the Eclectics for menstrual disorders, especially with nervousness and palpitations, considering it to be an emmenagogue, antispasmodic, nervine, laxative, and cardiotonic.[118] A number of Native American tribes used it for similar indications.[196,214] The Japanese prize their species of motherwort as an "herb of life," using it to enhance longevity.[195] Studies show mild sedative effects; direct myocardial action (including slowing of tachyarrhythmias)*; relaxation of vascular tone; lowering of lipids, inhibition of uterine fibroids; improvement of insomnia, muscle spasms, and headache; and protection during cerebral ischemia.[146,194,219,220]

Western botanical practitioners use motherwort for strengthening the heart and treating anxiety, premenstrual syndrome (PMS), menstrual problems, infertility, postpartum depression, irritability, and climacteric symptoms, especially when accompanied by palpitations; also to improve circulation, lower lipid levels, and reduce platelet aggregation.[194,221] David Hoffmann describes it as "a useful relaxing tonic for aiding in menopausal changes," and "an excellent tonic for the heart, strengthening without straining. It is a specific for over-rapid heartbeat brought about by anxiety."[135] Tori Hudson ND, a naturopathic physician specializing in women's health, adds it to her general menopause formula to control mood swings.[222]

Peony

Peony (also known as white peony) root has long been used in Chinese medicine and benefits a variety of gynecologic disorders, including amenorrhea, hypermenorrhea, and polycystic ovary syndrome (PCOS). Recent animal studies suggest peony root glycosides may also have antidepressant effects.[223-225] Specifically, the studies have demonstrated upregulation of brain-derived neurotrophic factor (BDNF) levels in a corticosterone-induced model of depression, as well as monoamine oxidase inhibition in mice.[226,227] Peony is ingested as a tea or tincture, and is often used in combination with other herbs.

Rhodiola

Rhodiola rosea originates from northern circumpolar or high altitude regions, and was traditionally used in Tibetan, Siberian, and Scandinavian cultures. In the Russian pharmacopoeia, it is indicated as an antidepressant, adaptogen, and nervous system tonic. Contemporary use in the form of tincture or capsules also includes supporting sport performance and immunity. Results from numerous rodent studies support antidepressant effects.[228,230] A phase III randomized controlled trial was conducted to determine the safety and efficacy of a standardized rhodiola extract in the treatment of mild to moderate depression. Patients were randomized into three groups: (1) 31 patients receiving 340 mg/day, (2) 29 patients receiving 680 mg/day, (3) 29 patients receiving placebo. Using the HAMD, the treatment groups showed improvement in depressive symptoms compared with controls.[231]

Rosemary

A randomized clinical study showed that smelling rosemary essential oil for 3 minutes resulted in a significant decrease in State-Trait Anxiety scores, and a reported feeling of more alertness, confirmed by appropriate EEG changes.[201,232] A murine study tested several rosemary fractions for their antidepressant effects. Results suggested that carnosol and betulinic acid could be responsible for the mood improvement effect of rosemary extracts.[233] In another study, investigators assessed the capacities of rosemary hydroalcoholic extract to reverse biochemical alterations associated with depression compared with fluoxetine. Using a variety of behavioral tests assessing cognitive function and exploratory behavior, rosemary extracts exhibited antidepressant effects. Changes in serum glucose level and hippocampal acetylcholinesterase activity were reversed by rosemary, whereas fluoxetine only affected acetylcholinesterase activity.[234] Herbalists use it widely in tea and tincture form, as well as aromatherapy (e.g., in baths) to relieve symptoms of depression and improve cognition. It also can be included in foods, particularly taken raw, steeped in olive oil to use on bread and salads, or cooked into soups.

Shatavari

Shatavari translates as "she who has a hundred husbands," and is a major Ayurvedic tonic adaptogen, traditionally used to promote physical and mental health, improve the body's defense mechanisms, and enhance longevity, especially for females; it is used for menopausal symptoms and for depression.[102,103] It is also used in TCM formulae for depression.[84]

---

*References 146,194,196,215-219.

Studies support its efficacy as an adaptogen, protecting against a variety of stressors.[98,102] Shatavari is used mainly by Ayurvedic practitioners. Anne McIntyre refers to it as the most important rejuvenative tonic for women and an excellent remedy in menopause that is calming and helpful to relieve stress and anxiety.[235]

St. John's Wort

St. John's wort's (Fig. 6-1) association with mood disturbance and the nervous system has a long historical precedence: medical use was documented by ancient Greek medical herbalists, including Hippocrates, who recommended it for "nervous unrest"; by Dioscorides and Galen for nerve pain; it is also used in Ayurvedic medicine.[141,196,236] The aerial flowering parts have been used in traditional European medicine for centuries internally to treat neuralgia, anxiety, neurosis, and depression.[196] The Eclectics used it internally to treat spinal injury pain, hysteria, and nervous affections with depression, and externally for pain, bruises, and sprains.[198]

Research and Studies

A number of studies have revealed that St. John's wort has a series of bioactive compounds with effects on a number of neurotransmitters, including serotonin, dopamine, norepinephrine, GABA, and glutamate.[237-239] It also affects the function of the HPA axis.[240] Reduced activity of the latter is known to be associated with atypical depression, somatoform disorder, neurasthenia, and fibromyalgia.[241] An interesting recent study investigated a number of extracts, found strong activity in all but one, and then discovered that the inactive extract lacked the flavonoid rutin; addition of rutin then resulted in a strong pharmacologic effect, comparable with that of the other extracts.[242] Hyperforin is considered to be one of St. John's wort's key active ingredients, and is detected in rodent brain tissue after oral administration of ethanol extracts.[243] Hyperforin alters sodium and calcium entry in TRPC6 (Transient receptor potential cation channel, subfamily C, member 6)-expressing cells, and researchers posit that this might be a mechanism of neuronal amine uptake inhibition. Hyperforin also induces neuronal axonal sprouting, like nerve growth factor in a TRPC6-dependent

manner.[244] However, the spectrum of CNS activities is felt to be caused by the synergy of its beautifully balanced components, rather than to a single "active ingredient."[150,179,245]

The major focus of contemporary investigation has been on St. John's wort's antidepressant activity, for which there is now considerable evidence. The first meta-analysis by Linde and colleagues in 1996 reviewed 23 randomized clinical trials, with 1757 outpatients with mild to moderate depression; *Hypericum* was found to be significantly superior to placebo, and efficacy was similar to standard antidepressants (TCAs).[246] Two more meta-analyses in 1999 and 2000 came to the same conclusions.[247,248] This was followed by a Cochrane Database review in 2000, involving 27 trials and 2291 patients, with the same findings; two meta-analyses, in 2001 and 2002, both finding St. John's wort to be significantly more effective than placebo for mild to moderate depression, similar to standard antidepressants (still TCAs); and two recent reviews with the same conclusions.[249,253] A 2008 update to the Cochrane review evaluated a total of 29 trials with 5489 patients, with 18 comparisons with placebo and 17 comparisons with standard antidepressants. After review, the following conclusions were drawn: *Hypericum* is superior to placebo in patients with major depression; *Hypericum* is as effective as antidepressants for depression with fewer side effects.[254]

One multicenter randomized, double-blind, placebo-controlled clinical trial was stopped early because convincing treatment efficacy could already be demonstrated; the conclusion was that *Hypericum* extract is an effective drug for the treatment of mild to moderate major depression.[255] A very large multicenter study of 2166 patients with mild to moderate depression, 75% of whom were women, with an average age of 50 years of age, were found to have clinically relevant improvement in symptoms with two dose levels of *Hypericum*, with 83% to 89% responding.[256] Another double-blind, randomized, placebo-controlled trial with 375 patients showed a significantly greater reduction in total score on the HAMD, and significantly more patients with treatment response or remission.[257] Two studies comparing *Hypericum* with SSRIs did not find a difference in efficacy between 900 mg/day of St. John's wort and 75 mg/day of sertraline (30 patients); compared with fluoxetine, *Hypericum* had significantly superior scores and responder rates (240 patients); however, there have been sharp criticisms of both studies.[258,259]

A double-blind 8-week clinical trial (n = 200) investigated the antidepressant efficacy of *Hypericum* extract as an extract compared with placebo. Utilizing the HAMD, efficacy of *Hypericum* was observed over placebo, particularly with hypersomnia symptoms (600 mg hypericum extract).[260] Another randomized controlled trial (n = 124) compared *Hypericum* to sertraline and placebo to treat depression over the course of 26 weeks. Using the HAMD, significant differences between the experimental and control groups were not observed at week 26 (900-1500 mg.).[261] Data from a 12-week clinical trial investigating the efficacy of *Hypericum*, citalopram, or placebo as acute treatment for minor depression did not reveal superiority of

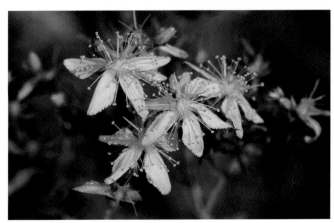

FIGURE 6-1 St. John's wort *(Hypericum perforatum)*. (Photo by Martin Wall.)

either intervention. Researchers observed a high placebo response from all outcomes measures.[262] A trial that was attempted by Massachusetts General Hospital, but that was closed prematurely by the sponsor, compared *Hypericum* 900 mg/day with fluoxetine 20 mg/day and placebo; data showed a trend toward significance for both *Hypericum* and fluoxetine.[263] A fifth trial (70 patients, randomized, controlled, double-blind) concluded that *Hypericum* is therapeutically equivalent to fluoxetine.[264] A 2008 study tested *Hypericum* for the prevention of depression relapse after recovery. It was executed in two phases: a 6-month continuation of 900 mg daily *Hypericum* treatment and 12 months of a maintenance dose. Using the HAMD and Beck Depression Inventory, *Hypericum* performed better than placebo and was well tolerated.[265] Additionally, a three-arm, double-blinded trial evaluated two *Hypericum* preparations (containing concentrations of 0.12% and 0.18% hypericin) for patients with minor depressive symptoms or dysthymia. Patients (n = 150) were randomized into two *Hypericum* extract and control groups, with HAMD scores taken at baseline and 3 and 6 weeks. Interestingly, the investigators found a discrepancy in responses between patients exhibiting dysthymic and nondysthymic tendencies, with the latter more responsive to *Hypericum* treatment. Secondary analysis using the Beck Depression Inventory found significant responses for both doses of *Hypericum* compared with placebo (270 mg).[266] Numerous additional clinical trials support the use of *Hypericum* for the treatment of depression.[267-270]

A recent open and uncontrolled outpatient study in Germany (n = 1778, 1541 completed) aimed to assess the safety and efficacy of *Hypericum* extract for mild to moderate depression over 12 weeks. Patients were evaluated every 4 weeks using a International Statistical Classification of Diseases and Related Health Problems (ICD)-10–derived symptom score and Clinical Global Impression scale. The majority reported improvement in symptoms. *Hypericum* extract was found to be effective and well tolerated with no reports of side effects or adverse reactions. (Extract dose was not disclosed.)[271] However, side effects have been observed in trials. A 2009 open multicenter study (n = 440 outpatients) evaluated the long-term effects of *Hypericum* extract in mild depression. Patients were treated with 500 mg of *Hypericum* extract daily for up to a year. Using the HAMD, depressive symptoms decreased from baseline over the course of treatment. Approximately 6% of patients exhibited adverse effects that may have been related to *Hypericum* treatment, with GI and skin complaints as some of the most commonly recorded.[272]

It is important to keep in mind that there is no difference in efficacy among the varied categories of antidepressants; they are all equally effective; they differ in type and severity of side effects.[67] It is useful when contemplating this mass of data to consider the results of a review conducted of clinical trial data for the nine antidepressant drugs approved by the Food and Drug Administration (FDA) between 1985 and 2000; this reviewed 10,030 patients with depression in 52 trials; the findings were that fewer than half (48%, 45 out of 93) of the antidepressant treatment arms showed superiority to

placebo.[273] A study on treatment for menopausal symptoms found that after 12 weeks of treatment, climacteric complaints diminished or disappeared completely in 76% (patient evaluation) to 79% (physician evaluation) of patients.[274] A sleep PSG study in healthy older women showed improved sleep quality (increased deep sleep without interference with REM sleep), no sedative effect, and improved well-being.[275] Other studies have shown possible effectiveness in reducing alcohol cravings; treating anxiety, PMS, stress, chronic fatigue syndrome, and obsessive-compulsive disorder; and improving learning and memory.[276-285] In addition, other documented activities include antiviral, antibacterial, antiinflammatory (i.e., cyclooxygenase-2 [COX-2]), and anticancer effects.[286-289]

Hypericum is used both as a simple extract and in formulae. Recent animal evidence suggests a potentiation effect when *Hypericum* is used in combination with passionflower.[290] A double-blind pilot study (n = 28) tested the use of a combination of *Hypericum* and kava kava for the treatment of depression and comorbid anxiety. The researchers began with a placebo run-in of 2 weeks, then utilized a crossover design administering *Hypericum* and kava kava against placebo over two 4-week phases. Utilizing the Beck Depression Inventory, *Hypericum* and kava kava significantly ameliorated symptoms of self-reported depression, but not anxiety or quality of life. The researchers speculated that the absence of anxiolytic effects may have been due presence of depression or inadequate kava kava dose (doses were not disclosed).[291]

A 1996 review of the side effects in clinical trials involving 3250 patients showed only allergic reactions (0.5%), GI upset (0.6%), and fatigue (0.4%); since then, side effects have been consistently reported to be far less severe or frequent than with standard antidepressant drugs, with no cardiac effects or sedation (i.e., no impairment of psychomotor performance, attention, or driving).[292-296] One review concluded that its tolerability is so much better than antidepressant drugs that it might be an especially useful option in older people.[297] In 1998, Hippius was able to state, "Overall, for a total of around 3.8 million patients treated during the period 1991 to 1996 … there have been only 32 spontaneous reports of side effects recorded by the German reporting system."[298] The issue of phototoxicity, which surfaced after several cases occurred during intravenous high-dose hypericin (presumed "active ingredient," not whole-herb extract), has been laid to rest by two careful studies showing that oral whole-herb extracts of *Hypericum* (i.e., LI 160), even in high doses (12 tablets a day, which is 10 times the usual dose), cause only limited photosensitivity. UVA sensitivity increased only after the highest dose; solar light sensitivity did not increase at all. This finding was replicated in a very recent study finding no phototoxic potential in humans in typical clinical doses (up to 1800 mg/day), confirming the prior review conclusion that it would require an oral dose of *Hypericum* 30 to 50 times greater than the recommended daily dose taken at one time to lead to severe phototoxic reactions in humans.[299-301]

HERBAL FORMULAE FOR TREATING DEPRESSION

Depression with Cognitive Dysfunction (i.e., Memory Loss)

St. John's wort	(Hypericum perforatum)	20 mL
Motherwort	(Leonurus cardiaca)	20 mL
Bacopa	(Bacopa monnieri)	20 mL
Eleuthero	(Eleutherococcus senticosus)	30 mL
Rosemary	(Rosmarinus officinalis)	10 mL
	Total: 100 mL	

This formula includes herbs with antidepressant and mentally stimulating effects and cerebrovascular blood flow–enhancing action to improve memory, learning, and mood.

Dose: 5 mL, twice daily. Use for at least 3 to 6 months for best results.

Tiger Today, Butterfly Tonight

(Modified depression formula from Amanda McQuade Crawford from *The Herbal Menopause Book.*)

Black cohosh	(Actaea racemosa)	25 mL
St. John's wort	(Hypericum perforatum)	25 mL
Eleuthero	(Eleutherococcus senticosus)	25 mL
Lavender	(Lavandula officinalis)	10 mL
Blue vervain	(Verbena officinalis)	10 mL
Licorice	(Glycyrrhiza glabra)	5 mL
	Total: 100 mL	

This formula is designed to regulate the hypothalamic-pituitary-adrenal (HPA) axis, improve stress adaptation responses, lift the spirits, directly treat depression, and help regulate hormonal activity.

Dose: 5 mL, twice daily. Use for at least 3 to 6 months for best results.

Interactions

A clinically relevant safety issue is that of interactions with other drugs. Recent work has documented that *Hypericum*, like many drugs and foods, potentiates several enzymes in the CYP series, affecting the metabolism of multiple categories of drugs, including lowering serum concentrations of warfarin, digoxin, theophylline, indinavir (i.e., HIV protease inhibitor), and cyclosporine and irinotecan (i.e., posttransplant immunosuppressants).[302-307] One case report described digoxin toxicity after stopping an herbal tea containing *Hypericum*.[308] Another study showed lowered plasma concentrations of simvastatin but not of pravastatin, caused by differences in Cytochrome P450 3A4 (CYP3A4) involvement.[309] It is important to remind ourselves that fluoxetine (and even grapefruit juice) is a potent inhibitor of CYP, which could increase levels of other drugs.[162]

The other issue involving drug interactions is the possibility of developing a potentially life-threatening serotonin syndrome (including agitation, hyperthermia, tachycardia, diaphoresis, rigidity) from adding St. John's wort to SSRIs. Please note that this is a known risk of SSRIs combined with other drugs, especially in older people. Several cases of this in older patients combining *Hypericum* with SSRIs have been reported.[310]

There are a small number of case reports of episodes of mania and hypomania in bipolar patients who use St. John's wort; caution is advised.[295] At least one component is measurable in breast milk.[311]

Prevalence of Use

St. John's wort is now the number one antidepressant prescribed by German physicians; almost 3 million prescriptions annually.[141,312] Even using standardized extract (the most expensive version) the cost is considerably less than the SSRIs.[387] Among botanical practitioners, it is used to lighten the mood, lift the spirit, relax tension and anxiety, and improve sleep and energy levels, especially for premenstrual dysphoric disorder (PMDD), PMS, menopausal symptoms, dysmenorrhea, and SAD.[150,179,313] In addition, it is used as an antiviral and antibacterial, and for nerve pain or trauma, wounds, and burns.[179]

Turmeric

Brain inflammation and microglial activation has been linked to a number of neurologic and psychological pathologies, including depression and chronic pain.[314] Turmeric downregulates several inflammatory pathways and may be implicated in treating inflammation-associated depression. Several in vivo studies support this use, but no clinical trials have been conducted to date. One mouse study tested antidepressant activity of three water-soluble curcumin formulations. Using the forced swim test, the preparations decreased immobility time, suggesting anxiolysis. Turmeric also increased serotonin and dopamine levels in the brain tissues.[315] Another mouse study (2008) found that turmeric extract modulates nitric oxide as a means of ameliorating oxidative damage.[316] An ethanolic extract of turmeric significantly reversed stress-induced increases in serum corticotropin-releasing factor and cortisol levels in two mouse studies.[317,318] A 2006 rodent study investigated whether curcumin treatment (2.5, 5, and 10 mg/kg, p.o. [by mouth]) affected behavior correlates of depression. Curcumin reversed changes in adrenal gland weight to body weight ratios, serum corticosterone levels, adrenal cortex thickness changes, and BDNF expression.[319]

NUTRITIONAL CONSIDERATIONS

Diet and nutrition can play a major role in depression, both as a cause and a treatment; it is the foundation of prevention.[312] There is ample research to document the nutritional inadequacies of the American population's diet and the contribution these deficiencies make to the worsening of depression.[168,320,321] Common deficiencies include vitamins A, C, D, E, and the B vitamins; the minerals calcium, magnesium, potassium, zinc, and selenium; fiber, complex carbohydrates, clean water, and essential fatty acids.[172] The opposite problem, that of dietary excesses, is contributing equally to the miserable nutritional situation.[172] Notorious excesses include caloric intake from excess carbohydrates, sugar, alcohol, and caffeine, all of which may contribute to depression.[172] Many nutrients have proven roles in both the etiology and treatment of depressive symptoms, most notably the B vitamins, but also vitamins D and E and the minerals calcium, iron, potassium, magnesium,[172] selenium, and zinc; and essential fatty acids, especially the omega-3s.*

The B vitamins function as a team, and work best when supplemented as B complexes rather than isolated B vitamins; this avoids potential neurotoxic side effects.[185,325] Good-quality high-potency multivitamins and multiminerals are cost-effective ways of achieving desired results and continuing to improve diet habits.[184,321]

Magnesium

Magnesium modulates glutamatergic pathways and may reverse stress-induced neuronal changes.[326,327] A 2013 systematic review on magnesium in the treatment of depression analyzed 21 cross-sectional studies, three clinical intervention trials, one prospective study, one case-only study, and one case series study. Reviewers concluded that higher dietary magnesium intake is likely associated with lower depressive symptoms.[328] A clinical trial of 23 elderly patients with type 2 diabetes and hypomagnesemia were randomized to receive 450 mg of magnesium or imipramine 50 mg daily during 12 weeks. Using the Yasavage and Brink score, the two groups exhibited comparable improvements in depressive symptoms.[329]

S-adenosylmethionine

A number of dietary supplements have been shown to improve outcomes in the treatment of depression. S-adenosylmethionine (SAMe) is an essential compound required by all body tissues; it has been used in Europe for decades, with extensive documentation of efficacy comparable to TCA drugs in clinical trials, including 13 RCTs and 1 meta-analysis.[312,321,324,330] A review of 28 high-quality SAMe studies for evidence on treatment of depression, osteoarthritis, and liver disease published by the Agency for Healthcare Research and Quality found SAMe superior to placebo in reducing symptoms of depression. It has been shown to boost levels of neurotransmitters, including serotonin, norepinephrine, and dopamine, and improve nerve cell function.[324] Improvements may begin within 2 weeks.[324,330] It requires adequate levels of B vitamins, especially folate and B_{12}.[324] Treatment dosage is 400 to 1200 mg/day. According to Low Dog, the patient should be started on 200 mg/day for 5 days, which is increased by 200 mg/day every 3 to 5 days. Side effects include GI upset, agitation, and insomnia. This supplement is contraindicated in patients with bipolar disorder.[9]

Omega-3 Fatty Acids

Omega-3 fatty acids may play an important role in the prevention and treatment of depression. A number of studies have suggested efficacy in the treatment of a variety of psychological disturbances and psychiatric disorders, ranging from impulsivity and aggression to PMS, postpartum depression, and general clinical depression.[331-334] Epidemiologically, there are lower rates of depression in cultures in which there is significant dietary (i.e., fish) consumption of omega-3 fatty acids compared with those cultures with less fish in the diet.[335] Unfortunately, few well-controlled studies have been conducted evaluating efficacy. However, given the potential overall benefits essential fatty acids on the nervous and cardiovascular systems, and the safety of supplementation, it seems reasonable to include essential fatty acids in a treatment protocol for depression.[9] Commercial supplements from fish oils have been found to be free of mercury and other heavy metal contamination by the FDA and consumer labs. The daily recommended dose is 1 to 3 g. Doses higher than his have not been found to have added benefits.

ADDITIONAL THERAPIES

It is crucial to initially address underlying issues contributing to depression and associated conditions, including psychosocial factors, lifestyle issues, and spiritual stressors. Simply substituting the prescription medication for an herbal medication does not qualify as "holistic" medicine. The preferred holistic strategy in all cases would be prevention, and the partial list of possibilities discussed in this section would be applicable to that aim as well as to treatment of an illness that results from failure of prevention.

Exercise

Exercise has been shown to be effective for both the treatment and prevention of depression, and the data are even stronger for women than men.[336,337] In treatment of older patients with major depression, supervised exercise was as effective as the antidepressant drug sertraline.[338] Moderate exercise was more effective than vigorous exercise in decreasing the anxiety and stress components of depression, and in improving self-esteem.[336] A randomized, placebo-controlled trial showed that a program as simple as a brisk 20-minute walk outdoors at a target heart rate of 60% max, 5 days a week (with increased light exposure and vitamins—see discussion later) was effective in improving mood, self-esteem, and sense of well-being, and decreasing depressive-symptom scores, and with an impressively high level of adherence by the study participants.[336] In multiple studies, exercisers' moods were found to be significantly more positive, regardless of menopausal state[144]; scores were lower on somatic symptoms and memory/concentration difficulties and significantly higher on well-being, positive mood, and libido.[172,339,340] In addition to aerobic exercise, strength training offers many of the same benefits.[184,341] Yoga and tai chi practices yield not only all the benefits of other exercise programs[324] but also improvement in flexibility and balance, and achievement of "relaxation/stress management" benefits; in addition, they may include a meditation component that enhances the latter effect.[312]

Relaxation and Stress Management

Relaxation training and stress management techniques have been demonstrated to be effective in many clinical studies, and should be considered in every prevention or treatment program.[77] Possible components include progressive

---

*References 172,184,185,320-324.

relaxation, abdominal breathing, meditation,[342] imagery, and biofeedback. Relaxation response (i.e., mental focusing, diaphragmatic breathing, breath awareness) has been shown in randomized, controlled prospective clinical trials to produce significant improvement in hot flashes, tension/anxiety, and depression.[172,343-345] Yoga and tai chi have profound effects via physical positions, breathing exercises, meditation, and spiritual practices; studies document successful outcomes in treatment of anxiety disorders, depression, PMDD, menopause, and sleep disorders.[105,324]

Light Therapy

Light therapy has been studied repeatedly and found to be effective not only for SAD but also for nonseasonal depressions and eating disorders.[312,336] This is consistent with data showing that in Finland and Sweden the best single predictor of general well-being was the amount of light and length of day; a London study of women without SAD found a stronger correlation between mood and outdoor light levels than with menstrual cycle phases.[336] Adding bright light to an exercise program gave better reduction of depressive symptoms than the same exercise program with normal lighting.[336] Light exposure in the morning has been shown to deepen sleep via reinforcement of circadian rhythms.[346] In the study by Brown and coworkers, walking briskly outdoors 5 days a week for 20 minutes (plus vitamins—see the following) resulted in a significant improvement in mood, self-esteem, and sense of well-being, and decreases in depressive-symptom scores, and with an impressively high level of adherence by the study participants.[336]

Counseling

The role of counseling in treatment of depression has been well substantiated in a variety of modes—individual, family, self-help, group, and sex therapies. It has been progressively marginalized in the orthodox medical community because drug prescription has become fashionable, but professional help sorting through the individual, family, societal, and planetary influences on our affective disorders can shorten the precious time we spend mired in psychic mud, freeing us to move again toward our life goals. Once again, it is important to stress that immediate, confirmed referral to a psychiatrist is mandatory in cases of suicidal ideation, paranoia, psychosis, or very severe depression.[68,322]

Many other possibilities also may be helpful, with a partial list including art therapy, music therapy, spirituality or religion, massage, laughter, hypnosis, solitude, journaling, self-nurturing, and acupuncture. An important and often-overlooked consideration is that of the influence of one's home and work surroundings on mood and health; attention to healing environments and to space-clearing techniques may contribute considerably to restoration of well-being.

It is not expected that anyone would incorporate all of these wildly varied types of approaches into a treatment strategy for depression. An informed practitioner should be able to suggest a varied and colorful palette of choices, based on careful evaluation of the individual, who can be assisted to select one or more that resonate with her own sense of self. Initial strategies should be reevaluated jointly by the individual and her practitioner, with additions and substitutions as needed, until the desired outcome is attained. At that point, a maintenance plan to prevent recurrence must be instituted to avoid contributing to the dismal relapse statistics.[70,347,348] Because humans are an integral part of a local and planetary ecosystem, all choices should be evaluated carefully for their potential to damage the health of humans, other species, or the ecosystem (i.e., Precautionary Principle).[349]

ANXIETY

Anxiety is defined as "excessive worry involving a variety of issues related to health, family, money, or work in which the concerns seem pervasive, repetitive and out of proportion to actual life circumstances."[350] Many individuals experiencing anxiety may fail to recognize the symptoms in themselves, and may present to a practitioner with the following signs and symptoms: easy fatigability, difficulty concentrating, irritability, muscle tenderness, muscle tension, restlessness, and sleep disturbance. The most frequently reported clinical symptoms of general anxiety are diaphoresis, headache, and trembling.[350]

General anxiety disorders are one of the most common medical conditions. According to the National Institute of Mental Health, the 1-year prevalence rate is 13.3% of the population.[71]

The pathophysiology of generalized anxiety disorder (GAD) is multifactorial and remains incompletely understood. Studies in humans and animals have attempted to pinpoint general areas in the brain that seem to play a critical role in anxiety, but consensus has not been reached. Functional imaging studies suggest that a number of areas in the brain of patients that have been diagnosed with GAD, including the occipital cortex, limbic system, and basal ganglia, show altered metabolism after benzodiazepine therapy.[351]

The binding functions of several neurotransmitter receptors appear deregulated in GAD and include the GABA-A and benzodiazepine receptors.[352] The noradrenergic system appears involved, but studies detailing the exact mechanism have not been consistent. However, higher levels of catecholamines have been correlated in anxiety,[353] as have elevated levels of the neurotransmitter 5-hydroxytryptamine. Other neuropeptides such as cholecystokinin, corticotrophin-releasing factor, and tachykinins (including substance P), as well as neuroactive steroids such as dehydroepiandrosterone (DHEA) are also implicated, but again, their relationship to GAD is not well defined.[351]

Numerous studies evaluating depression and anxiety in relation to gender have shown an increased rate of depression and anxiety in women over men beginning in adolescence, with a small peak just before menopause.[354,355] Although there seems to be some biochemical evidence for a hormonal role in the development of mood disorders, correlated increases during menopause do not appear evident. Several longitudinal studies in Europe and North America have observed cohorts of women through menopause and most studies have reported no increase in moderate or severe depression nor anxiety with menopause.[354] Factors correlated with increased anxiety in menopause are more strongly correlated with women who are more symptomatic[356] (e.g., experience more hot flashes and night sweats), have a prior history of mood disorders, lower socioeconomic status,[356] poor marital adjustment[357] unemployment,[356] and lower educational level.[358] Therefore experts in women's health have attributed anxiety in menopause to sleep deprivation as a secondary occurrence to night sweats and menopausally related discomforts, or personal perceptions involving the physiologic changes associated with menopause.[184] Sometimes, anxiety can be a secondary phenomenon accompanying depression.[359]

DIAGNOSIS

As with many psychological presentations the symptoms of anxiety can overlap with very serious medical conditions and a full medical workup by a health care professional is suggested to prevent overlooking this as a contributing factor. Table 6-5 presents a simplified list of common medical conditions associated with anxiety.

CONVENTIONAL TREATMENT APPROACHES

Many conventional medications are available for the treatment of anxiety. These include antidepressants such as TCAs or the newer SSRIs. The use of SSRIs has steadily increased from 2% in 1992 to 19% in 1997, to now between 1 in 4 and

1 in 6 women taking an antidepressant of some form. Loss of libido, restlessness, or sedation are frequent side effects for which this class of medications is often discontinued.[360] For short-term treatment, the use of benzodiazepines is a consideration, but they are associated with sedation, habituation (i.e., tolerance), and the potential for long-term cognitive deficits.

Another option is the medication buspirone. An azapirone, it is in a different pharmacologic class from the benzodiazepines. Buspirone has not been reported to be associated with tolerance. However, in comparison with the TCAs or SSRIs, its therapeutic effects are mild. Therefore it is considered useful for mild anxiety. It also takes approximately 4 weeks to reach a therapeutic level. In 4 of 11 placebo-controlled studies comparing buspirone with placebo or a benzodiazepine, after 4 weeks of treatment, buspirone showed no benefit.[360] Further discussions of these options are beyond the scope of this chapter; those interested in this aspect of treatment should consult a general psychiatric text.

THE BOTANICAL PRACTITIONER'S PERSPECTIVE

Herbalists have recognized a number of botanical preparations as nervines and anxiolytics, and categorized them as nerve tonics (i.e., preparations that tone or rehabilitate the nervous system), nerve sedatives (i.e., relax the nervous system), nerve stimulants (i.e., increase vitality without provoking the nervous system or creating agitation), or nerve demulcents (i.e., soothe and heal; may physically "protect" the nerve endings).[361] Use of the botanicals classified in this way may include a combination of botanicals in tincture or extract form from the different categories based on historical and anecdotal clinical experience of the practitioner. In other instances, treatment may include the use of a bath containing the herb(s) in combination with consumption of a tea or other form of oral preparation. Similarly, in many traditional cultures (e.g., Chinese, East Indian) preparations are used in combinations as formulae to support (regenerate), soothe, and calm with the common philosophic objective that treating a variety of facets of the disease or imbalance may hasten healing via synergism of the group of plants selected. This philosophy is different than the biomedical approach of using singular pharmacologic agents to treat an illness.

The herbs discussed in Table 6-6 are nervines, adaptogens, and anxiolytics. However, practitioners are encouraged to draw from a wide selection of herbs, including nervines, adaptogens, and sedatives to create an optimal formulation for each individual woman with anxiety.

Black Cohosh

Black cohosh has been used for more than four decades in Europe to treat symptoms associated with menopause, including anxiety in menopause.[362] Although it is reported to reduce the symptoms of menopause, which include hot flashes, mood disorders, diaphoresis, palpitations, and vaginal dryness, there

TABLE 6-5 Medical Conditions Often Associated with Symptoms of Anxiety	
Type of Condition	**Examples**
Cardiovascular	Acute myocardial infarction (i.e., heart attack)
	Angina
	Arrhythmias
	Hypertension
	Mitral valve prolapse
Endocrine	Hyperthyroidism
	Hypothyroidism
	Parathyroid disease
	Adrenal disorders
	Hypoglycemia
Gastrointestinal	Irritable bowel syndrome
Vitamin deficiency states	Vitamin B_{12} deficiency
Toxic conditions	Alcohol and drug withdrawal
	Mercury
	Arsenic
	Caffeine and caffeine withdrawal
Neurologic	Brain tumor
	Seizure disorder
Respiratory	Asthma
	Pulmonary embolism
	Chronic obstructive pulmonary disease

have been no trials showing its efficacy for anxiety alone. One study done in 1987 randomized 80 menopausal women to Remifemin (four pills daily), 0.625 mg of conjugated estrogens, or placebo for 12 weeks. The Kupperman Index and HAMD scores were significantly lower in the groups treated with black cohosh.[363] Borrelli and Ernst published a brief systematic review of controlled trials of black cohosh and its effects on menopausal symptoms. Four trials were included and the conclusion was that "the evidence was not compelling enough to support improvement."[364] However, many of the trials have been small with generally suggestive outcomes. In many of the studies, the standardized measurement used to assess symptom improvement was the Kupperman Index, which is considered outmoded as a standardized instrument for menopausal symptoms. The index omits some important symptoms classically associated with menopause, making the assessment of black cohosh in these studies harder to evaluate.[365] The use of this botanical primarily for anxiety in menopause is based primarily on traditional or theoretical use.

The mechanism of action for improvement of neurovegetative symptoms (including mood disorders) by black cohosh is not clear. Initially because of the reported presence of formononetin, estrogenic receptor binding activity with lowering levels of follicle-stimulating hormone (FSH) levels was considered the basis of the pharmacologic effectiveness of black cohosh.[21] The majority of subsequent studies both in animals and in vitro have demonstrated mixed results, and it is now believed that there is no estrogenic activity to black cohosh.[126,366,367] A recently identified compound found in black cohosh, fukinolic acid, has been shown to have weak estrogenic effects but this does not fully explain the estrogen-like activity of this botanical.[368]

Current recommendations for dosages range from 40 to 80 mg daily, although most clinical trials have used 80 mg daily. A recent clinical trial compared the efficacy of two different doses of a proprietary product of black cohosh (40 versus 127 mg daily), which showed similar efficacy profiles.[369] It is not clear if black cohosh is safe in individuals with hormone-sensitive conditions such as breast cancer or endometriosis because of the conflicting reports on estrogenic activity. The *ABC Clinical Guide to Herbs* states that "Despite earlier concerns about the possible estrogenicity of black cohosh, and thus a possible contraindication for women with estrogen-positive breast cancer ... it is clearly established that black cohosh is not estrogenic. Thus no such contraindication is warranted."[21] With overdoses, occasional GI effects[370] have been reported, as well as vertigo, headache, nausea, vomiting, impaired vision, and circulation.[362,370] There are no known drug interactions.[372]

Chamomile

Chamomile is a soothing, gentle, and calming herb used to alleviate nervous agitation and anxiety in people of all ages. The flowers soothe both the GI and nervous systems. Though it has a long history of use, studies are sparse. A randomized clinical trial (n = 57) investigated the effect of a 220 mg standardized chamomile extract in depressed patients with comorbid anxiety. Measured with the HAMD, the chamomile group exhibited statistically significant improvements in symptoms of anxiety and depression compared with placebo.[372] It is commonly consumed as a tea due to its sweet and palatable flavor, but is increasingly found in tincture combinations and encapsulated products. It is often used in combination with other calming nervine herbs, such as lemon balm and lavender. It is suitable for daily use. However, some people with

TABLE 6-6 Herbs for Anxiety

Therapeutic Goal	Therapeutic Activity	Botanical Name	Common Name
Relieve anxiety	Anxiolytic	*Actaea racemosa*	Black cohosh
		Lavandula officinalis	Lavender
		Passiflora incarnata	Passionflower
		Piper methysticum	Kava kava
		Valeriana officinalis	Valerian
Relieve anxiety	Nervine	*Avena sativa*	Milky oats
		Hypericum perforatum	St. John's wort
		Matricaria recutita	Chamomile
		Melissa officinalis	Lemon balm
		Scutellaria lateriflora	Skullcap
		Turnera diffusa	Damiana
Relieve anxiety	Sedative	*Corydalis ambigua*	Corydalis
		Eschscholzia californica	California poppy
		Humulus lupulus	Hops
		Passiflora incarnata	Passionflower
		Valeriana officinalis	Valerian
		Ziziphus spinosa	Ziziphus
Relieve anxiety	Adaptogen	*Withania somnifera*	Ashwagandha
Relieve palpitations associated with anxiety		*Leonurus cardiaca*	Motherwort

allergies to *Asteraceae* or daisy family plants should proceed with caution when using chamomile.

Kava Kava

Kava kava is an excellent alternative for those wishing to avoid using conventional medications. This plant, indigenous to the Pacific islands, has been used for many centuries by the local cultures as a part of celebrating special events and people.[373] Kava kava has been found to reduce anxiety in a number of small clinical trials. One systematic review assessed seven clinical trials evaluating the efficacy of kava kava in anxiety, and in all seven kava kava was found to be superior to placebo.[374] Major criticisms of these trials are that they have used small-size, ill-defined patient populations, or failed to meet the DSM-IV criteria for generalized anxiety. Several trials have been done specifically addressing anxiety in menopausal women. In these trials, not only was a reduction in anxiety statistically significant, but many of the neurovegetative symptoms associated with menopause were also improved.[375-377] The 2009 Kava Anxiety Depression Spectrum Study (KADSS) was a 3-week, placebo-controlled, double-blind, crossover trial (n = 60) that used an aqueous standardized extract of kava kava for the treatment of anxiety and depression. Using the HAMD, Beck Anxiety Inventory, and Montgomery–Asberg Depression Rating Scale, the kava kava extract was found to be significantly more efficacious ($p < 0.0001$) compared with controls. It was also well tolerated, with no adverse events or hepatotoxic effects observed. (Kava extract dose not noted.)[378]

The active constituents responsible for kava kava's effectiveness in reducing anxiety are the kavalactones. These are a group of 15 lactones, maximally concentrated in the lateral roots of the plant. These lipophilic compounds exert their effects in several areas: at the GABA-A receptors[379]; and at receptor sites that regulate serotonin,[380] noradrenaline,[381] and dopamine.[382] Kava kava also may act at the limbic structures, reducing anxiety without causing sedation.[383] However, the exact mechanisms of how kavalactones exert their effects have not been entirely determined. The actual lactone content in the root varies between 3% and 20%.[384] Until recently, the reported adverse effects of kava kava have been mild or negligible, except for a dermatologic condition reported with chronic use. This dermatologic disorder, called kava dermopathy, is only seen with prolonged and excessive use of kava (doses of 400 mg for more than 3 months).[385] It is reversible with reduced intake or cessation. Until the last several years, rare reports of drug interactions, mostly involving sedation, have occurred with the concomitant use of other pharmaceutical drugs that share similar mechanisms of action with the kavalactones. However, by 2002, approximately 28 cases of severe liver toxicity associated with kava kava intake were reported in Europe (four in Switzerland and 24 in Germany).[386] The adverse effects reported included cholestatic hepatitis, jaundice, increased liver enzymes, liver cell impairment, severe hepatitis with confluent necrosis, and irreversible liver damage requiring transplantation of the liver (four cases). In the United States, five cases of liver

dysfunction have been reported associated with the use of kava kava. The reviews of the adverse case reports emphasize that in many of the reports the individuals were concurrently using medications known to be hepatotoxic.[387] In several cases, other causes of hepatitis, such as viral infections or use of alcohol, could not be excluded. Currently, because of the recent adverse effect reports, kava kava has been removed from unrestricted use in several countries including France, England, Germany, and Canada.[21] In the United States in March 2001, the FDA issued a public warning in response to the hepatotoxic case reports.

Currently, the recommendations are a daily dose equivalent of 60 to 120 mg of kavalactones in a semisolid or dry extract (with not less than 30% kavalactone content).[21] Because of concerns over hepatotoxicity, it is recommended that those patients who have known liver disease, are taking hepatotoxic medications, or frequently using alcohol should be advised to consult a health care professional before considering use of kava kava. In light of the recent reports on hepatotoxicity, it has been advised that use beyond 1 month be monitored by a health care professional.[21] Consumers should be advised of the rare but potential risk for liver problems when kava kava is taken along with alcohol, barbiturates, drugs affecting mental activity, or other substances acting on the CNS; such combinations may increase inebriation or the effect of the drug.[21] Kava kava should not be used during pregnancy or while nursing.[370]

Lavender

Lavender has been used in aromatherapy as an anxiolytic.[388] There have been one randomized trial, two controlled trials, and one case series evaluating efficacy of lavender herb as an anxiolytic. The largest randomized trial, consisting of 122 ICU patients, used a lavender oil massage, grapeseed oil massage, or undisturbed rest for three sessions lasting 30 minutes, at least 24 hours apart. The finding showed initial benefit in the first session that dissipated in later sessions.[209] Another study demonstrated the anxiolytic effects of inhaled lavender in female college students (n = 42). Participants were studied during 4 weeks: a control week, a 60% lavender fragrance treatment week, a washout week, and a 100% lavender fragrance treatment week. Outcomes were self-reported and suggested beneficial effects on sleep patterns and overall mood after lavender treatment.[35]

In general, although the evidence for lavender as an anxiolytic aromatherapy agent is generally positive, the trials are considered flawed enough methodologically to make the evidence weak.[389] The mechanism of action for anxiolytic activity has been attributed to linalool. In mice, linalool was found to reduce motor activity because of a dose-related binding of glutamate. Glutamate is an excitatory CNS neurotransmitter.[390] Another rodent study investigated the effects of inhaled linalool on anxious and aggressive behaviors. After administration of linalool, mice displayed anxiolytic effects in the light/dark test, as well as decreased aggressive behavior.[391] However, there are over 100 constituents in lavender, including linalool, perillyl alcohol, linalyl acetate, camphor, limone triterpenes, coumarins, cineole, and flavonoids, which also may have some activity.[389] Lavender oil is quickly absorbed when topically applied and has a peak of 19 minutes; it disappears from the blood within 90 minutes.[392] In general, lavender is well tolerated with minimal adverse effects. There have been cases of mild[393] with topical use,[394] with oral use, CNS depression[395] with aromatherapy, and reversible neutropenia[396] with high oral doses of perillyl alcohol.

Lemon Balm

Lemon balm, named for its citruslike and uplifting flavor, is a gentle herb used in tea and tincture forms to calm anxiety, improve mood, and soothe nervous stomach disorders. One mouse study evaluated the effects of a lemon balm extract on anxious behavior. Using the elevated plus maze test, a significant and dose-dependent effect was observed.[397] A valerian and lemon balm combination was tested for anxiolytic effects in a double-blind crossover clinical trial (n = 24). On separate days separated by a 7-day washout period, participants received three separate single doses of a standardized lemon balm and valerian extract product—600 mg, 1200 mg, or 1800 mg—and a placebo. Mood alterations were assessed before administration and subsequently at 1, 3, and 6 hours postdose using a 20-minute version of the Defined Intensity Stressor Simulation (DISS) battery. The 600 mg dose of the combination ameliorated anxiety related to the administration of DISS. However, the 1800 mg dose showed an increase in anxiety in one testing session.[398]

Passionflower

Historical uses of passionflower have been as an analgesic, anticonvulsant, for chronic pain, perimenopausal hot flashes, and tension, to name a few.[399] It generally has been used in combination with other herbs, making it difficult to evaluate on its own. Few clinical trials have been done assessing its anxiolytic potential. One pilot evaluating passionflower (45 drops/daily) against oxazepam (30 mg/daily) for 4 weeks showed reduction in anxiety comparable with benzodiazepine. There were fewer difficulties with impairment in job performance noted in the passionflower arm.[400] Another trial with a mixture of passionflower, valerian, *Crataegus, Ballota, Cola,* and *Paullinia* showed improved HAMD scores compared with placebo for 28 days.[401] A 2-year multicenter study of nervous agitation in children (n = 115) found benefit from a combination of *Hypericum*, passionflower (*Passiflora incarnata*), and valerian root extracts. (Extract dose not provided.)[402] A 2007 Cochrane summary on the safety and efficacy of passionflower for treating anxiety disorders found too few studies to draw conclusions.[403] There are other botanical preparations that have a historic use for anxiety but do not have clinical trials evaluating efficacy. The basis for passionflower use with anxiety has been derived either from use in other traditional medical systems or use in Western herbalism.

Skullcap

Skullcap is used to sooth anxiety and emotional distress. A 2014 clinical trial tested the mood effects of skullcap on 43 healthy volunteers. Participants were randomized to receive 350 mg of skullcap or placebo three times daily for 2 weeks. The group was characterized as nonanxious using the Beck Anxiety Inventory. The authors observed a significant group effect where some participants moderate their opinions in order to go along with a majority view. Mood disturbance was assessed by the Profile of Mood States, and the skullcap group exhibited significant decreases compared with baseline scores and controls.[404] Skullcap (*Scutellaria lateriflora*) is not to be confused with Chinese skullcap (*Scutellaria baicalensis*), which has a very different therapeutic profile.

Valerian

Valerian's use as a sedative and sleep aid in Europe dates back to the time of Hippocrates.[389] It is currently used in Western botanical medicine as a sedative. Since 1982, there have been 20 clinical studies on valerian for insomnia ranging from 1 night to 4 weeks in duration. The majority of studies consistently report improvement of sleep with valerian. Five blinded or randomized clinical studies evaluated valerian for anxiety; two were combination preparations: most concluded that valerian significantly lowered the HAMD scores.[21,405] A major criticism of many of the studies were that they had inadequate descriptions of randomization and blinding, and in some there was inadequate power to statistically detect significant differences.[405-407] The studies ranged from 2 to 4 weeks with the doses ranging from 50 mg (in combination with other botanicals) to 300 mg daily. The mechanism of action with respect to action as an anxiolytic is attributed to the valepotriates and their breakdown products,[21] but valerian root contains as many as 150 compounds. Recently it is thought that synergistic action by multiple compounds may exert a sedative effect.[47] Valerian-treated mice exhibited higher hippocampal levels of 5-HT.[408] Animal models suggest that valerianic acid may inhibit enzymes that break down GABA, and that increased GABA levels may produce sedating or CNS–depressant effects.[409] Other animal studies suggested the involvement of metabotropic glutamate receptors (mGluRs) I and II.[410]

Valerian has a characteristic odor, attributed to isovaleric acid, that many find unpleasant. It is poorly absorbed by mouth. Mexican and Indian sources of valerian have reportedly high concentrations of valepotriates, which may be toxic and should be avoided.[411] General adverse effects have included headaches and stomach upset, but adverse reports are rare. In one case, a combination of valerian and skullcap plus other herbs, which may have adulterated the sample, caused an elevation of liver enzymes (i.e., hepatotoxicity). It was undetermined in this case whether valerian contributed to this pathology.[412]

ADDITIONAL THERAPIES

Mind–Body Medicine

Psychotherapy has been shown to be effective in the treatment of GAD, with or without medical intervention. Behavioral therapy and cognitive behavior therapy (CBT) are two commonly used techniques that allow patients to identify their behavioral patterns and learn to change their thinking, reactions, and behaviors to create new response patterns.

Relaxation Techniques

Numerous relaxation techniques can help patients identify and shift anxiety patterns. These include visualization, massage, aromatherapy, sound therapy, and hypnosis, to name a few. Biofeedback also has been shown to be useful in the treatment of anxiety disorders. Exercise also can be a beneficial relaxation technique for some patients.

 TREATMENT SUMMARY

Anxiety

- Consider botanicals as an alternative for some who cannot tolerate the adverse effects of prescriptive medicines or in those who prefer more natural remedies.
- Choose from a variety of nervine categories and specific herbs according to patient indications.

LOW LIBIDO AND SEXUAL DYSFUNCTION

Sexual relationships are some of the most important social and biological relationships in human life. Next to thirst, hunger and sleep, the sexual urge is the most powerful biological drive. This physiological instinct, so essential to the survival of the species, is one of the mainsprings of human motivation, and its fulfillment or disappointment is closely related to happiness or misery. Normal sexual function involves the successful integration of biological, psychological, and interpersonal influences.[413]

Binu Tharakan and Bala Manyam

"Female sexual response is a complex, nonlinear progression from desire to arousal to orgasm."[414] Sexual response in women is highly variable and multifaceted, including a complex interplay of physiologic, psychological, and interpersonal components.[415] It naturally fluctuates with stress, fatigue, the menstrual cycle, illness, and other factors (Table 6-7). Low libido becomes increasingly common during a woman's midlife (the fifties and sixties), and for a smaller percentage of women, as early as in their thirties. Female sexual dysfunction (FSD) is a medical condition defined as persistent or recurrent reduction in libido, aversion to sexual activity, difficulty becoming aroused, inability to achieve orgasm, or dyspareunia (i.e., painful intercourse) that a woman self-identifies as causing her personal discomfort or dissatisfaction with her sex life.[416] A variety of terms have been used to describe disorders of sexual desire and arousal, including sexual avoidance, low libido, inhibited sexual desire, hypoactive sexual desire, hypoactive sexual desire disorder (HSDD), female sexual arousal disorder, and sexual aversion disorder.[417]

It has been estimated, and widely purported, based on a study of sexual behavior in a demographically representative cohort of US women, that as many as 43% of women experience some form of sexual dysfunction, with one report estimating as high as 76% of women.[418-421] It has been suggested, however, that even the 43% figure is an overestimation, and that the entity FSD is an invention of the pharmaceutical industry for economic gain. According to a recent article in the *British Medical Journal*, "The marketing of a disease: female sexual dysfunction," "Widespread and growing scientific disagreement exists over both its definition and prevalence. In addition, the meaningful benefits of experimental drugs for women's sexual difficulties are questionable, and the financial conflicts of interest of experts who endorse the notion of a highly prevalent medical condition are extensive."[419]

In spite of some controversy over the extent or exact definition of FSD, the decline in libido in midlife that many women experience is a well-recognized phenomenon. Decreased sexual desire is one of the most common problems seen in a primary care or obstetrics and gynecology (OB/GYN) office, and is multifactorial in origin.[417,422] Reasons for decline in libido include[424]:

- Irregular ovarian function and declining hormone levels associated with perimenopause and menopause
- Changes in anatomy (e.g., vaginal prolapse, atrophy, or dryness), neurologic function, and vascular responsiveness
- Psychosocial issues related to sexuality, the sexual relationship, body image, or the changes that may accompany aging
- Relationship dynamics
- Personal sexual beliefs, expectations, and prior sexual experiences

TABLE 6-7	Factors Influencing Female Sexual Function
Factor	**Examples**
Biologic/ Physiologic factors	Neurologic disease
	Cancer
	Urologic or gynecologic disorders
	Medications
	Endocrine abnormality
Psychological factors	Depression/anxiety
	Prior sexual or physical abuse
	Substance abuse
Interpersonal factors	Relationship quality and conflict
	Lack of privacy
	Partner performance and technique
	Lack of partner
Sociocultural factors	Inadequate education
	Conflict with religious, personal, or family values
	Societal taboos

From Amato P: Categories of female sexual dysfunction, *Obstet Gynecol Clin North Am* 33:527–534, 2006.

Loss of libido can indicate the presence of underlying disorders; for example, diabetes, cardiovascular disease, pituitary tumors, depression, chronic pelvic pain, interstitial cystitis, and chronic renal disease.[414,424-426] Women whose partners have erectile dysfunction may suffer from increased rates of FSD.[427] Previous pelvic or bladder surgery may predispose women to sexual dysfunction. Many medications, including antihypertensives, antidepressants (especially SSRIs), and tranquilizers can adversely affect libido. Antihistamines can reduce vaginal lubrication and thereby affect sexual response and comfort. In women in their thirties and forties, declines in libido are more likely to have psychoemotional origins rather than physiologic underpinnings. For example, low libido in these groups may be a sign of relationship/marital discord or a reaction to negative sexual experience.[424] At any age, low libido is more likely to occur in those with poor physical and emotional health and is highly associated with negative experiences in sexual relationships and overall well-being.[418] Sexual dysfunction can be categorized into subtypes including HSDD, sexual arousal disorder, orgasmic disorder, and sexual pain disorder.[416,428,429]

Physiologic declines in reproductive function (i.e., menopause and the cessation of fertility) typically precede loss of sexual interest by a couple of decades; for many women, this is extremely frustrating because they enter a time in their lives when they first might be able to experience greater sexual freedom and lack of concern over unwanted pregnancy, and find themselves with low libido. Other women see menopause as a painful loss of their youth and femininity, negatively affecting their self-perception and their sexuality; others see (or use) loss of libido as an excuse to avoid sexual activity (e.g., in an unhappy marriage).[423] For some women and couples, loss of sexual interest may not be problematic at all, and unless there is an underlying disorder, this does not necessitate treatment.

FEMALE SEXUAL RESPONSE

In the 1960s, Masters and Johnson proposed a model of female sexual response that outlined a linear progression through four phases: excitement, plateau, orgasm, and resolution.[417] Kaplan updated this to a three-phase model consisting of desire, arousal, and orgasm, which forms the foundation of the DSM-IV classification of FSD. Basson and colleagues have more recently suggested a multifactorially stimulated, circular, psychophysiologic model that recognizes emotional intimacy and physical satisfaction as goals in the female sexual experience.[415,417,429] Classifications of FSD have been expanded to include psychogenic and organic causes of desire, arousal, orgasm, and sexual pain disorders.[416] An essential element of the FSD diagnostic system is "personal distress" as part of the criterion.[416]

The Physiology of Women's Sexual Response

The sexual response is a complex interplay of psychological, emotional, visual, "scentual," tactile, and physiologic stimuli.

Erotic feelings are coupled to vascular changes that are characteristic of female sexual excitement.

- Vasocongestion of deep vaginal tissues leads to secretion of clear, slippery vaginal mucus within less than a minute of sexual arousal. This fluid serves a lubricating function for penile movement, neutralizes normal vagina acidity, and supports sperm survival.
- Vasocongestion not only affects vaginal tissue, but also causes flushing across the chest, back, and neck in as many as 75% of women.
- Vasocongestion of the breast tissue causes engorgement of the areola and results in nipple erection characteristic of sexual arousal.
- The labia majora respond according to parity. In women who have not borne children, they become flatter and thinner during arousal and orgasm. Women who have previously given birth have an extensively developed vascular network in the labia majora, which becomes engorged to two to three times its normal size because of vasocongestion with arousal. The labia darken to a deep red or purple color during the height of arousal.
- The inner portion of the vagina distends as arousal continues, forming a receptacle for semen; the uterus becomes engorged and uplifted.
- The clitoris enlarges and becomes more sensitive to touch and pressure but is covered by the engorged prepuce. The clitoris appears and disappears under the prepuce as arousal continues. Immediately before orgasm the clitoris turns upward 180 degrees and retracts behind the symphysis pubis in a flattened position.
- During orgasm, the inner third of the vagina continues to distend while the pelvic floor muscles rhythmically contract. After orgasm, unless there are psychoemotional conflicts about the sexual experience, the resolution phase results in mental and physical relaxation, accompanied by a feeling of well-being.[424]

Phases of the Sexual Response

1. Desire and Arousal (sometimes referred to as Excitement)
   Activation of the CNS, desire, causes specific changes in blood flow-arousal. During the latter part of arousal—also called the plateau phase—the clitoris retracts, the labia becomes engorged, and muscle tension increases.

2. Orgasm
   During orgasm, muscular contractions of the levator ani muscles occur at precise intervals. Vaginal and uterine contractions occur followed by massive release of muscle tension.

3. Resolution
   Resolution is characterized as a gradual, pleasant diminishment of sexual tension and response, lasting a variable amount of time in different women.[423]

DIAGNOSIS

Lack of physician training in female sexual issues and sexual dysfunction commonly leads to an underrecognition of FSD.[417] Although numerous models and screening tools have been proposed, there is not a universally accepted tool to define FSD, and a combination of clinical evaluation, patient history, and screening surveys are used to establish a diagnosis.

CONVENTIONAL TREATMENT APPROACHES

Conventional treatment of FSD includes psychological and pharmacologic approaches, the latter primarily using hormone replacement therapy (HRT) (e.g., estrogen, androgens), sildenafil, and tiblone.[417,422] Many treatments that are used in practice are not supported by adequate evidence.[422,430] The adverse effects of HRT should be weighed against potential side effects and risks associated with use; the long-term use of testosterone in women has not been thoroughly investigated and can lead to symptoms of masculinization over time, including deepening of the voice and hair growth changes.[422,430] Local estrogen application relieves vaginal dryness and dyspareunia. The recent discoveries of the side effects of HRT necessitate careful evaluation of the indication for hormone therapy, and the duration of treatment is recommended to be as short as possible. Sildenafil has shown a positive effect on FSD only in women with arousal problems without desire problems.[430] There appears to be limited controlled research on the efficacy of psychophysiologic approaches to FSD.[431] Although psychological treatment for some subtypes of sexual dysfunction have been shown to be helpful, these are commonly overlooked or dismissed in the medical visit.

THE BOTANICAL PRACTITIONER'S PERSPECTIVE

Numerous herbal products on the market boast the ability to improve sexual function and treat sexual dysfunction, as evidenced by a visit to a local vitamin and supplement shop or health food store.[432] Rowland and Tai recently cataloged those botanical products offered at two major national health food chains and found that ginseng, muira puama, saw palmetto, *Tribulus terrestris, yohime,* and ginkgo were the most popular.[432] Of these, all are used for male dysfunction, and all but yohimbe are used for female dysfunction.[432] Other ingredients, to name a few of the dozens identified, include horny goat weed, kava kava, yerba mate, deer antler, guarana, nettles, sarsaparilla, and cayenne.[432]

Demand for products to treat sexual dysfunction is not a modern phenomenon—the history of herbal medicine is replete with herbal aphrodisiacs from charms and love potions to elaborate traditional medicines and elixirs.[433] Ayurvedic medicine contains ancient texts and treatises focused solely on the treatment of sexual dysfunction and the support and restoration of healthy sexuality and sexual pleasure.[413] Few studies have been conducted to validate botanical therapies for FSD, with a slightly greater number of studies available on the botanical treatment of male sexual dysfunction.[434] Conventional medicine also has focused more on the treatment of male sexual dysfunction. However, there is a rich materia medica of traditional herbs to consider in the treatment of decreased sexual desire, FSD, and some of the factors that contribute to sexual function difficulties such as vaginal dryness or anxiety associated with sexual activity and performance. Further, herbal therapies may have a role in the treatment of associated or other contributory problems such as fatigue and depression (see related chapters). Finally, TCM and Ayurvedic medicine offer several historically important female tonics. These are also included in the following discussion.

Proprietary Products

Several herbal products including ArginMax (a proprietary blend of L-arginine, ginseng, ginkgo, damiana, calcium, iron, and 14 vitamins), Zestra (containing borage seed oil, evening primrose oil, angelica root extract, and *Coleus forskohlii* extract), Kyo-Green (a powdered drink of barley leaves and wheat grass with antiinflammatory and antioxidant properties), and ginkgo (*Ginkgo biloba*) have been evaluated in peer-reviewed, published studies for the treatment of FSD.[435] Used daily, the supplements claims to enhance a woman's sexual response by increasing blood flow and promoting relaxation. In a double-blind, placebo-controlled study of women older than 21 years of age with an interest in improving their sex lives, 4 weeks of ArginMax use was associated with an improvement in sexual desire, sexual satisfaction, reduction of vaginal dryness, increased frequency of sexual intercourse, and improved clitoral sensation over placebo.[436] ArginMax improved sexual arousal and frequency of intercourse in a 2006 clinical trial of 108 women who were either premenopausal, perimenopausal, or postmenopausal. Using the Female Sexual Function Index, after 4 weeks of treatment premenopausal women reported significant improvement in level of sexual desire (72%; $p = .03$), satisfaction with overall sex life (68%; $p = .007$) and frequency of intercourse (56%; $p = .01$) compared with controls. Perimenopausal women experienced increased frequency of intercourse (86%; $p = .002$), satisfaction with the sexual relationship (79%; $p = .03$), and less vaginal dryness (64%; $p = .03$) compared with controls. Postmenopausal women primarily showed an increase in level of sexual desire, with 51% showing improvement, compared with only 8% in the placebo group.[437] In an open-label trial of women with lack of libido, 80% of the women reported improved sexual function after Kyo-Green use.[435] A double-blind clinical trial (n = 100) with Lady Prelox demonstrated efficacy in the treatment mild sexual dysfunction.[438]

The topical preparations Vigorelle (ingredients include damiana leaf, suma root, motherwort, wild yam, ginkgo, peppermint leaf, L-arginine, and vitamins A and C) and Pro Sensual (ingredients include mint, orange, and clove oils) claim to enhance a woman's sexual responses by increasing blood flow to her sexual organs. None have peer-reviewed data to support this claim.[435] I have no experience with these products and include them merely for the familiarity of the practitioner whose patients may be taking them or requesting information about them.

Decreased Libido

Damiana

Damiana is an herb with a long history of folk use as an aphrodisiac, particularly in Latin America, and it continues to be popular among herbalists today. The Aztecs described it as a sexual stimulant at least 300 years ago.[432] The herb is purported to have progestin receptor binding activity; however, it appears to be neither an agonist nor an antagonist; it may also exert some of its action via antidepressant and nervous system stimulant activity.[432,439] The evidence for its aphrodisiac properties are limited to in vitro or animal studies.[440]

Maca

The Quechua Indians of Peru's central highlands consider maca a highly nutritious food that promotes mental acuity, physical vitality, endurance, and stamina. It is also well-known as an aphrodisiac tonic that enhances sexual desire and performance, and is especially reputed to increase fertility. Maca is often eaten by Peruvian women wishing to get pregnant.[442] Dried maca root is rich in essential amino acids, iodine, iron, and magnesium, as well as sterols that may possess a range of activities, including aphrodisiac properties.[432] It has been used to treat menstrual and menopausal complaints as well. The evidence base for maca is growing but still preliminary. An uncontrolled pilot study tested two doses of dried maca root (1.5 g and 3 g, daily) on 20 outpatients with SSRI–induced sexual dysfunction. Outcomes were assessed using the Arizona Sexual Experience Scale and Massachusetts General Hospital Sexual Functioning Questionnaire. Subjects in the higher dose group (i.e., 3 g) experienced improved sexual function.[441] A 2010 systematic review evaluated four clinical trials of maca for the improvement of sexual function, but there were too few studies and limited evidence to present any conclusions.[443]

Tribulus

Tribulus terrestris has been widely used in Ayurvedic medicine as a sexual stimulant for both men and women to improve libido and performance. It is also popular among athletes for improving sports stamina and performance.[432] *T. terrestris* appears to support the production of steroid hormones, including DHEA and androstenedione, possibly explaining its reported effects.[432] It may stimulate luteinizing hormone (LH) production: in men, LH stimulates testosterone production in the testes; in women, LH stimulates estrogen production in the ovaries. However, these are speculative mechanisms.[432]

The effects of damiana, maca, and *T. terrestris* on sexual function are plausible; however, there is a paucity of studies, particularly studies relating to female sexual complaints. Side effects are not anticipated with use of these herbs, although very small amounts of cyanide have been detected in damiana and could cause renal or hepatic damage, although this is not reported in the literature.[432]

Ginkgo

Ginkgo is also used to treat sexual dysfunction in men and women. Study results have been mixed. In an open-label trial of women experiencing antidepressant-induced sexual dysfunction, ginkgo improved sexual function; however, there were no significant differences between ginkgo and placebo; both improved sexual function.[444] This study did show that women are more responsive to the sexually enhancing effects of the herb than men, with success rates of 91% compared with 76%.[445] A 2008 study investigated of the effects of both short- and long-term *Ginkgo biloba* extract (GBE) administration on subjective and physiologic (vaginal photoplethysmography) measures of sexual function in women with sexual arousal disorder. The first part of the study focused on acute effects of GBE on sexual arousal. The group of 99 subjects experienced a small but significant improvement in physiologic correlates of sexual arousal. In the second part of the study, 68 women with sexual dysfunction were randomized into four treatment groups: placebo, 300 mg of GBE daily, sex therapy, and sex therapy plus 300 mg of GBE daily. Ginkgo did not perform better than placebo on measures of sexual arousal, and sex therapy treatment groups exhibited significant improvements compared with controls and GBE.[446] It is postulated that the ginkgo's ability to improve peripheral vascular circulation may be the explanation for its supposed effects in improving sexual response.[432]

Additional Treatments

Warming and stimulating herbs, for example, cinnamon and ginger, are thought to stimulate sexual appetite, and are therefore commonly included in formulae intended to stimulate sexual desire.

The herb milky oats was used by the Eclectics to treat what was termed *sexual neurasthenia*, a lack of sexual energy causing lack of libido.

Vaginal Dryness

Vaginal dryness is most often a function of age and declining estrogen levels. It is also associated with cyclic fluctuations in hormonal cycles, candidiasis, inadequate intake of dietary essential fatty acids, and rarely, it is associated with the autoimmune condition Sjögren's syndrome. Intake of phytoestrogenic foods and herbs to support estrogen, as well as the use of topical emollients to moisten vaginal tissue locally and heal tissue that might be irritated or damaged by chronic dryness, may help to relieve vaginal dryness and more immediately relieve discomfort during sex. Treatments for vaginal dryness are elaborated on in the Vaginal Dryness and Atrophy section of this chapter. Shatavari root and Chinese asparagus, two herbs with very similar activity to one another, are used in Ayurvedic and Chinese medicine respectively to increase vaginal mucus. Long-term use along with other yin tonics can help to reestablish normal vaginal secretions. In TCM, Chinese asparagus is considered a yin tonic, as is licorice rhizome, which also may be considered for vaginal dryness. Licorice contains isoflavones, which act as phytoestrogens. Vulnerary herbs such as calendula and comfrey can be used topically in suppositories, ointments, or vaginal lubricant creams to relieve irritation and inflammation associated with vaginal dryness, and to promote tissue healing.

Depression and Sexual Dysfunction

Damiana is an herb with a long folk history of use as an aphrodisiac, particularly in Latin America. The herb is considered a phytoprogestin, and also may exert some of its action via antidepressant and nervous system stimulant activity.[439] Ginkgo extract claims include increased pelvic blood flow and nerve transmission. As mentioned earlier, ginkgo improved sexual function in an open-label trial; however, improvement was not greater than placebo.

Painful Intercourse

Painful intercourse can be caused by lack of lubrication, sexual trauma, vulvodynia, vaginismus, uterine fibroids, sexually transmitted diseases (STDs), cervicitis, and uterine prolapse, discussed in Chapter 12.

Orgasmic Dysfunction

Anorgasmia is an inability to achieve orgasm. Ginkgo and damiana should be considered for improving orgasmic function.[432] Muira puama has been suggested for improving low libido and anorgasmia in women; however, studies are limited. A study by Waynberg and Brewer demonstrated the prosexual effects of a commercial muira puama and ginkgo product (Herbal vX) in women complaining of low libido. Compared with pretest evaluation, 65% of the women reported improvements in frequency and intensity of sex drive, sexual fantasies, and ability to achieve orgasm. Side effects possibly include sour stomach and headache.[445]

Sexual Anxiety

Fear of not being loved, pregnancy, inadequacy, or acquiring STDs, previous sexual trauma, poor body image, lack of self-esteem, and guilt related to personal or religious beliefs

> ### BOX 6-2   Traditional Chinese Medicine and Low Libido
>
> According to Oriental medicine, the kidneys govern sexual vitality and mental energy. Aging; stress; overwork; loud noise; cold temperature exposure, especially to the lower back (e.g., from a draft); drinking and eating icy foods; overusing stimulants, including caffeine; and fatigue may exhaust the kidneys and libido.

about sex can all contribute to anxiety associated with sexual encounters. Herbs can help relieve the anxiety; however, counseling or therapy is needed to get to the root of the problem and provide behavioral modification techniques and new patterning. Milky oats, ashwagandha, and skullcap are all excellent nervous system tonics and restoratives that should be considered when there is anxiety related to sex. Passionflower also can be considered in formulae for anxiety.

Female Sexual Tonics

In Chinese medicine, herbs that build the blood (i.e., xue) are used to strengthen and nourish the female reproductive system.[447] Herbs in this category include processed rehmannia, dong quai, He Shou Wu, and white peony. Other female reproductive tonics include the classic Ayurvedic herb for women—shatavari—and the Chinese asparagus root, which possesses very similar activity. Epimedium is among the classic kidney tonics (Box 6-2) used in TCM for kidney deficiency and related sexual problems.

ADDITIONAL THERAPIES

Individual and relationship counseling, behavioral modification, and sex therapy are all important adjuncts to the treatment of debilitating sexual problems. There are innumerable resources, ranging from books and tapes to seminars designed to help improve women's understanding of their sexuality and thereby increase sexual pleasure and satisfaction. Competent and experienced sex therapists can help clients to identify effective resources.

Bone Health

OSTEOPOROSIS

Osteoporosis is the most common bone disease affecting humans, and it disproportionately affects postmenopausal women. It is defined as a skeletal disorder characterized by compromised bone density predisposing an individual to an increased risk of fractures; osteopenia is bone loss that is less advanced than osteoporosis and is a potential harbinger of osteoporosis.[1] Osteoporosis is now considered one of the most important diseases women face, affecting as many as 18% (approximately 12 million) of US women older than 50, with another 37% to 50% (approximately 5 million) having osteopenia.[1-3] Caucasian women are at greatest risk for osteoporosis, although all races are affected, as are men in lesser but still significant numbers.

Peak bone mineral density (BMD) is typically achieved by about age 30, after which time bone loss begins to outweigh bone formation, a process that accelerates with menopause. In the 5 to 7 years immediately after menopause, women may lose as much as 20% of their BMD, largely as a result of declining estrogen levels and the resultant loss of the positive effects of estrogen on bone formation and protection against bone loss.[3] Aging itself is also associated with changes that contribute to bone loss; for example, inefficient kidney function leads to poor calcium reabsorption, which in turn leads to hyperparathyroidism and increased bone mineral loss. By age 80, at which time risk of falls and fractures is markedly increased, women may have lost as much as 30% of their BMD.[1] The risk of osteoporotic fractures doubles every 7 or 8 years after age 50.[1]

Osteoporosis is often a silent condition; the first sign of the disease is commonly a fracture.[1,3] Major sites for osteoporotic fractures include the hip, wrist, and vertebrae; thoracic fractures lead to restriction of lung function and digestive problems. Most nonvertebral fractures occur as the result of a fall; however, vertebral fractures commonly occur spontaneously, often with simple activities such as stepping off a curb or sitting down in the seat of car, or without a provoking cause.

Fractures resulting from osteoporosis account for substantial morbidity and mortality.[4] As many as 25% of women who sustain a hip fracture will die within 1 year of the incident, and 50% of women who sustain a hip fracture do not

The editor wishes to thank *Botanical Medicine for Women's Health*, Edition 1 contributor, Robin DiPasquale, for her original contributions to this chapter.

return to their full functional status, becoming dependent on others for their daily needs, with 25% to 30% requiring long-term care.[1,3-5] In addition to the physical, emotional, and psychological costs to individuals, including loss of function, pain, dependence, and loss of self-esteem and negative changes in body image, this condition carries a considerable financial and social price for both family and society.[3,4] It is estimated that the directly attributable costs of osteoporosis in the United States may be as high as $10 billion annually, excluding the costs of long-term home care—a figure expected to grow as the US population ages over the next couple of decades.[2]

Osteoporosis is classified as either type 1 or type 2 osteoporosis, reflecting regional BMD loss, patterns of fracture, hormonal changes, and causal mechanisms.[2,3] Type 1 osteoporosis typically affects women within the first 10 years after menopause and is characterized by fractures that occur at sites rich in cancellous bone, such as crush fractures of the vertebrae and Colles' fracture of the distal forearm. Type 2 osteoporosis is associated with age-related changes, such as impaired vitamin D metabolism, osteoblast function, and bone formation; secondary hyperparathyroidism; vitamin D deficiency; and inadequate calcium intake, which occur as a late consequence of estrogen-deficiency osteoporosis. Type 2 osteoporosis is characterized by fractures at sites containing substantial portions of both cortical and cancellous bone including the hip, proximal humerus, proximal tibia, and pelvis. Anterior wedging of the vertebra of the dorsal spine is also common.[3]

RISK FACTORS

Risk factors for developing osteoporosis include:
- Family history of osteoporosis or hip fracture in a parent
- Advanced age (risk begins to increase after 50 years of age and is greatest at about 80 years of age)
- Low BMD (demonstrated by dual-energy x-ray absorptiometry [DEXA] scan—see Diagnosis)
- Prior fracture
- Thinness (body weight <127 lb [57.7 kg] or body mass index [BMI] <21)
- Smoking in any amount
- Low calcium or vitamin D intake
- More than two alcoholic beverages daily
- Oral or intramuscular glucocorticoid use for >3 months

- Low levels of physical activity
- Increased fall risk[1,4]
- Warfarin use >1 year[6]

Factors that increase fall risk include impaired vision, dementia, poor health or frailty, low physical activity, problems with balance, history of syncope or seizures, and history of recent falls.[1,4] Medications that increase fall risk include antihypertensives, anticholinergics, sedatives, and analgesics. Polypharmacy also may increase the risk of falls via potential drug interactions. The greater the number of risk factors, the greater the risk of falling, with four combined risk factors leading to an 80% increased risk of falling.[1]

A number of disease states and additional factors can lead to osteoporosis, commonly as a result of increased bone loss, or problems with mineral excretion, absorption, or deposition. Examples include but are not limited to:

- *Genetic disorders:* osteogenesis imperfecta; thalassemia; hemochromatosis
- *Calcium balance disorders:* hypercalciuria; vitamin D deficiency
- *Endocrinopathies:* cortisol excess; Cushing's syndrome; gonadal insufficiency; hyperthyroidism; type 1 diabetes mellitus; primary hyperparathyroidism
- *Gastrointestinal (GI) disorders* that prevent calcium absorption
- *Chronic renal disease*
- *Medications:* oral or intramuscular glucocorticoids for >3 months; excessive thyroxin intake; long-term phenytoin use; heparin; cytotoxic agents; gonadotrophin-releasing hormone (GnRH) agonists; immunosuppressives[1]

Bone health cannot be viewed in isolation from the environment in which we live. The depletion of vital nutrients in our food, sedentary lifestyles, and increased levels of stress all diminish bone density. Our elderly population is faced with the major challenge of being socially marginalized, frequently living alone, consuming diets inadequate in nutrients essential for bone health, and having few people to depend on for assistance getting up and down flights of stairs or other activities of daily living (ADL) that predispose them to risk of fracture.

It is significant to note that optimal bone building and prevention of osteoporosis begins in childhood, and is well under way in the teen years. Ninety percent of bone density is achieved by the age of 20, and bone remodeling continues to be optimal until about the age of 35. Education about osteoporosis prevention is ideally begun early in life when girls are still actively laying down vital bone matrix. Adolescents also face unique threats to bone health; for example, inadequate nutrition and consumption of large amounts of soft drinks that can compromise nutrition and predispose them to later development of osteoporosis.[7,8] A specific area of concern for development of healthy bones in adolescent girls is the attempt to conform to the cultural idealization of thinness, which leads to dieting, a decrease in caloric intake, and a decrease in nutrient intake. Emotional and psychological stress also may interfere with bone development in the teen years. Attention to lifestyle beginning at a young age may be among the most important strategies we take in the prevention of this devastating disease.

DIAGNOSIS

It is recommended by the North American Menopause Society that BMD be measured in[1]:

- Postmenopausal women with medical causes of bone loss regardless of age
- Postmenopausal women at least 65 years of age regardless of additional risk factors

In 1994, the World Health Organization (WHO) developed an international standard for evaluating bone strength.[9] The North American Menopause Society supports the WHO definition of osteoporosis in postmenopausal women as a BMD test score of less than or equal to standard deviations (SD) in the following: the mean at the total hip, femoral neck, or lumbar spine (posterior-anterior measurement, not lateral). The BMD test score is derived by comparing the current BMD of the patient to the mean peak BMD of a normal young adult population of the same gender. For women, the reference standard is white women age 20 to 29 years old, as this is the age at which physiologic bone density is at or near its peak. If the patient's body habitus (e.g., obesity) or medical conditions (e.g., arthritis) make such measurements difficult or invalid, then the density of the distal one third of the radius bone may be considered a valid diagnostic site.[1] Osteopenia, suggestive of early BMD loss, is defined as BMD 1.0 to 2.5 SD in the following mean. Osteoporosis is also clinically diagnosed regardless of BMD test score based on the presence of a fragility fracture.[1]

DEXA is the gold standard screening test for osteoporosis and for assessing BMD. A first DEXA is generally taken between the ages of 40 to 50 as a baseline. This baseline can then be referenced at further points along the menopausal transition. The National Osteoporosis Foundation recommendations for DEXA screening are:

- Postmenopausal women younger than 65 with one or more of the following risk factors:
  - Oral steroids use
  - Thyroid problems
  - Eating disorders
  - Amenorrhea 3 months or longer
  - Family history of osteoporosis
  - Smoking
  - Alcoholism
  - Very thin/small body frame
  - Low calcium intake
- Postmenopausal women who have had a past bone fracture
- Any woman older than 65 years old
- Premenopausal women with any of these risk factors

Serum and urine markers of bone turnover, although sometimes used to assess therapeutic response to treatment, are not reliable for the diagnosis of osteopenia and osteoporosis, and are not especially clinically useful.[1]

Monitoring weight and height is a simple, important clinical screening method for evaluating bone health. A decrease in height or weight, especially postmenopausally, may be indicative of decreasing BMD and should lead to further evaluation. Assessment for chronic back pain is also essential because this may be the only clinical indication of vertebral fractures. Kyphosis is an important indication of bone loss and possible vertebral fracture.

CONVENTIONAL TREATMENT

The primary goal in the prevention and treatment of osteoporosis is the deterrence of fractures via minimizing or stopping bone loss, maintaining bone strength, and reducing or eliminating factors that increase fracture risk.[1] Conventional medical approaches include nonpharmacologic and pharmacologic treatments. The treatment of secondary medical conditions (e.g., predisposing diseases, medications) that can lead to osteoporosis (see earlier discussion) is not discussed in the following.

NONPHARMACOLOGIC APPROACHES

Nutrition

Calcium

The role of calcium in establishing BMD during childhood and adolescence is well established, as is the important role of calcium supplementation during pregnancy and lactation. It is optimal to obtain calcium from dietary sources; however, because most diets do not supply an adequate amount, supplementation is advised at the recommended daily allowance (RDA) of between 1200 and 1500 mg daily from adolescence through perimenopause.[1]

Substantial epidemiologic data have been amassed assessing the relation between calcium intake and bone density. The efficacy of calcium supplementation to prevent and treat osteoporosis in later life has been controversial.[2] Most researchers and clinicians support a valuable role for supplementation.[1,2,6,10] Reviews of more than 20 studies on postmenopausal women have concluded that calcium supplementation can decrease bone loss by about 1% per year.[6] In a meta-analysis of 13 trials, calcium induced significant mean gains (or slowed loss) of 0.6% at the forearm, 3% at the spine, and 2.6% at the femoral neck. A more recent meta-analysis found that in 15 trials, calcium changes were 1.66% at the lumbar spine and 1.64% at the hip.[6] Case-controlled studies and some double-blind, placebo-controlled studies (but not all) have corroborated the finding that 500 to 1000 mg of daily calcium supplementation may offset postmenopausal bone loss for at least 3 years in women age 40 to 70 years old. Calcium-supplemented postmenopausal women also demonstrated lower levels of serum parathyroid hormone (PTH), decreased alkaline phosphatase concentrations, and urinary hydroxyproline excretion, all markers of bone turnover.[2,3]

The beneficial effect of calcium intake on bone mass may be greatest in older and late postmenopausal women, and in women with low baseline calcium intakes.[6] Calcium supplementation also appears to improve the efficacy of antiresorptive therapy, for example, hormone replacement therapy (HRT), on bone mass.[1,2,6,10] It is estimated that approximately 1500 mg per day of calcium would be needed to counteract bone loss associated with the estrogen depletion that occurs postmenopausally.[1,2]

Many forms of calcium supplements are available. Calcium citrate is the most bioavailable and leads to greater inhibition of PTH compared with calcium carbonate.[2] Also, the absorption of calcium citrate is independent of stomach acid levels, which commonly decline with age, whereas calcium carbonate requires adequate stomach acid for absorption and is thus better absorbed when taken with meals.[2] The primary advantage of calcium carbonate is that the amount of calcium per pill is higher; therefore fewer pills are required.

Food sources of calcium include dairy products, dark green leafy vegetables, tofu, sesame seeds, almonds, sardines (bones included), and seaweeds. Calcium absorption can be inhibited by foods high in oxalic acid (e.g., spinach) and phytate-rich foods, for example, wheat bran.[1] Calcium supplementation at the RDA is not expected to cause kidney stones; however, supplementation is contraindicated in women with renal calculi.[1]

Vitamin D

Vitamin D is actually a hormone precursor essential for the intestinal absorption of calcium and bone mineral deposition.[2] Genetics may play up to a 75% role in the ability to effectively synthesize vitamin D; this appears to contribute significantly to the 80% supposed role of genetics in determining peak BMD in children and young adults.[2] Vitamin D synthesis begins in the skin upon exposure to ultraviolet light; further synthesis occurs in the liver, and finally the kidney, where the active form, calcitriol, is produced. Aging can decrease the skin's ability to synthesize provitamin D, and age also tends to decrease time spent exposed to sunlight and consumption of milk fortified with vitamin D. Individuals living in northern latitudes are also more prone to vitamin D insufficiency caused by overall less sun exposure than those living in southern climates. Use of sunscreen further decreases vitamin D synthesis. A population-based cohort study in Sweden followed 61,433 women for 19 years to investigate the association between long-term dietary intake of calcium and risk of fracture and osteoporosis. Patterns of dietary calcium intake and incident fracture or osteoporosis were not clear, and positive correlations were not seen. However, with reduced vitamin D intake, the rate of fracture in the first calcium quintile increased.[11] In 2011, researchers hypothesized that dietary supplementation with combinations of vitamin D and phytochemicals (specifically resveratrol, genistin, and quercetin) inhibits bone loss and decreases adiposity better than controls or vitamin D alone. In a model of ovariectomized rats, a synergistic effect was observed with their coadministration through improved BMD, reduced body weight gain, and decrease in bone marrow adipocytes (2,400 IU/kg).[12]

Reduction of both hip and other nonvertebral fractures, as well as delays in bone loss, have been demonstrated in trials supplementing 700 to 800 IU of vitamin D with 500 mg calcium daily; thus many experts are recommending supplementation of 700 to 800 IU vitamin D daily with calcium for women older than 65 and for those at risk for osteoporosis.[3,4,6,10,13] Studies using vitamin D supplements alone have had less impressive results. Sources of vitamin D include sunlight, fortified dairy, fish liver oils, butter, and oily fish.[1]

At recommended doses, vitamin D is considered safe, well tolerated, and with no expected serious adverse effects.[2] Vitamin D analogs (see Calcitriol) have been shown to have greater benefit in osteoporosis.

Vitamin K

Vitamin K is a fat-soluble vitamin found in dark green leafy vegetables, fruits, and vegetable oils; small amounts are found in dairy products and grains; and a subset of vitamin K is found in fermented dairy and soy products, fish, meat, liver, and eggs.[6] Vitamin K is required for the synthesis of osteocalcin, the matrix that provides structure to bone, as well as for preventing excess urinary calcium excretion.[6] Studies have demonstrated that adequate vitamin K intake is associated with positive effects on bone turnover, and that daily supplementation is associated with a reduced postmenopausal bone loss, particular of the hip.[1,6] Caused by limited current evidence, there are insufficient data to recommend the required level of vitamin K supplementation for optimal bone health.[6] A daily dose of 1 mg of vitamin K (i.e., phylloquinone) is recommended based on a single trial using a 3-year supplementation of this dose with calcium and vitamin D; reduced hip bone loss was demonstrated.[1,6] A healthy diet, high in fruits and vegetables, ensures adequate vitamin K for most people.[6] Vitamin K supplementation interferes with the effectiveness of warfarin and is thus contraindicated for patients taking this medication.

Vitamin C

Vitamin C is an essential cofactor for collagen formation and synthesis of hydroxyproline and hydroxylysine. Low consumption of vitamin C has been epidemiologically associated with lower bone mass and a faster rate of BMD loss; however, there are no clinical trials evaluating the role of vitamin C in osteoporosis.[6] Recommended intake of five or more servings of fruits and vegetables daily should provide adequate vitamin C for bone health.

Fluoride

Since the late 1930s, it has been known that fluoride can increase BMD. It is now readily available in commonly ingested substances—fluorinated water, juices made with fluorinated water, toothpaste, and mouthwash, for example. It is highly absorbable in the stomach. In large doses, fluoride actually causes bone to become excessively brittle. However, supplemental doses of 50 mg per day, along with calcium supplementation, can promote bone strength and decrease vertebral and femoral osteoporotic fractures by increasing osteoblast recruitment, decreasing osteoclast activity, and by forming fluoroapatite—a more densely packed bone matrix than the normal hydroxyapatite.[2,14] Toxicity, skeletal problems, and GI side effects are dose dependent and are especially associated with plain fluoride and monoflurophosphate.[5] Slow release tablets do not cause GI side effects.

Magnesium

A 2014 clinical trial suggests that *Vitex* coadministered with magnesium may promote fracture healing in women. A group of 64 women with long bone fractures between the ages of 20 and 45 were randomized to receive either 4 mg *Vitex* extract plus 250 mg magnesium oxide, *Vitex* alone, magnesium alone, or placebo daily for 8 weeks. Treatment with *Vitex* and magnesium significantly enhanced the osteocalcin level. However, alkaline phosphatase activity did not improve (Vitex extract preparation details were not disclosed).[15]

Vitamin A

Excess consumption of vitamin A in the form of retinol equivalents (RE) at doses greater than 1500 mg daily has been associated with a doubling of the rate of hip fractures in one study in the United States and Sweden, but not in Iceland or other US studies. Beta(β)-carotene supplementation has not been associated with an increase in osteoporosis or other fractures.[6] Patients at risk for osteoporosis should avoid excessive supplementation with vitamin A from retinol.

Protein

The Framingham osteoporosis study, a longitudinal cohort trial, demonstrated that adequate protein intake in women older than 75 years of age could help minimize bone loss.[16] Also, in patients with a mean age of 82 years hospitalized for hip fracture, protein supplementation of 20 g per day has been shown to lead to improved clinical outcome and dramatically shorter hospital stays of a mean of 69 days versus 102 days for placebo.[1]

Isoflavones

A significant amount of data from numerous studies on cultured bone cells and rat models of postmenopausal osteoporosis support a significant bone-sparing effect of the soy isoflavones, genistein and daidzein; however, although a small number of human studies have shown promising results, these have been variable, with some authors reporting no benefits at all.[1] Human clinical studies have generally been of short duration and with relatively small sample sizes, making it difficult to observe significant and accurate bone changes.[17] Overall, the cumulative data suggest that diets rich in phytoestrogens have bone-sparing effects in the long term; however, the extent of the benefits and the exact mechanisms of action are currently undetermined.[17] No studies have been conducted to evaluate the effects of isoflavone intake on fracture rate.[17] Given the safety of legumes in the diet as a high-quality protein source and the possible benefits, it seems reasonable for menopausal women to include traditional soy products and other beans as a regular part of the daily diet.

Ipriflavone

Ipriflavone (IP) is a synthetic derivative of naturally occurring isoflavone, manufactured from daidzein. It has been shown to inhibit osteoclast formation without suppressing the rate of bone formation.[18] IP also shows bone-forming activity through proliferation of osteoblast cell lines and inhibition of parathyroid hormone activity.[19] More than 60 human study trials have been published in the last 10 years evaluating IP for prevention and treatment of osteoporosis, and it is a popular nonprescription supplement. Before 2001, many of the studies showed promising outcomes. Throughout nine Italian sites, 196 subjects were randomly assigned to either IP 200 mg TID with food or placebo. All subjects were also given 1000 mg per day of calcium carbonate or gluconolactate. BMD by x-ray of at least one SD in the following mean was a requirement for inclusion. After 2 years, the placebo group showed a decline in BMD, whereas the IP group maintained bone mass.[20] Two studies were able to show a slight increase, primarily in vertebral bone, when using IP, after 2 years and 1 year.[21,22] One additional study looked at 91 post-menopausal women who were divided into early menopause (<5 years) or late menopause (>5 years). After 6 months of treatment with IP, the late menopause group had a statistically significant increase in BMD at the lumbar spine but the placebo and early menopause group showed no statistically significant differences.

In 2001, the Multi-Center European Fracture Study, which consisted of four European sites, 205 and 52 Belgian subjects, 197 Danish subjects, and 20 Italian subjects, published its 3-year outcome. Women ages 45 to 75, with a natural menopause of at least 1 year and with BMD at least 2 SDs in the mean for perimenopause were given 200 mg of IP or placebo 3 times daily. All subjects were also given a 500 mg per day calcium supplement. BMD was determined by DEXA at onset and every 6 months throughout the 3 years; bone resorption markers were evaluated every 6 months as well. After 36 months, there was no statistically significant difference between the BMD and the bone resorption markers in the IP and placebo groups. Overall, there is conflicting data on the benefits of IP for prevention or treatment of bone loss. There are enough studies, however, showing that IP helps prevent bone loss at menopause to merit continued study.

IP is associated with a variety of side effects. GI symptoms have been reported and lesser side effects include rash, headache, depression, drowsiness, and tachycardia. In one study, a decrease in lymphocytes was shown during IP treatment.[23]

Questions have arisen as to the safety of long-term use of IP because of its estrogen-like effects. Two studies have demonstrated no changes in serum luteinizing hormone (LH) and follicle-stimulating hormone (FSH) levels, prolactin, and estradiol, nor changes in vaginal cytology between IP and placebo, with the estrogen arm of the study demonstrating a considerable increase in superficial vaginal cells.[24] The recommended dose is 200 mg three times daily, except in patients with renal insufficiency, in which case if creatinine clearance is between 40 and 80 mL per minute, the dose should not exceed 400 mg per day; if the creatinine clearance is less than 40 mL per minute, the dose should be no more than 200 mg per day. In one large study, IP use was associated with a significant incidence of lymphopenia, which resolved within 12 to 24 months of discontinuation of use.[24]

Exercise

A Cochrane Database Review of 18 randomized controlled trials (RCTs), including a total of 1423 subjects from North America, Europe, and Asia, reported that aerobics, weight bearing, and resistance exercises were all effective in enhancing the BMD of the spine. The analysis also showed walking to be effective in improving BMD of the spine and hip. The review results showed some evidence that the slowing of bone loss was most effective with exercise done for 1 year or longer.[25]

A second meta-analysis was undertaken looking at aerobic exercise on bone density at the hip in postmenopausal women. Six studies were evaluated with the conclusion that aerobic exercise has a moderately positive effect, with 67% of the exercise groups demonstrating benefits versus the nonexercise groups. It was noted, however, that the activity should probably be weight bearing to optimize bone density.[26]

Elite and professional athletes have demonstrated greater than 12% higher BMD of the hip and almost 9% greater BMD of the spine than controls, even many years after discontinuing competitive training.[2] The benefits of exercise appear to be independent of estrogen levels.[2] The Surgeon General's Guidelines for moderate physical exercise, written in 1996, recommends some form of workout 5 or more days per week with moderate intensity of the activity, including a slight increase in breathing and little or no sweating, for 30 minutes or more per session. It may be necessary for patients to start off more slowly, progressively increasing their time toward this goal. For elderly women with osteoporosis, moderate exercise also may play an important role in preventing fall risk by improving strength and balance, with up to a 75% reduction in falls according to the 2006 North American Menopause Society Position Statement on the Management of Osteoporosis in Postmenopausal Women.[1]

Smoking Cessation

Cigarette smoking is reported to have definite deleterious effects on BMD, increasing the risk of fractures.[1] Smoking cessation can be very difficult for patients to achieve, but given the availability of a range of tools and the numerous deleterious effects of smoking in addition to BMD loss, attention should be given to help willing patients achieve this goal.

Alcohol Reduction

Alcohol consumption of greater than seven drinks per week is associated with an increased overall risk of falls as established by the Framingham Heart Study.[1]

Pharmacologic Therapies

Following are the descriptions of the major categories of drug therapies that are generally recommended for osteoporosis treatment.

Bisphosphonates

Alendronate (Fosamax) and Risedronate (Actonel) are members of a class of antiresorptive drugs called bisphosphonates, approved in the United States for the treatment of osteoporosis and demonstrated to be effective in the prevention of vertebral and nonvertebral fractures. Bisphosphonates are a group of synthetic analogs of pyrophosphate that is absorbed into the hydroxyapatite of bone and known to act as nonhormonal inhibitors of bone resorption. In an RCT of more than 2000 women with previous vertebral fracture, alendronate reduced the risk of hip and wrist fractures by 50%.[27] Multiple other trials have found that at a dose of 10 mg daily, BMD is increased and risk and incident of fracture is decreased.

Esophageal and gastric irritation are common side effects of these medications, and patients are required to drink water and remain in an upright position for 30 minutes after ingestion to prevent irritation. Severe side effects include esophageal erosion and esophagitis.[28] Weekly dosage schedules are available for these drugs; all fracture data are from studies in which there was a daily dosing protocol.[1] This class of drugs is contraindicated in patients with a creatinine clearance of 30 mL per minute or greater. Discontinuation of therapy after 4 to 5 years of continuous use is followed initially by BMD stability but an eventual return to pretreatment levels over time.[1]

Calcitonin

Salmon calcitonin is an antiresorptive agent that acts by inhibiting osteoclast activity. Calcitonin may increase 1,25 (OH)2 D, as well as intestinal calcium absorption, all leading to an increase in BMD and reported reductions in vertebral fractures of up to 66%.[29] It may be administered either intranasally or by subcutaneous injection. In two studies, it was shown to reduce vertebral but not nonvertebral fractures.[4] It has a low side effect profile, although in one study it was shown to cause headache and increase menopausal symptoms.[4] Intranasal use has been associated with some GI discomfort, facial flushing, rash, and dry nasal mucosa.[24]

Calcitriol

Calcitriol is an analog of 1,25-dihydroxycholecalciferol or vitamin D_3, the active form of vitamin D. Vitamin D analogs have been found to be effective at reducing fractures compared with placebo and vitamin D in postmenopausal women.[4] One study suggested an increased risk of hypercalcemia with calcitriol compared with vitamin D; however, alpha (α)-calcitriol, another vitamin D analog, was not associated with this risk.[4]

Hormone Replacement Therapy

The beneficial effects of estrogen replacement therapy (ERT) on BMD and fracture prevention are well established.[1,3,4] Estrogen appears to act both directly and indirectly on bone. Direct action occurs through osteoblast stimulation and inhibition of osteoclast activity; indirect action occurs via antagonizing actions of estrogen on cytokines, which stimulate osteoclast activity.[2]

A 2002 meta-analysis of 57 RCTs found consistent improvements in BMD with estrogen replacement or estrogen and progesterone replacement therapies over placebo. In trials of 2 years of length, the mean difference in BMD was 6.8% at the lumbar spine and 4.1% at the femoral neck.[3] Although trials such as the Women's Health Initiative study and the Postmenopausal Estrogen/Progestin Interventions Trial have demonstrated the harmful effects of estrogen replacement, including increased incidence of cancer (with the exception of colon cancer) and cardiovascular disease, the benefits of

hormone replacement on BMD were clearly shown.[1,3,30] Of note is that rates of BMD loss do not differ significantly between women stopping HRT and women who never underwent treatment with HRT.

Until recently, the minimum effective dose of estrogen has been considered to be 0.625 mg/d conjugated equine estrogen (CEE), 0.05 mg/d transdermal estrogen, or equivalent. Recent promising research has demonstrated positive effects of estrogen on BMD with doses as low as 0.3 mg/d orally or 0.025 mg/d transdermally, with no changes in endometrial thickness, however, it is unclear whether, for most women, the potential risks of higher doses of HRT outweigh the benefits.[3,4]

Selective Estrogen Receptor Modulators

Selective estrogen receptor modulator (SERM) is a term for compounds that can bind to and stimulate estrogen receptors but whose effects on target tissue differ from those of estrogen.[2] Selective estrogen receptor modulation retains the action of estrogen on certain receptors, for example, in the cardiovascular system and skeletal systems, without activating uterine and breast estrogen receptors. Their development was pursued in the treatment of osteoporosis as an alternative to HRT, with its potentially serious adverse effects of breast and endometrial cancers. SERMs have been shown to selectively decrease bone resorption.[31] One of the most prescribed SERMs is raloxifene, which acts primarily as an antiresorptive, inducing a positive shift in calcium balance in postmenopausal women. Two large RCTs in postmenopausal women with osteoporosis found that raloxifene reduced vertebral fractures compared with placebo after 36 months but found no significant difference in nonvertebral fractures after up to 8 years. Another small RCT found no significant difference between raloxifene and placebo in fractures over 1 year. The two large RCTs found that raloxifene reduced the risk of breast cancer. The first large RCT found that raloxifene increased the number of women with venous thromboembolic events compared with placebo. The second large RCT found that raloxifene increased the risk of fatal stroke.[4]

THE BOTANICAL PRACTITIONER'S PERSPECTIVE

There is limited evidence of a role for botanicals in the treatment of osteoporosis; however, practitioners can play a significant role in promoting healthy lifestyle choices and changes that lead to prevention of the disease (Table 7-1). There appears to be some role for herbs that contain isoflavones and that act as SERMs. There is a vital folk tradition of using infusions and herbal vinegars to build bone; however, these products have not been evaluated for mineral content or clinical efficacy, although they largely appear harmless.

Phytoestrogens: Soy, Red Clover, and Alfalfa

flax

Phytoestrogens were discussed previously under nonpharmacologic interventions for osteoporosis. They are found relatively abundantly in legumes, especially in soy products, alfalfa, and

TABLE 7-1   Herbs Used in the Prevention of Osteoporosis

Therapeutic Goal	Therapeutic Activity	Botanical Name	Common Name
Reduce bone loss	Phytoestrogen	Glycine max	Soy
		Medicago sativa	Alfalfa
		Trifolium pratense	Red clover
Bone mineralization	Nutritive	Avena sativa	Milky oats
		Camellia sinensis	Green tea
		Equisetum arvense	Horsetail
		Taraxacum officinale	Dandelion leaf
		Urtica dioica	Nettles

red clover. Although studies have yielded mixed results, there appears to be some modest but beneficial protection against spinal bone loss with the incorporation of soy into the diet.[17] Red clover contains the isoflavone biochanin A, primarily in the foliage. Alfalfa is high in genistein, daidzein, and coumestrol. Freshly ground flax seeds are rich in lignins; about 1 to 3 tsp per day can be sprinkled on food after cooking or put into beverages such as juice or smoothies to provide a regular source of lignins in the diet. Lignins are also found in fresh fruits, vegetables, and whole grains. One study using Rimostil (a red clover product), which did not have a control group, randomized the patients into three dosage levels: 28.5 mg, 57 mg, or 85.5 mg of phytoestrogen per day. The BMD of the proximal radius, ulna, and bones of the wrist rose 4.1% in a 6-month period with the dose of 57 mg per day. The 85.5 mg per day group rose 3%, and the 28.5 mg per day group did not have a significant response.[32]

A 2007 multicenter, 2-year, double-blind clinical trial (n = 389) assessed the effects of 54 mg per day of pure genistin on bone metabolic parameters in postmenopausal women with osteopenia. Outcomes were assessed at baseline and 24 months and included femoral neck and lumbar spine BMD, along with serum alkaline phosphatase (ALP), insulin-like growth factor-1 (IGF-1), and uterine thickness. Women were randomized into either a treatment group or placebo control. All participants received calcium and vitamin D. In the genistin group, bone turnover significantly decreased, and increases in ALP and IGF-1 were observed compared with controls.[11] (Note that 18% of women in the genistin group withdrew as a result of unpleasant GI side effects, compared with a 9% withdrawal rate in the placebo group.)

A 2013 clinical tested the efficacy of an enzymatic soy isolate (DT56a, n = 27) compared with hormone therapy (n = 26) and placebo (n = 36) in alleviating postmenopausal symptoms. Outcomes were assessed through the Kupperman index, serum lipids and lipoproteins, calcium, BMD, endometrial thickness, and mammography at baseline and 12 months. The two treatment arms exhibited similar efficacy on measures of femoral bone density and performed better than controls.[33] Findings from a 3-year double-blind RCT suggested soy isoflavones to be moderately beneficial for midshaft femur volumetric BMD (vBMD). This three-arm trial randomly assigned healthy female volunteers to two soy isoflavone treatment groups (80 mg or 120 mg daily) or placebo. Primary outcomes were measured by vBMD and strength

(via peripheral quantitative computed tomography). In the soy isoflavone group, the 80 mg dose exhibited protective properties as bone turnover increased (p = 0.011). Treatment did not affect cortical BMD, cortical thickness, periosteal circumference, or endosteal circumference.[34] But some trial results have been negative. A 2011 double-blind trial evaluated soy isoflavones in the prevention of bone loss and other menopausal symptoms. A group of 148 women—aged 45 to 60 years, within 5 years of menopause, and with a BMD test score of -2.0 or higher—were randomized to receive either soy isoflavone tablets (200 mg) or placebo daily. Outcomes were measured by changes in the lumbar spine, total hip, and femoral neck BMD at the 2-year endpoint. Compared with baseline scores, no statistically significant differences were seen between the soy isoflavone and control groups.[35]

Black Cohosh

In two different animal studies in ovariectomized rats using extracts of black cohosh, positive results were seen in parameters that correlate with bone loss, pyridinoline and deoxypyrimidine rates, and osteocalcin and leptin rates. Further, in the study by Seidlova-Wuttke and colleagues, the black cohosh extract BNO 1055 exerted estrogenic activity in the bone but not the uterus. In the study by Nisslein and Freudenstein, results were found to be similar in quality and magnitude to raloxifene.[36-38] A triterpene-saponin fraction of black cohosh reduced the development of osteoporosis in ovariectomized rats, potentially by decreasing bone marrow fat and proinflammatory cytokines.[39] Additionally, a 2010 study in the same rodent model tested the healing capability of black cohosh compared with 17-a-estradiol after metaphyseal tibial-osteotomy and standardized T-plate-osteosynthesis. Black cohosh administration slightly improved trabecular bone formation, but the time course of fracture healing was not altered. Overall, black cohosh supplementation did not exhibit positive effects in severe osteopenic fracture healing as was seen in early postmenopausal osteoporosis in rats.[40] The same year, investigators compared the metaphyseal callus formation and fracture healing abilities of black cohosh versus estrogen in ovariectomized rats over a 5-week period. Osteoporotic metaphyseal fracture healing was improved more by estrogen than black cohosh in the 5-week period. Black cohosh administration was associated with a higher metaphyseal callus formation rate, whereas estrogen improved the bio-mechanical properties of the callus itself.[41] Another rodent study compared the efficacy of three cycloartane-type triter-penoids from black cohosh on bone resorption in vitro and bone loss in ovariectomized mice. In vitro, all three com-pounds suppressed both the formation and the resorbing activity of osteoclast-like cells (with a synergistic effect seen with their coadministration) and prevented the bone loss in ovariectomized mice without affecting uterine weight.[42] In a double-blind, placebo-controlled study on black cohosh on 62 menopausal women treated for 6 months with either placebo or BNO 1055, beneficial results were seen on bone parameters with no evidence of increased endometrial thickness.[36] Recent reports on black cohosh have specu-lated whether its mechanism of action was in part related to SERM activity; however, it is most likely that black cohosh exerts its influence through nonhormonal pathways, possi-bly through mechanisms involving neurotransmitters.[43]

Nutritive Herbs: Milky Oats, Horsetail, Nettles, and Dandelion Leaf

There is a rich contemporary folk herbal tradition of using nutritive herbs for the prevention and treatment of osteo-porosis via supplementation of minerals such as calcium, potassium, and silica. These preparations are typically taken as either foods or strong aqueous preparations (8- to 10-hour length for steeping decoctions), and also may be steeped in vinegar for an extended period of time and used by the tablespoon in salad dressings and over other foods. Four herbs particularly stand out as those included as part of the treatment protocol of osteoporosis given by contemporary herbalists and naturopaths: nettles, horsetail, milky oats, and dandelion. Although there have been no studies to demon-strate efficacy in osteoporosis prevention and treatment, they are considered relatively benign herbs and gentle tonics.

Nettles

Nettles are reported to be high in vitamins A (as carotenoids), B complex, C, D, K, and in the minerals calcium, magnesium, manganese, boron, chromium, phosphorus, iron, potassium, and silica, as well as chlorophyll. It is the upper part of the plant that is used, taken as a cooked green vegetable (not raw because of the stinging hairs!), as a strong infusion, or made into herbal vinegar.

Milky Oats

Oats contain vitamins B, C, D, E, K, and carotenes, as well as many minerals, including calcium, magnesium, chromium, and silica. The milky oat pods are harvested before their full maturity and are used as a tincture or infusion, although eat-ing oatmeal as a breakfast cereal is probably the most effective way to derive nutrients from this herbal food.[24]

Horsetail

Horsetail also has the common name scouring-rush because of its high silica content, which was considered by pioneers as abrasive enough to scour wood and pewter. This silica,

along with calcium, magnesium, bioflavonoid, carotenoids, chromium, potassium, iron, and copper, is only bioavailable at a certain stage of the plant's maturity (before the leaves open to an angle of 90 degrees). It is taken as a fresh infu-sion, a decoction, or a vinegar extract for optimal mineral extraction. Capsules can be used, and are best with freeze-dried plant material. The vinegar extract is made by chopping the fresh plant, filling a jar with the chopped plant material, pouring organic apple cider vinegar to cover the plant and fill the jar, and steeping for 2 to 3 weeks, shaking once daily. The herbal vinegar is strained from the plant material and stored in a cool dark place or refrigerated.

Dandelion

Dandelion leaves are rich in vitamins and minerals, as are many leafy greens. The leaves are especially rich in calcium, magnesium, manganese, boron, iron, and potassium. They are eaten raw in salads or steamed as a potherb. They also can be prepared as a vinegar extraction, along with horsetail, nettles, and many other leafy greens.

Ginseng

Ginseng is commonly used as an adaptogen to improve hypothalamus-pituitary-adrenal (HPA) axis tone and treat fatigue, depression, and poor memory and concentration. In one study, *Panax ginseng* restored BMD levels to that of baseline in a model of inflammation-induced osteoporosis in ovariectomized mice. (Preparation not noted.)[44] In another model of ovariectomized rats, ginsenoside normalized lum-bar vertebra and tibia BMD, and increased the number of osteoblasts, ALP activity, and cyclic adenosine monophos-phate (cAMP) concentration in cultured osteoblast cells.[45] In 2011, researchers found *Panax notoginseng* saponins pro-moted proliferation and osteogenic differentiation of rodent bone marrow stromal cells via upregulation of osteogenic marker gene expression and downregulation of adipogenic marker gene expression in a dose-dependent manner.[46]

Ginkgo

Ginkgo has been revered as a neuroprotective, antioxidant, and cardiovascular supportive herb. Recent animal evidence suggests it may also have a role in bone health and metabo-lism. In 2012, investigators found ginkgo extract to promote osteoblastogenesis and lower bone marrow adipogenesis in vitro.[47] In a 2013 rodent model of glucocorticoid-induced osteoporosis, ginkgo extract improved Bcl-2 and reduced Bax expression of osteoblasts in mandibular alveolar bone.[48] In another rodent model of glucocorticoid-induced osteo-porosis, ginkgo extract treatment was associated with a sig-nificant increase in the percentage of trabecular bone of the femur and alveolar bone of the mandible.[49] In a very similar study conducted the same year, ginkgo extract–treated oste-oporotic mice demonstrated a significant increase in mesial and distal periodontal bone support.[50] However, a 2008 study did *not* find ginkgo extract to benefit severe bone den-sity loss in ovariectomized rats, but it stimulated osteoblast differentiation and antiosteoclastic activity in vitro.[51]

Green Tea

Green tea may mitigate bone loss in elderly women and men and decrease risk of osteoporotic fractures. A 6-month randomized clinical trial (n = 171) tested the efficacy of green tea polyphenols (GTP) alone or with tai chi for the improvement of postmenopausal osteopenia. Outcomes were measured using bone turnover biomarkers bone alkaline phosphatase (BAP) and tartrate-resistant acid phosphatase (TRAP), calcium metabolism, and muscle strength. GTP supplementation, tai chi, and their combination increased BAP, improved the BAP:TRAP ratio, and improved muscle strength; it was also found to be well tolerated (500 mg daily green tea polyphenols).[52,53]

SUMMARY

Adequate nutrition and exercise from a young age are essential for the prevention of bone loss and maintenance of bone mass throughout the life cycle. Healthy living may therefore be the most important resource we have for osteoporosis prevention for future generations. Optimal nutritional intake, especially calcium, vitamin D, and protein throughout a woman's life are necessary for bone strength and health. Avoiding cigarette smoking and reducing risk factors for falls is also significant. Finally, a number of nonpharmacologic and pharmacologic strategies are available that can prevent BMD loss and improve bone strength, before, during, and after menopause.

Cardiovascular Health

PREVENTION OF CARDIOVASCULAR DISEASE

Cardiovascular disease (CVD) is the leading cause of major illness and death among women older than age of 50 in the United States, amounting to 2.5 million hospitalizations and 500,000 deaths each year.[1] Coronary artery disease (CAD), myocardial infarction (MI), and stroke (i.e., cerebrovascular accident [CVA]) are the most common disorders in this category of disease. According to the National Institute on Aging, one in ten women age 45 to 64 will suffer from CVD. Although women perceive a greater risk from breast cancer, the actual lifetime risk of death associated with breast cancer is 1 in 25, versus a 1 in 3 risk of death from CVD. More women die of CVD than from all cancers, accidents, and diabetes combined.[1] CVD occurs at a later age in women compared with men, and carries with it a worse prognosis. Approximately 80% of deaths from CVD in women younger than 65 years of age occur during the first MI, and 63% of these women never have a symptom before the fatal event. During the first year after an MI, 44% of those who survive die, and 64% never completely recover.[1,2]

Many risk factors, both modifiable and nonmodifiable, have been identified as contributing to CVD. The National Heart, Lung, and Blood Institute lists the following[2]:

- *Age:* After menopause, women lose the protective effects of estrogen and experience an increased risk of coronary disease. Estrogen also has been found to affect cholesterol levels, homocysteine levels (involved with inflammatory process), and clotting mechanisms, and it inhibits platelet aggregation and diminishes the viscosity of blood. In general, women experience coronary heart disease (CHD) 10 years later than men because they are protected by the effects of estrogen until after menopause.[1]
- *History of CVD, stroke, or peripheral vascular disease*
- *Family history of premature CVD*
- *Dyslipidemia:* According to the National Institute on Aging, cholesterol levels in women begin to rise somewhat after the age of 20, and again more rapidly after the age of 40. This increase in total cholesterol continues until the age of 60, with no observed difference by race or ethnicity. Women with high levels of high-density lipoproteins (HDLs) have lower risk for CHD, with HDL offering a greater predictive value for women than men. Elevated triglyceride levels also indicate an elevated risk for heart disease.[1,3]
- *Cigarette smoking:* Data from the Nurses' Health Study show that women who were heavy smokers had more than six times the risk of CHD than nonsmokers, and after quitting for 3 to 5 years, were able to reduce their risk of CHD to almost within the range for nonsmokers. Smoking has been found to decrease estrogen levels in women, along with the cardioprotective effects of this hormone.[3]
- *Hypertension:* This is the most significant risk factor for stroke, and also contributes greatly to risk of heart disease. Although rates of hypertension for all women has been declining, black women are more likely to suffer from this disorder than white, Asian, or Hispanic women.[3]
- *Diabetes mellitus:* This disease increases a woman's risk of heart disease by three times and is felt to reduce the protective effect of estrogen. Those women with diabetes who experience an MI are more likely to die, compared with women without diabetes or men.[1-3]
- *Obesity (especially central):* Obesity has been defined as a body mass index (BMI) >30. The proportion of women who fall into this category has been increasing steadily over the past 40 years, with an increase in prevalence among black women (37.6%) over white women (23.5%) in 1994.[3]
- *Lifestyle—diet, physical activity, psychosocial factors, alcohol:* A diet high in saturated and transsaturated fats is felt to increase the risk for CHD. Vigorous physical activity reduces cholesterol levels, obesity, and hypertension, and most likely contributes to decreased incidence of CHD through these mechanisms. Psychological factors that may contribute to CHD in women include stress and stressful life events, anger, hostility, hopelessness, depression, social support/networks, education, occupation and job control, and chronic fatigue.[3]
- *Homocysteine and C-reactive protein (CRP):* Increased levels of these biochemical markers have been associated with an increased risk of CVD.[2,3]

Modifiable risk factors include cigarette smoking, alcohol use, and lifestyle (diet, physical activity, and psychosocial factors). Nonmodifiable factors include age, gender, and family history.

The editor wishes to thank *Botanical Medicine for Women's Health*, Edition 1 contributor, Wendy Grube, for her original contributions to this chapter.

Symptoms

The major presenting symptom of CAD in women is angina, which may be accompanied by palpitations, shortness of breath, dyspnea on exertion, nausea, sweating, and fatigue. Associated CAD pain may occur in locations such as the jaw, arms and shoulders, or back. This profile of symptoms often leads to nonrecognition of their cardiac origin, leading to delayed medical recognition and treatment. Statistically, women receive less medical attention for their symptoms of coronary disease than men.[1]

Diagnosis

Unfortunately, the diagnosis of CAD usually follows symptoms of angina that occur after years of plaque development, or an acute cardiovascular event, such as an MI. In the past, women who presented with chest pain were evaluated less aggressively than men, most likely caused by an erroneous belief that angina in women was benign. In the contemporary medical system, a woman complaining of chest pain may expect to undergo the following:

1. *Detailed history and characteristics of the chest pain:* These include onset, location, duration, characteristics, concomitant symptoms, aggravating or relieving factors, and any self-treatment. Chest pain associated with angina is usually described as a feeling of retrosternal burning, heaviness, or a "crushing" sensation, which may radiate to the back, arm, neck, or jaw, lasting over 1 minute but less than 10 minutes. In the event of an MI, the pain is similar, but usually lasts 30 minutes to 2 hours, and may be associated with nausea and vomiting, sweating, dizziness, weakness, or shortness of breath. It may have occurred after an episode of physical exertion or anxiety, and is relieved by narcotic analgesics.[4]

2. *Focused examination:* This involves evaluation of all peripheral pulses, auscultation of the carotid arteries for bruits, awareness of any existing jugular venous distention, and recording of blood pressure while the patient is sitting, lying, and standing.[4]

3. *Diagnostic tests:* These usually include an electrocardiogram (ECG), nuclear scanning, and angiography to evaluate how many vessels are affected and to what degree. A "stress test" or exercise ECG may be used to evaluate the heart's ability to respond adequately to the increased oxygen demands required by vigorous physical exertion. Nuclear scanning measures an "ejection fraction," or the ability of the left ventricle to pump blood effectively. Angiography (i.e., cardiac catheterization), is the actual viewing of the coronary arteries via a catheter, through which stents or balloons can be placed to hold the artery open, or fibrinolytic medications can be distributed to unblock an affected artery. A comprehensive 12-lead ECG is used to look for diminished coronary artery blood flow (i.e., ischemia) or resulting injury to the surrounding cardiac tissue. Ischemia of heart tissue results in changes of the electrical conduction (i.e., depolarization and repolarization) of the cells. This creates an enlargement and inversion of the T wave on ECG. When actual injury occurs, there is visible ST-segment elevation, followed by a significant Q-wave after infarction (i.e., necrosis) occurs. The ECG is accompanied by serial cardiac enzyme levels, which can support the diagnosis of MI and assist in determining when the event occurred.[4]

If the woman is not experiencing an acute coronary event such as an MI, routine screening for risk factors will take place. This includes continued monitoring of blood pressure and identification of hypertension when it exists; and lipid testing to detect elevated total cholesterol and, more significantly, low-density lipoprotein (LDL) cholesterol, as well as triglycerides. At times, other potential risk factors may be screened for by checking serum homocysteine, CRP, or lipoprotein-a.[5]

CONVENTIONAL MEDICAL MANAGEMENT OF CAD

Management strategies for CAD (Table 8-1) revolve around the reduction of risk factors identified during the diagnostic process, and the prevention of an MI or sudden death.[4] These approaches include attempted correction of hypertension, dyslipidemias, elevated serum glucose levels in diabetics, and risk of thrombus formation.

Medications

Medications used for the management of CAD in women include diuretics for hypertension, exogenous hormones and statins for lipid improvement, insulin and oral hypoglycemics for blood glucose control, antiplatelet drugs to prevent thromboembolic events, β-blockers plus angiotensin-converting-enzyme (ACE) inhibitors to reduce morbidity and mortality related to MI, vasodilators to reduce afterload and/or preload, and calcium channel blockers with some of the aforementioned medications to relax peripheral vascular resistance. The overall goal is to relieve the work the heart has to do and maximize efficiency to reduce the oxygen consumption requirements of the heart.

Hormonal Replacement Therapy

Traditionally, the hormones most widely used and studied were conjugated equine estrogens plus medroxyprogesterone acetate, a synthetic progestin derived from wild yam. In the past, various observational studies indicated a 35% to 80% decrease in CAD in women using estrogen replacement therapy (ERT). However, the use of estrogen alone, without adding a progestin, in a woman with a uterus was found to increase her risk of endometrial hyperplasia and cancer. The Postmenopausal Estrogen/Progestin Interventions (PEPI) trial results showed beneficial effects of estrogen on HDL, LDL, and fibrinogen levels compared with placebo (in 875 healthy postmenopausal women).[6] A study using postmenopausal women with established heart disease, the Heart and Estrogen/Progestin Replacement Study (HERS), showed no significant differences between groups of women who used hormones and placebo in primary or

TABLE 8-1   Conventional Management of Coronary Artery Disease in Postmenopausal Women

Disorder	Management

Dyslipidemia
Goals:
  Women without CAD
  Low risk (<2 risk factors)
  LDL <160 mg/dL
  Ideal LDL <130 mg/dL
  Higher risk (≥2 risk factors)
  LDL <130 mg/dL
  Women with CAD
  LDL <100 mg/dL
  Other lipid goals:
  HDL >35 mg/dL
  Triglycerides <200 mg/dL
	Some studies have shown decreased incidence of CAD in women using HRT. HRT raises HDL cholesterol by 10% while decreasing LDL cholesterol by 10%; however, it also raises triglycerides by 25%, and carries up to a fourfold risk of a thromboembolic event, and a small early risk of MI and CVA. This risk of thromboembolic disease has been found in clinical trials to persist for 4 years after discontinuation of HRT use. Because of the lack of clinical evidence demonstrating cardiovascular benefit from HRT use, hormonal supplementation is no longer recommended for management of dyslipidemia.
	Pharmaceutical management includes statins, niacin, fibrate, or combination of the three:
	• LDL ≥ 190 mg/dL in postmenopausal women with <2 risk factors
	• LDL ≥ 160 mg/dL in postmenopausal women with ≥2 risk factors
	• Elevated triglyceride levels
	• Statins have shown a 29% risk reduction of CHD in women; however, adverse effects may include liver and renal dysfunction.

Hypertension Goal: <140/90 mm Hg Ideal: <120/80 mm Hg	Lifestyle modification is necessary, including weight loss, physical exercise, and moderation in alcohol and salt intake. Individualized pharmaceutical intervention is advised in the following instances: • BP elevation of ≥140/90 mm Hg after 3 months of lifestyle change • Systolic BP ≥160 mm Hg initially • Diastolic BP ≥100 mm Hg initially

Diabetes
Blood glucose goals:
  Preprandial: 80-120 mg/dL
  Bedtime: 100-140 mg/dL
  Hemoglobin A1C goal: <7%
	American Diabetes Association Diet
	Weight loss and physical exercise
	Pharmaceuticals (insulin or oral medication) as indicated to achieve blood glucose goals

Thromboembolic Events *Women with established CVD*	Atherosclerotic CVD: Use aspirin 80-325 mg a day Women who cannot take aspirin: Use antiplatelet medications
Reinfarction and Sudden Death, *Overall Mortality in Women After MI*	Hospitalized women with an evolving MI and no contraindications may start a β-blocker within hours of admission, or within the few days after the event, and should be continued indefinitely. Women with left ventricular dysfunction may be started on an ACE inhibitor for 6 weeks, and then stopped.

CAD, Coronary artery disease; *LDL,* low-density lipoprotein; *HDL,* high-density lipoprotein; *HRT,* hormonal replacement therapy; *MI,* myocardial infarction; *CVA,* cerebrovascular accident; *CHD,* coronary heart disease; *BP,* blood pressure; *CVD,* cardiovascular disease; *ACE,* angiotensin-converting-enzyme.

secondary cardiovascular outcomes after 4.1 years. HERS also indicated an increased risk of CVD events in the first year of HRT use, followed by less events in years 4 and 5.[7] The Women's Health Initiative (WHI), a National Institutes of Health (NIH)-sponsored multicenter study of healthy postmenopausal women, showed a significant increased risk of CAD, stroke, venous thromboembolism, and biliary tract surgery, and a nonsignificant risk of breast cancer, with HRT use. It is now recommended that HRT be prescribed for a short duration (3 to 5 years) for the control of vasomotor symptoms, and should not be used for primary or secondary prevention of CHD.[2]

Statins

Statins are drugs used to lower cholesterol and LDL levels, and are categorized as 3-hydroxy-3-methylglutaryl-coenzyme A (HMG-CoA) reductase inhibitors. They block the production of cholesterol in the liver and increase the speed of breakdown of LDL, resulting in LDL level lowering by 25% to 45%, triglycerides lowering by 10% to 30%, and HDLs increasing by 8% to 10%. They are also effective because of antiinflammatory effects. Common mild side effects include headache, myalgia, abdominal pain, and gastrointestinal (GI) symptoms such as dyspepsia, constipation, or diarrhea. Rhabdomyolysis and its associated renal dysfunction have been reported in 0.1% to

0.5% of patients using statins; elevated liver enzymes also may occur; and recent large studies conclusively link statins to causing diabetes and increasing risk of CVD in women.[7,8]

Hypoglycemics

Hypoglycemics include insulin and oral drugs used to lower serum glucose levels. Persons with type 1 diabetes lack endogenous insulin, and must be given exogenous insulin to prevent diabetic ketoacidosis and death. Persons with type 2 diabetes may have some endogenous insulin; however, they may suffer from insulin resistance. Oral agents act on glucose utilization and liver storage and production of glucose. Occasionally, persons with type 2 diabetes require insulin as well as oral agents. The goal of therapy is to normalize blood glucose levels, preventing the progression of the disease to target organs, such as the coronary arteries. The most common adverse effect is hypoglycemia.

Antiplatelet Drugs

Aspirin is the primary antiplatelet drug used to prevent clot formation in persons known to have CAD. It works by interfering with platelet aggregation. Common side effects include GI discomfort and bleeding. Warfarin or clopidogrel can be used if aspirin is contraindicated.[2] Antiplatelet medications are only recommended in patients with prior events or risk factors for disease; they are not recommended prophylactically for otherwise healthy individuals.

β-Blockers

In women who have experienced an MI, β-blockers are usually initiated within hours of the event unless contraindications exist, such as severe bradycardia, high-degree heart block, acute heart failure, asthma, or peripheral vascular disease. Essentially, these drugs decrease the workload of the heart by decreasing heart rate, conduction, velocity, and contractility. They effectively reduce angina and the incidence of rhythm disturbances, and also decrease blood pressure over time by diminishing peripheral vascular resistance. Passive bronchial constriction may occur because of β-adrenergic receptors located in the lungs being affected by this class of drugs. Effects on the liver include a rise in total cholesterol, decrease in HDL, and elevation of triglycerides. Decreased insulin secretion by the pancreas also may be an effect of β-blockers. Other adverse effects include urinary frequency, male impotence, and diarrhea.

Angiotensin-Converting Enzyme Inhibitors

ACE inhibitors are used in the case of heart failure, and function to reduce cardiac preload and afterload, as well as peripheral vascular resistance and blood pressure, through decreased sodium and water retention. They are started as soon as possible after an MI, with the goal of reducing the likelihood of heart failure or extension of the infarction. They are also used in the management of left ventricular dysfunction and heart failure. Common adverse reactions include hypotension and dry cough, with rarer effects, including rash (with captopril), neutropenia with high doses, renal impairment, and

concomitant collagen diseases. Angiotensin receptor blockers are used with similar effects to the ACE inhibitors, without the side effects; bradykinin, a vasodilator maintained by the ACE inhibitors, is not maintained by this latter class of drugs, and it is the effects of bradykinin in the lungs that are thought to cause cough.

Niacin

Niacin is considered one of the most effective drugs for elevating HDL cholesterol, and is commonly combined with statins to increase the rate of improvement in cholesterol levels. Flushing is the major side effect but can be minimized by taking a baby aspirin 30 minutes before taking niacin. Niacin is contraindicated in patients with liver disease, and may transiently lead to an elevation in liver function test results even in healthy patients. Niacin may make glycemic control more difficult in diabetic patients and may aggravate arthritis associated with gout.

Procedural Interventions

Procedural interventions for the treatment of CAD include percutaneous transluminal coronary angioplasty, with placement of a stent in the coronary artery to maintain patency of the vessel, combined with antiplatelet therapy and coronary artery bypass graft surgery.

THE BOTANICAL PRACTITIONER'S PERSPECTIVE

Heart disease is perhaps the most overt example of pathology representing a confluence of influences that conspire to create disease: diet, exercise, sleep, stress and coping mechanisms, spirituality, culture, family, and environmental conditions—all of which also can work in concert to affect healing.

Botanical medicine offers a number of herbs that have been used historically and traditionally for the treatment of CVD. Every medical and herbal student learns the story of William Withering, who learned of the cure for dropsy (i.e., edema caused by congestive heart failure [CHF]) from a local herb woman, and from which the modern mainstay drug digoxin was derived. However, determining the appropriate role for botanical therapies in treating the patient with CVD can be difficult. A number of herbs with cardiovascular effects have now been well studied, and have been found to improve cardiovascular wellness. Several have been demonstrated to have actions that parallel those of conventional pharmaceuticals, often with fewer adverse effects. For example, garlic, fenugreek, and guggul have demonstrated positive effects on cholesterol levels, whereas hawthorn has been shown to have positive inotropic effects and be beneficial in the prevention of CHF, and none have remarkable adverse effects associated with their use. However, whether these herbs are a suitable substitute for patients with heart disease is undetermined. There are, for example, a number of effective herbal diuretics, most notably dandelion leaf, which is rich in potassium and therefore may offer diuresis without potassium depletion. Unfortunately, its diuretic effects are more difficult to predict, control, and quantify than a standard pharmaceutical dose of a diuretic; therefore although pharmaceutical diuretics certainly have more side effects, they may be easier to control in terms of dose and results. Because the potential for interactions exists between herbs and drugs, and because the effects on both patient safety and medication efficacy—either of the herb or the drug—when taken combined is largely unknown, it is advisable not to combine the two. Therefore for patients dependent on medications for basic cardiac functioning, it is probably best to take a conventional pharmaceutical treatment route; however, for patients in need of CVD prevention, or with only mild disease (i.e., moderate hypertension) who wish to avoid medications, a trial of botanical medicines along with therapeutic lifestyle change might be entirely safe and appropriate. Such decisions need to be made individually for each patient. Close monitoring of patients is important.

The importance of therapeutic lifestyle changes in altering the course of CVD also cannot be overemphasized. Even walking briskly for as little as 3 hours per week can reduce a woman's risk of heart attack by about 40%.[9] Similarly, dietary changes, stress reduction, treatment for depression, and perhaps most significantly, smoking cessation, can be life-saving. Therapeutic lifestyle changes are always the first line approach in any nonemergent medical setting, as well as in the herbal clinic. The possible actions of herbs and their effects on the cardiovascular system are presented in Table 8-2 and are discussed in the following. This section focuses on those herbs used directly to prevent and treat mild CVD. Treatment of concurrent problems, for example, diabetes, polycystic ovarian syndrome (PCOS), or insulin resistance, which are known to increase risk of cardiovascular problems, is essential.

For botanical options for stress, readers are directed to other chapters for discussions on herbs for treating depression, relieving anxiety, promoting sleep, and improving the stress response.

Patients with a history of CVD, a suspected cardiovascular problem, or who are currently being treated for CVD, are advised to work in conjunction with a physician when using botanicals. It is generally recommended that cardiotonic herbs (e.g., hawthorn) and cardioactive herbs (containing cardioactive glycosides, e.g., lily of the valley) not be combined with cardioactive medications because of possible potentiation of actions.

Black Cohosh

Traditionally, black cohosh was used by the Eclectics for a wide range of disorders, including emotional complaints associated with the perimenopause, as well as cardiovascular symptoms such as palpitations, arrhythmias, and hypertension caused by "nervous stimulation" of the heart. It was used in the treatment for angina and cardiac arrhythmias.[10] Primarily used for management of vasomotor symptoms commonly associated with the perimenopause, black cohosh also appears to increase the blood flow through peripheral vessels at doses of 0.5 mg/kg.[10] Animal studies have demonstrated a dose-dependent hypotensive effect; however, this has never been observed in human studies.[10] The primary use of black cohosh in a contemporary herbal approach to CVD is in combination with other herbs for its anxiolytic effects, relaxation of nonpathologic palpitations, and for concomitant relief of menopausal complaints. It is commonly given in tincture or capsule form.

Coleus

Valued by herbalists for its hypotensive actions, coleus also may contribute to the prevention of CHD through its antiplatelet activity.[11] Its constituent forskolin has been subject to in vitro and in vivo (by injection) investigation and has demonstrated hypotensive activity, positive inotropic action

TABLE 8-2	Herbs Used in the Prevention and Management of Coronary Artery Disease in Women	
Therapeutic Activity	**Botanical Name**	**Common Name**
Anticholesteremic	Allium sativum	Garlic
	Commiphora mukul	Guggul
	Cynara scolymus	Globe artichoke
	Salvia miltiorrhiza (Danshen)	Chinese sage
	Trigonella foenum-graecum	Fenugreek
Antihypertensive	Allium sativum	Garlic
	Actaea racemosa	Black cohosh
	Coleus forskohlii	Coleus
	Viburnum opulus	Cramp bark
Positive inotrope, cardiotonic	Crataegus oxyacantha	Hawthorn
Antithrombotic	Allium sativum	Garlic
	Angelica sinensis	Dong quai
	Salvia miltiorrhiza (Danshen)	Salvia
Relieve palpitations	Leonurus cardiaca	Motherwort
	Crataegus oxyacantha	Hawthorn
Prevent CHF	Crataegus oxyacantha	Hawthorn
	Convallaria majalis	Lily of the valley

CHF, Congestive heart failure.

on isolated heart muscle, and increased cerebral blood flow with vasodilatation. No clinical studies have been conducted using coleus. Although a closely related species is used in traditional Ayurvedic medicine, this species is used only as a condiment.[12] Coleus extracts containing a quantified level of forskolin are recommended, and it is not advisable to use this herb with other cardiac medications or without the advice or a qualified practitioner.[12] It is used in the form of a hydroethanolic extract, and is generally included as less than 20% of an herbal formula.

Cramp Bark

Considered a "vasorelaxant," this herb has been identified as having possible usefulness as an adjunct in the treatment of hypertension.[11,13] No clinical trials have evaluated the effects of cramp bark on blood pressure or cardiovascular measures. It is a highly respected musculoskeletal relaxant and is commonly combined in formulae for the treatment of stress, chronic pain, and insomnia.

Dong Quai

Animal and in vitro studies have found that dong quai may exert a cardioprotective effect, increasing myocardial blood supply, decreasing myocardial oxygen consumption, and reducing oxidative damage to ischemic myocardial tissue. In addition, studies have shown that it can act to inhibit platelet aggregation, increase prothrombin time, decrease peripheral vascular resistance and arterial blood pressure, and inhibit experimentally induced arrhythmias and ventricular fibrillation. Butylidenephthalide and sodium ferulate have been found to inhibit platelet aggregation in vivo and in vitro, primarily by interrupting arachidonic acid metabolism. Ferulic acid has been shown to increase coronary blood flow in vitro, and sodium ferulate may have antiarrhythmic affects. In addition, butylidenephthalide has shown hypotensive effects in vivo. Most of these proposed cardiovascular and hemorrheologic effects of dong quai or its constituents are consistent with the Traditional Chinese Medicine (TCM) use of this herb to "quicken the blood." Only three human controlled clinical trials evaluating dong quai's effects on CVD were identified. The studies, of variable quality (e.g., one study lacks a placebo arm), show some vasodilatory effects and possible improvement in postischemic stroke neurologic and hematologic perameters.[14]

Fenugreek

A systematic review by Thompson Coon and Ernst identified five randomized clinical trials using fenugreek for control of hypertension. The trials involved a total of 140 patients; all but one trial was conducted in India. Although the methodological quality of the studies was considered generally poor in four of the trials, statistically significant reductions occurred in total serum cholesterol of between 15% and 33% compared with baseline. Commonly reported side effects included mild GI symptoms, although none was severe enough to cause participant withdrawal.[15] This herb, like the others in this section, should not be used with conventional cardiac medications.

Fenugreek has a pleasant taste to most, and is used as tea, in tinctures, finely ground in capsules, or even in foods.

Garlic

Garlic has an extensive reputation for prevention and treatment of cardiovascular disorders. The fresh or dried cloves are used. (The cloves are secondary bulbs and make up the larger bulb.)[16] Approved by the German Commission E for the prevention of dyslipidemias in the aging and the treatment of hyperlipidemia,[16] it is popularly used for the treatment of mild hypertension and the prevention of atherosclerosis and CAD. The primary active constituent is considered to be allicin, produced when the clove is chopped or crushed.[17]

Garlic has been shown to inhibit enzymes involved in lipid synthesis, decrease platelet aggregation, prevent lipid peroxidation of oxidized erythrocytes and LDL, increase antioxidant status, and inhibit ACE. Numerous studies point to the fact that garlic reduces cholesterol, inhibits platelet aggregation, reduces blood pressure, and increases antioxidant status.[18] Like statins, garlic appears to inhibit cholesterol biosynthesis through inhibition of HMG-CoA reductase.[18-25] A recent systematic review suggested a hypotensive effect in hypertensive but not normotensive patients using garlic.[26] A 2012 Cochrane review identified two randomized controlled trials using garlic with 87 hypertensive patients. The reviewers concluded that garlic can reduce mean supine systolic and diastolic blood pressure by approximately 10 to 12 mm Hg and 6 to 9 mm Hg, respectively, but the confidence intervals derived from available trial data are not precise. They also note that these alterations may be caused by normal blood pressure variations.[27] Forty-four percent of the clinical trials conducted since 1993 have indicated a reduction in total cholesterol, and the most profound effect has been observed in garlic's ability to reduce platelet aggregation.

Inconsistent results have been seen in the area of blood pressure and oxidative-stress reduction, with very few studies addressing these. Negative findings from some clinical trials may have resulted from variations in the garlic preparations used, short trial durations, and other methodological limitations.[18] Although the World Health Organization (WHO) cautions against the use of garlic in patients taking warfarin and other anticoagulant medications, clinical trials and adverse events reports thus far do not support these concerns. However, increased clotting time has been reported in patients taking garlic supplements; therefore it is recommended that garlic supplementation be discontinued for at least 1 week before any surgical procedures, and it is prudent for patients on anticoagulant therapies to avoid garlic other than in common food quantities.[28] One clinical trial of human immunodeficiency virus (HIV) patients (n = 9) on saquinavir found significantly decreased serum levels of the medication after garlic ingestion.[29]

Garlic breath and GI complaints are the most commonly reported adverse effects; contact dermatitis has been reported with prolonged exposure. The German Commission E and the European Scientific Cooperative on Phytotherapy (ESCOP) both state that there are no known contraindications to garlic use.[16,30] This herb, like the others in this section, should not be used with conventional cardiac medications. Garlic may be eaten fresh in the diet in any number of foods, or may be taken in a variety of extracts, capsules, or other products available on the market. Which products are most efficacious remains a matter of some debate, with several types of preparations yielding positive results in clinical trials.[28]

Ginseng

A recent randomized controlled trial tested red ginseng for menopausal symptoms and CVD risk factors. A group of 72 women was randomized to receive either 3 g red ginseng (standardized to 60 mg of ginsenosides) or placebo for 3 months. Menopausal symptoms were measured using the Kupperman index, and cardiovascular correlates were serum lipid testing, CRP, and carotid artery intima-media thickness. Kupperman index scores decreased significantly in the red ginseng group, as did LDL cholesterol and carotid intima-media thickness. No differences were observed with HDL cholesterol or CRP.[31] Another clinical trial (n = 64) suggests that American ginseng may reduce arterial stiffness in patients with type 2 diabetes and concomitant hypertension. Participants took 3 g of American ginseng daily as an adjunct therapy over the course of 12 weeks (Extract; further preparation details not provided).[32]

Globe Artichoke

Prized for centuries as a medicinal plant used to "tonify the liver," globe artichoke extracts have been shown to produce various pharmacologic effects, including marked choleretic activity and inhibition of cholesterol biosynthesis and LDL oxidation.[33] It is considered safe when used in food or therapeutic amounts, and is not known to interact with foods, drugs, or laboratory tests. The only adverse reaction noted is allergic response, primarily in persons allergic to the *Asteraceae/Compositae* family of plants. It is not recommended for use when there is obstruction of the bile duct, and should be used with caution when gallstones are present. Of two clinical trials (n = 187), one (n = 44) showed some reduction in total serum cholesterol in patients with a baseline of over 5.4 mmol/L, and the other showed reductions in total serum cholesterol of 18.5% for artichoke and 8.6% for placebo.[34] This herb, like the others in this section, should not be used with conventional cardiac medications.

Guggul

Resin from the guggul tree, a native of western India, has been used in Ayurvedic medicine since at least 600 BCE. In 1986, guggul oleoresin was approved in India for marketing as a lipid-lowering agent. Studies have shown that guggulsterones are antagonist ligands for the bile acid receptor farnesoid X receptor (FXR), which is an important regulator of cholesterol homeostasis.[35,36] A review by Thompson Coon and Ernst identified six randomized clinical trials of guggul, involving 388 patients with different diagnoses. Five of the studies were conducted in India and one in the United States; four were placebo controlled; and one compared guggul with two reference compounds. Results suggest reductions in total serum cholesterol from 10% to 27% compared with baseline levels.

A statistically significant decrease in lipid peroxide levels was reported in one study, with no corresponding change in the placebo-treated group.[15] Guggul is associated with numerous side effects, including abdominal discomfort, diarrhea, headache, hypersensitivity rash, nausea, and hiccups. The herb is typically recommended in a standardized form, guggulipid, standardized to 25 mg guggulsterones per tablet, with an oral dose of 75 mg in three divided doses daily, or two tablets twice daily.[37] It is estimated that the onset of action is approximately 2 to 4 weeks. The use of guggul may decrease the bioavailability of propranolol, diltiazem, and thyroid medication, and caution is advised with concomitant use.[37] This herb, like the others in this section, should not be used with conventional cardiac medications.

Hawthorn

Hawthorn, widely accepted in Europe as a treatment for mild CHF and minor arrhythmias, is one of the most important herbs in the materia medica for the prevention and treatment of CVD.[9] Some consider it so beneficial that is has been called a "food for the heart" and suggested that everyone over 50 should take hawthorn daily. Much like red wine and green tea, hawthorn is rich in flavonoids (with the glycosides catechin and epicatechin) and oligomeric proanthocyanidins (OPCs), although amines and triterpene saponins are found as well.[28,38] It is thought to possess cardiotonic, coronary vasodilatory, and hypotensive actions. Traditionally, hawthorn has been used in the treatment of heart failure, myocardial weakness, paroxysmal tachycardia, hypertension, and arteriosclerosis. The pharmacologic actions of the leaf with flowers include increase in cardiac contractility, increase in coronary blood flow and myocardial circulation, protection from ischemic damage, and decrease of peripheral vascular resistance.

There have been no reported adverse reactions to the use of berries. However, there have been reports of nausea and GI discomfort, as well as palpitations, headache, dizziness, sleeplessness, agitation, and some circulatory disturbances when preparations containing the leaves and flowers have been taken, even in recommended therapeutic doses.[38]

Presently, hawthorn is used as a cardiac tonic for mild heart disorders, including CAD, angina, arrhythmias, hypertension, myocardial weakness; and prevention of arterial degeneration, well supported by scientific literature. Hoffman combines hawthorn with lime blossom, mistletoe, and yarrow in a formula to manage hypertension and circulatory system disorders.[39] In addition to the use of this plant as a cardiac tonic, it has been traditionally used as a diuretic.

Current research supports the use of hawthorn extracts for the treatment of CAD and angina, ischemia-induced arrhythmias, dyslipidemias, hypertension, and early-stage CHF. Modes of action suggested by animal and in vitro studies include positive inotropic activity (increased cyclic adenosine monophosphate [cAMP], similar to cardiac glycosides); reduced peripheral vascular resistance and increased coronary and peripheral blood flow; increased integrity of vessel walls; decreased oxygen demand by the myocardium; protection against myocardial damage through antioxidative properties; protection against arrhythmias through lengthening the refractory period; and antiinflammatory effects. There is also some evidence through animal studies that hawthorn may lower serum lipid levels and improve hypertension, perhaps through the release of the potent vasodilator nitric oxide (NO). Inhibition of platelet aggregation has been an additional observed effect of hawthorn in vitro. Although most of the science we have on hawthorn is from animal and in vitro studies, there have been extensive human trials investigating the use of hawthorn in early CHF. Preliminary studies by the German pharmaceutical company Schwalbe using an extract of hawthorn leaves and flowers (WS 1442) indicated the product was safe and effective to treat CHF in humans. Standardized to contain 18.75% oligomeric procyanidins, this product was found to increase exercise tolerance and decrease symptoms of CHF. Zapfe, in a recent randomized, double-blinded, placebo-controlled study using WS 1442 on 40 patients (75% women) with New York Heart Association (NYHA) class II mild, chronic CHF, confirmed a 10% improvement in exercise tolerance compared with a 15% reduction in the placebo group.[28,38] This herb, like the others in this section, should not be used with conventional cardiac medications.

Hibiscus

Recent trial evidence suggests that hibiscus tea may benefit diabetic patients with mild hypertension. A group of 60 patients, who were not taking antihypertensive or antihyperlipidemic medicines, ingested either 1 cup of sweetened hibiscus tea daily or black tea as a control. After 1 month, patients who consumed hibiscus tea demonstrated a decrease in average systolic (but not diastolic) blood pressure.[40]

Lily of the Valley

Lily of the valley is a cardioactive herb mostly used in European herbal medicine.[41] Its actions are considered similar to those of digitalis, although it is significantly less cumulative and apparently has a vastly broader therapeutic window. The plant contains approximately 40 glycosides, the principal three being convallatoxin, convalloside, and lokunjoside.[41] Cardiac glycosides improve the efficiency of the myocardium without increasing the need for oxygen, thus lessening the workload on the heart. Although US herbal practitioners seem wary of its use because of concerns over potential toxicity, UK herbalists continue to use it, respectfully, primarily for the treatment of mild heart failure and bradycardia, considering it to complement hawthorn well.[42] It has a rapid onset and a very short half-life.[43] Evans reports that the toxicity of this herb is often overemphasized, citing publication in the United States of 2639 case reports of ingestion, with 6.1% of patients experiencing symptoms, but only three showing severe side effects.[44] Lily of the valley, however, can induce side effects associated with cardiac glycosides including nausea and vomiting, although reported to be rare and mild.[42] This is a scheduled herb in the United Kingdom, and should be prepared as a 1:10 tincture and given only in low doses. This herb, like the others in this section, should not be used with conventional

cardiac medications. This herb should be used only by a professional trained and skilled in its application, and in conjunction with medical evaluation of cardiac effects.

Motherwort

Ever since Gerard wrote his famous herbal text in the late sixteenth century, motherwort has had a reputation of usefulness in cardiac disorders, and although beneficial for men and women alike, has had an association as a "women's herb." Motherwort is approved by the German Commission E for heart palpitations occurring with anxiety. Direct myocardial action of motherwort was noted by Newall in 1992, with stimulation of both α- and β-adrenoceptors and inhibition of calcium chloride effects. Another exploratory study by Bradley noted alkaloids contained in this plant depress the central nervous system and lower blood pressure. No modern studies have evaluated this herb clinically. Overall, however, this herb is little studied. It is quite safe and may be used in tinctures for anxiety, palpitations, and as a general cardiotonic, the latter especially when combined with hawthorn. As tea, motherwort is quite bitter, but some herbalists prepare a motherwort-infused honey, a teaspoon of which can be added to other teas.

🍃 CHANGE OF HEART CORDIAL

This cordial was created by herbalist Amanda McQuade Crawford to safely prevent or reduce hypertension, calm heart palpitations, support the hormonal changes of menopause, and to calm and relax the nerves.

Combine:

Hawthorn tincture	(*Crataegus oxyacantha*)	4 oz
Motherwort tincture	(*Leonurus cardiaca*)	2 oz
Chaste berry	(*Vitex agnus-castus*)	2 oz
Blackstrap molasses		2 oz
Blackberry juice concentrate		2 oz
	Total: 12 oz	

Dose: 1 tsp, twice daily, diluted in water, juice, or tea; 12 oz will last 30 days.

Red Clover

Red clover isoflavone supplementation (80 mg) positively affected the lipid profile of women with increased BMI, evidenced by a 3-month clinical trial (n = 60) that demonstrated a significant decrease in total cholesterol, Low-density lipoprotein (LDL), and lipoprotein(a) LpA levels.[45]

Salvia (Danshen)

Danshen, the root of *Salvia miltiorrhiza,* has a long history of use in TCM as a blood-moving herb, activating circulation and dispersing "stasis."[46,47] It continues to be widely used in China and, to a lesser extent, in Japan, the United States, and other European countries for the treatment of cardiovascular and cerebrovascular diseases. In China, the specific clinical use is angina pectoris, hyperlipidemia, and acute ischemic stroke.[48] It is thought to be capable of improving microcirculation, causing coronary vasodilatation, suppressing the formation of thromboxane, inhibiting platelet adhesion and aggregation, and protecting against myocardial ischemia, and is used alone and in combination with other herbs for the treatment of CAD.[47] It is conspicuously advertised in the *Chinese Journal of Cardiology,* which is the official publication of the Chinese Society of Cardiology.[47] Animal experiments evaluating cardiovascular effects report prevention of intrauterine growth retardation (compound product), blood pressure reduction, reduction of LDL oxidation and atherosclerosis, prevention of oxidative stress, protection from liver fibrosis and renal failure, and vasodilatation.[49-54] Although the effects of danshen have not been investigated in human clinical trials, several herb–drug interactions have been reported in the literature: combining danshen with warfarin results in strong antiplatelet activity; it is also necessary to avoid combining danshen with anticoagulant therapies.[47,55] The traditional dose of dried root is 6 to 15 g daily in decoction.[46] Reported adverse effects are pruritus, gastric discomfort, and appetite reduction.[46] In addition to cautions regarding combining danshen with anticoagulant and antiplatelet medications (including aspirin), it should not be combined with benzodiazepines because of possible potentiation on depressant CNS effects. Because it is commonly included in TCM herbal formulae, and is even found in certain Chinese cigarette brands, practitioners should be aware that patients may be taking this herb and not be aware of it.[47,56]

 SHEN: THE HEART AND MIND IN TRADITIONAL CHINESE MEDICINE

In Traditional Chinese Medicine (TCM), there is the concept of Shen, which may be thought of as the mind or spirit, but which is said to reside in the heart. As women age, it is believed, their yin becomes more deficient, leading to perturbations of Shen, which might include symptoms such as insomnia, irritability, and heart palpitations. Such disturbances are preferably prevented, but are also treated with TCM formulae for the heart.

NUTRITIONAL CONSIDERATIONS

The American Heart Association (http://www.heart.org/HEARTORG/HealthyLiving/HealthyEating/Nutrition/The-American-Heart-Associations-Diet-and-Lifestyle-Recommendations_UCM_305855_Article.jsp#.V4XIIFcaf0c) considered the following guidelines as part of a heart-healthy lifestyle:

- Reducing saturated and transfatty acids in the diet
- Minimizing the intake of food and beverages with added sugars
- Emphasizing physical activity and weight control
- Eating a diet rich in vegetables, fruits, and whole-grain foods

- Avoiding use of and exposure to tobacco products
- Achieving and maintaining healthy cholesterol, blood pressure, and blood glucose levels

Eat, Drink, and Be Healthy: The Harvard Medical School Guide to Healthy Eating and colleagues, by Walter Willett and colleagues, is an excellent resource for patients learning how to eat well. Willett lays out the following seven "most important dietary changes" patients can make toward heart and overall health[57]:

- *Watch weight:* The healthier the body weight for that patient, and the more stable the body weight, the lower are a patient's chances of CVD, diabetes, and of being diagnosed with postmenopausal breast cancer, endometrium cancer, and colon cancer.
- *Eat fewer "bad fats" and more "good fats":* Reducing dietary fat is not enough to protect the heart. Fats from nuts, seeds, grains, fish, and liquid oils (including olive, canola, soybean, corn, sunflower, peanut, and other vegetable oils) are healthy choices that allow the body to increase HDL and reduce LDL—which increases cardiovascular health.
- *Eat fewer refined-grain carbohydrates and more whole-grain carbohydrates:* Eating whole-grain foods is clearly better for long-term good health and offers protection against diabetes, heart disease, cancer, and GI problems such as diverticulosis and constipation—the latter is a known risk factor for colon cancer.
- *Choose healthier sources of proteins:* The best sources of protein are beans and nuts, along with fish, poultry, and eggs.
- *Eat plenty of vegetables and fruits:* A diet rich in fruits and vegetables will lower blood pressure and protect against heart attack, stroke, GI problems, and reduce the incidence of aging-related problems such as cataracts and macular degeneration.
- *Use alcohol in moderation:* Evidence strongly indicates that one alcoholic drink, preferably red wine, per day for women and one or two a day for men will reduce the chances of having a heart attack or dying from heart disease by about a third; risk of ischemic stroke is also decreased. For those who prefer not to drink alcohol, or for medical or personal history reasons are unable to, similar benefits can be gained by exercise.
- *Take a multivitamin for insurance:* Several of the ingredients in a standard multivitamin—especially vitamins B_6 and B_12, folic acid, and vitamin D—are essential players in preventing heart disease, cancer, osteoporosis, and other chronic diseases. At about a nickel a day, a multivitamin is a cheap and effective genuine "life insurance" policy. It will not make up for the sins of an unhealthy diet, but it can fill in the nutritional holes that can plague even the most conscientious eaters. A retrospective study examined the association between multivitamin/mineral supplement use and CVD incidence or mortality in healthy adults using *National Health and Nutrition Examination Survey* (NHANES) II data and the 2011 National Death Index. These two

surveys collated data from over 10,000 US adults. Data suggests that multivitamin/mineral supplement use did not affect CVD mortality. However, upon examination of the length of time of use, a significant inverse association was observed for multivitamin/mineral supplement use of greater than 3 years with a 35% reduced risk of CVD mortality in women.[58] (This effect was not observed with men.)

Furthermore, recent data from the Nurses' Cohort Study, a longitudinal study, identified lifestyle factors associated with CVD risk. The results suggest that nonsmoking women with a BMI less than 25 who exercise at least 30 minutes daily and consume a Mediterranean-style diet have a significantly lower risk of sudden cardiac death.[58]

Antioxidants: α-Lipoic Acid, Vitamins C and E, and β-Carotene

Although studies to date have been inconclusive regarding the use of antioxidants in the prevention of atherosclerosis, because the physiology of the disease involves oxidation, mechanisms have been proposed by which these substances may be effective: removing reactive oxygen species and improving the endothelial NO bioavailability. A 40% reduction in CVD risk was found in women with high vitamin E intake in the Nurses' Health Study. In individuals with known CAD, a prospective study found vitamin E to reduce the risk of nonfatal MI. Another large prospective study, the α-Tocopherol, β-Carotene Cancer Prevention Study, failed to find a decrease in CAD in men taking B-carotene over an 8-year period of time. Physicians taking 50 mg of β-carotene every other day also had no decrease in CAD in the Physicians' Health Study.[59]

Magnesium and Potassium

Low serum magnesium has been associated with an increased risk of heart disease, particularly hypertension, ischemic heart disease, CHF, sudden cardiac death, atherosclerosis, and associated risk factors such as insulin resistance and diabetes. Daily supplementation of 400 mg is recommended, in addition to a magnesium-rich diet, and is especially important for patients on thiazide diuretics, which lead to urinary magnesium loss.

Potassium has overall protective effects on the cardiovascular system, lowers blood pressure, and prevents stroke. A diet rich in fruits and vegetables provides substantial potassium. Patients on high-sodium diets who are unable to reduce their sodium intake may receive additional protective benefits in cardioprotection by consuming a high-potassium diet.

Arginine

This semiessential amino acid appears to encourage production of NO derived in the endothelium. Animal studies so far have demonstrated the ability of L-arginine to prevent lesions from forming in the endothelium of vessels, as well as diminishing ischemic and reperfusion injury in acute MIs. In humans, is it associated with increased exercise capacity in persons with CAD, decreased anginal episodes, and may play a role in prevention of atherosclerosis.

 IS THERE MORE TO CHOCOLATE THAN GOOD TASTE?

Chocolate is now estimated to be the most significant source of dietary antioxidants in the Western world. A 100-g bar of milk chocolate contains 170 mg of flavonoid antioxidants, procyanidins, and flavonols. Cocoa is especially rich in flavonoids, and dark chocolate has the highest flavonoid content of all—comparable to green tea and red wine. Consumption of chocolate has been often hypothesized to reduce the risk of cardiovascular disease (CVD) because of chocolate's high levels of stearic acid and antioxidant flavonoids. However, debate still lingers regarding the true long-term beneficial cardiovascular effects of chocolate overall. A review from 1966 through 2005 for experimental, observational, and clinical studies of relations between cocoa, cacao, chocolate, stearic acid, flavonoids (including flavonols, catechins, epicatechins, and procyanidins), and the risk of CVD (coronary heart disease [CHD], stroke) yielded a total of 136 well-designed studies. The body of short-term randomized feeding trials suggests cocoa and chocolate may exert beneficial effects on cardiovascular risk via effects on lowering blood pressure, antiinflammation, antiplatelet function, higher levels of high-density lipoproteins (HDLs), and decreased levels of low-density lipoproteins (LDLs).

It appears that one of the great culinary pleasures in life may actually also be part of a heart-healthy diet: in moderation, of course![60]

Calcium

Researchers and clinicians that hypothesized that calcium supplementation may contribute to adverse cardiovascular outcomes. However, recent medical evidence suggests that calcium supplementation does not contribute to an increase in cardiovascular risk factors. A retrospective analysis of data from 2710 men and 1143 women ages 30 and older suggests that dietary calcium intake is not significantly associated with coronary artery calcium scores in either group. Further, there was no association observed with calcium intake and fasting glucose, insulin, or platelet aggregation.[61] Furthermore, a randomized controlled trial of 1471 postmenopausal women tested the effect of calcium supplementation and cardiovascular events. The women were randomized to receive 1 g of calcium citrate or placebo daily for 5 years. Women taking calcium had a twofold increase in MIs compared with women in the control group. However, when the researchers incorporated national health data for unreported cardiovascular events, the increase was no longer statistically significant.[62]

Coenzyme Q10

Coenzyme Q10 (CoQ10), a lipid-soluble antioxidant, may decrease oxidation of LDL cholesterol; it also plays an active role in the manufacturing of ATP, vital for energy in the myocardium. Human clinical trials show patients who received CoQ10 had better exercise tolerance and less angina. Cardiac function after coronary bypass graft surgery was better in those patients who received pretreatment with CoQ10 1 week before surgery.

Folic Acid and Vitamins B$_{12}$ and B$_6$

Necessary for the metabolism of homocysteine, folic acid and vitamins B$_{12}$ and B$_6$ may be crucial to minimize homocysteine-associated endothelial dysfunction.

Omega-3 Fatty Acids

Studies have indicated that omega-3 fatty acids may play a direct role in the reduction of atherosclerosis, with positive effects on endothelial function and vascular tone, even at physiologic doses. They are shown to inhibit platelet aggregation, lower levels of fibrinogen, and promote healthier endothelial function. The 5-year Japan Eicosapentaenoic Acid (EPA) Lipid Intervention Study tested EPA supplementation and its effect on cardiac events. Both men and women, exhibiting a serum total cholesterol level of ≥250 mg/dL, participated (mean age 61). The participants received either pravastatin 10 mg, simvastatin 5 mg, or those same statin doses with 1800 mg of EPA daily. After 5 years' duration, the EPA group exhibited a 19% reduction in cardiac events.[63] EPA and DHA are key Omega-3 fatty acids. The American Heart Association recommends at least two servings of fish weekly, particularly salmon. Mercury-free fish oil capsules are available for those concerned about mercury contamination in fish, a very legitimate concern; these are a safer option for pregnant women and children, who are advised not to consume fish regularly because of the high risk of receiving toxic levels of mercury through dietary intake.

Vitamin D

Data from the Framingham Offspring Cohort (1739 offspring of the original Framingham Heart Study) suggest an inverse relationship between 25-hydroxyvitamin D levels and cardiovascular risk.[64]

Grape Skin Products and Red Wine

Resveratrol, a grape skin extract found in grape products along with flavonoids and proanthocyanidins, has been found to contain antioxidant and antiinflammatory activity. It also has demonstrated the ability to inhibit platelet aggregation and promote vasodilatation.[59]

ADDITIONAL THERAPIES

Smoking Cessation

Perhaps the most significant contribution an individual can make to prevent CHD is the cessation of smoking (see risk factors for CHD).

Exercise

Individuals at risk for CHD need to establish an exercise program that is individually appropriate and feasible. Yoga, tai chi, aerobic walking, dancing, swimming, and many other types of exercise all provide physical activity necessary for cardiovascular fitness.

Mind–Body

Meditation and deep relaxation techniques assist in management of daily life stresses, which contribute to the development of CHD. Stress and depression are associated with an increased risk of heart disease.

Sleep

Longitudinal data from the Nurses' Health Study (comprising 84,003 female registered nurses) suggests that women who sleep less than 5 hours per night have a higher risk of hypertension compared with women who sleep 7 hours a night or longer. This was observed in women under age 50, and not in women between the ages of 50 to 59.[65]

CASE HISTORY

Carol is a 51-year-old mother of two children who experienced her last menstrual period 14 months ago. She experiences rare, mild hot flashes and no night sweats, but continues to be mostly troubled by palpitations associated with a feeling of anxiety. She has difficulty falling asleep most nights, stating that she lies in bed and cannot shut her mind off. She sleeps for 5 to 6 hours each night. Carol has been thinking about hormone replacement therapy (HRT), but is afraid because of her mother's history of embolic disease and hyperlipidemia. Carol's history is unremarkable for major acute disease, but positive for episodic migraine with visual field loss (occurred only premenstrually) and mild Raynaud's disease. Both of her parents have mild hypertension. Her mother also has elevated cholesterol and angina; osteoporosis with severe osteoarthritis; and a history of a thrombophilia, requiring lifetime anticoagulation.

Carol works full time as a nurse in a busy hospital clinic, and states she enjoys her job but is just too busy at times. She has one child in college and one in high school, both demanding considerable attention periodically. She also spends a great deal of her time caring for her mother, who has difficulty with ambulation because of severe degenerative joint disease from osteoarthritis. She is married, and relates a good supportive relationship with her husband. She does not smoke, and drinks about two to three glasses of white wine a week. She describes herself as "active, happy, but too busy and stressed. I worry a lot." She has no history of endocrine dysfunction; however, she has steadily been gaining weight (10 to 12 lb) since menopause, and is worried about a possible thyroid abnormality, even though all laboratory tests are normal.

Carol complains of episodic palpitations associated with a feeling of chest tightness. These occur about three to ten times a day, both day and night. A feeling of anxiety may accompany them. She denies shortness of breath, nausea, or diaphoresis. She also complains of chronic shoulder and neck tension, and occasional tension headache, which she treats with nonsteroidal antiinflammatory drugs (NSAIDs).

Medications/Supplements
Carol occasionally uses NSAIDs for headache and prophylactically for migraine (she is unable to use triptans because of the Raynaud's). She occasionally takes a multivitamin and uses echinacea at the onset of colds.

Diet
Carol eats mostly fast foods. She eats on the run. She often eats fried chicken sandwiches, French fries, and colas; she rarely has a salad. She does not have time to cook much during the week.

CASE HISTORY—cont'd

Assessment
1. Postmenopausal woman with:
   a. Palpitations
   b. Stress
   c. Insomnia
   d. Weight gain
2. History of migraines with focal neurologic symptoms
3. History of Raynaud's disorder
4. Family history of osteoporosis, thrombophilia, hyperlipidemia, and hypertension

Plan
1. Botanical Tincture Formula 1: Daytime

Hawthorn	*(Crataegus oxyacantha)*	40 mL
Motherwort	*(Leonurus cardiaca)*	20 mL
Skullcap	*(Scutellaria lateriflora)*	20 mL
Eleutherococcus		20 mL
	Total: 100 mL	

Dose: 5 mL, TID.
The formula is intended to provide gentle cardiac and nervous system support and help with stress relief.

2. Botanical Tincture Formula 2: Evening

Valerian	*(Valeriana officinalis)*	40 mL
Passionflower	*(Passiflora incarnata)*	40 mL
Kava kava	*(Piper methysticum)*	20 mL
	Total: 100 mL	

Dose: 5 mL, 30 to 60 minutes before bedtime.
This formula is designed to help reduce anxiety and tension, both emotional and musculoskeletal, and promote sleep.

3. *Supplements:* Daily multivitamin with adequate B vitamins and folic acid; fish oil capsules (omega-3 fatty acids); and concentrated blueberry extract daily (antioxidant).
4. *Diet modification:* Increase green, leafy vegetables, soy foods, and garlic in diet. Meats should be lean and broiled (not fried). Reduce overall carbohydrate load and add more vegetables in general. Substitute red wine for white, as long as no migraine results. Snacks should be fresh fruit and nuts.
5. *Exercise:* Start with walking for 30 minutes three times per week. Work toward a 15-minute-mile (i.e., aerobic) walk. Add simple upper body weight exercise with professional direction (i.e., gym or personal trainer). Consider yoga three times per week.
6. *Mind–body:* Advised meditation or relaxation exercises on a daily basis. Take warm baths with lavender essential oil (5 to 7 drops per bath) at bedtime, and write in a journal for stress relief each night around 30 minutes before bed.

Follow-up
Phone call in 1 week; return visit in 1 month. Carol experienced restful sleep within 2 days of beginning the botanical formulae. Within 2 weeks of regular use, she experienced significantly fewer palpitations, and less anxiety associated with her daily life and work. She walks only about two to three times a week because of the weather (it is winter), but is joining a gym for consistent exercise opportunities (mostly because of concern over her weight) and expert direction. She still struggles with her diet because of the time factor but is making adjustments gradually. After taking a class on relaxation techniques, she manages to incorporate this into her morning and evening schedule on a daily basis. She loves the baths, and journal writing has helped her to gain perspective on her life, use her creative writing skills, and prepare for sleep.

9

Menstrual Wellness and Menstrual Problems

The scientific study of menstruation has been hampered by the overpowering influence of traditions and social and cultural beliefs. We have all, men and women, been conditioned to view menstruation in a negative way. Perhaps, it is time to look at menstruation from another point of view. How many fine novels have been finished in a burst of creativity in the premenstrual period? How many great ideas have been born premenstrually?

Clinical Gynecologic Endocrinology and Infertility[1]

MENSTRUAL HEALTH AND THE NORMAL MENSTRUAL CYCLE

This section reviews the historical and cultural beliefs and attitudes surrounding menstruation; "the normal menstrual cycle"; and provides an overview of the menstrual irregularities and conditions presented later in this chapter. This section also looks at practical ways to promote menstrual health.

A BRIEF HISTORY OF MENSTRUATION IN CULTURE AND MEDICINE

Menstruation has historically been cloaked by religious, social, and cultural myths and meaning. Menstrual blood and menstruating women have been surrounded by fear, taboo,* restrictions, and worship since ancient times. Cultural views on menstruation are diverse. The Beng people of the Ivory Coast believed that "Menstrual blood is special because it carries in it a living being. It works like a tree. Before bearing fruit a tree must first bear flowers. Menstrual blood is like the flower."[2] In stark contrast it has been referred to as "the curse" by Judeo-Christians and is considered a sign of uncleanliness, or even evil, in some cultures.[3] Menstrual blood was used as a panacea, a medicinal ingredient, an ingredient in casting spells, and even as a pesticide capable of making caterpillars drop from plants and insects die in the fields.[4] Menstruating

women were variably considered to be possessed by evil spirits or magic.[5-7]

Medical attitudes regarding menstruation have fluctuated over the centuries, from menstruation and menstrual blood being perceived as a natural process—a woman's "flowers," as menstruation was described not only by the Beng but in the *Treatise on the Diseases of Women, and Conditions of Women,* part of the medieval compendium known as the *Trotula,* which remained the definitive text on women's medicine for several centuries—to something capable of poisoning men and deforming children, as described by Pliny and others.[2,7] Hildegard of Bingen, the famed German nun and healer (1098-1179) used the term *flowers;* however, she also attributes menstruation to "Eve's sin in Paradise," reflecting both positive and negative attitudes toward menstruation. Hippocratic and Galenic medicine viewed menstruation as the basis of women's unique physiology. It was considered a necessary and healthy purgation upon which the health of the entire female body was dependent. Menstruation was seen as women's inherent constitutional "coldness": the inability to "cook" nutrients thoroughly led to an accumulation of waste in the body that could only be gotten rid of through menstruation. Lack of menses (e.g., amenorrhea) was believed to lead to a pathologic systemic state. Normal menstruation, that is, the proper amount at the proper time, was considered to reflect a state of health.[2]

In contrast, however, around the first century BCE, Pliny, a physician and prolific medical writer, wrote that menstrual blood could drive men and dogs mad, make vines wither, sour wine, and discolor mirrors, among other powers.[5,7,8] Pliny's views, as well as others' of his time, represented menstruation as poisonous or noxious, views that would contribute to misogynist medical views of women that have persisted.[1,2,4]

---

* Interestingly, the word *taboo* is derived from a Polynesian word meaning both "sacred" and "menstruating."

The editor wishes to thank *Botanical Medicine for Women's Health,* ed 1 contributors to this chapter: Bevin Clare, Angela J. Hywood, Laurel Lee, Linda Ryan, Jillian Stansbury, and Ruth Trickey.

Democritus wrote that "usually the growth of greenstuff is checked by contact with a woman; indeed, if she is also in the period of menstruation, she will kill the young produce merely by looking at it."[6]

Negative attitudes about menstruation have not only influenced the practice of women's medicine, but also the medical education of women. Western medicine historically viewed menstruation as a disease and an opportunity to treat women as fragile and weak.[7] Well into the nineteenth century in the United States, the fact that women menstruated was considered proof of the inferiority of the female intellect. Menstruation was used as a justification for keeping women out of medical schools, based on the grounds that menstruating women needed increased rest—mentally and bodily.[5]

Women's health reform and self-help movements throughout the twentieth century have played a major role in transforming and reshaping women's, society's, and medicine's attitudes toward menstruation. It has become a more acceptable topic for conversation, evidenced in many ways, not in the least by the mention of menstruation on television sitcoms, the openness of menstrual products advertisements on television and in print media, and articles in popular magazines. This is a positive trend allowing women to more openly seek information and medical care about menstruation and menstrual concerns. However, advertising also directly contributes to the perpetuation of cultural menstrual taboos—that menstruation is "dirty," and suggestions that it should remain hidden. Educational films and advertisements from menstrual product manufacturers stress products' abilities to keep safe the secret that the girl is menstruating and to help her feel fresh and clean, perpetuating the message that menstruation is shameful and dirty.[9]

Women's own personal and cultural views on menstruation also vary substantially. Menstruation may be considered a happy event, or a sign of uncleanliness—both attitudes persisting even in a single culture.[10] A correlation has been asserted in feminist literature that a woman's attitudes toward menstruation and can influence her physical experience of menstrual symptoms.[7] In one study analyzing menstrual attitudes, women were asked to describe their menstrual periods. Terms were rated as positive (such as "red friend," "my buddy"), negative (such as "the curse," "pain in the ass"), or neutral (such as "period," "surfin' the crimson wave"). In the groups combined, most terms were either neutral (46%) or negative (37%). There was a tendency for women in the negative group to employ negative terms (52% of negative group women used solely negative terms versus 18% in the positive group), whereas 55% of women in the positive group employed neutral, not negative terms.[9] Women in the negative group used negative terms significantly more than did women in the positive group. Many women consider menstruation somewhat of an inconvenience, but nonetheless, a natural event. Increasingly, American women are reframing menstruation as a celebration of women's femininity and women's connection to the rhythms of the earth and the moon.

WHAT IS NORMAL MENSTRUATION?

Menstruation is a cyclic process occurring in most women between 12 and 50 years of age. It generally occurs without difficulty, although there may be some normal sense of inconvenience accompanying the period. The variation in the interval between menstrual periods, the duration of each menstrual period, the amount of blood loss, the associated discomforts or lack thereof, and the subjective psychoemotional experience of menstruation among women is so great as to make it difficult to define "normal menstruation." There is a range of normal variation.

It is necessary to determine whether a pattern, symptom, or concern is normal for the individual woman in the context of her own gynecologic and menstrual history, as well as against objective measures. Certain characteristics of menstruation can be a reflection of an underlying pathologic process or may predispose a woman to the development of chronic disease.[11] For example, metrorrhagia predisposes to anemia, and the irregular menstrual cycles associated with polycystic ovary syndrome (PCOS) (see Polycystic Ovary Syndrome) can predispose a woman to diabetes and consequently, heart disease. Women with long or highly irregular menstrual cycles have a significantly increased risk for developing type 2 diabetes mellitus that is not completely explained by obesity.[12] Persistent deviations from the woman's own norms, as well as major deviations from accepted standards, require further evaluation.

ONSET, FREQUENCY, AND DURATION OF MENSTRUATION

The onset of the first menses (i.e., menarche) typically occurs between the ages of 10 and 16 years old (see Puberty, Menarche, and Adolescence). The menstrual cycle is generally irregular and anovulatory for the first several years after menarche, reaching a regular length and duration by 5 to 7 years after menarche. Variations outside of this range are generally normal, but could be signs of precocious puberty or amenorrhea, or sometimes symptoms of underlying medical disorders (see Puberty, Menarche, and Adolescence, as well as Amenorrhea).

A woman will experience from 300 to 400 menstrual cycles in her lifetime. Cycle length is controlled by the rate and quality of follicular growth and development, which varies in individual women.[1] Based on several observational longitudinal studies of thousands of women around the world, it was determined that at age 25, 40% of women had 25- and 28-day cycles, and from ages 25 to 35 60% had 25- to 28-day cycles. The average cycle length is 26 to 34 days.[13] Only 0.5% of women experience cycles shorter than 21 days and only 0.9% experience cycles longer than 35 days. At least 20% of women experience irregular cycles.[1] The length of the follicular phase is the primary determining factor in cycle length.

Menstrual bleeding lasts 3 to 6 days in most women, although there is variation in cycle length from 2 to 12 days after the start of ovulatory cycles. Longer periods (>8 days) are associated with anovulation.[13] The heaviest flow is consistently on day 2 of the cycle. Normal blood loss is considered 30 to 80 mL. Small clots are considered normal; large clots may suggest the need for further evaluation.[7]

The duration and amount of bleeding declines slightly (by about a half a day per cycle) in women older than age 35. However, women approaching menopause often experience significantly heavier bleeding than younger women.[13]

Although some women describe their periods coming "like clockwork," most describe some amount of irregularity over the course of menstrual life cycle, even if it is only occasionally. The endocrine system is easily affected by numerous factors: stress, changes in amount of daily and nightly light exposure, sleep patterns, diet, travel, amount of exercise, illness, and so forth. It is normal for women to occasionally experience an irregular period, a lighter or heavier period, a "crampy" period, or even to miss a period in the absence of pregnancy or lactation. It is when irregularity recurs repeatedly, presents with an acute problem (e.g., sudden, heavy, or unremitting vaginal bleeding), or occurs in the absence of other explainable factors that one might suspect a disorder.

Women in their late thirties and forties often begin to experience some degree of irregularity of menstrual frequency, duration, and amount of blood loss because of a decline in ovarian function as they approach menopause. In their late thirties, women experience a shortening of their cycle because of increased production of follicle-stimulating hormone (FSH), a result of follicle numbers beginning to decline. However, between 2 and 8 years before menopause, the cycles again lengthen.[1] Approximately 50% of women experience a cycle of 120 days or longer in the year before menopause, and 20% experience a cycle of this length or longer within 2 to 4 years of their final period.[13] The average age of menopause in the United States is 51 years old.[14]

FREQUENCY AND TYPES OF MENSTRUAL DISORDERS

Menstrual dysfunction is defined in several ways: bleeding patterns, for example amenorrhea (i.e., lack of menstruations), menorrhagia (i.e., excessive bleeding during menstruation), or polymenorrhea (i.e., frequent menstruation); ovarian dysfunction, for example anovulation and luteal deficiency; pain (i.e., dysmenorrhea); and premenstrual syndrome (PMS) (Box 9-1). Irregular menstruation is estimated to affect from 2% to 5% of the general population, and up to 66% among athletes.[15] In the United States, approximately 2.9 million office visits are made annually by women ages 18 to 54 for menstrual problems.[7,16] Two thirds of these women contact a doctor regarding menstrual problems each year, and 31% report spending a mean of 9.6 days in bed annually. Among young women, dysmenorrhea is the most common cause of time lost from work or school. The costs of menstrual disorders to US industry have been estimated to be 8% of the total wage bill, and the effect is particularly acute in industries that employ women predominantly.[16] Interestingly, it is estimated that primitive hunter-gatherer women, over the course of an average lifetime, experienced only one-third as many menstrual periods

---

BOX 9-1 Terms and Definitions for Common Menstrual Disorders[7]

Amenorrhea: Absence of menses

Anovulation: Absence of ovulation

Dysfunctional uterine bleeding: Prolonged, excessive, irregular uterine bleeding in the absence of an organic disorder

Dysmenorrhea: Painful menstruation

Hypomenorrhea: Scant but regular menstruation

Intermenstrual bleeding: Bleeding at any time between normal menses

Menometrorrhagia: Irregular heavy bleeding

Menorrhagia: Prolonged, excessive, regular menstrual bleeding

Oligomenorrhea: Infrequent menstrual cycles, ≥35 days

Polycystic ovary syndrome: A syndrome resulting from androgen excess and anovulation; may lead to irregular menses

Polymenorrhea: Frequent menses, ≤21 days

Premenstrual syndrome: Cyclic recurrence of psychoemotional and physical disorders during the luteal phase of the menstrual cycle

---

as do modern women because of later age at menarche, earlier and more frequent pregnancies, and breastfeeding, suggesting that modern women experience a significantly greater lifetime exposure to estrogen, which may be partially responsible for increased health risks. Traditionally, factors such as later menarche, earlier first pregnancy, breastfeeding, and earlier menopause may have played a protective effect against, for example, breast and gynecologic cancers.[16] Menstrual disorders also predispose women to other risks, for example, anemia, osteoporosis, cancer risks, diabetes, and cardiovascular disease.

In spite of the significance of menstruation in women's lives and the high incidence of menstrually related health problems in society, there is surprisingly little epidemiologic evidence on menstrual disorders and associated risk factors, and no prioritization of research in this area.[11,16]

Subsequent sections of this chapter address these dysfunctions either individually or as part of a larger syndrome in which they occur.

FACTORS AFFECTING THE MENSTRUAL CYCLE

Numerous factors influence the menstrual cycle, including a woman's nutritional status, stress levels, body weight, exercise patterns, attitudes and beliefs about menstruation, and environmental and workplace exposures. Investigation into these can sometimes explain dysfunction; corrections can often restore physiologic and emotional balance. A holistic approach to preventing and treating menstrual dysfunction should always include consideration of possible social and lifestyle issues.

Diet/Nutrition

Menstruation is influenced by the amount of energy provided by the diet as well as by the types of foods consumed.

Lean women with a low body mass index (BMI), as well as obese women, have an increased likelihood of menstrual disorders. Women with highly restrictive dietary practices are more likely to experience menstrual dysregulation, particularly amenorrhea, anovulation, and a shorter luteal phase.[17-19] Recent studies suggest that reduced energy availability (i.e., increased energy expenditure with inadequate caloric intake) is the main cause of the central suppression of the hypothalamic-pituitary-gonadal (HPG) axis. As a consequence, not only will there be menstrual dysregulation but a higher potential for bone demineralization and increased risk of skeletal fragility, fractures, vertebral instability, curvature, and osteoporosis.[19,20] Thus the importance of treating underlying dietary imbalances that can cause menstrual dysregulation becomes more significant.

Dietary fat restriction is associated with amenorrhea even in normal weight, nonathletic women.[11] A raw foods diet is commonly associated with low BMI, weight loss, and amenorrhea. In one study of 279 women on a raw foods diet, 30% of women younger than age 45 experienced amenorrhea.[21] There is a common belief among adolescent girls and women that a vegetarian diet leads to weight loss; thus many adopt a vegetarian diet as part of an attempt to diet. It has been suggested that a vegetarian diet is associated with menstrual disorders, especially amenorrhea; however, it appears that healthy, weight-stable, vegetarian women consuming self-selected diets do not experience more menstrual disturbances than healthy, weight-stable nonvegetarians.[11,22] There does not appear to be a correlation between a higher intake of soy foods in the vegetarian diet and menstrual dysregulation, as has been commonly assumed.[22]

The consumption of fruits, fish, and vegetables plays a protective effect against dysmenorrhea in adolescent girls and women. The protective role of the fish seems to be because of omega-3 fatty acids. During menstruation, this fatty acid competes with the omega-6 fatty acids for the production of prostaglandins and leukotrienes. The prostaglandins generated from the omega-3 fatty acids lead to a reduction in myometrial contraction and vasoconstriction.[23]

Weight

Overall weight and changes in weight affect menstrual regularity. Ovarian suppression can occur as a result of sudden or moderate weight loss, leading to amenorrhea. This is most pronounced in cases of eating disorders and famine. This phenomenon is also seen in women who are 20% to 30% below their ideal body weight, which is common in athletes or women on restricted caloric intake diets.[11] Obesity, particularly truncal obesity, is also associated with menstrual disorders, notably amenorrhea associated with PCOS, and an increase in incidence of diabetes and long-term health consequences. It appears that at both ends of the extreme spectra of weight, women are likely to have the longest menstrual cycles and anovulation.[11,24]

Caloric restriction itself, even before there is a loss of weight, can result in menstrual dysregulation. It was demonstrated in one study that girls who skip breakfast experience a higher degree of dysmenorrhea than girls who eat an adequate daily breakfast.[25] The effects of body weight on menstrual function may be a result of nutritional status, caloric intake, stress, psychiatric disorders associated with weight problems, or the mechanics of body fat on steroid hormone synthesis and estrogen metabolism.[11] Significantly, excessive exercise with menstrual irregularity can be an important sign of an eating disorder, psychological restraint issues around food consumption, higher perceived stress, and low self-esteem.[17,26]

Exercise

Moderate exercise from a young age is essential for optimal lifelong health, including prevention of cardiovascular disease, osteoporosis, and depression. However, excessive exercise or exercise at elite levels for competitive athletes can predispose women to nutritional deficiency, inadequate energy intake, and low body weight, all of which increase risk of menstrual dysfunction. Women athletes have a higher overall incidence of menstrual disorders. Ballet dancers and runners have an increased rate of amenorrhea, anovulation, and luteal phase defects compared with nonathletes.[11] In one study examining the role of nutritional status, eating behaviors, and menstrual function in 23 nationally ranked female adolescent volleyball players, these women were found to be low in folate, iron, calcium, magnesium, zinc, B complex, vitamin C, and carbohydrate intake, compared with recommended daily allowances (RDA). Approximately 50% of the athletes reported actively "dieting." Past or present amenorrhea was reported by 17% of the athletes; 13% and 48% reported past or present oligomenorrhea and "irregular" menstrual cycles, respectively.[27] Among women age 29 to 31, daily vigorous sports activity was associated with increased cycle variability and cycle length. Even recreational exercise is associated with an increase in mean cycle length.[11]

Exercise is an independent factor separate from weight loss in relationship to cycle variation and presence of amenorrhea. Cessation of training even in the absence of weight gain can restore cycle normalcy. The most likely mechanism of cycle irregularity caused by moderate exercise is decreased gonadotrophin-releasing hormone (GnRH), gonadotropin, and serum estrogen levels, along with a possible physiologic stress response mechanism. However, because of the increased likelihood of aberrant eating patterns in amenorrheic athletes, inadequate caloric intake and a negative energy balance also may be causative.[11] With a societal emphasis on a lean body, many young women use exercise as a means of weight control, frequently combined with rigorous dieting patterns; thus exercise patterns should be evaluated in the context of ruling out eating disorders, and proper amounts of exercise encouraged to ensure its benefits.

Stress

Most women have experienced, at least once in their lives, the effects of stress on menstrual regularity: skipping a period or having a period come late or early during a particularly difficult time. There is some evidence regarding connections between socioemotional processes and menstrual functioning. Psychological stress is generally acknowledged in the medical literature to affect menstruation; however, studies on stress and menstrual function are limited, consisting mainly of studies of major life changes and catastrophic events such as war or imprisonment. Studies on the effects of girls leaving home to attend school, the military, or work suggest that separation from home and family increases the likelihood of amenorrhea, but these studies have lacked adequate comparison groups.[11] High levels of workplace demand, combined with low levels of perceived control, have been associated with a doubled risk for short menstrual cycle length (i.e., less than 24 days) Characteristics consistent with submission (i.e., introversion, anxiety, low perceived control, inhibition of aggression) have been shown to be elevated among women seeking treatment for hirsutism and irregular menses compared with women without such conditions. However, this association could reflect the socioemotional consequences of these medical problems and their associated features.[28]

It is no surprise that delicate hypothalamic-pituitary-adrenal (HPA) axis and endocrine functions might be disrupted by personal upheaval and stress. The mechanisms of stress- and anxiety-related menstrual changes have not been fully elaborated. However, it is suspected that both central psychogenic disturbances cause changes in the hypothalamus that consequently affect prolactin (PRL) and endogenous opiate levels; that leads to a systemic physiologic response, causing elevated basal cortisol levels and alterations in hypothalamic response, as well as changes in luteinizing hormone (LH) (i.e., a reduced pulsatile frequency).[11,29]

Attitudes and Beliefs About Menstruation

In a survey-based study of college-aged women (n = 327) those who had extremely negative or extremely positive early menstrual experiences were strongly associated with correspondingly negative or positive current menstrual attitudes. There were additional associations between early menstrual experiences and measures of body image and health behaviors. Positive group participants reported a more positive body image and better general health behaviors. Results suggest that early menstrual experiences may be related to menstrual experiences later in life.[9] Unfortunately, adolescent girls often receive inadequate information or negative messages regarding menstruation from an early age. Although they may receive information on the biological aspects of menstruation from parents, teachers, and other sources, they are often not prepared for the practical aspects of getting their periods, for example, what it feels like or how to take care of themselves while menstruating. Instead, girls are directly and indirectly instructed about largely negative cultural beliefs concerning menstruation and the ways in which they will be expected to behave to uphold these beliefs. Somatization of these beliefs may translate into increased difficulty in the menstrual experience, particularly in the form of dysmenorrhea or PMS. Women with negative menstrual beliefs are more likely to seek menstrual suppression through pharmacologic means.[9]

Environmental/Work Exposures

Women whose work requires large amounts of physical labor may experience weight loss and subsequent menstrual irregularity. Workplace stress and noise also may contribute to menstrual dysregulation. Occupational chemical exposure has clearly been demonstrated to act on the ovaries; cytotoxic agents, for example, can induce ovarian failure, including follicular loss, anovulation, oligomenorrhea, and amenorrhea.[11] Many environment pollutants to which women are nearly ubiquitously exposed are now also recognized to be endocrine disruptors.

Pheromones and Menstrual Synchrony

Studies on menstrual synchrony—when women who spend time in close proximity begin cycling together—have yielded conflicting results. Nonetheless, the phenomenon is well known among women who report menstruating at the same time, or close to, that of roommates, daughters, sisters, or close friends; hence it is casually referred to as "the dormitory effect." Animal and human studies have shown that social interactions can modify endocrine function. It is suspected that pheromones may reduce menstrual cycle variability among women and synchronize menstruation. Pheromones are airborne chemicals released by one individual that can affect another. Odorless compounds obtained from the axillae of women altered cycles of other women exposed to these compounds.[1] However, a wider range of environmental signals may influence menstrual synchrony.[11] One study on women's qualitative experience of menstrual synchrony suggests that the concept of menstrual synchrony frames menstruation as a natural, healthy phenomenon for women.[30]

Ethnicity

Ethnicity is a determinant of menstrual patterns. African American girls, for example, are significantly more likely than Anglo-American girls to experience heavy bleeding. It may be that stress accompanying socioeconomic differences plays a role in this difference.[31]

PROMOTING HEALTHY MENSTRUATION

The health care profession has an obligation to promote menstrual education. We must have an understanding of reproductive physiology in order to impart it to our patients, and we must be sensitive to the need to present a positive attitude regarding sexual and reproductive functions.

Clinical Gynecologic Endocrinology and Infertility[1]

Menstruation, in the absence of underlying pathology, need not be fraught with discomfort. Menstruation is something that girls should be taught about from the time they are young, including an understanding of what is happening to their bodies, how to eat, exercise, rest, and care for themselves to avoid what are often preventable menstrual complaints, and to embrace this aspect of their feminine experiences. Unfortunately, many girls and women, remain unaware of the effect that basic lifestyle factors can have on the menstrual cycle and suffer unnecessarily from what can be debilitating physical, emotional, and psychological symptoms. Although some menstrual disorders have complex pathophysiologic etiologies that do not simply respond to lifestyle modification, practitioners treating clients with common menstrual complaints should always take a multifactorial approach that includes education about possible lifestyle contributors. The discussion here focuses on basic lifestyle strategies that specifically relate to menstrual health, or eumenorrhea—a healthy menstrual cycle.

Diet, Nutrition, and Body Weight

The effect of insufficient dietary energy intake, inadequate nutrition, being underweight, being overweight, and dieting on menstruation was discussed in the preceding section. Not only are diet and nutrition determinant of menstrual cycle function and regularity but also menstrual dysregulation can be predictive of bone mineral density (BMD) and osteoporosis risk, diabetes, and cardiovascular disease. What type of diet then *promotes* healthy menstruation and reduces the risk of later disease development? A whole-foods–based, primarily organic diet with an emphasis on vegetarian protein sources (although not exclusively vegetarian), good-quality cold-water fish, whole grains, fresh fruits, nuts, vegetables, and good-quality oil is probably the optimal human diet. Particularly important in maintaining menstrual health seems to be maintenance of stable blood sugar and stable weight at an ideal individual level, and adequate intake of healthy fats. For women, diet and body weight are intimately tied to self-esteem and personal identity. The landscape upon which this plays out can be reproductive function. Therefore nutritional and personal counseling may play a part in the treatment of menstrual problems when nutrition, eating habits, or body image are issues.

Avoiding or at least reducing the amount consumed of certain foods also may improve menstrual symptoms. For example, one report found that women with PMS consumed 275% more refined sugar, 79% more dairy products, 78% more sodium, and 62% more carbohydrates than women without PMS. They also consumed 77% less manganese and 53% less iron than symptom-free women. Another study found that consumption of caffeine-containing beverages increased the incidence and severity of PMS in college-age women.[32]

Conversely, the inclusion of certain foods and nutrients may prevent or reduce symptoms. In many cultures it is believed that cold foods should be avoided and only warm foods consumed during the menstrual cycle to prevent dysmenorrhea. Calcium, vitamin B_6, magnesium, vitamin E, vitamin A, and essential fatty acid supplementation may be helpful for menstrual dysregulation. These are discussed under specific conditions in subsequent sections of this chapter. Not only is proper nutrient intake essential, but proper digestion and assimilation is necessary for nutrient absorption and use.

Many women experience premenstrual cravings, particularly for sweets. Ensuring adequate nutrition often reduces cravings; however, it is perfectly fine to indulge cravings if nutritional needs have been met and the woman is at a healthy weight. As with all things, moderation is the key. Chocolate is a popular premenstrual craving. Although the relationship between chocolate and menstrually related skin problems remains controversial, many girls and women self-report that a reduction in chocolate consumption improves acne. Dark chocolate is rich in beneficial antioxidants, and many women find a small amount to be stimulating and stress relieving.

Encourage: Adequate nutritional and energy (i.e., caloric, fat) intake, consumption of fresh fruits and vegetables, leafy green vegetables, whole grains, vegetarian protein sources, cold-water fish, nuts, good-quality oil (especially olive and walnut oils), and essential fatty acids; maintenance of healthy weight and stable blood sugar; and positive body image and self-esteem.

Discourage: Excessive consumption of refined flour products, sugar, caffeinated products, red meat, and dairy products; excessive dieting, dramatic weight loss, being underweight, and obesity.

Exercise

Exercise, especially when regular and frequent, can reduce both physical and emotional menstrual discomforts, improving mood and relieving physical symptoms. The mechanisms for this are not fully understood but may include a reduction in estrogen levels and catecholamine levels, improved glucose tolerance, and increased endorphin levels.[32] Moderate exercise also reduces the risk of bone demineralization associated with menstrual dysregulation, especially anovulatory cycles and amenorrhea. Excessive exercise, which is discussed in the preceding, should be discouraged, or at least nutritional and energy requirements should be met and healthy body weight maintained.[15,18,20] Yoga and many forms of dance include movements and stretches that can be specific for relieving pelvic tension and discomfort associated with dysmenorrhea. Forms of movement that help women to positively experience their body can be helpful in overcoming negative personal attitudes.

Encourage: Moderate amounts of exercise; weight-bearing exercise for bone health; exercise that promotes relaxation and pelvic movement such as yoga and dance; exercise that improves self-perception and body image; and positive body image and self-esteem. Exercise must be accompanied by adequate caloric intake and maintenance of healthy body weight.

Discourage: Excessive exercise; exercise as part of an attempt at caloric restriction in nonoverweight women; and rapid weight loss.

Stress

As discussed, stress can contribute to physiologic changes that lead to menstrual dysregulation, and menstrual dysregulation itself can increase a woman's stress levels. Women can be encouraged to manage time to reduce work load or personal stress, and seek outlets for stress such as meditation, yoga, journaling, counseling, or other healthy means. Learning self-empowerment techniques can be very useful for women with stress-related menstrual dysregulation. Adequate nutritional and caloric intake (especially avoiding hypoglycemia) can reduce stress and improve stress resistance. Reduction in caffeine consumption can also reduce stress. Getting adequate rest is essential. Herbal adaptogens and nervines can be used to improve stress resistance and promote relaxation. Improving attitudes about menstruation can reduce the perception of menstrual problems.[1]

Encourage: Stress reduction activities, positive self-image and self-esteem; seeking creative outlets for stress; healthy diet with adequate nutrient intake; ample rest and relaxation; yoga; meditation; and exercise.

Discourage: Negative self-talk; overwork; poor self-image; and poor menstrual attitudes.

Attitudes and Beliefs About Menstruation

How we perceive our menstrual cycles can affect how we feel when we menstruate. Talking with patients about their menstrual beliefs and attitudes can help clarify whether underlying negative beliefs might be playing a role. Sometimes simply educating a woman about menstruation can help dispel ideas of it as a "bad" or "unclean" event and improve a woman's acceptance of this natural process. Women may find that setting aside designated time for themselves just before or during the first couple of days of their menses can improve their sense of well-being. This may include time for a bath and a cup of tea, journaling, a long walk or hike, curling up in bed with a good book, or any number of activities that an individual woman finds relaxing and replenishing to her spirit. Women often report that the time around their menses is one of heightened intuitive perceptions. Women can be encouraged to record their thoughts, dreams, feelings, and so forth in a journal designated for this purpose. Creating menstruation as a time of personal feminine power, and one that includes space for the woman to explore her creativity and experience replenishment and solitude, can help reframe it from a negative to a positive experience, and this in itself may go a long way to improving menstrual problems. There are numerous books in the self-help and women's book market with ideas for celebrating menstruation, including celebrations of a girl's menarche to help her begin her menstrual journey with a healthy attitude and necessary knowledge and self-care skills.

Environmental Exposures

Forty years ago, biologist Rachel Carson, whose own life was lost to cancer, began the task of alerting the public to the serious and long-term risks of environmental contamination to biological organisms. This concern has been reiterated by such scientists as Sandra Steingraber and Theo Colborn, who have written extensively on the subject of environmental pollution on human health. Numerous chemicals have the ability to mimic estrogen (and likely other chemical messengers) in our bodies. They are part of a larger class of chemicals called xenobiotics, many of which are endocrine disruptors. Because of the massive role of estrogen in women's reproductive physiology, women are highly susceptible to reproductive problems from endocrine disruptors. The DES (diethylstilbestrol) tragedy is a striking example of the effects of endocrine disruption, including reproductive cancers, reproductive failure, and congenital deformities in children exposed during pregnancy.

Nothing short of massive industrial regulation and change in consumption patterns of modern society can turn the tide on this environmental and chemical tsunami. Even if production of all endocrine disruptors were to cease today, these chemicals are pernicious and persistent. They last indefinitely in the environment, and tend to sequester themselves in the fat tissue of living organisms. Breast milk is one of the most likely repositories for these toxins.

Women can do a great deal to minimize their exposure to endocrine disruptors. They are widely present in inorganic food sources and soft plastics. Eating organically is advisable. Dairy foods, because of their high fat content, much like breast milk, are also likely to be more highly contaminated, so it is best to consume only organic dairy products. Practitioners must advise patients about environmental safety issues and ideally, work to advocate for improved workplace and environmental conditions to reduce overall exposure.

Some concern has been raised that standard commercial menstrual products are contaminated with dioxin and/or other organochloride compounds that can lead to reproductive disease, most notably, cancers; asbestos, which is alleged to be included in these products to increase the amount of bleeding, requiring women to use more of the products; and rayon fibers that may cause toxic shock syndrome (TSS). There are numerous Internet articles dedicated to spreading warnings about this topic. The Food and Drug Administration (FDA) has posted a response to this concern in a paper, *Tampons and Asbestos, Dioxin, & Toxic Shock Syndrome,* segments of which are quoted subsequently.

According to the FDA, no evidence of asbestos in tampons has been found nor have there been reports of increased bleeding from tampon use. The FDA states that before any tampon is marketed in the United States, the FDA reviews its design and materials. Asbestos is not an ingredient in any US brand of tampon, nor is it associated with the fibers used in making tampons. Moreover, tampon manufacturing sites are subject to inspection by the FDA to assure that good manufacturing practices are being followed. Therefore these inspections would likely identify any procedures that would expose tampon products to asbestos. If any tampon product were contaminated with asbestos, it would be as a result of tampering, which is a crime. Thus far, the FDA has received no reports of tampering. Anyone having knowledge of tampon tampering is urged to notify the FDA or a law enforcement officer.

On the topic of dioxin, the FDA states that:

State-of-the art testing of tampons and tampon materials that can detect even trace amounts of dioxin has shown that dioxin levels are at or below the detectable limit. FDA's risk assessment indicates that this exposure is many times less than normally present in the body from other environmental sources, so small that any risk of adverse health effects is considered negligible. A part per trillion is about the same as one teaspoon in a lake fifteen feet deep and a mile square. No risk to health would be expected from these trace amounts.[33]

This information is less than reassuring given the limited amount that is known about endocrine disruptors, the very minute and nearly undetectable quantities required for a substance to act as an endocrine disruptor, and the very significant hazards from and persistence of dioxins in biological systems. The only acceptable exposure should be no exposure.

Tampons currently sold in the United States are made of cotton, rayon, or blends of rayon and cotton. Rayon is made from cellulose fibers derived from wood pulp. In this process, the wood pulp is bleached. At one time, bleaching wood pulp was a potential source of trace amounts of dioxin in tampons, but that bleaching method is no longer used. Rayon raw material used in US tampons is now produced using elemental chlorine-free or totally chlorine-free bleaching processes. Some elemental chlorine-free bleaching processes can theoretically generate dioxins at extremely low levels, and dioxins are occasionally detected in trace amounts in mill effluents and pulp. In practice, however, this method is considered to be dioxin free. Totally chlorine-free bleaching refers to use of bleaching agents that contain no chlorine. These methods are also dioxin free. Totally chlorine-free methods include, for example, use of hydrogen peroxide as the bleaching agent.

The Environmental Protection Agency (EPA) has worked with wood pulp producers to promote use of dioxin-free methods because dioxin is an environmental pollutant. Because of decades of pollution, dioxin can be found in the air, water, and ground. Therefore, whereas the methods used for manufacturing tampons today are considered to be dioxin-free processes, traces of dioxin may still be present in the cotton or wood pulp raw materials used to make tampons. Thus there may be trace amounts of dioxin present from environmental sources in cotton, rayon, or rayon/cotton tampons.[33] Regarding rayon and TSS, the FDA states:

> *Although scientists have recognized an association between TSS and tampon use, the exact connection remains unclear. Research conducted by the CDC suggested that use of some high absorbency tampons increased the risk of TSS in menstruating women. A few specific tampon designs and high absorbency tampon materials were also found to have some association with increased risk of TSS. These products and materials are no longer used in tampons sold in the United States. Tampons made with rayon do not appear to have a higher risk of TSS than cotton tampons of similar absorbency.*[33]

Many women, reasonably concerned about the risk of exposure to toxins in menstrual hygiene products, choose instead to purchase only disposable menstrual pads and tampons made from organic cotton and other organic fibers that are non–chlorine bleach manufactured. These offer the convenience of disposability and are more environmentally friendly than many of the larger commercial brands. Still, a smaller group of women prefer to use only washable cotton pads, menstrual sponges, and menstrual cups. Although less convenient than disposables, and possibly offensive to some women because they require handling of the menstrual blood, these are environmentally friendly choices. Careful cleaning of these products after use is essential to avoid risks of infection. In one study of colonization of microorganisms during menstruation among women using various menstrual products, cultures from those from users of sea sponges were found to have significantly higher colonization rates with *Staphylococcus aureus, Escherichia coli,* and other *Enterobacteriaceae.* The association of sea sponges with a high rate of *S. aureus* colonization suggests that they are not an alternative to tampons for women seeking to decrease the risk of TSS.[34]

Menstruation and Lunar Cycles

Circatrigintan cycles refer to those cycles that occur in monthly rhythms. The most common of these are menstruation and the lunar cycle, which have historically been considered to correspond. The average menstrual cycle duration is 29.5 days; the lunar cycle is 28 days. Menstruation is referred to as "the moon" in any number of languages, from French to Mandingo.

There is anecdotal evidence that moonlight can help to synchronize the menstrual cycle. The author was able to identify only one clinical trial evaluating this phenomenon. A double-blind, prospective study during the fall of 1979 investigated the association between the menstrual cycles of 305 Brooklyn College undergraduates and their associates and the lunar cycles. All subjects were 19 to 35 years old and using neither oral contraceptives (OCs) nor an intrauterine device (IUD). Approximately one third of the subjects had lunar period cycles (i.e., a mean cycle length of 29.5 ± 1 day). Almost two thirds of the subjects started their October menstrual cycle in the light half of the lunar cycle, significantly more than would be expected by random distribution. The author of the clinical trial concluded that there is a lunar influence on ovulation.[35]

Natural treatment for infertility sometimes includes recommendations for having the woman adjust the lighting in her bedroom so that she is only exposed to the natural lighting from the moon, or that she mimic the cycle of the moon using lighting in her room to correspond with the moon's cycles as a way to synchronize ovulation and menstruation with the lunar cycles.

SUMMARY

Given the number of menstrual cycles a woman will experience in her lifetime, menstrual wellness and comfort are certainly desirable goals. Approaches to promoting menstrual wellness and reducing problems may include improving nutrition, ensuring enough exercise, and improving self-esteem and body image to reduce women's tendencies to overdiet and overexercise. Conversely, obesity needs to be addressed, as does its opposite, being underweight, as both are associated with increased menstrual problems. Stress reduction, menstrual health education, and improving both women's individual and society's attitudes toward menstruation also may influence the psychological, physiologic, and endocrine factors that lead to menstrual dysregulation.

Environmental hazards that predispose us not only to such problems as hormonal dysregulation and menstrual complaints but also to serious and life-threatening conditions and reproductive disasters need to be addressed. The ancients linked the earth to women, with Gaia representing both. The health of women may ultimately be linked to the health of our environment. Therefore those concerned about women's health must necessarily also turn their attention to the health of our planet.

PUBERTY, MENARCHE, AND ADOLESCENCE

Puberty and adolescence have long been considered synonymous. They are, however, properly considered distinct entities with puberty defined as the sequence of physical, endocrine, and reproductive system changes that lead to the physical maturation of a girl into womanhood, and adolescence encompassing the psychological maturation that leads to readiness to assume adult responsibility.[14] Menarche is the onset of the first menstrual period.

The HPG axis is established in utero and is functional at a mature level before birth. The HPG axis becomes nearly dormant during early childhood (typically at 1 to 2 years of age) to be reawakened at the onset of puberty by a nocturnal pulsatile signal of LH that soon establishes a pulsatile pattern during the day as well. By an uncertain mechanism that may be associated with nutritional status in the female signaled by blood chemical information about carbohydrate or protein metabolism, there is a resurgence of not only LH but also GnRH and FSH. GnRH causes morphologic changes in the ovarian follicles and a subsequent increase in estrogen production (i.e., steroidogenesis). A positive feedback system is created between estrogen and GnRH that persists until maturation is adequate to trigger ovulation; eventually, when sexual maturation is complete, the ovary assumes the role that the HPG axis has played in the regulation of hormonal secretion and feedback.

Puberty extends over a period of approximately 4.5 years and is classically divided into four stages associated with landmarks in sexual development: (1) growth spurt, (2) thelarche, (3) adrenarche, and (4) menarche. It is triggered largely by genetics but also appears to be influenced by geography, level of light exposure, nutritional status, general health, and psychological factors.[1] Body weight may be a significant factor in the onset of puberty, with girls who weigh more exhibiting earlier signs.

Beginning between the ages of 9 and 13 years (mean age 11.2 years), and as early as 8 years in girls of African descent (the earliest onset of pubertal changes), girls begin to experience a growth spurt that will typically persist for the duration of puberty and slightly beyond. Other than in infancy, this is the most significant episode of physical growth a female will experience in her lifetime, with girls growing approximately 6 to 12.5 cm (2.5 to 5 inches) in height and gaining 3.5 to 4.5 kg (8-10 pounds) during this time. In addition to increased height, bone density increases (in the presence of optimal nutrition, significant for the long-term prevention of osteoporosis), internal organ size increases, and most dramatically, there is an overall increased deposition of fat with the percent

of body fat increasing from 15.7% to 26.7%. Human growth hormone (HGH), released by the pituitary gland, is instrumental in this pubertal growth spurt; insulin-like growth factors (IGFs) play an important role in the deposition of fat, thus leading to an increasingly mature female shape (i.e., hip and breast development). By just over age 17, at least 50% of women have achieved full adult height, but the velocity of the growth spurt significantly decreases after the menarche. Full development is nearly always achieved by age 21.

About a year after the growth spurt begins, breast development, or thelarche, becomes evident. Female breast development is a result of increased fat deposition and branching of the ductile system stimulated by increased estrogen secretion. Breast development represents the onset of maturation of secondary sex characteristics. Breast growth in puberty begins with breast budding. During this time, a small amount of glandular tissue develops; there is breast enlargement, caused by increased deposition of fat in the breast tissue. Eventually there is elevation of the areola and the nipple. Finally, after approximately 3 to 3.5 years, breast maturation leads to an adult breast contour with protrusion of the nipple from the areola and a flat continuity between the areola and the breast tissue.

Adrenarche, the development of pubic hair, occurs before or concomitantly with thelarche, although in 20% of girls it precedes breast development. Initial hair growth is only slightly pigmented, sparse, and fine, appearing on the labia majora. With maturation, the volume of hair growth increases and spreads to cover the mons pubis. The hair becomes more darkly pigmented, coarser, and less straight. After approximately 2 years, at which time axillary hair growth begins, the genital pubic hair achieves its characteristic curly appearance and is distributed triangularly with a horizontal border at the level of the pubic bone. Androgens are primarily responsible for hair growth. During these stages, vaginal acidity is increasing and there is an increase in the number of normal vaginal flora.

Menarche, the onset of menstruation, is the final stage in the process of puberty and occurs at a mean age in the United States of 12.2 years for African Americans and 12.8 years for Anglo-Americans. Menarche typically occurs 1 to 3 years after the onset of breast development. Initial menstrual cycles are anovulatory, with anovulatory periods lasting from 12 to 18 months. Fifty percent of girls with early onset of menarche typically have established ovulatory cycles after 1 year, whereas girls with late onset ovulation often take 8 to 12 years for all cycles to become ovulatory.[36] Menstrual cycles are typically variable for the first 2 to 3 years after menarche, but most cycles range from 21 to 45 days even in the first year of menstruation. Occasionally, cycles may be shorter or longer than this with no pathology. Menstrual bleeding generally lasts for 2 to 7 days. The individual's own pattern of normal cycles is typically established by the sixth gynecologic year.[36] The time leading up to menarche and the pubertal years is typically marked by varying levels emotional lability and behavioral changes, including "euphoria, depression, mood swings with paradoxical and hysterical reactions, crying with ease, and a negative attitude toward school."[37] Emotional and behavioral challenges usually taper off once the process of sexual maturation is completed and hormonal regulation is achieved.

SIGNIFICANCE OF AGE AT MENARCHE AND PATTERNS OF EARLY MENSTRUAL CYCLES ON LONG-TERM HEALTH

There has been media attention and concern given to the idea that girls appear to be entering puberty at earlier ages than has been the case historically. In fact, there is some disagreement in the literature as to whether this is the case. One author states that in Anglo-American females, the mean age of menarche has not changed in 50 years, although the author admits that population studies may obscure the actual rates; others state that evidence from the United States points to a decline in the mean age of menarche from 14.7 years at the turn of the century to age 12.8 at the end of the twentieth century.[36,37] These latter data are corroborated by European data that demonstrate a decline in age of menarche of 3 months per decade over the past 150 years.[41] All authors agree that earlier menarche is noted in girls living in urban environments and relate this to heavier than average weight compared with cohorts in rural areas. Increased rates of obesity and exogenous estrogens may indeed play a significant role in the early onset of menarche, and in addition to the risks associated with being overweight, may have implications for increased adult rates of breast cancer development. In fact, early age at menarche (<12 years) is a recognized risk for breast cancer, with risk declining by 10% for each year after that in which menarche is delayed.[38] This is primarily thought to be associated with greater cumulative exposure to estrogen and progesterone, especially estradiol. This risk may be reduced by the fact that girls who begin menstruating earlier are more likely to experience adolescent childbearing.

Conversely, girls with higher estrogen levels may be less predisposed to osteoporosis owing to increased bone density accumulation in the pubertal period, as evidenced by lower rates of osteoporosis among African American women compared with Anglo-American women. Adolescent girls with suppressed estrogen levels should be carefully monitored for bone density. Optimally all girls should consume high-calcium diets or take calcium supplements, particularly in the few years after menarche when bone density accumulation is as great as 10% to 20% and ensures as much as 10 to 20 years of protection against age-related bone mass loss.[1]

Age at menarche may be an indicator of nutritional status. Poor nutritional status or excessively low body fat percentage can lead to delayed menarche and may be a result of socioeconomic status, excessive exercise or athletic activity, or an eating disorder such as anorexia nervosa or bulimia. A vegetarian diet or low fat or carbohydrate (i.e., energy) intake also may lead to delayed menses. Unlike malnourished girls, nourished girls with delayed menses do not necessarily experience lower height by adulthood than girls with earlier-onset menstruation; however, compromised nutritional status requires social and medical attention. The fact that skeletal growth is still occurring throughout the teenage years underscores the importance of good nutrition. Girls with eating disorders are at risk for numerous medical complications and require counseling and intervention. It should be remembered that overeating and subsequent obesity is the most common malnutrition problem among adolescents in the United States and has been increasing in epidemic proportions. Girls with eating disorders critically need help with understanding how to nourish their bodies, but also need support in establishing positive body images and self-esteem. Adolescent pregnancy can also have a dramatic and deleterious effect on growth and development. If adolescent pregnancy is accompanied by being overweight, it can predispose the girl to problems with weight and diabetes later in life owing to alterations in growth hormone and insulin patterns. Health professionals counseling girls about their menstrual cycles have a tremendous opportunity to also counsel girls about nutrition, sexuality, lifestyle management, and a wide array of psychosocial issues that can affect their lives and long-term health.

TALKING WITH GIRLS ABOUT MENSTRUAL HEALTH AND HYGIENE

Although our culture has certainly become more open about menstruation, with overt menstrual product advertisement or mention of PMS being commonplace, many girls are still reticent when discussing the topic. Girls may be generally ignorant about what is happening to their bodies, and even the more knowledgeable girls may be uncertain about such things as maintaining menstrual health and hygiene.

Learning to chart her menstrual cycles can be an important first step in a girl's increased self-awareness and is also an important way to keep track of whether the cycles are regular and normal. Although cycles may be irregular for the first few years after menarche, this does not mean that all irregularity is normal or healthy. Even within patterns of irregularity, most menstrual cycles will range from 21 to 45 days with deviations slightly higher or lower than this on occasion. Most periods will last from 3 to 7 days. Wildly irregular cycles, excessively heavy periods, or oligomenorrhea can be indicative of serious health problems requiring further attention, including PCOS, thyroid disease, Cushing's disease, diabetes mellitus, premature ovarian failure, eating disorder—or exercise-induced amenorrhea, congenital adrenal hyperplasia, adrenal or ovarian tumors or prolactinomas, or other endocrine problems. Providing girls with calendars for recording their menstrual cycles and instructing them on how to do this, including recording the days they are menstruating (day 1 is considered the first day of the period and counting extends to the last day before the next period, whereupon the cycle starts again with day 1); symptoms they might have before, during, or after menstruation (e.g., mood alterations, headaches, fatigue); how long the bleeding lasts; and the amount of flow that is considered normal can provide them with important gynecologic information about themselves.

A blood loss of 30 mL per cycle is considered normal; a loss of greater than 80 mL is considered abnormal and puts a girl at risk for anemia. However, there is little value in milliliter measurement as this is virtually impossible to calculate. More useful is keeping track of the number of menstrual pads changed daily and their level of saturation. Typically, a girl can expect to change her pad three to six times per day. If the pad is oversaturated, she might not be changing pads frequently enough, the pads may be of the wrong size or fit, or they may be slipping in her underwear. If after ruling out these factors, there is concern over excessive menstrual flow, evaluate further. Educating the girl about proper use of pads, how often to change them, and also about the different types of available products (e.g., tampons) and their use can help a girl to be more comfortable during her menses and also prevent the embarrassment that could come from overflowing a pad. Many girls, especially athletes, are curious about the use of tampons. This is an area in which education is particularly important. Although all tampons must now meet FDA regulatory limits on absorbency, 50% of all reported cases of TSS still occur in menstruating women. Current FDA recommendations state that tampons should not be worn for 24 hours a day nor 7 days a week, and should be alternated with the use of pads.[36] Tampons should be changed at least every 4 to 8 hours; it is preferable to sleep with a pad rather than a tampon, and the last tampon at the end of menses must be remembered—it is relatively common for a girl or women to forget to remove a tampon at the end of the period. TSS should be treated as an acute medical emergency.

Encouraging girls to use the increasingly available selection of disposable menstrual hygiene products—both pads and tampons—made from organic cotton encourages the use of more environmentally friendly products. Most major health food stores carry a selection of good alternatives to conventional commercial products. Reusable fabric pads and menstrual cups are environmentally friendly alternatives to disposable products.

MENSTRUAL IRREGULARITIES AND DIFFICULTIES IN THE ADOLESCENT FEMALE

Adolescent girls, like women, commonly experience menstrual complaints, the most common for girls being dysmenorrhea, mood changes, and acne. Irregular or abnormal bleeding, particularly menorrhagia or amenorrhea, also may occur, and should be evaluated medically if persistent. Each of these complaints is addressed separately throughout this book. Additionally, a specific overview of these complaints in relationship to the special considerations of adolescent girls and the use of botanicals with adolescents is presented in the following. To avoid redundancy, only a brief discussion of the botanicals is provided in this section. More detailed herbal information is provided further in this chapter and throughout the text.

EMOTIONAL AND PSYCHOLOGICAL CHALLENGES IN ADOLESCENCE

Adolescence is a challenging and confusing time for even the most stable of girls. Hormonal changes and fluctuations and physical changes leading to the sexualization of the body, combined with confusing cultural messages about the role of the adolescent and sex, increasing pressures at school and the challenges of teen friendships, and problems at home (e.g., stress with parents, birth of a sibling, trouble with a sibling, parents experiencing marital discord or divorce, financial troubles, moving to a new location/home/school, death of an elderly relative such as a grandparent, or personal illness) can lead to enormous internal turbulence. It is critically important for girls at this age to have women confidants they can turn to for security, advice, reassurance, and accurate information. An anchor in the storm may be the best thing a teenage girl can have to help her stay healthy and focused on self-development rather than getting side-tracked by the many distractions available to adolescents. And this anchor needs to be available as early into puberty as possible—access to drugs and sexual experience starts in middle school for many US children. Health care providers can also provide an anchor for adolescent girls. One study, conducted in the late 1980s, looked at the major topics that teenagers wanted to discuss with their physicians. The top concerns expressed were: sexually transmitted diseases, birth control, fear of cancer, self-image, self-confidence, sexual function, and sexual abuse; yet most doctors were found only to discuss the topic of menstruation.[36]

By charting their cycles, girls can begin to identify patterns in their mood fluctuations and how they are associated with their menstrual cycle. This can help them to recognize their emotions as cyclical changes related to hormones and not something that is inherently wrong with them. Teaching girls the value of good nutrition (i.e., adequate protein and healthy carbohydrates; a good vitamin and mineral supplement; keeping sugar and caffeine consumption to a minimum; and keeping the blood sugar stable) can reduce mood swings and show them that they have some control over their emotional lives. Adequate sleep (teenagers may require as much as 12 hours per day!) and moderate exercise are also important for keeping emotions level and can support cognitive function. Journaling can be a useful tool for self-expression and may help girls to both record and vent some of the challenging emotions they feel and situations they face as they emerge into womanhood. Finally, if emotional or behavioral conflicts are significant, girls may benefit from or require counseling, as might the other family members. A healthy home life is an important stabilizing force as young girls turn into women and sort through their own identity, personal and social roles, relationships, and responsibilities.

HERBS AND ADOLESCENT GIRLS: SAFE USE VERSUS WRONGFUL ADVERTISING

In 2000, a national advertising campaign was launched for an herbal product called Bloussant Breast Enhancement Tablets. The fall 2001 issue of *Teen Vogue* and the September 2001 issue of *Seventeen* ran full and quarter-page ads, respectively, for this product. These advertisements fed into the already prevalent idea that bigger breast size is better, which led nearly 4000 females 18 and younger to have breast augmentation surgery in the year 2000 alone (representing 2% of all such surgeries that year), a 425% increase over 1997 rates. This represents a growing trend of misuse of herbal products by teenagers.[39] Marketing of herbal products to teens has become increasingly popular, and teens are receptive to this marketing: many of them believe that natural means safer.[40] In fact, the prevalence of use as determined by limited population surveys appears to mirror that of national use by adults, with nearly half of all teens surveyed reporting complementary and alternative medicine (CAM) use, and the use of herbal products at approximately 12%.[40-42] Teens primarily appear to base their use on perceived parental or friend use, and primarily appear to use herbs without parental knowledge.[42] Many are concurrently using other pharmacologically active substances, including medications, other herbal products, or recreational drugs or alcohol. Common conditions for which teens use herbal products include PMS, urinary tract infections (UTIs), obesity, pregnancy, and enhancement of athletic performance or stamina. Adolescent girls are more likely than boys to seek health care, including CAM therapies, although the rate of supplement use is higher for adolescent male athletes than their female athletic counterparts (29% vs. 12%).[40]

Because little to no clinical research has been done on the safety of botanical medicines in the distinct population of adolescent females, extra care should be taken during this period of rapid growth, development, and hormonal change. Further, the combined use of herbs and pharmaceutical drugs, not to mention recreational use of pharmaceutical or "natural" drugs, is also largely unstudied, and may be an area in which teenagers either experiment or unknowingly use potentially harmful combinations. Teens may therefore be at additional risk compared with the adult population when using herbal remedies. Much like with young children, pregnant women, and lactating women, additional precautions should be taken to minimize the use of botanical therapies that might inappropriately affect the endocrine system during this developmental stage. Adolescents should be educated and cautioned about the use of products such as those for breast augmentation and athletic enhancement, and should be advised about the hazards of using such herbs as ephedra or other stimulant herbs for athletic performance or weight loss. Finally, adolescents should be encouraged to seek the help of a qualified herbal practitioner when choosing to use herbs for the treatment of health problems, and should be told to inform their primary care provider of the use of any herbal products, particularly if being prescribed a pharmaceutical drug or medical treatment. Adolescents should be informed that natural does not mean safe and that there are potential hazards associated with the use of herbal products. Practitioners should not make the broad assumption that herbs that are safe for adult women are always and entirely safe for adolescent girls, considering the unknowns of herbs for this population; short-term therapies (i.e., for 3 months or less followed by a rest) may be preferable to using herbs for long courses of treatment. More research in this area is warranted.

COMMON PROBLEMS OF PUBERTY AND MENSTRUATION IN ADOLESCENT FEMALES AND THEIR BOTANICAL TREATMENTS

Mood Changes
The Botanical Practitioner's Perspective

Mood swings are common among adolescent girls and may be particularly prevalent in the week or days just before the onset of menstruation, not dissimilar to PMS, or they may occur more frequently and unpredictably than monthly or cyclically. Frequently, girls start exhibiting mood swings as early as age 11, which many parents assume to simply be a behavioral problem rather than recognizing the beginning of hormonally mediated mood changes. Mood swings may be extreme, ranging from hysteria to euphoria in a matter of moments. Dramatic behavior is not uncommon. Girls also may find that their cognitive functioning is not as sharp, in particular just before menstruation, which makes it more difficult to concentrate and perform in school, especially in the more linear subjects such as science and mathematics. Tests in school just before menstruation may be especially challenging for some girls. These emotional and cognitive changes are typically the result not only of hormonal influences but also of dietary inadequacies and sleep deficiency so common to adolescence. Declining blood sugar associated with hormonal changes, along with inadequate consumption of high-quality protein and carbohydrates, and an overreliance on simple sugar for energy can lead to marked decline in mood and concentration. Inadequate rest as a result of staying up late at night and getting up early for school can exacerbate poor mood or concentration problems (see Premenstrual Syndrome).

Adolescent girls are also subject to hormonal dysregulation that can lead to irritability, depression, and anxiety, as frequently occurs with PMS. This period of time can be trying for parents and is difficult for the girl herself, who may be unhappy and feel out of control. Therefore a great deal of support, encouragement, and reassurance may be needed as part of the health consultation. Conventional treatment relies on medication (e.g., birth control pills, antidepressants) to regulate hormones, mood, or both. In some cases medication may be appropriate, but counseling, lifestyle support, and appropriate nutritional and herbal supplements are preferable first-line approaches when possible versus starting an adolescent on a course of hormonal or psychiatric drugs, whose long-term effects in the adolescent population are also frequently not well studied or understood. If depression is severe or thoughts or fears of suicide have been expressed, psychological counseling and medical intervention are essential. See Table 9-1 for a summary of mood-changing herbs.

Discussion of Botanical Protocol

A number of herbs can be used to calm and nourish the nervous system. The gentlest of those that are used for promoting short- and long-term relaxation with a high safety profile when used in correct dosages include chamomile (Fig. 9-1), passionflower, and lavender, all of which are mild and nonaddictive. Ashwagandha

TABLE 9-1   Summary of Herbs Used for Adolescent Mood Changes

Therapeutic Goal	Therapeutic Activity	Botanical Name	Common Name
Promote relaxation; decrease emotional and psychological stress	Nervines	*Hypericum perforatum*	St. John's Wort
		Lavandula officinalis	Lavender
		Leonurus cardiaca	Motherwort
		Matricaria recutita	Chamomile
		Passiflora incarnata	Passionflower
		Verbena officinalis	Blue vervain
Support healthy HPA axis function	Adaptogens	*Bacopa monnieri*	Bacopa
		Eleutherococcus senticosus	Eleuthero
		Panax quinquefolius	American ginseng
		Schisandra chinensis	Schisandra
		Withania somnifera	Ashwagandha
Improve hormonal regulation	Hormonal regulators; hepatic tonics	*Paeonia lateriflora*	White peony
		Taraxacum officinale	Dandelion
		Vitex agnus-castus	Chaste berry
Improve nutritional status; nourish the blood; treat anemia	"Blood tonics"	*Angelica sinensis*	Dong quai
		Urtica dioica	Stinging nettle
		Withania somnifera	Ashwagandha

HPA, Hypothalamic-pituitary-adrenal.

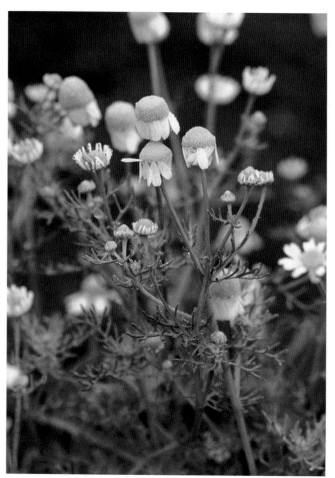

FIGURE 9-1 Chamomile *(Matricaria recutita).* (Photo by Martin Wall.)

is used over time as a tonic for the nervous system, and may exhibit beneficial effects on immunity and hemoglobin levels, and may have uterine antispasmodic activity as well, making it particularly beneficial when there is also dysmenorrhea.[43-46] For significant irritability and emotional lability many herbalists include the herbs motherwort or blue vervain in formulae. These bitter nervine herbs are applied in much the same principle as herbs for liver qi stagnation in Traditional Chinese Medicine (TCM), with the understanding that herbs that improve the smooth functioning of the liver (possibly through liver detoxification mechanisms) have a regulatory effect on the female endocrine system. St. John's wort is included when depression is a component of the emotional picture.[47] Additionally, bacopa, reputed for its ability to enhance cognitive function and retention of newly learned information, is used to improve concentration; dong quai is used in formulae when there is anemia.[46] *Vitex agnus-castus* is used when there is emotional lability associated with the menstrual cycle, particularly when there is also menstrual cycle irregularity.[43] It has a high safety profile, with no contraindications reported in the *German Commission E Monographs,* although it is generally considered contraindicated for use during pregnancy. Simultaneous use with hormone therapy and OCs is also contraindicated.[43-45,48] In rare cases, short-term use of *V. agnus-castus* has been seen clinically to worsen depression; if this is observed discontinue its use immediately.

Additional Therapies

Nutritional supplementation can play a pivotal role in the improvement of mood and cognitive function. In addition to taking a high-quality vitamin and mineral supplement (an adult dosage can be taken by girls 14 and older; younger girls can take a supplement designed for adolescents), adolescent girls can benefit from a high-quality essential fatty acid supplement containing both omega-3 and omega-6 fatty acids. The best supplements contain a combination of both plant-based

BOTANICAL PRESCRIPTION FOR ADOLESCENT MOOD CHANGES

A typical protocol for when there is slight menstrual irregularity, irritability, and emotional lability is as follows:

- Give *Vitex agnus-castus* (chaste tree) 5 mL, once daily (usually given in the morning).
- Also give the following formula:

Chamomile	*(Matricaria recutita)*	25 mL
Ashwagandha	*(Withania somnifera)*	25 mL
Passionflower	*(Passiflora incarnata)*	25 mL
Motherwort	*(Leonurus cardiaca)*	20 mL
Lavender	*(Lavandula officinalis)*	5 mL
	Total:	**100 mL**

Dose: 5 mL twice daily or 2.5 mL as needed throughout the day, not to exceed six doses.

If there is poor concentration or memory difficulty, take *Bacopa monnieri* (bacopa) 1:1, 5 mL one time daily or two 2.5-mL doses.

TREATMENT SUMMARY FOR ADOLESCENT MOOD CHANGES

- Calm and nourish the nervous system with herbal nervines including skullcap, chamomile, lemon balm, St. John's wort, milky oats, and passionflower.
- Treat depression with herbal antidepressants, appropriate nutrition, exercise, and counseling.
- Relieve stress and support adrenal function with adaptogens.
- Improve hormonal regulation through botanicals with endocrine effects and through improved liver function and bowel elimination (when there is hyperestrogenism).
- Enhance cognitive function and improve concentration with botanical agents and nutrition.
- Maintain stable blood sugar, mood, and cognitive function with adequate protein and complex carbohydrates.
- Include a high-quality essential fatty acid supplement containing both omega-3 and omega-6 fatty acids to improve mood, mental function, and skin problems.
- Supplement dietary iron.
- Encourage adequate rest.
- Provide opportunities for self-expression (e.g., journaling, art work) and physical activity to release tension (e.g., martial arts, running, swimming, boxing, yoga).
- Provide psychological counseling and medical intervention when necessary.

essential fatty acids (derived from evening primrose oil [EPO] or borage oil) and cold-water fish oil. Standard daily supplementation can improve mood and mental function, and can be helpful when skin problems are present (see Acne). Additionally, teenage girls who are menstruating need an adequate regular intake of dietary iron. If the diet is poor or there is heavy menstrual bleeding, dietary iron should be supplemented. Floradix Iron + Herbs is an excellent, highly absorbable, nonconstipating iron supplement derived primarily from

plant sources. It can be taken daily. Attention should be paid to adequate rest and opportunities for self-expression (e.g., journaling, art work) and physical activity to release tension (e.g., martial arts, running, swimming, boxing, yoga).

Dysmenorrhea in Adolescent Girls

Cramping and lower abdominal pain associated with the onset of menstruation are the most common complaints of adolescent girls, leading to missed days at school and self-medication with over-the-counter pain relievers, antiinflammatory drugs, and herbal products. In adolescents, dysmenorrhea is generally nonpathologic and coincides with ovulatory menstruation because progesterone secretion from the ovary is associated with uterine muscle contractility. It may coincide with or occur independently of PMS. Severe dysmenorrhea should be evaluated, particularly in sexually active girls, to rule out endometriosis, pelvic infection, or other problems (see Dysmenorrhea).

Conventional Treatment Approaches

Medical treatment for nonpathologic dysmenorrhea is generally medication for the symptomatic relief of discomfort.

The Botanical Practitioner's Perspective

Botanical medicines have a long history of use for the symptomatic treatment of dysmenorrhea and can be used as needed just before the onset of the expected cramping (i.e., 1 or 2 days before menstruation) and through the first day or two of menstruation, after which cramping usually ceases on its own. Practitioners also often suggest the use of antiinflammatory herbs and dietary strategies to help reduce the inflammatory processes caused by the increased prostaglandin production sometimes associated with menstrual cramps. Finally, herbalists may recommend herbs that help to stimulate pelvic circulation and relieve pelvic congestion to reduce ischemia and related pain.

Botanical Protocol

Cramp bark and black haw can be used interchangeably as single herbs for the symptomatic relief of uterine cramps.[49,50] Ginger is an antiinflammatory herb and traditionally used by herbalists for improving pelvic circulation.[8,43,50,51] It may be combined in tincture with other herbs or used alone beginning a few days before the expected menses and continued as needed. Dong quai also has demonstrated uterine antispasmodic activity.[46,47] Excessive use of either ginger or dong quai may increase uterine bleeding; their use should be avoided if there is menorrhagia. EPO is taken in capsules up to 1500 mg per day throughout the month or beginning in midcycle through the beginning of the menses. When there is significant cramping, white peony, an excellent uterine antispasmodic, and motherwort might be added to the formula, the latter as a uterine tonic and nervine antispasmodic.[46] See Table 9-2.

Additional Therapies

Increased arachidonic acid production is associated with increased inflammation and menstrual cramps. Reduction of

TABLE 9-2   Summary of Herbs Used for Adolescent Dysmenorrhea

Therapeutic Goal	Therapeutic Activity	Botanical Name	Common Name
Relieve uterine cramps	Antispasmodics Antiinflammatories	*Actaea racemosa* *Dioscorea villosa* *Leonurus cardiaca* *Matricaria recutita* *Viburnum* spp. *Zingiber officinale*	Black cohosh* Wild yam Motherwort Chamomile Cramp bark, black haw Ginger
Improve pelvic circulation		*Angelica sinensis* *Leonurus cardiaca* *Paeonia lateriflora* *Zingiber officinale*	Dong quai Motherwort White peony Ginger

*Recently concerns have been raised over hepatoxicity associated with black cohosh.

BOTANICAL PRESCRIPTION FOR ADOLESCENT DYSMENORRHEA

A typical formula for an adolescent with dysmenorrhea is as follows:

Cramp bark	(*Viburnum opulus*)	55 mL
Chamomile	(*Matricaria recutita*)	15 mL
Motherwort	(*Leonurus cardiaca*)	15 mL
Ginger	(*Zingiber officinale*)	15 mL
	Total:	**100 mL**

Dose: 2 mL repeated as needed up to every 20 minutes for 2 hours, or 2.5 mL up to one dose every 2 hours before and through the onset of menses.

Also: Evening primrose oil capsules, 1000 mg daily
Tea of chamomile or fresh ginger daily, as needed
Externally: Hot ginger fomentation over the uterus

TREATMENT SUMMARY FOR DYSMENORRHEA IN ADOLESCENT GIRLS

- Use botanical antispasmodics to reduce uterine cramping and pain: cramp bark, black haw, black cohosh, wild yam
- Use antiinflammatory herbs and dietary strategies to help reduce the inflammatory processes caused by increased prostaglandin production: ginger, evening primrose oil
- Use botanicals to stimulate pelvic circulation and relieve pelvic congestion to reduce ischemia and related pain: white peony, motherwort, dong quai
- Reduce arachidonic acid production through an antiinflammatory diet (e.g., reduction of red meat and dairy product consumption)
- Increase consumption of cold-water fish such as salmon and supplement with a high-quality fish oil (often combined with evening primrose or borage oil) to reduce inflammation and menstrual cramps
- Supplement with magnesium
- Exercise regularly, especially yoga poses for promoting pelvic circulation
- Use abdominal massage, hot packs, or ginger fomentations
- Take hot baths with relaxing essential oils such as lavender, rose, and sandalwood

red meat and dairy products in the diet may reduce the severity and frequency of menstrual cramps. Alternative sources of protein and calcium should be included in the diet to ensure adequate nutrition. Increased consumption of cold-water fish such as salmon and supplementation with high-quality fish oil (often combined with evening primrose or borage oil) also may help in the reduction of inflammation and menstrual cramps. Supplementation with magnesium was demonstrated in an open study to help improve uterine muscle activity and reduce symptoms.[50] Regular exercise with the addition of yoga poses for promoting pelvic circulation may be helpful. Abdominal massage, hot packs or ginger fomentations, and the use of hot baths with relaxing essential oils such as lavender, rose, and sandalwood can provide temporary comfort from menstrual cramps.

Menorrhagia in Adolescent Girls

The primary cause of menorrhagia (i.e., excessive menstrual bleeding ranging from heavy periods to hemorrhage, with durations of several days to several weeks), in adolescent girls is anovulatory cycles owing to hyperproliferation of the uterine endometrium in the absence of adequate progesterone. Menorrhagia can lead to acute and chronic anemia, weakness,

TREATMENT SUMMARY FOR MENORRHAGIA IN ADOLESCENTS

- Use uterine hemostatic herbs to control acute bleeding.
- Use *Vitex agnus-castus* daily for 3 months to stimulate ovulation in anovulatory cycles.
- Treat anemia with botanical agents and nutritional supplements.
- Vitamin A deficiency has been found to be an important factor associated with menorrhagia; vitamin A supplementation* may be effective in preventing excessive bleeding in some women. Some fish oil products contain substantial vitamin A and may be adequate for supplementation.

*Vitamin A is teratogenic and should not be taken as a supplement if pregnancy is suspected.

fatigue, and anxiety. Rarely menorrhagia can be caused by an uncommon congenital blood disorder called von Willebrand's disease (see Dysfunctional Uterine Bleeding).

Conventional Treatment Approaches

Acute treatment involves stabilization of bleeding, treatment of acute blood loss, and treatment of anemia. Treatment also includes use of hormone therapy to stabilize estrogen levels and provide progesterone to stabilize the endometrium.

The Botanical Practitioner's Perspective

Ovulatory cycles may be stimulated with regular use of *V. agnus-castus,* 5 mL once daily. Elevated prostaglandin E (PGE) may also lead to increased bleeding owing to reduced clotting and increased dilation of the blood vessels. Acute episodes of mild to moderate excessive bleeding may be controlled with uterine hemostatic herbs; significant excessive bleeding and hemorrhage requires medical intervention.

Botanical Protocol

Herbs may be used as hemostatics, progesterone production enhancers, and antiinflammatories in the reduction of PGE_2. *V. agnus-castus* is one of the primary herbs to be considered for stimulating the ovary and encouraging ovulation, thus increasing progesterone secretion. It should be given in a 3 to 5 mL daily dose.

Additional Therapies

As with dysmenorrhea, the addition of fish oils supplements may help in the reduction of menorrhagia.

Additionally, vitamin A deficiency has been found to be an important factor associated with menorrhagia. Vitamin A is a cofactor of 3-beta-hydroxysteroid-dehydrogenase in steroidogenesis, and deficiencies of this vitamin may result in impaired enzyme activity. The level of endogenous 17-β-estradiol appears to be elevated with vitamin A therapy, and in one study, menorrhagia was alleviated in more than 92% of patients.[53] Iron supplementation is essential because menorrhagia is regularly associated with anemia.

Amenorrhea in Adolescent Girls

Adolescent girls may experience either primary or secondary amenorrhea. Primary amenorrhea is the lack of menses by age 16; secondary amenorrhea is cessation of menses for three cycles or 6 months in girls or women who have previously menstruated. Primary amenorrhea is specific to adolescent girls and has a broad range of possible causes, requiring medical consultation.

Acne

Acne, often dismissed by the medical community as simply a consequence of adolescence, is actually the most common dermatologic condition, affecting at least 85% of all adolescents.[54] It not only has the potential to cause permanent physical scarring but may have a significant effect on psychoemotional and social well-being and quality of life (QOL). Acne in adolescents and adult women is addressed in the next section.

ACNE VULGARIS

Acne vulgaris, acne, is a common and chronic skin condition affecting the pilosebaceous unit. It affects 80% of people in the United States at some point in life, and at any given time in the United States affects an estimated 17 million people.[55] It is the most common dermatologic condition seen in clinical practice and leads to more dermatologic visits than any other skin condition, leading to absenteeism at school and work and millions of dollars in annual treatment costs.[56-58] At least 85% of adolescents and young adults are affected by acne. Not only does severe acne potentially cause permanent physical scarring; it has a significant psychosocial effect on the sufferer, sometimes dramatically reducing QOL, particularly, but not exclusively, in adolescent girls, where it can have a marked influence on self-esteem and lead to embarrassment, anger, anxiety, and depression.[54,59-61] Previously considered a condition of adolescence, it is now widely recognized to be a problem that can persist chronically or cyclically well into a woman's fourth decade of life.[62,63]

PATHOPHYSIOLOGY

The pilosebaceous unit consists of a hair follicle and its associated sebaceous gland. Acne is caused by the following constellation of four pathogenic factors at the pilosebaceous unit:

- Androgens act upon the sebaceous gland, causing increased sebum production.
- Impaired desquamation of the follicle leads to plugged pores and an abnormal pattern of follicular hyperkeratinization.
- Increased sebum supports the proliferation of bacteria, most commonly *Propionibacterium acnes.*
- Inflammatory mediators are released by *P. acnes* into the follicle and surrounding dermal tissue.[64-66]

During adolescence androgen levels increase, explaining the prevalence of acne during this time. However, elevated androgen levels are not always a finding; in 60% of women with acne, serum androgen levels are normal but there is significantly elevated 5-alpha (α)-reductase at the sebaceous gland, indicating a heightened sensitivity to androgen. This also may explain the persistent or recurrent acne that might occur well into a woman's forties.[1] Increased 5-α-reductase results in higher rates of conversion of androgens, specifically conversion of testosterone into its active metabolite dihydrotestosterone.[67] There is clearly an association between acne and menstruation with a premenstrual flare noted as common among 3394 women who completed a survey on the prevalence of acne in females in France.[68] Emotional stresses have also been demonstrated to increase acne outbreaks. Additionally, hyperandrogenic conditions including PCOS, 21-hydroxylase deficiency, adrenal androgen excess, and some medications (e.g., steroids) are clearly implicated causes of acne.[1,65,67,69-71] *P. acnes* converts sebum to free fatty acids, and individuals who are hypersensitive to these free fatty acids may experience the more uncommon forms of severe nodular acne.[67] Hyperinsulinemia also may play a role in the etiology of acne, evidenced by the increased glucose levels at the sebaceous gland of those with acne and the prevalence of acne and PCOS in those with hyperinsulinemia, although a causal association is not conclusive.

SIGNS AND SYMPTOMS OF ACNE

The characteristic clinical manifestations of *Acne vulgaris* are the appearance of comedones (i.e., blackheads) or pustules (i.e., whiteheads), typically appearing on the face, back, chest, and upper arms, the distribution of outbreaks making it among the most visible of dermatologic complaints. Inflammation may or may not be considerable. Diagnosis of hyperandrogenic and hyperinsulinemic states is essential to proper treatment. (See Polycystic Ovary Syndrome.)

DIAGNOSIS

A diagnosis of acne is made upon visual inspection and exclusion of other causes. Acne may be dismissed as an unimportant consequence of adolescence or cyclic hormonal fluctuation; however, this may be a gross underestimation of the significance of the problem.[54] In a 1994 study conducted by the American Medical Association (AMA), 89% of adolescent girls reported worrying about their complexion and 50% believed it was the first thing people noticed about them.[14] Therefore quick diagnosis and treatment from the time of onset of acne is important, particularly in the adolescent population when it tends to be the most severe and has the greatest social effect. Conventional therapy also calls for dermatologists to be adept at recognizing and treating resultant psychiatric disturbances in patients with acne.[57] Furthermore, the appearance of acne may be indicative of more serious problems, such as PCOS, which predisposes girls to obesity, diabetes, and cardiovascular problems.[71]

CONVENTIONAL TREATMENT

Acne vulgaris is not considered a curable disease by conventional medicine; however, symptoms are frequently well controlled and scarring prevented by a combination of systemic (i.e., internal) and topical therapies, with patients typically prescribed a combination of therapies as suggested by the causes and severity of the case.[56,72,73] Effective treatments are aimed at treating the four pathogenic factors mentioned in the preceding. Combination therapies are considered to be the most effective.[56] However, in mild cases, topical treatment sometimes may be adequate.[74]

Oral Contraceptives

OCs have demonstrable effects in improving hormonally mediated acne; however, women are often concerned about their side effects. Additionally, teenage girls may be concerned about social perceptions related to their use of OCs, including disapproval or misunderstanding of the reasons for the medication.[61] In addition to OCs, other androgen antagonists may be prescribed.[70] For a complete discussion of the treatment of PCOS, refer to that section of this text.

Oral Antibiotics and Retinoid Preparations

In addition to OCs, systemic treatments for acne include the use of oral antibiotics and retinoid preparations.[54,62,73,74] Isotretinoin is the only medication thus far to induce long-term, drug-free remission; however, its use internally has been clearly demonstrated to carry risks of teratogenicity. Therefore it cannot be used during pregnancy and ongoing negative pregnancy tests should be obtained when women of childbearing age use this drug. Isotretinoin treatments for clearing acne have been associated with marked improvement in QOL and psychological status in those with severe acne who have benefited from its use.[6] Unfortunately, there has also been substantial concern in recent years regarding its association with increased suicide rates among users.[54,74] Topical use is not associated with these risks and is considered effective and safe. Antibiotics can be effective at reducing inflammations; however, antibiotic resistance is emerging as a new and important concern in their use as first-line internal and topical therapies.[64] Internal therapies are aimed at reducing microbial colonization, treating hyperkeratosis, and reducing immune-modulated and inflammatory responses.[65]

Topical Treatments

Commonly prescribed topical treatments include retinoids, benzoyl peroxide, and antibiotics. Table 9-3 addresses the various systemic treatments currently in use, their actions, and their adverse effects. Conventional medical therapy for the treatment of *Acne vulgaris* may need to be maintained for months or well over a year. This is limited by the tolerability of systemic and local dermatologic agents, the stigma to adolescents of OC use, the long-term risks of OC and corticosteroid use, limited ability to control sebum production with medications, development of antibiotic resistance by *P. acnes,* and in women of childbearing age, interference of antibiotics with OCs and demonstrated teratogenicity of the most effective moderate to severe acne therapy—isotretinoin.

Botanical Treatment of Acne
Philosophic View

Botanical therapy for acne begins with the belief that the health of the skin is a reflection of the overall health of the organism. The skin, a major organ of elimination, is believed to bear an excess burden of elimination when other eliminatory and detoxification organs (e.g., bowels, lymph system, liver) are not functioning optimally or are overtaxed. Thus topical treatments are almost universally accompanied by systemic treatments that address the health of these other systems. An entire category of herbs, known historically and to this day as *alteratives* and referred to colloquially as *blood cleansers,* are included in the treatment of most skin condition for their perceived stimulatory effects on the lymph system and liver. Many herbalists rely on the use of gentle choleretics to stimulate bile flow and improve bowel regularity and frequency, and herbs to improve hepatic function, the long-term result of which is often found to be improved skin health. It is likely that the mechanisms of action include hepatic detoxification

TABLE 9-3	Common Pharmaceutical Systemic Approaches to Treating Acne[54,64-66]
Pharmaceutical Drug	**Action/Adverse Reactions**
Antibiotics: tetracycline, clarithromycin, clindamycin, doxycycline, erythromycin	Reduce microbial colonization; antiinflammatory for moderate to severe acne when topicals are not adequate alone. Adverse effects of oral antibiotic use include increased vaginal yeast infection, GI tract upset, decreased efficacy of OCs because of decreased intestinal absorption of estrogens caused by gut microflora disruption, and antibiotic resistance, an increasingly prevalent problem.
Hormonal drugs: oral contraceptives/antiandrogen therapy	Reverse hyperandrogenic states. Reduce hormonal pathogenesis associated with acne by lowering levels of circulating androgens; the only treatment effective at actually controlling sebum production. May also decrease adrenal and ovarian androgen production. Women using OCs are at risk for the well-documented common and serious adverse effects associated with their use. OCs containing androgenic progestins may aggravate acne. Spironolactone is the most commonly used antiandrogenic drug; it may cause menstrual irregularity and breast tenderness. Low-dose corticosteroids are sometimes used to control adrenal androgen production.
Isotretinoin (Accutane)	Strong antiinflammatory for severe inflammatory acne; only medication that addresses all four pathogenic factors simultaneously; produces significant reduction in sebum production. Known teratogen; may cause anemia or thrombocytopenia, adverse skin reactions (including pruritus, excessive granulation, secondary staphylococcal skin infection), nosebleeds, vaginal dryness, arthralgias, abnormal liver function tests, depression, and rarely, more severe problems.

GI, Gastrointestinal; *OCs*, oral contraceptives.

and a reduction in excess circulating hormonal load (i.e., excess estrogen, testosterone) via increased bile conjugation and intestinal elimination. Herbalists typically include botanical antimicrobials and antiinflammatories as topical and systemic therapeutic agents. Additionally, herbalists view the skin as the interface between the individual and the world, "being the vehicle through which we express, communicate, and perceive. Thus the psychological and spiritual aspects of an individual will affect and be affected by the skin."[2] This corroborates what medical science now recognizes as the effect of emotional stress on the health of the skin and the influence of skin problems on emotional health.

As more information on the role of herbs on endocrine functions emerges, herbs are increasingly being considered for treatment of hormonal dysregulation in acne, such as hyperandrogenism. Based on the suspected hormonal etiology of *Acne vulgaris* there clearly appears to be a role for herbal hormonal modulation as an alternative to OCs and corticosteroids. (See Polycystic Ovary Syndrome if this is a suspected or confirmed diagnosis of which the acne is symptomatic.) Hyperinsulinemia also should be evaluated for and treated if present because this may be a factor in hypersensitivity to androgens.

The botanical medicine practitioner takes a multifactorial approach by incorporating dietary and nutritional modifications, attention to the individual female's hormonal patterns, and the effects of stress on and from acne into a comprehensive treatment plan. Supporting evidence here focuses on herbs that directly target the skin through antiinflammatory, antimicrobial, or hormonal effects. Table 9-4 provides suggestions for adjunct therapies that might be considered in conjunction with these direct-acting agents; for example, the use of nervines or adaptogens.

It should be noted that immediate results are not expected when treating chronic acne. Improvement may take place over several weeks or longer, and when acne is associated with menstruation, over several cycles.

Discussion of Botanicals

Given the prevalence of skin complaints, there is a remarkable paucity of studies on botanicals for their treatment. The following discussion reviews the traditional and contemporary clinical uses of herbs for the treatment of acne.

Barberry Root: Internal. A 4-week randomized control trial (RCT) ($n = 49$) examined the effect of oral aqueous extract of barberry on *Acne vulgaris* in adolescents (ages 12 to 17) with moderate to severe acne. Outcomes were taken at baseline and weeks 2 and 4, and measures included total acne lesions and Michaelson's acne severity score. Using these parameters, statistically significant differences were seen in the treatment group compared with controls (600 mg daily).[75]

Burdock Root: Internal/Topical. A comprehensive database search for uses of burdock root yields a long list of articles demonstrating its historical and traditional use for the treatment of sores, boils, and abscesses. It is discussed in *King's American Dispensatory* as an alterative, aperient, and specific herb for impaired nutrition of the skin, specifically recommended for eczema, psoriasis, and dry scaly eruptions.[76] Burdock root is used as an alterative and gentle laxative. The root extract has mild antibiotic activity, attributed to its polyacetylene constituents, which, however, may not be present in commercially available dried material.[77,78] According to Wichtl, the European use of burdock as an herbal drug is nearly obsolete.[77] The German Commission E did not support its therapeutic use owing to insufficient evidence.[44] No clinical studies using burdock have been identified in the literature. Nonetheless, it remains widely used by herbalists as a decoction or tincture to be taken internally for the treatment of skin conditions, including acne. However, there is controversy among herbalists about its efficacy for skin conditions, and some have reported exacerbations of inflammatory skin conditions. It is typically used internally, although it may be used topically as well.

TABLE 9-4   Botanical Treatment Strategies for Acne

Therapeutic Goal	Therapeutic Strategy	Botanical Name	Common Name
Reduce inflammation	Antiinflammatories	*Glycyrrhiza glabra*	Licorice
		Hamamelis virginiana	Witch hazel
		Lavandula officinalis	Lavender
		Matricaria recutita	Chamomile
		Scutellaria baicalensis	Skullcap
Reduce local infection	Antimicrobials	*Echinacea* spp.	Echinacea
		Lavandula officinalis	Lavender
		Berberis aquifolium	Oregon grape
		Melaleuca alternifolia	Tea tree
Relieve stress, anxiety, tension, depression	Nervines, anxiolytics, antidepressants	*Hypericum perforatum*	St. John's wort
		Melissa officinalis	Lemon balm
		Scutellaria lateriflora	Skullcap
		Verbena officinalis	Blue vervain
Improve stress/adrenal response; enhance immunity	Adaptogens	*Withania somnifera*	Ashwagandha
Improve eliminative functions through lymphatic and hepatic systems	Alteratives, lymphagogues, choleretics, hepatics	*Arctium lappa*	Burdock
		Calendula officinalis	Calendula
		Galium aparine	Cleavers
		Rumex crispus	Yellow dock
		Scrophularia nodosa	Figwort
		Taraxacum officinale	Dandelion
		Trifolium pratense	Red clover
Hormonal regulation	Hormonal regulating herbs	*Vitex agnus-castus*	Chaste berry
Treat constipation	Aperients (mild laxatives)	*Linum usitatissimum*	Flax seed
		Rumex crispus	Yellow dock
		Taraxacum officinale	Dandelion
Topical applications	Antimicrobials; antiinflammatories	See earlier discussion	

Calendula: Internal/Topical. The effectiveness of calendula blossoms in the treatment of skin inflammations is well documented. Although the active principles have not been clearly defined, it contains both antiinflammatory flavonoids and retinoids.[44,77] Calendula, a bitter, cooling herb, exerts systemic antiseptic and antiinflammatory activity when used orally, and is considered specific for the treatment of sebaceous cysts and acne.[79,80] Limited uncontrolled studies on the antimicrobial activity of calendula have been conflicting and tend to discount its efficacy, although it has demonstrated antiinflammatory activity.[81] Its demonstrated effects include promoting epithelialization of surgical wounds and bactericidal action against *S. aureus*.[31] Herbalists continue to rely on it, finding it highly effective clinically for skin inflammation and infection, used both internally as a decoction and topically as a wash, steam, or fomentation. It is considered specifically when there are swollen lymph nodes, and used internally, is considered to promote lymphatic circulation and drainage.

Chamomile: Internal/Topical. Chamomile is indicated externally for treatment of inflammation of the skin and mucosa, used as a wash or steam. Its effects may be largely owing to the chamomile flavones (e.g., apigenin) that exert a local antiinflammatory effect with topical application. Apigenin is not only absorbed at the skin but also penetrates to deeper layers.[77] Although no reports on the use of chamomile for the treatment of acne were identified, several reports indicate beneficial effects from topical use of standardized chamomile creams in the treatment of eczema, with two trials showing chamomile cream to have equal or superior effects to topical steroidal and nonsteroidal antiinflammatory medications.[80,82,83] It is recommended in the *German Commission E Monographs* for inflammations and bacterial conditions of the skin.[44] No studies were identified on its specific use for acne. Allergic irritating skin reactions have been reported with the use of chamomile flowers topically, but such reports are very rare.[77] Internal use is appropriate as an adjunct treatment for stress and anxiety associated with acne.

Chaste Berry: Internal. Chaste berry is sometimes recommended for the treatment of acne, and in particular, menstrually or hormonally related skin problems.*

Its use for acne appears partly based on a study conducted in 1968 by Giss and Rothenberg demonstrating clinical effectiveness in a group of 118 men and women (70% were women, some with PMS), including recurrence of acne with lapses in herbal treatment and complete healing in 70% of patients who had previously been unresponsive to long-term conventional therapy.[86] Mills and Bone suggest the therapeutic efficacy seen in this study may be attributed to the mild antiandrogenic effects of *V. agnus-castus*, although this remains unknown.[52] Low Dog, however, argues that it

---

* 43,52,77,83-85.

seems illogical to give chaste tree for the treatment of acne given that acne seems to be aggravated in the progesterone dominant luteal phase of the menstrual cycle when *V. agnus-castus* appears to increase LH and progesterone levels.[83] Clearly, there is a great deal still not understood about the interactions of herbs with the endocrine system. *V. agnus-castus* has a good safety profile and may be of benefit in some women with acne; however, at this time there appears to be no scientific justification of its routine use as an acne treatment.

Chinese Skullcap: Internal/Topical. *Scutellaria baicalensis,* or "scute," is considered specific in TCM for clearing "damp heat," a category of diagnosis in which acne may commonly fall. It is clinically remarkable for reducing inflammation in dermatologic conditions and should be considered an important herb in formulations for treating acne and other skin conditions. It has also shown antimicrobial activity against a broad spectrum of microorganisms.[46] It can be used orally for its systemic antiinflammatory effects and topically in cream or wash form as a local antiinflammatory (Fig. 9-2).

Cleavers: Internal. Cleavers is used internally for the treatment of a wide range of skin conditions.[77,80] It is particularly indicated when there are enlarged lymph nodes, and for inflammatory, eruptive skin conditions.[78] Its use is based on traditional evidence.

Dandelion Root: Internal. Dandelion root is an alterative and perhaps one of the best-regarded tonics for the liver.[83] Traditionally, it has been included in formulae for skin conditions such as acne. No human clinical trials have been conducted to support the uses of dandelion root for skin conditions.[83,87] Its use as a bitter, cholagogue, and aperient to promote and enhance liver function, bile secretion, and bowel elimination, respectively, may suggest some of the mechanisms of action in treating acne.

Echinacea: Internal/Topical. Echinacea has been used traditionally to clear inflammatory skin problems. It was used in the treatment of boils, abscesses, and eruptive skin conditions. Echinacea is believed to exert its benefits in the treatment of skin conditions via enhancing the activity of the lymph system, which improves local elimination and reduces inflammation.[52] Echinacea also may be applied locally (i.e., topically) for inflammatory skin conditions. The polysaccharides are being investigated as possible active ingredients in its external activity.[77] Echinacea has demonstrated important immunomodulatory effects. In cell culture models of human bronchial epithelial cells and skin fibroblasts, a standardized preparation of *Echinacea purpurea* normalized IL-6 and IL-8 (CXCL8) levels.[88] It may be included in internal use formulae for chronic acne as a general antiinflammatory and immunotonic herb. Echinacea has been used successfully as a local antiinflammatory for minor wounds and may be considered as part of a rinse or cream-based topical preparation.[52]

Figwort: Internal. Figwort, an herb not commonly known outside of herbal and naturopathic practitioners, is an alterative used specifically in the treatment of skin

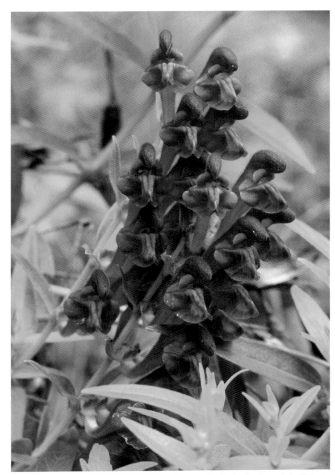

FIGURE 9-2 Chinese skullcap *(Scutellaria baicalensis).* (Photo by Martin Wall.)

conditions, usually reserved for those that are intractable, aggressive, or longstanding.[52] It is considered eliminative, having mild laxative, diuretic, and lymphatic activity. Hoffmann cites figwort as having cardiac stimulant activity, and cautions against its use in patients with tachycardia and those on cardiac glycosides, which it might potentiate.[78] It is otherwise unexpected to cause side effects when used at the recommended dosage.

Guggul: Internal. Guggul (equivalent to 25 mg guggulsterone) was found to decrease the number of inflammatory acne lesions by 68% in a small, randomized study (*n* = 20), compared with 65.2% with tetracycline (500 mg). The response in inflammatory lesions (e.g., papules, pustules, nodules, cystic lesions) was better than that in noninflammatory lesions (e.g., comedones). It is thought that the antilipolytic activity of guggulsterones reduces the output of sebum and inhibits the lipolysis of triglycerides to free fatty acids by bacteria.[89] The study design was not considered methodologically rigorous.[90]

Licorice: Internal. Licorice has demonstrated increased cortisol effects (primarily in ulcerative bowel conditions).[43,45,90-92] Glycyrrhizin, a saponin of licorice root, and its derivative, glycyrrhetinic acid (GA), have been found to inhibit 11-β-hydroxysteroid dehydrogenase, the enzyme that catalyzes conversion of cortisol to cortisone. One study found that 2% GA combined with hydrocortisone enhanced the local effects of the hydrocortisone. Because GA is already touted as a topical antiinflammatory for dermatitis and psoriasis, this may point to a potential concomitant use of GA with hydrocortisone, not only to enhance local effects but also to reduce systemic adverse effects with acne treatments.[93] It is used by herbalists as part of internal formulae for the treatment of acne and other inflammatory skin conditions. Licorice has not been directly studied for its effects in the treatment of acne; however, it should be considered for patients who wish to switch from corticosteroid treatments to a more natural approach to acne treatment, which should be done under the supervision of an experienced practitioner.[91]

Oregon Grape Root: Internal/Topical. Oregon grape root has a long history of use for the treatment of a variety of chronic skin conditions, including acne; it was listed as a bitter tonic in the *United States Pharmacopeia (USP)* until 1916 and the *National Formulary (NF)* until 1947; as discussed, this holds implications for its use in treating acne. One placebo-controlled clinical trial of nine male and female patients aged 12 to 30 years using a topical cream of 10% Oregon grape tincture in a 1:10 extract versus placebo, applied topically twice daily for 8 weeks, showed positive results: both groups demonstrated a reduction in skin oiliness and lesions, but only the Oregon grape group showed a decrease in sebum production. However, the study was considered too small and the preparation possibly too diluted to demonstrate a significant therapeutic effect.[94-96] Kraft lists Oregon grape as a primary treatment protocol for acne and seborrhea, citing its antiinflammatory effects.[97] Mitchell suggests that when thinking of Oregon grape, one should think of the skin-digestive system connection. He states that most cases of acne, eczema, and psoriasis are eased symptomatically by using this herb (Fig. 9-3).[98]

Tea Tree: Topical. Tea tree oil is a popular external application for skin problems. It has antibacterial and antifungal activity in vivo against a number of organisms, although its antiviral activities have not been conclusively demonstrated. An RCT of a 5% tea tree oil lotion demonstrated effectiveness as a topical antiseptic in the treatment of acne; it was slightly less effective than benzoyl peroxide in treating acne, although with fewer side effects. One hundred twenty-four patients were randomized to receive either tea tree oil or 5% benzoyl peroxide lotion for 3 months. Both groups showed improvement in the number of inflamed lesions, the number of noninflamed lesions, and skin oiliness. Side effects in the tea tree group included skin dryness, pruritus, stinging, burning, and redness.[77,99] A recent double-blind RCT tested the efficacy of a 5% topical tea tree oil gel in mild to moderate *Acne vulgaris*. Sixty patients with mild to moderate acne were randomized into treatment and placebo groups, and skin alterations were assessed using total acne lesions count (TLC) and acne severity index (ASI) every 15 days for 45 days. Statistically significant improvements in TLC and ASI scores were observed in the tea tree oil gel group compared with controls.[100] The *German Commission E Monographs* include skin inflammations and wound healing as indications for its use.[44] As with other essential oils, allergic dermatitis is a common side effect of tea tree oil, both from direct application to the skin (i.e., contact), inhalation of the vapors, and ingestion.[77,95] Skin irritation appears to increase with the age of the tea tree product, possibly as a result of oxidation products; thus product freshness and storage practices may influence the rates of dermatitis.[95]

Witch Hazel: Topical. The astringent and antiinflammatory herb witch hazel has been used successfully for the treatment of dermatologic conditions (i.e., inflammation, eczema) and may be used topically as a facial wash or in a cream base. Witch hazel distillate has demonstrated noteworthy effects in the treatment of topical inflammation after UV exposures, and witch hazel creams and ointments have shown antiinflammatory effects in patients suffering from atopic neurodermatitis, psoriasis, and eczema in a total of six different clinical trials.[92]

Yellow Dock: Internal. Yellow dock is a mild laxative, cholagogue, and alterative. Herbalists consider it a valuable herb in the treatment of chronic skin conditions, especially when there is accompanying constipation or digestive sluggishness.[80,98]

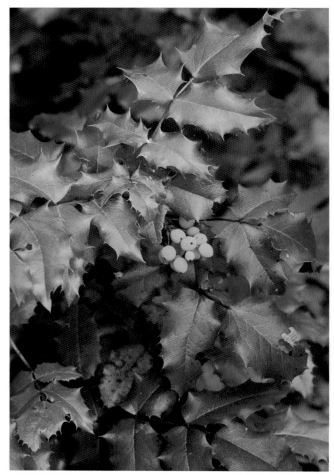

FIGURE 9-3 Oregon grape *(Mahonia aquifolium).* (Photo by Martin Wall.)

Topical Applications. The topical application of herbs for acne treatment relies on those that are antimicrobial, astringent, and antiinflammatory. Treatments may include the use of facial steams, washes, compresses, and creams. Topical use of neat (i.e., undiluted) essential oils is contraindicated owing to their irritating nature; their use may exacerbate the condition or cause tissue damage.

Differential Topical Treatment: Dry versus Oily Skin

Practitioners must be sensitive to the skin type and preferences of individual patients when choosing topical medications.[64] Agents containing a higher volume of alcohol may be preferable to patients with oily skin but drying to those whose skin is already dry. Conversely, patients with dry skin may prefer moisturizing bases such as creams, ointments, or oils.

Facial Steams

Hot facial steams are helpful for opening the pores and allowing delivery of antiseptic volatile oils to the affected areas. The patient is instructed to bring a large pot of water to a boil, and while doing so have ready a large bath towel, the necessary essential oils, and a trivet. The trivet is placed in a sink and when the water comes to a boil, the pot is placed on it. The lid is quickly opened, three to five drops of essential oil are added, and the lid quickly replaced. The patient is then to form a small tent over the head and sink and carefully remove the lid, allowing the steam to bathe the face. The face should be kept at least 18 inches from the pot and care must be taken to avoid burning from the steam. The steam exposure should be maintained for 3 minutes, after which the patient should rinse the face with cool water or an astringent herbal infusion (e.g., witch hazel distillate). Lavender, tea tree, and rosemary essential oils are all excellent antimicrobials and may be used alone or in combination. This treatment can be repeated several times weekly, and may be accompanied by systemic treatment. Herbalists often use lavender as a mild soothing topical antiseptic. Although no clinical trials using the extract or flowers have been identified, its aromatic nature enhances topical applications and inhalation of the essential oil has been shown to induce relaxation.[44,80] Witch hazel may be used as a cool rinse after the steam to tonify the pores. Additionally, the steam water can be substituted with an infusion of any number of botanicals for the skin, including a combination of the antiseptic and antiinflammatory herbs (e.g., calendula, chamomile, lavender, witch hazel) to which the essential oils are added.

Botanical Formulae for Acne

See Boxes 9-2 to 9-4 and 9-17.

Nutritional Considerations

Diet is an important part of any herbal treatment protocol. Cultures maintaining traditional diets other than Western diets clearly have lower rates of acne.[101,102] Optimal nutrition with an emphasis on foods and nutrients that promote skin health, as well as those that minimize the load on the

eliminative organs is recommended. Red meat should be minimized in the effort to reduce the overall inflammatory response. Specifically important is evaluating the diet for the presence of unhealthy oils and excessive refined carbohydrate intake.

BOX 9-2   Botanical Prescription for Acne Vulgaris

Tincture for Internal Use

Chinese skullcap	(Scutellaria baicalensis)	20 mL
Dandelion	(Taraxacum officinale)	20 mL
Echinacea	(Echinacea spp.)	20 mL
Licorice	(Glycyrrhiza glabra)	20 mL
Ashwagandha	(Withania somnifera)	10 mL
Oregon grape	(Mahonia aquifolium)	10 mL
	Total: 100 mL	

Dose: 3 mL two or three times daily depending on severity. Provide formula for 12 weeks, then reevaluate formula based on progress. The tincture can also be used at this dose during acute flare-ups only.

If acne is associated with the premenstrual period, give 5 mL *Vitex agnus-castus* each morning from the end of the menstrual period to the beginning of the next, for 3 consecutive months.

Rationale: Chinese skullcap, Oregon grape, echinacea, licorice, and ashwagandha appear in the formula for their alterative and antiinflammatory effects; Oregon grape and dandelion are choleretic, hepatic bitters; Oregon grape, echinacea, and licorice are antiviral, and licorice and ashwagandha are adaptogens included for general hypothalamic-pituitary-adrenal (HPA) support.

Rinse for External Use

Prepare a strong infusion using equal parts of the following herbs:

Calendula blossoms (Calendula officinalis)
Lavender flowers (Lavandula officinalis)
Rosemary leaf (Rosmarinus officinalis)
St. John's wort (Hypericum perforatum)
Witch hazel bark (Hamamelis virginiana)

Steam or wash the face or affected areas with hot water, then rinse the face or other affected areas once or twice daily with this infusion (either warm or at room temperature). Repeat daily as needed. This infusion also may be used as a warm compress rather than as a rinse.

BOX 9-3   Alterative Prescription for Treating Acne

Tincture for Internal Use

Echinacea	(Echinacea spp.)	25 mL
Cleavers	(Galium aparine)	25 mL
Dandelion root	(Taraxacum officinale)	25 mL
Red clover	(Trifolium pratense)	25 mL
	Total: 100 mL	

Dose: 5 mL twice daily.

BOX 9-4 Prescription for Constipation

Tincture or Infusion for Internal Use

Common Name	Scientific Name	Dried Herb	Tincture
Dandelion root	(*Taraxacum officinale*)	4 parts	40 mL
Yellow dock root	(*Rumex crispus*)	4 parts	40 mL
Anise seed	(*Pimpinella anisum*)	2 parts	20 mL
	Total: 10 parts		**100 mL**

Infusion Dose: Prepare as for standard infusion, one cup taken daily as warm tea in the morning.
Tincture Dose: 5 mL twice daily.

What to Expect with Treatment
Chronic acne typically requires 2 to 3 months of systemic and topical treatment before significant and consistent improvement is noticeable. Reduction in inflammation may be observable after several days of topical treatment with steams and skin rinses.

Warning Vitamin A in large doses (>5000 IU daily) is teratogenic. Supplementation in pregnant women or those planning to conceive should not exceed the normal amount present in a prenatal vitamin supplement and should only be taken as part of the prenatal vitamin. Extreme care should be taken in supplementation in those younger than 18 years old other than what is typical in a daily nutrient supplement.

TREATMENT SUMMARY FOR ACNE VULGARIS

- The skin is a reflection of overall health; thus herbalists take a systemic approach along with the use of local, topical applications.
- Digestive eliminative functions can be improved with the use of aperients such as dandelion root, yellow dock root, and flax seed and should be considered when acne is associated with chronic constipation or sluggish digestion (Box 9-4).
- Hormonal regulation is considered important when there is acne associated with menstrual problems and other hormonally related problems such as polycystic ovary syndrome (PCOS). Chaste berry is commonly used.
- Herbalists traditionally use herbs categorized as alteratives to improve lymphatic function and hepatic elimination, hormonal conjugation, and excretion. The most commonly used are burdock root, calendula, cleavers, yellow dock root, figwort, dandelion root, and red clover.
- An antiinflammatory diet is recommended and antiinflammatory herbs can be used internally and topically. These include licorice root, witch hazel, lavender, chamomile, and Chinese skullcap.
- Herbs can be used topically and internally to reduce infection and aid in reduction of inflammation. These include echinacea, lavender, Oregon grape, and tea tree.
- Stress can aggravate a tendency toward acne, and chronic acne can cause significant stress and depression. Herbal nervines, anxiolytics, and antidepressants can be included in formulae and include St. John's wort, lemon balm, skullcap, and blue vervain. Adaptogens can be used long term to improve the stress response, enhance immunity, regulate the hypothalamic-pituitary-adrenal (HPA) axis, and reduce inflammation. Ashwagandha should be considered. Other adaptogens are discussed in Chapter 5.
- Topical applications include washes, steams, and compresses. They are usually made up of antimicrobial and antiinflammatory herbs.
- Important nutritional considerations include an emphasis on optimal nutrition with good quality oils, brewer's yeast, vitamin A, zinc, vitamin B6, and vitamin C.
- Stress reduction and counseling can be beneficial in cases of severe and chronic acne.

Although there has been no scientifically proven correlation between chocolate consumption and acne, many adolescents and women report aggravated acne after consuming it in large amounts. Chocolate cravings also may indicate unmet nutritional needs, which should be met through diet and supplementation. Low Dog suggests that individuals should avoid those foods that they themselves believe to be aggravating.[83]

The following supplements have been shown to have a beneficial effect on acne:

- *Brewer's yeast:* 2 to 3 g three times daily may reduce insulin sensitivity and in one study showed a clinical improvement in acne patients. This supplement is contraindicated for those taking monoamine oxidase (MAO) inhibitors because concomitant use may cause hypertension.[66]
- *Vitamin A:* Retinoic compounds are a mainstay of acne treatment. Use of vitamin A as a treatment for acne may require intake of high (100,000 IU/day for 1 month followed by 25,000 to 50,000 IU per day for 3 months) and possibly unsafe dosages, leading to hypervitaminosis A and, if the use is prolonged, vitamin A toxicity. Kohani states that doses of 25,000 IU daily are safe and effective for acne treatment. Foods high in vitamin A (e.g., carrots, squash, sweet potatoes, apricots) can also be consumed as a regular part of the diet. Vitamin E assists in retinal regulation in humans and when combined with zinc may enhance the efficacy of the lower daily dose of vitamin A.[101]
- *Zinc:* Zinc is intrinsically important to the health of the skin, the healing of wounds, and to optimal immune functioning. There has been controversy over its effectiveness as an acne treatment, with some studies demonstrating effectiveness and others not showing benefit. The recommended dose for adolescents is 25 mg zinc picolinate twice daily for 2 weeks and then once daily for 2 months, taking care *not to exceed these recommended dosages.*[66,101]

- Vitamin B_6 (i.e., pyridoxine) has been shown to be beneficial when there is premenstrual aggravation of acne. Vitamin B_6 plays a role in steroid hormone metabolism and in animal studies B_6 deficiency appears to increase testosterone uptake and sensitivity.[101]
- Vitamin C has been suggested at a dose of 250 mg three times daily as a natural antiinflammatory.[101]

Additional Therapies

Hygiene

Although keeping the face clean can play an important role in maintaining healthy flora at the surface of the skin, over-cleansing of the face does not improve acne because poor facial cleansing does not cause it. In fact, excessive washing and scrubbing with abrasive cleansers can aggravate inflammation and damage the skin. Regular cleansing with antimicrobial soaps is also not recommended because they can encourage antibiotic resistance and destroy healthy skin flora, increasing susceptibility to secondary skin infections. Daily rinsing with warm water and a mild, natural ingredient soap, followed by a cool water rinse, is a good daily cleansing routine. Keeping the hair clean and off the face, keeping hands away from the face, and avoiding picking at pustules are all recommended. Avoid makeup that clogs the pores or is allergenic.

Stress Reduction and Counseling

The effect of acne on psychological and emotional health, and the influence of stress on acne, have both been made clear in this section. Stress reduction techniques and counseling can both be important parts of a treatment plan for those with acne, particularly adolescent girls, and particularly when acne is moderate to severe. Emotional and psychological support should not be overlooked.

▌AMENORRHEA

Amenorrhea is the absence of menses. It is divided into two categories: *primary amenorrhea*, the absence of menstruation by age 14 with no secondary sexual characteristics, or the absence of menstruation by age 16 regardless of the appearance of secondary sexual characteristics; and *secondary amenorrhea*, the absence of menstruation for a total of at least three previous menstrual cycle lengths, or at least 6 months in a previously menstruating woman in her reproductive years. Strict adherence to these criteria, however, should not lead to delay in medical evaluation in patients showing other signs of a medical condition warranting investigation.[1]

The prolonged absence of menstrual periods is considered normal only before puberty, during pregnancy, while breastfeeding, and after menopause. Primary amenorrhea is relatively uncommon, occurring in 0.3% of the population; secondary amenorrhea occurs in 1% to 3% of women; however, subgroups (e.g., college students, athletes) experience higher rates, the former as high as 5% and the latter as high as 66%. In most cases, patients with amenorrhea have simple problems that can be readily resolved; however, amenorrhea can be a challenging clinical situation caused by serious underlying conditions. It is completely normal for a woman to miss an occasional period. This can occur owing to stress, travel, illness, or minor or major changes that occur in the course of life (e.g., a breakup with a boyfriend, a move, a new job, a divorce).

PATHOPHYSIOLOGY

The absence of menstruation is a symptom of an underlying imbalance, disorder, or disease, rather than a disease in itself. The ability to menstruate is

"regulated by a complex mechanism that integrates biophysical and biochemical information composed of interactive levels of hormonal signals, autocrine/paracrine factors, and target cell reactions."
Clinical Gynecologic Endocrinology and Infertility[1]

Further, the ability to menstruate is dependent on a normal reproductive system. Genetic disorders, congenital abnormalities of the genital system (e.g., absence of the uterus or vagina, vaginal septum, cervical stenosis, imperforate hymen), endocrine disorders, pituitary or hypothalamic disorders, hyperthyroidism, hypothyroidism, defective enzyme systems, tumors, radiation or chemotherapy exposure, autoimmune diseases, smoking leading to premature ovarian failure, anorexia, abnormally low body fat or sudden weight loss (e.g., resulting from poverty, fad dieting, anorexia nervosa, bulimia, or very strenuous exercise), hypoglycemia, obesity, PCOS, emotional stress, medications, recent discontinuation of OCs, and past surgeries may cause amenorrhea. Most nonpregnant women with secondary amenorrhea have chronic anovulation, hypothyroidism, hyperprolactinemia, or weight loss and anorexia. Pituitary tumor is not uncommon in this category. Aside from pathologic and congenital etiologies of amenorrhea, eating disorders are a significant concern and common reason for lack of menstruation. Eating disorders can lead to severe and dangerous consequences and must be treated professionally as with any serious disease process.

SIGNS AND SYMPTOMS OF AMENORRHEA

Absence of periods may be accompanied by:
- Galactorrhea
- Symptoms of pregnancy
- Hirsutism (and other signs of androgen excess)
- Temperature intolerance
- Signs and symptoms of other disease

DIAGNOSIS

It is essential to take a comprehensive health and gynecologic history to include history of pediatric or adult cancer, thyroid or adrenal disorders, renal or liver disease, and history of exposure to medications, radiation, or chemotherapy. Pregnancy should be ruled out by pregnancy test rather than just by sexual history. An evaluation of recent or current stresses and lifestyle habits such as excessive exercise, dieting, or eating disorders is needed. A careful physical examination should assess for signs of congenital abnormality of the reproductive system. The patient should be assessed for the presence of galactorrhea, PCOS, and androgenization. Menopause should also be ruled out. Obstetric history must be reviewed, particularly for postpartum hemorrhage, which can lead to pituitary disease and resultant amenorrhea.

Other relevant tests include thyroid-stimulating hormone (TSH), PRL to rule out pituitary tumor, progesterone challenge, and estrogen challenge with progesterone withdrawal; the latter two tests to evaluate for anovulation and genital tract defects. Additionally, tests for ovarian and adrenal function, chromosomal disorders, autoimmune disease, anemia, and clotting disorders may need to be conducted. Brain magnetic resonance imaging (MRI) may be necessary to determine whether there is a pituitary tumor. Computed tomography (CT) or ultrasound scanning may be used to look for a tumor in the ovaries or adrenal glands (Box 9-5).

Differential Diagnosis

See Tables 9-5 and 9-6.

CONVENTIONAL TREATMENT APPROACHES

Treatment will vary widely depending on the cause of amenorrhea and may range from a dietary program to hormones or surgery.

Primary Amenorrhea

If a teenage girl has not started menstruating by age 16 and all test results are normal, an examination is performed every 3 to 6 months to monitor the progression of puberty. Progesterone and possibly estrogen may be given to start her periods. Estrogen is given to induce the changes of puberty in girls who have not developed breasts or pubic and underarm hair and cannot develop them spontaneously.

Secondary Amenorrhea

Treatment of secondary amenorrhea may include progesterone supplements (i.e., hormone treatment) and OCs (i.e., ovulation inhibitors). Dietary and exercise modifications may also be part of a treatment plan. In many cases, physicians will induce menstruation in nonpregnant women who have missed two or more consecutive menstrual periods to avoid increased risk of uterine cancer.

BOTANICAL TREATMENT OF AMENORRHEA

There is a long history of using herbs for the treatment of "retention of the menses," as amenorrhea is referred to in medieval botanical texts. Although it may appear that this was a convenient euphemism for herbal abortion prescriptions, there is evidence from classical texts such as the *Trotula* that such recommendations were also legitimately

---

BOX 9-5 Tests That May Be Considered When Evaluating Amenorrhea[103]

- ACTH (corticotrophin) and cortisol
- Chromosome analysis
- DHEA (dehydroepiandrosterone)-sulfate
- Human chorionic gonadotropin (hCG) level for pregnancy
- Imaging studies (head computed tomography [CT] or magnetic resonance imaging [MRI] scan, pelvic ultrasound)
- Laparoscopy
- Luteinizing hormone (LH) and follicle-stimulating hormone (FSH)
- Pap smear for maturation index
- Progesterone challenge
- Prolactin (PRL)
- Testosterone
- Thyroid-stimulating hormone (TSH), T3 (tri-iodothyronine), and T4 (thyroxine)
- Urine 17-ketosteroids

TABLE 9-5 Differential Diagnosis of Primary Amenorrhea

Athletic (hypothalamic) amenorrhea	Medications
Adrenal disease or dysfunction	Ovarian cysts, scarring, tumors
Autoimmune disease	Obesity
Chronic illness	Physiologic delay
Congenital abnormalities of the reproductive organs or sexual differentiation	Pituitary disorders/tumor
Cushing's syndrome	Polycystic ovary syndrome
Central nervous system disease	Prader-Willi syndrome; Turner's syndrome
Hyperprolactinemia	Psychiatric disorders including chronic stress, depression, emotional trauma, anorexia nervosa or other eating disorders
Hypothalamic disorders	Weight loss (sudden); eating disorders

---

TABLE 9-6 Differential Diagnosis of Secondary Amenorrhea

Conditions listed under Primary Amenorrhea	Menopause
Anovulation	Pituitary insufficiency (Sheehan's syndrome)
Autoimmune conditions	Post–oral contraceptive syndrome
Cervical scarring and stenosis	Pregnancy
Endometrial sclerosis	

intended for amenorrhea caused by a variety of etiologies. In fact, amenorrhea in the absence of pregnancy was considered a pathologic condition. Hippocrates and followers of the Hippocratic tradition believed that women eliminate harmful biological toxins through the process of regular menses. Amenorrhea was thought to lead to a dire pathologic build-up of these toxins; thus the largest percentage of prescriptions for women's diseases in most early medieval texts, reflecting the Hippocratic tradition, were "aids for provoking the menses."[3]

In the Eclectic literature, amenorrhea is often described as a cold, atonic condition requiring warming stimulants and tonifying herbs, for example, ginger Zingiber officinale (Fig. 9-4). It was described as sometimes being accompanied by a bearing down sensation or feeling of pressure, for which tonic, antispasmodic herbs were also given; for example, motherwort (*Leonurus cardiaca*) and black cohosh (*Actaea racemosa*). Contemporary practitioners recognize

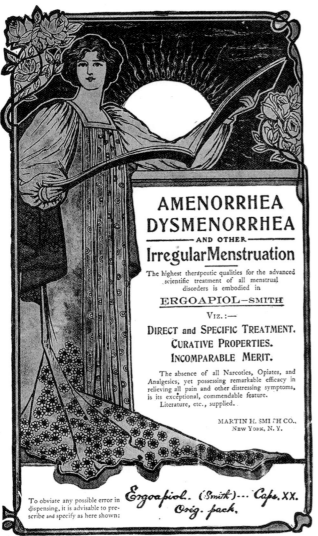

FIGURE 9-4 Amenorrhea/dysmenorrhea. Eclectic advertisement circa 1900.

that the cause of amenorrhea must be carefully identified to formulate an accurate and appropriate treatment strategy. Experimental evidence in primates indicates that corticotropin-releasing hormone (CRH) inhibits gonadotropin secretion, and this is the likely pathway by which stress interferes with reproductive function.[1] Stress-related amenorrhea is treated herbally with a combination of nervines and adaptogens. Targeting androgen excess and associated hyperinsulinemia is necessary in treating amenorrhea resulting from PCOS (see Polycystic Ovary Syndrome). Several studies have demonstrated reduction in PRL levels with chaste tree berry (*Vitex agnus-castus*), white peony (*Paeonia lactiflora*), and licorice (*Glycyrrhiza glabra*).[8] This may be considered with hyperprolactinemia in the absence of pituitary tumors. Amenorrhea associated with serious underlying disorders requires medical attention. Herbal treatments may be used as adjunct therapies in some of these cases. General botanical treatment strategies also include the use of herbs for promoting hormonal regulation, improving pelvic circulation and uterine tone (i.e., emmenagogues, warming pelvic circulatory stimulants, uterine tonics), and relieving pelvic tension (i.e., antispasmodics). Some of the effects of traditional actions of herbs on the reproductive organs have been associated with herbal activities on various prostaglandin receptors, α-adrenergic receptors, and H_1 receptors. Mills and Bone suggest that subtle hormonal effects are most likely responsible for the menstrual stimulating effects of herbs classified as emmenagogues.[52] Herbs may also be included to improve nutrition when women are energy deficient, underweight, or anemic (e.g., dong quai, ashwagandha, nettles, rehmannia, raspberry leaf).

Almost no clinical research has been done on botanical treatments for amenorrhea. There is a limited number of studies demonstrating efficacy in the treatment of amenorrhea with TCM protocol.[104,105] The majority of evidence supporting the efficacy of herbs in stimulating menstrual flow is derived from contemporary herbalists' clinical practice, and from the misuse of emmenagogues as abortifacients. According to toxicology reports, rue is the plant most commonly misused to induce abortion.[106] Herbalists do not routinely use this herb for the treatment of amenorrhea. Contemporary herbalists typically do not perform or endorse herbal abortion owing to the ethical and legal considerations; also because of the risks of the required volume of herbs and their toxicity in these doses, some of which are associated with a high morbidity and mortality rate.[52,106]

WEISS ON AMENORRHEA AND THE USE OF EMMENAGOGUES

According to Dr. Rudolph Fritz Weiss in his book *Herbal Medicine*, herbs tend to be more effective in treating secondary amenorrhea. Weiss points out that delayed puberty will generally not respond to botanical therapies; however, "medicinal plants get very good results in secondary amenorrhea and in oligomenorrhea." He adds that "Medicinal herbs ...

Continued

WEISS ON AMENORRHEA AND THE USE OF EMMENAGOGUES—cont'd

continue to have their place. Emmenagogues were very popular before hormone therapy. There remains the fact, based on experience, that emmenagogues will often restore normal menstrual flow and give very considerable subjective relief." All herbal emmenagogues are contraindicated in pregnancy.

In spite of lack of scientific evidence directly supporting the efficacy or safety of herbal emmenagogues, many women with nonpathologic bases for their amenorrhea prefer an herbal approach before using hormones for treatment, as do many women who have "just missed a period or two" and who do not technically have amenorrhea. The historical and clinical use of herbs for the treatment of amenorrhea suggests areas that warrant further study, particularly on the hormonal effects of these botanicals, and on the adjunct effects of herbs such as nervines for treatment.

Lifestyle modifications, for example, stress management or addressing weight gain or weight loss as necessary, are always included in a comprehensive treatment plan and may be suggested before initiation of herbal therapies. It is essential to rule out pregnancy before beginning an herbal program to "bring on" the menses; in high enough doses many are

potentially toxic to the fetus, and some may to act as abortifacients (Table 9-7).

Discussion of Botanicals
Blue Cohosh

Blue cohosh was used by northeastern indigenous American tribes to encourage menstruation and facilitate childbirth. The Eclectic physicians adopted blue cohosh as a treatment for a variety of gynecologic complaints, among them the treatment of amenorrhea, especially, but not exclusively, resulting from cold.[107] Felter describes *Caulophyllum* as an emmenagogue to be used where there is amenorrhea owing to pelvic congestion with irritation.[108] It was listed as an official emmenagogue in the *USP* from 1882 to 1905, after which it was dropped, and the *NF* from 1916 to 1950.[80,107] Eclectics relied on both the tincture of blue cohosh and a concentrated product of the glycosidic derivative *leontin*, which was particularly employed in the treatment of amenorrhea and was considered to give "excellent and quick results."[107] It was also used when there was excessive uterine, menstrual, or postnatal bleeding. Blue cohosh was also considered an antispasmodic and mild sedative in cases of anxiety and restlessness; however, it is not used for these indications in contemporary clinical practice. Herbalists today use blue cohosh for menstrual difficulties including amenorrhea and dysmenorrhea, whereas midwives widely use it to stimulate labor.[109] (See

TABLE 9-7   Summary of Botanical Treatment Strategies for Amenorrhea

Therapeutic Goal	Therapeutic Activity	Botanical Name	Common Name
Stimulate pelvic circulation; improve uterine tone; promote menstruation	Emmenagogues	*Angelica sinensis*	Dong quai
		Artemisia vulgaris	Mugwort
		Caulophyllum thalictroides	Blue cohosh
		Cinnamomum spp.	Cinnamon
		Gossypium herbaceum	Cotton root
		Leonurus cardiaca	Motherwort
		Zingiber officinale	Ginger
Treat hormonal dysregulation (e.g., hyperprolactinemia, insufficient progesterone)	Hormonal modulators	*Angelica sinensis*	Dong quai
		Glycyrrhiza glabra	Licorice
		Paeonia lactiflora	White peony
		Vitex agnus-castus	Chaste berry
Treat emotional and psychological stress and depression	Nervines	*Avena sativa*	Milky oats
		Humulus lupulus	Hops
		Hypericum perforatum	St. John's wort
		Leonurus cardiaca	Motherwort
		Matricaria recutita	Chamomile
		Melissa officinalis	Lemon balm
		Passiflora incarnata	Passionflower
		Scutellaria baicalensis	Skullcap
		Ziziphus spinosa	Ziziphus
Improve stress resistance	Adaptogens	*Eleuterococcus senticosus*	Eleuthera
		Panax ginseng	Ginseng
		Withania somnifera	Ashwagandha
Relieve pain/discomfort/pelvic pressure/ bearing down sensations accompanying amenorrhea	Antispasmodics	*Actaea racemosa*	Black cohosh
		Dioscorea villosa	Wild yam
		Leonurus cardiaca	Motherwort
		Viburnum spp.	Cramp bark, black haw
Improve general nutrition	Nutritive tonics Adaptogens	See Actions of Herbs See Adaptogens	

Chapter 15.) Blue cohosh is considered useful when there is uterine atony. Bone describes it as an ovarian tonic; however, this activity has not been demonstrated by scientific evaluation.[80] Its uterine-stimulating activity is justified by its chemical constituents, in vitro and in vivo studies, and clinical observation. Blue cohosh root contains the oxytocic quinolizidine alkaloids sparteine and N-methycystisine.[110,111] The liquid extract, hot water extract, saponin fraction, and isolated caulosaponin have all demonstrated utero-stimulant activity.[80] Toxicity symptoms (e.g., hyperthermia, hypertension, tachycardia, hyperventilation, diaphoresis, weakness) have been reported from excessive dosing in abortion attempts.[80] Blue cohosh is contraindicated for use during early pregnancy owing to potential teratogenicity, and throughout pregnancy because of abortifacient activity.

Chaste Berry

The Eclectic physicians used chaste berry as an emmenagogue, and contemporary herbalists continue to use it for a wide variety of menstrual irregularities, including amenorrhea.[112] The German Commission E approved it for irregularities of the menstrual cycle, premenstrual complaints, and mastodynia.[44] No specific studies were identified using chaste berry for the treatment of amenorrhea; however, it has shown menstrual regulating effects in a number of trials. Sustained use of *V. agnus-castus* over several weeks during the immediate postpartum period was associated with early return of the menses. McKenna and colleagues suggest that use of *V. agnus-castus* may be of benefit in restoring ovulation and the menstrual cycle in the lactating mother who is ready to resume regular cycles and to conceive another child.[43] [*Note:* This is an opinion that I corroborate from clinical use in my midwifery practice, where I have worked with women who have had lactation-related amenorrhea persisting between 10 and 18 months who wished to become pregnant with a subsequent child. Use of *V. agnus-castus* for 2 to 6 weeks, 5 mL twice daily, has resulted in resumed menstruation in several cases.] In vitro studies suggest a dopaminergic effect inhibiting release of PRL from the anterior pituitary gland, and several trials demonstrate regulation of the menstrual cycle, lengthening of the luteal phase of the menstrual cycle, and reduction of PMS symptoms.[80,113] An anecdotal report describes three patients with amenorrhea resulting from anorexia nervosa, hormonal imbalance, or idiopathic causes who were treated with 40 drops daily of 0.2% dried extract of *V. agnus-castus* fruit. Menstruation resumed in all three women after 5 weeks to 3 months. *V. agnus-castus* extract inhibited PRL release from rat pituitary cells; LH and FSH release were not affected.[113] Use of this herb is not recommended in conjunction with OCs, hormone replacement therapy (HRT), or progesterone drugs because it may interfere with these.[48,80]

Cotton Root Bark

Cotton root bark was historically used by indigenous North American tribes as an emmenagogue and abortifacient. Its use as an emmenagogue was adopted by the Eclectic physicians, and it was used as an abortifacient by southern physicians into the 1800s.[32,114] The plant has a profound history, reportedly used as an abortifacient by female slaves in the United States who were frequently victims of rape by their "masters," and consequently, experienced unwanted pregnancies.[32] The plant was marketed by Lloyd Pharmaceuticals and Eli Lilly as an oxytocic, emmenagogic agent. The *USP* listed cotton root as a parturient from 1860 to 1880. Cotton root is listed in the 1983 *British Herbal Pharmacopoeia (BHP)* as an emmenagogue.[115] The pharmaceutical agent *gossypol,* investigated for its male and female antifertility potential, as well as for anticancer activity, is derived from the cotton seed (and is now also synthetically produced). Animal and in vitro studies confirm the antifertility effects of gossypol observed in clinical trials. Use of gossypol (20 to 60 mg daily, or 0.6 to 0.8 mg/kg, for up to 6 months) has been associated with the risk of hypokalemia and possible permanent sterility. Less common adverse reactions that have been reported mainly in clinical trials with gossypol include mild leukopenia and thrombocytopenia, fatigue, dry mouth and skin, gastrointestinal (GI) distress, minor alopecia, and mild hepatotoxic effects. Cardiotoxic and hepatotoxic effects have been reported in animals and in vitro with gossypol. Altered hormone levels and other metabolic effects have been reported mainly in animals and in vitro but are also reported in human studies.[116] Gossypol is present in the seed in 0.5% concentration, and in lesser concentrations throughout the plant. Low Dog suggests it may actually induce amenorrhea and endometrial atrophy, thus resulting in infertility.[32] Gossypol has antiprogesterogenic activity; its action on the corpus luteum can cause abortion. Seed extract has demonstrated abortifacient effects in rat models, and marked malformations in uninterrupted pregnancies.[117] The root bark extract (not gossypol) is currently used by Western herbalists as an emmenagogue in cases of amenorrhea and as a uterine antihemorrhagic. Midwives occasionally use it as a labor stimulant in postdates pregnancies (see Chapter 20). No studies were identified in the literature on use of whole plant extracts; thus the safety of this herb cannot be accurately determined. It is clear, however, that this herb may have teratogenic effects if taken during early pregnancy, and may induce abortion or labor.

Dong Quai

Dong quai is one of the most important herbs used in TCM formulae for menstrual irregularities and amenorrhea. It has been used traditionally to treat conditions associated with the TCM diagnoses of "blood stasis" and "blood vacuity" (i.e., "emptiness," "deficiency").[118] Whole root has been shown to have a stimulatory effect on the uterus in vivo, and studies have demonstrated its ability to relax or coordinate uterine contractions depending on uterine tone. He and coworkers found a decoction of *Angelica sinensis* effective in treating patients with "energy-deficient" amenorrhea.[104] No other clinical studies have been done to substantiate its use in the treatment of amenorrhea.[80,118] Chronic and high-dose use of dong quai has been cited by herbalists as a cause of increased menstrual bleeding and increased period frequency; therefore many herbalists recommend its discontinued use during the menstrual period. It is regularly used by herbalists in Western herbal formulae to "move" the blood, improve nourishment, and stimulate the menses.

Ginger

In keeping with the belief that amenorrhea can be a result of "cold" conditions and brought on by exposure to cold, ginger is mentioned in the Eclectic text *Materia Medica and Clinical Therapeutics* (1905) as a treatment for congestive dysmenorrhea and amenorrhea.[114] It was recommended that tincture be taken diluted in hot water. Bone and Hoffmann also cite its traditional use as an emmenagogue.[78,80] Contemporary herbalists continue to incorporate fresh or dried ginger root into amenorrhea formulae as an adjunct herb, largely believed to increase pelvic circulation, warmth, and relaxation. It is also used topically over the lower abdomen as a fomentation. No studies have evaluated ginger's activity as an emmenagogue. Studies have demonstrated its safety and efficacy in tea and capsule forms in treating nausea and vomiting of pregnancy (NVP) even during first trimester pregnancy, suggesting that it does not have a directly abortifacient effect in modest, therapeutic doses.[77,119-121] However, it is recommended that doses not exceed 2 g of dried ginger daily during gestation.[120]

Motherwort

Motherwort was regarded by herbalists and the Eclectics as an emmenagogic agent to be used in cases of amenorrhea associated with nervous disorders. It was considered useful both internally and as a fomentation over the lower abdominal region.[122] Early research on the extract demonstrated mild uterine stimulatory and antispasmodic activity.[80] The German Commission E supports its use for nervous cardiac disorders, as an adjunct therapy in the treatment of hyperthyroidism, and mentions its traditional use for amenorrhea.[44] Motherwort is widely used by herbalists for a variety of menstrual disorders including dysmenorrhea, amenorrhea, and PMS; they find it a reliable uterotonic and nervine, especially when there is anxiety or irritability. Because of its bitter taste, it is primarily used in tincture form.

Mugwort and Artemisia Spp

Named for the Greek queen and healer Artemisia, who is credited with discovering the use of wormwood for women's health problems, and perhaps as a tribute to the Greek goddess Artemis, protector of women and children, members of the *Artemisia* family have been used for centuries for the treatment of amenorrhea and as abortifacients. In fact, several species are mentioned in ancient Greek sources.[123] *A. absinthium* (i.e., wormwood) was used as an oxytocic by Soranus and by Dioscorides to induce menstruation, abortion, miscarriage, and placental delivery. *A. arborescens* (i.e., southernwood) was considered an emmenagogue by Dioscorides, although not by Soranus. Pliny recommended it to be used as a sitz bath for "uterine inflammation." Galen also reported on the use of mugwort for amenorrhea.[3] It was popular in the sixteenth and seventeenth centuries for women's complaints, when it was referred to as *mater herbarum*.[123] The *BHP* lists *A. arborescens* as an emmenagogue.[115]

SAGE AND THE POWER OF HERBAL EMMENAGOGUES: A CAUTIONARY TALE

In the early years of my midwifery practice, about 20 years ago, I knew a midwife who conveyed the following story to me. She had become pregnant with her third baby while still breastfeeding her second child, then 10 months old. She was excited about the pregnancy but wanted to wean the older baby because she was fatigued. She had read in an herb book at her local health food store that sage was effective at drying up breast milk, so she decided to try this method to wean her baby. She obtained dried culinary sage and prepared a cup of tea using 1 tablespoon of the dried herb to 1 cup of boiling water. Approximately 30 minutes after drinking the tea, she experienced a sudden uterine hemorrhage that required an emergency dilation and curettage (D&C) at the hospital. She had miscarried. She had no prior history of miscarriage, and carried her next pregnancy to term with no complications. This reminder of the powerful nature of herbs instilled in me a great respect for using caution with even modest doses of possible emmenagogues during pregnancy—even seemingly benign culinary ones such as sage!

A. vulgaris (i.e., mugwort) was used traditionally as a treatment for amenorrhea and also dysmenorrhea, and it is the *Artemisia* species most likely to be used by herbalists in the United States today for gynecologic concerns.[77,78,124] In the Unani herbal tradition of India, single-dose mugwort decoctions (10 g) are dispensed for the treatment of amenorrhea, and this herb is also used in Ayurvedic medicine for "functional amenorrhea."[77] It is included in the German Commission E as an unapproved herb because of lack of therapeutic claims. Its gynecologic uses include menstrual problems and irregular periods, as well as promoting circulation and as a sedative; abortifacient action has been reported.[44] This intensely bitter herb is popular among grassroots women herbalists in the United States as an emmenagogue, and is often combined with other emmenagogic herbs such as pennyroyal herb, yarrow, and ginger in tea, taken hot.[125] Other *Artemisia* spp. are very high in the essential oil thujone, and may cause serious side effects if not used properly.[124] Mugwort contains only trace amounts of thujone and no side effects are expected when this herb is used in therapeutic doses. However, it may cause sensitization or allergic dermatitis, particularly in patients sensitive to the pollen in the *Asteraceae* family.[77,78]

Schisandra

Schisandra has demonstrated adaptogenic and tonic effects in experimental models and is sold in the United States as an adaptogenic tonic for decreasing fatigue and improving performance and endurance.[80,126] It is believed to strengthen uterine contractions and its use is cited in TCM to stimulate labor.[43,127] A 70% schisandra combination extract of the fruit suspension, fruit, and fruit coat demonstrated uterine stimulant activity in the pregnant, nonpregnant, and postpartum rabbit uterus, whereas a tincture administered to rabbits caused increased uterine tension and contractility. Its mechanism of action is not known. It appears to possess oxytocic effects; however, there are no endocrine receptor studies of this herb.[43] No clinical research has been conducted on its effects as an emmenagogue. McKenna and colleagues note that the effects of schisandra as an ovulation stimulator may have unpredictable effects on lactation-induced amenorrhea. Schisandra has a good safety profile when used in appropriate doses and with consideration of TCM contraindications (i.e., presence of excess heat, rash, early signs of a cough, epilepsy, excessive exercise, hypertension, intracranial pressure, excessive mental excitement, peptic ulcer).[43,126,127]

 A WORD ABOUT FALSE UNICORN: AN ENDANGERED SPECIES

Chamaelirium luteum, or false unicorn root, has traditionally been used by numerous native American tribes and the Eclectic physicians for the treatment of all manner of gynecologic conditions in which there was a lack of tone or vigor, and by the Eclectics to regulate glandular activity. It has traditionally been used as a stimulant for the treatment of amenorrhea.[82,107,127] False unicorn is popular on Internet chat groups for women seeking complementary and alternative medicine (CAM) therapies for the treatment of a variety of gynecologic difficulties, especially infertility. It is recognized as an ecologically at-risk botanical and it is very difficult to cultivate; thus its general use should not be widely recommended. Alternative herbs should be used when possible.

White Peony

Paeoniflorin, a constituent of white peony root, has demonstrated inhibition of testosterone synthesis in vitro without affecting estradiol synthesis. It reduces testosterone production by the ovaries but not the adrenal glands. In an ovariectomized model, oral administration of a combination of white peony and licorice increased dehydroepiandrosterone (DHEA) and serum estrogen concentration. It acts as a uterine smooth muscle relaxant in several animal species. In one case study, TJ-68, a Japanese traditional herbal formula containing *Paeonia lactiflora* and licorice, demonstrated effectiveness in treating risperidone-induced amenorrhea and hyperprolactinemia.[105] This combination, which consists of 6 g each of dried white peony root and licorice, has also demonstrated efficacy in clinical trials, lowering serum testosterone levels and inducing regular ovulation in one study, and improving testosterone levels and fertility in a group of PCOS patients.[80] In 2008, combination of white peony-glycyrrhiza decoction (PGD) and bromocriptine (BMT) demonstrated efficacy in attenuating risperidone-induced hyperprolactinemia in a small set of women (*n* = 20) currently experiencing oligomenorrhea or amenorrhea. The study utilized a crossover design. Women were randomized to receive either PGD (45g/d) or BMT (5g/d) for 4 weeks, followed by a 4-week washout, then another 4 weeks of the alternate treatment. PGD significantly decreased end-point serum PRL levels (comparable to BMT) without altering serum testosterone, progesterone, or estradiol.[128] It is commonly used by herbalists both in TCM formulae and in combination with Western

herbs in individualized patient prescriptions. The effects of this herb suggest it for treatment of amenorrhea, particularly in women with PCOS, although further research is required (Box 9-6).

 CAUTION AGAINST THE USE OF SEVERAL POPULAR HERBS TO BRING ON THE MENSES: RUE, PENNYROYAL, AND LIFE ROOT

American pennyroyal *(Hedeoma pulegioides)*: A member of the mint family; was considered specific by the Eclectics for "Amenorrhea of long standing, with pallor and anemia and dark circles around the eyes; the patient complains of languor, lassitude, takes cold easily, has pain in back and limbs."[44] It is probably the most notorious of the herbal emmenagogue-abortifacient genre of herbs owing to widely publicized adverse events and deaths caused by consumption of pennyroyal essential oil in attempted abortion. Pennyroyal oil is considered one of the most toxic of the essential oils because of the hepatic effects of pugelone, and the abortifacient dose is similar to the toxic dose.[48,123] The toxic effects of the oil have long been recognized: Felter stated in 1922 that "Oil of pennyroyal produces toxic effects when given in overdoses. A drachm caused severe headache, difficult swallowing, intense nausea, severe retching without emesis, intolerable bearing down, labor like pains, abdominal tenderness, constipation, dyspnea, semi paralysis of the limbs, and nervous weakness and prostration." Pennyroyal oil is no longer available in the herbal market because of its toxicity. In contrast, drinking the infusion of the leafy stems is considered safe.[48] However, there were two cases of acute liver damage reported in California in 1996 in infants given pennyroyal infusion; one case resulted in fatality.[48] The infusion was a popular diaphoretic among the Eclectics used for the treatment of acute colds.[82] It is popular among grassroots herbalists for the treatment of amenorrhea, generally combined with other emmenagogic herbs.

Ruta graveolens: Although rue is an effective emmenagogue, the furanocoumarin content of the plant presents a toxicologically known risk.[125] The German Commission E does not support its use, stating that the known risks outweigh the benefit of the plant.[44] Rue oil can cause contact dermatitis; phototoxicity, severe liver and kidney damage, and deaths of pregnant women attempting abortion have all been reported with its use. Therapeutic doses can cause melancholy, sleep disorders, dizziness, and spasms. The use of this herb is not recommended on the basis of significant safety concerns.

Senecio aureus, S. vulgaris, S. jacobaea: Mitchell references the use of *Senecio* species (i.e., ragwort) for the treatment of amenorrhea, dysmenorrhea, metrorrhagia, and menorrhagia.[98] Based on information in popular herb books for women's health, women may use this herb for a variety of menstrual disorders. However, such use is not recommended because of the contents of pyrrolizidine alkaloids (PAs) in *Senecio* spp., which has caused serious and occasionally fatal cases of venoocclusive disease in humans, and poisonings and deaths in animals. Bovine and equine poisoning with this herb, whether from grazing or feed contamination, has been widely reported in the literature.[48,126] I cannot recommend the use of this herb on the basis of significant safety concerns.

TREATMENT SUMMARY FOR AMENORRHEA

- Rule out pregnancy before starting any treatment.
- Proper diagnosis of the cause of amenorrhea is essential because causes may range from stress to hormonal dysregulation, which can be indicative of an underlying disorder such as polycystic ovary syndrome (PCOS). Primary versus secondary amenorrhea must also be determined.
- General botanical treatment includes the use of herbs for improving hormonal regulation, for example, chaste berry, when there is underlying hormonal dysregulation. Treatment of accompanying conditions (e.g., PCOS) should occur concurrently.
- Emphasis is placed on improving pelvic circulation and uterine tone via the use of warming pelvic stimulants, emmenagogues, and uterotonic herbs, as well as through pelvic movement and exercise, for example, belly dancing or yoga postures.
- Pelvic relaxation is effected through the use of antispasmodics.
- Stress-related factors contributing to amenorrhea are treated with a combination of nervines and adaptogens, for example, milky oats, hops, St. John's wort, motherwort, chamomile, passionflower, skullcap, eleuthero, ginseng, and ashwagandha.
- Adaptogens may be used to improve energy and nutrition when women are energy deficient, underweight, or anemic.
- Proper body weight should be achieved through attention to diet and avoiding excessive exercise. Body image issues sometimes can be addressed through counseling.

What to Expect with Amenorrhea Treatment

If amenorrhea is acute and owing to stress, travel, or other simple disruption of regular lifestyle rhythm, the use of emmenagogues and warming pelvic stimulants can bring on the menses within a couple of days of treatment. In chronic amenorrhea, duration of treatment is usually longer, commonly one or more expected menstrual cycles before the menses becomes regular. The treatment course will also depend on the nature of the underlying cause; for example, if it is PCOS, treatment will be ongoing and it may take 3 to 6 months to see lasting and significant effects.

BOX 9-6 Botanical Prescriptions for Amenorrhea

Tincture for Internal Use

Black cohosh	(Actaea racemosa)	20 mL
Dong quai	(Angelica sinensis)	20 mL
Motherwort	(Leonurus cardiaca)	20 mL
White peony	(Paeonia lactiflora)	20 mL
Ginger	(Zingiber officinale)	20 mL
		Total: 100 mL

Dose: 5 mL twice daily until the onset of the menses.

Rationale: White peony is included as a hormonal regulator; motherwort is a bitter nervine, acting on the liver and reducing stress, tension, and irritability; dong quai is a blood nourisher and antiinflammatory adaptogenic tonic. Both motherwort and dong quai are used to promote pelvic circulation and menstrual flow; black cohosh is an antispasmodic for the uterus, and ginger is antiinflammatory, antispasmodic, and increases pelvic flow. It also improves the taste of the formula and is an "activating" herb in the formula.

Sample Infusion for Amenorrhea

From *Herbal Remedies for Women* by Amanda McQuade Crawford

Eleuthero	(Eleutherococcus senticosus)	2 parts
Licorice root	(Glycyrrhiza glabra)*	2 parts
Motherwort	(Leonurus cardiaca)	1 part
Mugwort leaf	(Artemisia vulgaris)	1 part
Peppermint	(Mentha piperita)	2 parts
Skullcap	(Scutellaria lateriflora)	2 parts
		Total: 10 parts

Indications: Amenorrhea caused by stress.

To prepare: Infusion using 28 g (1 ounce)/750 mL (3 cups) water, steeped 10 to 15 minutes.
Dose: One cup three times daily for 10 to 12 days; then take a 1-week break. If menses does not occur, repeat using half the amount of herbs per 3 cups of water. Repeat for up to 3 months.

Rationale: Mugwort and motherwort are included for their specifically emmenagogic actions, whereas eleuthero is included as a nourishing and tonic adaptogen to regulate the hypothalamic-pituitary-adrenal (HPA) axis. Skullcap is a gentle nervine; mint is a digestive tonic and improves the flavor of the formula, as does licorice, which is also an antiinflammatory, adaptogen, and harmonizer of the entire formula.

Topical Applications
Ginger compress: Use in conjunction with internal treatment. Apply hot directly over the lower abdomen, several times per week until the onset of menses.

*If there is hypertension, omit the licorice and replace with 1 part each marshmallow and burdock roots.

Additional Therapies

It is essential to address lifestyle, dietary, and psychobiological factors when treating a patient with amenorrhea. Optimally, a patient should have at least 22% body fat, exercise within moderation, learn stress management, and not smoke. There is a substantial correlation between inadequate body weight, eating disorders, psychological disorders, and amenorrhea.

These conditions can lead to severe and even fatal consequences when left untreated. Excessive exercise, whether as part of an athletic training program, as a result of addiction to an "exercise high," or because of a body-image disorder, can result in amenorrhea and other medical consequences. Patients should be referred to physicians, therapists, and nutritionists as appropriate.

There are still many negative connotations about menstruation and female sexuality in our society. Interestingly, the earliest reported case of anorexia and amenorrhea occurred around the year 1000 in Portugal, when Wilgefortis, the King's seventh daughter, in protest of an undesired arranged marriage, went into intense prayer. Her anorexic state was accompanied by loss of her sexual characteristics, and she was released from the marriage. (She was instead crucified by her father!) She became a symbol of a woman who freed herself of her female problems and unwanted men, and later became a patron saint of women with sexual problems or problems associated with childbirth. The association between eating disorders and the desire to separate from sexual development at puberty is well recognized today.[1] It is important to refer patients for counseling to discuss issues of sexuality and menstruation when problematic. Explain to your patient that there is nothing bad or wrong about menstruating; that it is a healthy, normal, physiologic process.

DYSMENORRHEA

Dysmenorrhea literally means "difficult menstruation," and refers to painful menstruation. The pain may be of varying intensity, and is characterized by pelvic discomfort and menstrual cramps that may be wavelike or constant, and which may radiate to the lower back, legs, and vulva. Dysmenorrhea is frequently accompanied by additional symptoms including backache, headache, dizziness, nausea, vomiting, and diarrhea. Discomfort may begin 12 to 24 hours before menses and persist for the first 48 to 72 hours of the period. Estimates of adolescent girls and women experiencing dysmenorrhea range from 45% to 95% internationally, with debilitating to incapacitating dysmenorrhea occurring in approximately 7% to 15% of women. Dysmenorrhea is a major cause of work and school absenteeism, as well as a significant reason for regular use of analgesics and nonsteroidal antiinflammatory drugs (NSAIDs).

Dysmenorrhea is categorized as either primary or secondary dysmenorrhea. Primary dysmenorrhea is pain in the absence of organic pathology. It mostly affects young women, and has an onset after the beginning of ovulatory menstrual cycles. Secondary dysmenorrhea is associated with underlying pathology, for example, endometriosis or ovarian cysts. It typically occurs in the third and fourth decades of life, and presents with painful periods that often become increasingly severe. Dysmenorrhea is more prevalent in smokers. It typically improves in most women after a full-term pregnancy.

PATHOPHYSIOLOGY

Primary dysmenorrhea is caused by myometrial contraction induced by excessive cyclic prostaglandin $F_{2\alpha}$ ($PGF_{2\alpha}$) production in the secretory endometrium. Dysmenorrheic women appear to produce as much as seven times more $PGF_{2\alpha}$ than asymptomatic women. Excessive prostaglandin also leads to increased intrauterine pressure. Concomitantly, this same form of prostaglandin causes smooth muscle contractility in other muscles, leading to other symptoms associated with dysmenorrhea. The greatest menstrual release of prostaglandins occurs in the first 48 hours, the time of greatest symptom intensity. The cause of secondary dysmenorrhea is the presence of underlying pelvic pathology.

SIGNS AND SYMPTOMS

- Cramps, spasm, and nagging discomfort in the uterus, pelvis, and/or lower back accompanying menstruation
- Accompanying menstruation, pelvic heaviness, fullness, and aching that is typically worse when upright and active and remits somewhat with rest and reclining postures
- Headache, nausea, vomiting, or diarrhea may accompany dysmenorrhea

DIAGNOSIS

Primary and secondary dysmenorrhea are diagnosed by symptom picture, history of onset and occurrence, and the exclusion of underlying structural or pathologic abnormalities (Tables 9-8 and 9-9). Dysmenorrhea is markedly cyclical, with discomfort occurring just before or during the menstrual period.

Differential Diagnosis

See Tables 9-8 and 9-9.

TABLE 9-8 Differential Diagnosis of Primary Dysmenorrhea	
Bowel obstruction	Ovarian cysts
Constipation	Pelvic inflammatory disease (PID)
Endometriosis	Renal inflammatory and infectious disorders
Irritable bowel syndrome (IBS)	Renal colic
Intestinal ulcers	Uterine fibroids
Miscarriage	Urinary tract infection (UTI)
Musculoskeletal disorders	

TABLE 9-9 Differentiating Primary and Secondary Dysmenorrhea	
Primary Dysmenorrhea	**Secondary Dysmenorrhea**
Occurs after menarche with the onset of ovulatory cycles	Occurs in second to fourth decades of life
Occurs in relationship to the menses, usually just before and through the first 12-72 hours of the menses	May occur before, during, or after the menses
Typically improves over time	Typically worsens over time

The editor wishes to thank *Botanical Medicine for Women's Health*, ed 1 contributor to this chapter, Jillian Stansbury.

CONVENTIONAL TREATMENT

Conventional treatment options are the prostaglandin synthetase inhibitors (PGSIs), NSAIDs, and OCs.

Prostaglandin Synthetase Inhibitors

PGSIs prevent the synthesis of prostaglandin, thus reducing uterine hypercontractility, pressure, ischemia, and pain. Improvement also occurs in concurrent symptoms including backache, nausea, vomiting, dizziness, leg pain, insomnia, and headache. There is also a reduction in the amount of menstrual blood flow. PGSIs are quick acting, can be taken once symptoms have begun, and are effective in reducing pain in about 80% of dysmenorrheic women. Side effects include GI upset, edema, and skin rash.

Oral Contraceptives

OCs also work on the principle of decreasing prostaglandin production. Long-term OC use has side effects and is contraindicated in women who smoke, have high blood pressure, or have blood-clotting problems. Many women complain of unpleasant side effects with both short- and long-term use, especially weight gain and depression.

Nonsteroidal Antiinflammatory Drugs

Several families of NSAIDs are prescribed for the relief of dysmenorrhea, including indomethacin, ibuprofen, naproxen, and the fenamate drugs. Common names are easily recognizable and include such drugs as Advil, Motrin, and Aleve. Although these drugs may bring quick and temporary relief, they often require increasing doses to maintain efficacy, and sometimes eventually cease to bring relief at all. Gastric bleeding is a problematic side effect, and recent studies[128] have found a causal relationship between NSAID use and increased risk of heart disease, enough so that the FDA has added a black box warning to this commonly used drug class. Further, the combination of selective serotonin reuptake inhibitors (SSRIs) and NSAIDs may prove to be dangerous, with an increased risk of brain bleeding seen with this combination.

In all cases, although medication can bring needed pain relief, it does little to address the underlying causes of prostaglandin overproduction, thus offering little to improve the condition in any real or lasting way.

BOTANICAL TREATMENT OF DYSMENORRHEA

Botanical treatment is highly effective for treating the pain and reducing inflammation associated with both primary and secondary dysmenorrhea. The treatment of secondary dysmenorrhea requires attention to the underlying pathology.

Herbalists subdivide dysmenorrhea into two additional categories: congestive dysmenorrhea and spasmodic dysmenorrhea.[129] In the former, there is scant or difficult blood flow, a feeling of pressure, congestion, or dull aching in the pelvis, and a sense of stagnation or bogginess in the uterus. Treatment emphasizes the use of uterotonic and astringent herbs that promote uterine circulation, reduce uterine blood congestion and stagnation, and facilitate the expulsive action of the uterus.[129] Improving uterine blood circulation is also a conventional pharmacologic strategy, but the pharmaceutical agents commonly used may have side effects.[130] Herbs used may include blue cohosh, dong quai, ginger, and yarrow. Spasmodic dysmenorrhea presents with spastic, cramping pain. Treatment focuses on antispasmodics, anodynes, analgesics, and sedatives, commonly cramp bark and black haw, wild yam, and black cohosh. Most commonly, these strategies are combined in a composite approach.

Treatment with herbal antispasmodics and analgesics can bring significant prompt relief. The goal of the herbalist, however, is not to simply eliminate acute pain but to prevent chronicity of the problem. As with other conditions, the botanical practitioner applies a variety of therapeutic strategies to affect not only the local symptoms, but to reduce the systemic factors that lead to the symptoms. In the case of dysmenorrhea, herbs are incorporated for their antispasmodic, tonic, and analgesic effects, as well as for their ability to reduce excessive production and circulation of inflammatory mediators and normalize the hormones. Herbs are also incorporated to improve sluggish pelvic circulation and relieve engorgement and pressure. Herbalists take psychogenic factors into consideration, providing nervines and adaptogens when appropriate.[129] Hormonal dysregulation is evaluated and treated as necessary, as part of an overall protocol. Finally, if there is constipation, this is treated to reduce pelvic discomfort and pressure and prevent hormonal dysregulation via adequate bile–bowel axis elimination of estrogens.

Treatment of acute and chronic dysmenorrhea relies upon a combination of the most effective herbs for this condition. Although certain single herb drugs, such as cramp bark, may be used effectively for reduction of acute uterine spasms, a combination of uterine antispasmodics and tonics is usually prescribed. A number of herbs may actually act as both (e.g., cramp bark, black cohosh, blue cohosh), which may seem contradictory; however, uterine physiology actually depends on a coordinated action of the uterine muscles, based on adequate contractile and relaxation ability.[129] A number of herbs seem, by their clinical actions, able to effect regulation of uterine activity.

Herbs are given with a variety of scheduling approaches as appropriate for the woman's complaints, as follows:

- Throughout the month to treat chronic dysmenorrhea
- Every 3 to 4 hours for several days before the onset of the period to prevent or mitigate pain
- Frequently at the onset of the period to reduce acute pain. Treatment for acute pain is given in a schedule of frequent, small doses until relief is achieved, frequently as every 15 to 30 minutes if pain is severe (Table 9-10).

TABLE 9-10 Botanical Treatment Strategies for Dysmenorrhea

Therapeutic Goal	Therapeutic Activity	Botanical Name	Common Name
Relieve pain and relax cramping	Uterine antispasmodics; analgesics	Anemone pulsatilla	Pulsatilla
		Angelica sinensis	Dong quai
		Actaea racemosa	Black cohosh
		Corydalis ambigua	Corydalis
		Dioscorea villosa	Wild yam
		Foeniculum vulgare	Fennel
		Leonurus cardiaca	Motherwort
		Matricaria recutita	Chamomile
		Paeonia lactiflora	White peony
		Piscidia piscipula	Jamaican dogwood
		Viburnum prunifolium	Cramp bark
		Viburnum opulus	Black haw
	Antiinflammatories	Glycyrrhiza glabra	Licorice
		Zingiber officinale	Ginger
	Uterotonics	Achillea millefolium	Yarrow
		Caulophyllum thalictroides	Blue cohosh
		Leonurus cardiaca	Motherwort
		Mitchella repens	Partridge berry
		Rubus idaeus	Red raspberry
Improve pelvic circulation	Circulatory stimulants; "blood movers"	Angelica sinensis	Dong quai
		Paeonia lactiflora	White peony
		Zingiber officinale	Ginger
Support liver's function in hormonal conjugation, detoxification, and elimination	Hepatic alteratives	Arctium lappa	Burdock
		Mahonia aquifolium	Oregon grape
		Taraxacum officinale	Dandelion root
Relieve constipation	Aperients/laxatives	Rumex crispus	Yellow dock
		Taraxacum officinale	Dandelion root
Topical applications for pain relief		Heat	
		Ginger fomentations	
		Essential oil applications/baths: chamomile EO, caraway EO, fennel EO, peppermint EO	

EO, Essential oil.

Discussion of Botanicals
Black Cohosh
Black cohosh is spasmolytic and antiinflammatory to the smooth and skeletal muscles, making it particularly useful in the treatment of dysmenorrhea with associated aching discomfort in the lower back and legs. It was used by the Eclectics for this purpose, and continues to be used extensively for dysmenorrhea by modern herbalists as well.[76,80,122] The salicylates and gallic acid in black cohosh are analgesic and antiinflammatory; this may help to reduce prostaglandin excess if given before the period.[129,131] Ferulic and isoferulic acids are inhibitors of leukotriene production.[7] Black cohosh is approved by the German Commission E for the treatment of premenstrual complaints and dysmenorrhea.[44] Black cohosh is indicated for muscular pains, nervous tension, and has been noted to have antiinflammatory and analgesic effects.[80]

Blue Cohosh
Blue cohosh is indicated when there is dysmenorrhea owing to uterine atony. It was popular among the Eclectics and continues to be used by herbalists as a uterine tonic, promoting effective uterine contractions and relieving spasticity in conjunction with a uterine spasmolytic.[107,129] Blue cohosh is an emmenagogue and uterotonic. The quinolizidine alkaloids N-methylcysteine and sparteine are believed to be responsible for caulophyllum's oxytocic, stimulatory effect on the uterine muscle.[80] Its steroidal saponins, caulosaponin, caulosapogenin, and caulophyllosaponin also may have an effect on the uterus. Blue cohosh typically constitutes only a small fraction (i.e., 20%) of a formula owing to its potential hypertensive activity and toxicity.

Chamomile
Chamomile is an effective antispasmodic and antiinflammatory useful in the treatment of menstrual discomfort and bowel disorders.[77,80] Water extracts of chamomile have been shown to enhance uterine tone in isolated animal uterine samples. Other investigations have demonstrated chamomile to possess weak estrogenic and progesteronic activity. The antispasmodic activity of chamomile has been credited to a

number of flavonol glycosides. Apigenin is the most mentioned of the over 20 flavonoids, and currently thought to be the strongest antispasmodic agent in *Matricaria*. German studies have shown that the flavonoids in chamomile are a stronger antispasmodic than papaverine from the opium poppy. It is also a reliable nervine, used as a mild sedative. This makes it especially valuable in the treatment of dysmenorrhea with concurrent diarrhea, bloating, and gas, as well as anxiety and irritability. Weiss and Fintelmann recommend that the tea be sipped hot for rapid reduction of menstrual cramps.[121] It is not considered one of the stronger uterine antispasmodics; however, it makes an excellent addition to formulae, is a pleasant infusion to sip when there is pain, and has a marked effect on GI discomfort.

Chaste Berry

A 2014 clinical trial compared *V. agnus-castus* with ethinyl estradiol/drospirenone for the treatment of severe primary dysmenorrhea while assessing uterine artery blood flow via Doppler ultrasonography. Ninety women were enrolled in the study. Thirty remained controls, and sixty were randomized to receive ethinyl estradiol 0.03 mg/drospirenone or *V. agnus-castus* for three menstrual cycles. The outcomes were measured with visual analog scale (VAS) scores, the pulsatility index (PI), and the resistance index (RI) of the uterine artery. Mean PI and RI values in women with severe primary dysmenorrhea were significantly higher than in the control groups on day 1 of the menstrual cycle, but lowered during the course of treatment. No significant differences between treatment groups were observed (Preparation not noted).[132]

Corydalis

Corydalis is a highly effective analgesic that may be used in the treatment of congestive and spasmolytic dysmenorrhea. It has also demonstrated analgesic effects in the treatment of neuralgia and headache. The analgesic potency is considered to be 1% to 10% of that of opium.[46] Although not commonly known by Western herbalists as a treatment for dysmenorrhea, this herb should be considered for acute spasms associated with dysmenorrhea, and also may be of use in treating associated headache and musculoskeletal discomfort.

Cramp Bark/Black Haw

Cramp bark and black haw are considered by herbalists, midwives, and naturopathic physicians to be among the most important and reliable uterine antispasmodics and tonics.[49] They were extensively used by the Eclectics for dysmenorrhea, with numerous references throughout the Eclectic literature on their efficacy.[49,76,129,133] The actions of the herbs are so similar that they are frequently used interchangeably. Owing to slight variations in their chemistry, there may be minor differences in therapeutic effect and strength, but herbalists do not seem to consider these consequential. Both are considered effective uterine antispasmodics, used for sedating pain and relieving menstrual disorders, especially dysmenorrhea and amenorrhea.[49,77,129] They are also considered uterotonic. Studies have been limited. In vitro and in vivo experiments

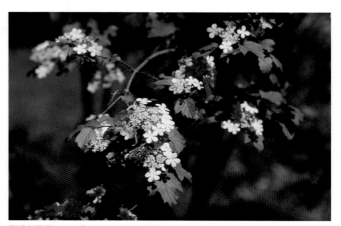

FIGURE 9-5 Cramp bark *(Viburnum opulus)*. (Photo by Martin Wall.)

have repeatedly demonstrated its effectiveness as a spasmolytic for the uterine musculature, an effect that is producible with oral administration.[49,77,80] The mechanism of action is unknown, but the herb is suspected to contain a number of constituents that act on the uterine musculature, most notably scopoletin and aesculetin, which are believed partly responsible for their spasmolytic activity.[77] Flavonoid constituents have also been identified, including amentoflavone. Amentoflavone has been noted to inhibit cyclic adenosine monophosphate (cAMP) phosphodiesterase in human platelets.[134] No clinical trials have been conducted using cramp bark or black haw. Cramp bark was listed as a sedative and antispasmodic in the *USP* from 1894 to 1916 and the NF from 1916 to 1960.[49,80] *V. opulus* and *V. prunifolium* are used in acute formulae, often combined with other sedating herbs, and are also used in formulae for longer-term treatment, combined with other uterotonic and hormone-regulating herbs (Fig. 9-5).

Dong Quai

Dong quai has been used in TCM for the treatment of gynecologic complaints, including dysmenorrhea, since at least the sixteenth century.[134] It is used for the treatment of the TCM diagnoses of "blood stasis" and "blood vacuity," which are associated with the Western diagnoses of amenorrhea, dysmenorrhea, uterine fibroids, and endometriosis.[49] In spite of its long history of use for these conditions, few clinical trials have been conducted. In a 1988 study, Gao et al administered either ligustilide (an isolated constituent believed responsible for uterine relaxant activity), 150 mg three times daily, or dong quai aqueous extract tablets, 2 g three times daily, for 3 to 7 days during menstruation to women with dysmenorrhea. The ligustilide group had an effectiveness rate of 77% compared with 38% for the dong quai extract. Reported side effects included nausea, dizziness, and an increase or decrease in menstrual flow. Dong quai's ability to relax smooth muscle is thought to be caused by its volatile oil–containing fraction, especially the phthalides. The aqueous extract, which contains ferulic acid, appears to act as both a uterine stimulant and relaxant.[49] Ligustilide inhibited spontaneous potassium (K^+) depolarization–induced contraction in rat uterine tissue in vitro, demonstrating multiple mechanisms of action and nonspecific antispasmodic properties.[135] Dong quai may also reduce tissue congestion through enhanced blood and lymph circulation. Animal studies have shown *A. sinensis* to have a general analgesic and antiinflammatory effect.[136] Dong quai also contains nicotinic acid, which is believed to have a blood vessel–relaxing or vasodilating action. The vasodilatory effects mentioned in the preceding also appear because of the coumarin compounds in dong quai. Many women have found dong quai to improve menstrual cramps. Interestingly, several studies have shown dong quai to act as a muscle relaxant overall, but to stimulate the uterus briefly before relaxing it.[137,138] This curious action is likely the result of two chemical constituents in *Angelica* spp. that have opposite actions on the uterus. Animal studies (i.e., rabbits, cats, dogs) have shown *Angelica* spp. to increase the "excitability" of the uterus. Like other muscles, uterine spasms may occur when the uterine muscle is out of shape.[139] Because dong quai dilates the blood vessels and improves circulation in the uterus, regular use can sometimes make menstrual flow heavier.[139] Many herbalists recommend that dong quai be stopped during the actual menstrual period in individuals prone to heavy menses.[112] Dong quai is typically used in combination with other herbs, and is rarely used singly. Bone suggests its use in combination with corydalis, white peony, and *Ligusticum* for the treatment of dysmenorrhea.[80]

Fennel

Fennel seeds have been used to promote menstruation, alleviate the symptoms of the female climacteric (i.e., during menopause), and increase libido. Fennel essential oil (FEO) also possesses emmenagogue and galactagogue properties. Seeds of fennel are used in folk remedies for treatment of dysmenorrhea. This traditional usage might be related to the antispasmodic effects of FEO.[130] Recent research on fennel oil shows promise in the treatment of dysmenorrhea. A 3-month, three-cycle clinical trial of 30 women with dysmenorrhea compared the efficacy of mefenamic acid with a 2% fennel seed essence extract. The first cycle was a control cycle with no medications administered; in the second cycle women were treated with the pharmaceutical drug; and in the third cycle women received the fennel extract. Results were based on a self-scoring system. Both treatment groups showed improvement in symptoms compared with the control cycle. Mefenamic acid had a more potent effect than fennel on the second and third menstrual days; however, the difference on the other days was not significant. No complications were reported in mefenamic acid treated cycles, but five people (16.6%) withdrew from the study owing to fennel's odor, and one person (3.11%) in the fennel group reported a mild increase in the amount of her menstrual flow. The authors of the study concluded that essence of fennel can be used as a safe and effective herbal drug for primary dysmenorrhea; however, it may have a lower potency than mefenamic acid in the dosages used for this study.[140] A 2014 clinical trial tested fennel for the treatment of symptoms associated with primary dysmenorrhea. Eighty women were randomized to receive either placebo or fennel capsules (30 mg) every 4 hours from 3 days before menstruation until day 5 of the menstrual cycle. Using the VAS, the McGill pain questionnaire, and three additional questionnaires, the fennel group exhibited less nausea and decreased duration of menstruation (Fennel capsule preparation details not noted).[141] In an in vitro study, administration of different doses, FEO reduced the intensity of oxytocin- and PGE_2-induced contractions significantly (25 and 50 μg/mL for oxytocin and 10 and 20 g/mL PGE_2, respectively). FEO also reduced the frequency of contractions induced by PGE_2 but not by oxytocin. LD_{50} (i.e., lethal dose in 50% of population) 1326 mg/kg of FEO was obtained in the female rats by using the moving average method.[130] Oral administration (200 mg/kg) of fennel seed methanolic extract exhibited inhibitory effects against acute and subacute inflammatory diseases and showed a central analgesic effect.[142] Estrogenic effects are attributed to the polymers of anethole (i.e., dianethole, photoanethole) and lend credence to claims of increased human milk production and promoting menstruation.[143]

Fenugreek

In addition to its use as a galactagogue, fenugreek may also benefit a number of menstrual complaints. A recent double-blind clinical trial found fenugreek seed to benefit symptoms of dysmenorrhea. The participants included 101 women of similar age, BMI, and baseline levels of menstrual cramp pain; they were randomized to receive either ground fenugreek seed capsules (900 mg) three times daily or placebo control for the first 3 days of menses for two consecutive cycles. VAS was used to assess pain during the first 3 days of menstruation. Both placebo and fenugreek treatment groups exhibited lower pain levels compared with baseline after 2 months, but the decrease observed with fenugreek was far more statistically significant (Fenugreek capsule preparation details not noted).[144]

Ginger

Ginger root is used both internally and topically as a warming circulatory stimulant and antiinflammatory in the treatment of dysmenorrhea. The Eclectics used it for this purpose, and it is a common ingredient in herbal formulae for menstrual cramps to this day, taken as a hot tea, tincture, fomentation, or hot bath. Further, its positive effects in relieving nausea have been repeatedly demonstrated, making it an especially useful herb when there is dysmenorrhea accompanied by nausea and vomiting. Ginger exerts antiinflammatory effects in the prostaglandin synthesis pathway, and its activity as a thromboxane synthetase inhibitor and prostacyclin agonist may be responsible for its analgesic effects in dysmenorrhea.[80] Recent clinical trial research corroborates its historical use. For a 2013 trial on the efficacy of ginger in the treatment of primary dysmenorrhea, 70 college students received either ginger or placebo capsules during the first 3 days of their menstrual cycles. After 2 months, the group receiving ginger capsules experienced significantly less menstrual pain as recorded by VAS, Likert, and Wilcoxor scales compared with placebo (Preparation not noted).[145] Another recent trial (n = 120 college students) similarly tested efficacy of ginger compared with placebo in the treatment of primary dysmenorrhea. The investigators used two protocols for administering ginger. In the first, ginger (500 mg) and placebo capsule were given 2 days before menstrual onset and continued through the first 3 days of the menstrual cycle. In the second, these were given only for the first 3 days of the menstrual period. According to VAS scores, there were statistically significant improvements in symptoms of pain for the ginger treatment groups, with the first protocol (5 days of administration) associated with less pain than the second.[146] Another clinical study that same year with 75 students tested two protocols of ginger against placebo capsules for dysmenorrhea. The first treatment group received 1 g of ginger root in warm water after meals twice daily, and the second group received ginger only during the first 3 days of the menstrual cycle. Using metrics of daily symptom calendars and Likert scales, the ginger groups appear to have exhibited statistically significant improvement in symptoms of dysmenorrhea compared with controls.[147] A 2009 double-blind clinical trial tested ginger against mefenamic acid and ibuprofen for menstrual pain. One hundred and fifty women with primary dysmenorrhea were randomized into treatment groups of either ginger (250 mg), mefenamic acid (250 mg), or ibuprofen (400 mg) four times daily for the first 3 days of the menstrual cycle. Outcomes were measured using a verbal multidimensional scoring system taken at baseline and after one menstrual cycle. End point scores indicated improvements compared with baseline, but no significant differences were observed between treatment groups (Preparation: dry rhizome powder).[148]

Jamaican Dogwood

Jamaican dogwood is a highly reliable and strong uterine antispasmodic and analgesic for the treatment of acute and severe dysmenorrhea. It is traditionally used for all manner of neuralgic and muscular pains and spasms.[80] It is especially indicated when there is sharp and nearly unremitting menstrual pain, or when pain is causing inability to work or sleep. Herbal literature commonly warns that this herb is toxic in large doses. Though this is not a problem at clinically recommended doses, recommended doses should not be exceeded.[80] Reported side effects include nausea, vomiting, and headache, although these are not commonly seen clinically.

Licorice

Herbalists often include licorice as an adjunct herb in formulae for dysmenorrhea, considering it a possible mediator of adrenal and sex hormones and inflammation. A number of studies have demonstrated prostaglandin inhibition and improvement in dysmenorrhea with the TCM formula Shakuyaku-Kanzo-To, which consists of equal parts of licorice and white peony (see White Peony).[149] These studies suggest the need for further research into the role of licorice in the treatment of dysmenorrhea.

Motherwort

Motherwort has been used traditionally for dysmenorrhea, both by herbalists and the Eclectics, and has demonstrated uterine spasmolytic and sedative effects.[77,80] Herbalists consider motherwort a uterine tonic as well, particularly valuable in improving uterine atony owing to pelvic congestion, improving circulation, and relieving vascular congestion. Motherwort may reduce pain via a reduction in endogenous inflammatory mediators, enhancing the synthesis of prostaglandins via prostaglandin E9-ketoreductase, important in the synthesis of the desirable PGE_2 series prostaglandins.[150] Motherwort may relieve vascular congestion in the pelvis and enhance general circulation. The constituent prehispanolone (i.e., a tetrahydrofuran) has been noted to inhibit platelet aggregation via platelet-activating factor (PAF) receptor antagonism.[151] Motherwort is a well-known childbirth and postpartum botanical because of its galactagogue and uterine tonic properties. Motherwort is a hypotensive nervine useful for headache, insomnia, and vertigo, as well as gynecologic and obstetric conditions.[152] It is specific for pelvic pain with concomitant heart palpitations, anxiety attacks, and stress. Motherwort may improve uterine tone through a slight stimulating action. Motherwort has been shown to stimulate both H_1 and α-adrenergic receptors.[153] Motherwort injections were recently shown to improve blood viscosity by decreasing platelet aggregation, fibrinogen content, and erythrocyte deformation. Lectins extracted from motherwort seeds are noted to affect red blood cell agglutination, and are credited with some of the blood flow–enhancing effects.[154] Another species, the Chinese *Leonurus heterophyllus,* is noted to contain a constituent able to bind to PAF receptors.[151] In addition to lectins, motherwort contains phytosterols, flavonol and iridoid glycosides, and the alkaloid leonurine.[155-157] Motherwort is reported to have a uterotonic effect throughout the European and Chinese literature and this is supported by modern animal research.[158] Leonurine has caught the attention of pharmaceutical researchers and is able to be synthesized. Synthetic leonurine has also displayed uterotonic activity in both in vivo and in vitro experiments.[159] It contains the alkaloids leonurine, leonurinine, and leonurinide.[155,160] Motherwort also contains volatile oils, tannins, and citric acid (Fig. 9-6).

Pulsatilla

Pulsatilla is considered specific for painful or inflammatory reproductive conditions, including dysmenorrhea.[80,124] Its sedative action is beneficial when there is nervous tension causing or accompanying dysmenorrhea, and it also exerts pronounced effects on uterine pain.[129] No pharmacologic or clinical trials were identified on this herb. Only the dried herb is used. The fresh plant contains an irritating component: protoanemonin. The German Commission E has not approved the use of pulsatilla species on the basis of lack of evidence of efficacy.[44] It warns against fresh plant use, which can cause severe irritation of the skin and mucosa, and in high doses can lead to renal and urinary side effects.[44,124] This plant is

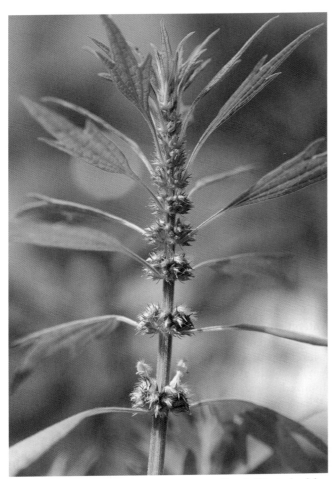

FIGURE 9-6 Motherwort *(Leonurus cardiaca).* (Photo by Martin Wall.)

teratogenic and abortifacient in cattle, and should not be used during pregnancy.[124]

Valerian

Valerian has long been used as an antispasmodic and sedative herb. A 2011 double-blind clinical trial evaluated the ability of valerian root to ameliorate menstrual pain in 100 college students. The valerian experimental group was administered 255 mg three times daily for the first 3 days of the menstrual cycle for two consecutive cycles, and the control group received placebo capsules. Outcomes were tracked using VAS and a multidimensional verbal scale taken at baseline and throughout the intervention. A significant difference in pain scores was observed between the groups, and valerian treatment was associated with decreased pain severity (Preparation not noted).[162] Valerian is used in both tincture and capsules, and is frequently combined with additional analgesic and antispasmodic herbs.

White Peony

White peony is an herb in TCM for the treatment of dysmenorrhea and muscle cramping. Paeoniflorin has exhibited smooth muscle relaxant ability in in vitro models (i.e., rat stomach and uterus) and it has demonstrated in vivo

analgesic and spasmolytic activity. Paeoniflorin also demonstrated inhibition of twitch responses in skeletal muscles, an effect that was potentiated in vitro and in vivo by the addition of glycyrrhizin from licorice.[46] Additionally, clinical trials have demonstrated positive results in the treatment of dysmenorrhea owing to "qi and blood stasis" (with licorice root); a reduction of serum and free testosterone in women with PCOS (with licorice); and an improvement in clinical symptoms and reduction in size of fibroids in an open study of 100 women (with *P. suffruticosa, Poria cocos, Cinnamomum cassia,* and *Prunus persica*).[46,161] Several clinical trials have been conducted with the TCM herbal medicine Shakuyaku-Kanzo-To for the treatment of dysmenorrhea. The formula consists of an equal amount each of white peony and licorice. It appears that this blend may exert its action against dysmenorrhea through preventing prostaglandin production.[149] This suggests that this herb and traditional herbal combinations may play a role not only in symptom reduction with primary dysmenorrhea but in treating the underlying causes associated with secondary dysmenorrhea. White peony may be used in decoction or tincture in traditional TCM formulae, or in combination with other herbs in Western botanical formulae.

Wild Yam

Wild yam has been used historically to treat spastic, dyspeptic pain of the abdomen, uterus, and gallbladder, and still finds popular use as such among herbalists. It was highly popular among the Eclectic physicians as an antispasmodic treatment for dysmenorrhea with spasmodic, colicky pains, for which it was given every few hours. Wild yam continues to be one of the primary uterine antispasmodics used for dysmenorrhea by contemporary herbalists.[129] No contemporary research is available on its effects on the uterine muscle. An in vitro analysis in 1916 failed to show effects on the uterine muscle.[32] A 1997 report demonstrated that diosgenin, a constituent in wild yam, exerts intestinal antiinflammatory activity when consumed as a dietary supplement (Fig. 9-7).[50]

Yarrow

Yarrow is used in traditional and folk herbal medicine to relieve menstrual pain. Wichtl compares its actions, both internally and topically, to chamomile flowers. Its sesquiterpene lactones lend antiphlogistic activity, whereas its spasmolytic activity is attributed to its flavonoids.[77] Research has been limited, but some investigations have shown yarrow to act as an antispasmodic and antiinflammatory, making it useful for pain and uterine cramps.[163,164] Yarrow may be taken at a low dose all month, or more aggressively for menstrual cramps when symptomatic relief is needed.

Other Herbs
Bromelain

Cervical application of bromelain (found in pineapple) improved symptoms in nulliparous women with severe primary dysmenorrhea. Bromelain was applied locally to the cervix in

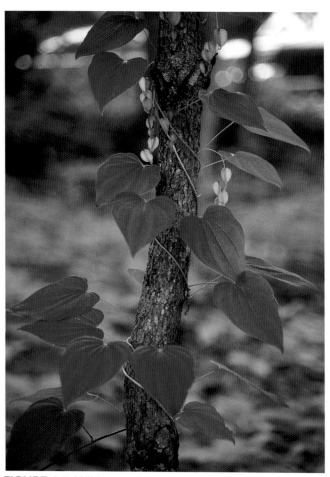

FIGURE 9-7 Wild yam *(Dioscorea villosa)*. (Photo by Martin Wall.)

a phosphate buffer solution (pH 5.6). The solution was slowly poured into the vagina via a rubber catheter attached to a 20-cc syringe with the patient in Trendelenburg position. The solution remained in the vagina for 10 minutes. After the application of bromelain, there was some degree of cervical dilatation in each patient. The uterine isthmus was affected dependent on the phase of the menstrual cycle. All patients obtained instantaneous relief of their primary dysmenorrhea. An unspecified number of patients with disabling dysmenorrhea was treated with solution of bromelain. Of 64 patients treated, 40 obtained immediate relief. Only fair to poor results were achieved in patients with secondary dysmenorrhea caused by other gynecologic diseases (Boxes 9-7 to 9-9).[7]

NUTRITIONAL CONSIDERATIONS

A multifactorial approach that incorporates an antiinflammatory diet and the use of essential fatty acids is an indispensable aspect of botanical treatment for chronic dysmenorrhea.

A diet rich in whole grains, plenty of fruits and vegetable, legumes, fish, and poultry can help to minimize dysmenorrhea.

Fish Oil Supplementation and the Antiinflammatory Diet

Supplementation of the diet with omega-3 fatty acids and following an antiinflammatory diet are indicated to reduce the production of the inflammatory prostaglandin-2 series (i.e., $F_{2\alpha}$). Arachidonic acid, which is present in animal fats and dairy products, is converted into $F_{2\alpha}$; thus a reduction in red meat and dairy products is recommended. Supplementation of omega-3 fatty acids can be accomplished by increasing the amount of cold-water fish in the diet to two to three times per week or adding a fish oil supplement to supply eicosapentaenoic acid (EPA) and docosahexaenoic acid (DHA). One placebo-controlled, crossover RCT of adolescent girls ($n = 42$) with primary dysmenorrhea showed improvement of subjectively rated symptoms in 73% of girls taking a fish oil supplement with 720 mg DHA, 1080 mg EPA, and 1.5 mg vitamin E (see Vitamin E) for 2 months.[32] A double-blind RCT demonstrated reduction in amount of analgesics needed in dysmenorrheal women after 45 and 90 days of treatment with an extract of Antarctic brill, compared with control and women taking omega-3 fish oil.[32,131] A recent four-arm clinical trial tested fish oil capsules and vitamin B_1 tablets in 240 high school females with dysmenorrhea. The participants were randomized to receive either vitamin B_1 (100 mg daily), fish oil capsules (500 mg daily), both, or placebo for two consecutive menstrual cycles. After a 2-month duration, the intensity and duration of pain significantly decreased in all treatment groups.[165] In another trial, 36 young women (ages 18 to 22) were randomized into placebo and treatment (15 mL fish oil/daily; 550 mg EPA, 205 mg DHA) groups. After 3 months with treatment, the regimens were exchanged per the crossover design. With primary outcomes measured via VAS, significant improvements in pain were reported over controls.[166] Salmon, tuna, and halibut contain linolenic acid, which helps to relax the muscles by manipulating production of the prostaglandin 1, 2, and 3 series; the antiinflammatory 1 and 3 series are increased and the proinflammatory 2 series is decreased. Seeds that contain linoleic acid such as pumpkin, flax, sesame, and sunflower also increase PGE_3 levels.[7] Mercury contamination in cold-water fish is likely to be significantly higher than in high-quality fish oil screened for heavy metals.

Magnesium

An open trial of a small group of women with primary dysmenorrhea who were given 4.5 mg oral magnesium pidolate 7 days before the onset of menses through day 3 of menstruation showed a reduction in dysmenorrhea with no reported side effects. Magnesium also had a therapeutic effect on back pain and lower abdominal pain on the second and third days of the menstrual cycle in women with primary dysmenorrhea who were given magnesium or placebo beginning the day preceding menstruation and on the first 2 days of the menstrual cycle. Magnesium is a cofactor in delta-6 desaturase, which is involved in antiinflammatory prostaglandins (i.e., PGE_1) and

---

BOX 9-7 Botanical Prescriptions for Dysmenorrhea

Tincture for Acute Menstrual Cramps[1]
Take for acute pain during menses. Can be taken for several days before anticipated onset of menses.

Cramp bark or black haw	(*Viburnum opulus* or *prunifolium*)	30 mL
Wild yam	(*Dioscorea* spp.)	20 mL
Motherwort	(*Leonurus cardiaca*)	20 mL
Black cohosh	(*Actaea racemosa*)	20 mL
Ginger	(*Zingiber officinale*)	10 mL
	Total: 100 mL	

Dose: 2 to 4 mL three times daily.

Rationale: Cramp bark and wild yam are employed for their antispasmodic effects. Motherwort is included in the formula for its supportive effects as a uterotonic, bitter nervine, and antispasmodic herb. Black cohosh provides analgesic effects, and ginger is included as an antiinflammatory. For severe cramping pain, take this tincture every 2 hours; add 1 mL Jamaican dogwood (*Piscidia piscipula*) every 2 hours, not to exceed six doses per day or more than 2 days.

Tincture for Acute Menstrual Cramps[2]
Take for *severe* acute cramps.

Cramp bark, black haw	(*Viburnum opulus* or *prunifolium*)	50 mL
Jamaican dogwood	(*Piscidia piscipula*)	30 mL
Corydalis	(*Corydalis ambigua*)	10 mL
Pulsatilla	(*Anemone pulsatilla*)	10 mL
	Total: 100 mL	

Dose: Take 1.5 mL every 20 minutes for six doses, or 2 mL every 30 minutes for four doses to relieve acute pain. This can be repeated twice daily at least 4 hours apart but should not exceed this dose.

Rationale: The herbs in this formula are included for their combined analgesic and antispasmodic effects.

Uterine Tonic Tincture
Use throughout the menstrual cycle to improve uterine tone and prevent recurrence of dysmenorrhea. Take for a minimum of three menstrual cycles for improvement.

Motherwort	(*Leonurus cardiaca*)	20 mL
White peony	(*Paeonia lactiflora*)	20 mL
Licorice root	(*Glycyrrhiza glabra*)	20 mL
Dong quai	(*Angelica sinensis*)	15 mL
Oregon grape root	(*Mahonia aquifolium*)	15 mL
Blue cohosh	(*Caulophyllum thalictroides*)	10 mL
	Total: 100 mL	

Dose: 3 to 5 mL three times daily.

Rationale: Motherwort is included as a uterotonic, antispasmodic, and bitter nervine; white peony licorice, and dong quai all possess antiinflammatory actions, whereas white peony and dong quai are also antispasmodic and are specific TCM herbs for dysmenorrhea. Oregon grape is used as a hepatic bitter to promote liver detoxification and as a choleretic to increase hormonal excretion via the bile–bowel axis. Blue cohosh is a specific uterine muscle tonic; licorice is also included in the formula as a harmonizer and to improve the taste.

BOX 9-8 Antispasmodic Oil for Topical Application

| Chamomile essential oil | Caraway essential oil |
| Fennel essential oil | Peppermint essential oil |

Place ½ tsp of each essential oil into a 4-oz squeeze bottle filled with olive or *Hypericum* oil. Massage 1 to 2 tsp into the lower abdomen and cover with heat for an analgesic, antispasmodic effect. To prevent a skin reaction, test a single drop of essential oil on the inner wrist and wait 5 minutes before applying essential oils to larger skin surfaces.

BOX 9-9 Hot Ginger and Chamomile Fomentation

Prepare a strong infusion of chamomile and ginger tea using 2 Tbsp chamomile blossoms and 2 Tbsp of fresh-grated ginger root per liter of boiling water. Steep 20 minutes and strain. Soak a cloth in the infusion, wring out, and apply as hot as can be tolerated. A hot water bottle and a warm towel can be applied over the fomentation to retain the heat. This can be repeated several times daily. Alternatively, the recipe can be doubled and added to a hot hip bath.

exerts a relaxing effect on skeletal and smooth muscle cramping. Magnesium is contraindicated in heart block and severe renal disease.[131] The recommended dose varies but is generally 300 to 600 mg three times daily for several days before the onset of the period.[32] Excessive doses can lead to serious toxicity.

Calcium

Two trials demonstrate the effectiveness of calcium in reducing cyclic uterine pain. Calcium supplementation was effective in reducing premenstrual pain (but not menstrual) in a prospective, randomized, double-blind, placebo-controlled, parallel-group, multicenter clinical trial of PMS. Subjects ($n = 497$) were given 1200 mg calcium or placebo daily for three menstrual cycles. Subjective rating scales of 17 symptoms revealed significantly lower scores for all pain measures in the treatment group during the luteal phase of the third menstrual cycle, whereas scores did not change significantly in controls. In a prospective, randomized, double-blind, crossover trial targeted at investigating PMS, calcium carbonate supplementation (1000 mg/day for 3 months) was effective in reducing menstrual pain compared with placebo.[131]

TREATMENT SUMMARY FOR DYSMENORRHEA

- Herbalists categorize dysmenorrhea into congestive and spasmodic types. Both can occur concurrently, but identifying the characteristic features of the complaint can help to narrow treatment choices.
- Treatment of congestive dysmenorrhea emphasizes the use of uterotonic and astringent herbs. Herbs used may include blue cohosh, dong quai, ginger, and yarrow. Uterine tonics are used to improve pelvic and uterine circulation, relieve local congestion, and improve pelvic tone. Examples include yarrow, blue cohosh, motherwort, partridge berry, and red raspberry leaf. Herbs to move the circulation include dong quai, white peony, and ginger.
- Spasmodic dysmenorrhea is treated with antispasmodics, analgesics, anodynes, and sedating herbs including cramp bark, black haw, wild yam, black cohosh, Jamaican dogwood, motherwort, dong quai, and pulsatilla, among many other choices.
- Emphasis is placed on reduction of inflammatory compounds that can cause dysmenorrhea. Antiinflammatory diet and herbs (i.e., licorice, white peony, ginger) can be beneficial, as can supplementation with omega-3 fatty acids with eicosapentaenoic acid (EPA), fish oils, or cold-water fish.
- Topical applications can be used for soothing pain relief, and include ginger fomentations, massage with warm essential oils, and hot baths with essential oils.
- Supplementation with magnesium, calcium, and vitamin E has demonstrated varying levels of improved outcomes.
- Stress management, yoga, and exercise have also been shown to be beneficial in the treatment of dysmenorrhea.

What to Expect with Dysmenorrhea Treatment

Acute treatment with analgesics, antispasmodics, anodynes, and sedatives can bring relief within 2 hours of the onset of treatment. Prevention of acute dysmenorrhea, if begun 3 to 5 days before the onset of menstruation, can similarly be quickly effective, with pain offset at the next menstruation. Treating chronic dysmenorrhea may require several months of use of antiinflammatory herbs and adherence to an antiinflammatory diet for women to be able to reduce dependence on acute pain relief treatment.

Vitamin D

A 2012 clinical trial investigated the therapeutic effects of a single high dose of vitamin D (i.e., 300,000 IU) in the treatment of dysmenorrhea-related pain compared with placebo. Study participants included 40 women (aged 18 to 40) who exhibited serum vitamin D <45 ng/mL for at least 4 consecutive months who were randomized to receive either the vitamin D dose or placebo before the anticipated onset of menses. The primary measured outcome was the intensity of the menstrual pain, with the secondary outcome as the use of NSAIDs during the study. After 2 months and two menstrual periods, the pain scores decreased 41% in the vitamin D group and there was no difference in the placebo group, with the greatest improvement in pain scores seen in women who exhibited the greatest vitamin D deficiency at baseline.[167]

Vitamin E

In a study of vitamin E for dysmenorrhea treatment, 68% of women ages 18 to 21 with spasmodic dysmenorrhea ($n = 100$) improved with 50 mg vitamin E three times daily after two cycles of treatment. After three cycles, 76% of the treated group had improvement; vitamin E can increase bleeding time, so use should be monitored in patients with blood-clotting disorders or those taking anticoagulant medication. See Fish Oil (preceding) for a combined study with vitamin E.[131]

ADDITIONAL THERAPIES

Aromatherapy

Aromatherapy with essential oils aids in overall relaxation and may be used to address dysmenorrhea and associated discomforts. A clinical trial tested the use of aromatherapy (i.e., lavender, clary sage, rose) on symptoms of dysmenorrhea in college students ($n = 67$) against placebo massage and controls. Menstrual cramp pain severity was assessed via VAS, and severity was assessed through a verbal multidimensional score system the first and second day of the menstrual cycle after treatment. The aromatherapy group exhibited decreased menstrual pain compared with placebo massage and controls.[168] Another clinical trial tested inhalation of lavender essential oil scent for relief of dysmenorrheal symptoms and potential effects on duration of menstruation. Ninety-eight college students were randomized to inhale the scent of either lavender oil on a sesame carrier base or placebo sesame oil. The women inhaling the lavender oil scent experienced significantly fewer symptoms of dysmenorrhea. The lavender group also demonstrated decreased menstrual bleeding, but this was not statistically significant.[169]

Stress Management and Visualization

Stress management and visualization can be used to address dysmenorrhea. Teaching patients skills in these areas can be a useful adjunct to other strategies. Counseling may be beneficial for some women.

Yoga, Exercise, and Massage Therapy

Light general exercise in the form of walking, stretching, and pelvic exercise can improve pelvic circulation and reduce dysmenorrhea, both preventatively and acutely. Excessive exercise should be avoided. A number of yoga asanas (i.e., poses) are specifically indicated for improving pelvic circulation and reducing dysmenorrhea. Receiving massage therapy can also promote general relaxation and reduce musculoskeletal and pelvic tension.

PREMENSTRUAL SYMPTOMS, PREMENSTRUAL SYNDROME, AND PREMENSTRUAL DYSPHORIC DISORDER

Is PMS due to an individual pathologic problem or is it due to cultural beliefs, beliefs that lead to the menstrual cycle being associated with a variety of negative reactions, or a combination of both? What if our societies and cultures had celebrated menstruation as a time of pleasure (and even public joy) rather than something private (to be hidden) and negative? Would we have PMS today? The answer may lie in the unravelling of the role of our shared beliefs about menstruation in society, rather than the functioning of those beliefs in individuals.[1]

Clinical Gynecologic Endocrinology and Infertility[1]

Premenstrual symptoms have been recognized at least since the time of Hippocrates; however, it was not until 1931 that the term PMS first appeared in the medical literature. By the 1950s, the term PMS was applied to the physical and psychological symptoms occurring for up to 2 weeks before menses with relief seen after the onset of the menstrual period. In the 1990s, criteria were included in the appendix of the *Diagnostic and Statistical Manual for Mental Disorders (DSM),* third and fourth editions, describing late luteal phase dysphoric disorder (LLPDD) and finally premenstrual dysphoric disorder (PMDD), a particularly severe form of PMS with an emphasis on the affective symptoms (Box 9-10). In April 2000, the American College of Obstetricians and Gynecologists (ACOG) published a practice bulletin on the topic of PMS that included criteria for diagnosis and recommendations for the treatment of clinically significant PMS (Box 9-11).[170,171]

PMS is characterized by a wide range of symptoms (Box 9-12) that recur in the luteal phase of the menstrual cycle

(1 to 2 weeks before the next menstrual period) and that cease soon after menstruation commences. Surveys estimate that 30% to 85% of women report at least one premenstrual symptom during each menstrual cycle.[172] In its milder form, PMS is estimated to affect approximately 40% of women of reproductive age; in its most severe form, it affects roughly 2.5% of women in this age group.[173] In 2% to 10% of cases, symptoms are significant enough to cause disruption in family, personal, or occupational function.[173] Between 3% and 8% develop a severe type of PMS termed *premenstrual dysphoric disorder* (PMDD).[174] PMDD is most likely to appear in the late twenties to midthirties. PMDD is primarily characterized by severe irritability, unprovoked anger, anxiety, and/or depression.[175]

Women can develop PMS at any time between puberty and menopause but tend to seek treatment more often in their thirties and forties. PMS symptoms do not persist after natural, surgical, or medically induced menopause.

More than the type of symptom, it is the timing during the menstrual cycle that is diagnostic of PMS and PMDD, although symptom severity (especially those related to

---

BOX 9-10 American Congress of Obstetricians and Gynecologists Diagnostic Criteria for Premenstrual Syndrome[171]

Patient reports one of the following affective and somatic symptoms during the 5 days before menses in each of three prior menstrual cycles:

Affective symptoms
- Anxiety
- Breast tenderness
- Confusion
- Headache

Somatic symptoms
- Abdominal bloating
- Angry outbursts
- Depression
- Irritability
- Social withdrawal
- Swelling of extremities
- Symptoms are relieved within 4 days of menses onset without recurrence until at least cycle day 13
- Symptoms present in the absence of any pharmacologic therapy, hormone ingestion, or drug or alcohol abuse
- Symptoms occur reproducibly during two cycles of prospective recording
- Patient suffers from identifiable dysfunction in social or economic performance

---

BOX 9-11 Diagnostic and Statistical Manual of Mental Disorders Fourth Edition Criteria for Premenstrual Dysphoric Disorder[176]

A. In most menstrual cycles of the past year, five (or more) of the following symptoms, which begin during the last week of the luteal phase (after ovulation) and end in the follicular phase (menses), were present most of the time and absent in the week postmenses. At least one of the symptoms must be 1, 2, 3, or 4.
   1. Markedly depressed mood; hopelessness; self-deprecating thoughts
   2. Marked anxiety, tension, feeling "keyed up" or "on edge"
   3. Marked affective lability (feeling suddenly sad or tearful; increased sensitivity to rejection)
   4. Persistent and marked anger, irritability, or increased interpersonal conflicts
   5. Decreased interest in usual activities
   6. Difficulty concentrating
   7. Lethargy, easy fatigability, or marked lack of energy
   8. Marked change in appetite; overeating or specific food cravings
   9. Hypersomnia or insomnia
   10. Sense of being overwhelmed or out of control
   11. Physical symptoms such as breast tenderness or swelling, headaches, joint or muscle pain, bloating, weight gain
B. The disturbance markedly interferes with work, school, usual social activities, and relationships with others.
C. The disturbance is not merely an exacerbation of the symptoms of another disorder, such as major depressive disorder, panic disorder, dysthymic disorder, or a personality disorder.
D. Criteria A, B, and C must be confirmed by prospective daily ratings during at least two consecutive symptomatic cycles.

BOX 9-12   Common Symptoms of Premenstrual Syndrome

Physical:
- Abdominal distention, bloating, and discomfort
- Abnormal appetite, craving sweet foods, alcohol, and/or fatty foods
- Altered libido
- Breast swelling, pain, discomfort, and/or breast lumps
- Change in bowel habit
- Cyclic weight gain
- Dizziness or fainting
- Fatigue and weakness
- Fluid retention
- Headaches
- Insomnia or excess sleepiness
- Joint pains and/or backache
- Palpitations
- Pelvic discomfort or pain
- Poor motor coordination
- Premenstrual acne/skin blemishes
- Tendency to have minor accidents
- Undesirable hair changes

Emotional and mental:
- Aggression
- Angry outbursts
- Anxiety
- Confusion
- Depression
- Feeling "overwhelmed" or "out of control"
- Forgetfulness
- Hyperreactiveness
- Irritability
- Lack of concentration
- Loneliness
- Mood swings/moodiness
- Negative affect
- Nervous tension
- Poor judgment
- Restlessness
- Tearfulness

mood changes) is the feature that distinguishes PMS and PMDD. Because PMDD differs from PMS in severity but not type of symptoms, there is considerable debate as to whether PMDD is a subset of PMS or constitutes a distinct entity. On the one hand, it has been suggested that PMDD is a media construct brought about by the popularization of PMS as a catchall diagnosis; on the other hand, it has been said that having a name and diagnosis for their intense premenstrual emotions actually provides a sense of relief and sanity to women with PMDD's characteristic symptoms. Women with PMDD have severe mood changes that occur premenstrually to the point of significant disruption in their abilities to perform daily tasks at work or in the home, unlike women with PMS, who may report the same symptoms but of a less disabling nature.[175] The mood changes seen in both PMDD and PMS must be differentiated from premenstrual magnification of an underlying psychiatric disorder or medical problem. Because differentiating between PMS and PMDD is difficult, and much of the literature considers PMDD a severe form of the psychoemotional manifestations of PMS, in this discussion PMDD is considered a subset of PMS (see Box 9-12).

PATHOPHYSIOLOGY

The precise etiology of PMS remains unknown; however, there are many proposed theories. These include:
- Abnormal hormone levels/hormonal imbalance, particularly excess estrogen; deficient progesterone; estrogen deficiency; endorphin/opiate deficiency; thyroid disorders
- Discrepancies in prostaglandins or neurotransmitters
- Latent hyperprolactinemia
- Disordered aldosterone function caused by excess estrogens
- Abnormal HPA axis functioning with diminished stress response and decreased cortisol response
- Nutrient deficiencies (especially B_6, vitamin E, vitamin A, calcium, and magnesium)
- Inappropriate diet (e.g., leading to blood sugar dysregulation; excessive caffeine intake)
- Environmental factors
- Stress (e.g., current relationship/marital/sexual difficulties; poor coping skills; workplace stress)
- Psychosocial factors (e.g., negative attitudes about menstruation, sense of personal disempowerment or low self-esteem, history of sexual abuse)
- Cultural factors (e.g., negative attitudes about menstruation, cultural expectation that menstruation is accompanied by unpleasant symptoms)[1,32,44,173,177-180]

In spite of these numerous theories, no physiologic mechanisms have been identified as definitive causes of PMS. Elimination of ovarian function by hysterectomy and bilateral oophorectomy or by medical suppression of the cycle results in complete suppression of premenstrual symptoms, implying that they are triggered by cyclical fluctuation in endogenous estrogens and progesterone. The mechanism underlying an abnormal response to these hormones in some women is not clear.[181] Studies have failed to demonstrate any consistent or remarkable hormonal differences throughout the menstrual cycle or specific to the luteal phase in women with and without symptoms, including estrogens, progesterone, testosterone, FSH, LH, PRL, endogenous opiates, and sex hormone-binding globulin (SHBG), both in terms of secretion and circulating levels.[1]

A recent hypothesis on the physiologic origins of PMS is that symptoms are related to central neurotransmitter changes occurring in response to normal fluctuations in hormone levels. Estrogens increase the production rate and receptor density of serotonin, dopamine, β-endorphins, and noradrenaline, whereas progesterone may have the opposite effect and reduce these neurotransmitters.[182-186] In part, this seems to be related to the effects of estrogens and progesterone on MAO; estrogens decrease MAO activity and progesterone increases MAO activity. In the presence of high levels of estrogens, the decreased activity of MAO reduces the catabolism of neurotransmitters and thus increases their availabilities in brain centers; conversely, high levels of progesterone (and progestogens) reverse this effect. It is hypothesized that women may have a greater susceptibility to changes in central neurotransmitters resulting from normal cyclical changes in sex steroids.[1] The largest body of evidence suggests that serotonin (5-HT) is the major neurotransmitter involved in PMS and PMDD, and that progesterone may be a key mediator of PMS. It has been found to increase 5-HT uptake in several brain regions, as well as increasing 5-HT turnover. Decreased 5-HT activity has also been observed in the late luteal phase of the menstrual cycle, and this has been implicated in increased appetite, psychomotor activity, and depression. Other aspects of central nervous system (CNS) physiology, including allopregnanolone, an allosteric receptor for gamma (γ)-aminobutyric acid (GABA) and a metabolite of progesterone, and the neurotransmitter glutamate are also responsive to cyclical variations in estrogen and progesterone, and may be collectively or independently responsible for dysphoria and PMS symptoms.[185,186]

Interest has also focused on serotonin and the positive results seen with the use of SSRIs. Women with PMS have been shown to have abnormal functioning of the serotonergic system that is related to altered serotonin levels and serotonin transmission.[187] The normal fluctuations in estrogen levels that occur in the second half of the cycle are thought to enhance or even trigger these abnormalities in susceptible women and lead to the alterations in mood seen in PMS. As described, increasing levels of estrogens in the luteal phase could inhibit the deactivation of noradrenaline and influence serotonergic pathways, thus contributing to symptoms of heightened mood such as aggression, irritability, and anxiety. Lower estrogen during perimenopause seems to contribute to depression and also seems to be influenced by altered serotonergic activity.

Symptoms are also said to develop among women with PMDD because of altered sensitivity to these central neurotransmitters, especially serotonin, triggered by changes in the normal circulating levels of estradiol and progesterone.[188] Earlier suggestions have centered on other hormonal causes of PMS, including an estrogen to progesterone ratio imbalance in favor of estrogen; or to problems with progesterone receptors such that the receptors do not transport progesterone into cells.[189,190] These theories have not borne out using biochemical assays, and have largely gone out of favor.

Disruption of the HPA axis has also recently been proposed as a cause of PMS and PMDD, and is an interesting and promising theory. It has been demonstrated that women with PMDD demonstrate a decreased effectiveness in their stress response, including a blunted cortisol response, blunted adrenal response, and decreased adrenal ACTH (i.e., corticotrophin) receptors compared with women who do not exhibit PMS symptoms.[191] These women have higher than normal circulating levels of allopregnanolone than their nonsymptomatic counterparts; however, they do not appear to break it

down to a usable form under conditions of stress, indicating a diminished stress response. Allopregnanolone is a neuroactive metabolite of progesterone and a barbiturate-like modulator of central GABA.[192] The importance of progesterone as a neuroendocrine modulator in PMS has not been fully explored. Animal studies demonstrate that stressors repeated at 3- to 5-week intervals can generate adrenal hyporesponsivity or hypocortisolism, which in turn may contribute to stress-related pathology. The role of repeated dysphoric episodes occurring on a monthly basis in PMS can be regarded as potentially affecting stress physiology. Women with PMS appear to have an abnormal response to normal levels of progesterone compared with nonsymptomatic women. Although the mechanism underlying the abnormal response to progesterone is unknown, as is the possible contribution of abnormalities in the stress axis to the symptomatology of PMS, recent data strongly suggest that PMS is characterized by stress axis physiology.[191,193]

The nature of PMS has been hotly debated and discussed, with opinions ranging from its etiology in biochemical imbalances to negative sociocultural issues influencing psychological expectations and biological responses to menstruation. Purely biochemical hypotheses may be criticized for pathologizing menstruation and ignoring social and cultural forces, whereas taking a purely sociobiological stance may ignore physical etiologies and suggest that women can merely reframe their attitudes toward menstruation and become symptom free. Many practitioners believe that the most effective approach is multifactorial and integrative, looking at biological, cultural, psychosocial, nutritional, and lifestyle factors that lead to premenstrual discomforts, PMS, and PMDD.[1,173] Further, it should be recognized that individual symptoms of PMS, for example, social withdrawal, may to a certain extent reflect a natural inclination toward solitude and quiet during what many women consider a more sensitive, creative, and intuitive time, and should not be pathologized.

DIAGNOSIS

Several sets of diagnostic criteria have been developed for PMS and PMDD (see Boxes 9-10 and 9-11). The American Psychiatric Association (APA), the National Institute of Mental Health (NIMH), and the ACOG have all established diagnostic guidelines (see the following discussion). The criteria from the APA are for PMDD. Because severity is subjective, it is difficult to definitively differentiate between premenstrual complaints, PMS, or PMDD—they represent a spectrum of symptom severity. The diversity of PMS symptoms and syndromes is great, and the validity of the *DSM-IV* descriptive entities, as well as their clinical relevance, should be seriously questioned, used as a guideline, and not be adhered to strictly.[194] At any given time, many individuals, both male and female, can identify symptoms in themselves that are characteristic of PMS/PMDD. PMS should not ultimately be considered a psychiatric disease but a constellation of symptoms that possibly occur as part of a complex interplay of biological, psychological, and societal factors.

BOX 9-13 Menstrual Symptom Diary

NAME:_____ Age:_____ Month:_____

Date																																			
Day of cycle	1	2	3	4	5	6	7	8	9	10	11	12	13	14	15	16	17	18	19	20	21	22	23	24	25	26	27	28	29	30	31	32	33	34	35	36
Menstrual flow																																				
PMS with mood changes																																				
Nervous tension																																				
Irritability																																				
Anxiety																																				
Insomnia																																				
Crying/sadness																																				
Depression																																				
Social withdrawal																																				
Lack of interest in life																																				
PMS with food cravings																																				
Craving sugar/carbs																																				
Headache/migraine																																				
Irritability if hungry																																				
Fatigue																																				
PMS with fluid retention																																				
Breast fullness																																				
Abdominal bloating																																				
Weight gain																																				
Swollen hands & feet																																				
PMS with pain																																				
Period pain																																				
Breast pain																																				
Aches and pain																																				
PMS with depletion																																				
Tiredness																																				
Mental fatigue																																				
Hot flushes																																				
Headaches/migraines																																				

Grading of menstruation
0-none
1-slight
2-moderate
3-heavy
4-heavy and clots

Grading of symptoms
0-none
1-mild-only slightly aware of symptom
2-moderate-aware of symptom, but does not interfere with activities
3-severe-continually aware of symptom, but not disabling
4-very severe-disabling and unable to function

The NIMH criteria require documentation of at least a 30% increase in severity of symptoms in the 5 days before menses over the 5 days before that. Using these two sets of criteria, approximately 5% of women are thought to experience disruptive PMS.[1]

A menstrual symptom diary that categorizes the classical symptoms of PMS is the preferred method to diagnose this syndrome (Box 9-13). The diary should be completed over at least two consecutive cycles and should show the typical variations in timing that suggest PMS—symptoms are absent for the week after the period, but appear at any time in the 2 weeks preceding menstruation, and then decline at the beginning or in the first days of the period. Symptoms should be apparent during at least two menstrual cycles for a positive diagnosis to be made.

Four distinct symptom patterns of PMS have been described (Table 9-11). These categorizations provide useful information to assist with refining the treatment plan, although they are somewhat arbitrary and there is significant overlap in symptoms.[32] Some women report greater symptoms around ovulation and the week after; others are symptomatic in the premenstrual week only; yet others report symptoms from ovulation through to the first days of the period.

There is evidence that women often do not consult a physician if they have moderate to severe PMS or PMDD symptoms. Physicians also frequently fail to ask women if moderate to severe premenstrual symptoms affect their mood and well-being. Thus the diagnosis of PMDD is often missed in primary care and gynecology settings.[186] Furthermore, whether or not a diagnosis is assigned may differ according the practitioner's gender; female physicians may be less likely to apply psychiatric labels to their female patients, and may be more apt to recognize contextual contributions to symptoms than male physicians.[195]

It should be remembered that whether a woman meets the criteria for a PMS or PMDD diagnosis is somewhat arbitrary. Lack of a diagnosable case should not be reason to invalidate a woman's experience of premenstrual symptoms and difficulties, nor should it be justification for withholding beneficial therapies. To deny women's experience based on lack of meeting diagnostic criteria would be to return to the days when it was suggested that premenstrual symptoms were merely psychosomatic, or "all in their heads." Helping women to understand that there are both physiologic and social underpinnings to their experiences can give a name to their experiences, and help them contextualize, rather than personalize, their premenstrual states, and begin to find solutions. Women presenting with symptoms who do not meet diagnostic criteria should be offered follow-up care, particularly in the case of possible PMDD.

DIFFERENTIAL DIAGNOSIS

PMS, PMDD, and premenstrual magnification of a preexisting complaint, such as depression, irritable bowel syndrome

TABLE 9-11 Premenstrual Syndrome Pattern Categories[1,32,193]

Pattern	Possible Cause	Characteristics/Symptoms
PMS-A: Anxiety	Estrogen excess and/or progesterone insufficiency HPA–related diminished stress response Neurotransmitter related effects from normal hormonal changes associated with menstruation	Anxiety Insomnia Irritability Emotional lability
PMS-C: Carbohydrate craving	Possible enhanced insulin binding effects	Sugar cravings Increased appetite (even ravenous) Headache Hypoglycemia Heart palpitations Sweating spontaneously
PMS-D: Depression	Estrogen leading to increased neurotransmitter degradation	Depression Despair Crying Feelings of hopelessness Fatigue Insomnia Apathy Low libido
PMS-H: Hyperhydration	Possible effects of increased aldosterone in the late luteal phase because of excess estrogen	Edema of hands and feet Weight gain Sense of "bloating" Clothes feel tighter Breast tenderness or sense of engorgement

PMS, Premenstrual syndrome; *HPA*, hypothalamic-pituitary-adrenal.

(IBS), or certain autoimmune conditions, can present or worsen premenstrually. Many other conditions, such as diabetes, anemia, and abnormal thyroid function or other endocrine abnormalities, might mimic some of the features of PMS without actually worsening premenstrually and also should be excluded as a cause of the symptoms. A completed menstrual symptom diary that does not reveal the previously described pattern is indicative of diagnoses other than PMS. PMDD presents with the characteristic symptoms of irritability, anger, internal tension, dysphoria, and mood lability and should be suspected when symptoms are rated as very severe on the menstrual symptom diary (grade 4).[196] It is important to note, however, that although the use of the prospective menstrual symptom questionnaire can provide useful information on the type of symptoms, it is not always a reliable indicator of symptom severity. Trials have shown that questionnaires can be used to differentiate between women with and without symptoms suggestive of PMS, but that they are not sensitive predictors of severity or reliable tools to make a definitive diagnosis of PMDD.[197] Differentiation between PMS and PMDD usually relies on the clinical judgment of the consulting practitioner in conjunction with an evaluation of the symptoms against the criteria described in the appendix to the 1994 *DSM-IV: Criteria for Premenstrual Dysphoric Disorder* (Box 9-11). Symptoms must be confirmed by prospective daily ratings during at least two consecutive symptomatic cycles. At least one of the symptoms must be severe depression, anxiety, mood lability, or anger, and the severity of the symptoms must be such that they disrupt daily life.

CONVENTIONAL TREATMENT APPROACHES

The medical treatment of PMS and PMDD includes OCs and other hormonal treatment strategies, NSAIDs, SSRIs, BMT, antidepressants, and diuretics, as well as concentrating on symptom relief with specific symptom-related drug treatments. Most of these methods have failed to demonstrate definitive benefits over placebo, with the exception of antidepressants (particularly SSRIs) and GnRH and other ovulation suppressants, which have demonstrable benefit.[187]

Hormonal Treatments

Of the hormonal medications used to treat PMS, some prevent ovulation, whereas others affect the hormonal profile. OCs improve PMS symptoms in some women, have no effect in others, and may worsen symptoms in some. A monophasic pill is the most suitable option for women who experience PMS with mood changes, whereas a triphasic pill is more suitable when women have physical symptoms of breast pain and swelling.[198] Danazol is also prescribed to manipulate hormones. When taken on a daily basis this drug suppresses ovulation and is used for the treatment of breast pain and PMS.[199,200] This is generally an unpopular treatment because of side effects; however, reported improvements include a reduction in breast pain, fatigue, food cravings, and anxiety.

GnRH agonists have been trialed, sometimes in combination with OCs for premenstrual symptoms.[201] These protocols, known as "add-back" therapy, require that a woman take the GnRH agonist combined with low doses of estrogens and progestogens. GnRH agonists alone are unpopular because many women are not prepared to exchange PMS for menopausal symptoms and reduced bone density; also GnRH agonists alone did not help mood symptoms.[202] Add-back therapy showed more promise. This treatment is controversial and is reserved for severe and intractable cases of PMS.

Ponstan (mefenamic acid) has been used to treat mood swings, fatigue, headache, and the general aches and pains that accompany PMS.[203] The use of these NSAIDs should be restricted to a 7-day interval, making them unsuitable for the many women who experience PMS for more than 7 days before their period.[204] NSAIDs do not reverse the prostaglandin imbalance that causes excessive menstruation, pain, or PMS, and have to be used indefinitely unless the causes of the imbalance are identified and rectified. This prospect is not appealing to many women, especially because these drugs have many side effects.

Diuretics

Diuretics will not improve most symptoms of PMS and have been shown to be useful only symptomatically for those women who gain weight premenstrually. Spironolactone has not demonstrated benefits over placebo in double-blind, placebo-controlled trials.[1]

Antidepressants

A number of recent trials have verified the effectiveness of the SSRIs in the treatment of severe PMS or PMDD. Fluoxetine, sertraline, and citalopram given throughout the menstrual cycle have been shown to be well tolerated and effective.[197,231] Some of the SSRIs, such as citalopram, have also been shown to be effective when used during the luteal phase of the cycle only.[206] Venlafaxine (Effexor), a new-generation antidepressant that selectively inhibits serotonin and noradrenaline reuptake, has been evaluated for effectiveness in the treatment of PMDD and has been shown to be more efficacious than placebo.[207]

Despite their effectiveness, the SSRIs have considerable side effects, including GI disturbances, headache, sedation, insomnia, weight gain, impaired memory, excessive perspiration, and sexual dysfunction. The tricyclic antidepressants have been used successfully, particularly nortriptyline and clomipramine. The benzodiazepine Alprazolam has also been suggested as a treatment for PMS and PMDD; however, dependence and tolerance occur quickly and make these types of drugs less attractive options for these conditions.

Dietary Supplements

Physicians have also prescribed vitamins B_6, A, and E; phenylalanine, L-tryptophan, calcium, magnesium; and herbal remedies, especially chaste berry extract. Among the treatment modalities that have not been shown to be effective in well-controlled studies are progesterone, thyroid hormones, lithium, and EPO.[187]

Surgery

Surgery to remove the ovaries is a controversial and radical option sometimes suggested; however, it is unacceptable to most women to trade the symptoms of PMS with those of premature menopause as well as the risk of loss of bone density; thus this option is reserved for severe and intractable cases.

BOTANICAL TREATMENT OF PMS AND PMDD

Botanical practice takes a multifactorial approach to PMS, addressing the patient's personal beliefs about menstruation, psychosocial situation, lifestyle factors, and incorporating a physiologic approach that treats both symptoms and underlying hormonal and HPA dysregulation. This integrative and comprehensive approach may be particularly relevant in PMS and PMDD because the condition is considered to have physiologic, psychological, and sociocultural origins.[173]

Physiologic treatment with herbs focuses on symptomatic relief (e.g., treatment of anxiety, irritability, depression, insomnia, acne, mastalgia, dysmenorrhea) for mild premenstrual complaints, and a combination of the aforementioned symptomatic relief, hormonal modulation, and improving physiologic and emotional stress response in PMS. PMDD is treated slightly more aggressively, with herbs included for hormonal and stress response dysregulation and mood dysphoria symptoms. Though some of these approaches are based on what are still theoretical grounds, a small number of trials and significant practitioner experience provide at least preliminary justification for these strategies.

For many women, a complex plan with a combination of herbal therapies is required to treat a constellation of symptoms; for example, when there are concomitant sugar cravings, dysmenorrhea, moderate to severe anxiety, or depression. Lasting improvements also require lifestyle, stress management, and personal/attitudinal changes. Patients should eliminate or at least minimize coffee, alcohol, and tobacco use, and should have a diet with frequent meals high in protein and low in refined sugar, and with optimal intake of vitamins and minerals. Excess sodium should be reduced when there is fluid retention, edema, or breast tenderness. Women should get regular exercise and maintain a healthy body weight for their heights, ages, and activity levels. Stress management techniques should be practiced regularly. Women who feel self-empowered and in control of their lives experience PMS symptoms with less frequency than other women; women should seek support and counseling to create the necessary lifestyle changes that improve self-esteem.[1,175]

The treatments discussed in the following are categorized by major PMS/PMDD symptoms. For comprehensive treatment of multiple symptoms, readers will want to refer to additional sections mentioned under the Botanical Treatment Summary for Premenstrual Syndrome—for example, insomnia, dysmenorrhea, acne, and mastalgia—and include protocol from those sections into multiherb formulae (Table 9-12).

Hormonal Modulation

Symptoms suggesting the need for hormonal modulation include:

- Mood swings
- Breast fullness or heaviness
- Fatigue
- Abdominal bloating

Hormonal modulation is a regular part of the treatment approach to PMS management. Chaste tree *(Vitex agnus-castus)*, taken daily throughout the cycle, is the principal herb used. Increased enterohepatic recycling of estrogens,

achieved through dietary modification and herbal bitters (see Bitters and Hepatic Tonics) is often also suggested.

Mood Changes

Symptoms suggesting the need to address mood include:

- Fatigue
- Feeling overwhelmed
- Anxiety
- Crying
- Depression
- Increased sense of vulnerability

TABLE 9-12   Botanical Treatment Summary for Premenstrual Syndrome

Therapeutic Goal	Therapeutic Action	Botanical Name	Common Name
Hormonal regulation	Hormonal modulators	*Vitex agnus-castus*	Chaste berry
Mood stabilization; improve stress response	Nervines	*Hypericum perforatum*	St. John's wort
		Lavandula officinalis	Lavender
		Leonurus cardiaca	Motherwort
		Matricaria recutita	Chamomile
		Passiflora incarnata	Passionflower
		Scutellaria lateriflora	Skullcap
		Valeriana officinalis	Valerian
	Adaptogens	*Eleutherococcus senticosus*	Eleuthero
		Panax ginseng	Ginseng
		Panax quinquefolius	American ginseng
		Rhaponticum carthamoides	Rhaponticum
		Rhodiola rosea	Rhodiola
		Schisandra chinensis	Schisandra
		Urtica dioica	Nettles
		Withania somnifera	Ashwagandha
	Antidepressants	*Hypericum perforatum*	St. John's wort
		Melissa officinalis	Lemon balm
		(See Adaptogens)	
	Anxiolytics	*Eschscholzia californica*	California poppy
		Lavandula officinalis	Lavender
		Leonurus cardiaca	Motherwort
		Matricaria recutita	Chamomile
		Passiflora incarnata	Passionflower
		Piper methysticum	Kava kava
		Scutellaria laterifolia	Skullcap
		Valeriana officinalis	Valerian
		Verbena officinalis	Blue vervain
		Withania somnifera	Ashwagandha
	Hormonal regulators	*Vitex agnus-castus*	Chaste berry
		Cimicifuga racemosa	Black cohosh
Regulate appetite; relieve sweets cravings; improve bowel function to reduce circulating estrogen load	Bitters	*Centaurium erythraea*	Centaury
		Gentiana lutea	Gentian
		Taraxacum officinale	Dandelion root
Relieve fluid retention; may improve edema and breast fullness/tenderness	Diuretics	*Taraxacum officinale*	Dandelion leaf
Relief of PMS headache	See Premenstrual Headache and Migraine		
Relief of menstrually related pain	See Dysmenorrhea		
Relief of mastalgia	See Benign Breast Disorders and Breast Pain		
Treatment of premenstrual acne	See Acne		
Promote improved sleep	See Insomnia		

PMS, Premenstrual syndrome.

- Insomnia
- Irritability and angry outbursts
- Lack of interest in daily life
- Nervous tension
- Sadness
- Social withdrawal
- Night waking

Many women respond to hormonal fluctuations with mild to severe mood changes, either with anxiety and heightened (negative) affect or classic depressive symptoms in which withdrawal and fatigue predominate. Perimenopausal women often experience heightened depressive symptoms owing to declines in estrogen and serotonin. PMS depression, irritability, and fatigue also may occur when a woman is postpartum, breast-feeding, overexercising, underweight, or under stress. Treatment concentrates on hormonal modulation, as well as the use of anxiolytic, antidepressant, nervine, and stress-modifying herbs (e.g., adaptogens).

Improve the Stress Response

Symptoms suggesting the need to modify the stress response include:

- Crying
- Fatigue
- Adrenal exhaustion
- Blood sugar dysregulation
- Labile mood
- Feeling out of control or overwhelmed
- Headaches or migraines
- Hot flashes and night sweats
- Mental fatigue
- Poor word finding, memory loss
- Other symptoms of stress, for example, hair loss and insomnia

Maladaptive stress response in women susceptible to PMS may be an important trigger for premenstrual mood difficulties. Decreased levels of plasma adrenocorticotropic hormones (i.e., ACTH) have been documented in PMS, and the suggestion that the dysphoria of atypical depressions such as postnatal depression, seasonal affective disorder, and PMS are caused by lower levels of CRH.[177,208] Herbal treatment for women who develop PMS in conjunction with exhaustion should combine hormone modulation with adaptogens, nervine tonics, and anxiolytic herbs to counteract the adverse effects of stress on the nervous system. Adaptogens not only assist in restoring a healthy response to stress but also have blood sugar regulatory effects (see Chapter 5 for more on adaptogens). Adequate rest, nutrition, and exercise can also improve stress response.

Premenstrual Pain

Symptoms suggesting the need for pain management include:

- Breast pain
- Headaches or migraines
- Dysmenorrhea
- Aches and pains

Some women experience increased sensitivity to pain premenstrually.

See related topics such as Premenstrual Headache and Migraine; Dysmenorrhea; and Benign Breast Disorder and Breast Pain for treatment options.

Sugar Cravings

Symptoms of PMS food cravings:

- Craving for sweets and refined carbohydrates
- Increased appetite
- Fatigue
- Headaches or migraines
- Irritability, especially when hungry

Sugar cravings are common before menses. Abnormal variations in blood sugar may be worsened by a magnesium deficiency, an imbalance in prostaglandins, or prolonged stress. Changes in serotonin levels are also associated with sugar and carbohydrate cravings. Herbalists often include bitters in herbal formulae for sugar cravings; however, the use of herbal treatments for PMS-C has not been evaluated. Herbal adaptogens have demonstrated the ability to regulate blood sugar, and may be of some help in premenstrual sugar cravings. Attention to diet may be the most beneficial approach, teaching women with PMS-C to maintain stable blood sugar by ensuring small frequent meals of high protein and high-quality complex carbohydrates, fresh fruits and vegetables, and high-energy snacks such as nuts and yogurt. Often when a high-quality diet is implemented, with the addition of a complex vitamin and mineral supplement, cravings dissipate. It is also perfectly reasonable for women who are within normal body weight and with healthy diets to indulge in a small amount of sweets premenstrually. When clients have chocolate cravings, encourage them to eat only very dark chocolate—it is much harder to overeat dark than milk chocolate. Nettle (Urtica dioica) is an herb often overlooked as an adaptogen; however, a number of herbalists specializing in women's herbal health care have found it remarkably effective in reducing sugar cravings when taken at the onset of a craving.

Premenstrual Syndrome with Fluid Retention

Symptoms of PMS with fluid retention:

- Breast fullness
- Abdominal bloating
- Weight gain
- Swollen extremities

Fluid retention is believed to be caused by an increase in circulating aldosterone levels. Aldosterone may be elevated in response to decreased progesterone secretion, elevated estrogens, magnesium deficiency, or stress. PRL also may be implicated when breast symptoms predominate. When fluid retention, bloating, breast soreness or heaviness, and weight gain are prominent symptoms, salt and high-sodium food (e.g., cheese) intake should be restricted and dietary potassium in the form of vegetables and fruits increased. Herbal diuretics may be considered, but diuresis, whether herbal or pharmaceutical, does not treat underlying causes. Chaste berry should be considered when there is suspected elevated PRL or fluid retention accompanied by mastalgia. However, herbal treatments for PMS-H have not been evaluated.

Premenstrual Dysphoric Disorder

Symptoms of PMDD:

- Nervous tension
- Irrational and angry outbursts
- Depression
- Insomnia
- Anxiety
- Agoraphobia
- Social withdrawal
- Lack of interest in daily life

The herbal therapies and additional treatments outlined throughout this section, particularly for PMS with mood changes, are applicable to PMDD, although more aggressive treatment may be necessary and more frequent follow-up conducted with the patient. Herbal strategies include hormonal regulation and use of nervines, adaptogens, antidepressants, and anxiolytics.

DISCUSSION OF BOTANICALS

Hormonal Modulation

Black Cohosh

Black cohosh has a history of use by the Eclectic physicians for premenstrual and menstrual complaints. Most research has evaluated black cohosh efficacy in perimenopause; it has demonstrated positive effects in the treatment of neurovegetative complaints, including hot flashes, sweating, sleep disturbances, and depression.[209-215] Black cohosh was initially thought to have estrogen-like effects via its ability to modulate estrogen receptors and called a phyto-SERM (selective estrogen receptor modulator), but it is now thought to have serotonergic or dopaminergic effects rather than estrogenic action. It may be beneficial in PMS patients with headache and those perimenopausal type of symptoms mentioned earlier that can occur premenstrually. The German Commission E approves the use of black cohosh for the treatment of premenstrual discomfort, dysmenorrhea, and neurovegetative symptoms of menopause.[44]

Chaste Berry

Chaste berry has been used traditionally, and is still commonly used in Europe and the United States, to relieve symptoms of a number of gynecologic disorders, including those attributed to PMS. The berries are the most popular part of the plant used and contain a wide range of potentially active constituents, including essential oils, iridoids, and flavonoids.[181] In humans, it has been shown (at doses of 120 mg/d) to reduce levels of FSH and increase LH, resulting in decreased estrogen and increased progesterone and PRL levels.[173] Several studies have shown reduction of PRL concentration after treatment with chaste berry. One proposed mechanism of action is that this herb (doses of approximately 480 mg/d) causes a decrease

in PRL, which leads to a reversal of LH suppression, allowing full development of the corpus luteum, increasing progesterone levels, and reducing symptoms of PMS. However, chaste berry also appears to have dopamine-agonistic properties at higher doses.

No long-term randomized trials have compared medical treatments (e.g., OCs, antidepressants) with chaste berry. Numerous trials have evaluated the efficacy of chaste tree in the treatment of PMS. A 2013 systematic review evaluated the safety and efficacy of chaste berry from 12 randomized clinical trials. For PMS, seven out of eight trials using chaste berry extracts improved PMS symptoms better than placebo, magnesium oxide, and pyridoxine. One trial reviewed found chaste berry to outperform fluoxetine for PMDD, but another reported the two to be equivalent in terms of efficacy. One trial investigating chaste berry and latent hyperprolactinemia observed effects superior to placebo in reducing TRH-stimulated PRL secretion, balancing luteal phase length, and increasing midluteal progesterone and 17-β-estradiol levels. Another trial found chaste berry to be equivalent to BMT for reducing serum PRL levels and alleviating cyclic mastalgia. Reviewers concluded adverse events associated with chaste berry use are mild and infrequent. Using the Cochrane risk of bias and the Jadad scale to assess methodological integrity, the reviewers judged the quality of evidence to be moderate to high.[216] A 2012 multicenter double-blind randomized trial ($n = 162$) investigated the clinical effects of 8 mg and 20 mg of chaste berry extract over three menstrual cycles. Using VAS to measure symptoms, significant effects were observed in the 20 mg group compared with the 8 mg group and placebo. A higher dose was tested at 30 mg, but no notable benefits were observed (Extract Ze 440).[217] In another clinical trial that same year ($n = 128$; active 62, placebo 66), participants recorded symptoms on a questionnaire at the commencement and conclusion of the study, with PMS symptoms rated using VAS. Forty drops of chaste berry extract were administered 6 days before menses for six consecutive cycles. Chaste berry extract was found to relieve PMS symptoms better than placebo (Further preparation details not provided).[218] A 2010 prospective double-blind randomized trial ($n = 67$) assessed the efficacy of chaste berry extract in treating PMS symptoms. Outcomes were measured using a premenstrual symptom diary (with a 60% reduction in sum scores defined as efficacy). The experimental group experienced reduced PMS symptoms (especially water retention and negative mood) compared with controls (Extract BNO 1095).[219] A 2009 randomized clinical trial investigated the effect of a combination of *Hypericum* spp. and chaste berry on premenstrual symptoms (particularly anxiety and dehydration) in perimenopausal women. Over 16 weeks, 14 women participated. Benefits over placebo were observed as measured by the Abraham's Menstrual Symptom Questionnaire (Preparation not provided).[220] Another 2009 double-blind, multicenter clinical trial (experimental $n = 108$, placebo $n = 109$) investigated the efficacy of chaste berry extract in treating PMS symptoms. Outcomes were measured using a premenstrual symptom diary, with scores taken at baseline and at termination (i.e., third cycle). The treatment group experienced a significantly lower final premenstrual symptom diary score than the placebo group (Extract BNO 1095).[221]

A multicenter study over 16 years assessed the efficacy of chaste berry (Agnolyt) in 1592 women suffering from PMS and related menstrual disorders.[222] In 90% of patients, the doctor's evaluation was good or satisfactory; 33% became symptom free; 51% recognized improvement but not complete alleviation. One third of those wanting to conceive became pregnant during treatment. A study involving 1500 women suffering from PMS were administered chaste berry extract. Of these women 1016 had corpus luteum insufficiency and 170 had fibroids. After treatment for an average of 166 days, 90% showed improvement in symptoms occurring on average 25 days after commencing treatment.[223]

A double-blind study involving 217 women tested *V. agnus-castus* against placebo for the treatment of PMS. For a period of 3 months, 105 women took chaste berry 300 mg tablets three times daily, whereas 112 women took placebos. The results of the study showed a dramatic improvement at the end of the first cycle for both groups with relative stability over the remaining two cycles. *V. agnus-castus* improved the symptom "feel jittery or restless," but there was a difference observed between placebo and the herb for other symptoms. Another study compared the efficacy of chaste berry to pyridoxine (B_6) in the treatment of PMS over three menstrual cycles. Ninety participants were given one capsule of Agnolyt (each capsule containing 3.5 to 4.2 mg of dried chaste berry). The other 85 participants were given placebo twice daily from day 1 to 15 and then 100 mg twice daily of pyridoxine from days 16 to 35. When assessed by patients and the investigators, the chaste tree group achieved a significantly greater improvement in typical PMS complaints such as breast tenderness, edema, inner tension, headache, constipation, and depression compared with pyridoxine. Both preparations were well tolerated with only mild reactions reported in a few patients. Five patients from the chaste tree group became pregnant.[224]

Another double-blind, placebo-controlled study examined the tolerability and efficacy of chaste berry extract for premenstrual mastalgia. The treatment or placebo was given over three menstrual cycles. Mastalgia during at least 5 days of the cycle before the treatment was the strict inclusion criteria. The results showed the intensity of the cyclical breast pain diminished in the chaste berry group and the herb was well tolerated.[225] In a prospective, multicenter trial the efficacy of a chaste berry was investigated in 43 patients with PMS. The patients took 20 mg *V. agnus-castus* extract daily for three menstrual cycles. Symptoms in three posttreatment cycles were compared with baseline cycles before administration of the herb. A menstrual distress questionnaire was the tool used for self-assessment. At the end of the study, symptoms were reduced in the late luteal phase by 47.2%. Although symptoms gradually returned after treatment cessation, a difference from baseline remained for up to three cycles.[226] A multicentric open trial investigated the efficacy and tolerance

of *V. agnus-castus* in 1634 patients suffering from PMS. A specific questionnaire was developed for determining the effect of chaste berry on the four characteristic PMS symptom complexes: depression, anxiety, craving, and fluid retention. After three menstrual cycles, 93% of patients reported a decrease in the number of symptoms or symptom complexes or even cessation of PMS complaints and 85% of physicians rated the treatment as good or very good. The severity and frequency of breast pain reduced after 3 months. The majority of patients assessed the tolerance of *V. agnus-castus* as good or very good. Adverse drug reactions were suspected in only 1.2% of patients, but none were serious.[44]

A randomized, double-blind, placebo-controlled trial compared chaste berry with placebo in 170 women with PMS over three menstrual cycles. Women undertook self-assessment of irritability, mood alteration, headache, breast fullness, and other menstrual symptoms and were also assessed for changes in clinical global impression. The study showed that chaste berry was an effective and well-tolerated treatment for the relief of PMS symptoms in 52% of the trial participants compared with 24% in placebo.[227]

As with all herbal remedies, a variety of chaste berry preparations are used that can differ substantially in terms of, for instance, concentration of active ingredients or bioavailability. Surveys of members of the National Institute of Medical Herbalists and the American Herbalists Guild showed that the tincture is the most popular preparation among herbalists, in a dose of 3 to 5 mL once or twice daily, but fluid extracts and powdered herb preparations are also used.[112,181] Chaste berry is approved by the German Commission E for irregularities of the menstrual cycle, PMS, and mastodynia (Fig. 9-8).[44]

Adaptogens

Although research has not been conducted specifically on the treatment of PMS with adaptogens, herbs in this category may have an important role to play in the treatment of affective mood symptoms and decreased stress resistance in the luteal phase of the menstrual cycle. For

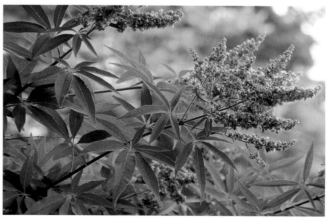

FIGURE 9-8 Chaste tree, chaste berry *(Vitex agnus-castus)*. (Photo by Martin Wall.)

example, ashwagandha is an important nervine tonic and anxiolytic for women and is used as an adaptogen during episodes of prolonged stress. It can be used as an adjunct to other herbal treatment to reduce the effects of stress-induced hormonal changes, and has mild musculoskeletal relaxing activity.[85,228] Numerous clinical studies have confirmed that *Eleutherococcus* has the ability to improve physiologic responses to stress.[52] Apart from improving exhaustion-induced PMS symptoms, it can be used to improve mood in conjunction with nervine tonics, and as an adrenal adaptogen to improve HPA axis activity. A discussion of adaptogens is found under Herbal Actions; thorough evidence for individual adaptogens is presented in Chapter 5. No clinical trials have evaluated the effects of adaptogens on PMS. Suggested adaptogens for PMS treatment include ashwagandha, ginseng, American ginseng, and eleuthero.

Anxiolytics, Nervines, and Antidepressants

Chamomile

A recent double-blind clinical trial tested the effects of chamomile extract (100 mg) and mefenamic acid (250 mg) taken three times daily for symptoms associated with PMS in 90 college-aged women. Using daily questionnaires, chamomile demonstrated more efficacy in attenuating the emotional correlates of PMS than mefenamic acid.[229]

Kava kava

Herbalists commonly use kava kava for anxiety and insomnia accompanying PMS. A systematic review and meta-analysis of the evidence for kava kava as an anxiolytic suggests that kava kava is effective compared with placebo.[230] Several small trials have demonstrated the efficacy of kava kava in treating menopause-related anxiety; however, no trials have evaluated kava kava for women with PMS symptoms.[173] Recently, concerns have arisen over the safety of kava kava owing to approximately 80 international case reports of hepatotoxicity allegedly related to kava kava consumption, leading several nations to ban kava kava sales. Although the evidence for kava kava-related liver disease is highly inconclusive, kava kava should not be taken by patients using other medications, known hepatotoxic substances, or with known liver disorders.[32]

Lavender

Lavender is an excellent herb for the anxiety, irritability, insomnia, and depression that accompany PMS. The essential oil constitutes 1% to 3% of the active components and has been shown to elicit feelings of happiness.[231] The *Complete German Commission E Monograph* states the indications for lavender as mood and sleep disturbances, restlessness, and intestinal conditions of nervous origin.[44] It can be taken as a tea or tincture, or the essential oil scent can be indirectly inhaled through a diffuser, in a bath, via application to a pillow on which the patient will sleep, or diluted for use in a massage oil.

Motherwort

Motherwort was used by the Eclectics and continues to be used by herbalists today for the treatment of nervous exhaustion, irritability, hysteria, and nervous excitability.[122] It is used clinically for the treatment of dysmenorrhea, and also has mild cardiotonic action, effectively reducing palpitations. Motherwort's combined actions make it a useful addition to PMS formulae, particularly when there is emotional lability and irritability, and if there is accompanying pain. It has a good safety profile. Because of its bitter taste, it is typically taken in tincture form. The German Commission E approves motherwort for nervous cardiac disorders.[44]

St. John's Wort

St. John's wort is prescribed for depressive symptoms of PMS or for PMDD. Trials have shown favorable results in depression, and St. John's wort has been compared favorably with both placebo and other antidepressants. A pilot study evaluating the effects of St. John's wort on PMS demonstrated significant improvement in all outcome measures, with over two thirds of the sample experiencing at least a 50% decline in symptom severity.[232] Antidepressant drugs for PMS are increasingly prescribed during the luteal phase of the cycle only; however, St. John's wort seems to be more effective when taken all month. In recent years, numerous double-blind, randomized trials have been conducted examining the efficacy of St. John's wort compared with placebo. Although one study failed to find any benefit over placebo, many others have found it to be an effective and well-tolerated herb for the treatment of mild to moderate depressive disorders.[233-235] In a large study of 2166 patients suffering from mild to moderate depression, between 83.7% and 88.6% improved after approximately 7 weeks of treatment. The drug tolerance was good or very good for 99% of all patients, and adverse drug reactions were only 0.41%.[236] A randomized, double-blind, placebo-controlled, crossover study ($n = 35$) investigated the use of *Hypericum* spp. 900 mg/day (standardized to 0.18% hypericin, 3.38% hyperforin) in PMS symptoms alleviation over four menstrual cycles. Measures included daily symptom report, State-Trait Anxiety Inventory (STAI), Beck Depression Inventory, aggression questionnaire, and Barratt Impulsiveness Scale. Plasma hormone (i.e., FSH, LH, estradiol, progesterone, PRL, and testosterone) and cytokine (i.e., IL-1, IL-6, IL-8, interferon-gamma [IFN-γ], and tumor necrosis factor-alpha [TNF-α]) levels were measured in the experimental and control groups. *Hypericum* spp. demonstrated statistically significant benefit in physical and behavioral PMS symptom alleviation ($p < .05$) compared with controls. No significant benefits were seen with mood, pain, plasma hormone, or cytokine levels.[237]

A number of trials have compared *Hypericum* with common antidepressant medications, usually with favorable results. One double-blind, randomized trial compared the efficacy and side effects of St. John's wort and the antidepressant sertraline in 87 patients with major depression.

Both treatments were effective and there were no important differences in changes in depression between the two groups at 12 weeks, with significantly more side effects in the sertraline group than in the St. John's wort group, suggesting St. John's wort is a good first-choice therapy.[238] Another trial compared St. John's wort, placebo, and sertraline. Neither sertraline nor St. John's wort were significantly different from placebo and neither was effective in moderately severe major depression, with 31.9% of the placebo-treated patients, 23.9% of the St. John's wort–treated patients, and 24.8% of sertraline-treated patients showing improvement.[239] Two randomized, controlled, double-blind trials compared St. John's wort and Prozac. In one, between 42% to 50% of the St. John's wort group and 52% to 58% of the Prozac group responded favorably, suggesting that St. John's wort is therapeutically equivalent to Prozac and is a rational alternative to synthetic antidepressants.[240] In the other trial, St. John's wort extract and fluoxetine were compared in 240 patients with mild to moderate depression. Both treatment groups were equivalent in terms of response, but the safety of St. John's wort was substantially superior to fluoxetine and fewer adverse events were reported.[241] A recent study examined the acute effects of St. John's wort on cognitive and psychomotor function compared with amitriptyline. Amitriptyline impaired performance on a battery of psychological tests, whereas St. John's wort had neutral effects on performance in these tests.[242]

Additional important nervines and anxiolytics for the treatment of anxiety, insomnia, and irritability associated with PMS include:

Blue vervain
California poppy
Chamomile
Passionflower
Skullcap
Valerian

These herbs are discussed elsewhere throughout this book.

Antiinflammatory Herbs
Evening Primrose Oil

Many practitioners use EPO for PMS believing that its effects on reduction in inflammatory prostaglandins (PGE_1) may improve PMS symptoms. Seven clinical trials have failed to find any improvement in PMS symptoms; however, it has been noted in the literature that small sample sizes in five of the trials may have prevented detection of modest benefit.[173] One paper reported positive outcomes for cardinal symptoms, but the trial had methodological flaws.[181] It is typically recommended at a dose of 2 to 3 g/d.[173]

Ginkgo

A placebo-controlled trial demonstrated statistically significant positive results in reduction of breast pain and fluid retention, but no other symptoms of PMS, after treatment for two cycles.[32,181] A recent single-blind, randomized, placebo-controlled trial ($n = 90$) in 2009 investigated the use of ginkgo leaf tablets in medical students. Subjects were administered 40 mg tablets 3 times daily. Using daily symptom rating forms, the ginkgo group reported a 23.7% reduction in symptoms, compared with 8.7% reported in the placebo group.[148] Constituents may play a role in antiinflammatory effects, antioxidant effects, or vascular smooth muscle relaxation. Further evaluation is needed to determine whether there is an important role for ginkgo in the treatment of these PMS symptoms.[173,181]

Bitters and Hepatic Tonics

Many herbalists consider the use of herbs that gently improve liver function important in formulae for hormonal regulation.

Herbal bitters, such as gentian, centaury, and dandelion, are commonly used and also may be used to regulate blood sugar fluctuations associated with functional (reactive) hypoglycemia and may improve symptoms when associated with PMS.[52]

🌸 TRADITIONAL CHINESE MEDICINE AND PRE-MENSTRUAL SYNDROME

When it comes to the treatment of premenstrual syndrome (PMS) in the clinic, many herbalists turn to the use of Traditional Chinese Medicine (TCM), which offers a unique perspective on possible etiologies and treatment. The predominant patterns associated with PMS are "liver qi stagnation" and "blood deficiency," to which women are considered especially susceptible because of monthly blood loss. Further, anger, frustration, and irritability may actually cause liver qi stagnation, making this a self-perpetuating problem. Although TCM prescribing is always based on physical examination and determination of the specific imbalances of the individual, several classic formulae may be more generically applied.

Xiao Yao Wan (Free and Easy Wanderer)
For liver qi stagnation: Indicated for premenstrual abdominal and breast distention, irritability, moodiness, depression, and clumsiness.

Ingredients: *Bupleurum falcatum* (9 g), *Angelica sinensis* (9 g), *Paeonia lactiflora* (12 g), *Atractylodes macrocephala* (9 g), *Poria cocos* (15 g), *Glycyrrhiza uralensis* (6 g), and *Zingiber officinalis* (three slices).

This formula is taken as a decoction or powder, and is available as a patent medicine. (See Selecting and Identifying Quality Herbal Products with TCM Patent Medicines.)

Angelica-White Peony-Rehmannia Decoction
For liver-blood deficiency: Indicated when there is depression, weepiness, slight abdominal and breast distention, fatigue, poor memory, poor sleep, mild dizziness, pale complexion, and scant periods. This formula is used to nourish the blood.

Ingredients: *Angelica sinensis* (9 g), *Paeonia lactiflora* (8 g), *Rehmannia glutinosa* (prepared 9 g), *Dioscorea opposita* (6 g), *Fructus corni officinalis* (4 g), *Alismatis orientalis* (4 g), *Moutan radicis* (4 g), *Poria cocos* (8 g), *Citrus reticulata* (4.5 g), *Bupleurum falcatum* (6 g), and *Albizia julibrissin* (9 g).

To be taken as a decoction throughout the menstrual cycle.

👤 CASE HISTORY: PREMENSTRUAL SYNDROME

Julie is a 42-year-old woman presenting with prolonged and severe premenstrual syndrome (PMS). She describes her moods as swinging violently just around her periods and says she is "unpleasant to be around, especially for her kids." On further questioning, she revealed a tendency to verbal abuse when premenstrual. She decided to have children late in life after a successful career and has had them close together so that the age gap is small. She is now a full-time mother and does not have the social or professional contacts she once enjoyed. Julie was seeking advice for self-diagnosed PMS but the severity of her symptoms indicated that a more appropriate diagnosis was PMDD. She had developed postnatal depression after the birth of her second child, but was offered little support from her medical practitioner who discouraged her from seeking counseling and put her on the antidepressant Prozac. She was taken off after a year but continued to have severe premenstrual mood changes, including depressive episodes, agoraphobia, low self-esteem, insomnia, and angry outbursts. This worsened as the children became older and, as she put it, "became more difficult to control." She described low energy levels, generalized body aching, poor adherence to a reasonable diet with abnormal sugar and salt cravings, headaches, and a tendency to catch numerous colds premenstrually. In addition, she developed stress and urge incontinence since the birth of her children. Although it was clear that counseling would go a long way to helping her deal with many of her emotional problems, she was unwilling to undertake this step and asked for herbal treatment instead. A treatment plan was discussed that consisted of hormone-regulating herbs combined with nervine tonics and nervine sedatives.

Her first treatment was as follows:
1. Chaste berry *(Vitex agnus-castus)* tablets 1000 mg, one tablet daily in the morning continued throughout the cycle
2. An herbal tincture:

Botanical Prescription 1

Ashwagandha	*(Withania somnifera)*	30 mL
Kava kava	*(Piper methysticum)*	30 mL
St. John's wort	*(Hypericum perforatum)*	20 mL
Lavender	*(Lavandula officinalis)*	20 mL
		Total: 100 mL

Dose: 7 mL twice daily

3. Fish oil capsules, 1000 mg, two capsules twice daily
She was asked to restrict stimulants, sugar, and salt; substitute refined carbohydrates with complex carbohydrates; have a higher-protein intake in the evenings; and increase her dietary intake of essential fatty acids. In addition, she undertook a regular regimen of pelvic floor exercises and restricted the number of times she passed urine by not voiding at the first urge to do so. She was also asked to keep a menstrual symptom diary for every day of the cycle.

At her next visit, Julie reported a marked change in her mood premenstrually, with improved sleep and better relationships with her children. Her bladder control had improved in that the urge incontinence was better, but she still suffered from stress incontinence. A referral was arranged for a physiotherapist specializing in bladder control and Julie also decided to see a counselor. Her herbal prescription was continued and she was also given magnesium and vitamin B complex to be taken for 10 days before her period. This regimen was continued for three cycles.

One of the main issues in PMDD is the long-term management, especially after postnatal depression. Herbal treatment for depressive mood change needs to be protracted in many cases and may need to be continued for up to a year or even longer. A holistic approach incorporating dietary and lifestyle changes in conjunction with effective counseling is necessary so that herbal medication can be stopped with a high degree of confidence that symptoms will not recur. In addition, hormonal symptoms must be addressed. It is common for some form of PMS to be an ongoing and major concern for women who have suffered from PMDD and postnatal depression, especially when they are in their forties when PMS can classically worsen anyway. In Julie's case, she had already tried antidepressants and was fearful that herbal treatments might cause her the same problem; that is, she would manage while on the treatment, but her mood would deteriorate once more when the herbs were ceased. The determining factor would be whether her mood changes and physical symptoms respond well to herbs and lifestyle changes. Good diet and regular exercise are essential.

Ongoing herbal treatment and supplements were:

Chaste berry	1000 mg	One tablet every morning for another 6 months
St. John's wort	1500 mg	Two tablets every morning for 6 months
Fish oils	1000 mg	One twice daily

Also included was an herbal mix of nervines for symptom control in the premenstrual week, which included:

Botanical Prescription 2

Ashwagandha	*(Withania somnifera)*	30 mL
Kava kava	*(Piper methysticum)*	30 mL
Lavender	*(Lavandula officinalis)*	20 mL
Milk thistle	*(Silybum marianum)*	20 mL
		Total: 100 mL

Dose: 5 mL daily for 10 days premenstrually.

NUTRITIONAL CONSIDERATIONS

Diet, nutritional supplements, and exercise have been studied for PMS, but not PMDD, albeit in a limited number of investigations.[170,172] In a comprehensive review of the literature on PMS and nutritional supplementation by Stevinson and Ernst, only 13 reliable RCTs were identified.[172] In spite of the lack of literature demonstrating efficacy of many of the dietary changes commonly recommended for PMS, strategies such as improving fiber intake; reducing harmful fats; improving the intake of good-quality fats, proteins, fruits, and vegetables; ensuring proper nutrient intake; and reducing the consumption of coffee, sugar, and refined carbohydrates are all beneficial health practices and seem wise to recommend. Calcium carbonate, 1200 mg per day in divided doses, has been found in two controlled studies to reduce PMS symptoms.[243,244] Magnesium supplementation was found to be effective for the treatment of PMS in one placebo-controlled trial.[245] Vitamin E, 400 units per day, may be minimally effective for PMS.[2] Vitamin B_6, 50 to 100 mg per day, may be effective for PMS based on meta-analysis of inconsistent data.[170] Dietary recommendations, such as avoiding salt, chocolate, caffeine, and alcohol, have never been subjected to either observational or controlled studies.[170] Low Dog cites a 1983 report that found that women with PMS consumed 275% more refined sugar, 79% more dairy products, 78% more sodium, 62% more refined carbohydrates, 77% less manganese, and 53% less iron than women without PMS.[32] A case-controlled study from within the Nurses' Health Study II cohort (1057 cases and 1968 controls) found an inverse relationship between dietary riboflavin and thiamine and PMS. No correlations between niacin, vitamin B_6, folate, or vitamin B_1 and incident PMS were observed.[246] These data tell us that dietary modifications may play a significant role in improving PMS symptoms. Surprisingly, no comprehensive dietary modification strategies for PMS treatment have been evaluated to date.[173]

Reduction in Coffee and Sugar

Coffee and sugar consumption is higher in women who experience PMS than in those who do not. Based on the findings from a 1983 survey and two trials demonstrating that regular caffeine consumption is associated with a higher incidence of PMS, many practitioners recommend the reduction of caffeinated products in susceptible women. Many women self-report that a reduction in coffee consumption improves their symptoms.[173,175] Heavy sugar consumption may increase sodium and water retention, and increase magnesium excretion.[32] Blood sugar imbalances as a result of high sugar consumption can also negatively affect mood and lead to further sugar cravings.

Calcium

Ovarian hormones influence calcium, magnesium, and vitamin D metabolism. Estrogen regulates calcium metabolism, intestinal calcium absorption, and parathyroid gene expression and secretion, triggering fluctuations across the menstrual cycle. Alterations in calcium homeostasis (hypocalcemia and hypercalcemia) have long been associated with many affective disturbances. A number of clinical trials have suggested a positive relationship between calcium supplementation and improved mood and somatic symptoms in PMS (including food cravings, water retention, pain, and negative affect), ranging from clearly beneficial to modest results.[244] Numerous researchers have concluded that unless contraindicated, calcium supplementation should be considered a sound treatment for PMS treatment. The recommended dosing schedule is 1200 to 1600 mg/day.[244,247]

Vitamin B_6

Pyridoxine deficiency is one hypothesized cause of PMS, and in Europe, B_6 supplementation is an accepted treatment.

Vitamin B_6 is prescribed for PMS symptoms based on the rationale that it demonstrates positive effects on the neurotransmitters serotonin, epinephrine, histamine, dopamine, and taurine.[173] Positive effects have been observed in most trials for PMS with B_6 doses ranging from 50 to 600 mg daily or when B_6 (300 mg) is given in conjunction with other nutrients and a healthy diet.[248-251] Two comprehensive literature reviews suggest that B_6 is better than placebo in improving PMS symptoms; however, owing to the nature of the trials, evidence of its value remains inconclusive.[32,172] Sensory neuropathy is unlikely to occur when vitamin B_6 is given at doses of 50 to 100 mg/day for short periods of no more than 6 months; nonetheless, practitioners should be aware of this possibility and inform their patients of toxicity symptoms.[252] Given its low cost and the relative safety of appropriate doses, supplementation of B_6 in the form of a multivitamin may be reasonable for women with PMS and a suboptimal diet.[32,251]

Magnesium

Three small RCTs evaluated the effects of magnesium supplementation on PMS symptoms. Two concluded that supplementation improved symptoms; in one trial overall scores were positive, and there was improvement in negative affect in the other trial. The only area of significance improvement was fluid retention. The third trial showed improvement in anxiety when combined with B_6.[172] In one trial, studies included data on $PGF_{2\alpha}$ levels in menstrual blood. Women taking magnesium demonstrated significantly lower inflammatory prostaglandins levels in their urine and reported a decrease in premenstrual pain. Magnesium is known to also promote muscle relaxation. A Cochrane database review on the literature on magnesium concludes that magnesium is more effective than placebo in the treatment of PMS-related pain.[173] Natural medicine practitioners typically recommend 400 to 800 mg/day.[32]

Tryptophan

There are some indications that premenstrual food cravings might be an attempt to increase the plasma ratio of tryptophan to other amino acids to improve symptoms via an increased central serotonergic activity.[253] There is also limited support (one placebo-controlled trial) for L-tryptophan, 6 g/day, from ovulation until day 3 of menses for the treatment of PMDD.[254] In addition, researchers have observed a reduction in premenstrual symptoms when women are given a dietary supplement that selectively increases tryptophan levels.[255] Dietary changes that can be reasonably expected to achieve a similar result include increased frequency of smaller volumes of food; no sugar or refined carbohydrates; and regular complex carbohydrate and protein intake at each meal with increased consumption of fish, legumes, egg, lean meat, and low-fat yogurt.

Essential Fatty Acids

Dietary or supplemental omega-3 essential fatty acids, generally in the form of fish oils, are beneficial in depression and doses of up to 4000 mg daily are advisable.[256,257]

Reduction in Saturated Fat Consumption

Reduction in saturated fat consumption is commonly recommended in the herbal and naturopathic communities based on the belief that reducing enterohepatic recycling of estrogens can improve symptoms of PMS, and can be achieved by a reduction in saturated fat consumption, views that are somewhat supported by early literature on excess estrogens.[258-260] However, this approach assumes that excess estrogen is an etiologic factor in PMS, which has not been conclusively demonstrated by biochemical assays.[1]

Increasing Dietary Fiber

As with the previous recommendation, an increase in dietary fibers is thought to reduce excess estrogen by a reduction in reabsorption of estrogens from the intestine; however, it is unclear how much of a role estrogen plays in PMS.[261-263] Vegetarians have significantly lower activity of the bacterial enzyme responsible for conversion of estrogen metabolites back into estrogens than meat eaters because they tend to have a higher fiber diet and a lower intake of fats. *Lactobacillus acidophilus* also reduces the activity of β-glucuronidase, suggesting a positive effect on estrogen excretion from eating yogurt and fermented milk products.[264,265] However, this practice has not been evaluated in the treatment of PMS, and like suggesting a low-fat diet, assumes that elevated estrogen level is part of the pathophysiology of symptoms.[32,173]

ADDITIONAL THERAPIES

Numerous nonpharmacologic therapies may be beneficial in the treatment of PMS, including supportive or psychological therapy, exercise, and dietary supplementation. The most extensively reviewed interventions and approaches are reviewed in Box 9-14.

Lifestyle
Exercise

Regular, moderate exercise improves mood and feelings of well-being. Women with PMS who exercise regularly and frequently have fewer symptoms than women who do not exercise. High exercisers experience fewer behavioral and mood changes, better concentration, and less pain.[172,266-268] One study of over 1800 women found that 50% used exercise as a self-help measure for alleviating PMS symptoms, and over 80% of these found it beneficial.[172] Aerobic exercise may help the physical symptoms of PMS.[266,269] Unfortunately, exercise is often overlooked as a treatment approach in conventional medicine.[172] Frequency of exercise, rather than intensity, appears more significant in prevention and alleviation of physical and psychoemotional symptoms.[32] The mechanism behind this is proposed to be a reduction in estrogens and catecholamine levels, leading to improved glucose tolerance and endorphin levels.[32] Regular exercise also may increase a woman's sense of personal control and self-esteem, also shown to lead to a reduction in symptoms.

> **BOX 9-14** **Summary of Nutritional and Additional Therapies for Premenstrual Symptoms, Premenstrual Syndrome, and Premenstrual Dysphoric Disorder**
>
> The interventions in this table are commonly recommended in clinical practice.
>
> **Diet and nutrition**
> - Reduction in coffee and sugar
> - Calcium
> - Vitamin B_6
> - Magnesium
> - Tryptophan
> - Essential fatty acids
> - Reduction in saturated fat consumption
> - Increasing dietary fiber
>
> **Lifestyle**
> - Exercise
> - Yoga
> - Massage therapy
> - Progressive relaxation and guided imagery
>
> **Psychosocial**
> - Cognitive therapies
> - Psychotherapy/counseling
> - Celebrating menstruation

Yoga

After a 10-month empirical study to evaluate the effectiveness of specific yoga postures in relieving PMS symptoms ($n = 40$), the authors found significant improvement of scores on self-reported menstrual distress scales in women in the yoga-trained group versus the control group, which did not undergo yoga training.[173]

Massage Therapy

One RCT evaluated the effects of massage therapy in improving PMS. Progressive relaxation was used as the control. Some improvement in PMS was seen over baseline after one cycle of treatment; however, the study methodologies did not include intergroup comparisons, so conclusive evidence cannot be inferred.[172] Although massage might not prevent PMS, it may improve symptoms; massage therapy has been demonstrated to reduce stress, so for women with a high stress component to their PMS symptoms or musculoskeletal discomforts, regular massage may be beneficial.

Progressive Relaxation and Guided Imagery

Eliciting the relaxation response is a safe and nonpharmacologic intervention in the treatment of PMS.[270] Women with PMS improved with progressive muscle relaxation in conjunction with guided imagery.[271] An interesting study of the use of foot, ear, and hand reflexology showed that those women who received pressure to actual reflex points responded significantly better than the women who were given treatment of incorrect reflex points.[272,273]

Psychosocial
Cognitive Therapies

Three published trials on cognitive therapy suggest that it is superior to a wait list (i.e., control) for improving premenstrual psychological and physical symptoms and functioning. Cognitive therapy was also found to be superior to group awareness and information-focused therapy.[170,274] Group coping skills training was found to be superior to relaxation training. However, relaxation therapy twice daily was found to be superior to daily PMS symptoms charting alone.[270] Diary symptom recording and communicating with family members about the connection between PMS and behavior are also considered supportive therapy, although they have not been well studied.[170]

Psychotherapy/Counseling

Women with low self-esteem, feelings of lack of control over their personal lives, and sense of personal disempowerment have a higher incidence of PMS symptoms. Psychotherapy and counseling have been shown to improve mild to moderate depression and anxiety as effectively as antidepressants. Various types of counseling and psychotherapy techniques are theoretically useful for women with PMS, although there have been few suitable studies to evaluate these techniques. One study looked at the effectiveness of cognitive behavioral therapy in PMS and found that it was useful in improving symptoms.[274]

PREMENSTRUAL HEADACHE AND MIGRAINE

Headaches and migraines are common conditions with substantial costs to individuals and society.[275] They are among the most common causes of emergency room visits and medical appointments, and also account for many lost days of school and work, and disruptions in family relationships.[276,277] In a survey of nearly 20,000 individuals, 53% reported that severe headaches caused substantial impairment in activities and required bed rest, and 51% reported that work or school activity was reduced by at least 50%.[277] Migraines cause more disability than tension headaches, with at least 20% of sufferers requiring at least 1 day of work absence per month, and cancellation of family and social activities.[278]

Data from several studies and surveys, including the American Migraine Study II, estimate the prevalence of migraine to be approximately 18.2% in females and 6.5% in males.[277,279] Before puberty, there is no gender difference in prevalence; however, after puberty, women experience them significantly more frequently. Menstrual migraine (MM) has an onset at menarche in 33% of affected women.[279,280] The female to male prevalence ratio is 2:1 at 20 years of age, and 3.3:1 between ages 42 and 44 years. This ratio decreases slightly but persists into menopause.[278] Prevalence is highest in middle life (ages 40 to 49).[277] In 7% to 14% of women with migraine, headache occurs only with menses. This is referred to as true menstrual migraine (TMM). Sixty percent of women with migraines throughout their cycle observe an association between increased headache onset and menses, referred to as *menstrual migraine* (MM), or menstrually triggered migraine.[1,278-280] In one study of 504 women with a history of migraine, 68.7% reported migraine occurrence with PMS, 29% reported menopausal symptoms, and 24.4% reported an association with OCs or HRT. Sixty-one percent reported experiencing migraine during pregnancy; 20.4% stated that they did not experience migraine during pregnancy. During pregnancy, headache symptoms improved in 17.8% of patients, remained unchanged in 27.8%, and worsened in 34%. Patients with onset of headache before age 20, or with menarche, are more likely to experience headaches with the menstrual cycle.[281] Although migraine prevalence typically decreases with advancing age, it may worsen at menopause.[279] Migraine prevalence appears to be higher in Anglo-Americans than African Americans and is inversely proportional to income status.[277]

The headache classification committee of the International Headache Society recognizes 13 distinct headache categories.[276] This chapter focuses on headache and migraine associated with the menstrual cycle. Menstrual headaches include all headaches temporally related to the menses, whether occurring before, during, or after the period.[1] Migraine headaches can be classified as *classic migraine* (i.e., associated with visual aura), *common migraine* (i.e., no aura), and *complicated migraine* (i.e., associated with dramatic transient focal neurologic characteristics such as blindness, unilateral paresthesias, and so forth).[1] Tension headaches are the most prevalent types of headaches, and can be episodic or may occur chronically and daily. When occurring daily, they may be associated with depression. As with these other headaches, tension headaches are more common in women than men.[276]

The term *menstrual migraine* has not been universally defined.[282] *True menstrual migraine* (TMM) is defined as migraine that occurs regularly 1 to 2 days before menses to day 3 of the menstrual cycle and at no other time.[275] Menstrual-associated migraine refers to attacks that occur at any time of the cycle, with increased frequency during menstruation.[275,279] Menstrual headache and migraine often occur in conjunction with other menstrually related symptoms, especially PMS, nausea, and dysmenorrhea; however, the presence of other symptoms is not a criteria for the diagnosis of a menstrual headache or migraine. MMs and TMMs are frequently longer in duration, intractable to regular migraine treatments, and are typically not associated with migraine aura, even in patients who at other times of the month experience aura with migraine; however, experience of migraine with aura is also increased 66% in the premenstrual and menstrual phase. Migraine and nonmigraine headaches are at least twice as common during the premenstrual and menstrual phases as between menses, and the highest incidence occurs on the day before and on the first few days of menstruation.[279]

PATHOPHYSIOLOGY

Headaches that specifically occur in relationship to the menstrual cycle, as well as menopause and pregnancy, appear to have their origins in the complex sex hormone fluctuations and interrelated neurotransmitter changes that occur during these times of intense hormonal change. The etiologies of PMS are similar to those implicated in premenstrual headache and migraine. [See Premenstrual Symptoms, Premenstrual Syndrome, and Premenstrual Dysphoric Disorder.] Estrogens and progestins have powerful effects on central serotonergic and other neurotransmitters and receptors.

Estrogen withdrawal in the luteal phase, particularly in women with elevated estrogen levels in the follicular phase, has been shown to precipitate migraine and may be the primary cause of migraine as opposed to sustained high or low levels of estrogens. Estrogens given premenstrually delay the onset of migraine without preventing the onset of menstruation.[278,279] Women with MMs may have higher baseline estrogen levels than nonsufferers, and thus the extent of the decline may be the causative factor.[278] 5HT levels are reduced during the luteal phase in MM sufferers, and may be caused by catabolic changes, reduced synthesis, or estrogen withdrawal, which is itself associated with decreased peripheral 5HT and increased blood vessel permeability to substance P, PRL, and neurotransmitters.[278]

Opioid responsiveness also changes premenstrually, and may be associated with premenstrual decreases in both pain and stress control.[278] The hormone-mediated effects on the rhythm of CNS neurons and the serotonergic pain-modulating systems appear to play an important role in the etiology of menstrually related headaches, as do the effects of progesterone metabolites on neurosteroids, particularly at the GABA receptors.[278,279] Progesterone metabolites (e.g., allopregnanolone) may modulate anxiety, pain, stress response, and depression in sensitive individuals through interactions with endogenous benzodiazepine receptors.[279,283] Declining progesterone levels owing to luteal phase insufficiency may be, in part, responsible for increased prevalence of headache and migraine during the luteal phase and early menstrual period. Increased inflammatory prostaglandins associated with menstruation may be implicated in the etiology of MM, TMM, and premenstrual headaches because of neurogenic inflammation. Other associated symptoms include cramping, diarrhea, nausea, fainting, flushing, and difficulty concentrating.[278,279]

Women with MMs also have decreased nocturnal urinary melatonin immunoreactivity, a marker for nocturnal melatonin secretion. Melatonin exhibits a circadian pattern, with low concentrations during the day and high concentrations at night. Melatonin promotes sleep and helps to establish patterns for biological rhythms, including hormone patterns. It may be that women with MM have delayed melatonin secretion or a sympathetic hypofunction, which has been associated with migraine.[279]

Pregnancy is associated with noncyclic rises in sex hormone levels; menopause is associated with noncyclic declining levels—both are associated with changes in previous migraine status.[280] Additionally, OC use during the reproductive years and HRT use in menopause may increase the intensity and prevalence of headaches in some women.[284]

Stress is also a common trigger of both headache (especially tension headache) and migraine. Migraine attacks frequently occur within 2 days of increased periods of exposure to stressors, or "daily hassles," defined as "the minor events of everyday life." Mood changes, including tension, irritability, annoyance, depression, or fatigue, significantly increase the likelihood of a migraine attack in women.[285] Stress has been demonstrated to exacerbate hormonally related stress intolerance, which in a vicious cycle can further dysregulate the endocrine system (i.e., stress can increase latent hyperprolactinemia); women with PMS symptoms may have endocrine and neurotransmitter-related reduction in stress tolerance.

In vitro fertilization and embryo transfer (IVF-ET) might also be associated with various degrees of headache, mostly observed in patients with a migraine headache background, and occurring specifically in the downregulation stage of treatment when very low levels of 17-β-estradiol are observed.[286]

SYMPTOMS OF MIGRAINE

- Unilateral or bilateral head pain that is aching, throbbing, stabbing, or burning
- May be preceded or accompanied by a visual "aura" or other visual disturbances such as flashing lights or visual field defects
- Extreme sensitivity to light, noise; craving for a dark, quiet environment
- Nausea, vomiting
- Pain aggravated by motion/movement
- Attacks may persist for 3 to 72 hours

DIAGNOSIS

History taking and review of a "headache diary" are the most accurate diagnostic tools for premenstrual headache and migraine; establishing the timing of headache/migraine allows for a definitive diagnosis. Possible serious underlying causes of headache should always be ruled out through differential diagnosis; however, insidious causes rarely cause headaches that occur with the periodicity of MM and TMM.

DIFFERENTIAL DIAGNOSIS

Less than 5% of headaches are the result of serious underlying causes.[276] Differentiation of TMM and MM is based on the appearance of TMM exclusively in the days immediately before or during the menstrual flow. Table 9-13 provides a differential assessment of headache patterns for migraine and tension headaches. Any headaches presenting with the warning signs in Box 9-15 require prompt medical evaluation.

TABLE 9-13	Differential Diagnosis of Tension versus Migraine Headache	
Symptom	**Tension Headache**	**Migraine**
Onset	Gradual, triggered by stress	May be precipitated by aura, patient may waken with headache; many women report that migraines commonly begin in the late afternoon
Duration	8-12 hours, but may be episodic or chronic (i.e., lasting days, weeks, or months)	Typically 8-12 hours but may last 3 hours to 3 days
Frequency	Variable from daily to only occasionally or rarely	1-2/month or less; some patients may have a migraine even weekly, but this is rare
Pain locus	Usually bilateral, frontal, or "hatband"	Generally unilateral but may switch sides or become bilateral
Type of pain	Constant, nagging, severe	Throbbing, moderate to severe
Triggers	Stress	Stress, menses, foods, alcohol, OCs, HRT, menopause, pregnancy
Accompanying symptoms	Light, noise	Nausea, vomiting, photophobia, phonophobia

OC, Oral contraceptives; *HRT,* hormone replacement therapy.
Adapted from *Women's Health: A Primary Care Clinical Guide,* ed 2, Stanford, 1998, Appleton and Lange.

BOX 9-15 Warning Signs for Dangerous Headaches[244]

If a patient reports any of these symptoms, immediate medical attention is advisable:
- No identifiable pattern of a benign headache
- Patient describes headache as "the worst headache ever"
- Vomiting without nausea
- Personality or consciousness changes
- Abnormality upon physical examination (e.g., fever, neck pain/stiffness, neurologic signs)
- Seizure activity
- Onset of headache with exertion
- Sudden change in headache pattern
- Worsening symptoms

CONVENTIONAL TREATMENT APPROACHES

Unfortunately, the treatment of migraine associated with changes in sex hormone levels is difficult and often refractory to conventional therapies.[284] The conventional medical approach includes a combination of preventative, nonpharmacologic, and pharmacologic interventions.

Prevention

Premenstrual migraine prophylaxis uses a combination of pharmacologic and nonpharmacologic measures, for example, stress reduction and pharmacologic agents. These are timed in accordance with the pattern of the headache diary; the use of preventative pharmacologic agents typically commences just before or with the onset of menses, with increasing doses of pharmaceutical agents as appropriate closer to the menses.[278] Specific interventions are discussed in the following. Prophylactic methods should be tried for several months to determine efficacy.[278]

Prevention also involves the avoidance of migraine triggers, which many migraine sufferers can self-identify or which they can learn to identify by keeping a headache diary that includes recall of associated factors.

Nonpharmacologic Treatment

- Stress management and behavioral modification techniques, for example, relaxation training, biofeedback, and cognitive-behavior approaches.[287]
- Physical therapies for the prevention of migraine, including acupuncture and cervical manipulation.[287]
- Avoidance of migraine triggers: In addition to stress, these include sleep deprivation, hunger, environmental factors, foods, fatigue, alcohol, caffeine, excess sleep, physical exertion, head trauma, travel, sexual activity, medications, smoking, and poor pillow placement.[32]
- Foods that have been implicated in migraine onset include: cheeses, chocolate, citrus, hot dogs, monosodium glutamate (MSG), aspartame, fatty foods, ice cream, and alcohol. Additionally, food allergies and sensitivities, as well as certain medications, may adversely affect serotonin levels and exacerbate the problem (Box 9-16).[32]

Pharmacologic Treatment

Conventional therapy relies heavily on pharmaceuticals to prevent or arrest headache/migraine.[288] The mechanism of action of medications proved effective in the treatment of migraines generally (not specifically MM or TMM) varies, and no single medication has demonstrated superiority. Mechanisms of action include specific serotonin receptor antagonism ($5HT$ and $5HT_2$), platelet antagonism (e.g., aspirin), hormonal intervention, prevention of vasodilatation or vasoconstriction, enhancement of serotonergic transmission, leukotriene antagonism, prostaglandin-mediated actions, and monoamine-mediated actions.[287] The most commonly used types of medications include:
- SSRIs
- NSAIDs
- Ergot alkaloids
- OCs

BOX 9-16   Common Migraine Triggers: Foods

Aged cheese
Alcohol
Avocado
Bacon
Bananas
Canned figs
Chicken livers
Chinese food (with monosodium glutamate [MSG])
Chocolate
Citrus fruits
Coffee (including decaf)
Dry soup mixes (and similar products with MSG)
Fermented sausages
Hot dogs
Nuts
Onions
Tea
Yogurt

Source: The National Headache Foundation, Chicago.

- Estrogen
- Progesterone
- Prostaglandin inhibitors
- Triptans (5HT agonists)

BOTANICAL TREATMENT OF HEADACHE AND MIGRAINE

The botanical approach to the treatment of headache and migraine, and specifically those that occur as a result of hormonal changes, includes:

- The direct use of herbal analgesics, sedatives, and antispasmodics for acute pain management and symptomatic relief
- The use of herbs to address endocrine-related dysfunction
- Treatment of chronic stress, affected mood (e.g., depression, anxiety, irritability), and sleep disturbances with adaptogens, nervine tonics, and herbal antidepressants
- Lifestyle modification to reduce exposure to triggers, including dietary modifications and stress reduction
- Dietary changes and nutritional supplements

The most commonly included herbs for the treatment of headache and migraine are listed in Table 9-14. Data in Discussion of Botanicals focuses on those herbs that have been specifically investigated for the treatment of headache.

DISCUSSION OF BOTANICALS

Hormone Modulators

Chaste berry

Chaste berry has been extensively studied for relief of PMS symptoms, including headache and migraine. A 2013 3-month open-label clinical observation evaluated chaste berry extract in the amelioration of premenstrual migraine frequency and duration ($n = 107$, 100 completed). Sixty-six percent experienced a reduction of PMS symptoms and 42% experienced fewer migraines by more than 50%.[289] Another RCT ($n = 128$; active 62, placebo 66) evaluated the effects of chaste berry in PMS symptoms compared with placebo. Participants recorded symptoms on a questionnaire at the commencement and conclusion of the study, with items rated using VAS. Forty drops of chaste berry extract were administered 6 days before menses for six consecutive cycles. Chaste berry extract was found to relieve PMS symptoms (including headache) better than placebo.[218]

Antiinflammatories

Butterbur

Butterbur, or *Petasites* spp., exhibits a marked antiinflammatory effect that has demonstrated efficacy in the prevention of both asthma and migraines.[32,290-295] Its activity is largely attributed to inhibition of leukotriene biosynthesis; however, it also may be related to effects on calcium channel regulation.[293] Data from clinical trials support its efficacy in migraine prophylaxis. Doses in clinical trials have included 25, 50, 75, 100, and 150 mg given twice daily, usually for 2 to 4 months. Trials have consistently demonstrated that *Petasites* spp. significantly reduced the number of migraine attacks and migraine days per month over placebo.[290-295] A 2012 report from the Quality Standards Subcommittee of the American Academy of Neurology and the American Headache Society published in *Neurology* summarized the evidence base for the use of NSAIDs and complementary treatments in episodic migraine disorders. Reviewing the evidence from 1999 to 2009, the authors cited ample evidence to support the efficacy of butterbur for migraine prevention.[296] In a study conducted by Lipton and colleagues, 245 patients in a 5-month study received either 50 mg, 75 mg, or placebo twice daily. The 4-month mean attack count was reduced by 48% in patients who received 75 mg twice daily, whereas those receiving 50 mg twice daily presented with a 34% reduction and those who took placebo, 26%.[293] In two controlled clinical trials, a total of 187 patients with migraine were exposed to doses of the special butterbur extract between 100 mg and 150 mg daily for at least 3 months. Compared with placebo, no significant differences were observed regarding adverse events rated to be at least possibly causally related to the product, except for mild GI discomforts, notably nausea and eructation (i.e., burping). These adverse effects were mild and transient; burping occurred in about 20% of study patients. A total of 188 patients (145 suffering from migraine, including 50 children and adolescents from 6 to 17 years of age) were treated with butterbur extract at various doses for several months in the framework of four postmarket surveillance studies, two of which have been finished.

A 2006 systematic review found that higher doses (150 mg) were more effective than moderate doses (100 mg) in preventing migraines.[297] In 2008, a small 8-week controlled trial evaluated the use of butterbur root extract against

TABLE 9-14	**Summary of Botanical Treatment Strategies for Headache and Migraine**		
Therapeutic Goal	**Therapeutic Action**	**Botanical Name**	**Common Name**
Reduce possible inflammatory response involved in headache etiology	Antiinflammatories	*Petasites hybridus*	Butterbur
		Tanacetum parthenium	Feverfew
		Zingiber officinale	Ginger
Relieve nausea; vomiting	Antiemetic	*Mentha piperita*	Peppermint
		Zingiber officinale	Ginger
Relieve headache/migraine pain	Analgesics	*Anemone pulsatilla*	Pulsatilla
		Corydalis ambigua	Corydalis
		Piscidia piscipula	Jamaican dogwood
		Piper methysticum	Kava kava
		Salix spp.	Willow
		Withania somnifera	Ashwagandha
Relieve stress, anxiety, musculoskeletal tension	Nervines/Antispasmodics	*Actaea racemosa*	Black cohosh
		Lavandula officinalis	Lavender
		Leonurus cardiaca	Motherwort
		Matricaria recutita	Chamomile
		Scutellaria lateriflora	Skullcap
		Verbena officinalis	Blue vervain
		Viburnum spp.	Cramp bark, black haw
Promote sleep	Sedatives	*Anemone pulsatilla*	Pulsatilla
		Corydalis ambigua	Corydalis
		Eschscholzia californica	California poppy
		Humulus lupulus	Hops
		Matricaria recutita	Chamomile
		Passiflora incarnata	Passionflower
		Piscidia piscipula	Jamaican dogwood
		Valeriana officinalis	Valerian
		Withania somnifera	Ashwagandha
Improve stress response	Adaptogens	*Eleutherococcus senticosus*	Eleuthero
		Panax ginseng	Ginseng
		Panax quinquefolius	American ginseng
		Rhaponticum carthamoides	Rhaponticum
		Rhodiola rosea	Rhodiola
		Schisandra chinensis	Schisandra
		Urtica dioica	Nettle
		Withania somnifera	Ashwagandha
Relieve depression and anxiety	Antidepressants/Anxiolytics	*Hypericum perforatum*	St. John's wort
		Passiflora incarnata	Passionflower
		Piper methysticum	Kava kava
		Scutellaria lateriflora	Skullcap
		Valeriana officinalis	Valerian
		Withania somnifera	Ashwagandha
Treat possible underlying hormonal dysregulation (e.g., estrogen withdrawal, luteal phase insufficiency)	Hormonal modulation	*Vitex agnus-castus*	Chaste berry
TCM approaches to headache/migraine related to hormonal changes	Treat blood deficiency; treat liver qi stagnation	See Premenstrual Symptoms, Premenstrual Syndrome, and Premenstrual Dysphoric Disorder	

TCM, Traditional Chinese Medicine.

placebo and music therapy for the prevention of migraine episodes in children (*n* = 58). At a 6-month follow-up, the butterbur group experienced fewer migraines than the placebo group (but not at the 8-week post treatment). The extract was well tolerated.[298] Excellent tolerability at

doses from 50 to 150 mg has been reported, even for children from 6 years of age. About 90% of study patients rated global tolerability to be "excellent" or "good." It is estimated that since 1992, approximately 450,000 individuals would have been exposed to the product according to sales figures, reflecting a total of approximately 75,000 patient years of exposure. A total of 75 reports of suspected adverse reactions from Germany and 18 spontaneous reports from other countries were received by the manufacturer from 1976 to June 30, 2002, representing a frequency of suspected adverse reactions of as low as 0.022%. Only 19 reports were determined to be possibly causally related to the administration of the butterbur root extract. The reported suspected adverse reactions with the highest frequency such as nausea, eructation, and stomach pain are considered a mild discomfort of the GI system. However, the frequency of these suspected adverse reactions is less than 0.01%. Therefore even the most frequently reported adverse reaction for the product can be assessed as "very rare."[292] Owing to the potential for hepatotoxicity from the pyrrolizidine alkaloid (PA) content of butterbur, only PA-free products (or those containing up to the detectable limit of 0.08 ppm) should be used, and the herb should be avoided during pregnancy and lactation.[32,295]

Feverfew

Feverfew is an aromatic plant with a traditional history of use for the treatment of gynecologic complaints, and a recorded history of use for headache since the 1700s.[32,299] It is one of the few herbs with substantial scientific evidence for its efficacy in migraine prophylaxis. Most RCTs and surveys of individuals using feverfew for migraine prevention have documented beneficial results.[300-302] Not only has feverfew demonstrated a reduction in migraine frequency and pain intensity, but also a profound reduction has been observed in typical accompanying symptoms, including vomiting, nausea, photophobia, and phonophobia.[301] A 2012 10-week, three-arm study tested a combination of feverfew and acupuncture in the QOL improvement in women experiencing chronic migraines. Primary outcomes were assessed using SF-36 QOL assessment score, and MIDAS (Migraine Disability Scale) and VAS were used to track secondary outcomes. A combination of acupuncture and feverfew performed better along these measures compared with single treatment groups (150 mg/day, preparation not disclosed).[303] A multicenter clinical trial (n = 60, 45 treatment and 15 control) tested a combination sublingual feverfew and ginger tablet against placebo in episodic migraine treatment. Participants used diaries to track migraine incidence and pain levels (on a 4-point scale) at 2 hours, and the feverfew/ginger group experienced less pain at that marker compared with controls (Dose and preparation not noted).[304] A small open-label pilot study (n = 12, 10 completed) tested a combination of feverfew and white willow (Salix alba) in migraine frequency, duration, and intensity. Participants took the treatment (300 mg of each botanical) for 2 weeks and recorded migraine frequency with other measures of duration and intensity. At 6 and 12 weeks, improvements were seen in all patients; 70% of participants reported a greater than 50% reduction in pain (Tanacetum parthenium 300 mg plus S. alba 300 mg twice daily, preparation details not noted).[305]

The combined data from six randomized clinical trials suggest that Tanacetum is an effective agent over placebo for preventing migraine, with only mild and transient side effects noted in a few cases.[306] A systematic review of feverfew as a migraine prophylactic reported that current data suggest efficacy, but also cited concerns over its cyclooxygenase-2 (COX-2)–inhibiting effects in cases of long-term use.[307] According to a subsequent systematic review by Pittler and colleagues using the Jadad scoring system, only four trials evaluating feverfew efficacy for migraine met strict methodological inclusion criteria. The review suggested that feverfew compared favorably with placebo; however, the trial with the highest methodological quality found no significant difference between the herb and placebo.[308] The mechanism of action remains uncertain, but it is suspected to have an antiinflammatory effect, possibly through its inhibition of granule secretion from platelets.[80] Feverfew does not, however, appear to interfere with normal clotting mechanisms.[32,80] Its pharmacologic activity is often attributed to its parthenolide content; however, although parthenolide may be a useful marker of activity in feverfew products, the active constituents have not yet been established.[299] Efficacy of ethanolic extracts has been questioned on the basis of clinical studies; preparations made from dried whole leaf are recommended.[299] No studies were identified that specifically evaluated this herb for the treatment of TMM or MM. T. parthenium also may reduce the severity of dysmenorrhea through antiinflammatory mechanisms. Feverfew is recommended by European Scientific Cooperative on Phytotherapy (ESCOP) for the treatment of migraine.[119] Long-term safety has not been questioned, and continuous consumption by large numbers of individuals over 10 years did not cause toxicity. Occasional mouth ulcers have been reported; however, in the one clinical trial in which this was evaluated, mouth ulcers were reported with greater frequency in the placebo group consuming cabbage leaves. Patients allergic to members of the daisy family (Asteraceae) should using caution with this herb.[299] Feverfew should not be used during pregnancy owing to purported emmenagogic effects (Fig. 9-9).

Antiemetics

Ginger

Ginger's use for the treatment of headaches and nausea dates back 2500 years in both China and India, and it is still used for headache treatment in these countries, as well as in East Africa.[309,310] Clinical trials have demonstrated the efficacy of ginger in the treatment of nausea generally, postsurgically, and during pregnancy (NVP), and its use for nausea and vomiting is supported by ESCOP and the German Commission E (the latter, however, does not recommend its use during pregnancy).[44,119,310-312] Ginger exerts an antiinflammatory effect through inhibition of cyclooxygenase and lipoxygenase enzymes of the prostaglandin and leukotriene synthesis pathways, and thus also may be of use in the prevention and relief of headache and migraine; however, it does not appear to exert direct analgesic effects.[312] One case report published in 1990 describes a case history of a 42-year-old woman who

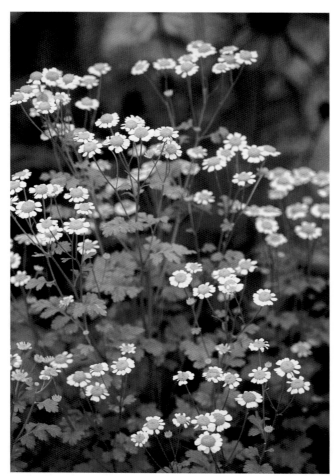

FIGURE 9-9 Feverfew *(Tanacetum parthenium)*. (Photo by Martin Wall.)

experienced an abortive effect on migraine taking 1.5 to 2.0 g/day of dried, powdered ginger root. The authors of the report attributed thromboxane and prostaglandin inhibition with the outcome.[313] A recent clinical trial (*n* = 100) tested ginger against acute migraine without aura. Patients were randomized to receive either ginger powder or sumatriptan. At 2 hours postheadache, both groups exhibited similar improvements in migraine intensity (Dose and preparation not noted).[314]

Peppermint

Peppermint is discussed in the next section on Analgesics.

Analgesics

Analgesics play an important role in the symptomatic management of headache/migraine pain. They can be taken before the onset of headache, or acutely during headache. Effectiveness depends on adequate dosing. The most effective dosing strategy is typically to take small frequent doses of herbal extract until relief is achieved, for example, 1 to 3 mL of a tincture every 15 to 30 minutes, and then to repeat as needed to sustain relief, usually for a maximum of 2 hours. If relief is not achieved after 2 hours, the formula can be

modified or the protocol can be repeated again after a break of 2 hours. If pain was successfully relieved but returns, the protocol also may be repeated after a rest of 2 hours. The protocol may be repeated up to three times daily. Caution is warranted with dosing for those herbs that have a toxic threshold. Note that doses that herbalists find clinically effective often exceed the recommended doses in safety charts. This is a confusing fact and often a conundrum for practitioners, who of course want to avoid toxicity for patients; there is also legal liability to prescribe within suggested parameters. Unfortunately, dosing charts are often based on theoretic toxic effects or limited safety and clinical studies, and are not entirely dependable as the final word on safety. Nonetheless, they are a useful guide within which a modicum of flexibility may be allowed to achieve clinical efficacy, based on the individual patient's size and weight, tolerance, age, and status (e.g., pregnancy, nonparturient).

Corydalis

Corydalis is used in TCM, and called yanhusuo. It is an effective analgesic, sedative, and hypnotic, useful in the treatment of headache, insomnia, and dysmenorrhea. Thus it is especially applicable for the treatment of headache and migraine associated with menstruation, and general menstrual pain. It combines well with antiinflammatory herbs, antispasmodics, and anxiolytics.[315] Its action is attributed to the alkaloid tetrahydropalmatine, which lends sedative, hypnotic, and tranquilizing properties.[124] The mechanism of action appears to be blocking of postsynaptic dopaminergic receptors, but the CNS effects also may involve serotonin and noradrenaline.[124,315]

Cramp Bark/Black Haw

Cramp bark/black haw are similar enough in effect to consider relatively interchangeable as spasmolytic and mild analgesic herbs. These salicylate-containing *Viburnum* spp. are generally considered for their effectiveness as uterine muscle relaxants in the treatment of dysmenorrhea (see Dysmenorrhea). Their mild sedating and general spasmolytic actions also make them invaluable in the treatment of mild to moderate headache, and combined with Jamaican dogwood, for temporary relief in case of migraine.

Jamaican Dogwood

Jamaican dogwood is a highly reliable analgesic, antispasmodic, and CNS–sedating herb, especially valuable in the treatment of headache, migraine, and dysmenorrhea, making it specific for women suffering from either or a combination. It is also used for cases of severe insomnia and anxiety.[32,80] It is quite a bit stronger than most of the other analgesic and sedative nervines; thus it is advised to stay strictly within the recommended dosing schedule. No clinical studies using this herb were identified.

Kava Kava

Kava kava is approved by the German Commission E for the treatment of nervous anxiety, stress, and restlessness.[44]

Its biological effects, owing to a mixture of compounds called kavalactones, are reported to include sedative, anxiolytic, antistress, analgesic, local anesthetic, anticonvulsant, and neuroprotective properties.[317] Kava kava's efficacy in the treatment of tension headache has not been evaluated specifically. However, it may be useful in preventing and treating underlying hyperexcitability and anxiety that appear to be triggers to tension headaches and MMs, and may provide reliable mild analgesic effects. The kavapyrones dihydromethysticin and dihydrokavain are muscle relaxants when given to animals. Animal and in vitro experiments support certain analgesic actions of kava kava. Both the aqueous and lipid-soluble extracts of kava kava were tested for analgesia in mice. Both extracts were shown to elicit an analgesic response. Kava kava is contraindicated in patients with liver disorders and should not be taken concurrently with pharmaceutical medications.

Peppermint

Peppermint oil has long been topically applied to the forehead and temples for the treatment of headache. *Mentha piperita* oil was equally effective as acetaminophen in relieving headache in a double-blind, placebo-controlled, crossover study with 40 patients. Each patient had four episodes of tension headaches. Topical peppermint oil application was equally effective as a 1-g oral acetaminophen dose in relieving headache, whereas their combination was significantly more effective than either treatment alone. The peppermint dose was 10% oil in ethanol applied to forehead and temples every 15 minutes for a total of three applications. Results were measured every 15 minutes for the first 60 minutes, at 15, 30, 45, and 60 minutes. Peppermint, acetaminophen, and their combination significantly reduced headache intensity compared with placebo; the combination resulted in the greatest reduction in pain and headache-related disability. No adverse effects were reported.[318] The effects of peppermint oil and eucalyptus oil preparations on neurophysiologic, physiologic, and experimental analgesimetric parameters were investigated in 32 healthy subjects in a double-blind, placebo-controlled, randomized crossover design. Four different test preparations were used. The test preparations were applied to large areas of the forehead and temples using a small sponge. The treatment effect of the preparations tested was evaluated by comparing baseline treatment measurements. The combination of peppermint oil, eucalyptus oil, and ethanol can increase cognitive performance and has a muscle-relaxing and mentally relaxing effect, but has little influence on pain sensitivity. However, a significant analgesic effect with reduction in sensitivity to headache is produced by the combination of peppermint oil and ethanol. The essential plant oil preparations often used in empirical medicine can thus be shown by laboratory tests to exert significant effects on mechanisms associated with the pathophysiology of clinical headache syndromes.[319] Additionally, peppermint has demonstrated significant clinical effects in the treatment of nausea. Most studies have looked at postoperative benefits, but given the frequency of nausea and vomiting accompanying migraine, its use as an antinauseant/antiemetic also may be well applied here.

Pulsatilla

Pulsatilla, or pasque flower, is a strong, effective, and potentially toxic analgesic and sedative herb. It is included in this discussion because experienced herbalists and naturopathic physicians may recommend it for severe and intractable pain and insomnia. It is also used in the treatment of dysmenorrhea; in vitro it has been shown to reduce uterine contractions.[32] In dried form, this herb is expected to cause little harm when used in the proper dosage range; however, excessive (undefined amount) doses of the herb may cause severe gastritis, kidney, or urinary tract irritation (see Appendix I). In its fresh form, pulsatilla can cause serious irritation and blistering of the oral, esophageal, and gut mucosa. Pulsatilla also may be adulterated by the presence of other more toxic species of *Pulsatilla*. Therefore this herb should be restricted to use ONLY by those trained in its use and familiar with its identification and contraindications. It is fully contraindicated during pregnancy and lactation.[44] This herb is also contraindicated in depression, psychosis, and in children. Its use with pharmaceutical analgesics is not recommended.[320] No studies using this herb have been identified. Its use is not recommended by the German Commission E.[44]

Willow

Willow (and other salicylate-containing herbs) has been used as an analgesic for at least 2000 years, recommended by physicians such as Paracelsus and Hippocrates all the way up to the Eclectic physicians. Native Americans used numerous willow species for their analgesic, anthelmintic, and hemostatic properties.[321] The modern history of use focuses on the discovery and isolation of salicin from its bark and leaves. Herbalists' popular use of willow and other salicylate-containing herbs such as wintergreen *(Gaultheria procumbens)*, meadowsweet *(Filipendula ulmaria,* formerly *Spirea* spp., from whence the word *aspirin* is derived), lavender *(Lavandula officinalis)*, and rosemary *(Rosmarinus officinalis)* as analgesics or antiinflammatories for mild headache (meadowsweet is not typically used for headache) is mostly extrapolated from traditional use and reinforced by knowledge of the herbs' salicylate contents.[322,323] Surprisingly, no clinical trials have been conducted to assess the efficacy of these herbs for the treatment of headache. Two randomized, double-blind, placebo-controlled clinical trials and two open trials have demonstrated the efficacy of willow in treating lower back pain and osteoarthritis.[32,119,324] Inhibition of platelet aggregation was evaluated in two randomized, double-blind placebo-controlled groups of patients with chronic low back pain. They were treated with willow bark equivalent to 240 mg of salicin (*n* = 19) or placebo (*n* = 16) for 28 days; a third group suffering from chronic ischemic heart disease was treated with 100 mg acetylsalicylate daily for the duration of the study period. Aristolochic acid (AA)–induced platelet aggregation was measured ex vivo in blood samples and was minimally inhibited by the willow bark, but to a much lesser extent than the acetyl-salicylic acid.[119] Salicin did not induce gastric lesions in rats at a dose in which a comparable amount of sodium salicylate did.[119] Wintergreen herbs and other salicin containing herbs are similarly expected to be safer than salicylic acid.[323] White willow bark is approved by the German Commission E for the treatment of headaches, rheumatic ailments, and fever.[44] It is contraindicated in those patients with known salicylate allergy or hypersensitivity, and in those with glucose-6-phosphate deficiency (G6PD) in whom it can cause hemolytic anemia, although allergic reactions are considered improbable.[77,320] Willow bark is high in tannins, and therefore may interfere with nutrient absorption if used for prolonged periods; theoretically, it may interfere with anti-coagulant therapy through potentiation. Its use in conjunction with pharmaceutical analgesics is not recommended.[320] However, salicylate-type side effects are not expected owing to the very low dose of salicylate provided by the herb. GI side effects may be owing to the presence of tannins.[77]

Nervines/Antispasmodics

Nervines and antispasmodics are used to reduce anxiety, emotional and musculoskeletal tension, and irritability, all of which have been shown to be headache and migraine triggers, and symptoms of PMS. Although few have been studied directly for their role in the treatment of headache and migraine, many play an adjunct role in combination herbal formulae for these problems. They also may be especially useful in promoting sleep in the event of headache, and improving sleep overall to prevent fatigue that accompanies sleep disorders and may produce the end result of headache or migraine. Examples of commonly used herbs for the treatment of headache are listed in Table 9-14.

Following are data on those nervines and antispasmodics that have been specifically evaluated for headache/migraine treatment.

Black Cohosh

Black cohosh was traditionally used for relief of a number of types of neuralgias, and many herbalists today include black cohosh in formulae in which there is emotional and/or musculoskeletal tension associated with gynecologic conditions. Research has focused on menopausal symptom relief and not on relief of premenstrual tension and headaches. Use of black cohosh to relieve menstrually related headaches is primarily based on case reports and traditional use. One double-blind, randomized, placebo-controlled trial evaluated a combination of soy, dong quai *(Angelica sinensis),* and black cohosh *(Actaea racemosa)* and found that the supplement successfully reduced migraine frequency. After a 4-week placebo run-in period, patients were randomized to receive either a phytoestrogen supplement (*n* = 20) containing 75 mg soy extract (40% isoflavones), 50 mg dong quai extract (standardized to 1% ligustilide), and 25 mg black cohosh (standardized to 8% triterpenes) or an identical-looking placebo (*n* = 18) twice daily for 24 weeks. Significant reductions in the primary outcome measure of mean number of MM attacks (weeks 9

to 24) was observed in the supplemented group compared with placebo. Secondary outcomes including frequency of any migraine attack (weeks 20 to 24), mean headache severity score (weeks 20 to 24), self-medicated triptans doses (weeks 20 to 24), and doses of analgesics (weeks 20 to 24) were all significantly reduced compared with placebo. Black cohosh has been demonstrated to have positive effects in the treatment of neurovegetative and psychological complaints associated with the hormonal changes of menopause, including sleep disorders and nervous irritability.[119] Onset of action is expected after 2 to 4 weeks of use, and it should be given a 12-week trial of use for maximal effects to be seen.[119] The German Commission E supports the use of this herb for the treatment of premenstrual discomfort, dysmenorrhea, and menopausal symptoms.[44]

Lavender

Lavender is considered a mild sedative for restlessness, nervous exhaustion, and sleep disorders, and is approved by the German Commission E for these purposes.[44] It is also a mild antidepressant and anxiolytic.[80,326] The scent of the flowers, whether as one takes the tea or the tincture diluted in water, is in itself uplifting.[80,327] Human and animal studies have indicated that linalool and linalyl acetate are the active sedating compounds.[77] Considerable evidence from case reports and studies suggests the effectiveness of lavender oil in the treatment of pain; however, these studies tend to be small, and were not rigorous or controlled.[327] Although not a primary treatment for headache, lavender makes an excellent addition to internal use formulae for headache and migraine, and is also useful as a topical application to the temples (see the following discussion) or in baths or other inhalation methods.

Sedatives

Botanical sedatives can be highly effective in promoting sleep and relieving pain during acute headache/migraine, especially when combined with analgesic and antispasmodic herbs. Many of the most appropriate sedatives for headache/migraine treatment are listed in Table 9-14.

Adaptogens

Stress and other affective moods are both a causative factor and a result of headache and migraine. Stress can lead to and exacerbate hormonal dysregulation. Adaptogens are especially appropriate for the long-term reduction and prevention of headache and migraine owing to stress, fatigue, irritability, and other affective moods, and should be considered whenever treating chronic premenstrual headache, MM, and TMM. They should be used long-term (for at least 12 weeks) before optimal results are evident. A number of adaptogens, for example, ashwagandha, also have mild sedative action and may be especially beneficial for treatment of headache and migraine. Adaptogens are listed in Table 9-14. Readers will want to refer to Chapter 5 for more data on adaptogens, as well as to discussions on adaptogens throughout this text.

BOX 9-17 **Nervine Prescription**

Tincture for Internal Use

Chamomile	*(Matricaria recutita)*	30 mL
Lemon balm	*(Melissa officinalis)*	30 mL
Blue vervain*	*(Verbena officinalis)*	30 mL
Lavender	*(Lavandula officinalis)*	10 mL
		Total: 100 mL

Dose: 2 to 5 mL three times daily, or 3 mL as needed.

These herbs can also be used as tea; taken one to two cups daily. Omit the vervain or motherwort if taken as a tea (both are bitter in tea).

*Blue vervain may be replaced with motherwort *(Leonurus cardiaca).*

Antidepressants/Anxiolytics

Like stress, anxiety and depression often accompany, precipitate, or are a result of headache and migraine. Therefore anxiolytic and/or antidepressant herbs should be included in herbal protocol when indicated. Many herbs have multiple effects; for example, kava is an excellent anxiolytic and mild analgesic, and St. John's wort used long-term is both a tonic nervine and antidepressant (Box 9-17).

External Treatments for Headache and Migraine
Peppermint and Lavender Oil Compresses

Dilute five drops each of peppermint and lavender essential oils in a bowl of cool water. Stir well to distribute the oil throughout the water, and dip a folded washcloth into the bowl. For pain and nausea, apply the cloth to the forehead and temples, and if desired, another to the back of the neck. If warm water is preferred, then it may be substituted. Relax the head on a pillow for 10 minutes and breathe deeply during the application. Repeat two to three times per day as necessary. Herbal baths with essential oil (e.g., lavender) can also be very relaxing, and used prophylactically or for acute care.

Warm Ginger Compresses

For women who prefer heat to cold, warm ginger compresses can provide modest temporary relief of pain and nausea. Grate 1 tablespoon of fresh ginger into a bowl of boiling water. Cover and let steep for 5 minutes. Dip a folded washcloth into the preparation and apply the cloth to the forehead and temples, and if desired, another to the back of the neck. Relax the head on a pillow for 10 minutes and breathe deeply during the application.

Tiger Balm Herbal Salve

Tiger balm is a topical medication used for almost a century to relieve pain and muscle tension. Tiger balm's active ingredients are camphor, menthol, cajuput, and clove oil. One RCT concluded that Tiger balm is as effective as any other commonly used analgesic.[328] Participants rubbed Tiger balm on their temples as soon as symptoms of headache presented. They repeated the application at 30 minutes and 1 hour.

Patients with severe migraine headache were excluded from the study.

NUTRITIONAL CONSIDERATIONS

Teach patients to:
- Avoid dietary triggers of headache/migraine (see Box 9-16).
- Maintain a diet that is low in proinflammatory precursors (e.g., arachidonic acid) by minimizing red meat and dairy (with the exception of some yogurt) and maximizing whole grains and complex carbohydrates, fish (especially cold-water fish such as salmon and tuna), poultry, vegetarian protein sources (legumes, tofu, tempeh), and plenty of fresh fruits and vegetables.
- Maintain well-regulated blood sugar by eating regularly (i.e., do not skip meals), getting adequate complex carbohydrates and snacking on healthful choices. Avoid excessive (i.e., more than two times per week) consumption of refined flour products and sugar, as well as excessive salt intake; the latter can lead to fluid retention and increased headache susceptibility.
- Minimize consumption of caffeinated products (e.g., coffee, black tea, soda, chocolate) (see Box 9-16).

Magnesium

Whether magnesium supplementation is beneficial in the prevention and treatment of migraine is inconclusive; however, several trials have suggested improvements with its use, especially for women who experience aura with MMs.[32] A 2008 double-blind RCT evaluated the prophylactic effects of 600 mg daily magnesium supplementation in migraine treatment. Thirty migraine patients (without aura) were randomized into treatment and placebo control groups. Statistically significant improvements in migraine frequency and duration were observed over controls, with beneficial effects noted in regards to cortical blood flow.[329] One study, reported in *Headache: The Journal of Head and Face Pain,* reported that the incidences of magnesium deficiency in women with MMs was 45%, compared with 15% in nonmenstrual attacks, 14% during menstruation without migraine, and 15% between menstrual and migraine. The authors concluded that the high incidence of magnesium deficiency and the elevated calcium to magnesium ratio during MM confirm previous suggestions of a possible role for magnesium deficiency in the development of MM.[330] This study also confirms older studies that point to magnesium supplementation as a further means for MM prophylaxis, and support the possibility that a lower migraine threshold could be related to magnesium deficiency.[331] Because magnesium supplementation is relatively safe and affordable, practitioners may feel that a trial of 200 mg magnesium salts twice daily or 400 mg four times daily is a sensible approach to migraine prophylaxis.[32,294]

Coenzyme Q$_{10}$

Coenzyme Q$_{10}$ is an essential element of the mitochondrial electron transport chain. A recent open trial by Rozen and coworkers assessed the efficacy of coenzyme Q$_{10}$ as a

BOTANICAL PRESCRIPTION FOR PREMENSTRUAL HEADACHE: PREVENTION

The following tincture can be taken throughout the month as a prophylactic remedy for headache/migraine. It can be accompanied by the next tincture for mild–moderate headache, as directed, for optimal prevention.

Tincture for Internal Use:

A general adaptogenic, antiinflammatory, and anxiolytic formula:

Ashwagandha	(*Withania somnifera*)	30 mL
Feverfew	(*Tanacetum parthenium*)	20 mL
Skullcap	(*Scutellaria lateriflora*)	20 mL
Chamomile	(*Matricaria recutita*)	15 mL
Ginger	(*Zingiber officinale*)	15 mL
		Total: 100 mL

Dose: 3 to 5 mL two or three times daily.

Variations

If there is anxiety, reduce chamomile and skullcap by 10 mL each and add 20 mL *Passiflora incarnata*. If there is depression, reduce chamomile by 10 mL, skullcap by 5 mL, and add 15 mL *Hypericum perforatum*.

Botanical Prescription for Premenstrual Headache: Acute

This tincture can be taken at the onset of an acute headache and throughout, or preferably, it can be taken for several days before the typical time of onset for prophylactic pain treatment.

Mild to Moderate Pain

Black cohosh	(*Actaea racemosa*)	30 mL
Cramp bark/black haw	(*Viburnum* spp.)	30 mL
Passionflower	(*Passiflora incarnata*)	20 mL
Motherwort	(*Leonurus cardiaca*)	20 mL
		Total: 100 mL

Dose: Prophylactically: 3 to 5 mL two to three times daily.

Acute pain: 2 to 5 mL every 1 to 4 hours, up to 30 mL daily of total tincture.

Severe pain: To the tincture, consider adding 2 mL *Piscidia piscipula* or *Corydalis*, repeated as needed up to four doses over an hour, not to exceed 2 hours.

Relaxation Tea

Chamomile	(*Matricaria recutita*)	4 parts
Lemon balm	(*Melissa officinalis*)	3 parts
Lavender	(*Lavandula officinalis*)	2 parts
Spearmint	(*Mentha piperita*)	1 part

Mix these dried herbs together. Steep 2 tsp per cup of boiling water for 10 minutes (cover while steeping). Strain, sweeten lightly if desired, and drink hot, up to 3 cups daily.

---

preventive treatment for migraine.[332] Thirty-two patients with migraine were treated with coenzyme Q_{10} at a dose of 150 mg/day. Thirty-one of 32 patients completed the study; 61.3% of patients had a greater than 50% reduction in number of days with migraine headache. The average number of days with migraine during the baseline period was 7.34 and this decreased to 2.95 after 3 months of therapy, which was a statistically significant response. Mean reduction in migraine frequency after 1 month of treatment was 13.1% and this increased to 55.3% by the end of 3 months. Mean migraine attack frequency was 4.85 during the baseline period and this decreased to 2.81 attacks by the end of the study period, which was a statistically significant response. There were no side effects noted with coenzyme Q_{10}. Coenzyme Q_{10} was recently assessed in a double-blind trial by Sandor and colleagues.[294] After 3 months, patients receiving 100 mg of coenzyme Q_{10} had less attacks per month, days with headache and days with nausea. A total of 47.6% of those receiving coenzyme Q_{10} had more than 50% reduction in the frequency of pain versus 14.3% in the placebo group. One patient in the active group withdrew from the study owing to cutaneous allergy.[294]

Riboflavin, Magnesium, and Feverfew Combination

A randomized double-blind placebo-controlled trial was conducted to determine the efficacy of a combination of riboflavin, magnesium, and feverfew for migraine prophylaxis. A compound providing a daily dose of riboflavin 400 mg, magnesium 300 mg, and feverfew 100 mg was administered. The placebo contained 25 mg of riboflavin. Previous studies of magnesium and feverfew for migraine prophylaxis have found conflicting results, and there has been only a single placebo-controlled trial of riboflavin. The study included a 1-month run-in phase and 3-month trial. The protocol allowed for 120 patients to be randomized, with a preplanned interim analysis of the data after 48 patients had completed the trial. Forty-nine patients completed the 3-month trial. For the primary outcome measure—a 50% or greater reduction in migraines—there was no difference between active and placebo groups, achieved by 10 (42%) and 11 (44%), respectively. Similarly, there was no significant difference in secondary outcome measures for active versus placebo groups, respectively, 50% or greater reduction in migraine days (33% and 40%); or change in mean number of migraines, migraine days, migraine index, or triptan doses. Compared with baseline, however, both groups showed a significant reduction in number of migraines, migraine days, and migraine index. This effect exceeds that reported for placebo agents in previous migraine trials.[359] Riboflavin 25 mg showed an effect comparable with a combination of riboflavin 400 mg, magnesium 300 mg, and feverfew 100 mg. The placebo response exceeds that reported for any other placebo in trials of migraine prophylaxis, and suggests that riboflavin 25 mg may be an active comparator.[333]

Magnesium, Coenzyme Q$_{10}$ Riboflavin, and Vitamin B$_{12}$ Combination

The therapeutic potential of magnesium, coenzyme Q$_{10}$, riboflavin, and vitamin B$_{12}$ can be cautiously inferred from some published open clinical trials; it should, however, be considered that double-blind randomized larger studies are needed to correctly estimate the effect of the placebo effect in these promising therapies.[334]

Vitamin D and Calcium

Two premenopausal women with a history of menstrually related migraines and PMS were treated with a combination of vitamin D and elemental calcium for late luteal phase symptoms. Both cited a major reduction in their headache attacks as well as premenstrual symptomatology within 2 months of therapy.[335]

Essential Fatty Acids

EPO is heavily promoted as a product for the treatment of PMS; however, trials have not demonstrated its benefits inconclusively. EPO contains two essential fatty acids—linoleic acid and γ-linoleic acid (GLA). Linoleic acid is needed for the synthesis of prostaglandin E, and GLA is needed for the synthesis of prostaglandin E$_1$. Results of uncontrolled studies suggest abnormal essential fatty acid metabolism as an underlying problem in PMS. Resultant low levels of prostaglandins E$_1$ may lead to increased sensitivity to PRL and consequently, the problems associated with PMS.[336] EPO is considered generally safe, although side effects of occasional nausea, indigestion, and headache have been reported, as has the rare risk of inflammation, thrombosis (i.e., blood clot), and immunosuppression (i.e., reduced resistance to infection) with prolonged use of GLA use.

ADDITIONAL THERAPIES

Exercise

Exercise is beneficial for stress reduction and promoting mood elevation, and thus is an excellent adjunct preventative therapy when headache/migraine is mood or stress induced. (See Premenstrual Symptoms, PMS, and PMDD.)

Body Work
Spinal Manipulation and Massage Therapy

Spinal manipulation has been evaluated and shows some benefit in the treatment of menstrual headache and migraine.[32,337] Subjectively, many individuals report that regular massage reduces stress, anxiety, and associated health problems, and thus is a commonsense therapy to include for the prevention of headache and migraine. However, there are minimal data pertaining to the benefits of these therapies for the treatment of these conditions.[288]

Behavioral Modification

Relaxation and biofeedback have also been shown to be effective in the treatment of tension headaches.[172,270]

Dysfunctional Uterine Bleeding

Dysfunctional uterine bleeding (DUB) is defined as excessive, prolonged, unpatterned endometrial bleeding in the absence of organic disease.[1,2] DUB is a subset of abnormal uterine bleeding (AUB), which encompasses all abnormal uterine bleeding regardless of cause.[3] After pathologic abnormalities, systemic disorders, or iatrogenic causes have been ruled out, *functional* (i.e., endocrinologic) causes are then considered; any remaining case of uterine bleeding is described by the term *dysfunctional uterine bleeding.*[4] Some authors further recommend limiting the definition of DUB to apply only to anovulatory cycles, allowing for medical differentiation of excessive bleeding in ovulatory cycles to be classified as *functional menorrhagia,* a condition that involves disturbances in endometrial tissue prostaglandin synthesis, other forms of uterine pathology, or systemic causes.[5,6] For the purpose of examining a broader spectrum of support options, this discussion addresses DUB as irregular uterine bleeding without organic pathology.

DUB is a common diagnosis. It is estimated that 5% to 10% of women experience some form of DUB in their lifetime. DUB occurs most commonly at the beginning and end of the reproductive years; 20% of cases occur in adolescent girls, and more than 50% occur in women older than age 45. It is estimated that 70% of DUB cases occur in anovulatory or infrequent ovulatory cycles. Irregular uterine bleeding accounts for 20% of all gynecologic visits. DUB may be accompanied by pain; can severely and negatively affect quality of life, including limiting activity; and can lead to fatigue and increased risk of illness if there is concomitant anemia.[7]

Most AUB is the dysfunctional type, but this diagnosis is made only when all other possibilities have been excluded. Primary presenting complaints may include:

- Menorrhagia (i.e., excessive bleeding, either in number of days, amount of blood, or both)
- Hypomenorrhea (i.e., scanty flow, brief number of days, or both)
- Metrorrhagia (i.e., bleeding that occurs at times other than the menses)
- Menometrorrhagia (i.e., excessive bleeding at irregular intervals)
- Oligomenorrhea (i.e., bleeding occurs infrequently; prolonged time between cycles)
- Oligohypermenorrhea (i.e., infrequent and heavy)
- Oligohypomenorrhea (i.e., infrequent and scant)
- Polymenorrhea (i.e., bleeding occurs often; less than 21 days between cycles)
- Amenorrhea (i.e., absence or suppression of menstruation)

Occasionally, patients also exhibit signs and symptoms of hypovolemia, such as hypotension, tachycardia, diaphoresis, and pallor. Iron deficiency anemia is a common consequence of excessive menstrual flow in quantity, duration, or frequency.[2]

Excessive bleeding can refer to amount or duration of blood loss. The average blood loss per normal menstrual cycle is 20 to 60 mL, with median expected blood loss of approximately 30 to 40 mL. Menstrual blood loss of 80 mL or more is considered excessive and increases the risk of iron-deficiency anemia.[8] This can initiate a chronic pattern of cyclical excessive bleeding because iron deficiency can be an etiologic factor in AUB.[9] Prolonged bleeding is defined as bleeding lasting longer than 7 or 8 days; however, 10 days has been suggested as the maximum duration that distinguishes normal from abnormal bleeding.[8]

Heavy but regular menstrual bleeding may occur in normally ovulating women, and is usually a result of minor hormonal disturbances.[10] Many women who present with complaints of excessive menstrual bleeding have blood losses within the normal range.[11,12] Conversely, in one study, 40% of women with excessive uterine bleeding (>80 mL) reported that their periods were normal or even light. Some women with light periods viewed their bleeding as severe.[2,13] Practitioners routinely assess menstrual blood loss by inquiring about the number of sanitary pads or tampons that are used during the menstrual period. This is the most practical method of evaluation, as volumetric measurement of actual blood loss is not feasible. A clinically objective measurement is to assess blood hemoglobin and serum ferritin levels. Two thirds of women with excessive menstrual bleeding develop iron-deficiency anemia.[14]

PATHOPHYSIOLOGY

Determining the ovulatory status helps narrow the etiologic possibilities contributing to DUB. Life stage may also provide some clues. A discussion of these factors follows (Box 10-1).

Additional factors that may influence the development of DUB and menstrual bleeding disorders include prenatal exposure to DES (diethylstilbestrol); body mass index (BMI)

The editor wishes to thank *Botanical Medicine for Women's Health,* ed 1 contributor to this chapter, Linda Ryan.

BOX 10-1　Overview of Possible Etiologies in Dysfunctional Uterine Bleeding

- Hypothalamic-pituitary-ovarian (HPO) axis disorder is most commonly seen in the postpubertal period when normal hypothalamic function is not yet well established.[7]
- Hormone imbalance owing to insufficient estrogen production, or disordered estrogen to progesterone ratio.[3]
- Hormone imbalance resulting in excess estrogen, either from endogenous production or exogenous sources. Women with higher levels of estrogens often have prolonged intervals of amenorrhea followed by excessive episodes of bleeding.[15]
- Vascular fragility in cyclic angiogenesis. The continuous estrogen stimulation leads to a vascular, friable endometrium that may bleed intermittently or slough at irregular intervals.[16-18]
- Iron deficiency.
- Stress.[19,20]
- Excessively overweight women often have high estradiol levels because fat cells produce the aromatase enzyme that causes the body to make more estrogen.[21] A recent study concluded that obesity has been found to increase endometrial thickness independently.[22] Excessive endometrial thickness commonly results in menorrhagia when the lining is shed.
- Liver clearance of hormones. If estrogen cannot be conjugated properly, it will not be excreted normally and levels will remain high.[3,19,23]
- Eating disorders: anorexia nervosa, bulimia. A study of 117 adolescent girls found a high percentage (43.7%) of those with menstrual dysfunction also had eating disorders.[24]
- Overexercise in athletes or overexercisers.[25]
- Disordered prostaglandins.[6,12,26]
- Increase in fibrinolytic activity within the uterine cavity.[12]
- Thyroid conditions.[27]
- Hypothyroidism. Reduced levels of sex hormone-binding globulin (SHBG) causes an increase in estrogen availability.
- Hyperthyroidism promotes increased conversion of androgens to estrogens.

and dieting; perceived stress (blood coagulation factor activity may decline when an individual is under prolonged stress); cigarette smoking; obesity; mild hypothyroidism; inherited bleeding disorders; IUD devices (unless they contain progesterone); and use of aspirin or oral anticoagulants.[8]

Ovulatory Dysfunctional Uterine Bleeding

In normal ovulatory cycles, progesterone production from the corpus luteum converts the estrogen-primed proliferative endometrium to a secretory endometrium, which sheds cyclically if pregnancy does not occur. Ovulatory DUB is less common than anovulatory DUB, and the bleeding, although abnormally heavy, is usually regular. Ovulatory DUB may be owing to abnormalities in the 2-week luteal phase of menstruation that occurs before menstruation. It can also result from an "atrophic endometrium" that can result from a high progesterone to estrogen ratio. A lack of cell-building estrogen

causes the endometrium to shed and bleed irregularly. This may occur in women who take over-the-counter progesterone creams or progesterone-only contraceptives.

Anovulatory Dysfunctional Uterine Bleeding

Any disruption in the cyclic release of gonadotrophin-releasing hormone (GnRH), follicle-stimulating hormone (FSH), or luteinizing hormone (LH) can result in anovulation. This is most often owing to immaturity of the hypothalamic-pituitary-ovarian (HPO) axis just after menarche and decreased sensitivity of the ovary to gonadotropin stimulation in perimenopausal women. Most anovulatory DUB is caused by estrogen withdrawal or estrogen breakthrough bleeding (EbB).

In anovulatory cycles, follicular growth occurs with stimulation from FSH; however, because estrogen levels remain below the threshold, there is a lack of LH surge and ovulation fails to occur. Consequently, no corpus luteum is formed and no progesterone is secreted. The endometrium continues its proliferative phase. When the follicle degenerates, estrogen levels drop and estrogen withdrawal bleeding occurs.[15] EbB may exhibit the pattern of normal menses; however, EbB generally occurs as scant (i.e., hypomenorrhea), irregular bleeding that may continue for a prolonged period. The low estrogen levels prevent excessive endometrial thickening between cycles, which accounts for the light-bleeding pattern.

EbB also occurs when unopposed estrogen levels are sustained, resulting in excessive endometrial proliferation and thickness. In the absence of progesterone, the endometrium does not develop the spiral arterioles of the secretory phase and the endometrial tissue eventually becomes fragile and breaks down erratically.[4,19,29]

SUMMARY OF ETIOLOGIES AS ASSOCIATED WITH LIFE STAGES

Adolescence

Owing to immaturity of the HPO (hypothalmic-pituitary-ovarian) axis there is a pattern of erratic ovulation in adolescents. FSH acts on ovarian cells, producing estrogen; however, either the estradiol concentrations are not high enough to stimulate positive feedback of LH release, or the hypothalamus-pituitary (H-P) complex fails to trigger the LH surge. Inadequate LH to induce ovulation results in the absence of luteal phase progesterone. This leads to a prolonged proliferative phase of the endometrium, resulting in excessive thickness. Uncoordinated sloughing of the endometrium occurs either in response to estrogen withdrawal or owing to insufficient blood supply for the excessive endometrial tissue. There is usually prolonged bleeding owing to a lack of chemical mediators (i.e., prostaglandins, thromboxane) that normally contribute to cessation of menses in the normal cycle. The presence of these chemicals is relative to the secretion of progesterone.[3]

Reproductive Age

Women of reproductive age more commonly experience DUB associated with ovulatory cycles that exhibit a luteal phase defect. The hormones do not support an adequate corpus luteum; therefore, progesterone secretions are insufficient. One study found that 70% of luteal phase defect patients had excessive prolactin levels.[30] Cycles are usually regular, but bleeding is prolonged and/or excessive. Low estrogen production and the consequent poor endometrial development typically results in estrogen withdrawal bleeding. In these cases, there are rising estrogens that are not enough to trigger LH, but are enough to inhibit further FSH release, which, in turn, inhibits estrogen production by the ovaries. Excess, sustained estrogen levels resulting from anovulation is commonly associated with oligomenorrhea followed by acute, heavy EbB. An additional consideration for DUB in the reproductive years is excessive exercise. Studies of female athletes demonstrate a correlation between inadequate LH secretion by the pituitary gland and excessive exercise.[31]

Polycystic Ovarian Syndrome

Polycystic ovarian syndrome (PCOS) can contribute to DUB in women of reproductive age. In this condition, there is a hypersecretion of LH and suppression of FSH, which results in chronic anovulation. PCOS is associated with insulin resistance; common clinical presentations include hirsutism (from excess androgen production), acne, elevated lipids, male-pattern baldness, and truncal obesity.

Other factors contributing to DUB in women of reproductive age include:
- Hypothyroidism
- Hyperthyroidism
- Diabetes mellitus
- Androgen excess disorders

Perimenopausal Years

During this stage, the ovaries become less responsive to gonadotropins and the production of active follicles declines. In addition, the active follicles produced do not secrete sufficient estrogen to trigger the LH surge needed for ovulation and corpus luteum formation. DUB at this stage may be attributable to this anovulatory pattern.[32] Approximately 50% of all cases of DUB occur in women aged 40 to 59 years old.[7]

Postmenopausal Years

In the absence of exogenous hormone therapy, postmenopausal bleeding is abnormal and women presenting with such should be investigated for neoplastic lesions.

DIAGNOSIS

DUB is a diagnosis of exclusion. To accurately evaluate this condition it is important to determine when the menstrual pattern changed, determine whether or not pregnancy or pelvic infection is present, and particularly to document the frequency, duration, and amount of bleeding. Initial testing may include complete blood cell count, prothrombin time, activated partial thromboplastin time, iron profile, serum creatinine, thyroid-stimulating hormone (TSH) level, factor VIII level, von Willebrand factor antigen, ristocetin cofactor,

platelet aggregation studies, a Pap smear, and a pregnancy test. Standard invasive diagnostic tests include the combination of hysteroscopy and curettage or guided biopsy, with the exception of adolescent patients, who generally do not require invasive diagnostics.[1,11] In women of childbearing age who are at high risk for endometrial cancer, the initial evaluation includes endometrial biopsy; saline-infusion sonohysterography or diagnostic hysteroscopy is performed if initial studies are inconclusive or the bleeding continues. Women of childbearing age who are at low risk for endometrial cancer may be assessed initially by transvaginal ultrasonography. Postmenopausal women with AUB should be offered dilatation and curettage (D&C); if they are poor candidates for general anesthesia or decline D&C, they may be offered transvaginal ultrasonography or saline-infusion sonohysterography with directed endometrial biopsy.[33]

DIFFERENTIAL DIAGNOSIS

Disorders that need to be excluded are:
- Pregnancy; hydatidiform mole
- Coagulation defects—adolescents with acute menorrhagia have a 20% to 30% incidence of a coagulation disorder, such as von Willebrand's disease, idiopathic thrombocytopenic purpurea (ITP), or leukemia[14]
- Trauma to the vulva, vagina, or cervix
- Organic pathologies, such as diabetes mellitus, hypothyroidism, hyperthyroidism, hypertension, liver or adrenal disorders, or thrombocytopenia
- Carcinomas of the reproductive organs
- PCOS
- Medications, such as low-dose estrogens, exogenous progestins or over-the-counter (OTC) progesterone creams, anticoagulants, nonsteroidal antiinflammatory drugs (NSAIDs), or aspirin
- Infections, such as cervicitis, sexually transmitted diseases (STDs), or salpingitis
- Structural disorders, such as leiomyomas, endometriosis, or polyps
- Drugs or nicotine
- High stress levels
- Obesity
- Excessive exercise[7]

CONVENTIONAL TREATMENT APPROACHES

Women with DUB are currently treated with a variety of approaches, including expectant management, iron replacement, medical therapy, and surgery. Surgery for DUB is generally reserved for situations in which the condition is life threatening, medical therapy is not effective or is not tolerated by the woman, or surgery is the woman's preference or the surgeon's recommendation. Types of surgery include hysterectomy and endometrial ablation (EA). EA is the targeted destruction or removal of the endometrium, leaving the uterus otherwise intact, and is performed using either hysteroscopically directed techniques (i.e., hysteroscopic EA or HEA) or a specialized device without hysteroscopic guidance (i.e., nonhysteroscopic EA or NHEA).[34] Hysterectomy carries a high complication rate but is associated with a high satisfaction rate.[35] EA therapy is an alternative to hysterectomy and allows for reduced surgical and recovery times, and does not require removal of the uterus.[2]

Medical therapies may include:
- Gestagens, estrogens, or combinations thereof.
- If contraception is needed, ovulation inhibitors are chosen.
- Nonsteroidal antirheumatics or antifibrinolytics are used if there are contraindications to the use of hormone therapy.
- Antifibrinolytic agents are used to prevent the proteolysis digestion of fibrinogen to fibrin and thus prevent the breakdown of blood clots. Aprotinin, isolated from bovine lung tissue, is a naturally occurring inhibitor of serine proteolytic enzymes.
- NSAIDs are used to decrease the production and use of prostaglandins.
- Iron supplementation and antiprostaglandin medications are recommended during bleeding episodes.
- Intravenous Premarin is given every 4 hours until the bleeding stops.
- High-dose estrogen therapy addresses DUB by maintaining the endometrial lining.
- Prostaglandin synthetase inhibitors (PGSIs), a nonhormonal treatment, is associated with a 20% to 50% reduction in bleeding.[2]
- The levonorgestrel intrauterine contraceptive device may be recommended.

Invasive therapies include:
- Hysteroscopy
- D&C
- EA
- Hysterectomy[36]

One study concluded that because none of the treatments for dysfunctional bleeding is superior to one of the others, and all treatments have advantages and disadvantages, counseling of patients with dysfunctional bleeding should incorporate a comprehensive review of the many options available to evaluate quality of life and risk to benefit ratio in relationship to patient preferences.[35] Surgical therapies generally may be avoided with appropriately applied hormonal therapies, particularly progesterones, and NSAIDs, allowing surgical intervention to be used in only severe, unresponsive, or life-threatening cases.[34,37]

WARNING! Severe bleeding can be life-threatening and must be treated acutely as an emergency.[38] Bleeding in excess of two menstrual pads soaked in 30 minutes is considered a hemorrhage and medical care should be sought. If there is excessive bleeding accompanied by orthostatic hypotension or a hematocrit less than 25%, hospitalization is required.

BOTANICAL TREATMENT OF DYSFUNCTIONAL UTERINE BLEEDING

Because DUB is a physiologic rather than a pathologic problem, it is reasonable to attempt botanical and adjunct complementary therapies such as nutrition, stress reduction, and weight management before using more aggressive therapies. Once a diagnosis of DUB has been confirmed (i.e., underlying pathology has been ruled out) the primary botanical treatment goals are:
- Normalization of excessive or prolonged bleeding
- Correction of anemia or underlying nutritional deficiency
- Reduction of stress if stress related
- Correction of hormonal dysregulation

DUB treatment approaches can be divided into two categories:
1. Treatment of acute, non–life-threatening bleeding episodes
2. Treatment/prevention of chronic DUB

The role of the herbalist in cases of DUB is to address the primary complaints while working to restore hormonal balance. It is necessary to have an understanding of the underlying hormonal dysfunction to devise an appropriate therapeutic strategy. This can best be established by evaluating the woman's gynecologic and menstrual history, assessing her life cycle (i.e., postmenarchal, reproductive age, perimenopausal, postmenopausal). In most cases, the client will present with a diagnosis of DUB established by conventional diagnostic techniques. If this has not been done, it is strongly advised that the client have the condition medically investigated to rule out potentially grave pathology.

A systematic approach to choosing the most appropriate herbs for each individual case is to determine the key actions needed and to use those herbs known to reliably exert those actions. These herbs are then put into a formula (typically a tincture) according the specific needs of the individual client. Frequently, a client is given a formula to use in case of mild to moderate acute bleeding along with the formulae needed for addressing underlying dysfunction. Herbs may be used as hemostatics, progesterone production enhancers, and antiinflammatories in the reduction of PGE_2 (Table 10-1).

DISCUSSION OF BOTANICALS

The following discussion highlights several key herbs commonly used in the treatment of DUB. They specifically target hormonal and menstrual cycle regulation, and the treatment of mild to moderate acute excessive bleeding. Most evidence for antihemorrhagic activity is based on traditional use. Strategies for hormonal regulation can be used to treat DUB when there is a physiologic correlate (e.g., the use of chaste berry for DUB when it is related to luteal phase insufficiency). Readers should refer to the sections on PCOS, anemia, adaptogens, and nervines for additional and adjunct herbal treatments.

Of note, dong quai is used in Traditional Chinese Medicine (TCM) formulae for conditions such as amenorrhea, irregular menstruation, menorrhagia, metrorrhagia, infertility,

TABLE 10-1 Botanical Treatment Summary for Dysfunctional Uterine Bleeding

Therapeutic Goal	Therapeutic Action	Botanical Name	Common Name
Control of acute and excessive uterine bleeding	Antihemorrhagic, uterine astringents	Achillea millefolium Capsella bursa-pastoris Hamamelis virginiana Panax notoginseng Trillium erectum	Yarrow Shepherd's purse Witch hazel Tienchi ginseng Birthwort, birthroot, bethroot
Hormonal regulation, especially of estrogen to progesterone ratio	Hormonal modulatory herbs	Actaea racemosa Chamaelirium luteum* Dioscorea villosa Foeniculum vulgare Vitex agnus-castus	Black cohosh False unicorn Wild yam Fennel Chaste berry
Promote uterine tone and efficient evacuation of uterine endometrium during menstruation	Uterine tonics	Angelica sinensis Caulophyllum thalictroides Chamaelirium luteum* Rubus idaeus	Dong quai Blue cohosh False unicorn Red raspberry
Promote normal levels of estrogen and progesterone; improve luteal function and luteal phase of the cycle	Ovarian tonics	Caulophyllum thalictroides Paeonia lactiflora Chamaelirium luteum[28,37]	Blue cohosh White peony False unicorn*
Address iron-deficiency anemia[7]	Nutritive	Angelica sinensis Rehmannia glutinosa Urtica dioica Withania somnifera See Iron deficiency anemia	Dong quai Rehmannia Nettle Ashwagandha
Reduce underlying stress	Nervines, sedatives, hypnotics	See Nervines in Chapter 3	
Restore/improve HPA axis function	Adrenal restoratives and tonics	Eleutherococcus senticosus Glycyrrhiza glabra Panax ginseng Schisandra chinensis Turnera diffusa Withania somnifera	Eleuthero Licorice Ginseng Schisandra Damiana Ashwagandha
Treat chronic UTI; vaginal infection	Antimicrobials, urinary antiseptics		
Optimize the liver's ability to metabolize and eliminate hormones as part of improving hormonal dysregulation Also see PCOS	Hepatic herbs	See Actions of Herbs	

HPA, Hypothalamic-pituitary-adrenal; *UTI,* Urinary tract infection; *PCOS,* Polycystic ovarian syndrome.
Chamaelirium luteum, or false unicorn, is an endangered plant and should not be used unless from a cultivated source. It is included here for historical purposes, and to encourage cultivation of this valuable gynecologic herb.

dysmenorrhea, PMS, and menopause, and also as a general female reproductive tonic.[38] It has been shown to *inhibit* platelet aggregation and inhibition, *increase* prothrombin time, and has been known clinically to *increase* uterine bleeding. This should only be used with caution for patients with DUB.[39,40] Should there be increased bleeding with use of this herb, it should be discontinued.

Botanicals for Hormonal Regulation
Chaste Berry

Herbalists have traditionally used chaste berry for a range of gynecologic applications, especially menstrual disturbances. Contemporary herbalists consider chaste berry an important herb for conditions resulting from unopposed estrogen, luteal phase defects, or latent hyperprolactinemia.[41] Bone

specifically suggests the use of chaste berry for metrorrhagia from functional causes, menorrhagia, and polymenorrhea.[39] Increased serum prolactin levels are associated with menstrual irregularities. In vivo and in vitro experiments with chaste berry have demonstrated that extracts possess dopaminergic, prolactin-inhibiting activity, and thus suggest a role for the treatment of menstrual dysregulation.[40] Positive results on the treatment of secondary amenorrhea were seen in early clinical studies. In a clinical study of 52 women with luteal phase defects owing to latent prolactinemia, statistically significant changes were seen in the group taking the chaste berry extract. The prolactin release was reduced after 3 months, shortened luteal phases were normalized and deficits in the luteal progesterone synthesis were eliminated.[42] A study examined the use of *Vitex agnus-castus* for menorrhagia and polymenorrhea over a 2-year period. Fifty-one women participated in the study, and of these, 64% reported an improvement, which was noted within 2 to 3 months of commencing treatment. No side effects were reported.[43] A partially homeopathic preparation (containing *V. agnus-castus, Caulophyllum thalictroides, cyclamen, Ignatia, iris,* and *Lilium tigrinum* in 53% ethanol) was effective in treating 13 women with hyperprolactinemia and menstrual cycle disorders, including secondary amenorrhea, polymenorrhea, menorrhagia, ovulation bleeding, and metrorrhagia. At the start of the study, 12 patients' baseline prolactin levels ranged between 41.4 ng/mL and 93.5 ng/mL, and one was 514.9 ng/mL. Patients received 30 drops (equivalent to 33.4 mg *V. agnus-castus*) of the preparation twice daily for 3 months. Prolactin levels significantly decreased in all patients over the course of treatment; in eight cases prolactin levels returned to normal or high normal. At the end of the study, all cases of DUB were resolved. No adverse effects were reported.[44] The German Commission E approved the use of chaste tree fruit for menstrual irregularities.[45]

White Peony

See Polycystic Ovarian Syndrome for a discussion of this herb.

Uterine Hemostatics
Erigeron

Erigeron, or Canada fleabane, is a classic Eclectic herb for the treatment of uterine bleeding; it is still in use by herbalists, although not widespread.[46,47] It was described by Ellingwood as the agent to be given in cases of "postpartum hemorrhage, abortion with alarming flow, menorrhagia with profuse flow of bright-red blood, dysmenorrhea with blood clots, bloody lochia increased by movements" and numerous other hemorrhages, as well as for diarrhea.[47] Use is based purely on historical evidence and contemporary clinical observation. Use of this herb has not been evaluated by the German Commission E nor the American Herbal Products Association.[38,45]

Shepherd's Purse

This herb has a long history of use as an astringent and antihemorrhagic, and was specifically used for heavy uterine bleeding.[48] Nineteenth-century American Eclectic physicians used shepherd's purse to treat hematuria and menorrhagia.[47] During World War I, this herb was used to stop hemorrhaging when other medicines were not available. Use in treatment of heavy menstrual bleeding seems justified through empirical evidence. The hemostatic action of the extract may be because of a peptide with oxytocin-like activity; however, its use for severe uterine bleeding is not recommended owing to unreliability. Interestingly, one study noted that the maximum activity of shepherd's purse extract was attained only 3 months after the manufacture date.[49] Clinical studies that correlate with pharmacologic studies of humans have not been conducted. Ex vivo studies demonstrated accelerated blood coagulation; however, a 1969 in vivo experiment did not demonstrate hemostatic activity.[39] Studies have shown that *Capsella bursa-pastoris*

exerts a strong contractile effect on the uteruses of guinea pigs. Clinically observed hemostatic action also may result from high oxalic and dicarboxylic acids; these phytochemicals have been shown to have a beneficial effect in the control of hemorrhage.[50] Because of its high oxalate content, care is advised for people with renal stones.[51] Shepherd's purse has been shown to be an important biomarker of environmental heavy metal contamination because it appears to absorb heavy metals in large concentrations; therefore, care should be taken with long-term use.[52] The Commission E approved the internal use of shepherd's purse for symptomatic treatment of menorrhagia, metrorrhagia, and hematuria, and topically for nosebleeds, superficial skin wounds, and bruising (Fig. 10-1).[45]

Tienchi Ginseng

Tienchi ginseng has been used traditionally in TCM for traumatic injury, bruising, and hemorrhage, and is included in protocol for uterine bleeding and menorrhagia. A comprehensive medical database search yields numerous studies evaluating the adaptogenic, antioxidant, immunologic, and cardiovascular effects of *Panax notoginseng* and its saponins and ginsenosides. No studies of effects on uterine bleeding were identified. An animal study was conducted comparing the hemostatic activity of various *P. notoginseng* preparations in 62 male Wistar rats by administration of placebo (wheat flour), and alcohol, hydrophilic (i.e., water), and lipophilic (i.e., hexane) extracts of notoginseng.[53] Rats were divided into five groups, and their tails were transected 5 mm from the tip. The alcohol extract group had the shortest bleeding time, which was significantly shorter than that of the control, placebo, and lipophilic extract groups. Alcohol extract provided better hemostatic effects than no treatment, placebo treatment, and treatment with lipophilic extract. Bone cites shortened clotting time in rabbits and good effects in visceral bleeding with tienchi.[46] *P. notoginseng* has traditionally been given as a powder or tablet in an emergency to be taken with red wine. It is an ingredient in the traditional trauma formula Yunnan Baiyao.

Witch Hazel

Tannin-rich witch hazel is considered an astringent and hemostatic herb, and has been used traditionally for menorrhagia and metrorrhagia (Fig. 10-2).[23] The German Commission E and European Scientific Cooperative on Phytotherapy (ESCOP) monographs approve the use of this herb only for topical anti-inflammatory, astringent, and local hemostatic effects (e.g., for hemorrhoids). No studies were identified using witch hazel for the treatment of uterine bleeding. Oak bark (*Quercus* spp.) has been used in much the same way, and similarly has no studies relating its use to uterine bleeding; however, its internal use is approved by the German Commission E for the treatment of diarrhea.[45]

Yarrow

Yarrow has been used traditionally as a hemostatic and antihemorrhagic by both herbalists and the Eclectics.[39,46,48]

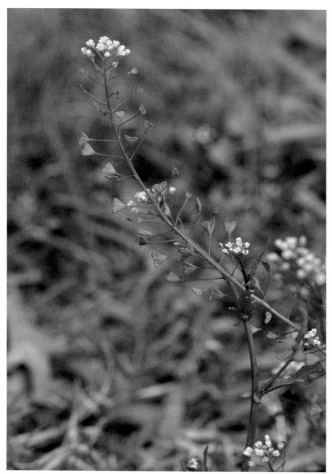

FIGURE 10-1 Shepherd's purse *(Capsella bursa-pastoris).* (Photo by Martin Wall.)

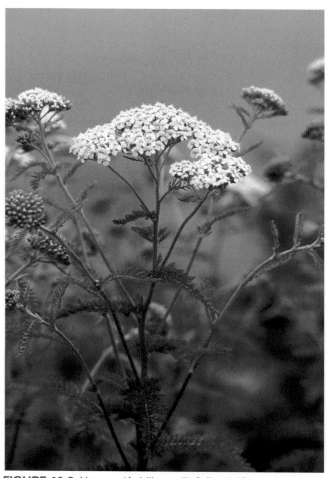

FIGURE 10-3 Yarrow *(Achillea millefolium).* (Photo by Martin Wall.)

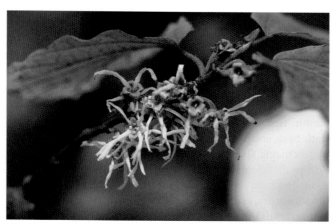

FIGURE 10-2 Witch hazel *(Hamamelis virginiana).* (Photo by Martin Wall.)

Midwives and herbalists consider yarrow infusion one of the most reliable herbal uterine hemostatics available, employing it for DUB, uterine bleeding, hematuria associated with urinary tract infection (UTI), and heavy bleeding with inevitable miscarriage. No studies were identified using yarrow for uterine bleeding (Fig. 10-3).

Other Uterine Hemostatics

The following herbs are also commonly used as uterine hemostatics/antihemorrhagics. Their use is based on traditional and empiric evidence and they are considered reliable and effective:

- Bayberry bark *(Myrica cerifera)*
- Lady's mantle *(Alchemilla vulgaris)*
- Oak bark *(Quercus* spp.)

Bayberry bark tincture is widely used by midwives for mild postpartum bleeding, generally in combination with equal parts of fresh shepherd's purse tincture.

NUTRITIONAL CONSIDERATIONS

Vitamin K

Vitamin K is a cofactor for the enzyme responsible for chemical reactions that maintain blood clotting factors: prothrombin; factors VII, IX, and X; and proteins C and S. Because vitamin K is supplied in the diet and by synthesis of intestinal bacteria, deficiencies are not common. Menorrhagia can be a symptom of vitamin K deficiency. Women at greatest risk for deficiency are those with poor diet, malabsorption, and liver or biliary diseases. Vitamin K is found in broccoli, Brussels

SAMPLE FORMULA FOR HORMONAL DYSREGULATION WITH LUTEAL PHASE DEFECT

Chaste berry	Chaste berry (Vitex agnus-castus)	30 mL
Eleuthero	(Eleutherococcus senticosus)	20 mL
White peony	(Paeonia lateriflora)	20 mL
Schizandra	(Schizandra chinensis)	20 mL
Licorice	(Glycyrrhiza glabra)	10 mL
	Total: 100 mL	

Dose: 5 mL twice daily for up to 3 months; longer if needed.

Add nervines to protocol in a separate formula, or substitute *Schizandra chinensis* with 20 mL *Scutellaria lateriflora.*

SAMPLE GREAT FLOOD FORMULA FOR ACUTE UTERINE BLEEDING

This formula is an effective uterine hemostatic for *mild to moderate* bleeding only. For continuous or heavy bleeding, or any bleeding that soaks more than two menstrual (maxi) pads in 20 minutes, seek emergency medical care.

Yarrow	(Achillea millefolium)	30 mL
Shepherd's purse	(Capsella bursa-pastoris)	30 mL
Ladies' mantle	(Alchemilla vulgaris)	30 mL
Cinnamon	(Cinnamomum zeylanicum)	10 mL
	Total: 100 mL	

Dose: Take 2.5 mL repeated every 15 minutes for up to 2 hours until bleeding abates. If bleeding continues beyond 2 hours or at any time becomes heavy, seek medical care. This formula can be taken preventatively immediately upon the start of menstruation during days 1 and 2.

CASE HISTORY: DYSFUNCTIONAL UTERINE BLEEDING

Kate is a 47-year-old female, gravida 2, para 2. Weight is excessive for height (185 lbs. 5′ 4″). Primary complaint is erratic, occasionally excessive menstrual bleeding. She was diagnosed with dysfunctional uterine bleeding (DUB) by her obstetrician/gynecologist (OB/GYN), who recommended hysterectomy and hormone replacement. Although she has no plans to have additional children, she is uncomfortable with the options presented to her.

Kate describes her cycle as erratic for the past 7 or 8 months (31 to 52 days), with some menses with very light flow and acute onset of excessive flow four of the past six cycles. Heavy days require 8 to 10 pad changes. Cycle lasts at least 7 to 10 days. Previous menstrual history was 28 to 31 days with normal flow for a maximum of 5 days. She denies any discomfort from cramping.

Additional complaints:
- Excessive stress owing to full-time job (high school math teacher), caring for elderly parent, financial difficulties, and "no time for herself"

- Constipation
- Fatigue, extreme at times
- Sleep onset insomnia
- Joints ache upon rising
- Bruises easily

Herbal Prescription for Dysfunctional Uterine Bleeding
Uterine Antihemorrhagic Herbal Formula
Tincture:

White peony	(Paeonia lactiflora)	40 mL
Tienchi ginseng	(Panax notoginseng)	40 mL
Shepherd's purse	(Capsella bursa-pastoris)	20 mL
	Total: 100 mL	

Dose: 5 mL in water qid at first indication that menses is about to start; continue until bleeding is controlled.
Also:
- *Vitex agnus-castus:*
  Dose: 3 mL once per day upon rising, starting on day 5 of menses and continuing until the start of the next menses; repeat each cycle.

- *Eleutherococcus senticosus* tablets:
  One tablet three times a day
- Dietary recommendations:
  Boost iron levels, address low fiber intake and hypohydration, reduce proinflammatory prostaglandin production with dietary increase of eicosapentaenoic acid (EPA) and fish, eliminate hydrogenated products, address blood sugar management, and reduce caffeine intake. Include dietary phytoestrogens (e.g., soy, flax seed, red clover, fennel teas).

At 3 weeks, patient reported reduced constipation and that her period was lighter than previously. At 8 weeks, patient reported having a "tolerable" cycle at 34 days with a lighter flow lasting 6 days. She also reported an improved sense of well-being. For persistent sleep difficulties, she was prescribed a tablet formula of valerian, *Ziziphus spinosa*, and passionflower extracts to be taken as two tablets before bed; one additional tablet should be taken if not asleep within 1 hour. At 12 weeks, the patient reported an "almost normal" cycle starting at 30 days. Her heaviest flow on day 2 required only four pads, and the menses lasted for only 5 days. Patient reported good sleep for several consecutive days with improved energy levels. She has taken up a low-impact aerobics class and has lost 8 pounds over the past 6 weeks. Constipation returns occasionally, especially with stress, and she does not routinely use the flax meal preventatively. Practitioner plans to continue *V. agnus-castus* for several more cycles and to begin weaning patient off antihemorrhagic herbs as improvements become consistent, but to have them on hand for use if needed.

TREATMENT SUMMARY FOR DYSFUNCTIONAL UTERINE BLEEDING

- Hemostatic and uterine tonic herbs are used to modulate mild to moderate acute episodes of excessive bleeding. Examples include yarrow, shepherd's purse, witch hazel, and tienchi ginseng. See Great Flood Formula.

Continued

- Use botanicals to normalize hormonal function and the hypothalamic-pituitary-ovarian (HPO) axis; chaste berry is a classic example. Other herbs may include peony, black cohosh, and fennel. Herbalists commonly include herbs for the support of liver function and proper bowel elimination as part of a plan to regulate hormonal activity.
- Nutritive herbs should be included when there is anemia. Dong quai, rehmannia, nettles, and ashwagandha should be considered.
- Chronic excessive bleeding can lead to significant stress; therefore, nervines and anxiolytics can be included in formulae. Examples are passionflower, motherwort, skullcap, and kava kava. Adaptogens can play a role in helping to regulate the hypothalamic-pituitary-adrenal (HPA) axis, and also may be included.
- Associated or underlying causes such as urinary tract infection (UTI) and vaginal infection should be addressed.
- The diet or supplementation should provide adequate vitamins A, C, E, and K, essential fatty acids, and iron, all of which play an important role in the regulation of hemostatic function and the prevention of anemia.
- Reduction of inflammation through an antiinflammatory diet and the addition of essential fatty acid (EFA)–rich foods and supplements may reduce the production of endogenous inflammatory compounds and thus play a role in the prevention and treatment of dysfunctional uterine bleeding (DUB).

What to Expect with Dysfunctional Uterine Bleeding Treatment

Acute treatment with uterine hemostatic herbs is often effective for mild to moderate bleeding within a couple of hours of beginning treatment. Experienced practitioners also may find success with more severe bleeding, but this should only be undertaken with proper knowledge and medical supervision.

For chronic episodes of acute bleeding, as well as chronic bleeding, it can take several months to regulate hormones, achieve adequate control of bleeding, and prevent recurrence of episodes. In many cases, small gains will be seen in the first couple of months of treatment, and the practitioner may feel the need to revise the formula to achieve more specific goals as care progresses. For example, in a woman with cramping, mood swings, and irregular DUB, one might achieve improvement in two of the three complaints using a single formula, and then decide to modify the formula to focus on the complaint that remains outstanding or is the most pronounced. Modification of formulae over the course of care is very common with herbal medicine.

Many women, particularly in the perimenopausal years, will achieve a high degree of success in modulating excessive bleeding; however, they may keep a formula on hand, such as Great Flood, should there be an unexpected episode of uterine bleeding as hormones shift into a menopausal state.

sprouts, spinach, cauliflower, green leafy vegetables, and egg yolks.[54]

Essential Fatty Acids

As with dysmenorrhea, the addition of cold-water fish to the diet and fish oil supplements may help in the reduction of menorrhagia via reduction of inflammatory mediators in the prostaglandin pathway, in turn promoting the production of antiinflammatory prostaglandins.

Vitamins C, A, and E

Include nutrients to address integrity of the microvascular and macrovascular systems: whole-food sources of vitamin C (with bioflavonoids), vitamin E, and beta-carotene (instead of preformed vitamin A). Additionally, deficiency of vitamin A has been found to be an important factor associated with menorrhagia. Vitamin A is a cofactor of 3-beta (β)-dehydrogenase in steroidogenesis and deficiencies of this vitamin may result in impaired enzyme activity. The level of endogenous 17-β-estradiol appears to be elevated with vitamin A therapy, and in one study, menorrhagia was alleviated in more than 92% of patients (see Menarche: Adolescent Menorrhagia).

Iron

Iron supplementation is essential when there is anemia. Iron supplements are notoriously hard to digest and poorly bioavailable. Floradix Floravital Iron + Herbs is an excellent source of bioavailable iron primarily derived from fruit and botanical sources. Take with vitamin C to enhance absorption (see Anemia).

Additional Therapies

Stress reduction strategies can be incorporated to address stress associated with this condition. An exercise program appropriate for individual lifestyle and ability may improve pelvic circulation, hormonal regulation, and decrease menstrual irregularities.

Breasts, Uterus, and Pelvis

UTERINE FIBROIDS

Uterine fibroids (properly called leiomyomata or myomas) are solid, well-defined benign monoclonal tumors of the smooth muscle cells of the uterus (Fig. 11-1).[1,2] They range in size from microscopic to many pounds in weight, and may be singular or clustered. Multiple myomas in the same uterus are not clonally related.[3] Fibroid size is described in comparison to a pregnant uterus (e.g., a fibroid the size of a 16-week pregnancy). As many as 20% to 40% of all women develop fibroids by age 40.[1] Approximately 17% of all hysterectomies performed in the United States are for uterine myomas, with a peak incidence of surgery occurring for women around age 45, making fibroids the primary annual cause of premenopausal hysterectomy in the United States.[3,4] They are rare in a premenarchal young women and shrinkage typically occurs in postmenopausal women with the natural decline in estrogen levels, unless stimulated by exogenous estrogen (i.e., xenoestrogen or foreign estrogens, usually a result of environmental exposure, for example, from pesticides or plastics).[1] For unknown reasons, fibroids are two to three times more common in African American women than Anglo-American, Asian, and Hispanic women.[1,3] Fibroids are classified according to their site of growth in the uterine or surrounding tissue as submucosal, intramural, and subserous (see Fig. 11-1). They also may occur in the cervix (i.e., cervical fibroids), between the uterine broad ligaments (i.e., interligamentous fibroids), or they may be attached to a stalk (i.e., pedunculated fibroids) and protrude into the uterine cavity (i.e., pedunculated submucosal fibroids) or through the cervix.[1,3]

The exact etiology of uterine fibroids remains undetermined.[5] Leiomyomas are hormone dependent. This is evidenced by the facts that they develop during hormonally active years and decline during menopause; fibroid tissue has an increased number of estrogen and progesterone receptors; fibroid tissue is hyperestrogenic, hypersensitive to estrogen, and does not possess the normal regulatory mechanism that limits estrogen response; the peak mitotic activity occurs during the luteal phase; and they respond to treatment with gonadotropin-releasing hormone (GnRH) agonists.[3,6-8] Growth factor also plays a role in leiomyomata

development.[3,9] As estrogen and progesterone levels rise, insulin is released, causing the transient hypoglycemia commonly experienced premenstrually. When plasma glucose levels fall, pituitary growth hormone is released, exerting bodywide effects. Its action on hepatocytes causes the release of insulin-like growth factors (IGFs). In a study by Vollenhoven et al, it is postulated that the net effect of these changes increases the bioavailability of free (i.e., bioactive) IGF, which may play a major role in promoting fibroid growth.[9] A further study by De Leo and Morgante states that concentrations of epidermal growth factor, insulin-like growth factor 1 (IGF 1), and platelet-derived growth factor AB (PDGF-AB) are present in myomatous tissues together with their receptors.[6] Prolactin also may be a factor. Leiomyomata express a number of hormones, including parathyroid hormone–related protein (i.e., a growth factor), prolactin, and IGF.[3]

Factors that might increase fibroid development and growth include:

- Increased lifetime estrogen exposure caused by early age at menarche, fewer pregnancies, increased follicular phase, or obesity[2,4]
- Exposure to exogenous estrogens (e.g., environmental exposure, such as plastics, pesticides, hormones through meat and dairy; or medical exposure, such as hormone replacement therapy [HRT])
- Poor enterohepatic estrogen clearance
- Hypertension[2]
- Pelvic inflammatory disease[2,4]
- Intrauterine device (IUD) use with infectious complications[2,4]
- Perineal talc use[2,4]

The use of oral contraceptives (OCs) is not associated with any changes in fibroid size, and may even be protective; however, one study reported a slight increase in risk with a history of OC use beginning in the early teenage years.[2-4]

PATHOPHYSIOLOGY

Myoma risk is inversely related to increasing parity and age at last pregnancy, and is decreased by smoking (because of its inhibition of estrogen) and increased by obesity (likely because of increased estrogen levels) and hypertension.[1-3,10] Fibroids occur in 1% to 2% of pregnancies. However, it is uncertain whether this relationship is entirely causal. Infertility, as well as early pregnancy loss, may be caused by mechanical obstruction

The editor wishes to thank *Botanical Medicine for Women's Health*, ed 1 contributors to this chapter: Isla Burgess, David Winston, Suzanna M. Zick, and Amanda McQuade Crawford.

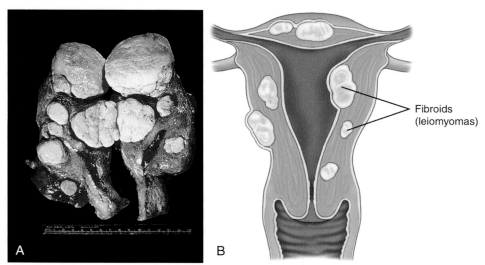

FIGURE 11-1 Uterine fibroids. (From Salvo S: *Mosby's pathology for massage therapists,* St. Louis, 2004, Mosby.)

of implantation or distortion of the cervix or endometrium. Once a pregnancy is established, it is rare for myomata to interfere with its progress, and most proceed uncomplicated. However, a higher rate of cesarean section has been noted, and premature labor may result from very large myomata.[1] Degeneration of fibroids caused by hemorrhagic infarction may rarely occur during late pregnancy and is marked by pain, and also may be accompanied by rebound tenderness, fever, nausea, vomiting, and leukocytosis.[3] Treatment consists of rest and analgesia; surgery is a last resort.

Anemia and fatigue can be caused by excessive blood loss associated with fibroids. Pressure on the bowel or bladder can cause constipation, urinary frequency, and dyspareunia. Large fibroids may mask the diagnosis of serious gynecologic neoplasm. Rapidly growing fibroids may indicate a more serious pathology such as leiosarcoma and should be investigated. Malignancy is rarely associated with uterine fibroids; however, they occur with increased frequency in endometrial hyperplasia and are associated with a fourfold increased risk of developing endometrial cancer.[1]

SYMPTOMS

Most women with myomas are asymptomatic, never knowing that they have them unless informed of such by gynecologic examination. This was discovered based on ultrasound and autopsy results that revealed that many more women had fibroids than had ever been diagnosed or treated for symptoms.[2] The most common symptoms are menorrhagia and the physical effects caused by large myomata, such as increased pelvic pressure, frequent urination, difficulty with defecation, and dyspareunia with deep penetration.[1,3,5] Abnormal uterine bleeding is present in about 30% of all patients, and periods are typically heavy and prolonged, often with premenstrual and postmenstrual spotting.[2,4] Uterine bleeding caused by myomas can be associated with significant social, emotional, financial, and medical difficulties; women's concerns should

be addressed. Some women experience dysmenorrhea.[2] Metrorrhagia may occur, but should be evaluated with an endometrial biopsy to rule out other endometrial disease.[4] About 2% to 10% of women experience infertility as a result of fibroids, ostensibly caused by abnormal uterine tubal motility, interference with sperm movements, or abnormal uterine blood flow.[3,11] Fibroid degeneration, torsion, or compression of a nerve against the pelvis caused by encroachment by a fibroid can lead to significant pain.[4,11]

DIAGNOSIS

Diagnosis can be determined by:
- Pelvic bimanual examination: Large fibroids (greater than a 12- to 14-week gestation) can be manually palpated and felt as an enlarged uterus, lump, or mass.
- Ultrasound scan: It is useful to monitor size and growth rate of fibroids. Repeat scans should be done during the same phase of the menstrual cycle.
- Laparoscopy: This is important if the mass is indistinguishable from the ovaries.

The differential diagnosis includes[1]:
- Ovarian neoplasm
- Tubo-ovarian inflammatory mass
- Diverticulum inflammatory mass
- Endometrial carcinoma

CONVENTIONAL TREATMENT

Unless fibroids are symptomatic, observation is the most prudent form of treatment and no other intervention is necessary.[1,4] GnRH agonists (e.g., leuprolide) have been used effectively to control symptoms and reduce myoma size through suppression of estrogen and progesterone production.[3,12] Mean uterine size decreases 30% to 64% after 3 to 6 months of treatment, and symptoms associated with fibroids are alleviated as a result. Possible side effects include hot flashes, headache, vaginal dryness, vaginitis, decreased libido, joint and muscle stiffness, and depression, and 30% of patients continue to have light, irregular vaginal bleeding.[3,12] Local allergic reaction occurs in about 10% of patients.[3] Bone loss occurs but is reversible, and a small number of women (2%) experience major vaginal hemorrhage 5 to 10 weeks after treatment commences. Steroid add-back therapy has been investigated to prevent bone loss in women requiring long-term GnRH therapy; however, because of the risk of osteoporosis, long-term therapy is inadvisable.[3,12]

Surgery should be reserved for women who are past childbearing, who are heavily symptomatic and not responsive to drug therapy, or who have suspected malignancies. Women wanting to preserve childbearing ability should be given the option of conservative therapy. GnRH therapy may be prescribed as pretreatment for surgical procedures to reduce fibroid size and bleeding. Myomectomy may be performed vaginally, hysteroscopically, or laparoscopically, and when performed skillfully, improves symptoms in 80% to 90% of patients. Between 15% and 30% experience fibroid regrowth after 5 years. Uterine scarring may occur from the procedure and affect fertility.[12] Endometrial ablation and uterine artery embolization (UAE) are additional options.[13,14] UAE is increasingly popular, and appears generally safe, but it is uncertain how long the treatment lasts and whether future fertility may be affected. The procedure involves injection of polyvinyl or gelatin particles into the uterine arteries to cut off blood supply to the fibroids, which leads to shrinkage over the next 3 to 12 months. Approximately 85% of patients gain relief from the procedure, which has been performed since 1995. However, it is not risk free. Adverse outcomes include infection, bleeding, and formation of emboli, as well as future fertility problems. For women intending to become pregnant in the future, myomectomy may still be the most certain conventional surgical intervention.[14] Hysterectomy is generally recommended when women are past childbearing age, are symptomatic, if malignancy is suspected, or if other therapies are ineffective.[1,3,12]

BOTANICAL TREATMENT

Among Western herbalists specializing in gynecologic complaints, there is a common perception that although symptoms of uterine fibroids are not difficult to control with botanical medicines and their growth can be arrested, they are difficult to eliminate entirely unless the fibroid is small at the onset of treatment (i.e., smaller than 12-week size). Many women are content to have symptom control over pharmaceutical or surgical intervention, as long as the fibroids present no mechanical problems.[15] Traditional Chinese Medicine (TCM) has clearly defined diagnostic constructs, many herbal formulae, and well-developed adjunctive treatment protocols (e.g., acupuncture, moxibustion) for treating uterine fibroids and has claimed success in entirely eliminating uterine fibroids.

Western herbal treatment protocols include a variety of strategies (Table 11-1). These include weight reduction, which promotes hormonal balance, specifically through the elimination of estrogens by enhancing liver detoxification

mechanisms; promoting pelvic circulation and simultaneously controlling bleeding if necessary; and general improvement of uterine tone. These are integrated with the general recommendation to avoid excess exposure to xenoestrogens (i.e., environmental estrogens) and reduce overall estrogen levels, exposure to both being a risk factor for the development of uterine fibroids. Women with fibroids report greater frequency of red meat and pork intake, and less frequent green vegetable, fruit, and fish consumption.[4] Although there is little correlation between the development of uterine fibroids and cancer, numerous studies have demonstrated a connection between diet, estrogen levels, and hormone-dependent cancers, as well as a protective effect of fruits and vegetables against cancer.[4] No studies have evaluated the effects of US dairy consumption and the development of uterine fibroids. However, an association between dairy intake and increased risk of ovarian cancer has been reported.[16,17] Herbalists recommend that patients avoid foods that increase risk, and emphasize intake of those shown to facilitate estrogen biotransformation, for example, by increasing dietary fiber and regular intake of complex carbohydrates found in vegetables and grains.[11,18,19] Botanical strategies are aimed at reducing the estrogen burden through liver detoxification and improved elimination, promoting gynecologic health in general by improving pelvic circulation, reducing symptoms, and controlling fibroid size.

TCM treatment for fibroids has been evaluated through several preliminary studies, which are presented in the following section. Western botanical protocol for the treatment of uterine fibroids has not been subjected to controlled trials.[4] The Western botanical information presented in this chapter reflects the opinions of herbalists practicing in the United States, United Kingdom, Canada, Australia, and New Zealand, regarding the efficacy and safety of the primary herbs used to treat myomas. Given the general safety of the botanicals being discussed, and the lack of noninvasive long-term effective medical treatments for fibroids, it seems that investigation of the primary Western herbal protocols cited in Table 11-1 is warranted. Nervines, laxatives, adaptogens, and other herbs included in fibroid protocol are discussed elsewhere throughout this text. Stress reduction should not be overlooked as part of the treatment protocol for women with symptomatic fibroids because chronic uterine bleeding can cause emotional, social, financial, and medical consequences.[2]

Traditional Chinese Medicine Treatment
Cinnamon and Peony

TCM has numerous well-developed treatment protocols and formulations, some of which have been used for several centuries for promoting gynecologic health in general and for treating uterine fibroids specifically. For a more comprehensive review of the Chinese treatments for gynecologic problems, readers are referred to the primary TCM literature. Generally speaking, TCM views uterine myomas as a result of poor circulation of chi (i.e., energy) and blood through the pelvic region. Many formulae are designed to dispel pelvic stagnation and increase the flow of blood to uterine and ovarian tissues and facilitate the smooth flow of blood

TABLE 11-1   Botanical Treatment Strategies for Uterine Fibroids

Therapeutic Goal	Therapeutic Activity	Botanical Name	Common Name
Hormonal regulation; increased hormone biotransformation, conjugation, and improved elimination; displace endogenous estrogen with estrogen receptor competitors	Cholagogues Hepatic detoxification stimulants	*Berberis vulgaris*	Barberry
		Camellia sinensis	Green tea
		Chelidonium majus	Chelidonium
		Hypericum perforatum	St. John's wort
		Schisandra chinensis	Schisandra
	Hormonal modulators	*Actaea racemosa*	Chaste tree
		Vitex agnus-castus	Black cohosh
	Phytoestrogens/ SERMs	*Glycine max*	Soy
		Trifolium pratense	Red clover
	Laxatives (i.e., bulk, anthraquinone)	*Linum ussitissimum*	Flax seed
		Rumex crispus	Yellow dock
		Taraxacum officinale	Dandelion root
Improve uterine tone, reduce menorrhagic bleeding (Also see Dysfunctional Uterine Bleeding)	Uterine tonics	*Caulophyllum thalictroides*	Blue cohosh
		Leonurus cardiaca	Motherwort
		Mitchella repens	Partridge berry
		Rubus idaeus	Red raspberry
		Viburnum opulus	Cramp bark
Improve uterine tone, reduce menorrhagic bleeding (Also see Dysfunctional Uterine Bleeding)	Uterine astringents	*Achillea millefolium*	Yarrow
		Alchemilla vulgaris	Lady's mantle
		Capsella bursa-pastoris	Shepherd's purse
		Cinnamomum spp.	Cinnamon
		Erigeron canadensis	Canada fleabane
		Geranium maculatum	Cranesbill geranium
		Hamamelis virginiana	Witch hazel
		Myrica cerifera	Bayberry
		Rubus idaeus	Red raspberry
		Trillium erectum	Birthroot, birthwort, bethroot
Relieve pelvic stagnation and blood stasis; improve uterine circulation	Uterine circulatory stimulants	*Angelica sinensis*	Dong quai
		Cinnamomum cassia	Cinnamon
		Paeonia lactiflora	White peony
		Paeonia suffruticosa	Peony
		Prunus persicae	Peach
		Zingiber officinalis	Ginger
Treat dysmenorrhea	Uterine antispasmodics See Dysmenorrhea		
Treat anemia	Iron-rich supplements and herbs See Iron Deficiency Anemia		

SERM, Selective estrogen receptor modulator.

via menses. A classic TCM formula used for relieving blood stagnation is Cinnamon Twig and Poria Pill (Gui Zhi Fu Ling Wan), consisting of: *Cinnamomum aromaticum* twigs, *Poria cocos, Paeonia lactiflora* root, *Paeonia suffruticosa* root, and *Prunus persica* seed. It should also be noted that in TCM, each herbal formula has specific diagnostic criteria for which it is used, as well as clear contraindications and cautions. For maximum efficacy in using TCM protocols, a qualified herbal TCM practitioner should be consulted. In addition to herbal protocol for promoting gynecologic health and specifically treating uterine fibroids, TCM also employs numerous other modalities, which may include

walking to promote circulation in general and abdominal circulation specifically, moxibustion, acupuncture, external application of compresses, and other such adjunctive therapies. Specific lifestyle recommendations also can be given such as the avoidance of cold foods and drink (in TCM coldness is said to cause congealment and stagnation) and constrictive clothing.[20]

Several studies have looked at the efficacy of the Cinnamon Twig and Poria Pill formula noted in the preceding section for the treatment of uterine fibroids. Specifically, the studies investigated the effectiveness of the Japanese version of this formula, Keishi-Bukuryo-Gan (KBG) in an open study on 110 premenopausal women with symptomatic uterine fibroids measuring less than 10 cm in diameter. They were treated with 22.5 g/day of a freeze-dried decoction of the herbs for 12 weeks. Twenty-one women were considered "normal" and 47 women much improved by the end of the trial. This herbal formula is frequently used to treat a range of gynecologic disorders including dysmenorrhea, cervical erosion, ovarian cysts, chronic salpingitis, and endometriosis, to name a few conditions.[15] There is research to suggest that the *Paeonia* spp. in this formula may act as a luteinizing hormone (LH)–releasing hormone (LH-RH) antagonist with weakly antiestrogenic effects in the presence of estrogen.[21] In another study, the authors applied individualized TCM formulations and treatments to treat 223 cases of uterine fibroids with a reported 72% reduction of menorrhagia in 160 women complaining of this symptom, 58% improvement in backache, and an overall effectiveness rate of 92.4%. Myomas were eliminated in 29 of 223 patients and markedly diminished in 42 patients. In 32 patients, no changes were seen, and there were no positive results in 12.5% of patients.[15]

In an interesting study by Mehl-Madrona et al, an integrated TCM-Western medicine pilot study was conducted to compare the cost and efficacy of a set of therapies typically used by complementary and alternative medicine (CAM) practitioners and conventional medicine on the ability to reduce uterine fibroid size. All patients were premenopausal and age 24 to 45 years, educated, employed, and from a socioeconomic bracket that allowed them to pay cash for all treatments. None were on pharmaceutical treatment or hormonal contraceptives at the time of the study and all received a pelvic ultrasound before and 6 months after treatment. Sonograms were obtained on patients who dropped out of the study as well, so sonograms were available on all patients. Uterine fibroids measured at least 6- to 8-week pregnancy size, with palpable fibroids 2 to 3 cm in diameter. Inclusion in the study required hemoglobin greater than 8 g/dL, with fibroid growth of less than 6 cm/year. CAM treatment included a combination of nutritional, herbal, acupuncture, bodywork, and psychological interventions. Acupuncture and herbal protocols were selected individually for the patient, using formulae and points traditionally indicated for the patient's patterns: symptoms, constitution (based on TCM pulse and tongue diagnosis), and condition. The comparison group used progestational agents, OCs, and nonsteroidal antiinflammatory drugs (NSAIDs). The results of this study demonstrated no statistically significant difference in change of symptoms between the two groups when measured after 6 months of treatment. Both experienced improvement in symptoms and fibroid size. Patients in the treatment group considered the pilot study a success because they were able to achieve results equivalent to pharmaceutical interventions using nonconventional methods.[15]

Hormonal Modulators
Chaste Berry

Chaste berry is the primary herb employed by herbalists and integrative medicine practitioners for hormonal modulation in the botanical treatment of fibroids.[4,22] It acts as a dopamine agonist, resulting in a reduction in prolactin release.[23] Prolactin may play a role in fibroid growth. No scientific evidence in the literature has been found for the use of chaste berry specifically in the treatment of fibroids, and although its use may result in reduction of apparent estrogen excess caused by relative progesterone deficiency, increased progesterone levels have been shown to result in increased mitotic division in fibroid tissue. Wuttke et al, studied the putative estrogenic effects of a chaste berry extract and found it contained substances that replaced radiolabeled estradiol from a cytosolic estrogen receptor (ER) preparation, and appeared to be agonistic to ER-beta (β). However, because the uterus expresses ER-alpha (α), no effects on the uterine expression of estrogen were expected or have been experimentally observed.[23]

Black Cohosh

A double-blind randomized controlled trial (RCT) tested the uterine fibroid–reducing effects of an isopropanolic black cohosh extract (i.e., Remifemin) against tibolone. The group of 244 women (ages 40 to 60, experiencing menopausal symptoms via the Kupperman Index) were randomized into equal groups ($n = 122$) to receive daily doses of either 40 mg Remifemin or 2.5 mg tibolone for 3 months for treatment of menopausal symptoms. The investigators then tested the herbal product in the women experiencing at least one uterine fibroid in the study ($n = 62$), who were subsequently randomized to receive 40 mg Remifemin ($n = 34$) or 2.5 mg tibolone ($n = 28$). Fibroid size was measured by transvaginal ultrasonography. In the Remifemin group, median fibroid size decreased by 30% ($p = .016$) whereas an *increase* by 4.7% was observed in the tibolone group. The percentage of volume change, mean diameter change, and geometric mean diameter change was also significantly altered in the Remifemin group compared with the tibolone group.[24]

Phytoestrogens and Selective Estrogen Receptor Modules

Phytoestrogens are plant compounds with a similar molecular shape and structure to endogenous estrogen molecules, and which can bind competitively to ERs, preventing the binding of more potent estrogen and estrogen metabolites (see Part V).[25] They appear to behave similarly to selective estrogen receptor modulators (SERMs). Low Dog explains their potential clinical application in conditions of estrogen excess, in relationship to the role of phytoestrogens in breast cancer treatment:

By binding to estrogen receptors in the premenopausal woman, phytoestrogens "turn down" estrogen production through negative feedback at the level of the hypothalamus and pituitary gland … when endogenous estrogen levels are high, phytoestrogens may have an antiestrogenic activity by preventing estrogen from binding to the estrogen receptor through competitive inhibition.[26]

Legumes, including soybeans and red clover, are rich in phytoestrogens.[27] In a study by Liu et al, methanol extracts of red clover (*Trifolium pratense*), chaste berry, and hops

(*Humulus lupulus*) showed significant competitive binding to both ERα and ERβ. In the same study, dong quai (*Angelica sinensis*) and licorice (*Glycyrrhiza uralensis*) showed weak ER binding, whereas black cohosh did not exhibit any competitive binding. Controversy abounds as to the mechanisms of action of black cohosh, which do not appear to be directly phytoestrogenic.[28] Current research is suggesting a dopaminergic or serotonergic effect for this botanical.[26,28] The application of phytoestrogens may be a promising area for further investigation for the botanical treatment of fibroids, and should be considered in the development of botanical protocols.

Hormone Excretion and Biotransformation

More than 50% of all estrogen metabolism and conjugation occurs in the liver, suggesting a basis for the belief among herbalists that herbs that improve liver function may increase estrogen excretion and either treat or lower the risk for uterine fibroids.[4,22] Herbalists commonly include liver-specific herbs in formulae for treating fibroids. Several herbs actively affect phase 1 and phase 2 liver detoxification systems and cytochrome P450 (CYP), an enzyme system partially involved in the metabolism of estrogen. These effects and their relationship to uterine fibroid treatment, if any, have not been formally investigated but are often applied by modern herbal practitioners in putatively reducing estrogen burdens. Cholagogues, herbs that stimulate the release of bile from the gallbladder, also may be useful for clearing estrogen through increased bowel clearance resulting from their indirect laxative action. Examples of cholagogues include bayberry and *Chelidonium* spp.[22]

Uterine Tonics, Astringents, and Hemostatics

Because bleeding is a common symptom of uterine fibroids, numerous antihemorrhagic herbs are used in botanical medicine protocols (see Dysfunctional Uterine Bleeding).[22] Yarrow dried plant infusion is perhaps one of the most widely used uterine antihemorrhagics, reliably reducing acute uterine bleeding; conversely, it promotes menstrual flow when suppressed. It has been used since ancient times as a styptic.[26] Either dry or fresh plant can be used as a tea or tincture. Many herbalists believe that yarrow herb taken as tea is more quickly effective for stopping acute uterine bleeding than other preparations. Other traditionally used uterine antihemorrhagic herbs include lady's mantle, shepherd's purse (fresh only), cranesbill geranium, witch hazel, bayberry, red raspberry, and bethroot. These are all generally taken in tincture form in 2- to 4-mL doses repeated every 15 minutes as needed until bleeding subsides, or combined into larger formulae for the treatment or prevention of chronic menorrhagia. Shepherd's purse in particular has been used traditionally as a uterine antihemorrhagic. The 1986 Commission E monograph recommends daily oral doses of 10 to 15 g of crude herb (or equivalent in extract) for mild gynecologic bleeding.[29] Extracts of the drug contain a hemostyptic action, likely owing to the presence of a peptide that has demonstrated oxytocin-like activity in vitro.[29,30] Many modern Western herbalists believe that it is imperative to prepare shepherd's purse from fresh, not dry, plant material.

The mechanism of action of lady's mantle lies in its high tannin content, indicating it for bleeding, diarrhea, and wound healing, a likely mechanism for many of the other herbs used as uterine antihemorrhagics.[30] The combination of *Cinnamomum* and *Erigeron* was relied upon by the Eclectics for uterine hemorrhage, and is still employed by midwives today for the treatment of nonemergency postpartum bleeding, and by herbalists for the treatment of menorrhagia.[31,32] Red raspberry leaf is typically used more as a long-term uterine tonic than to arrest acute bleeding. Blue cohosh has been used historically for its uterotonic actions. It is listed in the 1918 *US Dispensatory* for the treatment of menorrhagia and dysmenorrhea, and is still widely used by herbalists for these conditions.[33]

🌿 GREAT FLOOD FORMULA (TINCTURE)

Yarrow	(*Achillea millefolium*)	30 mL
Shepherd's purse	(*Capsella bursa-pastoris*)	30 mL
Ladies' mantle	(*Alchemilla vulgaris*)	30 mL
Cinnamon	(*Cinnamomum zeylanicum*)	10 mL
	Total:	**100 mL**

Dose: Take 2.5 mL repeated every 15 minutes for up to 2 hours until bleeding abates. If bleeding continues beyond 2 hours or at any time becomes heavy, seek medical care. This formula can be taken preventatively immediately upon the start of menstruation during days 1 and 2.

WARNING: Soaking more than two maxi-pads in 30 minutes is considered a uterine hemorrhage. If this occurs seek medical care immediately.

Antioxidants
Green tea

A 2013 pilot study tested the efficacy of green tea extract in the treatment of symptomatic uterine fibroids and in patients' overall quality of life (QOL). Thirty-nine women between the ages 18 to 50 who had at least one fibroid lesion 2 cubic cm or larger were randomized to receive either 800 mg of green tea extract (45% epigallocatechin gallate [EGCG]; 95% total polyphenols) or placebo control (i.e., 800 mg of brown rice) for 4 months. Fibroid size was monitored by transvaginal ultrasonography taken at baseline and end point, and QOL assessed using the symptom severity and QOL questionnaires at each monthly visit. Blood loss was monitored by visual assessment and menstrual log. Using the student's T-test, statistically significant reductions in fibroid volume (32.6%, $p = .0001$) were seen compared with placebo controls, where fibroid size actually increased over the trial duration. Green tea extract treatment was also associated with a reduction in symptom severity (32.4%, $p = .0001$), correlates of anemia, and improvement in QOL (18.53%, $p = .01$) compared with controls. The treatment was also well tolerated.[34] As an isolate, EGCG exhibited antiproliferative effects on cultured human leiomyoma cells in a dose- and time-dependent manner in vitro. EGCG also upregulated genes associated with TGF-B, and downregulated NF-kB-dependent pathway. It also decreased PCNA, CDK4, and BCL2 expression and increased BAX expression in a dose-dependent manner.[35]

Relieving Uterine Stasis: Circulatory Stimulants

Improving pelvic circulation and relieving stasis is a common approach to fibroid treatment in both Western and traditional Chinese herbal medicine, based on the belief that relieving stagnation and congestion in the pelvis will facilitate the removal of blockages and growths (e.g., fibroid tissues), remove wastes, and promote greater health and nourishment of the pelvic organs in general.[11,18,20] Decreasing pelvic stagnation is also thought to help reduce uterine hemorrhage. Ginger and cinnamon are both traditionally used to increase circulation to the reproductive organs. Further, cinnamon has been used historically to reduce uterine bleeding, making it specific for the treatment of uterine fibroids with menorrhagia or metrorrhagia.[31,32] White peony, an ingredient in Keishi-Bukuryo-Gan (KBG), discussed in the preceding, is a common herb used in TCM for the treatment of women's disorders, including menstrual dysfunction and uterine bleeding.[36] Red peony is often combined with white peony and peach seed to dispel blood stasis and conditions associated with it, including excessive uterine bleeding, particularly with the presence of thick, purple clots.[36]

CASE HISTORY: UTERINE FIBROIDS

> Latisha, a 44-year-old café worker, presents with irregular heavy bleeding, strong mood swings, and insomnia. Uterine myomata had been diagnosed by ultrasound and are easily palpable at rest. She has overwhelming sweet cravings premenstrually, poor dietary habits, and no exercise. She is currently using a women's multivitamin and ferrous gluconate tablets, but no other treatments. She experiences some flatulence associated with certain foods and regular constipation, especially when she "forgets to eat." She has had several miscarriages, two terminations, and one live birth. Christine works late nights, does not sleep well, and describes herself as "living on her nerves." Uterine fibroids are causing discomfort at night. She drinks several cups of coffee and several glasses of wine daily. Her blood pressure is 110/65. She describes herself as happy at home and likes her work but realizes it affects her health. Menstrual irregularities have developed over the past 5 years.
>
> **Treatment Protocol**
> - For promoting hormonal regulation:
>   *Vitex agnus-castus* (chaste berry) tincture
>   *Dose:* 2.5 mL each morning and evening
>
> - As a uterine tonic:
>
> | Raspberry | (Rubus idaeus) | 30 mL |
> |---|---|---|
> | Lady's mantle | (Alchemilla vulgaris) | 25 mL |
> | Nettle | (Urtica dioica) | 20 mL |
> | White peony | (Paeonia lactiflora) | 15 mL |
> | Ginger | (Zingiber officinale) | 10 mL |
> | | **Total: 100 mL** | |
>
> *Dose:* 3 mL twice daily for 3 months.

> She was also given a series of dietary guidelines (as described under Additional Therapies) and prescribed a strong chamomile infusion before bed. Her menstrual cycle became more regular over the proceeding 3 months, with a significant reduction in bleeding (1.5 days of medium to heavy bleeding reduced to mild to moderate).
>
> After 3 months the protocol was modified to:
> - For promoting hormonal balance:
>   *Vitex agnus-castus* (chaste berry) tincture
> - As a uterine tonic and to promote pelvic circulation:
>
> | Red raspberry leaf | (Rubus idaeus) | 40 mL |
> |---|---|---|
> | White peony | (Paeonia lactiflora) | 40 mL |
> | False unicorn* | (Chamaelirium luteum) | 15 mL |
> | Ginger | (Zingiber officinale) | 5 mL |
> | | **Total: 100 mL** | |
>
> *Dose:* 3 mL twice daily.
>
> She was told to take yarrow tea and was also given a botanical tincture for promoting sleep, to be taken 20 minutes before bed and repeated as needed because her insomnia was still problematic:
>
> | Ashwagandha | (Withania somnifera) | 40 mL |
> |---|---|---|
> | Lemon balm | (Melissa officinalis) | 30 mL |
> | Hops | (Humulus lupulus) | 15 mL |
> | Valerian | (Valeriana officinalis) | 15 mL |
> | | **Total: 100 mL** | |
>
> *Dose:* 5 mL each time.
>
> Her blood loss continued to be well controlled; she was sleeping better, experienced reduced sugar cravings, and was eating better. She felt light-headed just before and during her period but without extreme mood swings. She had no sensation of the fibroids at all when at rest. A reduction in symptoms of fibroids does not necessarily mean a reduction in fibroid size, but this does appear to have been the case with Christine. Without a follow-up ultrasound, this conclusion is unsupported.

*False unicorn is an at-risk species

NUTRITIONAL CONSIDERATIONS

Obesity/Weight Management

Obesity is a risk factor for fibroid development. Therefore dietary and lifestyle strategies should be aimed at weight reduction and healthy weight maintenance.

Xenoestrogens/Endocrine Disruptors

Avoid xenoestrogen ingestion from pesticide and herbicide residue by eating organically cultivated foods and avoiding foods in plastic containers. Xenoestrogens are found most concentrated in the fat of meat, farmed fish, and nonorganic dairy products.[12] Eating primarily organic meat, dairy, and produce, washing fruits and vegetables thoroughly before eating, and minimizing the use of soft plastics, such as for food storage, can help reduce xenoestrogen intake.

Estrogen Biotransformation and Diet

Metabolism and detoxification of estrogen in the body ultimately determines its biological effects. Estrogen biotransformation occurs mainly in the liver through phase 1 (i.e., hydroxylation) and phase 2 (i.e., methylation and glucuronidation), allowing estrogen to become a water-soluble, excretable compound.[11] This is predominantly excreted by the liver in bile (see Dietary Fiber). Phase 1 detoxification yields three estrogen metabolites with highly variable biological activity: 2-hydroxyestrone (2-HE), 16-alpha-hydroxyestrone (16α-HE), and 4-hydroxyestrone (4-HE). 2-HE is a beneficial estrogen metabolite in that among its effects, it competitively binds estrogen sites, blocking more potent estrogens. Conversely, 4-HE and 16α-HE are potent estrogens that may promote the growth of estrogen-sensitive tissue.[11] Dietary consumption of cruciferous vegetables, such as broccoli and cabbage, as well as green tea, garlic, and rosemary, can increase the amount of 2-HE by modifying CYP activity in phase 1, and they have antioxidant effects as well.[11,37]

Dietary Fiber

Once estrogen metabolites are excreted by the liver in bile, the metabolites are soaked up by fiber in the small intestines and excreted via defecation. If the diet lacks fiber, bile, along with the estrogen metabolites, are reabsorbed, adding an unnecessary estrogen burden to the body. Soluble fiber such as the lignins found in flax seeds also increases sex hormone–binding globulin (SHBG), decreasing the amount of available active estrogen because estrogen bound to SHBG is rendered inactive.[11] *Brassicae* vegetables such as cabbage and broccoli contain indole glucosinolates, which when chewed, are degraded by a plant enzyme into a variety of indole structures. When degraded in the body, these structures induce CYP expression (i.e., CY1A1) in hepatic and extrahepatic tissue, leading to greater conversion of 2-HE and decreasing the availability of E1 for conversion to 16-HE, thereby reducing the estrogen burden overall.[26] This is partly associated with the anticancer effects of these foods.

Dietary Antioxidants

The conversion of estradiol to catechol estrogens via 4-hydroxylation stimulates an oxidant stress response induced by free radicals. This activity is markedly increased in fibroid tissue. Therefore daily intake of foods containing the vitamins A, C, and E; the minerals zinc and selenium; and a range of phytochemicals would be appropriate supportive treatment, as would inclusion of antioxidant adaptogen herbs.

ADDITIONAL THERAPIES

Exercise not only encourages weight reduction but also improves pelvic circulation, promotes uterine muscular tone, promotes regular bowel elimination, and reduces stress. Herbalists often recommend specific yoga postures or Kegel exercises to assist in improving pelvic circulation.[38] Vigorous walking, hip circling, pelvic thrusts, and belly dancing can all be useful to improve pelvic circulation.

🌿 TREATMENT SUMMARY: UTERINE FIBROIDS

- Achieve a healthy body weight and distribution.
- Promote hormonal regulation and elimination of excess estrogen. Avoid excess environmental and dietary estrogen exposure.
- Encourage an antiinflammatory diet low in red meat and dairy products and high in fresh fish, green vegetables, and fresh fruit.
- Improve uterine tone and circulation with herbs and exercise (e.g., specific yoga postures, belly dancing).
- Treat/prevent acute and chronic symptoms, such as bleeding and pain with appropriate botanicals.
- Treat anemia if necessary.
- Supplement with vitamins A, C, and E, and the minerals zinc and selenium.

What to Expect with Treatment

- Expect an immediate reduction in acute pain within 1 to 2 hours of the onset of treatment with analgesic, antispasmodic, and sedative herbs, and a reduction in bleeding within 1 to 4 hours with the use of herbal astringents and antihemorrhagic herbs.
- Expect an overall reduction in symptom occurrence within two menstrual cycles after the onset of treatment.
- Expect to begin to see reduction in fibroid size within 3 to 6 months of onset of treatment.
- Fibroids may not be eliminated entirely but can be reduced significantly enough to prevent symptoms and mitigate the need for pharmaceutical and surgical interventions.
- If after two menstrual cycles symptom relief is not beginning to be achieved, the botanical protocol and other strategies, as well as patient commitment, need to be evaluated and formulae possibly modified.

FIBROCYSTIC BREASTS AND BREAST PAIN

Benign breast conditions are a common finding in clinical practice, with fibrocystic breast changes and fibroadenomas occurring in 60% to 90% of all women.[39] The hallmark of fibrocystic breast changes is that the cysts fluctuate in size and shape, may entirely disappear and reappear cyclically, and are associated with hormonal changes in the menstrual cycle. Women with this condition describe their breasts as feeling lumpy, "ropey," and tender. The changes occur bilaterally. Fibroadenomas are mobile, solid, firm, rubbery masses that typically occur singly, and are not usually painful (Fig. 11-2). They are second only to fibrocystic changes as the most common of the benign breast conditions, and are commonly found in women in their twenties. Breast tenderness that accompanies the menstrual cycle is known as cystic mastalgia.[40,41] Cyclic mastalgia may be associated with other premenstrual complaints. The terms *benign breast disorder* and *benign breast disease* are unfortunate misnomers because these occurences are neither a disorder nor a disease. In only a small percentage of cases are the atypical ductal and lobular hyperplasias associated with increased risk of breast carcinoma. Practitioners consulting with women for fibrocystic breast changes and other findings must be sensitive

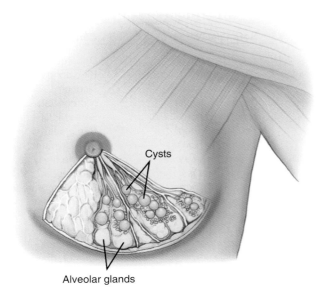

FIGURE 11-2 Comparison of normal and fibrocystic breast tissue. (From Salvo S: *Mosby's pathology for massage therapists*, St. Louis, 2004, Mosby.)

to a patient's increased anxiety about finding a breast lump, and provide clear information and calming reassurance both during the examination and while the patient awaits tests results if any were deemed necessary.

PATHOPHYSIOLOGY

Fibrocystic breast changes are an exaggerated response to cyclic ovarian hormones.[41] The etiology of fibroadenomas and cyclic mastalgia may also be hormonal, though in some cases, the cause of a fibroadenoma may be unclear. When this occurs in women older than 30, removal of the mass is generally recommended.

DIAGNOSIS AND DIFFERENTIAL DIAGNOSIS

There are two primary aims when arriving at a diagnosis of fibrocystic breasts. The first is to rule out breast cancer, and the second is to determine whether benign breast symptoms warrant treatment. A careful history, physical examination, and cancer risk assessment are indicated (Box 11-1 and Table 11-2).[39] A thorough breast examination is best performed after the menses because examination before menses (i.e., when the pain is likely to be most acute) can obscure problematic lumps caused by normal breast tissue proliferation and nodularity from normal hormonal changes. If a suspicion of breast cancer remains after the history and physical, further diagnostic tests should be performed as appropriate.[39] Diagnosis of fibrocystic breasts can be made on the basis of cancer exclusion. For women experiencing symptoms including pain, tenderness, swelling, inflammation, or nipple discharge, the comprehensive history and physical can be used to determine whether the problem is cyclic or noncyclic in nature and whether it is associated with other

BOX 11-1 Clinical Features of Benign Breast Changes

Breast tenderness and swelling
Nodularity
Breast pain (i.e., mastalgia)
Lumps
- Gross cysts
- Galactoceles
- Fibroadenomas
Nipple discharge
Breast infections
- Lactational or postpartum mastitis
- Acute mastitis associated with macrocystic breasts
- Chronic subareolar abscess

TABLE 11-2 Risk for Development of Breast Cancer by Type of Benign Breast Disease

Histologic Pattern	Approximate Relative Risk of Developing Breast Carcinoma	Proportion of Benign Lesions*
Nonproliferative changes	No increased risk	70%
Proliferative disease without atypical hyperplasia	Twofold increased risk	27%
Proliferative disease with:	Fivefold increased risk	3%-4%
Atypical hyperplasia	Fivefold increased risk	
Atypical lobular hyperplasia	Twofold increased risk	
Atypical ductal hyperplasia		
Proliferative disease with atypia and family history†	Elevenfold increased risk	3%-4%

*As determined by biopsy.
†Family history limited to mother, daughter, or sister with breast cancer.

signs and symptoms, including fever or premenstrual mood swings. It is also important to gently move aside the breast tissue and examine the chest wall and muscle to determine whether breast pain or muscle pain is the proper diagnosis.[42] Depending on the associated signs and symptoms, a diagnosis, including breast infection, muscle sprain/strain, premenstrual syndrome, or noncyclic mastalgia can be determined.

CONVENTIONAL TREATMENT

Conventional treatment for fibrocystic breasts includes encouraging women to wear loose-fitting brassieres, decrease caffeine consumption, and stop smoking. There is also a pharmacologic focus on hormonal modulation, including OCs, prolactin antagonists, and antiestrogen agents; diuretics for moderate premenstrual mastalgia; and analgesics such as ibuprofen, salicylates, and

TABLE 11-3   Summary of Botanical Treatment Strategies for Treatment of Fibrocystic Breasts

Therapeutic Goal	Therapeutic Activity	Botanical Name	Common Name
Hormonal modulation	Herbs with putative or known hormonal activity	Angelica sinensis	Dong quai
		Caulophyllum thalictroides	Blue cohosh
		Glycyrrhiza glabra	Licorice
		Leonurus cardiaca	Motherwort
		Smilax ornata	Sarsaparilla
		Trifolium pratense	Red clover
		Verbena officinalis	Blue vervain
		Vitex agnus-castus	Chaste berry
Hormonal modulation	Essential fatty acids	Linum usitatissimum	Flax seed
		Oenothera biennis	Evening primrose
Enhanced clearance of estrogen by liver and bowel; improvement of liver function	Aperients Cholagogues Hepatics	Calendula officinalis	Calendula
		Ceanothus spp.	Red root
		Chelidonium majus	Celandine
		Chionanthus virginicus	Fringe tree
		Mahonia spp.	Oregon grape
		Taraxacum officinale	Dandelion root
Relief of local congestion and swelling through lymphatic clearance (topical/internal)	Lymphatics	Galium aparine	Cleavers
		Phytolacca americana	Poke root

acetaminophen for pain.[39,40] Hormonal therapies often carry unwanted side effects, including weight gain, lipid profile changes, depression, and abnormal bleeding.[39] Although OCs reduce symptoms in up to 90% of women, symptoms return upon discontinuation.[39] Danazol, which suppresses the pituitary ovarian axis by inhibiting the output of both follicle-stimulating hormone (FSH) and LH from the pituitary gland, is also used for mastalgia. Its side effects include virilization, muscle cramps, creatine phosphokinase (CPK) elevations, and liver damage. Bromocriptine is also used for breast pain and nodularity but has several common side effects, including nausea, giddiness, and postural hypotension.[39] Reduction in dietary fat intake has been shown to reduce cyclic mastalgia. Elevated high-density lipoprotein cholesterol and dietary fat intake in women with cyclic mastopathy.[43]

BOTANICAL TREATMENT

Botanical treatment for fibrocystic breasts has not been widely subject to scientific evaluation, in spite of this being a commonly treated condition in the herbal clinic. Treatment aims primarily at hormonal regulation through direct (i.e., hypothalamic-pituitary-adrenal [HPA] and hypothalamic-pituitary-ovarian [HPO] axes) and indirect (i.e., improved hormonal biotransformation and excretion) actions, and reduction of local congestion and symptomatic pain relief through topical applications (Table 11-3). The liver plays a central role in metabolizing and detoxifying sex hormones.[37] Consequently, herbal practitioners typically include herbs that are known or thought to enhance hepatic detoxification functions in formulae for treatment of fibrocystic breasts.[37] Such herbs, many of them considered "bitters," include dandelion root, burdock root, licorice root, Oregon grape root, fringe tree, motherwort, blue vervain,

and celandine. These botanicals are usually included in ranges of 5% to 20% of the formula in tincture or decoction forms. Although there has been little investigation of such herbs to establish their pharmacologic or physiologic action for such use, they are nonetheless a common part of the protocol for many gynecologic concerns, including benign breast complaints, and their role in formulae should be considered and further evaluated.

Chaste Berry

Chaste berry is extensively recommended by herbal practitioners for cyclic breast pain and fibrocystic breasts, both when it presents independently and when associated with premenstrual syndrome (PMS). This traditional use is supported by clinical trials. Chaste berry may be used singly or in combination with other herbs that enhance hormonal regulation and hormone metabolism (e.g., herbs that promote liver function and hormonal conjugation and elimination). A 2013 systematic review evaluating 12 randomized controlled trials (RCTs) concerning chaste berry and PMS symptom alleviation cited one trial that found chaste berry to be equivalent to bromocriptine for reducing serum prolactin levels and alleviating cyclic mastalgia.[44] There have been three placebo-controlled, double-blind, RCTs examining the effects and safety of a proprietary chaste berry extract–containing solution (i.e., Vitex agnus-castus) on cyclic mastalgia. VAC is sold as Mastodynon, and manufactured by Bionorica Arzneimittel GmbH (Neumark/Opf. Germany).[45] It contains 32.4 mg of chaste berry fruit extract per 60 drops as well as a mixture of homeopathic ingredients, including Caulophyllum thalictroides, cyclamen, ignatia, iris, and lilium. This product is available as both a tablet and a liquid extract in Germany. German drug indications for the product include menstrual disorders based on a temporary or permanent corpus luteum insufficiency, infertility resulting from corpus luteum insufficiency, and menstrually related complaints, including mastodynia.[46] All three of the studies used the liquid solution, which contained 53% (volume to volume ratio [v:v]) alcohol, although the study by Wuttke et al, also used the tablets.[45,47] All three studies defined cyclic mastalgia as having at least 5 days of breast pain the previous cycle and treated women for three menstrual cycles with 30 drops two times daily of VAC (1.8 mL/ equivalent to 32.4 mg extract of chaste berry drug). Researchers found that both the severity (assessed on a 1- to 100-mm visual analog scale [VAS]) and presence of breast pain (as measured by women's diaries) were significantly improved in the women who were assigned to the chaste berry groups compared with placebo after the first month of treatment. Although pain intensity was reduced by 30% in the chaste berry group compared with 11% in placebo after one cycle, pain intensity was even more reduced at the end of the second month of treatment, with 53% of women receiving chaste berry having decreased severity of breast pain compared with 25% of the placebo group ($p = .006$).[45] No further improvement was obtained with longer treatment periods. However, to reduce the number of days with severe pain, women needed to receive VAC for three to four cycles before they had significantly fewer days with breast pain compared with the placebo group ($p = .21$).[45,48] Two of the studies also measured serum hormone levels including estradiol, progesterone, FSH, LH, and basal prolactin levels at baseline and in the premenstrual weeks of cycles 1, 2, and 3.[47,49] One study found a significant rise in prolactin levels and a decrease in progesterone levels,[49] whereas another study found no effect on FSH, LH, and progesterone, but did see a decrease in estradiol levels and a significant decrease in basal prolactin levels with 3.7 ng/mL tablets and 4.35 ng/mL liquid extracts compared with placebo.[47] Adverse events were rare and did not differ from placebo in any of the RCTs.

Dong Quai and Blue Cohosh

Along with chaste berry, dong quai and blue cohosh are commonly employed by herbal clinicians to modulate hormone levels. Blue cohosh, as part of the German herbal formulation Mastodyn (reviewed in the preceding), may provide some of the therapeutic benefit of that formulation. However, to date, no studies have demonstrated that blue cohosh has any effect on hormonal levels. Dong quai in vitro can weakly bind to estrogenic receptors and induce progesterone receptors. However, it did not stimulate vaginal cells or increase endometrial thickness and had no estrogenic effect, showing no transactivation of either ERαs or ERβs.[28,50,51] Additionally, dong quai showed no significant effect on either hormonal levels or symptoms in an RCT in menopausal women.[52,53] Consequently, dong quai appears to have a limited, if any, effect on hormone levels. In a recent study, dong quai was found to have significant antiinflammatory effects because of one of its constituents, ferulic acid.[54] Although this study is preliminary, it may explain an alternative mechanism through which dong quai could be helping to decrease mastalgia in women with fibrocystic breasts. According to TCM theory, dong quai dissolves blockages and relieves blood stagnation, and is thus a common ingredient in formulae for mastalgia.

Flax Seed and Evening Primrose Oil

Flax seeds are the richest source of plant-based omega-3 fatty acids, with α-linolenic acid (ALA) being the primary fatty acid (18:3n-3).[55] These fatty acids are considered strongly antiinflammatory, being precursors for the antiinflammatory series prostaglandins (PGE_3). Flax seeds are also rich in fibers called lignins. Like isoflavones in soy and other foods, lignins and their associated phenolic compounds are classified as phytoestrogens.[56,57] Flax seeds are an especially rich source of dietary lignins, with 75 to 800 times more than any other food source.[55,58] Research has shown lignins to be a promising agent for binding excess sex hormones, including testosterone and estrogens. Through both its antiinflammatory and possible antiestrogenic effects researchers believe that flax may prove a beneficial treatment for fibrocystic breasts. One study examined the effect of eating one muffin daily supplemented with 25 g of ground flax seeds in 127 women with mastalgia.[59] Women experienced a significant reduction of symptoms; however, the full results of this study were never published and thus it is unknown how long women needed to take the flax seed–enriched muffins, what symptoms were reduced, what the degree of symptom reduction was, or if there was any placebo control to assess for the considerable level of spontaneous remission (60% to 80%) of symptoms in women with breast pain over time.[59] The recommended dose of flax oil to treat and prevent mastalgia and nodularity is two to four 500-mg capsules twice daily or 1 to 2 tablespoons of the oil daily. One to three grams daily is the recommended dose of ground seeds.[60]

Evening primrose oil (EPO) is a rich source of omega-6 essential fatty acids (EFAs). EFAs are precursors to either series 1 or 2 prostaglandins, depending on substrate availability. The more omega-6 EFAs there are in the diet, the more likely it is for the inflammatory series prostaglandins to be made; conversely, the less omega-6 EFAs there are in the diet, the more likely it is for antiinflammatory series 1 prostaglandins to be produced. Because of EPO's potential antiinflammatory properties, two randomized placebo-controlled, double-blind clinical trials and one open-labeled trial of EPO in both cyclic and noncyclic mastalgia have been conducted. One double-blind, placebo-controlled randomized study in 73 women with either cyclic or noncyclic mastalgia found that 1000 mg of EPO or placebo three times daily over 3 months significantly reduced symptoms of pain and tenderness in the women who received EPO compared with placebo.[61] In a similar study, 291 women with severe persistent breast pain given either placebo or 1000 mg EPO three times daily for 3 to 6 months found that 45% of women with cyclic pain taking EPO improved. Further, 27% of women with noncyclic breast pain improved compared with 9% in the placebo group.[62] In a nonrandomized open-labeled study, 94 women with cyclic and 32 women with noncyclic mastalgia received 3 g of EPO for at least 4 months. Severity of pain was diminished in a "clinically useful" manner in 58% of the women with cyclic mastalgia and 38% of the women with noncyclic mastalgia taking EPO.[12,40,53] Unfortunately, all three of these studies are difficult to assess because of lack of reporting of how pain and symptoms were measured and how great the effect, and thus how clinically relevant the effect of EPO was in women with breast pain.[42] A 2010 four-arm RCT ($n = 85$ women from two medical centers in the US) tested the use of vitamin E, EPO, and a combination of the two against placebo for the treatment of cyclic mastalgia. Women were randomized into one of four groups: vitamin E (1200 IU daily), EPO (3000 mg daily), vitamin E (1200 IU daily) plus EPO (3000 mg daily), or double placebo for a total of 6 months. Outcomes were measured as reduction in breast pain via modified McGill Pain Questionnaire at baseline and end point. The drop-out rate was high ($n = 41$ completed) and observations were analyzed using intent-to-treat analysis. Using these statistical strategies, differences in worst-pain improvement were seen with the vitamin E, EPO, and vitamin E plus EPO treatment groups compared with placebo. However, results from a two-sample t-test showed a nonsignificant decrease in cyclical mastalgia for the three treatment groups.[63] A typical dose of EPO is 1500 mg daily.

Red Clover

Red clover is rich in isoflavones, especially genistein and daidzein. Genistein and daidzein have weak estrogenic effects, which have led researchers to hypothesize that genistein may compete with stronger endogenous estrogens such as estradiol for ERs; although what effects this may have on breast tissue is unclear at this time. One unpublished study found that a red clover extract had a significant effect on improving mastalgia. No further information is available concerning this trial.[64]

Topical Applications
Castor Oil

Herbalists and naturopaths commonly recommend placing an absorbent cloth saturated with heated castor oil over the affected area of the breasts. The hot compress is typically applied for 1 hour for up to 5 days per week. The oil may be further medicated by the addition of essential oils as mentioned under poke root.

Poke Root

Poke root has traditionally been used to stimulate the immune system, relieve lymph congestion, and resolve lumps and cysts, and by extension, has been widely applied topically for the treatment of fibrocystic breasts. Poke root oil is applied topically by rubbing in a small amount (i.e., 1 tsp) of the oil throughout the affected breast(s) for at least 5 nights per week for 1 to 2 months. The addition of five to seven drops each of rose, geranium, and sandalwood essential oils makes the oil slightly more stimulating to the local circulation and also adds a pleasant scent to the oil. All parts of the poke root plant are toxic and can lead to contact dermatitis or even toxicity from handling large amounts. Internal use is not recommended without the supervision of a qualified practitioner.

BOTANICAL PROTOCOL FOR THE TREATMENT OF FIBROCYSTIC BREASTS

Use the following combined protocol for at least 3 months for optimal results.

I. Prepare the Following Tincture

Burdock root	(Arctium lappa)	20 mL
Calendula	(Calendula officinalis)	20 mL
Chaste berry	(Vitex agnus-castus)	20 mL
Dandelion root	(Taraxacum officinale)	20 mL
Sarsaparilla	(Smilax ornata)	20 mL
	Total:	**100 mL**

Dose: 5 mL twice daily for 3 months.

This tincture formula and infusion combination is designed to optimize liver function and promote the conjugation and elimination of excess estrogen and regulation of hormones.

II. Topical Application
- Ginger and poke root compress

Prepare a strong infusion of ginger root using 2 tablespoons of fresh grated ginger root to 1 cup of liquid. Add 1 teaspoon of poke root tincture to the infusion, stir thoroughly, and soak a towel in the hot liquid. Apply for 15 minutes, redipping the towel in the hot liquid to keep the compress hot. Repeat three or four times weekly for 3 months. The poke root may be omitted if practitioners are uncomfortable including it because of concerns about toxicity associated with the herb.

III. Nutritional Considerations

Eliminate caffeinated products. Reduce dairy consumption and exposure to environmental estrogens. A diet rich in essential fatty acids may be beneficial in hormonal regulation.

Vitamin E: 400 to 800 IU daily
Vitamin B$_6$: 50 to 100 mg daily

CASE HISTORY: CYCLIC MASTALGIA

Tanya, a 47-year-old perimenopausal woman, presented with increasingly painful cyclic mastalgia occurring 2 to 3 days before the onset of menses. Her pain had begun 2 years prior during a stressful time in her life at which time she also started having mild menstrual irregularities and bloating around the time of her periods. At that time, she started eating red meat again regularly and drinking several cups of caffeinated beverages daily. Tanya walks and rides an exercise bike 30 minutes daily five times weekly and has recently joined Weight Watchers and started eating cold-water fish three to four times weekly, as well as increasing her vegetable and fruit intake after finding out that she had high cholesterol (total cholesterol 251). She is drinking three to six glasses of water per day. She has some problems sleeping because of pain in her left hip and a history of gastroesophageal reflux disease (GERD), and was recently diagnosed with mild depression. Tanya has a history of numerous sinus infections and vaginal yeast infections. She is taking Effexor (150 mg daily) for depression. Physical examination of the breast revealed bilateral tender spots on left lower quadrant that felt like "bags of lentils." Patient claimed that she was aware of

Continued

these areas because of self-breast examination and that it appeared to worsen around the time of her menstrual cycle.

She was prescribed the following tea to take after supper to help her sleep:

Passionflower	(Passiflora incarnata)	2 parts
Chamomile	(Matricaria recutita)	2 parts
Skullcap	(Scutellaria lateriflora)	1 part

Dose: Infuse 1 level tablespoon of dried herbs per cup of boiling water, covered, for 15 minutes. Strain. Drink 2 cups within 2 hours before going to bed.

For her mastalgia and menstrual irregularities, she was prescribed the following tincture:

Dong quai	(Angelica sinensis)	40 mL
Chaste berry	(Vitex agnus-castus)	20 mL
Burdock root	(Arctium lappa)	20 mL
Cleavers	(Galium aparine)	20 mL
	Total: 100 mL	

Dose: 3 mL in water three times daily.

She returned 4 weeks later saying that her sleep had greatly improved. She also said that her GERD was about 75% improved. She estimated that she had about a 25% improvement in breast pain and tenderness. Her menstrual irregularities had not changed. The patient then returned 8 weeks later, and reported about a 75% improvement in breast tenderness and pain. She said that her last period was less irregular and closer to "being on time." Her sleep remained improved.

NUTRITIONAL CONSIDERATIONS

Elimination of Coffee, Tea, and Other Caffeinated Products

An association between caffeine, or methylxanthines, and fibrocystic breast disease has been reported but remains controversial. In one study of a group of 102 women who had mammograms performed to measure the level of fibrocystic breast disease, a strong correlation was found with both caffeine and total methylxanthine ingestion and fibrocystic breasts as determined by a series of questionnaires.[65] Similar results were found in a large case control study of 634 women.[66]

Other studies, however, have found only weak associations. Normal fluctuations in hormonal effects on breast tissue and difficulty in consistently measuring caffeine or methylxanthine intake make it difficult to conclusively demonstrate a causal relationship.[67,68] In a review of the literature presented on AltMedDex, the following studies are cited. A controlled clinical trial showed no clinically or statistically significant effects of alcohol- or methylxanthine-free diets on signs and symptoms of fibrocystic breast disease. One-hundred-sixty-two women with clinical and thermographic diagnoses of fibrocystic breast disease completed the study with evaluation at 6 months. It was concluded that abstinence from alcohol- or methylxanthine-containing beverages is not likely to

substantially reduce severity of fibrocystic breast disease within a few months.[69]

A case control study examined the relationship between coffee consumption and the development of benign breast disease by analyzing 854 cases of histologically diagnosed benign breast disease and 1748 control subjects. No association between coffee consumption and benign breast disease was found; neither was a dose–response relationship between methylxanthine consumption and benign breast disease development noted. These results suggest no association between caffeine intake and the development of benign breast disease.[70] In a randomized study, 158 women with breast concerns were divided into two groups; one group abstained from consumption of methylxanthine-containing foods and beverages. The second group (controls) had no dietary restrictions. The patients were reexamined at 4 months for palpable breast findings. One-hundred-forty patients completed the study. There was a statistically significant decrease in clinically palpable breast findings in the abstaining group compared with controls, but the absolute change was minor and may be of little clinical significance. This study offered little support for the claim that caffeine-free diets are associated with clinically significant improvement in benign breast disease.[71] In a study of 66 patients, restriction of dietary caffeine ingestion caused improvement in fibrocystic breast disease. Graphic stress telethermometry (GST) was performed as an objective monitor for fibrocystic breast. At baseline, an average score of 83.5 on GST was observed in these women. After dietary methylxanthine restriction, these scores were observed to be an average of 69.5 at 2 months and 55.5 at 6 months. Forty-two of the 66 patients had decreases in GST scores of more than 20 points at 6 months. Eighty-five percent of the patients showed improvement in GST patterns at 6 months, 15% of patients showed no change, and none showed worsening in GST patterns. Subjectively, at 6 months 22 of 66 patients reported marked improvement, 30 of 66 moderate improvement, 6 of 66 mild improvement, and 8 of 66 no change in symptoms of fibrocystic breast disease. At pretreatment, 78% of patients had 2+ or 3+ nodularity on palpation. At the 6-month examination, 89% of patients had no or 1+ nodularity on palpation (91% had improvement, 9% had no change, and none had worsening). In 85 US women with clinical and mammographically confirmed fibrocystic disease, complete abstention from methylxanthine consumption resulted in complete resolution of fibrocystic breast disease in 82.5% and significant improvement in 15% of the patients studied.[72]

Vitamin E and B₆ Supplementation

Supplementation with vitamin E (400 to 800 IU) may be beneficial for reducing mastalgia and nodularity of fibrocystic breasts; supplementation with pyridoxine (vitamin B_6/50 to 100 mg) may reduce breast tenderness and pain.[73,74] Women are also encouraged to increase dietary fiber and complex carbohydrates, reduce dietary fat to 15% to 20% of their diet, and move toward a more plant-based diet rich in phytoestrogens. A recent review examined various dietary therapies and their potential effects in treating fibrocystic breasts.[40] The review found that some dietary therapies, including vitamins E and B_6, do not have adequate evidence to support their use in fibrocystic breasts. Studies were either of poor quality or had too few study participants to make definitive conclusions. Because of the dynamic nature and very high placebo response (20%) in fibrocystic breast complaints, only well-designed studies with large numbers of participants can address the efficacy of these treatments. Indeed, better-designed studies of vitamin E have all showed no significant effect on any parameter of fibrocystic breast. Studies on reducing caffeinated products from the diet have been variable, some showing positive outcome, others showing no benefit at all. This review found no studies that had examined the effect on fibrocystic breasts of low-fat diets, increased dietary fibers, soy isoflavones, or a more plant-based diet. However, there are considerable mechanistic data, including increasing unabsorbable estrogen conjugates for excretion, reducing the recirculation of estrogen, and positively affecting bowel microflora populations that support the use of these dietary strategies. The general health benefits of adjunct therapies such as adding vitamin E, reducing poor-quality fat intake, or reducing caffeine consumption suggest that these may be worthwhile strategies to try.[40]

ADDITIONAL THERAPIES

Exercise

It is important to evaluate whether women with breast pain are exercising appropriately and properly. Some women who believe that they are experiencing breast pain or tenderness are instead having chest wall pain, often resulting from inappropriate or overexercise, especially strength-building exercises that emphasize the pectoral muscles.[41] No studies have examined the effect of any type of exercise on the symptoms or nodularity of fibrocystic breasts. Consequently, it is difficult to know what duration, type, or frequency of exercise would most benefit women with fibrocystic breasts.

Supportive Clothing

Inadequate support of the breasts is thought to lead to suspensory ligament strain, which may cause or contribute to pain and tenderness.[59] No randomized controlled studies have examined breast support and its relationship to breast pain.

Stress Reduction

No studies have examined the effect of stress, anxiety, depression, or sleep disturbances on fibrocystic symptoms. However, many other pain syndromes, including fibromyalgia and vulvar pain, are closely associated with levels of distress in a woman's life.[75] No RCTs have been conducted using acupuncture for fibrocystic breast symptoms; however, several open-label trials have found that up to 95% of women's mastalgia was improved after acupuncture treatment.

🌿 TREATMENT SUMMARY FOR FIBROCYSTIC BREASTS AND BREAST PAIN

- Reduce endogenous and exogenous estrogen load through dietary modification, reduction in environmental exposure, and botanical modulation of the hypothalamic-pituitary-adrenal (HPA) and hypothalamic-pituitary-ovarian (HPO) axes and biotransformation of hormones. Examples of herbal actions to accomplish this include adaptogens, hormonal modulators, cholagogues, and aperients.
- Use selective estrogen receptor modulators (SERMs) to competitively bind estrogen receptors (ERs).
- Relieve excess congestion in breast tissue via stimulation of local lymphatic drainage with lymphatics as well as diuretics to help eliminate excess fluids.
- Use topical applications for symptomatic pain relief and to stimulate local circulation and lymphatic flow.
- Avoid the use of caffeinated products, including coffee, black tea, chocolate, and caffeinated sodas.
- Supplement with vitamins E and B_6.
- Make certain that exercise is appropriate and not causing chest wall pain or strain.
- Make sure that the patient wears adequate breast support and appropriately sized brassieres.
- Acupuncture may be beneficial for relieving symptoms of fibrocystic breasts.

ENDOMETRIOSIS

Endometriosis is one of the most common gynecologic problems in the United States and a leading gynecologic cause of both hospitalization and hysterectomy.[26,76,77] Women with symptomatic endometriosis face chronic and sometimes debilitating pain; asymptomatic and symptomatic women alike may experience significant fertility problems caused by this condition. The least-biased estimate for the overall prevalence of endometriosis in reproductive-age women is about 10%.[78] Endometriosis is defined as the presence and growth of endometrial tissue in locations outside of the uterus. These cells may appear on the ovaries, fallopian tubes, bowel, bladder, peritoneal tissue, ligaments, or other structures in the abdominal cavity, and rarely may occur at other sites, including the nasal and respiratory passages leading to nosebleeds or pink frothy sputum at the time of the menses. Displaced endometrial tissue responds to cyclic hormonal changes, proliferating and shedding outside of the uterus. The bleeding is accompanied by inflammation caused by irritation of local tissue, such as the peritoneum. Recurrent inflammation can cause scarring and adhesions that can cause pain and dysfunction of other affected sites. Endometriosis is common in women between menarche and menopause, and is associated with as many as 25% of cases of infertility; however, causality has not been definitively established.[3,78]

Endometriosis occurs across all socioeconomic and ethnic populations, is more common in women who experience early menstruation and fewer than two pregnancies, is associated with menstrual cycle length greater than 30 days, and is more prevalent in women with IUD use greater than 2 years (Box 11-2). Studies demonstrate that women

BOX 11-2   Risk Factors for Endometriosis

Possible Risk Factors

Early menarche (i.e., before age 12)
Heavy bleeds >7 days
Intrauterine device (IUD) use
Dilation and curettage (D&C) history
Fewer than two pregnancies
Family history
High stress, especially linked to relationships or sexuality
High fat intake, especially heated fats and fried foods

Risk-Reducing Factors

Full-term pregnancies
Breastfeeding
Avoiding caffeine and alcohol
Regular exercise (timing and type are important)

who have experienced repeated vaginal and uterine infections have higher rates of endometriosis than the general population.[3] Women with a mother or sister with endometriosis are more likely to suffer from severe endometriosis, suggesting a genetic predisposition; however, milder forms do not always have familial association. The literature is conflicting on the relationship between OC use and the risk of endometriosis. A 1993 review by Vercellini et al. showed that four prospective investigations found a nonsignificant reduction in risk of up to 20%.[79] Of three case control studies, two suggested an increased risk and one indicated a reduced risk of developing endometriosis with OC use. The 1994 analysis of the Oxford Family Planning Association OC study found a significantly reduced risk of endometriosis in current OC users. The researchers found that OCs were associated with a 60% reduction in endometriosis. The risk of endometriosis was significantly related to age, with the highest risk occurring at ages 40 to 44 years compared with women ages 25 to 29 years. On the other hand, the risk of endometriosis was elevated among women who formerly used the pill by almost twice the rate of women who had never used OCs.[80-82]

Multiple theories exist on the etiology of this condition, including retrograde menstrual flow, lymphatic flow theory, and de novo origin. In fact, Konickx et al. propose that mild endometriotic lesions are common and to some extent normal at varying times in all women, and that it is symptomatic, aggressive, or deeply infiltrating endometriosis that should be considered a disease.[83] Retrograde menstrual flow theory describes menstrual or endometrial tissue flowing backward through the fallopian tubes and into the abdominal cavity. Lymphatic flow theory suggests the spread of endometrial tissue throughout the body via the lymphatic system. Some researchers postulate that coelomic metaplasia, a de novo origin, might be induced by pathologic processes as a result of chemical exposure. A role for oxidative stress has also been suggested as one of the contributing factors for the development of endometriosis, possibly as part of a conglomeration of factors

that pair immunologic and inflammatory factors in its etiology.[84,85]

There is substantial evidence that immunologic factors play a role in the pathogenesis of endometriosis and endometriosis-associated infertility, and that there is a bidirectional relationship between the endocrine and immune systems.[86] In early endometriosis, elevated levels of inflammatory mediators such as cytokines, lymphocytes, and macrophages can be identified in the peritoneal fluid. Immune alterations include increased number and activation of peritoneal macrophages, decreased T-cell reactivity and natural killer cell cytotoxicity, increased circulating antibodies, the presence of auto-antibodies, and changes in the cytokine network. Decreased natural killer cell cytotoxicity leads to an increased likelihood of implantation of endometriotic tissue. In addition, macrophages and a complex network of locally produced cytokines modulate the growth and inflammatory behavior of ectopic endometrial implants.[84,87-89] There also may be a positive correlation between immunosuppression and disease progression in the presence of established disease.[90,91] Further, women with endometriosis appear to have higher rates of atopic conditions and susceptibility to opportunistic infections (e.g., candidiasis) than women who do not have endometriosis.[92]

Environmental exposures appear to play a certain role in the development of endometriosis via endocrine disruption. Studies demonstrate a link between dioxin exposure and the disease, with increased dioxin-like compounds found in the serum of women with peritoneal endometriosis and deep endometriotic (i.e., adenomyotic) nodules. A search of the BIOSIS database for endometriosis and dioxin yielded over 50 studies. The development of this condition is likely a result of the interplay of numerous factors; thus it has been concluded by many researchers that endometriosis is most likely a condition with complex multifactorial origins.

SYMPTOMS

The following symptoms (Box 11-3), alone or in constellations, should alert a woman and her practitioner to the possibility of endometriosis: premenstrual pain, dysmenorrhea, dyspareunia, generalized pelvic pain throughout the month without other explanation, atypical periods, nausea, vomiting, exhaustion, bladder problems, frequent infections, dizziness, painful defecation, rectal pain, lower backache, irritable bowels, or infertility. The far-reaching nature of these symptoms and their possible association with other conditions helps to explain why this condition is difficult to diagnose. Dysmenorrhea and painful intercourse become even more suggestive of endometriosis if they begin after a history of relatively pain-free menstruation and intercourse. Severity of pain is not indicative of the severity of the condition, with the exception of severe pain, which is associated with extensive endometriosis and adenomyosis (i.e., deeply infiltrating endometriosis.)[3,83] Other causes of pelvic and abdominal pain or bleeding must be ruled out.

BOX 11-3 Common Symptoms of Endometriosis

Abdominal pain
Back pain
Depression
Frequent or constant pain that is over site
Infertility
Insomnia, lethargy
Later on, pinched nerve pain
Ovulation pain
Pain on intercourse
Pain with bowel movement or urination
Pelvic burning and aching not limited to menstruation
Premenstrual syndrome (PMS) with dysmenorrhea and infertility
Rarely, bleeding after bowel movements or after intercourse
Referred pain in distant sites, especially shoulder blades or top of collar bone
Swollen abdomen; intestinal gas

DIAGNOSIS

Endometriosis is most commonly seen in women 30 to 40 years old and is rarely found in postmenopausal women. Endometriosis has been thought not to occur before menarche; however, the rates of this condition are increasing among teenagers.[3] The site of lesions, although widely variable, is generally the posterior cul-de-sac or the ovaries. Diagnosis is based on pelvic examination, diagnostic ultrasound, or laparoscopy, with definitive diagnosis based on laparoscopy. Cancer antigen-125 (CA-125) is a serum antigen found in endothelial cervical cancer that can also be elevated in women with endometriosis. The diagnostic importance of the test for endometriosis is still uncertain; however, there appears to be some predictive value demonstrating which women might benefit from specific treatments on the basis of CA-125 levels, and CA-125 levels may indicate whether improvement is occurring.[93] Endometriosis is staged based on the location(s) of the endometrial tissue as follows:

- Stage I, or minimal, disease (i.e., superficial endometriosis, filmy adhesions)
- Stage II, or mild, disease (i.e., superficial and deep endometriosis, filmy adhesions)
- Stage III, or moderate, disease (i.e., superficial and deep endometriosis, filmy and dense adhesions)
- Stage IV, or severe, disease (i.e., superficial and deep endometriosis, dense adhesions)

CONVENTIONAL TREATMENT APPROACHES

Medical treatment of endometriosis includes both pharmaceutical and surgical approaches. Pharmaceutical treatments provide only suppression of the disease; they do not exact a cure.[3] Decisions regarding treatment are based on endometriosis severity and staging, symptom picture, and ultimately, the woman's needs and goals, for example, desire for children in the future.[94] For women experiencing mild or no symptoms and for women who are close to menopause, the appropriate treatment may be to do nothing.[83] For women with mild to moderate symptoms, and those who desire pregnancy, the appropriate pharmacologic therapy should be considered, and if necessary, can be combined with conservative surgery.

It should be noted that, in spite of medical treatment, endometriosis has a high recurrence rate of 5% to 20% unless total hysterectomy and bilateral oophorectomy are performed. With pharmacologic interventions, pain typically resumes upon cessation of medications, although initially with pain that is less intense than before treatment. Pain relief, pregnancy rates, and recurrence rates are similar with all treatment methods. The goal of pharmaceutical treatment is to interrupt patterns of endometrial stimulation and bleeding.[94] Pharmaceutical options include NSAIDs and hormonal therapies (e.g., progestins, GnRH analogs [GnRH-As], danazol, and OCs). NSAIDs (e.g., ibuprofen, naproxen) may be prescribed for mild to moderate pain. They are relatively safe for short-term symptomatic relief; however, long-term use can lead to health consequences, including gastrointestinal (GI) bleeding, and should be avoided in patients with a history of peptic ulcer disease or renal failure. It should be noted that none of these therapies demonstrates significant benefit over the others, and all are associated with a high recurrence rate (20% to 50%) upon discontinuation of the therapy.[94]

Progestins (e.g., medroxyprogesterone acetate [Depo-Provera]) suppress the response of endometrial tissue to cyclic hormones, leading to atrophy of this tissue and decreased pain. They are typically better tolerated than OCs, with fewer side effects, and are less costly than danazol and GnRH-As. This is often considered the pharmaceutical treatment of choice for endometriosis, although the Food and Drug Administration (FDA) no longer supports the use of Depo-Provera for this purpose. Side effects include weight gain, fluid retention, and breakthrough bleeding. Depression is a common significant side effect of medroxyprogesterone use. In high doses, medroxyprogesterone can adversely affect lipid profiles, and may lead to a state of hypoestrogenism, with subsequent potential for bone loss. OCs are used to control pain in women not desiring pregnancy. The combined effect of estrogen and progesterone is to induce a state of "pseudopregnancy," and appears to lead to a 90% rate of improved symptoms with long-term use. Side effects include all those typically associated with general OC use. Danazol, a synthetic testosterone, is used for the treatment of mild to moderate endometriosis in women who desire fertility but not necessarily in the immediate future. It induces a state of "pseudomenopause," eliminating midcycle FSH and LH surges. Once considered the optimal treatment for endometriosis, it is now considered no more effective than any of the other pharmaceutical treatments. Possible side effects include weight gain, fluid retention, fatigue, decrease in breast size, hirsutism, atrophic vaginitis, hot flashes, muscle cramps, emotional fluctuations, voice changes, spotting, and decreased high-density lipoprotein (HDL) cholesterol levels. In some patients it may cause hepatocellular damage; thus is contraindicated in patients with liver disease, and liver enzymes should be monitored in all patients during treatment. It is also contraindicated in patients with a history of hypertension, hyperlipidemia, congestive heart failure, renal impairment, and pregnancy.[3,26,94,95] GnRH-As (e.g., Leuprolide) also cause a suppression of endometriosis via a pseudomenopausal state. GnRH treatment does not carry the same risks of negative effect on serum lipids and lipoproteins compared with danazol; however, it does interfere with calcium metabolism via stimulation of a hypoestrogenic state, and thus can cause osteoporosis. Even after only 6 months of use, a 6% to 8% loss in trabecular bone has been observed. It can take up to 2 years after cessation of treatment to replace this bone loss; thus a treatment is usually restricted to 6-month durations.[3,96]

Surgical options include conservative surgery (i.e., destruction and removal of endometriomas but maintaining reproductive function) and radical surgery (i.e., hysterectomy, generally accompanied by bilateral salpingo-oophorectomy). Conservative treatment involves the removal of endometriotic lesions and restoration of normal anatomic relationships via removal of adhesions to the greatest extent possible, with the goal of pain relief, and possible restoration of fertility when achieving pregnancy is desired and has been impaired by the condition. In approximately one fourth of women treated surgically, however, there is no improvement in fertility even if the disease was considered mild. Procedures include knife excision, laser surgery, electrocautery, curettage, and laparotomy. The worse the disease, the worse the statistics for conceiving after surgery.[97,98]

Recurrence of endometriosis after surgery is dependent on the skill of the surgeon and extent of disease, and as with other endometriosis treatments, rates may be as high as 20%. Hysterectomy will not remove lesions outside the uterus and is not considered a successful treatment when used primarily to reduce the symptom of chronic pelvic pain (CPP). Surgery carries the risk of complications, especially adhesion formation and continuing pain. The total rate at which symptoms of CPP returned after drug treatment is estimated to be 5% to 15% at the end of 1 year, or up to 50% at the end of 5 years. Nonetheless, the risks of surgery or medication may be justifiable for severe pain that does not respond to other methods, especially if menopause is not expected for some time. There is a concern that diagnostic microsurgery may aggravate or cause the transfer of viable endometrial cells into general or lymphatic circulation, thereby causing the very condition being identified. Because of this, some wary clients choose natural treatment approaches for the condition without a certain diagnosis, believing that if the signs and symptoms respond, the holistic prescription was correct for the presumed diagnosis.

BOTANICAL TREATMENT

Herbalists share the conventional medical perspective that endometriosis has multifactorial causes. The botanical approach, however, takes into consideration immune dysregulation, inflammation, hormonal dysregulation, diet and nutritional status, lifestyle, exposure to exogenous estrogens, and the woman's emotional and psychological mechanisms for coping with this condition as components of a whole picture. Given that nonradical medical treatments for endometriosis

are purely suppressive rather than curative, the high recurrence rate of endometriosis upon cessation of pharmaceutical treatment, and the potential for drug-related or surgical side effects, botanical medicines may provide women with a safe alternative for symptomatic pain relief, reduction of inflammation, prevention and reduction of recurrent vaginal and pelvic infections, stress reduction, and improvement of overall immunologic health (Table 11-4). By applying a comprehensive natural health care protocol, many cases of endometriosis can also be resolved. The herbal approach should also include as part of the protocol herbs that address concomitant discomforts arising from the condition, such as irritable bowel complaints or depression.

Many herbs have multiple actions. Varying degrees of success have been obtained when improving as many of the known cofactors as possible. However, the mechanisms behind the success of herbal protocol are not well elucidated nor understood, and clinical successes are inconsistent. In fact, many Western herbalists consider endometriosis hard to completely "cure," and ultimately focus on symptom control and overall health improvement. There are well-developed treatment protocols for the treatment of endometriosis in TCM that have been associated with successful treatment. By applying a comprehensive natural protocol, endometriosis may be entirely resolved in some cases, and made significantly less problematic in many. The following section discusses the general Western botanical treatment approaches for endometriosis as well as a brief overview of TCM approaches. Fertility treatments appear in a chapter devoted to that subject. Also see chronic pelvic/vaginal pain, vaginal infection, dysmenorrhea, and other relevant topics under separate headings.

The following factors have been noted in endometriosis patients, but this does not explain why all patients with SOME of these findings do not necessarily have the other syndromes associated with these factors (e.g., PMS):

- Estrogen excess
- Progesterone deficiency
- Magnesium deficiency
- EFA deficiency
- High stress (often complicated by hypoglycemia)
- Hormone imbalance other than progesterone to estrogen ratio
- Excess dietary caffeine
- Excess alcohol consumption

Attention to these factors may help some women with symptom reduction and regression of size and infiltration of endometriotic tissue.

DISCUSSION OF BOTANICALS

For many women with endometriosis, pain is the single most debilitating aspect of this condition (other than chronic fertility problems in women desiring pregnancy). Therefore pain management should be an important focus in the care of women with this condition. Herbalists reliably employ a number of herbs for the treatment of pelvic and abdominal pain, many of which have a long history of traditional use for painful gynecologic conditions. These herbs can be used

TABLE 11-4 Botanical Treatment Strategies for Endometriosis

Therapeutic Goal	Therapeutic Activity	Botanical Name	Common Name
Pain relief	Analgesics Anodynes Sedatives	*Anemone pulsatilla* *Angelica sinensis* *Actaea racemosa* *Corydalis ambigua* *Eschscholzia californica* *Matricaria recutita* *Paeonia lactiflora* *Piper methysticum* *Piscidia piscipula*	Pulsatilla Dong quai Black cohosh Corydalis California poppy Chamomile White peony Kava kava Jamaican dogwood
Pain relief	Antiinflammatory	*Angelica sinensis* *Calendula officinalis* *Camellia sinensis* *Echinacea* spp. *Glycyrrhiza glabra* *Hypericum perforatum* *Matricaria recutita* *Oenothera biennis* *Paeonia lactiflora* *Prunus cerasus* *Rehmannia glutinosa* *Tanacetum parthenium* *Zingiber officinale*	Dong quai Calendula Green tea Echinacea Licorice St. John's wort Chamomile Evening primrose White peony Cherry Rehmannia Feverfew Ginger
Pain relief	Antispasmodics	*Actaea racemosa* *Dioscorea villosa* *Matricaria recutita* *Paeonia lactiflora* *Viburnum opulus* *Viburnum prunifolium* *Zingiber officinale*	Black cohosh Wild yam Chamomile White peony Cramp bark Black haw Ginger
Immunologic support; reduction in fatigue, depression, and concomitant psychoemotional symptoms	Immunostimulatory Adaptogens	*Angelica sinensis* *Astragalus membranaceus* *Calendula officinalis* *Cordyceps sinensis* *Echinacea* spp. *Eleutherococcus senticosus* *Panax ginseng* *Panax quinquefolius* *Picrorhiza kurroa* *Rhaponticum carthamoides* *Rhodiola rosea* *Schisandra chinensis* *Thuja arbor-vitae* *Withania somnifera*	Dong quai Astragalus Calendula Cordyceps Echinacea Eleuthero Ginseng American ginseng Picrorhiza Rhaponticum Rhodiola Schisandra Thuja Ashwagandha
Improve pelvic circulation and tone; reduce size and extent of endometriotic tissue	Emmenagogues Uterotonics	*Achillea millefolium* *Alchemilla vulgaris* *Caulophyllum thalictroides*	Yarrow Lady's mantle Blue cohosh
Hormonal regulation: Indirect via enhanced clearance of estrogen by liver and bowel, improved hormone metabolism by liver, and improvement of healthy hepatic function	Hepatic trophorestoratives Aperients Cholagogues Hepatics	*Calendula officinalis* *Chionanthus virginicus* *Curcuma longa* *Rosmarinus officinalis* *Schisandra chinensis* *Silybum marianum* *Taraxacum officinale*	Calendula Fringe tree Tumeric Rosemary Schisandra Milk thistle Dandelion
Hormonal regulation: Direct via known or putative hormonal actions	Hormonal regulators	*Gossypium herbaceum* *Verbena officinalis* *Vitex agnus-castus*	Cotton root Blue vervain Chaste tree
Improve pelvic and abdominal lymphatic circulation; enhance immunologic function	Lymphatics	*Calendula officinalis*	Calendula
Stress relief	Nervines	*Leonurus cardiaca* *Verbena officinalis*	Motherwort Blue vervain

Also see chapters discussing vaginal infection, dysmenorrhea, urinary tract infections, and fertility problems for additional protocols.

singly but are generally used in various combinations with other herbs in these categories, or as part of a larger protocol. Analgesic herbs are used for generalized or local pain of an aching or sharp quality and include black cohosh, black haw and cramp bark, chamomile, corydalis, pulsatilla, dong quai, ginger, and Jamaican dogwood. Corydalis, Jamaican dogwood, and pulsatilla are especially dependable for moderate to serious pain. Pulsatilla is considered specific for ovarian pain.[22] Antispasmodics are typically used for cramping pain, but also may be used for sharp or dull pain, aching, and drawing pains in the lower back and thighs; herbs include wild yam, *Viburnum* spp. (i.e., cramp bark, black haw), black cohosh, chamomile, and ginger. Dong quai's traditional TCM uses for gynecologic conditions, specifically for conditions of blood vacuity and stasis, the latter of which endometriosis may be considered among, along with its antispasmodic, antiinflammatory, and immunomodulatory qualities, make it an important herb to consider.[26,54,99] Many antispasmodics and antiinflammatories, such as wild yam, *Viburnum* spp., ginger, and chamomile are specific not only for uterine pain, but also for intestinal, bowel, and urinary pain and irritability, making them uniquely suitable for endometrial pain and accompanying bowel and bladder discomforts. This is important to keep in mind because the pain of endometriosis is related to irritation of tissue by endometrium outside of its normal site in the uterus. Sedatives are useful when there is the need to induce deep rest or sleep to obtain pain relief, and include California poppy, a combination of black cohosh and cramp bark, or a combination of cramp bark and Jamaican dogwood. Valerian and hops are also useful sedatives. The successful use of these herbs for pain depends largely upon adequate dosing and frequency of administration.

🌿 FORMULAE FOR DYSMENORRHEA

Formula for Treatment of Mild to Moderate Pain Associated with Dysmenorrhea

Black cohosh	(*Actaea racemosa*)	20 mL
Cramp bark	(*Viburnum opulus*)	20 mL
Chamomile	(*Matricaria recutita*)	15 mL
Dong quai	(*Angelica sinensis*)	15 mL
Wild yam	(*Dioscorea villosa*)	15 mL
Licorice	(*Glycyrrhiza glabra*)	10 mL
Ginger	(*Zingiber officinale*)	5 mL
		Total: 100 mL

Dose: 2.5 to 4 mL every 2 to 4 hours during episodes of endometrial discomfort. This can also be given 3 mL three times daily prophylactically for women who experience predictable cyclic pain associated with endometriosis.

Formula for Treatment of Moderate to Severe Pain Associated with Dysmenorrhea

Black cohosh	(*Actaea racemosa*)	25 mL
Cramp bark	(*Viburnum opulus*)	25 mL
Wild yam	(*Dioscorea villosa*)	20 mL
Corydalis	(*Corydalis ambigua*)	15 mL
Jamaican dogwood	(*Piscidia piscipula*)	15 mL
		Total: 100 mL

Dose: For severe, acute pain take 2.5 mL every 15 minutes until pain begins to subside, or for up to 2 hours consecutively, then reduce dose to 2.5 to 5 mL every 2 to 4 hours as needed.

Sedative Formula for Severe Pain Associated with Endometriosis

Cramp bark	(*Viburnum opulus*)
California poppy	(*Eschscholzia californica*)
Jamaican dogwood	(*Piscidia piscipula*)

Dose: Combine equal parts of the listed liquid extracts and take 2.5 mL every 15 minutes for 1 hour to induce sleep.

Immunomodulation

The exact immunologic underpinnings of endometriosis remain uncertain. There appears to be a complex interplay of hyperimmune, autoimmune, and hypoimmune function at work, either variably or concurrently leading only to the clear understanding that there is some level of immune dysregulation that accompanies this condition. The most appropriate response seems to be twofold: (1) to look at the unique constellation of symptoms presented by each individual woman, for example, whether she is depleted and susceptible to frequent colds and repeated vaginal infections or chronic atopic conditions—and to treat accordingly, and (2) to provide botanicals that support immune regulation—notably, the adaptogens. For women who evidence a state of immune depletion in combination with endometriosis some amount of immunostimulation may be appropriate to bolster the overall immune response, and may be provided through the use of herbs such as echinacea, astragalus, or *Picrorhiza kurroa* in combination with adaptogens such as ashwagandha, American ginseng, rhaponticum, or rhodiola. Such women also may benefit greatly from medicinal mushrooms such as reishi and *Cordyceps* for immune support. For women with signs of hyperimmunity, atopic conditions such as eczema or chronic rhinitis, or autoimmunity, the use of immunosupportive antiinflammatory adaptogens, such as licorice, ashwagandha, and American ginseng, may be most appropriate. It is unknown and a matter of great debate as to whether immunostimulating herbs such as echinacea and astragalus are safe and appropriate for use when there is autoimmunity.[22] Using adaptogens for treating endometriosis makes sense in that their actions simultaneously influence and restore normalcy to the functions of the immune system and the HPA axis, both of which appear to have dysregulated function in this condition. The uterine endometrium is a complex structure of interspersed glandular tissue and endometrial stroma, closely associated with lymphoid tissue.[86] The inclusion of herbs that are traditionally thought to improve lymphatic circulation, such as calendula, echinacea, cleavers, and poke root, are commonly included in botanical protocol for endometriosis.

Antiinflammatories and Antioxidants

Inflammation is a hallmark of endometriosis, and as discussed, free radical damage may be part of the etiology of this disorder. It has been suggested that growth factors and inflammatory mediators produced by activated peritoneal leukocytes participate in the pathogenesis of endometriosis by facilitating endometrial cells growth at ectopic sites.[86] Elevated levels of inflammatory cells and mediators such as peritoneal macrophages, prostaglandins, proteolytic enzymes, complement fragments, interleukin-1 (IL-1), and tumor necrosis factor (TNF) have been identified in the peritoneal fluid of patients with endometriosis.[86] Numerous herbs that have been used traditionally for inflammatory types of conditions demonstrate significant antiinflammatory and antioxidant effects and should be considered for use in formulations for treatment and symptomatic relief, along with herbs whose use for inflammation is only recently being discovered. These are discussed in the following.

Devil's Claw

Devil's claw is native to southern Africa and was named after the small hooks that cover its fruit. It has been used in Western herbal medicine for over a century to alleviate pain and inflammation associated with arthritis, headache, and back pain. Devil's claw contains iridoid glycosides, of which harpagoside is notable for limiting the release of inflammatory cytokines. In a recent pilot study on the use of devil's claw in the treatment of endometriosis symptoms, 12 patients took 400 mg of encapsulated extract 4 times daily for 12 weeks. Half of the group reported a reduction in pain after 4 weeks of treatment (specifically, dysmenorrhea and dyspareunia), and all patients felt that the treatment improved symptoms and overall QOL after 8 weeks (Extract preparation details not provided).[100] The root can be found in tinctures or capsules.

Dong Quai

Dong quai has antispasmodic, analgesic, and tonic effects, and has demonstrated significant antioxidant and free radical scavenging actions, partially through inhibition of anion radical formation. Limited animal and in vitro studies have reported on the specific immunomodulatory effects of dong quai, including a stimulation of phagocytic activity and IL-2 production, and an antiinflammatory effect. There is evidence to suggest that the polysaccharide fraction of dong quai may contribute to these effects. Immunostimulatory and antiinflammatory effects have also been documented for isolated ferulic acid. Dong quai has been traditionally used in Chinese medicine for the treatment of "blood stasis," which encompasses a diagnosis of endometriosis.

Echinacea

Echinacea is widely used by herbalists for its immunostimulatory and antiinflammatory effects to support and promote the body's natural immune responses.[26,101,102] Antioxidant effects appear to include free radical scavenging mechanisms and transition metal chelating, whereas immunostimulating effects include enhanced phagocytosis, and the stimulation of cytokine and immunoglobulin production.[30,103]

Feverfew

Feverfew has been used for the treatment of menstrual complaints since at least the time of the ancient Greeks. In fact, its botanical name may reflect such use—*parthenos* means "virgin" in Greek.[104] It is mentioned by the Eclectic physicians for use in the treatment of menstrual irregularity.[105] Feverfew also has been used for the treatment of other inflammatory conditions, including headache, fever, psoriasis, and arthritis. Although studies have not been done on the use of this herb in the treatment of endometriosis, and indeed, it is not widely discussed for such use even in the herbal literature, its pharmacology and actions as an antinociceptive and antiinflammatory suggest that consideration of such use is warranted.[106] Feverfew has exhibited inhibition of prostaglandin synthetase, which inhibits the conversion of arachidonic acid (AA) to inflammatory prostaglandins, inhibits mast cell degranulation and subsequent histamine and serotonin release, and has shown inhibition of other inflammatory cytokines such as tumor necrosis factor alpha (TNF-α), IL-1, nuclear factor kappa B (NFκB) and interferon-gamma (IFN-γ), as well as inhibiting peritoneal cyclooxygenase (COX) in animal models.[103]

Ginger

Herbalists use ginger root as an antiinflammatory and antispasmodic herb for the treatment of numerous painful inflammatory conditions from arthritis to dysmenorrhea.[107,108] No studies have been identified for its use for painful gynecologic complaints. One trial of 120 women reported ginger to be an effective antiemetic for the treatment of postoperative nausea, with specific trials demonstrating its efficacy in reducing postlaparoscopic gynecologic procedures. However, two other trials demonstrated either no effect compared with placebo, or negative effect (i.e., increased nausea) with increased doses of ginger.[103] Ginger remains popular among Western and TCM herbalists as an antispasmodic treatment for dysmenorrhea.[26] It is taken in tincture form in combination with other herbs, in infusions, and also used externally as a poultice and in baths for pelvic discomfort.

Gotu Kola

Numerous studies support the traditional uses of the popular Ayurvedic herb gotu kola as a wound healing, antiinflammatory, and antimicrobial herb. Additionally, it has been demonstrated to have antiproliferative and antioxidant effects, and to prevent the formation of keloid scar tissue.[109-113] Its use as a neurogenerative and neurotrophorestorative adaptogen makes it particularly useful in the treatment of stress disorders, and may play some role in its mediation of other effects.[114] Given the association of these actions with the clinical and etiologic picture of endometriosis, this herb deserves consideration as part of a protocol for this condition both when botanical treatment is the primary modality and to heal from surgical intervention and reduce adhesion and scar formation. Gotu kola is typically used in combination with other herbs as part of a comprehensive formula.

Green Tea

Green tea is rich in polyphenolic compounds, with catechins as its major component. Studies have shown that catechins possess diverse pharmacologic properties that include antioxidative, antiinflammatory, anticarcinogenic, and antibacterial effects. Tea catechins are well absorbed in the GI tract; thus drinking unfractionated green tea is the most simple and beneficial way to consume this herb.[115,116]

Licorice, Calendula, and St. John's Wort

Licorice root *(Glycyrrhiza glabra)* and calendula blossoms *(Calendula officinalis)* are used by herbalists as antiinflammatory herbs, and may frequently be included in formulae for treating endometriosis. The aim of one recent study was to investigate whether standardized hydroalcoholic plant extracts such as calendula, St. John's wort, plantain *(Plantago lanceolata),* and licorice can suppress the activities of 5-lipoxygenase (5-LO) and cyclooxygenase-2 (COX-2), key enzymes in the formation of proinflammatory eicosanoids from AA. The researchers concluded that licorice extract might be a potential drug possessing antiinflammatory activity devoid of the most troublesome (gastric) side effects seen for drugs used as COX-2 and 5-LO inhibitors. They purported that St. John's wort, plantain, and licorice extracts can be added to an already impressive list of botanicals with antiinflammatory activity.[117]

Peony and Rehmannia

Two herbs commonly used in TCM formulae, peony and rehmannia, have demonstrated significant antiinflammatory and antispasmodic activity. Both are specifically recommended by Mills and Bone for endometriosis, whereas Low Dog discusses the use of peony in the traditional Japanese medicine Shakuyaku-Kanzo-To (which also contains the antiinflammatory *Glycyrrhiza uralensis*).[22,26,114] Studies using the latter formula have demonstrated prostaglandin production inhibition in the uterine myometrium via phospholipase A2 inhibition, whereas other studies have demonstrated AA inhibition, platelet-activating factor (PAF) inhibition, reduction in free radical formation, and smooth muscle relaxation. Note that nearly all of the studies use these herbs in traditional formulae rather than in isolation, and that studies are conducted in animal models, and have focused on arthritis, ulcers, and other chronic inflammatory conditions. Licorice, a potent antiinflammatory, is frequently included in TCM formulae that also contain peony and rehmannia, as is dong quai when these herbs are used for gynecologic conditions. It must be remembered that in TCM, herbs are not prescribed on the basis of a disease entity or a pharmacologic expectation of efficacy, but rather on an individual diagnostic approach using traditional parameters and categories.

Sour Cherries and Raspberry Fruit

Although not part of a traditional botanical approach to gynecologic problems, interesting new data suggests that sour cherry anthocyanins may have a beneficial role in the treatment of inflammatory pain. The antihyperalgesic effect may be related to the antiinflammatory and antioxidant properties of anthocyanins, and was found comparable to the commercial antioxidants and superior to vitamin E at a test concentration of 125 µg/mL.[118] Anthocyanins from raspberries *(Rubus idaeus)* and sweet cherries *(Prunus avium)* demonstrated COX-1 and COX-2 inhibitory activities comparable to those of ibuprofen and naproxen at 10 µM concentrations.[119] The value of these findings in endometriosis is not known, but perhaps this is a worthy reminder that a diet rich in deep-colored berries and other fruits and vegetables may hold a key to improving health and preventing disease.

Hormonal Modulation

Predicated on the belief that steroid hormones are the primary regulators of the growth and activity of ectopic endometrial tissue, therapies aimed at hormonal modulation have been the foundation of conventional therapy for endometriosis, and have also featured prominently in botanical protocol.[86] Unfortunately, even less is known about the effects of botanical therapies on the endocrine system than about pharmaceutical medications. The goal of pharmaceutical therapies is to create an acyclic, low-estrogen environment that prevents bleeding, leads to atrophy of ectopic implants, and possibly minimizes retrograde bleeding. However, endometrial tissue may be histologically different than normal uterine endometrial tissue, and may respond differently to hormonal stimulation. Again, much remains unknown about this enigmatic condition.[86] Several botanicals are frequently used as hormonal modulators, in conjunction with other herbs discussed in this chapter. Little research is available on their application in endometriosis. But as part of a comprehensive protocol, many herbalists and naturopathic physicians report positive outcomes for achieving the goals established earlier in this paragraph. There is also some small discrepancy in the herbal literature as to which herbs should be avoided because of potential exacerbating hormonal effects. For example, Mills and Bone caution against the use of what they refer to as "estrogen promoting herbs" such as false unicorn *(Chamaelirium luteum)*, the use of which should primarily be avoided in clinical practice because of its endangered status, and wild yam *(Dioscorea villosa)*; however, wild yam is used widely for abdominal and pelvic cramping pain associated with the condition, whereas the late Silena Heron included these in endometriosis protocol and authors Hobbs and Keville, in *Women's Herbs, Women's Health*, mention wild yam as an antispasmodic specifically for endometriosis.[22] There would potentially be numerous plants in this category, ranging from fennel and hops to common foods such as legumes, most of which are rich in phytoestrogens, which would need to be avoided on this presupposition. One study on the estrogenic contents and activity of commonly used herbs found that soy, red clover, licorice, hops, and fo-ti have a large amount of measurable estrogen bioactivity not previously reported. Chaste tree berry, black cohosh, and dong quai did not have measurable activity with the methods used in the study.[120] Confusion stems largely from the fact that so much remains unknown about the endocrine effects of botanicals, and until more information is available, rational conclusions are hard to draw, suggesting that caution and observation of clinical response are required. Women with a predisposition to estrogen-dependent cancers are probably wise to avoid unnecessary and excess consumption of herbs with estrogenic effects. However, it should also be considered that herbs that competitively bind with ERs might displace endogenous estrogen with weaker, plant-based estrogens, decreasing a woman's overall estrogen response.

Black Cohosh

Black cohosh is widely used as an herb for the treatment of many women's health concerns, including climacteric symptoms, neurovegetative menopausal symptoms, and discomforts associated with PMS. Although no studies have been identified addressing black cohosh and endometriosis treatment, recent trial evidence suggests a role for the herb in managing the side effects of conventional medical treatment. A clinical trial of 116 women tested the efficacy of an isopropanolic extract of black cohosh (i.e., Remifemin) compared with tibolone for the treatment of perimenopausal symptoms induced by postoperative GnRH, which is a therapy for endometriosis. The black cohosh extract exhibited comparable reduction in perimenopausal symptoms to tibolone, and with fewer adverse effects (20 mg Remifemin twice daily).[121]

Blue Vervain

Blue vervain (Fig. 11-3) has a long history of use in traditional European herbalism as an emmenagogue and galactagogue, and a contemporary popularity among herbalists experienced in women's reproductive care for its regulating effects on gynecologic complaints, particularly for irritability associated with PMS. A BIOSIS database search and extensive review of the herbal literature references yields very little data on the medicinal uses of this plant, although historical references to its use as a treatment for rheumatism were identified.[30,122] A single study from 1974 on the effect of this herb on the uterus and its interactions with prostaglandins was identified but not obtainable. According to studies cited in Wichtl et al, hot water extracts of European verbena stimulates LH and FSH secretion. Other noted endocrine effects include antithyrotropic and abortifacient effects via inhibition of human chorionic gonadotropin (hCG). Verbena has also demonstrated immunomodulatory effects, primarily through inhibition of phagocytosis by human granulocytes.[30] The German Commission E cites its uses, among other things, for irregular menstruation, nervous disorders and exhaustions, and complaints of the lower urinary tract; however, the efficacy for these claims remains unsubstantiated.[30] Many herbalists consider it an excellent herb for "sluggishness of the liver," and attribute its hormonal action to stimulated liver function and subsequent actions on hormonal metabolism and elimination. It is typically used as a small part of a larger general formula aimed at treating underlying causes of endometriosis.

Chaste Berry

Chaste berry has a reputation for its ability to regulate female menstrual cycles and relieve complaints and complications

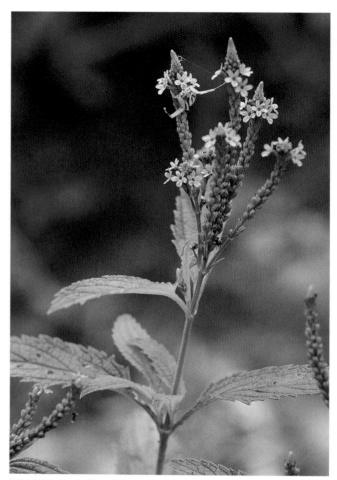

FIGURE 11-3 Blue vervain *(Verbena officinalis)*. (Photo by Martin Wall.)

stemming from dysregulation of sex hormones. Clinical trials support the use of *Vitex agnus-castus* for menstrual irregularities (e.g., secondary amenorrhea, oligomenorrhea, polymenorrhea), and relief of PMS symptoms, mastalgia, latent hyperprolactinemia, and infertility caused by luteal phase dysfunction.[123] The effects of *V. agnus-castus* on estrogen levels remains uncertain, with one study (the full details of which were undisclosed) demonstrating its ability to elicit estrogen-like effects (e.g., increased uterine growth) in ovariectomized rats, and another reporting decreased estradiol levels, whereas other studies have reported no effects or were inconclusive.[123] Its efficacy in the treatment of endometriosis, for which is it widely used by herbalists, is supported by clinical observation, with no research identified for its use for this condition.

Cotton Root

Cotton is predominantly used as a uterine tonic and to stimulate uterine contractions. Gossypol, the active ingredient in the roots and seeds of cotton, has been used in the treatment of gynecologic disorders ranging from uterine myomas to menopausal bleeding, based on the discovery that regular cooking with cottonseed oil over long periods of time leads to amenorrhea and endometrial atrophy in females. Several studies over a 15-year period have demonstrated short-term efficacy of up to almost 90% in the treatment of endometriosis, and long-term effectiveness after 1 to 3 years of 54% to 63%. Treatment is typically accompanied by amenorrhea persisting for up to 6 months in 80% of women, and up to 1 year in 16% of women, with 4% experiencing amenorrhea lasting longer than 1 year.[124] Gossypol is reported to antagonize the actions of estrogen and progesterone, and may mimic a pseudomenopausal state.[124] A frequent side effect of gossypol treatment is hypokalemia, which is treated with administration of slow-releasing potassium salts. High-dose programs can lead to elevated liver enzymes, nausea, edema, and palpitations, as well as possible rash, reduced appetite, fatigue, and possible inhibition of thyroid function and mitochondrial energy metabolism. This compound is not available in the West, and would be considered a pharmaceutical drug rather than a botanical product were it made so. Studies on the use of cotton root bark, used as a partus-preparator, emmenagogue, and abortifacient by Western herbalists, for endometriosis have not been conducted.

Pine Bark Extract

A recent clinical trial tested a proprietary pine bark extract (i.e., Pycnogenol) against a GnRH agonist (i.e., leuprorelin acetate) in the treatment of endometriosis. Fifty-eight women surgically diagnosed with the condition were randomized into treatment groups (i.e., Pycnogenol, 60 mg daily, $n = 32$) and positive controls (i.e., leuprorelin acetate, standard treatment, $n = 26$). Patients were examined at 4, 12, 24, and 48 weeks for "endometriosis signs and symptoms" as well as CA-125 and serum estrogen levels. The treatment group exhibited a consistent but slow decrease in symptom scores and CA-125, but no changes in serum estrogen. The positive control group experienced a quicker decrease in symptom scores accompanied by a significant rebound at week 24. The positive control group also showed a reduction in CA-125, but these levels rebounded as well. Patients with smaller endometriomas responded more favorably to both treatments. The results suggest Pycnogenol to be a promising and longer-lasting alternative to GnRH agonist treatment.[125]

St. John's Wort

According to modern clinical research, St. John's wort is commonly used for the treatment of mild to moderate depression and additionally has been shown to exhibit antiviral activity. In traditional herbal medicine, currently and historically, it is used internally for anxiety and as a general nervous system tonic; externally it is used as a primary application for scrapes and burns. Recent concerns regarding the interaction between St. John's wort and numerous pharmaceutical drugs have led to a host of contraindications for use of this herb. One such contraindication is the use of OCs because it has been shown to induce the activity of CYP 3A4 and increase the clearance of numerous drugs and steroids, such as cortisol and ethinyl estradiol.[126] This interaction suggests the potential for use of St. John's wort to positively interfere with estrogen binding in states of estrogen excess, for example, in endometriosis. A limited number of studies have evaluated the estrogen-binding capacity of St. John's wort extracts. One study by Simmen

et al, found that estrogen binding was 50% inhibited by the bioflavonoid I3,II8-biapigenin at micromolar concentration in the central nervous system (CNS).[127] Use of St. John's wort to deliberately modulate estrogen levels represents a potentially novel application for this botanical. This herb should also be considered in endometriosis treatment for its beneficial role in the treatment of mild to moderate depression, which may accompany this condition in women who suffer with it chronically.

Hepatics, Aperients, and Cholagogues

The use of herbs to improve hepatic function and affect the improved metabolism and elimination of excess hormones has been discussed throughout this text. Herbs for these purposes are commonly included in many gynecologic formulae in which there is estrogen dominance or excess, including endometriosis. Popular choices include calendula, fringe tree, tumeric, rosemary, schisandra, milk thistle, and dandelion root. Mechanisms of action are not clearly elucidated for many of these herbs, but likely include increased bile release, leading to enhanced bowel elimination of estrogens, increased CYP activity, and improved liver health through antioxidant activity.

Uterotonics and Emmenagogues

Although the effect of uterotonic herbs, commonly included by herbalists in formulae for endometriosis, on endometrial tissue outside the uterus is dubious, uterotonic herbs may play a role in reducing retrograde menstruation via tonic and expulsive action, or other unknown mechanisms, for example, unidentified hormonal actions. Herbs that are commonly included as uterotonics in endometriosis formulae include blue cohosh, Lady's mantle, and yarrow.

CASE HISTORIES: ENDOMETRIOSIS

Endometriosis Patient 1

Lori, 35, is a highly stressed lawyer who smokes and experiences moderate to severe pain associated with endometriosis. She plans to quit smoking as soon as she gets a new job, marries, and moves this year. She hopes to have children soon after.

Tincture Formula I (Ovulation Through End of Menses)

Black haw	(Viburnum prunifolium)	25 mL
Blue vervain	(Verbena officinalis)	25 mL
Chaste berry	(Vitex agnus-castus)	12.5 mL
Corydalis	(Corydalis ambigua)	12.5 mL
Milky oats	(Avena sativa)	12.5 mL
Yarrow	(Achillea millefolium)	12.5 mL
		Total: 100 mL

Dose: 5 mL diluted in ¼ cup water three times daily.

Tincture Formula II (End of Menses to Ovulation)

St. John's wort	(Hypericum perforatum)	30 mL
Chaste berry	(Vitex agnus-castus)	25 mL
White peony	(Paeonia lactiflora)	20 mL
Calendula	(Calendula officinalis)	12.5 mL
Partridge berry	(Mitchella repens)	12.5 mL
		Total: 100 mL

Continued

CASE HISTORIES: ENDOMETRIOSIS—cont'd

Dose: 5 mL diluted in ¼ cup water three times daily.

Endometriosis Patient 2
Karen is a 21-year-old with no previous history of reproductive problems. After acute abdominal pain she was diagnosed with endometriosis by ultrasound, but decided against medication or surgery. She has abdominal pain and bloating, with spotting and heavy menstruation.

Tincture Formula I (Ovulation Through End of Menses)

Cramp bark	(Viburnum opulus)	25 mL
Blue vervain	(Verbena officinalis)	25 mL
Ashwagandha	(Withania somnifera)	25 mL
Chaste berry	(Vitex agnus-castus)	12.5 mL
Black cohosh	(Actaea racemosa)	12.5 mL
		Total: 100 mL

Dose: 5 mL diluted in ¼ cup water three times daily.

Tincture Formula II (End of Menses to Ovulation)

Chaste berry	(Vitex agnus-castus)	20 mL
Milk thistle	(Silybum marianum)	20 mL
Wild yam	(Dioscorea villosa)	20 mL
Blue cohosh	(Caulophyllum thalictroides)	20 mL
Sarsaparilla	(Smilax ornata)	10 mL
Partridge berry	(Mitchella repens)	10 mL
Valerian	(Valeriana officinalis)	10 mL
		Total: 110 mL

Dose: 5 mL diluted in ¼ cup water three times daily.

NUTRITIONAL CONSIDERATIONS

Fatty Acid Supplements

In addition to a balanced whole foods diet, use high-quality oils and minimize consumption of caffeine, sugar, alcohol, red meat, and large amounts of dairy. Also avoid excess refined carbohydrates, and address hypoglycemia with frequent small meals and snacks with high protein and complex carbohydrates. Adequate consumption of EFAs is important; encourage two to three servings of salmon or other high-quality cold-water fish per week. Fatty acid–mediated mechanisms have demonstrated decreased cytokine-induced adhesion molecule expression, thereby reducing inflammatory leukocyte–endothelium interactions and modified lipid mediator synthesis, influencing the transendothelial migration of leukocytes and leukocyte trafficking in general. Even the metabolic repertoire of specific immunocompetent cells such as cytokine release or proliferation is modified by n-3 fatty acids. Beyond this, fatty acids regulate lipid homeostasis, shifting the metabolic pathways toward energy supply, thus optimizing the function of immune cells. Because of the regulatory effect on different processes of inflammatory and immune cell activation, n-3 fatty acids provide positive effects on various states of immune deficiencies and diseases with a hyperinflammatory character, among which selected examples are presented.[128]

Choose between:*
EPO: 3 g/day (may be cost prohibitive to some)
Omega-3: 600 mg EPA
Flax oil: ⅛ tsp to 1 Tbsp daily
Flax seed oil starting at ⅛ tsp doses, up to 1 tsp per dose or more as individuals can tolerate.

B vitamin supplementation may assist in hepatic metabolism of estrogens and are recommended as part of an overall multivitamin and mineral supplement.

Melatonin

A phase 2 clinical trial tested melatonin for the treatment of endometriosis. Forty women were randomized into equal placebo control and 10 mg melatonin treatment groups for a period of 8 weeks. The main outcomes were pain scores determined by VAS. The treatment group demonstrated a 39.80% reduction in daily pain and a 38.01% reduction in dysmenorrhea (both with 95% confidence interval [CI]). Melatonin also reduced brain-derived neurotrophic factor (BDNF) levels and improved sleep quality.[129]

N-acetylcysteine

A 2013 observational cohort study tested N-acetyl-cysteine (NAC) for endometriosis treatment. Patients were selected for inclusion that had diagnosis confirmed by ultrasound, had not received hormonal treatment in the previous 2 months, and were scheduled for laparoscopic surgery in 3 months. Ninety-two women met the criteria and were randomized to receive 600 mg NAC 3 times daily for 3 consecutive days per week ($n = 47$). The control group ($n = 45$) did not receive any treatment (but the physicians were blinded). After 3 months of observation and examination, the NAC group experienced a mean decrease in cyst diameter (−1.5 mm), whereas controls experienced a significant increase. Twenty-one NAC-treated women reported a reduction in pain, and eight women experienced a complete disappearance in cysts. Additionally, 24 women in the treated group cancelled surgery because of decrease in cysts or pain (versus one woman in the control group), and there were eight subsequent pregnancies in the treated group (six in the control group).[130]

ADDITIONAL THERAPIES

Lifestyle Management

Provide counseling to address psychosocial issues; suggest stress reduction techniques (e.g., yoga, meditation, counseling, visualization).

Exercise

Regular exercise, such as yoga, to reduce pelvic tension and improve suppleness, as well as relieve general tension and fatigue, should be encouraged.

---

*When taking fatty acid supplements, it is important to increase antioxidant intake.

TREATMENT SUMMARY FOR ENDOMETRIOSIS

- Improve nonspecific immunity with adaptogens and immunomodulators.
- Reduce inflammation.
- Improve organ and tissue health where possible using uterine tonics.
- Decrease exposure to xenoestrogens.
- Decrease relative excess of estrogen.
- Increase liver function for hormone metabolism, from cholesterol synthesis to steroidal catabolism.
- Manage pain using antispasmodics.

CHRONIC PELVIC PAIN

CPP is defined as pelvic pain lasting longer than 6 months. Some authors add the additional criteria that the pain be noncyclic.[131] It is one of the most common presenting complaints in gynecologic practice, affecting as many as one in seven American women. CPP causes up to 10% of outpatient gynecologic visits, accounts for 20% of laparoscopies, and results in 12% (75,000/year) of all hysterectomies performed annually in the United States.[132] Estimated annual direct medical costs for outpatient visits for CPP in the United States among women 18 to 50 years old is estimated to be $881.5 million. It is often an extremely frustrating condition for both patient and care provider because in many cases an etiology cannot be identified and there is no apparent pathology. Treatment of presumed underlying conditions is frequently ineffective, and the "pain itself becomes the illness."[132] Because the cause often cannot be identified, CPP is frequently attributed to psychogenic causes. Although these may play a role in CPP for some women with lack of an identifiable cause, this does not necessarily equate with a psychosomatic origin for this complaint.[133]

Common causes of CPP include endometriosis, pelvic inflammatory disease (PID), adhesions, ovarian remnant syndrome, pelvic congestion syndrome, and cyclic uterine pain, which may be caused by primary or secondary dysmenorrhea, uterine myomata, and adenomyosis. History of psychosexual trauma is common in women diagnosed with CPP.[134] CPP is frequently associated with systemic inflammation, including autoimmune diseases. Peritoneal chronic inflammation is sometimes also associated. A study of chronic pain reveals that the immune system is intimately involved in the production, conduction, and exacerbation of pain and of its clinical features, such as hyperalgesia and allodynia.[135]

Not all pelvic pain is of gynecologic origin; other conditions must be ruled out. Genitourinary pain (e.g., because of interstitial cystitis, urethral syndrome, or overactive bladder), GI pain (e.g., irritable bowel syndrome [IBS], bowel obstruction, bowel neoplasm), and neuromuscular pain are also common causes of CPP. CPP may be intermittent or continual. Pain is affected by physical and mental fatigue, as well as stress. It may lead to depression and anxiety, dyspareunia (i.e., painful sex/intercourse), difficulties with sleep, decreased ability to work and enjoy normal activities, and may be a contributing factor in job loss, relationship dysfunction, and divorce.[136-138]

SYMPTOMS

Symptoms associated with CPP include:
- Anxiety and depression
- Constipation or diarrhea
- Dysmenorrhea
- Dyspareunia (i.e., painful and difficult intercourse/vaginal penetration)
- Family/relationship problems
- Fatigue
- Leg pain radiating from the groin
- Loss of interest in social activities
- Lower back pain and a feeling of heaviness in the lower abdomen
- Menstrual irregularity
- Persistent pain despite multiple treatments
- Reduced libido
- Sleep disruption
- Spasms of the vaginal and/or pelvic floor muscles
- Substance use/abuse

DIAGNOSIS

Diagnosis of CPP is based on identifying the underlying cause(s). It also may be a diagnosis of exclusion, with no identifiable etiology. Careful attention should be paid to the history and physical examination, particularly a thorough pelvic examination to evaluate for tenderness, pelvic mass, adhesions, or prolapse. Testing may include ultrasound, laparoscopic examination, pregnancy test, complete blood count (CBC), vaginal and cervical cultures, Pap smear, evaluation for GI disorders, and urologic examination.

DIFFERENTIAL DIAGNOSIS

Differential diagnosis in CPP is really a matter of identifying the possible causes of pain (Table 11-5), treating the etiology, and addressing the pain and concomitant symptoms. In patients younger than 30 years of age, the most common causes of pelvic pain include endometriosis and PID; in older women, causes most likely include uterine myoma, adenomyosis, or pelvic relaxation. It is critical to rule out any serious or life-threatening causes, as well as to assess for depression, anxiety, and serious mental health disorders.

CONVENTIONAL TREATMENT APPROACHES

The choice of medical treatment for CPP depends on the etiology of the pain, thus necessitating careful diagnosis. Treatment of underlying conditions is the primary treatment strategy. However, in one third of cases, no etiology is identified. Sympathetic and supportive care is critical, with reassurance and validation of the woman's symptoms essential, especially in the absence of an identifiable cause.[133] The pain should be treated as a real problem. Multidisciplinary team management of CPP may be the most productive strategy, including the expertise of a gynecologist, a psychologist with expertise in sexual and relationship counseling, and also possibly an acupuncturist for pain management, in addition to the appropriate specialists for the underlying cause.[133,139] Treatment with medication includes the use of NSAIDs, antidepressants for depression and sleep disorders, and hormonal therapies (e.g., OCs for management of cyclic pain or GnRH-As for pain associated with endometriosis or uterine fibroids). Trigger point injections of local anesthetics has proved helpful for prolonged pain relief in some patients, as has transcutaneous electrical nerve stimulation (TENS) therapy.[140] Acupuncture has been used with good results in the treatment of dysmenorrhea, and may be beneficial in pain reduction for CPP.[140] Immune modification using steroids and disease-modifying antirheumatic drugs, such as hydroxychloroquine, are known to inhibit inflammatory cells and cytokines, such as IL-1, IL-6, and TNF, which are responsible for pain and tissue damage. These drugs are found to be effective in the treatment of CPP of an inflammatory nature and for symptomatic chronic inflammation of the vagina.[135,140] Surgical interventions include laparoscopy for the lysis of pelvic adhesions or removal of endometrial tissue,

or hysterectomy. Although hysterectomy without an associated pathology has not proved effective, it is nonetheless indicated as a reason for hysterectomy in 10% to 15% of those performed in the United States.[133] According to one study, 25% of hysterectomy patients reported persistent pain 1 year after surgery.[132]

BOTANICAL TREATMENT

Effective botanical treatment of CPP requires a clear understanding of possible etiologies and the appropriate treatment of the underlying cause of the pain. For patients with diagnosed gynecologic conditions associated with pelvic pain, readers are referred to the relevant chapters in this textbook, such as dysmenorrhea, interstitial cystitis, uterine fibroids, endometriosis, and so forth. Treatments discussed in the following may be used as adjunct palliative therapies for pain, inflammation, and concomitant symptoms in these conditions.

In the absence of a clearly identified pathology, the practitioner can approach treatment symptomatically via specific botanical treatments for pain reduction, and attempt to address mechanisms that may be associated with CPP, for example, inflammation. One theory of CPP that was popular among physicians in the early- and mid-twentieth century, and that is still considered a possibility, is that of "pelvic congestion syndrome."[8,132,140,141]

TABLE 11-5	Common Causes of Chronic Pelvic Pain		
Classification	**Conditions**	**Classification**	**Conditions**
Gynecologic	Abortion	Musculoskeletal/	Arthritis
	Adhesions	Neurologic	Coccydynia
	Adnexal torsion		Conus medullaris lesions
	Chronic salpingitis		Degenerative joint disease
	Dysmenorrhea		Fibromyalgia
	Ectopic pregnancy		Fractures
	Endometriosis		Lower back problems
	Mittelschmerz		Multiple sclerosis
	Pelvic congestion		Nerve entrapment syndromes
	Pelvic infection		Neuromuscular disorders
	Ruptured ovarian cyst		Pelvic floor spasm
	Salpingitis		Poor posture
	Uterine fibroids		Vertebral disk disorder
	Uterine prolapse/pelvic relaxation	Psychogenic	Abuse
Gastrointestinal	Appendicitis		Clinical depression
	Chronic appendicitis		Hypochondriasis
	Constipation		Pain medication seeking
	Diverticulosis		Physical or sexual abuse
	Enterocolitis		Premenstrual dysphoric disorder
	Gastroenteritis/Spastic colon		Psychiatric disorders
	Inflammatory bowel disease		Psychosocial stress
	Irritable bowel syndrome		Sleep disturbances
	Neoplasia		Substance abuse
	Ulcerative colitis	Other	Calcium/magnesium deficiencies
Urologic	Chronic cystitis		Hyperparathyroidism
	Detrusor hyperactivity		Trauma
	Interstitial cystitis		
	Ureteral calculus		

Data from Forrest D: Common gynecologic pelvic disorders. In Youngkin E, Davis M, editors: *Women's health: a primary care clinical guide*, Stamford, 1998, Appleton and Lange, pp 313–362; Ryder R: Chronic pelvic pain, *Am Fam Physician* 54(7):2225–2232, 1995; Ostrzens A: *Gynecology: integrating conventional, complementary, and natural alternative therapy*, Philadelphia, 2002, Lippincott Williams & Wilkins.

Women with this syndrome, which is poorly defined, are thought to exhibit many of the symptoms associated with CPP, including aching and dragging sensations in the lower back, lower abdomen, and pelvis, dysmenorrhea, and dyspareunia. The theory of pelvic congestion parallels Chinese medical theory regarding various forms of gynecologic pain. Pelvic vascular congestion is thought to be a dynamic vascular process, similar to migraine headache, with drug inducible (i.e., dihydroergotamine [DHE] injection) reversibility of vascular dilatation.[140] As with CPP, symptoms are commonly accompanied by depression, fatigue, and insomnia. Upon pelvic examination or laparoscopy, the uterus may be found to be enlarged and tender and the pelvic vessels engorged. However, there is no direct correlation between vessel engorgement and pain; some women have either pain without engorgement or vice versa.[8] Herbalists may include herbs in a formula to tonify and astringe the uterus and pelvic vessels, ostensibly to reduce pelvic congestion. Psychogenic causes may contribute to CPP. Although this should not be overemphasized, it should also not be overlooked. Chronic pain can affect nearly every aspect of a patient's life: physically, mentally, emotionally, socially, and even economically. Because chronic pain can lead to depression and anxiety, as well as to sleep disturbance, which can create a vicious cycle of psychoemotional upset and increased pain, care should be taken to approach pain holistically. Include herbs in the protocol that are restorative to the nervous system, for example, adaptogens and nervines, and when needed, anxiolytics or antidepressants.

IBS and inflammatory bowel syndromes are highly associated with CPP. Herbs commonly used for the treatment of CPP are listed in Table 11-6. Many of these herbs are discussed elsewhere in this book.

Analgesia

The history of botanical medicine reveals many herbs that have been used for the treatment of a variety of types of pain.[142] Many traditional medicines have actions such as inhibition of PAF, COX, prostaglandin formation, or AA pathways.[143] Although not typically as fast acting as conventional medications, repeated appropriate dosing over a short period of time, such as 1 to 2 hours, and continued as needed, often leads to satisfactory temporary alleviation of pain. Several herbs are reputed for their efficacy in the treatment of pain of gynecologic origin, as well as more generally (see Dysmenorrhea).

Black Cohosh

Black cohosh has historically been used by northeastern Native American tribes as an analgesic and as an emmenagogue.[144] The Eclectics used a resin of black cohosh specifically as a uterine tonic and in the treatment of dysmenorrhea and a number of other painful spasmodic or cramping gynecologic complaints.[145] It was also used in the treatment of deep muscle drawing in the legs, loins, and back, dull aching of the bowels, ovarian pains of a dull, aching quality, dragging uterine pain, and delayed menses with dull pain and

TABLE 11-6 Botanical Treatment Strategies for Chronic Pelvic Pain

Therapeutic Goal	Therapeutic Activity	Botanical Name	Common Name
Pain relief	Analgesia	*Actaea racemosa*	Black cohosh
		Anemone pulsatilla	Pulsatilla
		Corydalis ambigua	Corydalis
		Eschscholzia californica	California poppy
		Piper methysticum	Kava kava
		Piscidia piscipula	Jamaican dogwood
		Viburnum spp.	Cramp bark, black haw
		Also see Dysmenorrhea	
Relief of pelvic muscle spasm	Antispasmodics	*Achillea millefolium*	Yarrow
		Actaea racemosa	Black cohosh
		Angelica sinensis	Dong quai
		Cannabis spp.	Marijuana
		Dioscorea villosa	Wild yam
		Leonurus cardiaca	Motherwort
		Paeonia lactiflora	White peony
		Rehmannia glutinosa	Rehmannia
		Viburnum spp.	Cramp bark, black haw
		Zingiber officinale	Ginger
		Also see Dysmenorrhea	
Treatment of depression and anxiety	Antidepressants Anxiolytics	*Hypericum perforatum*	St. John's wort
		Lavandula officinalis	Lavender
		Leonurus cardiaca	Motherwort
		Matricaria recutita	Chamomile
		Melissa officinalis	Lemon balm
		Piper methysticum	Kava kava
		Also see Chapter 11	

Continued

TABLE 11-6	Botanical Treatment Strategies for Chronic Pelvic Pain—cont'd		
Therapeutic Goal	**Therapeutic Activity**	**Botanical Name**	**Common Name**
Nervous system support	Adaptogens	*Cordyceps sinensis*	Cordyceps
		Eleutherococcus senticosus	Eleuthero
		Panax quinquefolius	American ginseng
		Rhodiola rosea	Rhodiola
		Withania somnifera	Ashwagandha
		Also see Stress, Adaptation, the Hypothalamic-Pituitary-Adrenal Axis and Women's Health	
Reduce inflammation	Antiinflammatories	*Angelica sinensis*	Dong quai
		Glycyrrhiza glabra	Licorice
		Oenothera biennis	Evening primrose oil
		Paeonia lactiflora	White peony
		Salix spp.	Willow
		Tanacetum parthenium	Feverfew
		Zingiber officinale	Ginger
Digestive support; treatment of IBS and inflammatory bowel syndrome	Antispasmodics	*Achillea millefolium*	Yarrow
		Dioscorea villosa	Wild yam
		Matricaria recutita	Chamomile
		Mentha piperita	Peppermint
	Astringents	*Achillea millefolium*	Yarrow
		Hydrastis canadensis	Goldenseal
	Carminatives	*Matricaria recutita*	Chamomile
		Mentha piperita	Peppermint
		Pimpinella anisum	Anise
	Demulcents	*Althea officinalis*	Marshmallow
		Ulmus rubra	Slippery elm
	Laxatives	*Glycyrrhiza glabra*	Licorice
		Rumex crispus	Yellow dock
		Taraxacum officinale	Dandelion root
Treat insomnia/sleep disorders	Anxiolytics	*Anemone pulsatilla*	Pulsatilla
	Nervines	*Piper methysticum*	Kava kava
	Sedatives	*Eschscholzia californica*	California poppy
		Also see Chapter 5	
Treat possible pelvic congestion syndrome	Uterine tonics	*Aesculus hippocastanum*	Horse chestnut
	Venotonics	*Alchemilla vulgaris*	Lady's mantle
		Caulophyllum thalictroides	Blue cohosh
		Hydrastis canadensis	Goldenseal
		Mitchella repens	Partridge berry
		Rubus idaeus	Red raspberry
		Viburnum spp.	Cramp bark, black haw

IBS, Irritable bowel syndrome.

muscle soreness. Felter specifically describes a condition called "rheumatism of the uterus" for which this herb was prescribed.[105] The plant's antiinflammatory and analgesic properties are attributed to its aromatic acids, which appear to inhibit prostaglandin production. The herb is approved for use in Germany for the treatment of premenstrual discomfort and menstrual cycle pain.[26]

California Poppy

California poppy (Fig. 11-4) traditionally has been prescribed for reducing pain and producing calm sleep without the potential dangers of conventional opiate drugs. It may be useful for

painful conditions in which there is irritation or stimulation of afferent pain fibers, in disturbed sleep, and for anxiety.[114] Its medical use as an analgesic and sedative in the United States dates as far back as the late nineteenth century, even being included in the Parke-Davis catalog for these purposes, and as an excellent alternative to morphine without its side effects.[114,145] Today, California poppy is widely used by herbalists in tincture form. Pharmacologic data demonstrate sedative activity in vivo, as well as gamma (γ)-aminobutyric acid (GABA)-ergic activity, sedative and anxiolytic action, and dose-dependent analgesia (i.e., when administered by injection). In two controlled clinical trials, standardized extracts of California poppy

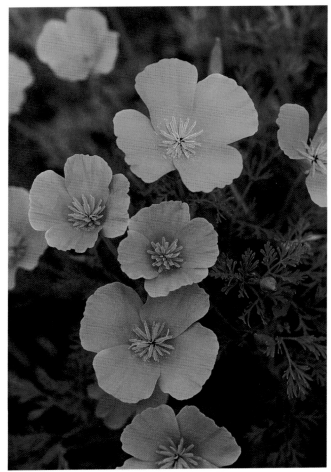

FIGURE 11-4 California poppy *(Eschscholzia californica).* (Photo by Martin Wall.)

and *Corydalis cava* demonstrated normalization of disturbed sleep without carryover effects or addiction.[114]

Corydalis

The Chinese botanical corydalis is a strong and reliable analgesic. It is commonly used for headache, lumbar pain, abdominal pain, joint pain, menstrual pain, and other neurologic pain, making it specific for the symptoms associated with CPP. Alcohol and acetic acid extractions are the strongest, although powdered herb is considered effective as well. The mechanism of action of analgesia is thought to be inhibition of the reticular-activating system in the brainstem. Corydalis can increase the pain threshold significantly. Continuous use of corydalis results in tolerance and may theoretically lead to a cross-tolerance to morphine.[146,147] However, from a Chinese medical perspective the effects of corydalis are more than palliative because it is used to help promote pelvic circulation and therefore may treat underlying pelvic congestion. The alkaloids in this herb have sedative and hypnotic effects and act synergistically with barbiturates.[146] Chinese pharmaceutical companies have produced several preparations from corydalis alkaloids for use as analgesics. The available preparations include a 30-mg tablet containing all alkaloids

and a 10% tincture used in doses of 5 mL three times daily.[146] Overdose leads to muscle relaxation and CNS depression. Corydalis is contraindicated in pregnancy.[32,146,147]

Cramp Bark and Black Haw

Cramp bark and black haw were similarly used for the treatment of pelvic pain, particularly of a spasmodic nature, and specifically when accompanied by a sensation of dragging pressure in the groin and drawing pain in the legs.[32,145]

Jamaican Dogwood

Jamaican dogwood is a reliable analgesic and spasmolytic herb with mild sedative properties. It was prescribed by the Eclectics for neuralgias, spasmodic complaints, migraines, dysmenorrhea, nervous tension, insomnia, and nervous excitability, although Felter cautioned about potential toxic effects (including convulsions) in large doses.[105] Ellingwood elaborated on its effects in quieting uterine pains of labor, promoting rest, and having a specifically relaxing influence in addition to its general analgesic effects. He stated that the herb "acts in close harmony with the vegetable uterine remedies, promoting the influence of Macrotys [*Actaea racemosa*-black cohosh], the viburnums … pulsatilla and dioscorea among others."[31] The spasmolytic activity of Jamaican dogwood may be attributable to its isoflavone constituents; however, this plant has been only minimally studied.[147] Combined in equal parts with cramp bark or black cohosh, I have found it a highly effective treatment for gynecologic and pelvic pain of neuromuscular origin, for dysmenorrhea, endometrial pain, urinary tract infection (UTI), and other pelvic pain. It also may be used postsurgically as an alternative to conventional pain medications. Regarding its toxicity, it is advisable that the recommended dosage range not be exceeded and that the herb not be used by pregnant women or patients with bradycardia or cardiac insufficiency (see Appendix I).[114]

Kava Kava

Kava kava has been used traditionally as a muscle relaxant and to reduce anxiety, and may be considered for the treatment of muscle spasms associated with CPP. Both aqueous and lipid soluble extracts of kava have demonstrated antinociceptive activity through nonopiate receptor mechanisms.[149] It is commonly used by herbalists for the treatment of pain as well as anxiety.

Pulsatilla

Pulsatilla (Fig. 11-5), also called pasque flower, has analgesic and sedative properties. It is listed in the *British Herbal Compendium* for the treatment of painful spasmodic conditions of the female reproductive systems and dysmenorrhea. It is generally used in tincture form. Fresh herb contains potential irritant and toxic compounds; therefore only dried plant should be used, and the herb should not be used during pregnancy. Overdose can lead to gastric irritation, coma, and convulsions; thus it is essential that patients stay within the proper dosage range, and use be monitored by an experienced practitioner.[26,114] This herb is more commonly prescribed by naturopathic practitioners than herbalists in the United States, although it is also used by European herbalists.

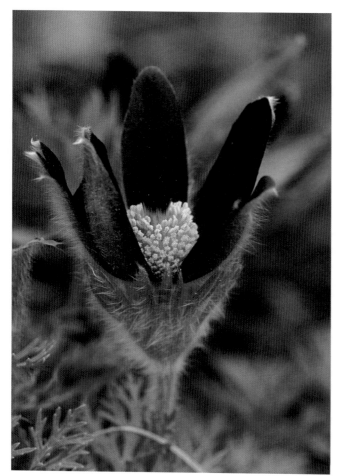

FIGURE 11-5 Pulsatilla *(Anemone pulsatilla).* (Photo by Martin Wall.)

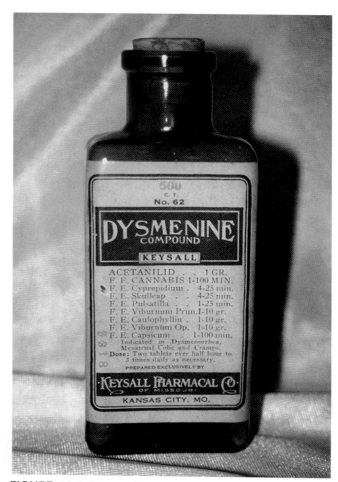

FIGURE 11-6 Dysmenine compound; old pharmacy bottle. (Photo by Ethan Russo.)

Black Cohosh, Cramp Bark, and Black Haw

Black cohosh, cramp bark, and black haw are traditionally used as uterine antispasmodics and analgesics, and are discussed throughout this text for these properties. This three-herb combination administered as a tincture is especially effective for the treatment of pelvic aching and pain.

Dong Quai and Peony

Dong quai and peony, in addition to their significant analgesic and spasmolytic actions, are considered herbs that "move blood" and relieve stasis or stagnation in TCM.[97,150-152] The TCM concept of uterine stasis is consistent with the Western concept of pelvic congestion syndrome described in the preceding. Additionally, these herbs, often used together in combination, and often with the addition of licorice (*Glycyrrhiza glabra* or *G. uralensis*) are considered effective for the treatment of a number of gynecologic conditions that may be involved in the etiology of CPP, such as dysmenorrhea, polycystic ovarian syndrome (PCOS), and uterine fibroids. The Japanese traditional formula TJ-68, Shakuyaku-Kanzo-To (Chinese: Shao-Yao-Gan-Cao-Tang), which contains concentrated white peony root and licorice, has been approved by the Japanese government for clinical use in the treatment of pain and acute muscle spasm, including dysmenorrhea.[114]

Marijuana

One herb not available widely (or at least, legally available) for clinical use that has clinically demonstrated significant uterine antispasmodic and analgesic effects is *Cannabis indica,* more commonly referred to as marijuana. This controversial medicinal plant and recreationally used herb has a long history of use for relief of uterine spasms and dysmenorrhea, considered by the Eclectics to be a "soothing uterine tonic."[31] In fact, its use is ancient, with references and artifacts of its use found widely in Middle Eastern, Ayurvedic, and Semitic writings, continuing through to its medical use in Europe well into the late nineteenth century; it was used to treat a variety of gynecologic and obstetric conditions including, but not limited to, dysmenorrhea. A pharmaceutical product from the late nineteenth century, Dysmenine Compound, produced by the Keysall Pharmical Company, Kansas City, MO, contained *Cannabis, Cypripedium, Scutellaria, Pulsatilla, Viburnum prunifolium, Caulophyllum, Viburnum opulus,* and *Capsicum* (Fig. 11-6). The compound was indicated for dysmenorrhea, menstrual colic, and cramps.[153] Indeed, this formula is not very different from one that might be prescribed by herbalists today (see sample formulae in the following) without the now illegal cannabis and the ecologically endangered lady's slipper orchid *(Cypripedium).* Although it is not possible to prescribe this herb clinically given the current legal–medical climate surrounding its use, it is worthwhile to note its use and possible beneficial effects; these have likely not escaped the notice of those who manage to procure it for self-medication of chronic or cyclic pelvic pain. Russo et al in *Women and Cannabis: Medicine, Science, and Sociology,* provide substantial evidence of its use. They cited Grinspoon and Bakalar's 1993 book *Marihuana, The Forbidden Medicine,* a discussion of numerous case studies of women using cannabis effectively to treat PMS, menstrual cramps, and labor pain; when used at low doses, there were not cognitive impairments. They also cited an Australian study of the uses of cannabis for obstetric and gynecologic complaints in which 51% of respondents indicated use for PMS or dysmenorrhea. Discussing this herb's appropriate use with patients, outside the context of prescribing or condoning its use, is therefore possibly important and appropriate. The mechanisms of action appear to be primarily through antiinflammatory activities. An interesting approach for inflammation-mediated pelvic pain is the use of the seeds of the hemp plants, which are notably rich in gamma (γ)-linolenic acid—something found to be low in women with PMS and dysmenorrhea. In one study, a daily dose of 150 to 200 mg of γ-linolenic acid over 12 weeks greatly improved PMS–related symptoms; this dose could be provided by a 5-mL daily dose of hemp seed oil.[153]

Motherwort

Motherwort *(Leonurus cardiaca)* is a classic herb for the treatment of pelvic pain. Its actions appear to modulate both relaxant and contractile activity of the uterus, perhaps with an overall effect of regulating a balance between the two for effective uterine muscle activity. The commonly used Western species *L. cardiaca* has barely been evaluated for its effects in gynecology, whereas Chinese species have been evaluated in several investigations and have been found to have stimulating effects on the myometrium in vivo. The effect on the uterine smooth muscle may be related to alteration of the ion concentration in relation to myoelectric activity, resulting in the increase of myoelectric activity of pace setter cells as well as in the acceleration of depolarization of spike activity.[154] Leonurine, a plant alkaloid present in Chinese motherwort, has demonstrated some efficacy as a vascular smooth tone inhibitor, possibly through inhibition of Ca^{2+} influx and the release of intracellular Ca^{2+}.[155] It is uncertain whether these findings and effects can be extrapolated to effects on uterine vascular tone. Other studies have demonstrated interesting effects on mediators of the inflammatory and coagulation pathways in relationship to coronary blood flow and alleviation of stasis; this may have some correlation to the use of this herb in both TCM and Western herbal medicine to alleviate pelvic congestion (in TCM "blood stasis" or "stagnation"). In one study of 105 patients, 94.5% showed improvements in reduction in blood viscosity and fibrinogen content, important for healthy blood flow and also in preventing release of inflammatory compounds associated with clot formation.[156] A Russian study reported on the soporific activity of a combination of equal parts of valerian, motherwort, and hawthorn (*Crataegus* spp.) in tincture form. This combination prolonged the soporific effect of sodium ethaminal.[157] The effects of motherwort *(L. cardiaca)* for the treatment of spasmodic uterine pain and pelvic congestion are predicated on historical and contemporary clinical use, for which it remains a popular choice in gynecologic formulae.

Wild Yam and Ginger

Wild yam and ginger are considered important herbs to include in the treatment of CPP, especially when it is associated with irritable bowel–type complaints. They are both effective for treating spasmodic uterine complaints and, in the case of ginger, inflammation; they exert these actions in the digestive system, thus addressing what may be causal associations or concomitant conditions that are mutually exacerbating.[26,114] These herbs may be used in combination in capsule or tincture form, and may be included in formulae with other herbs.

Yarrow

Yarrow, a favorite herb of many herbalists, has the interesting characteristic of being considered an effective antispasmodic for painful, cramplike conditions of psychosomatic origin in the lower pelvis in women when used as a sitz bath.[101] It is also used for dyspeptic complaints, including mild, spastic discomforts of the GI tract. This combination of qualities makes it a particularly interesting herb to consider for the treatment of CPP, especially when of psychogenic origin or when occurring in conjunction with or as a result of irritable bowel disorders.

Antidepressants and Anxiolytics

Herbs of note that possess both antidepressant or anxiolytic activity, as well as analgesic or antispasmodic activity, include St. John's wort, kava kava, motherwort, and ashwagandha, the latter of which is also a respected adaptogen and whose analgesic effects are discussed elsewhere in this text. Gentle nervines that are commonly used as adjunct teas in the treatment of mild depression include chamomile, lemon balm, and lavender. Lavender also may be used externally in baths for its soothing aromatherapeutic effects, as well as for mild topical analgesia for the vulva.

Adaptogens

The use of adaptogens in the treatment of CPP is primarily for the reduction of stress and anxiety, modulation of inflammation, and improvement of sleep disorders. They are part of a long-term treatment plan rather than quick-acting for specific symptoms (see Chapter 5). Ashwagandha has specific analgesic activity, and is among the most specific of choices for CPP.

Antiinflammatories
Dong Quai

Dong quai possesses antispasmodic, analgesic, antiinflammatory, antioxidant, uterine tonic, and specific immunomodulatory effects. Immunostimulatory and antiinflammatory effects have been attributed to isolated ferulic acid. It has been used traditionally in Chinese medicine for the treatment of "blood vacuity" and "blood stasis," which may be considered related to CPP.[99]

Evening Primrose Oil

It is thought that the use of EPO, with its high γ-linoleic acid content, may preferentially promote the synthesis of antiinflammatory prostaglandin series over inflammatory prostaglandins. One critical review of the effects of EPO for the treatment of PMS concluded that there was no benefit. However, in a study of women ($n = 40$) who experienced symptoms of IBS just before and at the onset of menstruation, 53% reported an improvement in symptoms, whereas no improvement was seen in the placebo group. Improvement generally took 2 to 3 months to become apparent. Blood analysis at the beginning and end of treatment revealed significant improvement in fatty acid imbalances in the EPO–treated group.[149]

Feverfew

Feverfew has exhibited inhibition of prostaglandin synthetase, preventing the conversion of AA to prostaglandins; it inhibits mast cell degranulation and subsequent histamine and serotonin release; and it has shown inhibition of other inflammatory cytokines such as TNF-α, IL-1, NFκB, and IFN-γ, as well as inhibiting peritoneal COX in animal models.[103] These effects suggest possible application of this herb to treat pain related to inflammation in CPP.

Ginger

Herbalists commonly use ginger root as an antiinflammatory and antispasmodic herb for the treatment of pelvic pain and congestion, as an infusion, and also in hip baths and hot compresses over the affected area. No studies have been identified for its use for gynecologic complaints. Ginger remains popular among Western and TCM herbalists as an antispasmodic treatment for dysmenorrhea; however, no clinical trials have been done to evaluate its efficacy.[26] Ginger's historical use for treatment of digestive disorders may be applicable for women with concurrent abdominal discomfort resulting from digestive complaints.

Licorice

Licorice root is commonly included in formulae when an antiinflammatory herb is indicated. It may be considered to have effective antiinflammatory activity without many of the most troubling side effects seen for drugs used as COX-2 and 5-LO inhibitors.[117] However, high doses of licorice may exacerbate hypertension.

Peony and Rehmannia

Two herbs commonly used in TCM formulae, peony and rehmannia, have demonstrated significant antiinflammatory and antispasmodic activity.[22,26,114] Studies using a traditional formula containing both herbs have demonstrated prostaglandin production inhibition in the uterine myometrium via phospholipase A2 inhibition, whereas other studies have demonstrated AA inhibition, PAF inhibition, reduction in free radical formation, and smooth muscle relaxation. Note that nearly all of the studies use these herbs in traditional formulae rather than in isolation, and that studies are conducted in animal models, and have focused on arthritis, ulcers, and other chronic inflammatory conditions. Licorice is frequently included in TCM formulae that also contain peony and rehmannia, as is dong quai when these herbs are used for gynecologic conditions.

Uterine Tonics: Venotonics

Treatment of pelvic congestion syndrome incorporates a combination of therapeutic actions, including antiinflammatory, uterine tonics, and vascular tonics. Uterine tonics, which historically have included herbs such as blue cohosh, goldenseal, lady's mantle, motherwort, partridge berry, red raspberry leaf, cramp bark, and black haw, are thought to exert their efforts by improving the overall tone of the uterine smooth musculature and vasculature. Goldenseal, for example, typically regarded for its antimicrobial effects, was used extensively by the Eclectics for the treatment of uterine bleeding resulting from a variety of conditions, including endometriosis, fibroids, and changes associated with menopause.[145] Although no clinical studies have been conducted using the whole herb, in vitro trials using berberine, one of the primary alkaloids in goldenseal, have demonstrated both stimulant and inhibitory activity of uterine smooth muscle.[22] Aqueous extracts of red raspberry leaf also have demonstrated both stimulatory and inhibitory effects on uterine smooth muscle.[114] In fact, this paradoxical effect is seen with several of the herbs commonly used as both uterine tonics and spasmolytics, for example, cramp bark and black haw. It is thought that the effect of these dual activities is a normalization of uterine activity and the promotion of smooth, nonspasmodic uterine muscle activity, thus improving tone and reducing pain.[158,159]

Several herbs with venotonic activity should be considered for the treatment of pelvic congestion in CPP. Most notable are blue cohosh and horse chestnut. Blue cohosh has demonstrated uterine tonic and vasoconstrictive activity, and continues to be used in many gynecologic formulae in which a uterine tonic is required. Historically, it has been used for labor induction, amenorrhea, dysmenorrhea, menorrhagia, and to induce abortion.[160,161] Blue cohosh is listed in the *British Herbal Pharmacopoeia* (1983) as a spasmolytic and emmenagogue.[161] It also may be used as an ovarian tonic and for the treatment of a variety of menstrual complaints, including menorrhagia, amenorrhea, dysmenorrhea, and pelvic congestion syndrome.[8]

Horse chestnut is used to improve circulation through vascular tonification, to improve venous tone in venous insufficiency, for the relief of aching discomfort in the lower limbs associated with varicosities, and for complaints associated with chronic venous insufficiency (CVI).[22,106,163] Traditionally, it was used in the treatment of neuralgia and "conditions of venous congestion particularly with dull, aching pain and fullness."[22] Horse chestnut extract is the third most widely sold herbal product in Germany, where it is used long-term in clinical practice, apparently without adverse effects.[106] There appears to be very low risk associated with proper administration, although it is recommended that only product standardized to its presumed active ingredient, escin (i.e., aescin) be used, and not to exceed 12 weeks at recommended doses.[163] Adverse effects from use of horse chestnut seed extract have included GI upset and calf spasm most commonly, with headache, nausea, and pruritus occurring less commonly. Overall, adverse effects are extremely rare; occurring at a rate of less than 0.6% in more than 5000 subjects in an observational study.[163]

FORMULAE FOR CPP TREATMENT

The following is a small selection of possible formulae to illustrate formulation strategies for CPP treatment. These various formulae can be used concurrently, or elements from several may be combined to create a unique formula for individual patients. Other herbs discussed earlier may be substituted if they are more specifically indicated to a particular patient's presenting picture. Further, CPP treatment, as discussed, almost invariably requires readers to refer to other relevant sections of this book for treatment options, for example, dysmenorrhea or interstitial cystitis.

🌿 FORMULAE FOR CHRONIC PELVIC PAIN

General Tincture for Chronic Pelvic Pain: Uterine Tonic/Antispasmodic

Blue cohosh	(Caulophyllum thalictroides)	20 mL
Cramp bark	(Viburnum opulus)	20 mL
Peony	(Paeonia lactiflora)	20 mL
Motherwort	(Leonurus cardiaca)	15 mL
Horse chestnut	(Aesculus hippocastanum)	15 mL
Yarrow	(Achillea millefolium)	10 mL
		Total: 100 mL

Pelvic Analgesic and Antispasmodic Tincture: Moderate to Strong Pain

Cramp bark	(Viburnum opulus)	40 mL
Wild yam	(Dioscorea villosa)	20 mL
Jamaican dogwood	(Piscidia piscipula)	15 mL
Corydalis	(Corydalis ambigua)	15 mL
Yarrow	(Achillea millefolium)	10 mL
		Total: 100 mL

Dose: 2.5 mL taken as needed, up to 6 doses per day. DO NOT EXCEED THIS DOSE.

Immune Support and Stress Reduction Tincture

Ashwagandha	(Withania somnifera)	30 mL
Milky oats	(Avena sativa)	20 mL
Blue vervain	(Verbena officinalis)	20 mL
Licorice	(Glycyrrhiza glabra)	15 mL
Lemon balm	(Melissa officinalis)	15 mL
		Total: 100 mL

Dose: 5 mL twice daily for 3 to 6 months.

This formula exemplifies the use of both adaptogens and gentle nervines to create a formula for everyday use to improve nervous irritability, reduce anxiety, and improve well-being. The formula is also antiinflammatory.

Insomnia/Sleep Disturbance Formula
See Insomnia.

DIETARY CONSIDERATIONS

Dietary changes are indicated when the client suffers from digestive complaints such as constipation, bloating, flatulence, being overweight, lethargy, excessive fatigue, or irritability accompanying CPP.[132] Achieving an optimal weight and stable blood sugar may lead to improvements in digestion and mood, and increasing dietary fiber and fluids can lead to reduction in constipation and bloating.[132] Additionally, a Mediterranean-type diet with the addition of high-quality EFAs can reduce the production of inflammatory mediators, and thus be beneficial in chronic pain reduction. Consider calcium and magnesium supplementation for relief of muscle spasm.

ADDITIONAL THERAPIES

Muscle Relaxation and Reeducation, Biofeedback, and Electrical Stimulation

Muscle tension in the pelvis, hips, and lower back may be caused by or lead to CPP. Helping a woman to identify and relax tension, become aware of and adjust her body mechanics and standing and sitting posture, and wear appropriate shoes to minimize postural problems can help to reduce pain caused by structural imbalances. Pelvic relaxation training techniques should be taught and practiced regularly. Much of this can be done at home, but physical therapy can be helpful if there is limited joint movement or muscular problems. Prolonged sitting or standing can aggravate CPP, so patients may need suggestions and supportive counseling for modifying jobs or activities that require positions that exacerbate the problem. Exercises such as running or high-impact aerobics also may be aggravating, and should be replaced with gentler, relaxing forms of exercise, for example, walking, tai chi, yoga, or dance.[164] Physical therapy for the treatment of musculoskeletal problems or postural problems can be beneficial for women with CPP.[165]

🌿 EXTERNAL TREATMENTS FOR CHRONIC PELVIC PAIN

Ginger-Yarrow Sitz Bath
Ingredients
Fresh ginger root: 4-in. section, grated
  Dried yarrow blossoms: 1 oz

Instructions
Bring 2 quarts of water to a boil in a large pot and remove from heat source. Add the ingredients and cover tightly. Allow to steep for 20 to 30 minutes. Fill bathtub to patient's waist height with water that is as hot as patient can comfortably tolerate. Strain the liquid into the tub, discarding the spent herbal matter. Soak. Repeat regularly as needed.

Medicated Analgesic Massage Ointment
To 2 ounces of a premade unmedicated ointment base add:
  15 mL tincture of *Viburnum opulus*
  10 mL tincture of *Capsicum*
  5 mL tincture of *Lobelia inflata*
  Mix thoroughly (product may occasionally require mixing before use). Apply to lower back, pelvis, and backs of thighs as needed. Avoid contact with mucous membranes and eyes because contact will cause burning.

Biofeedback machines can be effective in helping women to identify and improve the effectiveness of pelvic muscle relaxation techniques for acquired muscle tension. The woman is instructed to visualize and practice muscle relaxation techniques while using a biofeedback device for feedback on the relaxation efforts.

Electrical stimulation using vaginal, rectal, or surface electrodes is used to produce rhythmic contraction and relaxation of the pelvic floor muscles. Electrical stimulation may give immediate reduction in the level of pain early in treatment, restore more normal muscle activity patterns over time, and also may help to disperse inflammatory mediators caused by chronic muscle spasm.[166-168]

Uterine Displacement–Mayan Uterine Massage

It has been suggested that uterine retrodisplacement can lead to symptoms of CPP.[132] Although the role of pelvic tension and improper posture in the etiology of CPP is accepted, conventional medicine does not address the potential for uterine displacement, other than prolapse associated with pelvic relaxation as an etiologic factor. Mayan uterine massage is a practice introduced into the United States by Rosita Arvigo after dedicated study with a Belizean shaman who specialized in this technique. Ms. Arvigo trains and certifies people in this technique and it has grown in popularity because of many anecdotal reports of success for the treatment of vague but sometimes debilitating complaints such as CPP, as well as for many other gynecologic problems. The treatment is predicated on the belief that uterine displacement, which may occur as a result of childbearing, poor posture, sedentary lifestyle, and improper carrying and work habits can lead to significant pelvic congestion, gynecologic, nervous, circulatory, and digestive problems. No studies have been done to objectively demonstrate efficacy. The practice appears generally noninvasive (it is an intervention); however, it should not be used for pregnant women.

TREATMENT SUMMARY FOR CHRONIC PELVIC PAIN

- Symptomatic pain relief can be achieved with herbal analgesics and antispasmodics. Sedatives can be used if pain interferes with sleep.
- Anxiety and depression commonly associated with CPP can be treated with botanical anxiolytics and antidepressants, which may be combined with herbs for pain relief and sleep promotion.
- Reduce inflammation with herbs and an antiinflammatory diet, including EFA supplementation.
- Treat underlying or associated digestive problems such as bloating, constipation, or IBS.
- Treat underlying or associated gynecologic or menstrual problems, for example, ovarian cysts, dysmenorrhea, or endometriosis.

- Treat underlying or associated urinary problems such as UTI or interstitial cystitis.
- Treat pelvic congestion syndrome with herbs that stimulate pelvic circulation.
- Use external treatments such as sitz baths and massage with analgesic essential oils to improve pelvic circulation and relieve pain.
- Employ muscle relaxation techniques, pelvic muscle reeducation, biofeedback, or electrical stimulation to retrain muscle patterns and relieve pain.
- Mayan uterine massage may be a helpful technique for relieving pain and pelvic adhesions or uterine displacement.
- Achieve a healthy body weight, good posture, and adequate exercise.
- Supplement with calcium and magnesium for relief of muscle spasms.

CERVICAL DYSPLASIA: BOTANICAL AND NATUROPATHIC APPROACHES

Cervical dysplasia describes cervical cells with an atypical appearance, loss of uniformity in cell structure, and loss of their normal architectural orientation. Each year between 250,000 and 1 million women in the United States are diagnosed with cervical dysplasia. It can occur at any age, but the mean ages are 25 to 35 years old. Atypia and dysplasia can be caused by inflammation, cervical intraepithelial neoplasia (CIN), or carcinoma in situ (CIS) (see Staging Box). Atypical cervical cells can be a precursor to invasive cervical cancer. Mild dysplasia is the most common form of cervical dysplasia, and up to 70% of these cases regress on their own, the cervical tissue returning to normal without treatment. Moderate and severe dysplasias are less likely to resolve spontaneously and have a higher rate of progression to cancer. The greater the abnormality of the cells as determined by staging, the higher the risk for developing cervical cancer. Cervical cancer is the third most common gynecologic malignancy in US women. Cervical dysplasia is inversely related to the age of first intercourse; it is directly related to the number of sexual partners in the woman's lifetime, and the risk increases for the sexual partners of men whose previous partners had cervical cancer. The development of cervical dysplasia and cervical cancer is strongly associated with infection by human papillomavirus (HPV). There are many different types of HPV that are classified as high risk, most notably types 16 and 18. Contributing factors in the transformation of cells from dysplasia to neoplasm are smoking, poor diet, OC use, chronic cervicitis, herpes virus infection (HSV), human immunodeficiency virus (HIV), exposure to DES (diethylstilbestrol), immune suppression, and exposure to environmental carcinogens. A discussion of the benefits and risks of the HPV vaccine is beyond the scope of this book.

STAGING OF CERVICAL DYSPLASIA

The Bethesda System was developed by the CDC and NIH as a comprehensive, standardized scheme for classifying Pap smear results. It uses the term squamous intraepithelial lesion (SIL) to describe abnormal changes in the cells on the surface of the cervix. Changes are classified on a scale of low grade to high grade. It has largely replaced previous grading systems.

Bethesda System
- ASCUS (atypical squamous cells of undetermined significance): borderline, some abnormal cells
- LGSIL (low-grade squamous intraepithelial lesions): mild dysplasia and cellular changes associated with HPV
- HGSIL (high-grade squamous intraepithelial lesions): moderate to severe dysplasia, precancerous lesions, and carcinoma in situ (preinvasive cancer that involves only the epithelium)

DIAGNOSIS

Cervical dysplasia is typically asymptomatic and most commonly discovered upon routine Pap smear. In contrast, cervical cancer may be asymptomatic or present with abnormal vaginal bleeding. Pap testing has significantly reduced mortality from cervical cancer, a privilege of developed nations that if made available worldwide would nearly obliterate this disease. Current guidelines recommend that all women older than age 21 have a Pap test done every 1 to 5 years, depending on individual risk factors, medical history, and previous Pap smear and HPV testing results. With routine Pap smears, advanced morbidity and mortality from cervical cancer should be entirely preventable, particularly because it is a slowly progressing cancer, allowing plenty of time for detection and treatment. Sadly, 50% of all women diagnosed with cervical cancer have not had a Pap smear in longer than 10 years. Any suspicious lesion should be biopsied directly. Colposcopy-directed biopsy usually provides enough clinical evidence for an accurate diagnosis. The diagnosis of cervical dysplasia is largely anxiety provoking for women because of the association between dysplasia and carcinoma. Therefore it is important that practitioners take the time to thoroughly explain to each woman the level of concern that is warranted by her degree of dysplasia, and compassionately review options with her.

CONVENTIONAL TREATMENT APPROACHES

Medical treatment depends on the severity of the lesions. For women with preinvasive cervical disease, treatment options include laser therapy, cryotherapy, loop electrical excision procedure (LEEP), and conization biopsy. Most physicians have abandoned laser and cryosurgery because of the inaccuracy of treatment compared with LEEP. The depth of the treatment and amount of collateral tissue damage is easier to control with a LEEP. The LEEP removes tissue precisely and cauterizes simultaneously. Cone biopsy is the removal of a cone-shaped amount of cervix the depth of the entire cervix. In both the LEEP and the cone biopsy the physician is trying to obtain clean borders, meaning that there is no evidence remaining of cervical dysplastic cells. If the woman has progressed to cervical cancer treatment, it usually consists of a total hysterectomy and/or radiation treatment.

Conventional treatment is an efficient solution, usually covered by insurance. However, conventional treatments often cause permanent scarring and do not address potential underlying causes. Scarring can interfere with women's ability to conceive by obstructing the endocervical canal with scar tissue, and damaging cervical crypts that are important in providing proper nutrition for advancing sperm and the proper formation of cervical mucus. The scarring also may interfere with cervical dilatation in labor. Further, conization can occasionally lead to incompetent cervix during pregnancy, necessitating cervical cerclage, in which a suture is inserted into the cervix to allow the woman to maintain pregnancy and prevent premature labor.

Because of the risks associated with sexually transmitted infections and subsequent cervical dysplasia, current sexual partners should be screened and treated for HPV as necessary. Adolescent girls should be educated about the risk factors for developing cervical dysplasia. The sociologic components of women's health also cannot be ignored. A history of sexual abuse, for example, is not an uncommon clinical finding in women with a history of cervical dysplasia.

BOTANICAL AND NATUROPATHIC TREATMENT

Intrinsic to both herbal and naturopathic treatment of cervical dysplasia is the belief that conventional therapy alone does not address a woman's underlying propensity to dysplasia, nor does it address preventable causes. This is significant because the 5-year return rate with conventional therapies is as high as 75%.

In contrast to conventional approaches, botanical and naturopathic treatments attempt to address multifactorial causes, treating the woman, not just her cervix. A disadvantage is that natural medicine protocols are demanding, inconvenient, and potentially costly, requiring multiple office visits. Naturopathic and botanical medicine practitioners emphasize a number of therapies including the use of immune-enhancing, antiinflammatory, hormone-regulating, and antiviral botanicals both for internal and topical treatments.[26,169] Adaptogens often feature prominently in a botanical program to address immune and endocrine function. Stress can depress immune response, which can increase viral activation. Recent lifestyle changes or stressors, even as seemingly benign as exposure to increased amounts of sunlight, may suppress the immune system sufficiently to cause viral activation.[170] Environmental causes of gynecologic disease—ranging from exposure to excess exogenous estrogens to stress—must be addressed in the long-run for the benefit of all women. (See Endometriosis for a brief discussion of the role of exogenous estrogens on gynecologic health.)

Herbal and naturopathic treatment for the treatment of cervical dysplasia should occur in the context of a complementary relationship with a conventional care provider and in conjunction with appropriate medical care, rather than as a substitute. The development of cervical cancer from dysplasia is highly preventable with proper integrated conventional and natural medical treatment.

An Herbalist's Approach to Cervical Dysplasia

Because mild cervical dysplasia has a high rate of spontaneous regression, one approach of botanical practitioners is to encourage watchful waiting and use antiviral and immune-supportive herbs and supplements internally to boost immunity and topically to reduce viral proliferation and inflammation and promote tissue healing.

For persistent or more than mild cervical dysplasia, experienced gynecologic botanical practitioners favor the use of conventional procedures in combination with the postprocedural use of herbal suppositories and internal therapies to enhance immunity, reduce inflammation, and promote healing.

Because stress may play a contributory role in immune and endocrine dysregulation, and is often a consequence of a diagnosis of cervical dysplasia, long-term use (i.e., 3 to 6 months) of adaptogens is also commonly recommended. Topical herbal applications consist of insertion of a medicated suppository 5 nights per week for as many as 12 weeks, with a repeat Pap test at the end of 12 weeks. Several companies sell preformulated suppositories (see Resources at the end of this chapter). Alternatively, practitioners can make suppositories for patients using a suppository mold, or make a mold available to patients who wish to prepare their own. General instructions for preparing suppositories can be found in Chapter 3, with specific recipes for dysplasia treatment in the following pages. They can be prepared in large batches and kept refrigerated for use as needed. If after 3 months of botanical treatment the dysplasia has not improved or has progressed, further medical treatment should be pursued.

Although there are many similarities between botanical and naturopathic treatment of cervical dysplasia, the two approaches diverge over the use of escharotic treatments, a popular naturopathic approach. Escharotics can be caustic and irritating, and are much less controllable and reliable than the LEEP. The experience of herbalists using escharotic treatments does not endorse their use. There is no evidence for the efficacy of escharotic treatments for cervical dysplasia, and side effects seen with the LEEP, such as cramping and abdominal pain, may also be seen with escharotics. Additionally, escharotic treatment used topically on other tissue (e.g., for the treatment of breast tumors or skin cancers) has been associated with significant tissue damage in some cases. One observational study reports on dermatologic cases in which four patients had used escharotics in the treatment of basal cell carcinomas (i.e., skin cancer) in lieu of the recommended conventional treatment. One patient had a complete clinical response but had a residual tumor on follow-up biopsy. A second patient successfully eradicated all tumors but experienced severe scarring. A third patient disagreed with the physicians regarding her care and was lost to follow-up. One patient presented with a basal cell carcinoma that "healed" for several years after treatment with an escharotic agent but recurred deeply and required extensive resection. The lesion eventually metastasized. The researchers concluded that physicians should advise their patients against the use of escharotics. Low Dog states that although at this time there is only anecdotal evidence of the efficacy of escharotic treatments for cervical dysplasia, and because several of the herbs typically used possess antiviral and antiinflammatory

effects, further research is warranted.[26] Many licensed naturopaths specializing in the treatment of gynecologic complaints report excellent results and a high level of safety when using these preparations. No evidence for efficacy or safety for cervical dysplasia was identified in the literature.[26] Naturopathic protocols including the use of escharotics are described in detail in *Women's Encyclopedia of Naturopathic Medicine* by Tori Hudson. It remains a popular alternative that women may seek or be offered through their naturopathic care provider; in general I do not endorse their use. Nonetheless, their use is popular among naturopathic physicians, and women may choose this option when looking for alternatives to conventional medical treatments. Thus practitioners should be aware of their use.

Herbs commonly used internally and topically, both for herbal and naturopathic treatments, are listed in Table 11-7. Evidence and discussion of adaptogens is found elsewhere in this volume.

Botanical Treatment Program for Cervical Dysplasia
Internal Formula for Immune Support: Antiviral, Antiinflammatory, and Adaptogenic Effects

Reishi mushroom	(*Ganoderma lucidum*)	30 mL
Echinacea	(*Echinacea* spp.)	25 mL
St. John's wort	(*Hypericum perforatum*)	15 mL
Ginseng	(*Panax ginseng*)	15 mL
Licorice	(*Glycyrrhiza* spp.)	15 mL
		Total: 100 mL

Dose: 4 mL twice daily for 12 weeks, or as needed for the duration of treatment.

Suppository for Cervical Dysplasia/HPV Infection

Ingredients:
- ¼ cup cocoa butter
- ¼ cup coconut oil
- 1 Tbsp calendula oil or tincture
- 1 tsp each: thyme essential oil, lavender essential oil, and echinacea tincture
- 1 Tbsp each: dried goldenseal root powder and marshmallow root powder

Preparation instructions: See Suppositories and Pessaries in Chapter 3

Use: Insert one suppository on each of 5 consecutive nights per week for up to 12 weeks. It is advisable to wear a disposable cotton menstrual pad nightly during use, as the suppository will melt and leaking can cause staining of bedding or nightwear.

Combine the preceding protocol with the dietary and nutritional strategies described in the following as part of the naturopathic program. After 12 weeks, recheck the cervix with a Pap smear. If the degree of dysplasia has improved, repeat protocol for 8 to 12 additional weeks and recheck the cervix. If there has been no improvement, but also no worsening, make sure the patient has followed the protocol and repeat, modify the herbal protocol, or proceed with conventional medical care.

Alternatively, the naturopathic protocol can be followed as a botanical and nutritional protocol, omitting the escharotic

TABLE 11-7	Botanical Treatment Strategies for Cervical Dysplasia		
Therapeutic Goal	**Therapeutic Activity**	**Botanical Name**	**Common Name**
Reduce viral infection	Antimicrobial	*Calendula officinalis*	Calendula
Prevent neoplasia	Antitumorigenic	*Commiphora molmol*	Myrrh
Reduce cervical inflammation	Antiviral	*Echinacea* spp.	Echinacea
and heal tissue		*Ganoderma lucidum*	Reishi
		Hydrastis canadensis	Goldenseal
		Lavandula officinalis	Lavender
		Lomatium dissectum	Lomatium
		Origanum vulgare	Oregano
		Melaleuca alternifolia	Tea tree
		Sanguinaria canadensis	Blood root
		Thuja occidentalis	Thuja
		Thymus vulgaris	Thyme
		Usnea barbata	Usnea
	Antiinflammatory	*Althea officinalis*	Marshmallow
	Demulcent		Pineapple (i.e., bromelain)
	Proteolytic	*Ananas comosus*	Calendula
	Vulnerary	*Calendula officinalis*	Licorice
		Glycyrrhiza glabra	Goldenseal
		Goldenseal (Hydrastis Canadensis)	
	See Chapter 12: Human Papillomavirus and Genital Warts		
Support immune response and HPA regulation	Adaptogens	See Chapter 5: Stress, Adaptation, the Hypothalamic-Pituitary-Adrenal Axis and Women's Health	

HPA, Hypothalamic-pituitary-adrenal.

treatment and using either the suppository described in the preceding or those described in the following.

Supplementation with vitamin C, beta-carotene, folic acid, selenium, zinc, vitamin E, calcium, and magnesium are commonly recommended. EFAs are also advised.

Low Dog states that a multivitamin with folate and B vitamins may be especially indicated for women with cervical abnormalities, citing one study evaluating the relationship between individual nutrients and persistent HPV infection that showed circulating levels of vitamin B_{12} were inversely correlated with persistent HPV infection after adjusting for numerous factors, and another study demonstrating that low serum homocysteine levels were highly predictive of invasive cervical cancer risk, possibly suggesting folate, B_{12}, or B_6 insufficiency.[26]

Discussion of Botanicals
Blood Root

The blood-red color of the sap from the roots of blood root led to its traditional use as a blood purifier. It was used as an emmenagogue, in the treatment of respiratory conditions, as a strong emetic, and for the treatment of fungal infections and ulcers.[171] By the eighteenth century, blood root was used topically to treat indolent chancres and tumors as an ingredient in the popular "black salve," an escharotic treatment that was used topically for the treatment of tumors.[26] Extracts of sanguinarine, an alkaloid from the herb, have been shown to possess antiinflammatory, antimicrobial, antioxidant, antiviral, antiproliferative, and apoptotic activities, and are under active research for the treatment of cancer.[172,173] Sanguinarine, an alkaloid compound found in blood root, is a potent inhibitor of NFκB activation.[26,172,173] Sanguinarine is an ingredient in

dental hygiene products, for example, toothpaste, used for its antiplaque activity and in the treatment of gingivitis. There is controversy over the safety of its use in dental products, with contradictory research over whether it may cause malignant cell change and lead to the development of leukoplakia.[174-180] Most studies have concluded that the extract is safe for dental use; however, at least one study concludes that it should not be used until safety can be established. One study on reproductive and developmental toxicology conducted by orally administering blood root extract to rats and rabbits concluded that the oral intake of blood root extract has no selective effect on fertility or reproduction of fetal and neonatal development in either group.[181] The question of safety and effects of the herb on the oral mucosa remains relevant because the application to the cervix is similar in terms of direct treatment of epithelial tissue. The form used in black salve is the whole plant extract rather than the isolated alkaloid for which cautions have been raised. At this time, evidence regarding the internal use of this herb for cervical dysplasia treatment is lacking, and serious caution is suggested regarding its topical use. I do not recommend use for the treatment of cervical dysplasia.

Broccoli Sprouts, Diindolylmethane, and Indole-3-Carbinole

Diindolylmethane (DIM) is metabolized from indole-3-carbinol, a compound found in cruciferous vegetables. Current research suggests that DIM may function as a chemopreventive agent. A murine study demonstrated that DIM inhibited the formation of E6/E7 oncogene–induced cervical lesions.[182] Another study observed apoptotic effects of dietary indole-3-carbinol in cervical cancer cells in vitro.[183] A recent pilot study tested DIM to treat CIN grade 2 or 3. Sixty-four patients scheduled for LEEP were administered a 12-week course of DIM (2 mg/kg daily) or placebo, with evaluations occurring every 3 to 4 months for 1 year. The measurements included Pap smear, HPV test, colposcopy, biopsy, and physical examination. At the 6-month follow-up, 85% of subjects did not require LEEP based on improving global assessment. However, no statistically significant differences were observed between the DIM and placebo group.[184]

Bromelain

Bromelain is a complex mixture of proteinases derived from pineapple stems and fruit. Beneficial therapeutic effects of bromelain have been demonstrated in vitro, and in animal and human inflammatory disease models, including treatment of arthritis and inflammatory bowel disease, among others.[185,186] Bromelain inhibits plasma exudation through inhibiting the generation of bradykinin at the inflammatory site via depletion of the plasma kallikrein system, and possibly through other mechanisms, such as inhibition of the AA pathway.[187-189] Beneficial antiinflammatory effects have also been observed in patients suffering from HIV and cancer.[190-193] In one randomized study, 36 patients with *Chlamydia* infections were assigned either to a tetracycline-HCl plus bromelain (250 and 40 mg, respectively, four times per day) or a doxycycline (100 mg, twice daily) treatment for a period of 14 days. After 7 days, the pathogen was eliminated in 66.7% of the patients treated with tetracycline plus bromelain and in 55.6% of the patients receiving doxycycline. After the completion of the course of therapy, an infection with *Chlamydia* was no longer detectable in any patient of the two groups. The clinical effectiveness of the two therapies was considered to be good or very good in all cases. Adverse effects occurred in 11% (tetracycline plus bromelain) and 16% (doxycycline) of the patients. Treatment of the sexual partner with antibiotics was also considered essential to the success of the study.[194] Bromelain is an important proteolytic ingredient in the treatment of cervical dysplasia.

Calendula

Calendula flowers are indicated for the topical treatment of minor inflammations of the skin and mucosa, to assist in the healing of minor wounds, and for the treatment of burns.[101,103] The most common topical applications include infusions used as washes, oil-based extractions, ointments, and the succus, or juice, which is high in enzymatic activity.[103,160] Hydroalcoholic extracts have demonstrated antibacterial and antifungal activity, as well as high virucidal action.[27,30] Calendula extracts have shown specific activity against HSV, HIV, and *Trichomonas*.[103,195] Antiinflammatory and wound-healing effects have been demonstrated in vitro and in vivo, with topical antiinflammatory effects attributed to the effects of the polysaccharide fractions of the plant.[196-198] Other important compounds are thought to be the major antiinflammatory triterpenoid esters in the flower heads: faradiol-3-O-laurate, palmitate, and myristate.[147,199,200] In one study, freeze-dried extracts of St. John's wort, calendula, chamomile, and plantain were found to suppress both inflammatory effects and leukocyte infiltration in animal models.[201] Wound-healing effects also have been attributed to the angiogenic activity of the herb.[29] Calendula succus is used as a wash in the escharotic treatment, and as an ingredient in other topical applications for the treatment of cervical dysplasia, particularly in suppositories

for vulnerary and antiinflammatory effects after invasive gynecologic procedures (e.g., biopsy, LEEP). Calendula is used topically to hasten healing by reducing inflammation through an increase in granulation. No studies were identified using calendula for the treatment of HPV infection. Some concern exists as to whether use of calendula can lead to sensitization and potential for developing contact dermatitis; however, this risk appears to be insignificant, and in fact, the herb has been found to be highly effective for the prevention of acute dermatitis of grade 2 or higher in patients undergoing postoperative irradiation for breast cancer.[202] Known sensitivity to the *Composita* family can theoretically pose this risk; however, adverse effects from topical use have not been widely observed despite its widespread use.[103]

Green Tea

Research suggests that green tea extract and EGCG may inhibit expression of hypoxia-inducible factor (HIF)-1alpha protein induced by HPV-16, as well as vascular endothelial growth factor (VEGF) protein and messenger ribonucleic acid (mRNA) expression in cervical carcinoma cells in a dose-dependent manner.[203] Two recent clinical trials further suggest that green tea extracts may be effective in treating genital warts.[204,205]

Goldenseal

Goldenseal is one of the five top-selling herbs in the United States, yet little scientific evidence is available regarding its efficacy.[163] Many herbalists consider goldenseal an indispensable antimicrobial herb, in addition to being antiinflammatory, immune enhancing, and antiproliferative, effects largely attributed the herb's berberine content.[149] These actions form the basis for its topical use in the treatment of cervical dysplasia. Although no research has been done specifically on the treatment of HPV with goldenseal, the herb has shown broad antimicrobial effects, with specific effects against *Chlamydia, Staphylococcus aureus, Escherichia coli, Vibrio cholerae, Trichomonas vaginalis, Giardia lamblia,* and *Helicobacter pylori,* as well as other organisms.[206-209] It has also demonstrated antifungal effects against numerous organisms, including *Candida albicans.*[163] Its antiinflammatory effects are attributed to its ability to interfere with the AA pathway and COX generation, particularly COX-2 regulation and inhibition of phospholipase enzymes.[26,163] Berberine was demonstrated in vitro to have antiproliferative effects via inhibition of protein, deoxyribonucleic acid (DNA), RNA, and lipid synthesis in specific tumor cell lines; however, these effects were not borne out in vivo. Berberine extracts were able to induce apoptosis during S-phase of the cell cycle, and have demonstrated the ability to activate antitumor macrophages, in addition to several other anticancer in vitro effects.[163] In a study of the immunomodulatory effects of 6 weeks of orally administered goldenseal, the treated group showed an increase in the primary immunoglobulin M (IgM) response during the first 2 weeks of treatment, suggesting that goldenseal may enhance immune function by increasing antigen-specific immunoglobulin production.[210] Although direct effects against HPV are unknown, use of this herb in suppositories may be effective for reducing comorbid infection, allowing the body to direct its immune activity against the HPV; through eliminating overgrowth of pathogenic microorganisms, goldenseal may allow the body to restore a healthy vaginal environment that may be less likely to support the growth of HPV. As with other herbs, goldenseal's antiinflammatory effects may be beneficial in reducing cervical irritation or inflammation that might contribute to the development of dysplasia.

Licorice

Licorice is used in the treatment of cervical dysplasia, both topically and orally, for its antimicrobial, antiinflammatory, immunomodulating, and antitumorigenic effects. It has been shown to inhibit prostaglandin and leukotriene synthesis in a similar way to corticosteroids such as prednisone.[211] It has also demonstrated specific antiviral activity against a range of viruses associated with chronic illness and latent infection. In one study, treatment of cells latently infected with Kaposi's sarcoma–associated herpes virus (KSHV) with glycyrrhizic acid (GL), a component of licorice, reduced synthesis of a viral latency protein and induced apoptosis of infected cells. This finding suggests a novel way to interrupt latency.[212] GL demonstrated activity against Epstein-Barr virus (EBV) replication in superinfected cells in a dose-dependent fashion in a novel way that differed from that of the nucleoside analogs that inhibit viral DNA polymerase.[213] The mechanism underlying licorice's antiviral and antitumorigenic effects is poorly understood. One study looking at mechanisms was able to demonstrate that glycyrrhetinic acid (GA), an aglycone of GL, stimulates nitric oxide (NO) production and is able to upregulate isoform (iNOS) expression through NFκB transactivation in macrophages.[214] In vitro studies have demonstrated activity against HIV virus.[215]

Licorice and its extracts have been shown to improve immune function in HIV patients by stabilizing helper and T-lymphocyte counts in comparison with the control groups in one study.[216] In another study, it increased T-helper cell levels, improved helper to suppressor cell ratios, improved liver function, and stopped the progression of HIV-positive patients to AIDS in comparison with the control group that did progress on to AIDS.[217,218] In yet another study, it showed a reduction of P24 antigen, an indicator of viral load.[219] The antiviral properties of these compounds have been found to be effective in hepatitis B and C, where IV administration has resulted in up to 40% going into complete remission.[220] Topical use of licorice extract on herpes reduces the healing time and pain associated with both genital herpes and cold sores.[221] Another component of licorice, deoxoglycyrrhetol (DG), also showed a remarkable improvement in antiinflammatory, antiallergic, and antiulcer activities in animal experiments. Immunomodulating effects of GL, GA, and DG derivatives, which induce IFN-γ and some other cytokines, have been demonstrated in relation with their antiviral activities.[222] Glycyrrhizin has been used for the treatment of chronic viral hepatitis. One study evaluated the mechanism by which glycyrrhizin inhibits complement. Glycyrrhizin inhibited the cytolytic activity of complement via the activation of both the classical and alternative pathways, whereas it had no effect on immune adherence, suggesting that it blocks C5 or a later stage of the complement cascade. Further analysis revealed that glycyrrhizin inhibits the lytic pathway in which the membrane attack complex (MAC) is formed. This

mechanism suggests that glycyrrhizin may prevent tissue injury caused by MAC not only in chronic hepatitis, but in many autoimmune and inflammatory diseases as well.[223] Topical treatment of herpes simplex virus blisters with licorice extract may improve healing and prevent recurrence.[163] Although no studies were identified on the treatment of HPV with licorice or its extracts, other viral studies, as well as the herb's traditional uses, suggest that investigation into such use may be promising.

Lomatium

Lomatium has been used historically by Native Americans, mostly as a treatment for respiratory illness.[224] It is considered antiviral, antibacterial, and antiseptic; it is commonly used by naturopathic physicians and taken internally for the treatment of cervical dysplasia. Lomatium has demonstrated in vivo and in vitro efficacy against HPV and HSV and has been investigated for its effects against HIV.[225-227] Its use has been described for the treatment of "slow" viruses with accompanying immune depression, and may commonly be combined with other herbs with immune-building effects.[228] Lomatium is also used topically for gum and mouth inflammations and as a douche for vaginal infections.[229]

Marshmallow

Marshmallow root (Fig. 11-7) is a polysaccharide-rich herb, loved by herbalists for its soothing, demulcent properties.[26] The mucilaginous quality of aqueous extracts and moistened powdered herb provides a protective, soothing coating to mucosa; thus it is commonly included in preparations for throat, GI, and vaginal mucosal irritation.[103] Several studies have found the herb efficacious in combination with other specific herbs for the treatment of cough, and the herb is approved for use by the German Commission E for the treatment of irritation of the oral and pharyngeal mucosa and mild inflammation of the gastric mucosa.[101] The root also exerts immune-enhancing and antibacterial effects.[26]

Myrrh

The tincture and powdered forms of this herb are used topically for the treatment of inflammatory mucosal conditions, usually of the oral and pharyngeal mucosa but also as an ingredient in vaginal suppositories. Local anesthetic, antibacterial, and antifungal activities also have been ascribed to the sesquiterpene fraction of the herb.[30] It is a common ingredient in oral hygiene preparations, for example, ointments, dentifrices, and toothpastes.[30] It is approved by the German Commission E for the topical treatment of mild inflammations of the oral and pharyngeal mucosa.[101] Low Dog states that "No data have been found to document antiviral activity [of myrrh], but in light of the antiseptic, cytoprotective, and antiinflammatory effects of the herb it may offer some benefit" in the treatment of cervical dysplasia.[26]

Oregano and Thyme

Both oregano and thyme essential oils are regularly included in vaginal suppositories for the treatment of vaginal infections, including HPV infection. They are also used topically as antimicrobials against numerous bacterial and fungal infections, for which they are considered highly effective ingredients.[230-232] One study reports on the efficacy of thyme as an antibacterial; in another study oregano and clove oils were diluted and examined for their activity against enveloped and nonenveloped RNA and DNA viruses. Olive oil was also included as a control. Viruses were incubated with oil dilutions and enumerated by plaque assay. Antiviral activity of oregano and clove oils was demonstrated on two enveloped viruses of both the DNA and RNA types and the disintegration of the virus envelope was visualized by negative staining using transmission electron microscopy.[232,233] Care should be taken in the topical use of essential oils; used undiluted (i.e., neat) they can be irritating to sensitive tissues such as cervical or vaginal mucosa.

Reishi

Reishi (Fig. 11-8) is a medicinal fungus with a long history of use as a Chinese folk medicine for promotion of health and longevity. Numerous in vitro and animal studies have demonstrated antitumor and immunomodulatory effects of reishi mushrooms.[234] Clinical evidence furthermore suggests reduced wart recurrence after the use of immunostimulatory substances.[235] An OVID search for this herb yielded over 900 papers reporting on in vivo and in vitro effects. A wide range of antitumor and immunomodulatory mechanisms have been purported and observed with the water extract and the polysaccharide fraction, as well as the alcohol extract or the triterpene fraction; mechanisms include enhanced function of antigen-presenting cells and the mononuclear phagocyte system, humoral immunity, and cellular immunity.[236,237] Evidence is emerging on the effects of reishi against HPV. In vitro, the extract exhibited anti–HPV-16 activity in vitro by the suppression of tE6 oncoprotein.[238] An aqueous extract also inhibited the growth and proliferation of HPV–infected cervical cells. It also induced apoptosis and cell cycle arrest in HeLa, SiHa, and C-33A cancer cell lines.[239]

Reishi polysaccharide peptide (Gl-PP) has demonstrated antitumor effects in mice and potential antiangiogenesis; a reduction of Bcl-2 antiapoptotic protein expression; and an increase of Bax proapoptotic protein expression; therefore inducing cell apoptosis might be one of the mechanisms of action in inhibition of human carcinoma cells. High doses of Gl-PP resulted in a decrease in the secreted VEGF. Taken together, these findings support the hypothesis that the key attribute of the antiangiogenic potential of Gl-PP is that it may directly inhibit vascular endothelial cell proliferation or indirectly decrease growth factor expression of tumor

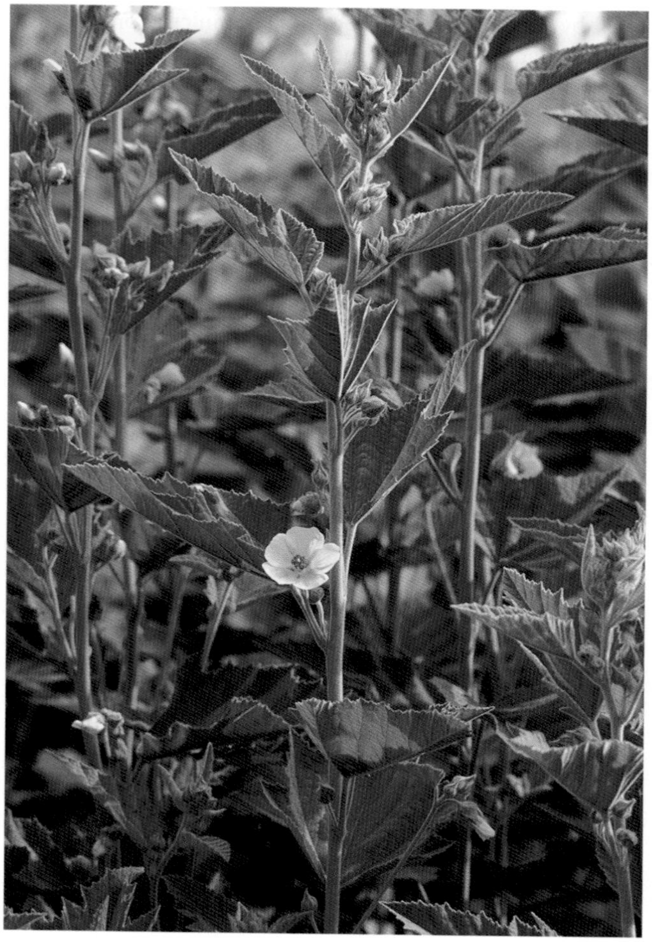

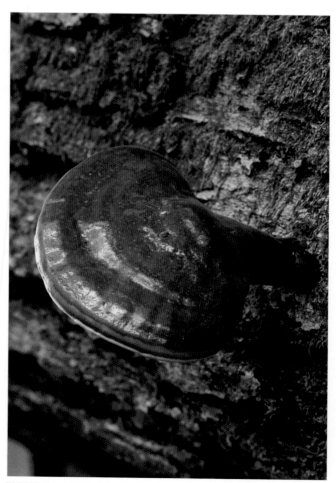

FIGURE 11-7 Marshmallow *(Althea officinalis)* (Photo by Martin Wall.)

FIGURE 11-8 Reishi *(Ganoderma lucidum).* (Photo by Martin Wall.)

cells.[240] It has been demonstrated that *Ganoderma lucidum* induces apoptosis, inhibits cell proliferation, and suppresses cell migration of highly invasive human prostate cancer cells PC-3.[241] Experimental results on cell-mediated immunity showed that *G. lucidum* could increase the percentage of CD5+, CD4+, and CD8+ T-lymphocytes. Experimental results on humoral immunity in horses showed that *G. lucidum* could help horses to produce a significantly higher quantity of specific antibodies in a shorter time.[242] Although the pharmacology and clinical application of water extracts of *G. lucidum* have been extensively documented, less is known regarding its alcohol extract. In one study, the antitumor effect of an alcohol extract was investigated using MCF-7 breast cancer cells. The extract inhibited cell proliferation in a dose- and time-dependent manner, which might be mediated through upregulation of p21/Waf1 and downregulation of cyclin D1. Furthermore, this compound can directly induce apoptosis in MCF-7 cells, which might be mediated through upregulation of a proapoptotic Bax protein and not by the immune system. There are likely multiple mechanisms underlying the antitumor effects of *G. lucidum*.[243] *G. lucidum* also demonstrated antioxidant activity, free-radical scavenging, and chelating abilities.[244]

Thuja

Thuja is used by many herbalists and naturopathic physicians for the treatment of genital and anal warts, and is commonly recommended in the naturopathic treatment of cervical dysplasia for its antiviral activity.[160] The main constituent is an essential oil consisting of α- and β-thujone, the content of which varies proportionally with the amount of ethanol used in producing the plant extract. If consumed internally, thujone can be neurotoxic, convulsant, and hallucinogenic. Long-term or excessive use of thujone-rich products can cause restlessness, vomiting, vertigo, tremors, renal damage, and convulsions.[245] Internal use of thuja decoctions and even very small doses of thuja oil (i.e., 20 drops per day for 5 days) as an abortifacient has been associated with neurotoxicity, convulsions, and death.[160] Additionally, thuja is associated with a substantial risk of inducing fetal malformation, and is absolutely contraindicated for use in pregnancy.[160] No research on the short- or long-term topical use of this herb was identified. Ingestion of thuja cannot be recommended because of potential for toxicity.

Turmeric

Turmeric and one of its chief constituents, curcumin, may benefit women with HPV. A group of 287 women with HPV was randomized into four groups to be treated with vaginal Basant cream (containing extracts of curcumin, reetha, amla and aloe vera), vaginal placebo cream, curcumin vaginal capsules, and placebo vaginal capsules respectively. After 30 days of consecutive application, the women with Basant cream treatment demonstrated the highest HPV clearance rate (87.7%). Curcumin was associated with a 81.3% HPV clearance rate, and the clearance rate in the control groups was 73.3%.[246]

SUMMARY

A number of conditions of the reproductive organs can be treated with botanical medicine. Table 11-8 includes a summary of the herbs used to treat these conditions.

TABLE 11-8 Condition/Botanical Medicine Summary Table					
	Benign Breast Disorder	Cervical Dysplasia	Chronic Pelvic Pain	Endometriosis	Uterine Fibroids
Achillea millefolium			X	X	X
Actaea racemosa			X	X	
Aesculus hippocastanum			X		
Alchemilla vulgaris			X	X	X
Althea officinalis		X	X		
Ananas comosus		X			
Anemone pulsatilla			X	X	
Angelica sinensis	X		X	X	
Astragalus membranaceus				X	
Berberis vulgaris					X
Calendula officinalis	X	X		X	
Camellia sinensis				X	X
Cannabis spp.			X		
Capsella bursa-pastoris					X
Caulophyllum thalictroides	X		X		X
Ceanothus spp.					X
Chelidonium majus					X
Chionanthus virginicus	X			X	
Cinnamomum spp. and *Erigeron*					X
Commiphora mol mol		X			
Curcuma longa				X	
Cordyceps sinensis			X	X	

Continued

TABLE 11-8   Condition/Botanical Medicine Summary Table—cont'd

	Benign Breast Disorder	Cervical Dysplasia	Chronic Pelvic Pain	Endometriosis	Uterine Fibroids
Corydalis ambigua			X	X	
Dioscorea villosa				X	
Echinacea spp.		X		X	
Eleutherococcus senticosus	X	X	X	X	X
Eschscholzia californica			X	X	
Filipendula ulmaria			X		
Galium aparine	X				
Ganoderma lucidum		X			
Geranium maculatum					X
Glycyrrhiza glabra	X	X	X	X	
Gossypium herbaceum					
Hamamelis virginiana					X
Hydrastis canadensis		X	X		
Hypericum perforatum		X	X	X	X
Lavandula officinalis		X	X		
Leonurus cardiaca	X		X	X	X
Linum usitatissimum	X				X
Lomatium dissectum		X			
Mahonia aquifolium	X				
Matricaria recutita			X	X	
Melaleuca alternifolia		X			
Melilotus officinalis	X				
Melissa officinalis			X		
Mentha piperita			X		
Mitchella repens			X		X
Myrica cerifera					X
Oenothera biennis	X		X	X	
Origanum vulgare		X			
Panax ginseng				X	
Panax quinquefolius	X	X	X	X	X
Paeonia lactiflora			X	X	
Phytolacca americana	X				
Picrorhiza kurroa				X	
Piper methysticum			X	X	
Piscidia piscipula			X	X	
Rehmannia glutinosa				X	
Rhaponticum carthamoides	X	X	X	X	X
Rhodiola rosea	X	X	X	X	X
Rosmarinus officinalis				X	
Rubus idaeus			X		X
Rumex crispus					
Sanguinaria canadensis		X			
Schisandra chinensis	X	X	X	X	X
Silybum marianum				X	
Tanacetum parthenium			X	X	
Taraxacum officinale	X			X	
Thuja occidentalis		X		X	
Thymus vulgaris		X			
Trifolium pratense	X				
Trillium erectum					X
Ulmus rubra			X		
Usnea barbata		X			
Verbena officinalis	X			X	
Viburnum opulus			X	X	
Viburnum prunifolium					
Vitex agnus-castus	X			X	
Withania somnifera	X	X	X	X	X
Zingiber officinale			X	X	

Vaginal and Sexually Transmitted Infections

VULVOVAGINITIS AND COMMON VAGINAL INFECTIONS

The normal vaginal environment is a dynamic milieu with a constantly changing balance of *Lactobacillus acidophilus* and other endogenous flora, glycogen, estrogen, pH, and metabolic byproducts of flora and pathogens.[1] *L. acidophilus* produces hydrogen peroxide that limits the growth of pathogenic bacteria.[2] Disturbances in vaginal ecology can allow the proliferation of vaginitis-causing organisms.

The term *vulvovaginitis* encompasses a variety of inflammatory lower genital tract disorders that may be secondary to infection, irritation, allergy, or systemic disease.[3] Vulvovaginitis is the most common reason for gynecologic visits, with over 10 million office visits for vaginal discharge annually.[4] It is usually characterized by vaginal discharge, vulvar itching and irritation, and sometimes vaginal odor.[5] Up to 90% of vaginitis is secondary to bacterial vaginosis (BV), vulvovaginal candidiasis (VVC), and trichomoniasis. The actual prevalence and causes of vaginitis, however, are hard to gauge because of the frequency of self-diagnosis and self-treatment.[1] In one survey of 105 women with chronic vaginal symptoms, 73% had self-treated with over-the-counter (OTC) products and 42% had used alternative therapies. On self-assessment, most women thought they had recurrent vulvovaginal candidiasis (RVVC), but upon diagnosis, only 28% were found positive for RVVC. Women with a prior diagnosis of VVC, however, were able to accurately self-diagnose up to 82% of the time based solely on symptoms.[6] This may be an overestimate; in another study (via a questionnaire) of 634 women, only 11% were able to accurately recognize the classic symptoms of VVC.[6] Another study of women who thought they had VVC also found that self-assessment had limited accuracy, with only 33.7% of women with self-diagnosed yeast infection having microscopically confirmable cases.[7]

Two thirds of patients with vaginal discharge have an infectious cause.[2] However, the presence of some amount of vaginal secretions can be normal and varies with age, the menstrual cycle, pregnancy, and the use of oral contraceptives (OCs).

Antibiotics, contraceptives, vaginal intercourse, receptive oral sex, stress, and hormones (e.g., hormone replacement therapy [HRT], endogenous hormonal dysregulation) can lead to overgrowth of pathogenic organisms.[1] Chemical vulvovaginitis can be caused by colored and perfumed soaps, toilet paper, bubble baths, panty liners, tampons, sanitary pads, and douches. Latex condoms, topical antifungal agents, and preservatives and other agents in lubricants can cause allergic reactions leading to vulvovaginitis.[2] Gastrointestinal (GI) dysbiosis, in other words disruption in the health of the intestinal microbiome, can lead to disruption in vaginal ecology; an example is the result of antibiotic use. In menopausal women or those on antiestrogen therapies, decreased estrogen levels may lead to atrophic vaginitis, which if asymptomatic generally requires no treatment. Forty percent of postmenopausal women, however, are symptomatic; symptoms are readily treatable with topically applied lubricants and the use of estrogen replacement therapies by topical or oral administration.

Although vaginal complaints may commonly be treated based on symptoms, studies have demonstrated a poor correlation between symptoms and diagnosis.[8,9] Therefore the most accurate diagnoses and thus the most appropriate treatments can best be made with testing methods specific for individual organisms. Acute singular episodes of vaginal infections are referred to as uncomplicated, whereas recurrent vaginal infections are considered complicated. Complicated cases are often more severe, resistant to treatment, and may be associated with underlying systemic causes, for example VVC, uncontrolled diabetes, or immunosuppression.[2]

The remainder of this section presents separate discussions of the most common vaginal infections (Table 12-1), followed by a discussion of the botanical treatment of vaginal infections. Table 12-2 provides a general overview of common causative organisms, agents, and conditions involved in vulvovaginitis. It should be remembered that multiple causes of vaginitis may occur concurrently.[2]

BACTERIAL VAGINOSIS

BV is a common form of infectious vaginitis caused by the polymicrobial proliferation of *Gardnerella vaginalis*, *Mycoplasma hominis*, and other anaerobes. It is associated with loss of normal lactobacilli.[2] BV accounts for at least 10% and as many as 50% of all cases of infectious vaginitis in women of childbearing age.[1,7] Determining the presence of BV can be difficult, however, because as many as 75% of women are asymptomatic.[1]

The editor wishes to thank *Botanical Medicine for Women's Health*, Edition 1 contributors to this chapter: Bevin Clare, Lise Alschuler, Christopher Hobbs, and Roy Upton.

TABLE 12-1   Differential Symptoms and Signs of Common Vaginal Infections

	Bacterial Vaginosis	Vulvovaginal Candidiasis	Trichomoniasis
Discharge color	Thin, off-white discharge	Curdy whitish to yellowish-white discharge	Yellow-green or colorless copious discharge
Discharge odor	Malodorous with a characteristic "fishy" odor that may be increased after sexual intercourse	May have no odor, or odor may be reminiscent of yeasted bread	Malodorous
Physical findings	Discharge and odor may be apparent; discharge may be adherent to vaginal walls; tissue typically appears normal	Vulvovaginal redness, swelling, and fissures; discharge appears thick, whitish, and adherent to vaginal walls	Vulvovaginal redness, swelling; "strawberry" cervix; frothy and purulent discharge is visible
Vaginal pH (normal <4.5)	High (>4.5)	Normal	High (>4.5)

Adapted from Egan M, Lipsky M: Diagnosis of vaginitis, *Amer Fam Phys* 62(5):1095–1104, 2000.

TABLE 12-2   Common Causative Organisms, Agents, and Conditions Involved in the Etiology of Vulvovaginitis

Organism/Agent/Condition	Examples
Bacterial vaginosis	*Gardnerella vaginalis, Mycoplasma hominis,* other anaerobic microorganisms
Vulvovaginal candidiasis	*Candida albicans, Candida tropicalis, Candida glabrata,* other *Candida* species
Trichomoniasis	*Trichomoniasis vaginalis*
Chemical vulvovaginitis	Feminine hygiene products: tampons, sanitary pads, douches; latex condoms, spermicides, colored and perfumed soaps, toilet paper, bubble baths
Allergic vulvovaginitis	Latex condoms, topical antifungal agents, preservatives and other agents in lubricants
Atrophic vulvovaginitis	Estrogen deficiency caused by menopause, antiestrogenic therapies, or hormonal dysregulation
General causes/factors that might lead to or increase susceptibility to vulvovaginal infection and VVC	Antibiotics, oral contraceptives, diaphragms, spermicide, IUDs, frequent vaginal intercourse, receptive oral sex, stress, public hot tubs, hormones (e.g., imbalanced endogenous hormones, HRT), uncontrolled diabetes mellitus, immunosuppression (e.g., HIV/AIDS, steroids), pregnancy; sexual abuse must be ruled in girls or young women with vulvovaginitis or recurrent vaginal infections

VVC, Vulvovaginal candidiasis; *IUD,* intrauterine device; *HRT,* hormone replacement therapy; *HIV,* human immunodeficiency virus; *AIDS,* acquired immunodeficiency syndrome.

Symptoms

Some or all of these symptoms may be present in women with BV:
- Milky, homogenous discharge
- Possible vaginal irritation
- Malodorous vaginal discharge (characteristic "fishy" odor)

BV is also commonly asymptomatic.

Diagnosis

Diagnosis is based on the Amsel criteria and is considered 90% accurate with three or four of the following findings: the presence of milky, homogenous discharge; vaginal pH greater than 4.5; positive whiff test ("fishy" odor to the vaginal discharge); and the presence of clue cells on light microscopy of vaginal fluid. Odor is a symptom that is frequently associated with BV; this is caused by amines produced from the breakdown products of amino acids produced by *Gardnerella vaginalis* in the presence of anaerobic bacteria. This also results in a rise in vaginal pH.[2]

Risks for Developing Bacterial Vaginosis

Numerous factors, described in Table 12-3, are associated with the development of BV. It is uncertain whether BV is a sexually transmitted disease (STD). The prevalence is higher in women with multiple sexual partners and in women seeking the services of STD clinics. Treatment of sexual partners of women with the infection has not definitely proved to be

TABLE 12-3 Factors Associated with the Development and Pathophysiology of Bacterial Vaginosis

Type of Risk Factor	Examples
Personal risk factors	Use of: tampons, sponges, douches, intrauterine devices, sex toys Sexual practices: new or multiple sexual partners, receptive oral sex, latex condoms, contraceptive methods such as cervical cap, IUD, or spermicide Other risk factors: antibiotic use, oral contraceptive use, smoking
Microbial factors	Initiating infectious agents; possibly a sexually transmitted infection Decline in lactobacillus numbers Rise in pH Lack of hydrogen peroxide produces lactobacillus strains

beneficial; however, urethral smears of male partners often show typical BV morphocytes.[1,2,5]

Risks Associated with Bacterial Vaginosis

BV in pregnancy appears to be a risk factor for second trimester miscarriage, premature rupture of the membrane, premature labor, chorioamnionitis, and postcesarean and postpartum endometritis.[10,11] Women with BV have an increased incidence of abnormal Pap smears, pelvic inflammatory disease (PID), and endometritis. Further, the presence of BV in women undergoing invasive gynecologic procedures may increase the risk of serious infections including vaginal cuff cellulitis, PID, and endometriosis.[1] Eliminating BV appears to decrease the risk of acquiring human immunodeficiency virus (HIV) infection; thus it is suggested that women with BV be treated regardless of whether they are symptomatic.[5]

Conventional Treatment of Bacterial Vaginosis

Centers for Disease Control and Prevention (CDC) guidelines recommend the treatment of all women with symptomatic BV.[5] Conventional treatment of BV is metronidazole, orally (Flagyl) or vaginally (MetroGel), or clindamycin. Proper treatment typically results in an 80% cure rate at 4 weeks, with recurrence rates of 15% to 50% in 3 months.[2] Treatment failure may be caused by lack of successful recolonization of hydrogen peroxide–producing strains of lactobacillus, antibiotic resistance, and possibly reinfection by male partners.

Metronidazole is also the prescribed treatment during pregnancy; however, it is contraindicated in the first trimester because of theoretic risks of teratogenicity. Thus, many pregnant women prefer to avoid exposure altogether.[10,11] Clindamycin is used as an alternative.[1] Evidence on the use of antibiotics in pregnancy to reduce the risk of preterm labor and its associated morbidities is somewhat conflicting. A Cochrane review concluded that no evidence supports the screening of all women for BV, and the guidelines of the American College of Obstetricians and Gynecologists (ACOG) also does not recommend screening in asymptomatic patients.[12,13] According to a 2005 systematic review, no evidence supports the use of antibiotic treatment for either BV or *Trichomonas vaginalis* (see later discussion) for reducing preterm birth in low- or high-risk women.[14] Nonetheless, CDC guidelines (2002) still recommend treating all pregnant women with BV with metronidazole or clindamycin.[5]

VULVOVAGINAL CANDIDIASIS

VVC, commonly referred to as *yeast infection,* is the second most common cause of vaginitis in the United States. Approximately 75% of all women will experience an episode of VVC in their lifetime, with RVVC occurring in 5% of women.[1,3] It is most commonly caused by the fungus *Candida albicans;* however, other *Candida* species, such as *C. tropicalis* and *C. glabrata,* are becoming increasingly common, possibly because of increased use of OTC antifungals; they are also typically more resistant to antifungal treatments.[1] OTC antifungal treatments are among the top 10 selling OTC medications in the United States with an estimated $250 million in annual sales.[6] Establishing *Candida* spp. as a cause of vaginitis can be difficult because 50% of all women have *Candida* organisms as part of their normal vaginal flora.[1] VVC is not considered an STD, and conventional medical practice does not include treatment of male partners unless they are uncircumcised or presenting with inflammation of the glans penis.[1] RVVC is defined as four or more episodes annually.[2] Recurrence may be a result of associated factors, intestinal microorganism reservoir, vaginal persistence, or sexual transmission.[1] Genital candidiasis is associated with antibiotic use, OCs, HRT, and other drugs that change the vaginal environment to favor proliferation of *Candida* spp. Vaginal yeast infections are also more common during pregnancy and menstruation, and in diabetics. Drugs and diseases that suppress the immune system can facilitate infection.

Causes and Risk Factors for Developing Vulvovaginal Candidiasis

Reported risk factors include:
- Recent/repeated antibiotic use
- Diabetes mellitus
- HIV infection/acquired immunodeficiency syndrome (AIDS)
- Increased estrogen levels (e.g., hormonal dysregulation, HRT)
- Pregnancy
- Hyperglycemia

Additional factors may include anything that disrupts the normal balance of vaginal flora (Table 12-2).

Symptoms

Women with VVC often develop mild to severe itching and irritation of the vulva and may have a vaginal discharge characteristically curdlike in appearance with a mild yeastlike odor. The vulva may be red, inflamed, and swollen and the tissue may become raw and fissured, particularly from scratching to relieve itch, which should be discouraged. Note that these symptoms are not specific only to VVC, and therefore other causes should also be ruled out. Physical findings in women with VVC include vulvar or vaginal erythema, edematous labia minora, appearance of vaginal thrush, and normal pH.

One or more of these symptoms are typically reported by patients with VVC:

- Vulvovaginal pruritus
- Vulvovaginal irritation
- Vulvovaginal swelling
- Dysuria
- Thick, whitish vaginal discharge
- Possible odor to vaginal discharge (characteristic "yeasted bread–like" odor)

Diagnosis

Definitive diagnosis of VVC can be based on positive microscopic findings.[6] Cultures are expensive, but obtaining a positive fungal culture can be important for the diagnosis and effective treatment of RVVC.[6] Candida vaginitis is associated with a normal vaginal pH (≤4.5). Identifying *Candida* by culture in the absence of symptoms is not an indication for treatment because it is a part of the normal endogenous flora.

Conventional Treatment Approaches of Vulvovaginal Candidiasis

Uncomplicated VVC is intermittent and infrequent, and in 80% to 90% of cases results in resolution of symptoms and negative culture after a short course of topical azole drugs.[5] Examples of azole-containing antifungal creams include: clotrimazole, miconazole, ketoconazole, and fluconazole. These are currently available OTC. The duration of treatment with these preparations may be 1, 3, or 7 days. Alternatively, ketoconazole, fluconazole (Diflucan), itraconazole, or nystatin can be taken orally. Self-medication with OTC preparations should be advised only for women who have been diagnosed previously with vaginal *Candida* infection and who have a recurrence of the same symptoms. Any woman whose symptoms persist after using an OTC preparation or who has a recurrence of symptoms within 2 months should seek medical care. Treatment with azoles results in relief of symptoms and negative cultures among 80% to 90% of patients who complete therapy. Topical agents usually are free of systemic side effects, although local burning or irritation may occur. A maximum of 7 days of topical therapy is recommended during pregnancy. Oral agents lead to better compliance but have a greater risk for systemic toxicity, and occasionally may cause nausea, abdominal pain, dizziness, rash, or headaches.[15] Therapy with the oral azoles occasionally has been associated with abnormal elevations of liver enzymes. Occasionally, women who take OCs must stop using them for several months during treatment for vaginal candidiasis because they can worsen the infection.

Women who are at unavoidable risk of vaginal candidiasis, such as those who have an impaired immune system or who are taking antibiotics for a long period of time, may need an antifungal drug or other preventive therapy. For women with complicated VVC (RVVC), a longer duration of therapy may be recommended, followed by a 6-month period of maintenance therapy.[5] Azole drugs may significantly interact with a number of drugs (e.g., astemizole, cisapride, H$_1$ antihistamines; interactions have been associated with cardiac dysrhythmia) owing to potent inhibition of cytochrome P450 3A4, which leads to increased bioavailability of the interacting drug.[2]

TRICHOMONIASIS

Trichomoniasis vaginalis is a motile, flagellate protozoan. It is the third most common cause of vaginitis. Every year, approximately 180 million women worldwide are diagnosed with this infection, accounting for 10% to 25% of all vaginal infections.[1] Current belief is that *T. vaginalis* is almost exclusively acquired through sexual contact.[2] Male sexual partners are infected in 30% to 80% of cases.[1]

Symptoms

Symptomatic infection causes a characteristic frothy, green, malodorous discharge with a high pH (can be as high as 6.0).[5] Additionally, there may be soreness and irritation in and around the vulva and vagina, dysuria, dyspareunia, bleeding upon intercourse, inability to tolerate speculum insertion because of pain, or a superficial rash on the upper thighs with a scalded appearance. The cervix may have a characteristic appearance, called petechial strawberry cervix, in up to 25% of cases.[1] Chronic asymptomatic infection can exist for decades in women; an infection also may present atypically.[2] In men, infection is mostly asymptomatic, or there may be a thin white or yellow purulent discharge with dysuria (i.e., nongonococcal urethritis).[2,5]

Diagnosis

Trichomoniasis can be diagnosed on the basis of simple microscopy, pH evaluation, and amine tests.[2] However, in as many as 50% of cases, microscopy yields negative findings in spite of strong evidence of *T. vaginalis* infection. In these cases, polymerase chain reaction (PCR) can be used to obtain a definitive diagnosis; however, it is more costly.

Risk Factors Associated with the Development of Trichomoniasis

Smoking, intrauterine device (IUD) use, and multiple sexual partners all increase the risk of contracting *T. vaginalis*.[1] Statistically, women who smoke cigarettes and use illicit drugs, less educated teenagers, and those of low socioeconomic groups are more likely to be colonized with this organism, as are women who have had more than five sexual partners in the past 5 years, have a history of gonorrhea or other STDs, and who first have intercourse at an early age.

Risks Associated with Trichomoniasis Infection

Trichomoniasis is associated with and may act as a vehicle of transmission for other STDs, including HIV.[1,2,7] It is also associated with an increased risk of premature rupture of the membrane, premature birth, and low birth weight.[2,5]

Conventional Treatment of Trichomoniasis Infection

The CDC treatment guideline for *T. vaginalis* infection is oral metronidazole, which has a cure rate of 90% to 95%. Unlike with other vaginal infections, treatment is recommended regardless of whether a woman is symptomatic.[7] Treatment success may be increased with treatment of sexual partners. Sex is to be avoided until the patient and any sexual partners are cured. Follow-up is considered unnecessary in patients who are initially asymptomatic or who become asymptomatic after treatment is completed. Oral metronidazole is recommended for treatment of symptoms in pregnant women.[5] Treatment during pregnancy has not been shown to reduce the risk of preterm delivery.[7] Also, as stated, physicians and pregnant women may be hesitant to use this drug during pregnancy owing to potential risks of teratogenicity. A recent Cochrane review found no benefit from antimicrobial treatment for *T. vaginalis* during pregnancy; in fact, the largest trial was stopped early because of increased risk of preterm labor with metronidazole treatment.[14] As this is the only medication used to treat *T. vaginalis*, hypersensitivity and drug resistance are potential obstacles to therapy. Increasing dosage may overcome resistance, and a desensitization protocol is used in cases of hypersensitivity to the drug.[7] Additionally, other drugs are available in Europe but have not yet been approved by the Food and Drug Administration (FDA) for use in the United States.[7]

THE BOTANICAL PRACTITIONER'S PERSPECTIVE

Research and clinical experience indicate that women commonly seek OTC and alternative therapies for the treatment of vaginal infections and vulvovaginitis (Table 12-4). In one study, 105 patients with a mean age of 36 years and 50% with college degrees, referred by their gynecologists for evaluation of chronic vaginal symptoms, were interviewed about their OTC and alternative medicine use in the preceding year. It was found that 73% of patients had self-treated with OTC antifungal medications or povidone-iodine douching and 42% had tried alternative therapies including acidophilus pills orally (50%) or vaginally (11.4%), yogurt orally (20.5%) or vaginally (18.2%), vinegar douches (13.6%), and boric acid (13.6%).[16]

Vulvovaginitis may simply be an acute response to a temporary period of imbalance or recent exposure to precipitating factors, such as a period of stress at school or work, excessive consumption of sugar or alcohol at holiday time, or increased sexual activity with condom and spermicide use, affecting

TABLE 12-4	**Botanical Treatment Strategies for Vulvovaginitis**		
Therapeutic Goal	**Therapeutic Activity**	**Botanical Name**	**Common Name**
Eliminate/reduce infection	Antimicrobial	*Allium sativum*	Garlic
		Arctostaphylos uva ursi	Uva ursi
		Mahonia aquifolium	Oregon grape
		Calendula officinalis	Calendula
		Coptis chinensis	Goldthread
		Glycyrrhiza glabra	Licorice
		Hydrastis canadensis	Goldenseal
		Melaleuca alternifolia	Tea tree
		Origanum vulgare	Oregano
		Thymus vulgaris	Thyme
		Usnea barbata	Usnea
Reduce swelling and irritation	Antiinflammatory	*Althea officinalis*	Marshmallow
		Lavandula officinalis	Lavender
Reduce swelling and irritation	Demulcent	*Althea officinalis*	Marshmallow
		Symphytum officinale	Comfrey
		Ulmus rubra	Slippery elm
Heal and repair tissue	Vulnerary	*Althea officinalis*	Marshmallow
		Calendula officinalis	Calendula
		Symphytum officinale	Comfrey
		Ulmus rubra	Slippery elm
Reduce vaginal discharge	Astringent	*Arctostaphylos uva ursi*	Uva ursi
Improve vaginal lubrication and treat vaginal atrophy	Demulcent/emollient	See Chapter 23.	
Improve vaginal lubrication and treat vaginal atrophy	Phytoestrogen	See Chapter 23.	
Improve immunity and resistance	Adaptogens	See Chapter 5.	

proper balance in local flora. In such cases, simple lifestyle modifications combined with topical applications are often adequate treatments. Recurrent vulvovaginitis may be part of a larger picture of chronic lifestyle imbalance, underlying conditions that disrupt the vaginal flora (e.g., bowel dysbiosis, hormonal dysregulation) or exposure to any of the many instigating causes mentioned earlier in this chapter (see Table 12-2). Complicated, recurrent vulvovaginitis can be more difficult to treat but can often be effectively addressed with a combination of local and systemic strategies and removal of underlying causes. Patients with intractable vulvovaginitis should be evaluated for serious underlying conditions such as immunosuppression or diabetes mellitus, and any botanical treatment should occur in conjunction with appropriate medical care. Although there is evidence in the medical literature to suggest that, with the exception of trichomoniasis, it is not necessary to treat sexual partners, empirical evidence from botanical clinical practice suggests that recurrence is less likely when all partners are treated. This should not be surprising, as with most vaginal infections, it has been found that men do harbor organisms in the urethra.

The goal of the botanical practitioner is to reduce or eliminate factors that encourage infection or overgrowth of pathogenic organisms, restore the normal vaginal environment and its flora, and relieve symptoms associated with infection. This chapter does not address hormonal dysregulation that may be associated with vulvovaginitis.

Antimicrobial Therapy

Antimicrobial herbs are used as primary treatments in cases of vulvovaginitis when caused by infections. For acute infections, they are generally used solely as topical applications. For recurrent cases, external application is combined with oral use. Internal treatment should focus on immunosupporting and antimicrobial botanicals, including echinacea, garlic, goldenseal, Oregon grape root, Pau d'Arco, astragalus, and various medicinal mushroom species such as maitake and reishi. Also see Chapter 5 for a discussion on adaptogens and immune support.

Numerous herbs have exhibited both broad spectrum and specific antimicrobial activities. Although treatment approaches vary with each of the different infectious causes of vulvovaginitis, antimicrobial herbs are usually applied generically regardless of the infectious agent. There appears to be little, if any, risk of resistance with herbal treatments; however, labs specializing in delivering services to complementary and alternative medicine (CAM) practitioners sometimes do sensitivity and specificity testing for natural agents with screening for vaginal infections. This is unnecessary except in chronic, recurrent, or intractable cases.

Garlic

Garlic is a popular antimicrobial botanical treatment for vaginal infections, effective when applied in fresh, whole form. A single clove is peeled and inserted whole at each application, usually at night, and left in during sleep. It is sometimes dipped in a small amount of vegetable oil to ease insertion. It also may be wrapped in a small piece of gauze or with a piece of string with a tail left hanging to ease removal. Otherwise,

it can be removed manually. In vitro, garlic has demonstrated antimicrobial effects against a wide range of bacteria and fungi, including *Escherichia coli, Proteus, Mycobacterium,* and *Candida* species.[17] In a study by Sandhu and colleagues, 61 yeast strains, including 26 strains of *C. albicans,* were isolated from the vaginal, cervix, and oral cavity of patients with vaginitis and were tested against aqueous garlic extracts. Garlic was fungistatic or fungicidal against all but two strains of *C. albicans.* In another in vitro study, an aqueous garlic extract was effective against 22 strains of *C. albicans* isolated from women with active vaginitis. Oral garlic may be less effective. A recent clinical trial did not find any benefit to oral garlic tablets over placebo (Dose not noted other than "3 tablets daily").[18] At body temperature, garlic had mostly fungicidal activity; below body temperature, the action was mostly fungistatic.[19,20] Cases of irritation and even chemical burn have been reported after prolonged application of garlic to the skin or mucosa.[21]

Goldenseal, Goldthread, and Oregon Grape Root

Goldenseal, goldthread, and Oregon grape are all herbs that contain the alkaloid berberine, a major active component possessing antimicrobial activity.[22] In vitro studies demonstrate a rational use of the herb for its antibacterial properties.[23,24] Berberine has demonstrated specific activity against *C. albicans* and *C. tropicalis,* as well as to a species of trichomoniasis, *T. mentagrophytes,* among other pathogens.[21,23] These herbs have been used historically and in modern herbal medicine with good reliability for the treatment of a variety of infectious conditions, both internally and topically. Goldenseal is considered by many herbalists to be the most effective of the three herbs. It is commonly included, as is Oregon grape root, as an ingredient in topical preparations for the treatment of vaginitis, added in powder or tincture form to suppositories; powder can be inserted vaginally in 00-size capsules. Internal use of goldenseal, in addition to specific antimicrobial activity, may enhance immune response via stimulation of increased antibody production and may be suggested for oral use in intractable cases.[25] Goldthread has demonstrated significant antimicrobial activity against a wide range of *Candida* spp.[26]

Oral consumption of these herbs is generally contraindicated for use in pregnancy. Goldenseal root is an endangered North American plant. Therefore only cultivated root should be purchased for use. Oregon grape and goldthread can be substituted with confidence.[26]

Note: Berberine-containing herbs stain fabrics a very distinctive yellow color. Patients using any of these herbs in suppositories or other external treatments should be advised to avoid staining towels, clothing, and bed coverings. It is advisable to insert suppositories before bed, and to wear a menstrual pad to protect bedding.

Licorice

Licorice root is one of the most widely used herbs for the treatment of a range of inflammatory conditions. It has demonstrated effectiveness as a demulcent in the treatment of oral, gastric, and respiratory tract conditions, including ulcers and inflammation.[21] Although no research was identified on the use of this herb for vulvovaginitis, its effects on other mucosa would seem to substantiate this application. Additionally, licorice alcohol extracts have shown effectiveness against *E. coli,* and *Candida* and *Trichomoniasis* species in vitro. Alcohol extracts can easily be added to suppository blends for topical application.

Oregano and Thyme

The antimicrobial properties of essential oils have been known since antiquity. In vitro testing of essential oils against a wide variety of microorganisms showed thyme and oregano to possess the strongest antimicrobial properties among many herbs that were tested.[27] Thyme essential oil has also found to be specifically effective against *Candida* spp.[28,29] Direct application of undiluted oil (i.e., neat oil) is not recommended because it is too caustic to the skin and sensitive mucosa. Rather, a small amount of essential oil can be added to suppository blends, diluted tincture may be added to peri-washes and sitz baths, and tea of these herbs may be used as a base to which other herbs may be added for peri-washes and sitz baths. See sample formulae in this chapter and Chapter 3.

Tea Tree

Tea tree oil (TTO) is derived from the leaves of the tea tree (Fig. 12-1), a native to Australia; there is a history of use of the leaves for the treatment of colds, coughs, and wounds by indigenous Australians, who spoke of healing lakes in which leaves had decayed. The medical use of the oil as an antiseptic was first documented in the 1920s, and led to its commercial production, which remained high throughout World War II.[30] Legend has it that it was provided to Australian soldiers fighting in World War II for use as an antiseptic and that harvesters were exempt from enlisting.[30] Reports of the effectiveness of TTO appeared in the literature from the 1940s through the 1980s, with a significant increasing interest in the medical value of TTO seen in the 1990s to the present, corresponding with interest in CAM generally. Current research, presented in a thorough review by Carson and colleagues, supports its use as an antibacterial and antifungal, as well as an antiinflammatory.[30] Limited studies have been done on TTO's use as an antiviral, but a few trials have indicated possible activity against enveloped and nonenveloped viruses.[30] A broad range of bacteria have demonstrated in vitro susceptibility to TTO, including those known to be associated with BV. A case report in which a woman successfully self-treated with TTO–containing suppositories also supports the use of TTO in BV.[31-36] At concentrations less than 1%, TTO may be bacteriostatic rather than antibacterial.[30] Several studies have demonstrated efficacy against *C. albicans;* however, to date no clinical trials have been done. Terpinen-4-ol exhibited the same antimicrobial effects as TTO in azole-susceptible and azole-resistant human pathogenic *Candida* species in a rodent model of vaginal infection.[37] A rat model of vaginal candidiasis supports the use of TTO for VVC.[31] Numerous TTO studies have focused on it's antimicrobial effects.[33,36,38,39] Two studies demonstrated antiprotozoal activity of TTO, one specifically supporting anecdotal evidence that TTO is effective against *T.*

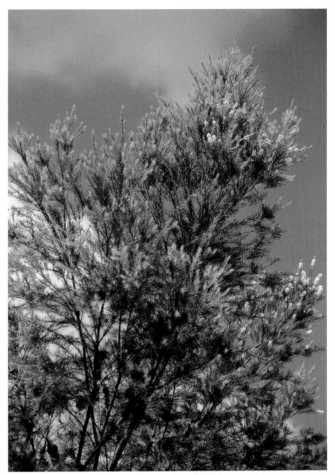

FIGURE 12-1 Tea tree *(Melaleuca alternifolia).* (Photo by Martin Wall.)

vaginalis. The mechanisms of antimicrobial action are similar for bacteria and fungi and appear to involve cell membrane disruption with increased permeability to sodium-chloride and loss of intracellular material; inhibition of glucose-dependent respiration; mitochondrial membrane disruption; and inability to maintain homeostasis.[34,40-42] Perhaps what has attracted the most interest about this herb is that it has demonstrated activity against antibiotic-resistant bacteria. Its use in Australia since the 1920s has not led to the development of resistant strains of microorganisms, nor have studies that have attempted to induce resistance, with the exception of one case of induced in vitro resistance in *Staphylococcus aureus.*[43,44]

Usnea

Usnea lichens (Fig. 12-2) have a history of use that spans centuries and countries from ancient China to modern Turkey, from rural dwellers in South Africa to modern day naturopathic physicians and herbalists in the United States.[45,46] The lichen is rich in usnic acid, which has demonstrated in vitro antimicrobial activity against bacteria, viruses, and protozoa. Additionally, it exhibits antiinflammatory and analgesic activity.[26] Alcohol extract may be added to a suppository blend or diluted in water or tea (1 Tbsp of tincture per cup of liquid) for use as a peri-wash or in sitz baths.

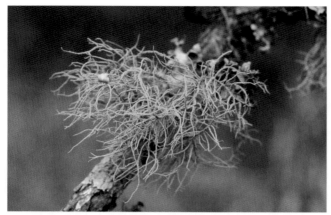

FIGURE 12-2 Usnea *(Usnea barbata).* (Photo by Martin Wall.)

Uva Ursi

Uva ursi or bearberry is used by midwives as a topical anti-septic and astringent to relieve vulvar and urethral irritation associated with vulvovaginitis. Leaf preparations have shown antimicrobial activity against *C. albicans, S. aureus, E. coli,* and other pathogens.[21] For vulvovaginitis, it is used topically as a peri-rinse or in sitz baths.

Symptomatic Relief and Tissue Repair

Irritation and superficial damage from vulvovaginitis can lead to significant discomfort as well as fissures and rawness of the vaginal tissue. The use of herbs as topical agents for reducing inflammation, irritation, and for promoting healing are an important part of any herbal protocol for this condition. Tissue repair is also especially important because inflamed and fissured vaginal tissue increases a woman's susceptibility to secondary infection; notably, HIV. Herbs commonly used to promote local tissue repair and reduce discomfort fall into several categories including antiinflammatories, vulneraries, demulcents, and astringents. Antiinflammatories relieve local swelling, irritation, and pain; vulneraries work to heal wounds and irritated tissue; demulcents cool and soothe irritated tissue; and astringents tonify tissue and create a protective barrier on the surface, reducing further insult. Astringents can also be effective in drying up excessive secretions. Some of the many herbs with topical antiinflammatory effects to consider using include licorice, marshmallow root, and lavender, all of which may be used in various combinations and preparations with other herbs to treat vaginitis.

Calendula

Calendula has demonstrated efficacy in the treatment of wounds, promoting tissue regeneration and reepithelialization, and has also shown some antimicrobial activity (see the preceding). It is soothing as a tea, oil, or diluted tincture (1 Tbsp tincture to ¼ cup of water), and is an important ingredient in topical vulvovaginitis preparations.[47] European Scientific Cooperative on Phytotherapy (ESCOP) recommends calendula for the treatment of skin and mucosal inflammation and to aid wound healing.[48]

Comfrey Root

Comfrey root (Fig. 12-3) has a very long history of folk use for healing damaged skin, tissue, and broken bones. It is highly

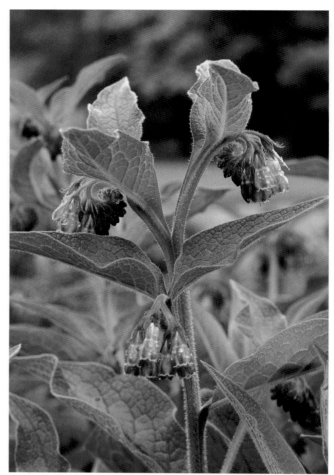

FIGURE 12-3 Comfrey *(Symphytum officinale).* (Photo by Martin Wall.)

mucilaginous. It is thought that allantoin and rosmarinic acid are the constituents mainly responsible for comfrey's healing and antiinflammatory actions.[49] Comfrey is indicated for topical use only. Use on broken skin or mucosa should be minimized but is reasonable for short durations (1 to 2 weeks at a time), and should not exceed 100 µg of pyrrolizidine alkaloids with 1,2 unsaturated necine structure daily for a maximum of 4 to 6 weeks annually.[50] Comfrey infusion may be added to a peri-rinse or sitz-bath blend, or comfrey oil or finely powdered herb may be added to a suppository blend.

Lavender

Lavender has a folk tradition of use for topical treatment of mild wounds, for which it is still included by herbalists and midwives in topical preparations for vulvovaginitis.[49] Additionally, its fragrance imparts a pleasant scent to herbal preparations. It may be used as a peri-rinse or sitz bath in tea form or using diluted tincture, or several drops of essential oil may be added to rinses, sitz baths, or suppositories.

Marshmallow Root

Marshmallow is demulcent and vulnerary. Marshmallow root contains a mucilage that covers the mucosa, protecting it from local irritation.[48] Topical application is soothing in sitz baths and peri-rinses, and the powdered herb, finely ground, helps give herbal suppositories firmness. Slippery elm bark powder can be substituted for marshmallow root powder in suppository blends.

Topical Preparations for Treating Vulvovaginitis
Sitz Baths, Peri-Washes, and Suppositories

The most common forms of topical applications used in the treatment of vulvovaginitis are sitz baths, peri-washes, and suppositories. Instructions for each of these preparations are found in Chapter 3.

Sitz baths may be done either in a bath tub with the water filled to hip height or in a purchased sitz bath, which is a small basin that fits over the bowl of the toilet and which may be purchased at most pharmacies. When prepared with antiinflammatory and antimicrobial herbs, they provide a soothing relief to vulvar/urethral irritation. The bath water and herbs should be used only once, and prepared fresh each time. The water may be hot or tepid, according to the patient's comfort.

For a soothing sitz bath, combine equal parts of dried thyme, calendula, lavender, and uva ursi leaf. Place 1 ounce of the herb blend into a quart glass jar or pot with a close-fitting lid. Cover with 1 quart of boiling water, close the vessel, and steep for 30 minutes. Strain the entire contents into a sitz bath and fill with water to the desired level. Add 2 tablespoons of sea salt per bath and soak. Repeat up to twice daily for 2 weeks.

Peri-rinses provide an excellent alternative to sitz baths if there is a lack of time to soak, and also make a soothing, antiseptic rinse after using the toilet. They can be done anytime during the day if vulvar itching or irritation becomes uncomfortable (or unbearable as some women find it does!). The same infusion described for sitz baths can be used to fill peri-bottles—small, pointed-top squeeze bottles also available at most pharmacies. The peri-bottle can be kept filled and left near the toilet. Add 1 tsp of sea salt to each bottle. Use as frequently as needed, patting dry after each rinse.

Suppositories prepared with a blend of herbs specific for vulvovaginitis can provide effective, soothing relief, heal tissue, and have antiseptic action. They can either be custom-purchased through naturopathic pharmacies or made by the practitioner or the patient. Although this may cause some inconvenience, they can be prepared in large batches and kept in the freezer for many months and the refrigerator for many weeks, ready for use. Please see Chapter 3: Suppositories and Pessaries for more instruction.

An effective suppository blend for BV and candidiasis includes a vulnerary herb, antimicrobial herbs, and a demulcent herb in a base of cocoa butter and coconut oil. The following is a highly reliable formula:

1 cup cocoa butter
½ cup coconut oil
3 Tbsp calendula oil
2 tsp thyme oil
1 tsp lavender oil
4 Tbsp marshmallow root powder, finely ground
2 Tbsp goldenseal root powder

Suppositories are applied nightly for 7 to 14 days. It is advisable to wear a light pad and old underwear while sleeping because the suppository will melt at body temperature. The oils and herbs may stain bedding or clothes.

WHY DOUCHING IS NOT RECOMMENDED

Women commonly douche because of the misperception that it "cleans out" the vaginal canal and can thus cure vaginal infections. A systematic review found that although douching may provide some symptomatic relief and initial reduction in infection, it may lead to rebound effects and other complications in the long run. Povidone-iodine preparations, a common over-the-counter choice for self-treatment, have been demonstrated to cause a rebound effect in which a higher than normal bacterial colonization is seen within weeks of last douching, which could actually increase the risk of bacterial vaginosis. Routine douching for hygiene has been shown to double the risk of acquiring vaginitis. Douching of all types can lead to increased risks of pelvic inflammatory disease (PID), endometritis, salpingitis, and ectopic pregnancy.[20]

CHRONIC VULVOVAGINITIS AND INTESTINAL PERMEABILITY

The roles of intestinal dysbiosis and permeability (i.e., leaky gut syndrome) should not be overlooked in the etiology of chronic or intractable cases of vaginitis. The body's ability to maintain control over the volume of microorganisms present in the intestinal and vaginal tracts is intimately connected to the health of the bowel and bowel flora. If the body is unable to sustain a healthy balance of microorganisms, those that normally inhabit our bodies without causing harm can overproliferate or migrate, becoming pathogenic. This is often the case with chronic vaginal infections. Further, when the body is in a chronic state of immune-mediated response and inflammation, normally controlled organisms may become opportunistic. Thus a first line of botanical treatment for chronic vaginal infections, especially candidiasis, is improving the integrity of the bowel mucosa and helping to restore normal bowel flora. The former is done with many of the same antiinflammatory, antimicrobial, and vulnerary herbs already mentioned, and a few additional botanicals. The most important of these include chamomile, marshmallow root, calendula, slippery elm, goldenseal, Oregon grape root, *Dioscorea villosa* (wild yam), and licorice root. These may be administered as teas, tinctures, or capsules. Essential fatty acids of both the omega-3 and -6 varieties should be supplemented for their antiinflammatory action. Probiotics (see the following discussion) are useful in restoring gut flora and can be taken as a supplement or as live, active culture yogurt.

Nutritional Considerations: Lactobacillus/Yogurt

The goal of treatment with lactobacillus supplements or yogurt, taken orally or applied vaginally, is recolonization of the vagina (and bowel with oral intake) with adequate numbers of healthy flora capable of controlling and resisting pathogenic infection. The success of this treatment requires products that contain the proper lactobacillus species and that these species be active. Additionally, oral yogurt therapy requires the survival of lactobacilli through the GI system and digestive processes; it is thought that vaginal recolonization occurs as a result of migration of the microorganisms from the anus to the vaginal introitus.[20] Effective oral and topical yogurt therapy also requires that the lactobacilli be able to adhere to the vaginal epithelium. *L. acidophilus* is poorly adherent to the vaginal walls, and it also is not a major rectovaginal species. Although two clinical trials have demonstrated significant efficacy with oral and/or topical use, the use of other species of lactobacillus, such as *L. crispatus, L. jensenii, L. rhamnosus,* and *L. fermentum,* may be more effective.[21,51] A randomized crossover study with a washout period by Shalev and coworkers studied the effects of oral yogurt prophylaxis on a group of women (*n* = 46) with BV (*n* = 20) and candidal vaginitis (*n* = 18) or both (*n* = 8). The study showed a significant decrease in BV and no significant decrease in candidal infection. Only 28 participants were still enrolled in the study at 4 months and only 7 completed the protocol.[52] In an open crossover trial by Hilton and associates, a randomized group of women (*n* = 33) with RVVC were assigned to either a 6-month protocol of daily oral intake of *L. acidophilus* containing yogurt or a yogurt-free diet. In the yogurt group, a threefold decrease was seen in candidal infections, substantiated by wet mount and potassium hydroxide. Interestingly, although only 13 women completed the yogurt treatment, 8 women in the yogurt arm refused to switch over to the yogurt-free diet.[52] Patients with lactose intolerance may experience GI complaints from oral yogurt intake. Topical treatment of BV with yogurt has been evaluated in several studies. In an unblinded study of 84 pregnant women with BV a program of yogurt douching twice daily for 7 days (*n* = 32) compared with acetic acid tampons (*n* = 20) or no treatment (*n* = 20), it was found after 2 months of treatment that 88% of women in the yogurt group and 38% of women in the acetic acid group compared with 5% of women in the no treatment group were BV free[20]. A multicenter, placebo-controlled randomized controlled trial (RCT) looking at the effects of lactobacillus vaginal tablets combined with estrogen as a delivery agent on BV demonstrated a 75% cure rate at 2 weeks and an 88% cure rate at 4 weeks compared with a 25% and 22% respective cure rates at corresponding times in the placebo group.[20]

Empiric evidence from herbal and midwifery practice suggests that live active culture yogurt may be more effective than acidophilus tablets or capsules, although any of the options is potentially effective. It also provides some immediate relief of burning and itching to inflamed tissue. The easiest way to apply it is in the shower, placing one foot on the edge of the tub and using two fingers to insert the yogurt vaginally and around the vulva. Do not place fingers back in the yogurt after applying; rather place the appropriate amount (2 to 3 Tbsp) in a small container. The yogurt should be left on for 3 to 5 minutes, and then rinsed off, repeating up to two times daily depending on the severity of the infection and irritation. Repeat for up to 2 weeks, although treatment is often effective within several days.

Additional Therapies

Boric Acid

Boric acid is a common OTC treatment for VVC and RVVC that is both self-prescribed and recommended by health practitioners.[1,20,53] Although it has not been widely studied, four studies have shown positive outcomes, even compared with conventional antifungal therapy, and it is considered an effective therapy for the treatment of vaginal candidiasis.[1,18,20,53,54] In one study, 92 women with chronic mycotic vaginal infections had microscopic examination of the vaginal discharge during prolonged therapy with antifungal agents and boric acid[54]. A microscopic picture unique to chronic mycotic vaginitis was observed, representing the cytologic reaction of the mucous membrane to chronic yeast infection. This diagnostic tool proved extremely effective in detecting both symptomatic and residual, subclinical mycotic infection and provided a highly predictive measure of the probability of relapse. The ineffectiveness of conventional antifungal agents appeared to be the main reason for chronic mycotic infections. In contrast, boric acid was effective in curing 98% of the patients who had previously failed to respond to the most commonly used antifungal agents and was clearly indicated as the treatment of choice for prophylaxis.[54] In a double-blinded, randomized study, 108 VVC–positive college students used boric acid or nystatin capsules once daily for 2 weeks. Boric acid cure rates were 92% at 7 to 10 days posttreatment and 72% at 30 days, a statistically significant improvement over the nystatin capsules, which only had a cure rate of 64% at 7 to 10 days posttreatment, and 50% at 30 days posttreatment.[55] In a case series of 40 patients with vulvovaginitis, 95% of patients remained symptom-free at 30 days post–boric acid treatment; in another study, boric acid was tested against an azole-resistant strain of yeast, more commonly seen in women with recurrent yeast infections, and yielded clinical improvement occurred in 81% of cases, with mycological eradication in 77% of the women.[20,56,57]

The standard recommended dose and application is 600 mg of boric acid placed in a size 0 gelatin capsule and inserted vaginally. For acute treatment, one capsule is inserted nightly for 14 days, followed by a maintenance treatment of twice weekly insertion.[20,54] Some women report mild to moderate burning as the capsule dissolves. If intercourse occurs during the treatment period, males may report dyspareunia.[20] Serious side effects have not been reported from treatment.[54] Boric acid, available in drug stores, can be considered a safe, effective, accessible, and affordable treatment for vaginal candidiasis.

General Suggestions

Reducing exposure to the personal, sexual, chemical, and allergenic factors described in the preceding can be beneficial in preventing and reducing vulvovaginitis and infection. Wearing clean cotton underwear or "breathable" fabrics, changing underwear more often if there is copious vaginal discharge or dampness, sleeping without underwear, wearing loose-fitting pants, and observing hand-washing before and after genital contact may reduce the incidence and frequency of vulvovaginitis.[53] Wearing a thong may cause irritation or facilitate the transmission of anorectal organisms to the vulvovaginal area. Regular bathing and showering with gentle soap, keeping the vulvar area dry, and regular use of sitz baths also may be helpful, the latter particularly in candidal vulvovaginitis.

Sex Education and Empowerment

It is optimal for women to abstain from sexual activity while undergoing treatment for vulvovaginitis. Not all women feel comfortable addressing intimate sexual matters with their partners; therefore it may be important to help patients develop skills and confidence to tell partners what they need, encourage partners to obtain treatment when relevant, and make healthy sexual lifestyle choices that prevent infection.

🌿 TREATMENT SUMMARY FOR VULVOVAGINITIS

- Healthy vaginal flora and bowel flora must be promoted when there is chronic vulvovaginitis.
- Avoid precipitating factors, for example, anything that might trigger chemical or allergic reaction or mechanical irritation (e.g., tampons, sexual activity) (see Table 12-2).
- For infectious vulvovaginitis, consider antimicrobial herbs including calendula, garlic, goldenseal, oregano, thyme, tea tree, Pau d'Arco, marshmallow, lavender, and Oregon grape root.
- For relief of irritation, itching, and inflammation, use topical applications of calendula, marshmallow, comfrey, and lavender for their soothing, healing properties. Healing tissue can also reduce the spread of opportunistic infections such as human immunodeficiency virus (HIV).
- Use topical or oral preparations containing live, active acidophilus cultures to restore normal bowel and vaginal flora.
- For chronic, recurrent vulvovaginitis, consider adding internal treatment for immune supporting and antimicrobial activity, including echinacea, goldenseal, Oregon grape root, and medicinal mushrooms. Also see Chapter 5 for a discussion on adaptogens and immune support.
- The role of intestinal permeability or "leaky gut syndrome" and other bowel disorders should be evaluated in the treatment of chronic vulvovaginitis.
- Limit or eliminate refined flour, refined sugar, dairy products, fruits, and fermented foods.
- Supplement with 5 to 10 mg of zinc daily in intractable cases of yeast infection.
- Use boric acid capsules as suppositories, especially for intractable BV.
- Loose-fitting clothing made of natural fibers should be encouraged, especially during sleep.
- Avoid douching.
- Educate patient about vaginal hygiene and personal empowerment regarding healthy sexual behavior.
- When appropriate and possible, treat sexual partners.

HUMAN PAPILLOMAVIRUS AND GENITAL WARTS

Condylomata acuminata, commonly referred to as genital warts, is a highly infectious STD caused by the infectious agent human papillomavirus (HPV). More than 20 types of HPV have been identified as infective. Of these, types 6 and 11 typically produce visible genital warts. Warts typically occur at multiple sites in the urogenital, perineal, and perianal regions. They appear as soft, moist, small pink or gray polyps, although they can also appear flat and smooth or granulated. Polyps may enlarge to form pedunculated clusters the size of which can become so large as to affect urination, defecation, and normal vaginal delivery. Genital warts may be painful, friable, and pruritic; however, the majority are asymptomatic.

HPV types 16, 18, 31, 33, and 35 are strongly associated with cervical neoplasia, cervical intraepithelial dysplasia, and squamous cell carcinoma. Up to 80% of sexually active adults in the United States carry HPV; however, only 5% develop HPV lesions or cervical dysplasia. The outcome of HPV exposure depends on a number of factors, for example, HPV type, host immunity, and smoking status. The risk of infection increases with the number of sexual partners and is associated with unprotected sexual intercourse. Condoms are not adequate protection against transmission. Conditions of immunodeficiency, epithelial injury of the genital area, and pregnancy all increase the risk of HPV infection.

It is suspected that HPV remains dormant in the body once contracted; therefore the goal of treatment is to minimize visible lesions and prevent progression to neoplasia, rather than eradicate the virus.[53]

DIAGNOSIS

Diagnosis of genital warts typically occurs during a woman's routine screening health examination. The health care provider may visibly assess HPV infection if characteristic lesions are present. Genital warts must be differentially diagnosed from the flat-topped *condyloma lata* of secondary syphilis. A diagnosis made by inspection can be confirmed by biopsy. Biopsy is indicated only if the diagnosis is uncertain, if the lesions do not respond to standard therapy, if the disease worsens during treatment, if the patient is immunocompromised, or if the warts appear to be pigmented, indurated, fixed, or ulcerated (i.e., signs of neoplasia or squamous cell carcinoma). Endocervical warts can be detected via colposcopy.

Although there are HPV nucleic acid tests available to identify the viral type, these tests are not routinely ordered. There are, in fact, no data that support the use of type-specific HPV nucleic acid tests in the routine diagnosis or management of genital warts.[58] The HPV nucleic acid tests are available primarily for research purposes and to determine possible risk for carcinoma in high-risk individuals.

HPV is classified as clinical, subclinical, or latent, depending on the extent or absence of lesions.

CONVENTIONAL TREATMENT APPROACHES

The primary goal of conventional approach to HPV, aside from prevention with the HPV vaccine, the pros and cons of which are beyond the scope of this book, is removal of visible symptomatic warts. Most patients respond to conventional treatment

with wart-free periods. Without treatment, warts will spontaneously resolve, remain unchanged, or grow in size or number.
The factors influencing these outcomes are not known. The
main benefit of treatment is symptom improvement. A secondary likely benefit of treatment is the reduced risk of infectivity
and decreased likelihood of complications associated with HPV
infection. Current conventional treatment options do appear to
reduce HPV deoxyribonucleic acid (DNA) and thus infectivity.
However, successful treatment of genital warts does not eradicate
infectivity or the risk of recurrences of the disease. There are several standard, accepted conventional treatments.

Determination of the type of treatment is made after evaluation of wart size, location, morphology, patient preference, cost
of treatment, adverse effects, and provider preference. Generally,
a course of applied treatments is required to remove genital
warts. First-line therapy for HPV may consist of the application
of 0.5% podophyllotoxin (Podofilox 0.5% solution or gel) one to
four times. Podophyllotoxin is an antimitotic agent. This treatment has been shown to be effective in 70% to 90% of men or
women with exposed and accessible genital warts.[59,60] This treatment is typically well tolerated and self-administered, and produces minimal local irritation. Ten percent to 20% podophyllin
resin ethanolic solution has also been used topically. However,
podophyllin resin is less effective than podophyllotoxin. In one
study, 94% of patients treated with podophyllotoxin were cured
versus only 29% of patients treated with podophyllin resin.[60]
Additionally, podophyllin resin is commonly associated with
local inflammation, erosion, pain, and burning. Finally, concern
exists about the systemic absorption of the podophyllin resin and
its systemic toxicity, particularly in pregnant women.

An alternative to podophyllotoxin is topical application
of trichloroacetic acid (TCA) or bichloracetic acid (BCA).
TCA and BCA are caustic agents that coagulate proteins,
thus destroying the wart. A health care provider applies these
agents. Treatment is repeated weekly until the lesions resolve.
This treatment is generally effective but can cause inflammation at the site of application. If pain develops, soap or sodium
bicarbonate must be applied to neutralize the acid.

Cryotherapy is another common treatment for exposed
genital warts. Cryotherapy with liquid nitrogen or cryoprobe is
typically done weekly or biweekly. Cryotherapy causes thermal-
induced cytolysis. This therapy can be quite effective if
applied properly; however, overtreatment can cause localized
pain and blistering. Conversely, undertreatment is ineffective.
Typical second-line therapeutic interventions include surgical removal of warts. There are several techniques of surgical removal. All techniques require local anesthesia. Surgical
removal is a one-time treatment. However, surgery is more
expensive and requires more time than medical treatment
options. Surgical treatment of genital warts is usually reserved
for patients with a large number of lesions or for patients who
have not responded to other treatments. Another second-line
therapy is the intralesional injection of interferon (IFN).
Many trials have confirmed the efficacy of this treatment. It
causes the disappearance of all visible warts in approximately
43% of patients and visibly shrinks visible warts in an additional 25%.[61] However, IFN therapy is expensive and requires
three treatments each week, usually for 4 to 6 weeks.

All conventional treatments are somewhat limited in
their efficacy. To increase efficacy, it is common for health
care providers to use combination therapy. However, combination therapy increases adverse effects. For this reason,
some providers prefer to use different therapies sequentially.
Warts that are not easily accessible, such as those located on
the cervix, in the anal canal, or in the urethral meatus, are
more difficult to treat. Liquid nitrogen or TCA (or BCA) are
common treatments for warts located in these areas. Cervical
warts must be closely monitored and high-grade squamous
intraepithelial lesions (HGSIL) must be excluded before treatment for warts is begun. An important and universal aspect
of the treatment of any type and location of genital warts is
to examine and treat the sexual partners of the patient. In
addition, women with genital warts should receive STD and
Pap screenings annually until normal Pap tests have occurred
for 36 consecutive months after treatment. After this time, a
woman may elect to receive Pap screenings every 36 months.
Women who are found to have HPV but who do not have any
visible warts are not candidates for treatment because there
are no treatments that are known to eradicate the infection.
These women should, however, obtain annual Pap screenings.
Additionally women with a Pap test indicative of low-grade
SIL or ASCUS (i.e., atypical squamous cells of undetermined
significance) should obtain HPV DNA testing. If high-risk
types of HPV DNA are found, these women should have a
colposcopy and biopsy to assess for more extensive dysplasia.
Gardasil, an HPV vaccine, has recently been released and is
recommended for women ages 14 to 26 years of age for the
prevention of HPV infection, and thus is expected to lower
cervical dysplasia and cervical cancer rates.

THE BOTANICAL PRACTITIONER'S PERSPECTIVE

The herbalist's approach to genital warts may be in conjunction with or in place of conventional treatment, with appropriate conventional attention to cervical (and anal) cancer risk. A
comprehensive botanical approach supports the body's inherent abilities to resist infection and uncontrolled cellular proliferation caused by the virus. Herbs with antiviral actions are
key components of the botanical protocol. Herbs with immunostimulatory actions, particularly activation of cell-mediated
immunity, are of specific importance. Adaptogens (see Chapter
5) are also ideally included in a comprehensive botanical protocol to further support the immune system.

DISCUSSION OF BOTANICAL PROTOCOL

Treatment of HPV can be approached topically alone, but it is
optimal to boost overall resistance using a combination of topical and internal therapies (Table 12-5). For topical treatment,
undiluted botanical extracts can be directly applied to warts
using a cotton swab several times daily (use a fresh cotton swab
for each application) for 6 to 12 weeks, as needed. Suppositories
can be inserted vaginally or rectally for warts in those areas.
They should be inserted nightly five times per week for 6 to 12
weeks. The patient should be reevaluated periodically for HPV.

PROTOCOL FOR THE TREATMENT OF HUMAN PAPILLOMAVIRUS

Topical Treatment

Option 1. Combine the following tinctures and apply to lesions two to three times daily with a cotton swab for 6 to 12 weeks:

Thyme	(Thymus vulgaris)	30 mL
Goldenseal	(Hydrastis canadensis)	20 mL
Myrrh	(Commiphora molmol)	20 mL
St. John's wort	(Hypericum perforatum)	20 mL
Thuja	(Thuja occidentalis)	10 mL
	Total: 100 mL	

Option 2. Combine the following tinctures and apply to lesions two to three times daily with a cotton swab for 6 to 12 weeks:

Tea tree	(Melaleuca alternifolia)	30 mL
Goldenseal	(Hydrastis canadensis)	20 mL
Oregano	(Origanum vulgare)	20 mL
Lemon balm	(Melissa officinalis)	20 mL
Licorice	(Glycyrrhiza glabra)	10 mL
	Total: 100 mL	

Note that applying undiluted tincture to sensitive mucosa can cause a burning sensation. If this is too irritating to the patient, first apply a small amount of calendula oil to the surrounding area, and then apply tincture carefully on the lesion.

Option 3. For suppositories, use either combination of the previous tincture combinations in a suppository recipe. See Chapter 3 for general suppository instructions.

Combine external treatment with the following internal treatment.

Antiviral Tincture: Internal Treatment

Combine the following tinctures:

Astragalus	(Astragalus membranaceus)	25 mL
Reishi	(Ganoderma lucidum)	25 mL
Ashwagandha	(Withania somnifera)	25 mL
Echinacea	(Echinacea spp.)	15 mL
Usnea	(Usnea barbata)	10 mL
	Total: 100 mL	

Dose: 5 mL twice daily for up to 6 months for acute cases; 3 mL daily for maintenance and prophylaxis for up to 6 months posttreatment for an acute case

TABLE 12-5   Botanical Treatment Strategies for Human Papillomavirus

Therapeutic Goal	Therapeutic Activity	Botanical Name	Common Name
Reduce viral infection	Antiviral	Allium sativum	Garlic
Prevent neoplasia	Antimicrobial	Astragalus membranaceus	Astragalus
Reduce cervical inflammation and heal tissue	Antitumorigenic	Calendula officinalis	Calendula
		Commiphora molmol	Myrrh
		Echinacea spp.	Echinacea
		Ganoderma lucidum	Reishi
		Hydrastis canadensis	Goldenseal
		Hypericum perforatum	St. John's wort
		Lavandula officinalis	Lavender
		Lomatium dissectum	Lomatium
		Melaleuca alternifolia	Tea tree
		Melissa officinalis	Lemon balm
		Origanum vulgare	Oregano
		Thuja occidentalis	Thuja
		Thymus vulgaris	Thyme
		Usnea barbata	Usnea
Improve overall immune response via HPA axis support	Adaptogens	See Chapter 5 for a discussion of adaptogens.	

HPA, Hypothalamic-pituitary-adrenal.

Astragalus

Astragalus has been used for centuries in Chinese medicine as a qi tonic, specifically for strengthening what is called the *wei qi* or the protective energy of the body. It has long been used to build energy, increase general immunity, improve digestion, and improve longevity. Herbalists and naturopathic doctors commonly use astragalus for its immunostimulatory effects. Oral doses of astragalus have been found to increase immunoglobulin E (IgE), IgA, and IgM antibody levels and lymphocyte levels in humans.[62] Of particular relevance to the treatment of genital warts was an RCT involving 531 patients with chronic cervicitis secondary to HPV, cytomegalovirus (CMV), and herpes simplex virus (HSV) infections. This trial demonstrated that a liquid extract of astragalus root potentiated recombinant IFN in the treatment of cervicitis, particularly when resulting from HPV infection.[63] In addition to the immunostimulatory effect of astragalus, people who take it often experience increased physical stamina, increased mental alertness, and decreased fatigue.

Echinacea

The purified polysaccharide from *Echinacea purpurea*, arabinogalactan, has been found to increase T-cell proliferation and the production of IFN by macrophages.[64] Additionally, unpurified fresh pressed juice of *E. purpurea* has been shown in vitro to induce macrophages to produce cytokines, which in turn create an antiviral effect against viruses, including the herpes virus. Clinical trials of echinacea are of mixed results. As an example, a yearlong prospective, double-blind, placebo-controlled crossover trial (*n* = 50) examined the efficacy of a tablet form of *E. purpurea* (i.e., Echinaforce) in the clinical course of genital herpes. The study found no statistically significant benefit in the clinical course of frequently recurrent genital herpes.[65] It is possible that this study failed to show benefit because of insufficient dosing and/or the use of a tablet form of echinacea. Certain constituents in the echinacea species, namely alkenes and amides, possess potent antiviral activity (including against HSV). Ethanol extracts of these constituents and these extracts of echinacea have been shown to have the most potent antiviral activity.[66] Although clinical trials have not yet conclusively demonstrated significant antiviral and immune stimulation, previous and current naturopathic and herbal practice demonstrate these effects and hence many modern herbalists and naturopathic doctors use echinacea as part of their treatment of HPV.

Green Tea

A 2008 RCT (*n* = 503) randomized women and men with HPV into two treatment groups with standardized green tea extract (i.e., Polyphenon E at strengths of 10% and 15%) and one group with a control ointment. Patients applied the ointments three times daily and were assessed twice weekly for symptoms and adverse events until wart clearance or 16 weeks. In the Polyphenon E 15% group, 53% of patients experienced complete clearance, along with 51% of patients in the Polyphenon E 10% group and 37% in the control group. Women were more successfully treated than men (i.e., 60% of women experienced complete eradication compared with 45% of men). The treatment was well tolerated.[67] A similar study was conducted the same year. A group of 502 patients with external genital and perianal warts was randomized to receive sinecatechins ointment at 15% or 10% concentrations or a matching vehicle control three times daily until clearance for a maximum of 16 weeks. Like the previous study, 12-week follow-ups were conducted to evaluate incidences of recurrence. Clearance of warts was observed in 57.2% and 56.3% of the sinecatechins ointment 15% and 10% groups, respectively, compared with 33.7% for vehicle (*p* < .001), with improvements seen in week 4 forward. The treatment groups exhibited fewer recurrences than controls, and the treatment was similarly well tolerated.[68]

Goldenseal

Although no research has been done specifically on the treatment of HPV with goldenseal, the herb has shown broad antimicrobial effects that suggest this herb may be beneficial as part of a topical herbal application for this infection.

Lemon Balm

Acutely, lemon balm extract is applied topically for its virostatic action. Lemon balm has demonstrated effects against a number of viruses, including HSV and influenza. Virostatic effects are attributable to the glycoside-bound phenol carboxylic acid and its polymers. These constituents block cellular receptors responsible for viral adsorption, and thus viral replication.[69] Additionally, oxidation products of caffeic acid, found in lemon balm, inhibit protein biosynthesis in vitro, which may account for the antiviral activity of topical application.[70] These in vitro data have been confirmed in at least three human trials. One of the more recent trials was a prospective, double-blind, randomized trial (*n* = 66). The treatment group applied a standardized lemon balm cream—1% Lo-701 dried extract from *Melissa officinalis* leaves (70:1)—four times daily to an active *Herpes labialis* lesion over a 5-day period. All patients suffered from recurrent *H. labialis*. However, there was a significant decrease in the intensity of herpetic symptoms by day 2 of treatment between the active versus the placebo group (*p* = .042).[71] Lemon balm also has anxiolytic and sedative actions.[72]

Licorice

Although no studies were identified on the treatment of HPV with licorice or its extracts, other viral studies suggest, as well as the herb's traditional uses, that investigation into such use may be promising.

Oregano and Thyme

Both oregano and thyme essential oils are regularly included in vaginal suppositories for the treatment of vaginal infections, including HPV infection. One study reports on the efficacy of thyme as an antibacterial, and in another study oregano and clove oils were diluted and examined for their activity against enveloped and nonenveloped ribonucleic acid (RNA) and DNA viruses. Olive oil was also included as a control. Viruses were incubated with oil dilutions and enumerated by plaque assay. Antiviral activity of oregano and clove oils was demonstrated on two enveloped viruses of both the DNA and RNA types and the disintegration of virus envelope was visualized by negative staining using transmission electron microscopy.[73,74] Care should be taken in the use of essential oils topically; used undiluted (i.e., neat) they can be irritating to sensitive tissues such as cervical or vaginal mucosa. Tincture may be applied directly.

Thuja

Thuja (Fig. 12-4) is used for the treatment of genital and anal warts, and is commonly recommended in the naturopathic treatment of cervical dysplasia for its antiviral activity.[75] The main constituent is an essential oil consisting of alpha (α)-thujone and beta (β)-thujone, the content of which varies proportionally with the amount of ethanol used in producing the plant extract. If consumed internally, thujone can be neurotoxic, convulsant, and hallucinogenic. Long-term or excessive use of thujone-rich products can cause restlessness, vomiting, vertigo, tremors, renal damage, and convulsions.[76] Internal use of thuja decoctions and even very small doses of thuja oil (e.g., 20 drops per day for 5 days) as an abortifacient has been associated with

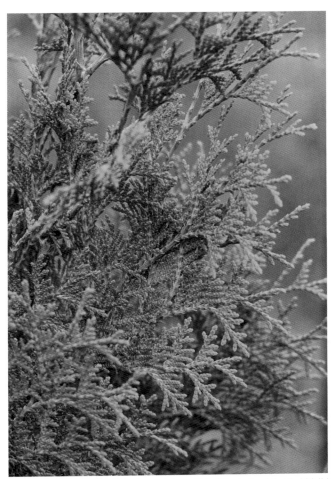

FIGURE 12-4 Thuja *(Thuja occidentalis)*. (Photo by Martin Wall.)

neurotoxicity, convulsions, and death.[75] Additionally, thuja is associated with a substantial risk of inducing fetal malformation, and is absolutely contraindicated for use in pregnancy, even topical use.[75] No research on the short- or long-term topical use of this herb was identified. Ingestion of thuja cannot be recommended because of its significant potential for toxicity.

Usnea

Usnea lichens have a history of use that spans centuries and countries from ancient China to modern Turkey, from rural dwellers in South Africa to modern-day naturopathic physicians and herbalists in the United States.[45,46] The lichen is rich in usnic acid, which has demonstrated in vitro antimicrobial activity against bacteria, viruses, and protozoa. Additionally, it exhibits antiinflammatory and analgesic activity.[26] Alcohol extract may be added to a suppository blend or diluted in water or tea (1 Tbsp tincture per cup of liquid) for use as a peri-wash or in sitz baths.

NUTRITIONAL CONSIDERATIONS

The nutritional supplements recommended in the treatment of cervical dysplasia (see Chapter 11) are recommended when treating HPV infection.

 TREATMENT SUMMARY FOR GENITAL WARTS

- Apply antiviral botanical agents directly to affected sites using a cotton swab. Use suppositories for cervical, vaginal, or rectal lesions.
- Support the body's inherent resistance using herbs with antiviral and immunostimulatory actions.

CASE HISTORY

Mary, a 27-year-old female patient, presented for her annual gynecologic examination and Pap smear. She had no menstrual or vaginal symptoms. She was currently not sexually active but had recently ended a 2-year, monogamous, heterosexual relationship. Her Pap smear revealed cervical atypia (ASCUS, i.e., atypical squamous cells of undetermined significance). The patient was counseled about her management options, ranging from colposcopy to wait-and-retest in 3 months. The patient was very anxious but chose to wait and have her Pap redone in 3 months. The second Pap demonstrated cervical ASCUS once again. The patient was extremely anxious about this result and wanted to be tested for HPV. She refused a biopsy. An HPV nucleic acid test was done that revealed the presence of noncancerous HPV. At this point, the patient continued to refuse colposcopy; however, she wanted to be on active treatment. She willingly agreed to engage in active naturopathic treatment for 3 months and then to undergo a repeat Pap smear. The following treatments were recommended to the patient:

- Increased consumption of dark leafy greens and broccoli to at least three servings weekly.
- Engage in relaxation activities regularly (the patient chose to attend a yoga class).
- Folic acid: 10 mg p.o. daily

Tincture Formula

Echinacea	(*Echinacea* spp.)	40 mL
Licorice	(*Glycyrrhiza glabra*)	20 mL
St. Johns wort	(*Hypericum perforatum*)	20 mL
Lemon balm	(*Melissa officinalis*)	15 mL
Thuja*	(*Thuja occidentalis*)	5 mL
		Total: 100 mL

Dose: 5 mL three times daily

The patient was diligent with her protocol and tolerated treatment well. A repeat Pap smear done after 3 months of treatment was normal. The patient discontinued the folic acid and herbal tincture after this normal Pap smear result. A subsequent Pap smear 6 months later was also normal. All subsequent Pap smears up to the most recent one, done 24 months after her initial atypical Pap smear, have been normal (i.e., no atypia present).

*To avoid possible toxicity resulting from thuja, replace with 5-mL thyme *(Thymus vulgaris)* tincture.

HERPES

HSV is a member of the human herpes virus group that includes HSV-1, HSV-2, and Epstein-Barr virus (EBV). HSV is a recurrent viral infection that remains dormant in the nervous system with periods of reactivation characterized by individual or multiple clusters of fluid-filled vesicles at specifically affected sites. HSV-1 and -2 are the main types of herpes virus seen in general clinical practice. HSV-1 typically manifests above the waist and is referred to as *Herpes labialis* because of it primarily appearing on the lips in the form of cold sores. HSV-2, *Herpes genitalis,* typically appears on the genitals, although it also produces skin lesions. The vesicles rupture, leaving small, sometimes painful ulcers, which generally heal without scarring, although recurrent lesions at the same site may cause scarring. Coinfection with HSV-1 and -2 increases the frequency of HSV-2 outbreaks. Orogenital sex can lead to cross-contamination of these sites, with oral herpes being more likely transmitted to the genitals than the other way around. The incubation period for HSV-1 is 3 to 7 days and 3 to 5 days for HSV-2.

Approximately 75% of individuals in the United States are infected with HSV-1, and about 25% with HSV-2, with an estimated incidence of 500,000 to 1 million new cases annually.[77-79] Independent predictors of HSV-2 infection include sex (i.e., women are more likely to become infected and have more frequent outbreaks, whereas men are more likely to transmit infection), increased age, poverty, cocaine use, and multiple sexual partners.[77] Since the late 1970s, seroprevalence has quintupled among white teenagers and doubled among whites in their twenties. The virus is spread through contact with the lesions and through viral shedding. Sexual contact is the primary method of contamination; however, kissing and other contact with sores or shed viruses in an asymptomatic individual can lead to infection. Casual contact, such as sharing of a drinking glass or cigarette, has also been known to lead to infection. Ninety percent of affected individuals are unaware they have herpes.[80] HSV-2 infection significantly increases susceptibility to HIV infection.

Immunologic changes of pregnancy, particularly depression of T-cell response, appear to make pregnant women more susceptible to a number of viral infections, including HSV.[81] Primary herpes outbreaks in pregnancy, especially during the third trimester, pose great danger to a newborn, causing significant morbidity and mortality. Antibodies to HSV-2 have been detected in about 20% of pregnant women, with only about 5% aware they have herpes (see Herpes Simplex Virus in Pregnancy).

Prevention is always the best treatment. Practicing safe sex on all occasions regardless of whether lesions are visible, and avoiding contact with active lesions is essential. HSV may be shed in the saliva and genital secretions of asymptomatic individuals. Active lesions shed between 100 and 1000 times the amount of virus. Minor injury, for example, irritation from vaginal *Candida* infection, may increase the likelihood of viral transmission. Condoms do not guarantee protection, but do significantly reduce HSV-2 transmission, especially to women.[82] The virus is commonly passed from a person who does not know they have the virus because they have never had any symptoms.

PATHOPHYSIOLOGY

HSV travels along the peripheral nerve axons to the nerve cell bodies in the dorsal root ganglia and can exist in the paraspinous ganglia indefinitely, sometimes in a completely inactive state. The virus can be reactivated and begin replicating in response to such factors as stress, depression, and anxiety, trauma to mucosa, fever, exposure to ultraviolet light (i.e., sun exposure), menstruation, poor sleep, spicy food, immunodeficiency, and other unknown factors. Migration to mucosal surfaces by way of the peripheral sensory nerves can lead to a cutaneous outbreak of lesions, which are often painful. Although the virus usually becomes dormant after an outbreak and before the next outbreak, if it occurs, an infected person, even if asymptomatic, can still pass the virus to another person. Asymptomatic viral shedding is common and occurs in cycles. Therefore transmission of infection is possible at any time regardless of the presence of active lesions. The possibility of transmission between an infected and uninfected person in a monogamous relationship increases at the rate of about 10% a year. Women who have regular herpes outbreaks, or who have a sexual partner who has active outbreaks, should have routine Pap smears because herpes may predispose women to cervical cancer. Recent research suggests possible long-term consequences of harboring chronic HSV infection, such as development of rheumatoid arthritis.[83]

SYMPTOMS

The first episode of herpes after initial infection is known as the primary outbreak, characteristically appearing with flulike symptoms such as fever, headache, and swollen lymph glands in the groin (Table 12-6). Primary outbreaks can last 2 to 3 weeks and can be severe enough in rare cases to require hospitalization. Recurrent herpes outbreaks are commonly heralded by a prodromal stage with characteristic feelings of tingling or itching in the genital area or around the mouth, pain and tingling in the groin, and possibly in the buttocks and backs of the thighs. Virus is already present on the skin in the prodromal phase, so this is considered a contagious phase although blisters are not yet visible. The prodromal phase typically lasts 1 to 3 days; the following vesicles, lesions, and scabbing last for up to 10 days before complete healing has occurred. Recurrent outbreaks are often mild and may present with pruritus, local tingling or pain, slight vaginal discharge but present with no generalized systemic symptoms. Small sores or vesicles can occur anywhere on the skin or mucous membranes of the mouth or anogenital region, and are most common around the mouth and genital area. The vesicles break and become wet, finally crusting over. Healing is complete when new skin is

TABLE 12-6   Symptoms of Herpes According to Type of Outbreak

Category	Clinical Manifestation
Primary outbreak	• This is the initial outbreak after infection; if patients do not notice vesicles, a primary outbreak may be dismissed as "flu." • Characterized by systemic infection, commonly with fever and aching • May last 2-3 weeks • Frequently accompanied by lymphadenopathy • Appearance of vesicle clusters on an erythematous base that develop into ulcers that crust over and heal • Severe primary outbreak can cause serious infection, including encephalitis, and may require hospitalization • Immunocompromised patients may develop especially severe symptoms
Recurrent episodes	• Symptoms of tingling and itching or perineal aching may precede the appearance of vesicles and last 1-3 days. Note that virus is already present on the skin during this stage. • Vesicles appear and last up to 10 days until full healing.
Subclinical infection	• Asymptomatic with viral shedding

Adapted from Roe V: Living with genital herpes: how effective is antiviral therapy? *J Perinat Neonat Nurs* 18(3):206–215, 2004.

formed under the scab, which falls off. Rarely, focal necrosis, ballooning degeneration of skin cells, and other histopathologic changes can result.

Most patients are mistakenly thought to be silent carriers. At least 90% of HSV-2 carriers are ignorant of their conditions with up to 60% to 75% having unrecognized signs and symptoms of genital herpes. Commonly, symptoms are falsely attributed to other more casual urogenital problems. Because herpes is a self-healing condition, with symptoms easily controlled with topical nonspecific agents, the diagnosis is not frequently made. The following are examples of the conditions to which female patients attribute what are actually symptoms of genital herpes outbreaks[84]:

- Vaginitis
- Allergies or reactions to medications, toilet paper, sanitary pads or other menstrual products, soaps, condoms
- Lack of lubrication during sex
- Excessively frequent sexual intercourse
- Irritation from tight jeans, g-strings, bicycle seats
- Urinary tract infections
- Vaginal dryness
- Shaving burns
- Reactions to hair removal products
- Hemorrhoids or anal fissures

DIAGNOSIS

When a patient presents with clusters of painful vesicles and inflammation of the surrounding area, herpes should be considered. The standard test for HSV infections is viral culture of vesicular fluid. Direct immunofluorescent staining with conjugated monoclonal antibodies to HSV is faster, more expensive, and only about 80% to 90% as accurate as viral culture. PCR is the most accurate and most expensive test.[85]

Diagnosis in the neonate can be difficult at first because symptoms are sometimes nonspecific (e.g., fever, lethargy), with no other outward signs of infection. Less than 50% of newborns with disseminated disease or encephalitis have skin lesions.[86] If diagnosis is delayed, damage to the central nervous system (CNS) or internal organs can be significant.

CONVENTIONAL TREATMENT APPROACHES

Antiviral therapy with drugs that selectively inhibit viral replication, including acyclovir, famciclovir (Famvir), and valacyclovir (Valtrex), is the standard treatment. Acyclovir has been on the market for longer than 20 years and has a reasonable safety profile, even when given during pregnancy. Teratogenicity has not been demonstrated, even during the first trimester. Famciclovir and valacyclovir are more absorbable and higher blood levels can be sustained, although their safety, especially during pregnancy, has not been as thoroughly tested as acyclovir.[79] Studies suggest that prophylactic administration of acyclovir during pregnancy can reduce shedding, shorten the duration of shedding, and reduce the cesarean rate, although these findings were small and not conclusive. The usual dose of acyclovir is 60 mg per kg of body weight per day in three doses intravenously for 14 days for localized skin disease, and 21 days for more severe infections.[87] Acyclovir has been associated with numerous side effects in its various dosage forms, including nausea and vomiting, diarrhea, headache, dizziness, fatigue, skin rash, edema, inguinal lymphadenopathy, anorexia, leg pain, medication taste, and sore throat from short-term oral administration; and nausea and vomiting, diarrhea, headache, dizziness, insomnia, irritability, depression, rash, acne, hair loss, arthralgia, fever, palpitations, sore throat, muscle cramps, menstrual abnormalities, and lymphadenopathy with long-term use.

HERPES SIMPLEX VIRUS IN PREGNANCY

It is estimated that 20% to 25% of pregnant women have genital herpes. With recurrent herpes, less than 0.1% of babies will contract the infection. Primary herpes outbreaks pose a much greater risk to the fetus/neonate with transmission rates as high as 50%. In asymptomatic cases the risk of transmission at birth is about 0.04%; in symptomatic cases, the risk is about 5%.

Primary herpes infection in pregnancy is associated with miscarriage, premature labor, intrauterine growth retardation, and neonatal infection. Neonatal infection most frequently occurs during labor and is associated with increased neonatal death, brain damage, seizures, cerebral palsy, blindness, and deafness.[88] Neonatal herpes affects about 1 in 15,000 newborns and the prognosis for disseminated disease with encephalitis is poor.[89] Because 90% of cases of neonatal herpes are a result of direct contact with lesions in the birth canal, cesarean section is routinely performed as the mode of delivery in active herpes outbreaks at the time of labor. Neonates are treated with acyclovir or vidarabine, but this treatment is less effective once the infection has spread to the brain and internal organs.[90]

More recently, experiments have looked at using acyclovir for herpes prophylaxis in late pregnancy. Treatment has been shown to reduce recurrences after a primary infection, and reduce asymptomatic viral shedding as well as need for cesarean delivery; however, prophylaxis only partly prevents neonatal herpes infection because it is not applicable to patients with no known clinical history (but may carry and transmit the virus).[89,91]

THE BOTANICAL PRACTITIONER'S PERSPECTIVE

HSV infection is a major global health problem, and its association with HIV infection makes it imperative to develop effective prevention and treatment strategies. The efficacy of many topical pharmaceutical agents in treating herpes has been somewhat disappointing and inconsistent, and additionally, they are costly.[92,93] Patients are often looking for safe and effective alternative measures to reduce the frequency of outbreaks and shorten their duration. It is also important to look for agents that will be effective at preventing the virus from inculcating into nerve cell bodies, proliferating, and taking up host residence. Botanicals represent a promising area for research.[16] Unfortunately, at present there are few well-designed human clinical trials looking at the effects of herbs on HSV. However, a number of botanicals have demonstrated antiherpetic activity in vitro, offering some validation of the traditional use of herbs for infection. Several herbs have been shown to be topically healing for wounds, and as discussed in Chapter 5, have demonstrated efficacy in improving immune response and reducing stress. These latter categories are listed in Table 12-7 with brief descriptions of their applications to HSV treatment, but discussions of these herbs are found elsewhere throughout this book.

Clinically, patients using a combination of botanical and nutritional therapies report reduced frequency, severity, and length of outbreaks. Herbalists have found botanical medicines effective at relieving symptoms associated with outbreaks, preventing outbreaks, and reducing the frequency of outbreaks (Table 12-7). Some patients have reported going 10 years or more without an outbreak, even with a history of regularly recurrent outbreaks. Similarly, pregnant women have been shown to cease to have recurrent outbreaks during gestation, even with a history of regular recurrence in prior pregnancies (see Case History: Herpes Simplex Virus 2 in Pregnancy). It is unknown how botanicals affect asymptomatic shedding.

 ## CASE HISTORY: HERPES SIMPLEX VIRUS 2 IN PREGNANCY

Caroline is a 38-year-old mother of two children born by cesarean section because of history of recurrent herpes simplex virus 2 (HSV-2) outbreaks, including at the time of delivery in both previous pregnancies. Currently 22 weeks pregnant with her third child, she is already being told by her obstetrician that she has almost no chance of a vaginal birth given the likelihood that she will again experience an outbreak close to labor given her frequently recurring outbreaks, sometimes as often as every 2 to 3 weeks. She is very discouraged by this because she found recovery from the cesarean sections challenging, and she would prefer to have a vaginal birth. She has been told by a birthing center that if she can remain free of herpes for several weeks before and at the time of labor, they will support her desire for a vaginal birth, barring other problems. At the time, Caroline was working as a nurse, doing many night shifts to bring in extra money for her family and to have time available in the daylight hours for her daughter. She was chronically stressed and exhausted, and the anxiety about the potentially impending cesarean was exacerbating her stress level. She was eating a lot of fast foods, especially in the evening at the hospital, and drinking coffee regularly to combat fatigue. Her marriage and home life were otherwise good, and she was committed to making personal and dietary changes to see if she could prevent herpes outbreaks.

Caroline immediately went on a high-lysine and low-arginine diet; cut back her night hours, switching to weekends with the plan to phase out working by the middle of her third trimester (she had planned to stop working then anyway); committed to stop drinking coffee; and began the following herbal protocol:

- Infusion of equal parts of echinacea and burdock roots, two cups daily, prepared by steeping 28 g of herb (1 oz) in 1 L of boiling water for 2 hours
- Nervine tea, two cups daily, consisting of chamomile, lemon balm, and lavender
- 2000 mg daily, vitamin C
- Alternating applications of vitamin E and antiviral tincture (i.e., lemon balm, licorice, thyme, and St. John's wort in a witch hazel extract base) should tingling or lesions become apparent

Caroline had an outbreak 1 week after the initial visit, at 23 weeks of pregnancy. This was not surprising, given that she had been under prolonged stress and had worked an especially long weekend, and had only just started the herbal protocol. This was the last outbreak she experienced during the pregnancy, and cultures at 38 and 40 weeks yielded negative results. Caroline gave birth vaginally, at the birthing center, after 3 days of difficult labor and antibiotics for prolonged rupture of membranes. She experienced a vaginal yeast infection after the birth but felt this was a mild inconvenience compared with the recovery she previously experienced postcesarean.

Symptomatic relief can be directed at systemic manifestations during a primary outbreak, mostly via analgesics to relieve discomfort and antivirals to control the degree of infection, and can be used topically to speed the healing of lesions and relieve discomfort associated with both primary

TABLE 12-7 Botanical Treatment Strategies for Herpes Simplex Virus 1 and 2

Therapeutic Goal	Therapeutic Activity	Botanical Name	Common Name
Pain relief for systemic aching and discomfort in primary outbreak	Analgesic	*Actaea racemosa*	Black cohosh
		Corydalis ambigua	Corydalis
		Piscidia piscipula	Jamaican dogwood
		Viburnum spp.	Cramp bark and black haw
Reduce systemic viral replication, inhibit viral attachment to cells; topical antiviral activity	Antiviral	*Aloe vera*	Aloe
		Calendula officinalis	Calendula
		Echinacea spp.	Echinacea
		Ganoderma lucidum	Reishi
		Glycyrrhiza glabra	Licorice
		Hypericum perforatum	St. John's wort
		Melissa officinalis	Lemon balm
		Salvia officinalis	Sage
		Thuja occidentalis	Thuja
		Uncaria tomentosa	Cat's claw
Wound-healing agents to promote granulation of new, healthy tissue	Vulnerary	*Aloe vera*	Aloe
		Calendula officinale	Calendula
		Symphytum officinale	Comfrey
Relieve local pain	Topical analgesic	*Hypericum perforatum*	St. John's wort
		Mentha piperita	Peppermint
		Piper methysticum	Kava kava
Relieve local pain	Antiinflammatory	*Glycyrrhiza glabra*	Licorice
		Hypericum perforatum	St. John's wort
		Lavandula officinalis	Lavender
		Scutellaria baicalensis	Chinese skullcap
		Symphytum officinalis	Comfrey
Dry weeping lesions	Astringents	*Hamamelis virginiana*	Witch hazel
		Plantago spp.	Plantain
		Quercus alba	White oak bark
Dry weeping lesions	Antimicrobial powder	*Commiphora molmol*	Myrrh
Enhance immune response, increase general resistance	Immunomodulation	*Andrographis paniculata*	Andrographis
Enhance immune response, increase general resistance	Adaptogens	*Eleutherococcus senticosus*	Eleuthero
		Panax ginseng	Ginseng
		Panax quinquefolius	American ginseng
		Rhaponticum carthamoides	Rhaponticum
		Rhodiola rosea	Rhodiola
		Schisandra chinensis	Schisandra
		Withania somnifera	Ashwagandha
Improve stress response	Adaptogens	*Eleutherococcus senticosus*	Eleuthero
		Panax ginseng	Ginseng
		Panax quinquefolius	American ginseng
		Rhaponticum carthamoides	Rhaponticum
		Rhodiola rosea	Rhodiola
		Schisandra chinensis	Schisandra
		Withania somnifera	Ashwagandha
Improve stress response	Nervines	*Avena sativa*	Milky oats
		Eschscholzia californica	California poppy
		Lavandula officinalis	Lavender
		Leonurus cardiaca	Motherwort
		Melissa officinalis	Lemon balm
		Passiflora incarnata	Passionflower
		Scutellaria lateriflora	Skullcap
		Turnera diffusa	Damiana

and recurrent episodes. A number of herbs have been shown to have beneficial effects in supporting and enhancing immunity. Because host immune response plays a role in the outcome of herpes infection, with the immune system modulating infection both in the nervous system and the periphery, prevention focuses on supporting optimal immune response using adaptogens and the use of antivirals to reduce viral attachment and proliferation.[94] Additionally, herbs that improve the stress response (i.e., adaptogens) and relieve stress (i.e., nervines) are important because stress is both a known precipitating factor for outbreaks and suppressive of immune function (see Chapter 5).

Analgesics

Analgesic herbs are used internally, typically as tinctures, either singly or in combination, for the symptomatic relief of generalized discomfort and aches in uncomplicated primary herpes outbreaks and for aching discomfort in the prodromal phase of recurrent outbreaks. Black cohosh, an antispasmodic and mild analgesic, was historically used specifically for aching, drawing discomfort in the buttocks and the backs of the thighs.[95] Cramp bark and black haw are reliable antispasmodic herbs with analgesic effects. Corydalis and Jamaican dogwood have strong analgesic and sedating effects.

Antiviral Botanicals

The following herbs represent a selection of botanicals used for internal or topical antiviral therapy. All have shown some measure of antimicrobial activity in various studies and are a promising area of research for herpes treatment. Specific studies of the effects of herbs on HSV are presented in the following. These herbs may be used singly, but more commonly are used by herbal practitioners in combination with other antivirals, or in comprehensive, multiherb, multieffect formulae.

Aloe

Aloe has long been used by herbalists as a topical healing agent for wounds, burns, irritated skin, and sores. Two studies were conducted by Syed and colleagues examining the efficacy of topical *Aloe vera* treatments on men experiencing primary outbreaks of genital herpes. In the first study, 120 men were randomized into three parallel groups receiving either 0.5% in hydrophilic cream, aloe vera gel, or placebo three times daily for 2 weeks. The shortest mean duration of healing occurred with aloe cream, followed by gel and then placebo with healing times of 4.8 days, 7.0 days, and 14.0 days, respectively. Percentages of cured patients were 70%, 45%, and 7.5%, respectively.[96] In the second study, 60 men were randomized into two groups receiving 0.5% aloe extract in a hydrophilic cream base or placebo. The trial had comparable favorable results to the previously discussed trial.[97] Additionally, in vitro testing has demonstrated virucidal effects of anthraquinones and anthraquinone derivatives such as emodin, a component of aloe.

Cat's Claw

The use of cat's claw, *una de gato,* by traditional healers of tropical South America extends back in history for an unknown length of time as part of oral tradition. It was used as an antiinflammatory,

antitumor, and antirheumatic, and to treat conditions including gastric ulcers, fevers, diarrhea, fertility, and female genitourinary cancers. It is also used in the treatment of disharmony between body and spirit, or what we might call anxiety.[21] Inhibition of HSV-1 and -2 was demonstrated in vitro by a standardized extract of cat's claw. *H. genitalis* was significantly more susceptible to inactivation by the extract than *H. labialis*.[21] Cat's claw appears to selectively modulate ovarian hormone function and therefore should be used with care in women with hormonal dysregulation, particularly progesterone insufficiency. It is completely contraindicated in pregnancy.[21] The herb has demonstrated significant in vitro and in vivo immunostimulatory, immunoregulatory, immunosuppressive, and antiinflammatory effects, specifically, enhanced lymphocyte production and inhibition of tumor necrosis factor alpha (TNF-α) in a dose-dependent manner.[21] Therefore it is cautioned that any patients on immunomodulating therapies (e.g., immunosuppressant, hyperimmunoglobulin therapy, receiving vaccinations) avoid the use of cat's claw; caution should also be exercised in patients with autoimmune conditions. Use of cat's claw–containing products is entirely contraindicated during pregnancy and lactation; however, it has been used traditionally in the immediate postpartum period for recovery after childbirth, and may facilitate milk supply through estrogen modulation.[21]

Echinacea

Echinacea is a popular herb used to prevent and mitigate viral infections, and also to prevent recurrent infection. It is commonly used as a tincture or decoction as part of a protocol for HSV infection. In one study, *E. purpurea* polysaccharides decreased the latency rate in HSV-1–infected mice when applied before infection.[98] Midwives rely on it in pregnancy as one of the antivirals considered safe to use during that time. In a 5-month uncontrolled clinical study of 4598 patients, a salve prepared from the juice of the aerial portion of *E. purpurea* was reported to have an 85% success rate in the treatment of a number of inflammatory skin conditions, among them Herpes simplex eruptions.[21] Echinacea is used by herbalists during pregnancy for the prevention of herpes outbreaks. Longitudinal use of echinacea in pregnancy was evaluated for safety and outcomes by Gallo and coworkers. In a prospective study, 206 Canadian women already taking echinacea-containing products were compared with a matched cohort not taking echinacea. The products mostly contained *E. angustifolia* and *E. purpurea,* although one respondent took *E. pallida.* Thirty-eight percent took the tincture at a dose of up to 30 drops daily and 58% took tablets or capsules at a dose of 250 to 1000 mg/day. Echinacea use was primarily in the first trimester (54%); 8% used echinacea during all three trimesters. There were no statistical differences between pregnancy outcomes in the two groups, nor were there statistically significant differences in the neonates.[99]

Lemon Balm

Lemon balm (Fig. 12-5) has classically been used as an uplifting herb for the treatment of stress and anxiety. Rich in volatile oils, in vitro and clinical research conducted over the past decade has demonstrated impressive

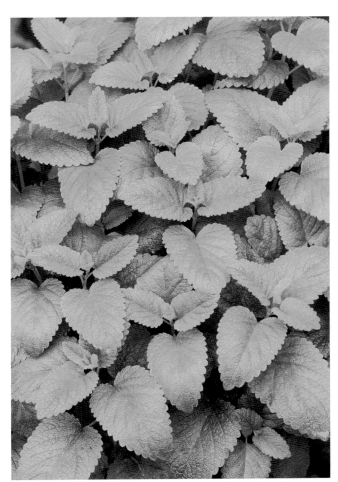

FIGURE 12-5 Lemon balm *(Melissa officinalis)*. (Photo by Martin Wall.)

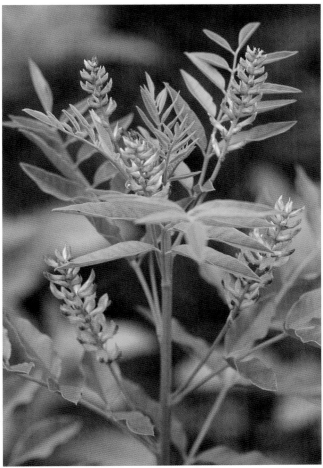

FIGURE 12-6 Licorice *(Glycyrrhiza glabra)*. (Photo by Martin Wall.)

results using lemon balm ointment as a local therapy in the treatment and prevention of herpes outbreaks.[48,100,101] In one study, four different concentrations of volatile oils extracted from lemon balm were examined for effects against HSV-2. At concentrations of 200 µg/mL, replication of HSV-2 was inhibited, indicating that the *M. officinalis L.* extract contains an anti–HSV-2 substance.[100] In another experiment, lemon balm extract inhibited virucidal activity and inhibited attachment of HSV-1 to host cells in vitro, even against acyclovir-resistant strains.[102-104] Another study, a double-blind, placebo-controlled, randomized trial, was carried out with the aim of proving efficacy of standardized and highly concentrated lemon balm cream for the therapy of HSV-1. Sixty-six patients with a history of recurrent HSV-1 (at least four episodes per year) in one center were treated topically; 34 of them with lemon balm cream and 32 with placebo. The cream had to be smeared on the affected area four times daily over 5 days. A combined symptom score of the values for complaints, size of affected area, and blisters at day 2 of therapy was formed as the primary target parameter. A significant difference seen in the combined symptom score on the second day of treatment is of particular importance because symptoms are usually worst at that time. In addition to reducing the duration of the healing period, the treatment led to prevention of spreading of the infection and had a rapid effect on common herpes symptoms including itching, tingling, burning, stabbing, swelling, tautness, and erythema. Some indication exists that the intervals between the periods with herpes might be prolonged with balm mint cream treatment. There is little reason to expect the development of resistance to treatment.[101] Commercial lemon balm extract concentrated creams for topical use are available over the counter and in herbal pharmacies.

Licorice

Numerous in vitro and in vivo studies have shown licorice preparations to have antiviral, antiherpetic, antiinflammatory, antiulcer, anticarcinogenic, and a wide variety of immunomodulating effects.[105,106] Licorice root (Fig. 12-6) is taken singly or in combination as a tea, tincture, or powdered extract in capsules or tablets. It is also applied topically for local relief of swelling and irritation. The herb is indispensable for its inhibitory effects on the virus, its antiinflammatory effects to reduce pain and swelling of lesions, and its immunomodulatory effects to enhance host resistance and reduce episodes of active lesions.[107] Glycyrrhizic acid has demonstrated lipoxygenase, cyclooxygenase, and protein kinase C inhibition. Active fractions include triterpenoids like glycyrrhizin (GR) and its aglycone glycyrrhizic acid, polyphenols, and immunomodulating heteropolysaccharides.[108,109] Licorice extract inhibited the growth and cytopathology of herpes, as well as inactivating HSV particles irreversibly. In vivo, GR administered intraperitoneally increased the survival rate of mice that were infected by HSV-1 with herpetic encephalitis by 2.5 times (37.5%-39.0% to 81.8%-83.3%). GR also reduced HSV-1 replication in vivo.[110] Glycyrrhizic acid inhibits the growth of several DNA and RNA viruses in cell cultures and inactivates HSV-1 irreversibly.[107] A recent study shows that treatment of cells latently infected with Kaposi's sarcoma–associated herpes virus (KSHV), a member of the herpes family, with glycyrrhizic acid reduces synthesis of a viral latency protein and induces apoptosis of infected cells, suggesting a novel way to interrupt latency.[111]

Reishi

Considered an adaptogenic and immunomodulating herb, reishi has a number of studies that demonstrate activity against HSV. One study looking at the mechanisms of action of reishi against HSV-1 and -2 found that the *Ganoderma lucidum* proteoglycan (GLPG), obtained by liquid fermentation of the mycelia, works by inhibiting viral replication by interfering with the early events of viral adsorption and entry into target cells.[112] Two protein-bound polysaccharides, a neutral protein-bound polysaccharide (NPBP), and an acidic protein-bound polysaccharide (APBP), isolated from water soluble substances of reishi were also found to be effective against HSV-1 and -2. APBP was found to have a direct virucidal effect on HSV-1 and -2. APBP did not induce IFN or IFN-like materials in vitro and is not expected to induce a change from a normal state to an antiviral state. APBP in concentrations of 100 and 90 µg/mL inhibited up to 50% of the attachment of HSV-1 and -2 to cells and was also found to prevent penetration of both types of HSV into cells. These results show that the antiherpetic activity of APBP seems to be related to its binding with HSV–specific glycoproteins responsible for attachment and penetration, and APBP impedes the complex interactions of viruses with cell plasma membranes.[113] Virucidal effects of reishi extracts have also been identified by other researchers.[114,115] A study by Oh and colleagues demonstrated potent synergistic antiviral effects against HSV-1 and -2 showed when combining APBP and acyclovir, suggesting the development of APBP as a new antiherpetic agent.[116] Reishi has also demonstrated beneficial effects in the treatment of herpes zoster, reducing postherpetic neuralgia.[117] Reishi is usually taken as a decoction or tablet. Although tinctures are also available, the polysaccharides are likely more bioavailable in whole or water-extracted forms.

Sage and Rhubarb Combination

Essential oil–rich herbs, for example, thyme *(Thymus vulgaris),* tea tree, and lemon balm, and anthraquinone-rich herbs such as aloe and St. John's wort, all contain antimicrobial activity, some specifically against HSV. A combination ointment containing sage (Fig. 12-7) and rhubarb extracts, the former essential oil–rich and the latter anthraquinone-rich, and a product containing sage alone, were evaluated for their efficacy against

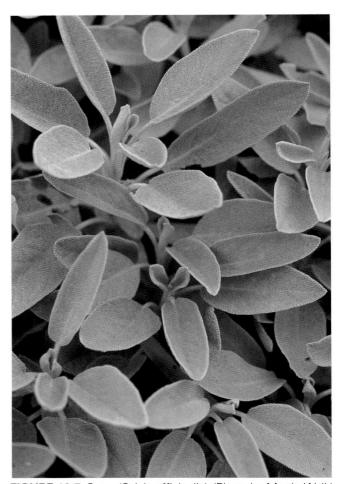

FIGURE 12-7 Sage *(Salvia officinalis).* (Photo by Martin Wall.)

HSV. They were be evaluated by intention-to-treat analysis. The dried rhubarb extract used was a standardized aqueous-ethanolic extract according to the *German Pharmacopoeia* and the dried sage extract an aqueous extract. The reference product was Zovirax cream, with the active ingredient acyclovir. A total of 149 patients participated: 145 (111 females, 34 males) of whom 64 received the rhubarb-sage cream, 40 the sage cream, and 41 Zovirax cream. The mean time to healing in all cured patients was 7.6 days with the sage cream, 6.7 days with the rhubarb-sage cream, and 6.5 days with Zovirax cream. There were statistically significant differences in the course of the symptoms. For the parameter *swelling,* at the first follow-up visit there was a significant advantage for Zovirax cream compared with sage cream, and for the parameter *pain,* at the second follow-up visit there was a significant difference in favor of the rhubarb-sage cream compared with the sage cream. The combined topical sage-rhubarb preparation proved to be as effective as topical acyclovir cream and tended to be more active than the sage cream.[92]

St. John's Wort

Hypericin and related compounds have been shown to have selective activity against viruses, both in vitro and in vivo, including HSV-1 and -2.[118,119] A prospective double-blind placebo-controlled study of St. John's wort extract compared with placebo was conducted in 110 patients with HSV-2. Patients were given a 90-day treatment protocol of 300 mg three time daily, and 600 mg three time daily on the days of herpes outbreaks. Symptoms were significantly and equally reduced compared with placebo, including severity of episodes, size of affected area, and numbers of vesicles.[21] Similar trials conducted by Koytchev and colleagues and Mannel and coworkers have yielded similar positive results.[21,120] Herbalists include St. John's wort in protocols for both internal and topical use for its positive effects on the nervous system, antiviral activity, and topically in tincture or salve for its mild vulnerary and antiinflammatory actions.

Tea Tree

Tea Tree Oil (TTO) has broad spectrum antimicrobial effects in vitro, and is specifically active against HSV. One in vitro study looked at the effects of both TTO and eucalyptus oil (EUO) against HSV-1 and -2.[121] At noncytotoxic concentrations of TTO, plaque formation was reduced by 98.2% and 93.0% for HSV-1 and -2, respectively. Noncytotoxic concentrations of EUO reduced virus titers by 57.9% for HSV-1 and 75.4% for HSV-2. Virus titers were reduced significantly with TTO, whereas EUO exhibited distinct but less antiviral activity. To determine the mode of antiviral action of both essential oils, either cells were pretreated before viral infection or viruses were incubated with TTO or EUO before infection, during adsorption, or after penetration into the host cells. Plaque formation was clearly reduced when HSV was pretreated with the essential oils before adsorption. These results indicate that TTO and EUO affect the virus before or during adsorption, but not after penetration into the host cell. Thus TTO and EUO are capable of exerting a direct antiviral effect on HSV. Although the active antiherpes components of TTO and EUO are not yet known, their possible application as antiviral agents in recurrent herpes infection is promising.[121] A clinical trial by Carson and associates focused on the effects of topical application of TTO on recurrent *H. labialis* (RHL). Patients age 18 to 70 years (*n* = 18) with a self-reported history of RHL completed the study. Patients who had antiviral therapy in the previous month, long-term steroid therapy, immunocompromised status, pregnancy, lactation, or known TTO allergy were excluded. Participants presented as soon as possible after onset of a herpes outbreak and randomly received and applied either 6% TTO in an aqueous gel base or placebo gel five times daily and recorded treatments and any adverse effects in a diary. Subjects were assessed in the clinic daily except Sundays, with swabs collected for culture and PCR evaluation for HSV. Visits continued until vesicles were completely healed (i.e., reepithelialized) and PCR was negative for HSV DNA on two consecutive days. Investigators were blinded to which patients were using which gels. Parameters measured included reepithelization time, time to crust formation, duration of detectable virus by laboratory methods, and virus titer. Although most of the parameters did not reach statistical significance, reepithelialization time with TTO was reduced compared with other common topical treatments. The authors stated that the study size may have been too small to draw complete conclusions, and that the study may have been confounded by the fact that eight of the nine patients in the

TTO group began the study in the vesicular stage compared with only six in the placebo group. Nonetheless, they concluded that TTO may be a useful and more affordable acceptable alternative to patients and poses little risk of causing resistance.[30]

Immunomodulation and Adaptogenic Support

Andrographis

Andrographis, an Asian herb used in Ayurvedic medicine and Traditional Chinese Medicine (TCM), has been used traditionally as an antiinflammatory, hepatoprotective, antiviral, antioxidant, and immune-enhancing herbal medicine.[122] In vitro and in vivo studies demonstrate immune-enhancing activity and immunomodulating effects, including its ability to stimulate both antigen-specific and nonspecific immunity, to reduce inflammation, to relieve fever and sore throat, and to reduce incidence of common cold and upper respiratory infection in children and adults.[123-125] Andrographalide, a constituent of the herb, has demonstrated anticancer activity. One study demonstrated specific anti–HSV activity using isolate diterpenes from the herb.[126] Western herbal medicine uses this herb in combination with other immunomodulating herbs, and in multieffect comprehensive formulae for patients who experience recurrent herpes outbreaks and who also have a tendency toward frequent colds and infections, and who also may be run down and depleted. It is excellent combined with adaptogens for overall immune support.

Eleuthero

Eleuthero is an important traditional medicine in China and Russia; it is used to stimulate the immune system, for prophylaxis of infectious diseases, and to enhance stamina and performance. It is mentioned repeatedly in the literature for its antiviral effects.[127] An in vitro study by Glatthaar-Saalmuller and colleagues demonstrated specific activity against HSV. Given the ability of this herb to support general immunity, it is recommended in the prevention of recurrent herpes outbreaks, particularly for patients exhibiting general susceptibility to infection, and when fatigue or stress precipitate episodes. It is regularly given in tincture or encapsulated forms, most often combined with other adaptogens, antivirals, and nervines. See Chapter 5 for a larger discussion in adaptogens and this herb.

Reishi

Reishi is an important adaptogen and immunomodulating herb. It was previously discussed extensively for its specific activities against HSV. The combination of immune supportive and anti–HSV activity makes this herb especially important to consider for patients who have recurrent herpes infection in the context of overall susceptibility to infection, fatigue, and general depletion.

Nervines

HSV outbreaks can be precipitated by stress. Nervines are therefore an important part of the treatment protocol in patients in whom stress is a chronic underlying factor. Not surprisingly, this may be the case for many individuals. Therefore herbalists routinely include herbs that nourish the nervous system—nervous trophorestoratives (i.e., nervines)—with the aim of reducing stress, improving sleep, and promoting a sense of well-being in herbal protocol to prevent recurrent HSV. Nervines work more directly on the nervous system than adaptogens, which improve stress response through their actions on the hypothalamic-pituitary-adrenal (HPA) axis. A combination of adaptogens and nervines is excellent for both short- and long-term tonification of the nervous system. The herbs in this section are discussed more thoroughly in chapters on anxiety and insomnia. A brief description to help differentiate when each nervine might be selected follows.

California Poppy

California poppy is the most sedating of the herbs in this section. Traditionally, it has been used to treat pain, neuralgia, anxiety, stress, depression, migraines, and to promote sleep. It was used by medical practitioners in the late nineteenth century for its soporific and analgesic effects, with a liquid extract sold as a product by Parke-Davis.[47] A hydroethanolic extract has demonstrated affinity for the benzodiazepine receptor, and the sedative, anxiolytic effects of the herb were inhibited by a benzodiazepine receptor antagonist.[26] It should be considered when there is the need to promote sleep during periods of serious stress that threaten to precipitate a herpes outbreak. It also can be used as a muscle relaxant for general aches and pain during a primary herpes outbreak. It can be taken as a tea, but is commonly prescribed as a sedative in tincture form to be taken in small repeated doses every 15 to 30 minutes for 2 hours before attempting to sleep. California poppy is not addictive and does not cause the adverse effects associated with opiates.

Damiana

Damiana is a nervine tonic with an affinity for the reproductive system. A South and Central American native herb, it has been used traditionally as an herb for nervous debility, an aphrodisiac, for menstrual disorders, an emmenagogue, and for bladder irritability. It should be considered when there is nervousness, anxiety, and depression, as well as sexual dysfunction. It is a mild stimulating tonic for the nervous system. It was official in the *National Formulary* from 1916 to 1942 as a stimulant and laxative.[47] It was described by Ellingwood as a valuable nerve tonic, particularly when there is sexual debility, and by Hoffmann as an excellent tonic for the nervous system. No clinical studies on this herb have been identified.[128,129]

Lavender

Lavender has a long history of use as a gentle sedative and antispasmodic, used to treat nervousness, restlessness, nervous exhaustion, sleep disorders, depression, and headache.[26,49] In Tibetan medicine, the flowers are used for the treatment of psychosis. Aromatherapy uses lavender oils to promote calm and relaxation in forms available for inhalation including diffusers, pillow sprays, and bath oils. Herbalists may employ it in its aromatherapy forms alone or in combination with either tea, in which it is pleasant tasting, or tincture form. Lavender is commonly combined with chamomile and lemon balm for a gentle but effective calmative tea. In higher doses, a tincture combination of these same herbs is more sedating and can promote a relaxed sleep.

Lemon Balm

This herb has been used historically to lift the spirits, hence its nickname "the gladdening herb." Surprisingly, little research has been conducted on its calming, sedating effects. The German Commission E supports the use of lemon balm for nervous sleeping disorders.[50] ESCOP lists its indications for internal use as tenseness, restlessness, and irritability.[48] Given its antiviral effects, it is commonly included in general formula for internal use in addition to topical use for treating HSV.

Milky Oats

Milky oats are considered a nervine tonic to be used when there is nervous exhaustion and related conditions including insomnia, chronic anxiety and stress, excitatory states, general debility, and depression.[47,50] Herbalists use milky oats to calm and regenerate the nervous system. A number of clinical trials demonstrate efficacy in the treatment of nicotine and opium addiction using extracts of the green milky oats.[47] It is typically taken for several months for maximum effects, and is considered nourishing rather than sedating. Tinctures should be made from fresh milky oats rather than dried tea.

Motherwort

Motherwort is widely regarded for its quick action as a calmative when there is nervousness, irritability, and anxiety. The German Commission E supports its use for nervous cardiac conditions and thyroid hyperfunction; however, its use as a nervine is derived from empirical and historical use.[49,50] Herbalists specializing in women's health favor it for irritability associated with hormonal changes, for example, in the treatment of premenstrual syndrome (PMS) or postnatal irritability, suggesting possible use for irritability and stress associated with menstruation, a known combination of precipitating factors for herpes outbreaks.

Passionflower

Passionflower is a highly valued calmative nerve used for nervous restlessness, as a gentle sedative for sleep difficulties, and to reduce anxiety, neurasthenia, and nervous disorders. It is gentle enough to be favored for use in children.[49,50,130] ESCOP supports its use for tenseness, restlessness, and irritability with difficulty falling asleep.[48] Animal experiments corroborate traditional use for its sedative activity and extracts have demonstrated effects on electroencephalogram (EEG) that support sedative action; however, because the herb is nearly always used in combination with other sedative herbs, no single-herb studies have been conducted that give proof of its efficacy as a monopreparation.[49] The herb may be taken as a tea or tincture, the latter preferred by herbalists for maximum efficacy. Numerous preparations containing passionflower, both as monopreparations and combinations, are available as sedative formulae in Germany. It is commonly combined with valerian root (*Valeriana officinalis*) and hops strobiles (*Humulus lupulus*).

Skullcap

Hoffmann describes skullcap as perhaps the most relevant nervine available to us in the Western materia medica.[129] It's an excellent nervous trophorestorative used to soothe tension and restore calm. It is not immediate acting, and is generally used long-term (up to 6 months) for optimal effects in the treatment of nervous conditions associated with exhaustion and in the treatment of PMS. A double-blind, placebo-controlled study of healthy subjects demonstrated noteworthy anxiolytic effects.[131] The identification and quantification of the flavonoid baicalin in a 50% ethanol extract; its aglycone, baicalein, in a 95% ethanol extract; the amino acid gamma (γ)-aminobutyric acid (GABA) in aqueous and ethanol extracts; and glutamine in an aqueous extract was performed using high-performance liquid chromatography (HPLC). Anxiolytic activity is suggested because baicalin and baicalein are known to bind to the benzodiazepine site of the GABA$_A$ receptor and because GABA is the main inhibitory neurotransmitter.[132] Skullcap is generally recommended as a tea or tincture, usually in combination with other herbs such as lavender, passionflower, and lemon balm; however, it also may be taken singly.

Vulneraries and Antiinflammatories

Vulneraries are herbs used to promote wound healing. Among herbs commonly used to heal herpes blisters are those mentioned earlier in this chapter, such as aloe, lemon balm, St. John's wort, sage and rhubarb combination; additionally, calendula and comfrey root may be used. Calendula, an herb long relied on for its wound-healing and antimicrobial abilities, has been shown to decrease rate of cutaneous herpes lesions when combined with acyclovir versus acyclovir alone.[133] Comfrey is primarily used as an antiinflammatory and to heal wounds, ulcers, and sores.[49] Any of these herbs may be used topically at the onset of blisters or once they have begun to crust over, and should be applied two to four times daily using a clean cotton swab for each application. Aloe may be used in the form of gel or cream, comfrey is used as a cream or ointment, and calendula and the others may be used in the form of tincture, oil, ointment, cream, or salve.

Topical Analgesics

A number of herbs have shown analgesic effects with topical application. Two studies specifically looked at topical pain management with herpes zoster, a relative of HSV that causes painful outbreaks along nerve dermatomes and often leads to significant postherpetic neuralgia. Both 100% geranium oil and peppermint oil, applied directly to the affected area, have demonstrated analgesic effects in a clinical trial and a case report, respectively. Geranium oil relieved pain dramatically in 25% of patients whose pain after shingles had lasted for 3 months or more and was not relieved by standard pain medications such as acetaminophen (Tylenol) or meperidine (Demerol). Fifty percent of patients showed some relief, and 25% did not benefit.[134] Other herbs used for topical analgesia include kava kava and St. John's wort.

Astringents

According to Schulz and colleagues, virtually all substances with a protein-coagulating, astringent action can improve symptoms associated with herpetic lesions.[130] Those herbs commonly relied on as astringents include witch hazel extract; plantain leaf poultice, salve, or tincture; and white oak bark tincture. Many patients find witch hazel easily acceptable and accessible because it can

be used in the readily available drug store form of the extract for external use. Witch hazel is approved by ESCOP and the German Commission E for use as a treatment of mild skin injuries and local inflammation of the skin and mucosa.[49,50] Plantain is approved by ESCOP for temporary, mild inflammations of mucosa (oral and pharyngeal are specified) and by German Commission E for inflammatory alterations of the skin.[49,50]

NUTRITIONAL CONSIDERATIONS

Reduce Arginine and Increase L-Lysine

In vitro evidence supports increasing dietary lysine and decreasing dietary arginine to prevent recurrent herpes outbreaks. Arginine is necessary for replication of HSV; it may actually stimulate cell replication, whereas L-lysine blocks arginine activity. L-lysine is shown in studies to decrease the severity of outbreaks and reduces recurrence, although it does not necessarily have an effect on healing time. Supplementation of 1 g daily is recommended preventatively or 1 g three times daily during an outbreak in addition to dietary modification.[125,135] Because of concerns over prolonged lysine supplementation and the risk of developing atherosclerosis, dietary adjustments may be optimal versus regular lysine supplementation, which can be reserved for acute need.[125] Nuts, a chief source of arginine, provide important and healthy fats to the diet; therefore it is not desirable to eliminate them entirely, especially during pregnancy. Moderation is advisable. Pregnant women should consult with their midwife or obstetrician when modifying their diet to ensure optimal health for themselves and their babies. See Box 12-1 for foods high in arginine and lysine. Lysine supplementation is not contraindicated during pregnancy.

 BOTANICAL TREATMENT PROTOCOL FOR RECURRENT HERPES SIMPLEX VIRUS

Combine the following botanical therapies both for internal and topical treatment as appropriate for specific patients' needs.

This symbol *** in front of internal protocol in the following indicates that the formula is not considered safe for use during pregnancy. Special pregnancy protocols are noted as such. Topical protocol can be used freely during pregnancy, although thuja should be omitted even for topical use in pregnancy.

***Immune Supporting/Antiviral Tincture

For patients prone to regular recurrent outbreaks give the following formula as a prophylactic agent to boost the immune system and for its antiviral effects, for use daily. For patients with only periodic and predictable outbreaks, such as during periods of stress after the holidays or during examinations or deadlines, give the following formula for 6 weeks before the time of anticipated stress and continue for 2 weeks after the stressful event or period. For women susceptible to herpes outbreaks at the time of menstruation, give daily until recurrent outbreaks become infrequent, and then take two to three times weekly.

Continued

BOTANICAL TREATMENT PROTOCOL FOR RECURRENT HERPES SIMPLEX VIRUS—cont'd

Ashwagandha	(Withania somnifera)	20 mL
St. John's wort	(Hypericum perforatum)	20 mL
Licorice	(Glycyrrhiza glabra)	15 mL
Lemon balm	(Melissa officinalis)	15 mL
Echinacea	(Echinacea spp.)	15 mL
Andrographis	(Andrographis paniculata)	15 mL
	Total: 100 mL	

Dose: 5 mL twice daily

***Herbal Infusion or Tincture (Alternative to Immune Supporting/Antiviral Tincture)

Adapted from Amanda McQuade Crawford, *Herbal Remedies for Women.*

Common Name	Botanical Name	Dried Herbs	Tincture
St. John's wort	(Hypericum perforatum)	3-½ parts	35 mL
Calendula	(Calendula officinalis)	2-½ parts	20 mL
Damiana	(Turnera diffusa)	1 part	10 mL
Echinacea	(Echinacea spp.)	2 parts	15 mL
Eleuthero	(Eleutherococcus senticosus)	½ part	10 mL
Pulsatilla	(Anemone pulsatilla)	½ part	10 mL
		Total: 100 mL	

To prepare infusion: Steep 28 g (1 oz)/1 L of boiling water for 20 minutes. Strain.

Dose: Infusion: 1 teacup three times daily

Tincture: 5 mL three times daily

Take 5 days weekly for 1 to 3 months to reduce frequency and severity of outbreaks.

For both of the preceding formulae, if menstrual hormone irregularity triggers or exacerbates herpes outbreaks, give 5 mL of *V. agnes-castus* tincture daily, preferably in the morning, for 3 to 6 months.

Antiviral Formula for Use During Pregnancy

Most of the antiviral herbs discussed in this chapter have not been proven safe for use during pregnancy. However, suppression of herpes simplex virus (HSV) outbreaks is particularly important during pregnancy owing to the potential consequences to the fetus of exposure to lesions during vaginal delivery, and risks to the mother of a cesarean delivery as the alternative. It has been the experience of many midwives who, using a combination protocol of a simple internal antiviral formula, topical applications, and dietary and lifestyle modifications (e.g., stress reduction), can reduce the frequency of outbreaks during pregnancy and prevent the need for cesarean section. The following protocol is reliable and the herbs not contraindicated during pregnancy. The case history at the end of this chapter illustrates the successful treatment of HSV-2 during pregnancy.

Prepare the following herbs as an infusion:

Echinacea root	(Echinacea angustifolia or purpurea)	6 parts
Lemon balm	(Melissa officinalis)	4 parts

Steep 28 g (1 oz) of herbs per L of boiling water for 1 hour. Strain and drink two cups daily during the first trimester; increase to four cups daily during the third trimester. Use other formulae in this chapter, both internally (i.e., nervine formula) and topically, along with the dietary considerations.

Nervine Formula

For patients with stress-induced HSV outbreaks, also give the following formula either daily on an ongoing basis, or for several weeks before and during times of anticipated stress.

Milky oats	(Avena sativa)	30 mL
Passionflower	(Passiflora incarnata)	30 mL
Blue vervain	(Verbena officinalis)	20 mL
Lavender	(Lavandula officinalis)	20 mL
	Total: 100 mL	

Dose: 3 to 5 mL two to three times daily, based on severity of stress

Topical Treatment

Herbs from the following topical formulae can be combined or treatments can be alternated for various effects, for example, using tincture to heal lesions twice daily alternated with topical application of herbs to dry lesions.

For painful lesions:

Mix the following combination in a 1-oz. amber or cobalt glass bottle. Shake hard before each use to mix the tinctures and oil. Apply using a cotton swab two to four times daily:

Kava kava tincture	10 mL
Licorice tincture	10 mL
Peppermint or geranium oil	20 drops

To speed healing and as a topical antiviral:

Mix a combination of equal parts of the following tinctures in a 1-oz. amber or cobalt glass bottle. Apply using a cotton swab two to four times daily:

St. John's wort	(Hypericum perforatum)
Thuja	(Thuja occidentalis)
Lemon balm	(Melissa officinalis)
Calendula	(Calendula officinalis)

Alternatively, use lemon balm or St. John's wort ointments, available over the counter in shops that retail herbal products, or simply use witch hazel extract that is available at regular pharmacies.

Omit thuja during pregnancy. Replace with licorice or lavender tincture.

For weeping lesions:

Option 1: Mix equal parts of powders of myrrh and goldenseal and apply several times daily by packing the powder onto weeping ulcers. Note that goldenseal powder may well stain clothing, so caution should be taken to avoid contact with garments, for example by using a panty liner in the underwear.

Option 2: Apply witch hazel extract onto weeping ulcers using a cotton swab, repeating two to four times daily.

To heal tissue once sores have begun to crust over:

Use a vulnerary salve containing comfrey, lemon balm extract, calendula, and an essential oil such as geranium or peppermint to quickly heal tissue.

Also see Nutritional Considerations for a high-lysine, low-arginine diet, and avoid outbreak triggers.

Zinc

Supplementation with 25 mg of zinc daily has been shown to inhibit HSV replication in vitro and clinically has led to complete suppression of an outbreak or resolution within 24 hours. It also stimulates cell-mediated immunity, and decreases frequency and reduces severity of outbreaks. Supplementation is suggested for 6 weeks with 250 mg vitamin C. Topical use of zinc sulfate solution (0.01% to 0.025%) improves healing of HSV-1 blisters and prevents recurrence. Internal use of zinc as a supplement is not recommended during pregnancy.[125]

Vitamin C

Supplementation with 1000 mg vitamin C with bioflavonoids daily during the prodromal phase and then 5000 mg divided into five doses daily for 3 days after the onset of symptoms was shown to reduce blister healing time in HSV-1 from 10 days in the placebo group to 4.4 days in the group receiving supplementation.[125] Pregnant women should not exceed 4000 mg vitamin C supplementation daily, including vitamin C that is in a prenatal vitamin.

Vitamin D

A 2011 mouse study found that vitamin D_3 alleviated HSV-1–induced Behçet's disease–like inflammation, potentially by downregulation of toll-like receptor (TLR2 and TLR4) and modulation of serum interleukin-6 (IL-6) and TNF-α.[136] No human studies have been done, but vitamin D has been associated with both important immune system and mood benefits, and is safe for most women to include dietarily at 1000 to 2000 units of vitamin D_3 daily. Serum vitamin D (i.e., 25-hydroxy-vitamin D) levels can be tested easily and a supplementation dose recommended accordingly to keep the serum level at at least 40 ng/mL daily.

Vitamin E

Topical use of vitamin E oil shortens healing time and significantly reduces pain associated with HSV-1 lesions. A combination of coenzyme Q10 (CoQ10), vitamin E, selenium, and methionine was tested for efficacy in immune defense against HPV (Trial 1, $n = 68$), HSV ($n = 60$), and herpes zoster ($n = 29$) in two separate trials. The treatments lasted for 90 days and were tested against acyclovir as a positive control, with viral DNA levels assessed by PCR. Quicker healing times in the nutraceutical groups were observed compared with controls (Dose not provided).[137] Vitamin E oil can be applied two to four times daily with a cotton swab.

ADDITIONAL THERAPIES

Chronic stress has the most significant effect on recurrent HSV, even more so than acute stress.[125] Regular practice of mind–body therapies that help to relieve stress are important in the prevention of recurrent HSV for many patients. Examples include meditation, yoga, biofeedback, and massage.

Patients can expect to shorten the duration, frequency, and severity of herpes outbreaks in as quickly as 24 hours with aggressive topical treatment in outbreaks that are caught early. Prevention of recurrence of herpes can be achieved quickly with the addition of dietary and lifestyle modifications accompanied by nervine, adaptogen, and antiviral therapy, both internally and topically as appropriate and indicated. Some patients may continue to experience periodic and infrequent outbreaks during times of heightened stress, but these can largely be ameliorated with adherence to botanical and dietary protocol. Some patients experience complete remission of the virus, and may go indefinitely, even more than a decade, without a sign of an outbreak.

HUMAN IMMUNODEFECIENCY VIRUS INFECTION AND BOTANICAL THERAPIES

An estimated 19.2 million women worldwide are living with HIV infection or AIDS. Since the early 1990s, the proportion of AIDS cases in females aged 13 to 49 years has tripled from 7% to 25%. Appropriate treatment is essential to the wellness and longevity of HIV/AIDS patients. Conventional medical treatment, for example highly active antiretroviral therapy (HAART), which consists of a combination of antiretroviral therapies, including protease and reverse transcriptase inhibitors, is showing tremendous promise.[138] Numerous HIV patients also use complementary and alternative therapies such as herbs and nutritional supplements in conjunction with their medical treatment, or in some cases, in lieu of conventional therapies. This section looks at the statistics and demographics of CAM use for HIV/AIDS, reasons for use, risks and benefits associated with use, and provides a brief review of the literature based on two major reviews conducted by other researchers. There is a tremendous paucity of evidence on botanical therapies for HIV/AIDS; however, there is also a tremendous amount of human experience in the HIV community regarding natural therapies that may support conventional treatment, and also may eventually point the way to more effective integrative therapies.

A comprehensive overview of HIV/AIDS is beyond what can be adequately covered within the scope of this book. The author hopes that this section will provide a glimmer of insight into the nature of CAM use by individuals with HIV/AIDS and elucidate the need for both practitioner understanding of patient motivation for using CAM therapies with HIV/AIDS, and the tremendous need for further research in this area.

COMPLEMENTARY AND ALTERNATIVE MEDICINE USE IN THE HIV/AIDS POPULATION

In general, chronic disease is a positive predictive factor for CAM use; however, people with HIV are more likely to use CAM than those with other serious illnesses, including cancer.[139] Patients with chronic illness are highly likely to turn to CAM therapies, sometimes with a sense of desperation, seeking a sense of control over their health and anything that will improve quality of life and reduce discomfort.[140] It is imperative that medical practitioners understand their patient's desire to use CAM therapies as part of their overall treatment, and help patients to obtain reliable, accurate information. These patients may be especially vulnerable to hype and scams in their deep desire to alleviate their suffering and improve their health. Misinformation about what therapies to use can be a problem. A study by Mills and colleagues illustrates the potential for misinformation and unnecessary products expenditure to patients.[141] Four male research assistants, posing as asymptomatic HIV–positive individuals, inquired of employees of all retail health food stores in a major Canadian city (32 stores) as to what is recommended for their condition. Eight store employees (25%) offered no advice; eight (25%) inquired whether the subjects were currently taking medications; six (19%) suggested visiting a physician; and eight (25%) suggested visiting a CAM provider. A total of 36 different products (mean 2.3 per employee) were recommended with considerable variability in product evidence and cost. There was considerable heterogeneity in advice on natural products provided by employees of natural food stores and, in general, these individuals had limited formal training in CAM. The products they recommended had limited evidence supporting their efficacy and in some instances were potentially harmful and had considerable costs. It is important for practitioners to develop patient education resources on CAM safety and efficacy, and for these to be made available in a variety of community settings in which HIV–positive patients might seek such information.[142]

Several studies have looked at the overall population demographics of individuals with HIV/AIDS using CAM.[138,139,143-149] These studies have shown that at least 50% and as many as 68% of individuals with HIV/AIDS have used a CAM therapy at least once, and many use them regularly as part of, or in conjunction with, HIV/AIDS treatment. Only a limited number of studies have investigated CAM use specifically among women with HIV/AIDS. Women in this population reporting CAM use are generally older than 35 years of age, have a higher degree of education, and are more likely to be uninsured than those not using CAM therapies. Women living with HIV for greater than 4 years are significantly more likely to be CAM users than those with shorter disease duration.[138] Meneilly and coworkers reported that HIV–positive Caucasian women were more likely to use botanical therapies than African American or Hispanic women with HIV/AIDS.[150] In a study of 391 women of mixed ethnicity 18 to 50 years old with HIV/AIDS, about 60% of women reported using at least one CAM therapy. Approximately 16% reported using herbs, 22% used dietary supplements, 27% practiced religious healing, 10% used bodywork (e.g., massage, yoga), and 1% practiced some type of psychic healing.[138] In another study, 53% of patients had recently used at least one type of CAM. Of these, 27% had used therapies with the potential for adverse effects and 36% had not discussed such use with their health care provider, a common problem with CAM use. Patients with a greater desire for medical information and involvement in medical decision making and with a negative attitude toward antiretroviral drugs were more likely to use

CAM. Only 3% used CAM instead of conventional therapy.[144] Patients in one survey ($n = 180$) saw CAM providers with greater frequency than primary care physicians and nurse practitioners, and were likely to report CAM therapies to be either "extremely" or "quite a bit" helpful.[143]

WHY ARE HIV/AIDS PATIENTS TURNING TO COMPLEMENTARY AND ALTERNATIVE MEDICINE THERAPIES?

Most people with HIV/AIDS report using CAM therapies to manage health complications, especially control of conventional medication side effects, which can be significant enough to reduce compliance with conventional therapy.[147] Many also report using CAM to cope with emotional issues such as depression and stress. Pain management is a significant reason for CAM use among HIV/AIDS patients.[149] Pain may result from direct effects of HIV on the peripheral nervous system or CNS, immune suppression and resulting opportunistic infections, antiretroviral medications, and common problems unrelated to HIV disease or treatment, such as lower back pain.[149]

Additional reasons for CAM use among those with HIV/AIDS include symptom management; as a way to prevent disease progression; to forestall beginning the use of conventional therapies (often while monitoring for disease progression); to gain freedom from medical regimens; and to avoid stigmas associated with the use of conventional therapy such as the self-perception of "being diseased," feeling dependent on conventional medications, or having to publicly and thus visibly fill prescriptions, take medications, or get medical care where they might be seen by those who know them.[151] A recent Canadian study reports that people with HIV/AIDS are drawn to CAM as a health maintenance strategy, a healing strategy, an alternative to Western medicine, as a way of alleviating the side effects of drug therapies, a strategy for improving quality of life, a coping strategy, and as a statement of political resistance.[152]

Approximately 50% of CAM users are what has been referred to as "pragmatic users."[151] This means that although they use CAM often, their use is limited to short durations and specific reasons such as stress or treatment of a cold. Interestingly, many individuals express interest in using CAM, but may choose not to for a variety of reasons, including cost, skepticism, lack of confidence in CAM therapies, inability to comply with complex protocols, lack of knowledge on how to obtain reliable information, lack of scientific data, and concerns about interactions with medications.[151] It appears that reducing viral load or "curing" HIV/AIDS is not a primary motivation, and in fact, in the underground HIV/AIDS community it seems that improving quality of life, maintaining optimal health in spite of the diagnosis, and preventing disease progression are the goals of CAM use, as well as management of drug side effects and so forth as already stated.

Desire to support a positive self-perception appears to be a reason that some individuals with HIV/AIDS seek CAM.

Patients report that conventional medical visits often leave them feeling medicalized and diseased, whereas CAM therapists, such as acupuncturists, are more likely to reinforce a positive approach to disease management and instill greater hope that the patient can achieve some sense of well-being in the context of having HIV/AIDS.[139]

BENEFITS OF COMPLEMENTARY AND ALTERNATIVE MEDICINE THERAPY

Perhaps most significantly, patients have reported that the use of CAM therapies enables them to remain on conventional treatment protocol, which is often accompanied by minor to debilitating side effects including fatigue, nausea, diarrhea, vomiting, anemia, neuropathy, and pancreatitis.[139] Foote-Ardah found that patients were using acupuncture for relief of neuropathic pain, Chinese herbs for nausea, and marijuana to improve appetite and weight gain.[139] The psychoemotional well-being and sense of empowerment reported by individuals using CAM therapies for the treatment of HIV/AIDS, as well as the increased ability of patients to comply with pharmaceutical regimens as a result of using CAM, represents an important benefit as long as the CAM therapies do not interfere with the medication or are not themselves harmful. This in itself should be a central reason for conventional practitioners to support their patient's choice to use CAM therapies with no demonstrated harm, and should encourage research on the safety and efficacy of botanicals used as adjunct therapies for associated complaints of HIV/AIDS patients and for side effects of HIV/AIDS pharmacotherapy, as well as herb–drug interactions. Clearly a combination of the two models is desired by the majority of HIV patients and may represent a simple, safe, and empowering method of treating minor to major complaints and side effects and lending a sense of empowerment to those who may otherwise feel entirely dependent on medical care and with very few medical options.

RISKS OF COMPLEMENTARY AND ALTERNATIVE MEDICINE USE IN HIV/AIDS

The major risks of using botanicals for HIV/AIDS and AIDS–related conditions are inherent risks of using unsafe therapies, foregoing use of conventional treatment in favor of therapies that may be ineffective, delaying necessary medical therapies for too long, and interactions that may interfere with the efficacy or safety of conventional therapies. Further, unnecessary cost to the patient may be considered an associated risk. For some, the use of CAM to forestall beginning conventional therapy, in conjunction with evaluation of CD4 counts, has allowed them to maintain a sense of autonomy from medical dependence for as long as possible, and has been met with positive outcomes, including delayed disease progression.[139] Other patients, however, have not fared as well, with attempts to avert medication with CAM therapies leading to the development of serious opportunistic infections.[139] Unfortunately, very little is known about the safety and efficacy of combining herbs and conventional HIV/AIDS pharmaceutical therapies, both directly for the reduction of viral load or enhancement of immunity, or for the treatment of side effects of medications or conditions associated with HIV/AIDS, such as fatigue, other infections, and depression.

EFFICACY OF BOTANICAL THERAPIES IN HIV/AIDS

There is an astounding paucity of research on the efficacy and safety of botanical therapies used for the treatment of HIV/AIDS. Two comprehensive reviews of the literature were identified, one by Mills and colleagues on CAM therapies and one by the Cochrane Collaboration specifically on botanical therapies. Mills and colleagues only identified three botanical trials that met their inclusion criteria. Two of the trials were of Chinese herbal preparations, the other of an extract of the boxwood plant (*Buxus sempervirens*). Another trial looked at the effectiveness of *Capsicum* on AIDS–related peripheral neuropathy.[153]

The Cochrane Collaboration review identified a total of nine randomized placebo-controlled clinical trials that met their inclusion criteria, involving 499 individuals with HIV or AIDS. A total of eight different herbal medicines were evaluated in these trials.[154] Herbal medicines were defined as preparations derived from plants, and could be extracts from a single herb or a compound of herbs. It should be noted that these are generally not herbal products that one can simply purchase at a natural foods store or obtain through a local herbalist. They are often more closely akin to pharmaceutical products. These were compared with no intervention, placebo, and antiretroviral therapies. Outcome measures included mortality, HIV progression, new AIDS–defining events, number and types of adverse events, immunologic indicators (i.e., CD4 and white blood cell counts), viral load, and psychological status and quality of life. With limited exception (e.g., diarrhea), most of these trials looked at herbs and HIV/AIDS directly, rather than at supportive therapies for specific symptoms or associated problems, such as ginger for nausea or marijuana for appetite stimulation.

IGM-1 (Chinese Herb Combination)

In a 1996 study by Burack and coworkers, 30 patients with at least two HIV–related symptoms were randomly assigned to receive herbs (*n* = 15) or placebo (*n* = 15). The product, IGM-1, is a standardized preparation of 31 Chinese herbs developed by one of the investigators. Of 31 herbal ingredients in the 650-mg tablet, those present in high concentration included *Ganoderma lucidum, Isatis tinctoria, Astragalus membranaceus, Andrographis paniculata, Lonicera japonica, Millettia reticulata, Oldenlandia diffusa,* and *Laminaria japonica*. Overall life satisfaction appeared to be improved in patients treated with herbs compared with placebo. Patients receiving herbs reported a reduced number of symptoms. There was no significant reported difference in overall health perception, symptom severity, absolute CD4 count, anxiety, or depression between the two groups. No adverse events were reported or identified in any of the patients randomized to herbs.[154,155]

"35" Chinese Herb Combination

In a 1999 study by Weber and associates, HIV–infected adults (*n* = 68) were randomized to receive a preparation of 35 Chinese herbs (*n* = 34) or placebo (*n* = 34). The preparation includes *Ganoderma lucidum, Isatis tinctoria, Millettia reticulata, Astragalus membranaceus, Tremella fuciformis, Andrographis paniculata, Lonicera japonica, Aquilaria agallocha, Epimedium macranthum, Oldenlandia diffusa, Cistanche salsa, Lycium chinense fructus, Laminaria japonica, Angelica sinensis, Polygonum cuspidatum, Panax quinquefolius, Schisandra chinensis, Ligustrum lucidum, Atractylodes macrocephala, Rehmannia glutinosa, Salvia miltiorrhiza, Curcuma longa, Viola yedoensis, Citrus reticulata, Paeonia lactiflora, Polygonum multiflorum, Eucommia ulmoides, Amomum villosum, Glycyrrhiza uralensis, Prunella vulgaris, Cordyceps sinensis, Pogostemon cablin, Crataegus cuneata, Massa medica fermentata, Hordeum vulgare,* and *Oryza sativa*. Of those who completed the study (24 in the herb group and 29 in the placebo group), there were no significant differences in CD4 cell counts and HIV-1 RNA load. There were no significant differences between the groups regarding new AIDS–defining events, number of reported symptoms, psychosocial measurements, or quality of life. There were more adverse effects in the herb group (19 out of 24) than in the placebo group (11 out of 29). Adverse events included diarrhea, increased number of daily bowel movements, abdominal pain, constipation, flatulence, and nausea. There was no evidence of toxicity from the study drugs, based on hematologic and blood chemistry analysis. The deaths of two patients in the herb group were attributed to severe immunodeficiency and preenrollment history of multiple severe opportunistic complications and not to the herbal preparation.[154,156]

SPV30: Boxwood

In a pilot trial in France, 43 asymptomatic HIV patients with CD4 cell counts between 250 and 500/mm³ were divided into an SPV30 (*n* = 22) or placebo (*n* = 21) group. Patients receiving SPV30 were less likely to progress to AIDS–related complications or to decrease to a CD4 cell count of below 200/mm³. There was a significant increase of CD4 cell count in people treated by SPV30 after 30 weeks compared with placebo. Based on these findings, 145 previously untreated participants with asymptomatic HIV infection and decreased CD4 cell count (250 to 500/mm³) were randomized to SPV30 990 mg/day (*n* = 48), SPV30 1980 mg/day (*n* = 49), or placebo (*n* = 48).[157] There was a tendency for AIDS–defining events such as candidiasis, herpes zoster, weight loss, and diarrhea to occur less frequently in the SPV30 groups than in the placebo group (Relative risk (RR) 0.12, 95% confidence interval (CI) 0.01 to 1.08; *p* = .06). There was no significant difference between either SPV30 990 mg/day or SPV30 1980 mg/day and placebo with respect to CD4 cell counts and viral load. The trial did not observe serious adverse effects, and biochemical parameters did not show abnormal changes in the participants.[154,157]

SP-303

SP-303 is a product containing a proanthocyanidin oligomer isolated and purified from the latex of *Croton lechleri*. Fifty-one patients with AIDS and diarrhea were randomized to either SP-303 or placebo. SP-303 reduced stool weight and abnormal stool frequency. The product was well tolerated and there were no adverse events reported in either group.[154,158]

The authors of the Cochrane review concluded that there was insufficient evidence to support the use of herbal medicines in HIV–infected individuals and AIDS patients.[154] It must be remembered that only a very few of the large number of herbs that are used for HIV/AIDS have been subject to any evaluation.

SAFETY ISSUES WITH HERBS AND HIV/AIDS THERAPY

There is no comprehensive list of herbs to be avoided by HIV/ AIDS patients. The efficacy and safety of standard HIV/AIDS pharmacotherapy is dependent on many delicate and complex mechanisms (e.g., cytochrome P450 metabolism), which may be affected by any number of substances, including botanical medicines. Several herbs are known to significantly interfere with the CYP450 system, most notably St. John's wort, which is contraindicated with HIV/AIDS pharmacotherapy. Although there is only very low-level evidence that herbal products might interfere with protease inhibitors, garlic and St. John's wort may reduce HIV drug concentrations and lead to drug failure.[153] Caution and knowledge of potential interactions are needed when combining HIV/AIDS therapies and herbal medicines. Cooperation between conventional and CAM practitioners in the treatment of HIV/AIDS patients may help to increase the efficacy and sustainability of treatment protocol for patients, as well as minimizing unwanted effects.

OVERVIEW OF IMMUNOMODULATING HERBS COMMONLY USED IN HIV/AIDS

Herbs used in the treatment of HIV/AIDS are focused on improving the integrity of the immune system. The following herbs are presented merely on an informational basis. They are generally used for tonic purposes, taken in any number of forms from concentrated extracts to use in soups. They are considered to have a high safety profile, although little research has been conducted on the effects of these herbs clinically in individuals with HIV/AIDS using conventional pharmacotherapy. Readers can refer to other topics in this textbook for HIV– and AIDS–related conditions, for example, nausea and vomiting of pregnancy for common anti-nausea herbs; vaginitis; insomnia; anxiety; or depression. Anecdotally, many HIV/AIDS patients have reported that, in conjunction with conventional therapies, various combinations of the following herbs and others, along with heavy nutritional supplementation programs, have vastly improved their quality of life.

Astragalus

Astragalus (*Astragalus membranaceus*) is the one of the most widely used immune-tonifying herbs of Chinese medicine. It is primarily used as a lung tonic, and may be helpful in increasing resistance against respiratory infections. It is also used as a digestive tonic. It has been shown to potentiate both thymus and spleen function, and to augment both humoral and cell-mediated immunity. Most studies evaluating the effects of astragalus on immunity have used cancer models and patients undergoing chemotherapy. The quality of astragalus products varies greatly. At least nine different species and one other genus (*Hedysarum*) of plant are traded as astragalus, but not all contain the primary marker compound astragaloside IV.

Atractylodes

Atractylodes (*Atractylodes lanata*) is much like astragalus in improving digestive and assimilative functions. It increases energy and has specific and nonspecific immune-stimulating activity. It can increase phagocytic activity, increase white blood cell counts, increase lymphocytic transformation, promote cellular immunity in general, and significantly increase IgG activity. It is also high in vitamin A.

Codonopsis

Codonopsis (*Codonopsis pilosula*) is used similarly to ginseng as a tonic. It can increase both red and white blood cell counts and hemoglobin, increase phagocytic activity, and promote lymphocytic transformation. It has also been reported to increase T-cell production.

Eleuthero

Eleuthero (*Eleutherococcus senticosus*) has primarily been valued for its adaptogenic properties and its ability to increase nonspecific resistance to physical and psychological stresses. Eleuthero increases macrophage activity in lymph tissue.

Licorice

Extracts of licorice (*Glycyrrhiza uralensis*) are widely used as part of an AIDS protocol in many clinics. Anti–AIDS activity that has been reported include reversal in P-24 antigen, reduction in the progression from AIDS-related complex (ARC) to AIDS in hemophiliacs, increases in overall lymphocytes, increase in natural killer (NK) cell activity, and a dose-dependent reduction in viral replication. Preparations used clinically include oral administration of crude licorice extracts as well as intravenous preparations. Although generally safe, excessive amounts of glycyrrhiza can cause fluid retention, heart palpitations, and contribute to hypertension.

Ligustrum

Ligustrum (*Ligustrum lucidum*) is widely used in China as an adjunctive therapy to chemotherapy and radiation therapy used in the treatment of cancer. It stimulates hematopoiesis and has been shown to restore immune functioning to almost normal in cancer patients. Ligustrum specifically promotes lymphocytic transformation, increases leukocytes, and may decrease the immunosuppressive side effects of radiation and azidothymidine (AZT).

Reishi

Reishi *(G. lucidum)* is one of the primary herbs of choice in any immune deficiency disease. It possesses a broad spectrum of immunostimulating activities, as well as antiinflammatory and antiallergenic properties. Reishi contains more than 100 oxygenated triterpenes, many of which exhibit a marked effect on the activity of NK cells. It has been widely used for a variety of infectious diseases such as bronchitis and hepatitis. It stimulates phagocytosis, increases T-cell activity, and is a treatment for viral hepatitis. Reishi has been reported to increase CD4 cells in vivo. It is also used as an effective antidepressant.

Shiitake Mushroom

Shiitake mushrooms *(Lentinus edodes)* are rich in immunostimulating polysaccharides and seem to exhibit a primary healing effect on the liver, being widely used for hepatotoxicity, hepatitis B, and cirrhosis. For this purpose, a high-tech extract of the immature mycelium has been used. It is rich in a broad spectrum of amino acids and B vitamins. One constituent, lentinan, has been shown to possess a 97% inhibition rate against sarcoma 180 growth, and 80% inhibition of Ehrlich's sarcoma in vitro.

SUMMARY

A number of vaginal infections and STDs can be treated with botanical medicine. A variety of strategies are used, including antimicrobial herbs, immunomodulating herbs for chronic recurrent infections, topical applications, and even botanicals for supporting the nervous system for stress-related infections. Table 12-8 includes a summary of the herbs used to treat these conditions.

TABLE 12-8   Condition and Botanical Medicine Summary Table

1.1	Analgesic	Antiinflammatory	Antimicrobial	Astringent	Demulcent	Immunomodulator	Nervine	Vulnerary
Actaea racemosa	X							
Allium sativum			X					
Aloe vera		X			X			X
Althea officinalis					X			
Andrographis paniculata			X			X		
Arctostaphylos uva ursi			X					
Astragalus membranaceus						X		
Avena sativa					X		X	
Berberis aquifolium			X					
Calendula officinalis		X	X					X
Commiphora molmol			X					
Coptis chinensis			X					
Corydalis	X							
Echinacea spp.			X			X		
Eleutherococcus senticosus						X		
Eschscholzia californica	X						X	
Ganoderma lucidum						X		
Glycyrrhiza glabra		X		X	X			X
Hamamelis virginiana		X						
Hydrastis canadensis			X					
Hypericum perforatum							X	
Lavandula officinalis			X				X	
Leonurus cardiaca							X	
Lomatium dissectum						X		
Melaleuca alternifolia								X
Melissa officinalis		X					X	
Mentha piperita								
Origanum vulgare								
Panax ginseng						X		
Panax quinquefolius						X	X X	
Passiflora incarnata			X					
Piper methysticum		X						
Piscidia piscipula	X	X						
Plantago spp.					X			
Quercus alba				X				
Rhaponticum carthamoides								
Rhodiola rosea						X		X
Salvia officinalis			X					
Schisandra chinensis						X		
Scutellaria lateriflora							X	
Symphytum officinale						X		X
Thuja occidentalis							X	
Withania somnifera	X					X	X	

Common Urinary Tract Problems

URINARY TRACT INFECTION

Urinary tract infection (UTI) refers to the presence of microbes anywhere in the urinary tract, ranging from the distal urethra to the kidney. UTI in the kidney is called *pyelonephritis;* in the bladder, *cystitis;* and in the urethra, *urethritis.* Infection is usually caused by bacteria, particularly *Escherichia coli,* which accounts for 85% to 90% of all UTIs, but also may be caused by other bacteria, viral, and fungal infections. *Klebsiella, Proteus,* and *Pseudomonas* are commonly associated with UTI, particularly in recurrent cases. Urine itself is normally sterile, but the moist environment of the peri-urethral area, the proximity of the urethral orifice to the rectum, and the short length of the urethra provide a conducive environment for the growth and ascension of potential uropathogenic microorganisms into the urinary system. The presence of bacteria in the urine is called *bacteriuria.* In nonpregnant women bacteriuria in the absence of symptoms is not considered an indication for treatment; however, during pregnancy, bacteriuria is associated with increased risk of pyelonephritis as well as prematurity and possibly other complications; therefore UTI in pregnancy requires special consideration.[1-3]

URINARY TRACT INFECTION INCIDENCE AND ETIOLOGY

It is estimated that several hundred million women suffer from UTI annually, with costs to health care providers amounting to over $6 billion annually worldwide, a figure that may even be an underestimate.[4] Additional costs to society of UTI are tremendous in terms of the personal suffering of millions of women annually, lost work days, and childcare costs. Over 56% of women will experience a UTI in their lifetimes, and among those experiencing uncomplicated acute UTI, as many as 20% will have a recurrence within 6 months. Overall UTI recurrence rate is between 27% and 48%.[4] Even with treatment, symptoms typically last for an average of 6 days, with nearly 2.5 days of limited activity. The rates of UTI are slightly higher in young, sexually active women because of mechanical factors affecting the urethra and the presence of uropathogenic organisms. UTI rates increase during

The editor wishes to thank *Botanical Medicine for Women's Health,* Edition 1 contributors to this chapter: Eric L. Yarnell and David Winston.

pregnancy and with age, the former because of the mechanical pressure of the growing uterus on the ureters and bladder preventing complete voiding, and the latter because of declining estrogen levels, declining mucin (i.e., a surface coating of the bladder epithelium that prevents bacterial adhesion), inability to void completely, incontinence, inadequate nutrition, the occurrence of other diseases, and excessive catheter use as a result of medical procedures.

RISK FACTORS FOR URINARY TRACT INFECTION

A number of common factors appear to increase the risk of developing a UTI. As mentioned, sexual activity is associated with a higher incidence of symptomatic UTI; however, risk only seems to be increased in the presence of uropathogenic microorganisms, either from a woman's own reservoir of bowel microbes, or those passed from a sexual partner. Urinating after sexual activity decreases the rates of infection. Evidence suggests that host genetic factors influence susceptibility to UTI. A maternal history of UTI is more often found among women who have experienced recurrent UTIs than among controls.

Susceptible patients may have a genetically increased number of receptors on uroepithelial cells to which bacteria may adhere. Additionally, nonsecretors of specific blood group antigens, which are glycoproteins, are at increased risk of recurrent UTI. Mutations in host genes integral to the immune response (interferon receptors and others) also may affect susceptibility to UTI.[3] The use of oral contraceptives (OCs) doubles the risk of UTI compared with no birth control, and the use of diaphragms and spermicides doubles the rate of UTI compared with OCs. Sexually transmitted infections and vaginitis can cause urethritis. Dehydration can increase bacterial growth, leading to UTI. A history of antibiotic use is common in women with a UTI; a possible mechanism that has been suggested is disruption of the vaginal flora and consequently overgrowth of pathogenic organisms. An interesting correlation exists between recurrent UTI and exposure to cold. A case-controlled study demonstrated a higher rate of UTI in women who reported cold hands, feet, or buttocks than controls. In a nonrandomized crossover study, cooling the feet of 29 healthy women with a history of recurrent UTI led to the development of UTI in five participants, compared with no UTI development in the control group.[1]

SYMPTOMS

UTI is commonly divided into lower UTI (i.e., urethritis and cystitis) and upper UTI (i.e., pyelonephritis), each with differing symptoms and treatments. Urethritis usually presents with a gradual onset, urethral irritation and inflammation, possible changes in voiding patterns and dysuric symptoms, as well as possible vaginal discharge or bleeding.

The most common symptoms of cystitis are frequent, painful urination, the urgent need to urinate, suprapubic pressure, and malaise, with up to 40% presenting with blood in the urine (i.e., hematuria). Some women may exhibit mild to moderate vaginal bleeding associated with UTI. Cystitis often has a sudden onset. Pregnant women may present with contractions and suprapubic pain, with dysuria possibly having been mistaken for normal polyuria of pregnancy. Women with lower UTI often complain of feeling achy, crampy, or "just not feeling well."

Pyelonephritis commonly has a gradual onset, although it can seem sudden if preceded by lower UTI, and is associated with not only urinary symptoms, but generalized symptoms such as fever, chills, nausea, malaise, and mild to extremely severe lower to middle back discomfort. Patients with pyelonephritis may appear quite ill. It is critical to differentiate between the symptoms of cystitis and pyelonephritis because the latter requires more aggressive treatment and carries greater risks, particularly during pregnancy (Box 13-1). Cystitis may resolve spontaneously; however, effective treatment lessens the duration of symptoms and reduces the incidence of progression to upper UTI. Pyelonephritis is associated with substantial morbidity. Complications include acute papillary necrosis with possible development of urethral obstruction, septic shock, and perinephric abscess. Chronic pyelonephritis may lead to scarring with diminished renal function.

DIAGNOSIS

Diagnosis is based on a combination of clinical symptoms, physical examination, and laboratory findings. Diagnostic testing methods include urinalysis and culture and sensitivity.

BOX 13-1 Differential Diagnosis of Cystitis and Pyelonephritis

Cystitis
  Sudden onset typical
  Dysuria and symptoms associated with urination
  No fever, chills, nausea
  No costovertebral angle (CVAT) tenderness (i.e., flank pain)
  White blood cell (WBC) count normal
Pyelonephritis
  Gradual onset typical
  Symptoms associated with urination may or may not be present
  Fever, chills, nausea
  CVAT tenderness (i.e., flank pain)
  WBC count elevated

Adapted from Youngkin EQ, Davis MS: *Women's health: a primary care clinical guide*, Stamford, 1994, Appleton and Lange.

A proper urine specimen is obtained via a midstream catch. Vaginal cultures may rule out sexually transmitted disease and vaginal infection.

Differential Diagnosis

Primary differential diagnoses include urethritis, cystitis, and pyelonephritis.[2] In women with recurring infection, it is important to differentiate between relapse and reinfection. Additional considerations for acute or chronic UTI include[5]:

- Asymptomatic bacteriuria
- Chancroid
- Constipation
- Diabetes
- Dysfunctional uterine bleeding
- Dysmenorrhea
- Endometriosis
- Gonorrhea
- Interstitial cystitis (IC)
- Ovarian cysts
- Pelvic inflammatory disease
- Pregnancy
- Renal calculi
- Sexual assault
- Toxic shock syndrome
- Vaginitis
- Vulvovaginitis

CONVENTIONAL TREATMENT APPROACHES

An oral antibiotic effective against gram-negative aerobic coliform bacteria, particularly *E. coli*, is the principal treatment in patients with UTI. A 3-day course is typical in patients with an uncomplicated lower UTI or simple cystitis with symptoms for less than 48 hours. A bladder analgesic may be given if the patient has intense dysuria. Increased fluid intake is often recommended to promote dilute urine flow. Pregnant, otherwise healthy women with no evidence of an upper UTI may be treated with a 7- to 10-day course of a cephalosporin, such as cephalexin, even in the absence of upper urinary tract signs. Pregnant women are typically treated for all episodes of bacteriuria, even in the absence of symptoms. Upper UTI requires antibiotic treatment and may require intravenous (IV) therapy and hospitalization. In most cases, pyelonephritis responds to antibiotic treatment in 48 to 72 hours.[5] Therapeutic approaches to treatment and prevention of urogenital infections have remained essentially unchanged for years. Antibiotics and antifungals remain the mainstay of therapy. Several antibiotic therapies have become less effective because of antibiotic resistance; the use of antibiotics in pregnancy often leads to vaginal yeast infection, requiring treatment.[6]

Lifestyle changes may be recommended, such as teaching the client to void at the first urge to urinate, void after intercourse, drink adequate fluids, and avoid contraceptives associated with high UTI risk. Estrogen cream may be recommended for older women.[1,2] Other risk factors may include use of menstrual pads (i.e., rather than tampons); wiping the anogenital region from back to front after a bowel movement (front to back is the proper motion); wearing nonabsorbent underpants or pantyhose; and bubble baths with irritating soaps; however, none of these factors have been found to be significant in clinical trials.[1] Increasingly, conventional practitioners are recommending the use of cranberry juice and vitamin C for UTI treatment. These are discussed under The Botanical Practitioner's Perspective.

THE BOTANICAL PRACTITIONER'S PERSPECTIVE

Botanical medicine provides an excellent alternative to antibiotic use for reducing the duration and symptoms of lower UTI, preventing progression to upper UTI, and preventing recurrence. Lower UTI in nonpregnant women is often easily treated with simple protocol. Because of the risks associated with untreated pyelonephritis, it is recommended that patients with upper UTI be referred for medical care, and that botanical interventions be used in the context of complementary care. Care of pregnant women requires specific expertise in midwifery or obstetrics, as well as knowledge of herbs that are contraindicated in pregnancy, and must be done in consultation with an obstetric care provider. This section provides guidelines for the treatment of uncomplicated cystitis (Table 13-1).

Botanical treatment of lower UTI incorporates the use of urinary antiseptic and antimicrobial herbs with demulcent herbs (Table 13-2). Additionally, a diuretic may be included to assist the body in its attempt to increase the delivery of fluids through the bladder. Herbs for cramping and aching may be included if needed. Herbs are used in the context of an overall protocol to increase fluids and diuresis and to relieve offending lifestyle causes (e.g., chronic vulvovaginitis, overgrowth of uropathogenic bowel flora, or use of birth control methods or sexual habits that may contribute to the problem). Rarely UTI can lead to vaginal bleeding that is sometimes copious. If this occurs, seek medical care.

Although not discussed in this chapter, herbal care also incorporates strategies for improving overall immunity in women with chronic recurrent UTI.

Cranberry

The use of cranberries (Fig. 13-1) for the treatment of UTI dates back to the mid-nineteenth century when German chemists discovered that consumption of the berries produced a bacteriostatic acid in the urine. By 1900 in the United States, it was postulated that eating cranberries acidified the urine and prevented UTIs.[7] This mechanism of action has been questioned because studies have failed to consistently show

TABLE 13-1	**Sample Botanical Protocol for Cystitis**		
Days	**Herbs**	**Supplements**	**Other**
1-2	Prepare the following decoction either as a hot or cold water infusion: • 6g Uva ursi leaf (*Arctostaphylos uva ursi*) • 6g Marshmallow root (*Althea officinalis*) • 2g Dandelion leaf (*Taraxacum officinalis*) • 500 mL water Steep and strain. *Dose:* ½-1 cup every 4 hours depending on severity of UTI. This preparation will keep refrigerated for 24 hours. 3 mL echinacea tincture every 2-4 hours, depending on severity of UTI. If there is discomfort and cramping associated with UTI in a nonpregnant patient, 3 mL each of cramp bark and wild yam tinctures may be mixed with the echinacea and the dose increased to 5 mL every 2-4 hours.	500 mg vitamin C every 4 hours	• Every 2 hours, drink 6-8 oz of spring water • Every 2 hours, drink 6-8 oz of unsweetened cranberry juice. (The juice can be cranberry-apple for palatability, but should contain no added sugars.) The patient is taking 6-8 oz of fluid per hour to increase urinary volume and flush the urinary tract. • Probiotic supplement • Urinate at first urge • Avoid sexual activity during treatment • Reduce dietary sugar intake other than fresh fruit • Address/reduce any risk factors that might be present as discussed earlier in the chapter
3-4	If symptoms have lessened, continue protocol but decrease all doses to ½ of the original volume. If symptoms have not lessened, continue as for days 1-2, taking one 00-sized capsule of baking soda with each dose of the uva ursi–containing infusion.	If symptoms have lessened, continue protocol but decrease all doses to ½ of the original volume. If symptoms have not lessened, continue as earlier.	If symptoms have lessened, continue protocol but decrease all doses to ½ of the original volume. If symptoms have not lessened, continue as earlier.
5-7	If symptoms have lessened or have disappeared, continue protocol but decrease all doses to ¼ of the original volume. If symptoms have not lessened, seek medical care.	If symptoms have lessened, continue protocol but decrease all doses to ½ of the original volume.	If symptoms have lessened, continue protocol but decrease all doses to ½ of the original volume.

TABLE 13-1   Sample Botanical Protocol for Cystitis—cont'd

Days	Herbs	Supplements	Other
8-14	UTI frequently recurs in the weeks after treatment. This is most commonly a problem with antibiotic treatment, but even with herbs, prophylaxis is preferable to retreatment. On days 8-14, maintain all day 5-7 treatments, but omit the uva ursi blend infusion from the protocol. Repeat days 5-7 for several days if patient notices any inkling of recurrence. Patients with a tendency to UTI can periodically repeat days 3-7 without the uva ursi blend infusion as prophylaxis on a semiregular basis, for example, for 1 week per month. In many cases this prevents recurrent episodes entirely.		

UTI, Urinary tract infection.

TABLE 13-2   Botanical Treatment Strategies for Simple Lower Urinary Tract Infection

Therapeutic Goal	Therapeutic Activity	Botanical Name	Common Name
Reduce infection	Antimicrobial	Achillea millefolium	Yarrow
		Arctostaphylos uva ursi	Uva ursi
		Calendula officinalis	Calendula
		Echinacea spp.	Echinacea
		Lavandula officinalis	Lavender
		Thymus vulgaris	Thyme
		Vaccinium macrocarpon	Cranberry
Relieve spasm in urinary tract smooth muscle	Antispasmodic	Achillea millefolium	Yarrow
		Actaea racemosa	Black cohosh
		Dioscorea villosa	Wild yam
		Piper methysticum	Kava kava
		Viburnum opulus	Cramp bark
		Viburnum prunifolium	Black haw
Relieve pain	Analgesic	Anemone pulsatilla	Pulsatilla
		Corydalis ambigua	Corydalis
		Eschscholzia californica	California poppy
		Piper methysticum	Kava kava
		Piscidia piscipula	Jamaican dogwood
		See Endometriosis, Chronic Pelvic Pain for discussions of analgesic herbs	
Soothe urinary tract irritation and inflammation	Demulcent Antiinflammatory	Althea officinalis	Marshmallow
		Solidago virgaurea	Goldenrod

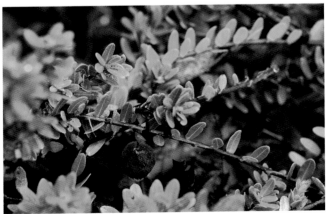

FIGURE 13-1 Cranberry *(Vaccinium macrocarpon).* (Photo by Martin Wall.)

acidification of the urine with consumption of cranberry juice. There are mixed results regarding the effect of cranberry juice, fruit, and extract on urine pH. It appears that cranberry does not consistently lower urine pH and it is uncertain whether any reduction in urine pH that does occur has an antibacterial effect.[8] However, the use of cranberry products continues to be a popular and empirically efficacious means of preventing and treating uncomplicated lower UTI. It is now accepted that the primary mechanism of action of cranberries is caused by two compounds in cranberries that each prevent fimbriated *E. coli* from adhering to uroepithelial cells in the urinary tract.[9-11] These compounds are also found in blueberries, which may also be used as part of the prevention and treatment of UTI.[12] Although cranberry has primarily been used against uropathogenic *E. coli*, recent evidence from in vitro studies suggests that it may have activity against other uropathogenic organisms, and also against *Helicobacter pylori*, which is responsible for gastric ulcers.[13] Cranberry also may prevent the formation of biofilms on epithelial mucosa—reservoirs of bacteria that are difficult to effectively treat with antibiotics.[8]

🌿 TOPICAL TREATMENT FOR URETHRITIS

Prepare a peri-urethral rinse:

   7 g dried calendula blossoms

   4 g dried lavender blossoms

   3 g dried thyme leaf

   Steep in 1 L of boiling water for 30 minutes. Cover while steeping. Strain and place in a peri-bottle to which has been added 1 tsp sea salt. Instruct patient to rinse the peri-urethral area with the tea after each urination and bowel movement (after wiping) and then pat dry gently.

   Alternatively, the mix could be prepared by adding 1 Tbsp of calendula tincture and 5 drops each of thyme and lavender essential oils to 1 cup of warm water with 1 tsp sea salt; use as per the instructions of the previous peri-rinse.

Based on a comprehensive review of the literature by the Cochrane Collaboration, there is some evidence from two good-quality randomized controlled trials (RCTs) that cranberry juice may decrease the number of symptomatic UTIs in women over a 12-month period. Based on the literature, there have been problems with noncompliance over long periods of administration, probably because of the taste of some cranberry products or possibly other side effects; and the optimum dosage and administration methods (e.g., juice or tablets) are unclear, necessitating further properly designed trials.[14] However, clinical experience with cranberry juice products in herbal practice suggests that compliance problems can be overcome by using palatable products. In two good-quality RCTs, cranberry products significantly reduced the incidence of UTIs at 12 months compared with placebo/control in women. One trial gave 7.5 g cranberry concentrate daily (in 50 mL); the other gave 1:30 concentrate given either in 250 mL juice or tablet form. There was no significant difference in the incidence of UTIs between cranberry juice versus cranberry tablets.[14] A subgroup analysis of an RCT evaluated the preventative capacities of cranberry juice (i.e., UR65) in cases of recurring UTIs. Outpatients were randomized into groups of 125 mL daily cranberry juice treatment (*n* = 55) and placebo control (*n* = 63). The primary outcome was UTI recurrence. The cranberry group experienced significantly less relapses than the controls (29.1% and 49.2%, respectively, according to subgroup analyses), and women older than 50 years of age were the most responsive to cranberry treatment.[15]

A pilot study (*n* = 20) explored the antimicrobial activity of a commercial cranberry preparation in urine samples. The study was conducted in two parts. In the first part, participants collected the first morning urine before ingesting 900 mg of cranberry and then at 2, 4, and 6 hours after ingestion. For the second part, participants collected urine on two consecutive days: day 1, when no cranberry was ingested; and on day 2, when cranberry was ingested. Specimens were then inoculated with *E. coli*, *Klebsiella pneumoniae* or *Candida albicans*. Colony-forming unit (CFU) were then compared with those in the specimens collected at 2, 4, and 6 hours postingestion. If there was a ≥50% reduction in CFU, the cranberry met the criteria for antimicrobial activity against the respective strains. In phase 1, 7 of 20 subjects had antimicrobial activity against *E. coli*, 13 of 20 against *K. pneumoniae*, and 9 of 20 against *C. albicans*. In phase 2, 6 of 9 subjects had activity against *K. pneumoniae* (Preparation not disclosed).[16] A liquid cranberry concentrate (i.e., UTI-STAT with Proantinox) was tested in women with recurrent UTIs. Twenty-eight women (average age 46.5 ± 12.8 years; data from 23 were used) who had experienced 2.78 ± 0.73 UTIs in the past 6 months were allocated into dosage groups: 15, 30, 45, 60, and 75 mL daily for 12 weeks. The study primarily evaluated safety, tolerability, and maximum tolerable dose (via blood/urine samples as baseline and weeks 4 and 12). UTI recurrence and quality of life (QOL), as measured by the Medical Outcomes Study short form 36-item questionnaire, were deemed secondary end points. At the conclusion of the study, participants reported reduced anxiety, higher QOL, and only two patients reported a UTI recurrence.[17]

A prospective pilot trial in Prague (*n* = 288) tested the use of cranberry extract capsules for the prevention of postgynecologic surgery (i.e., hysterectomy and/or anterior vaginal repair) UTIs. The investigators did not find evidence that women treated with cranberry experienced less UTIs. However, the capsules were administered for only 9 days (4 days before and 5 days after surgery). The preparation of the cranberry capsules and proanthocyanidin content is also unclear (dose information: [equiv. 17,000 mg of fresh fruit]).[18] A 2009 RCT tested cranberry extract against trimethoprim in the prevention of recurrent UTIs in older women (*n* = 137). Women who experienced two or more antibiotic-treated UTIs in the previous 12 months were eligible for inclusion and randomized to receive 500 mg cranberry extract or 100 mg trimethoprim daily for 6 months. Patients taking trimethoprim experienced slightly less recurrent UTIs than the cranberry group. There were more patient dropouts and adverse effects reported in the trimethoprim group. The onset of UTI did not differ between the two groups.[19]

A pilot study in 10 Greek postmenopausal women tested the efficacy of 400 mg of cranberry extract twice daily for 6 months to prevent recurrent UTI. Inclusion criteria were at least three documented UTIs in the previous year or at least two UTIs in the last 6 months before the start of the study. Outcomes were assessed by urinalysis at baseline and at every month for the duration of the study. During the treatment, none of the women experienced a UTI and nearly all exhibited sterile urine cultures. Three women experienced gastrointestinal (GI) upset and had to reduce the dose.[20]

A 2008 three-arm RCT tested cranberry juice in the prevention of asymptomatic bacteriuria and symptomatic UTIs in pregnant women (*n* = 188, 38.8% withdrew because of GI upset). The women were randomly allocated into three groups: cranberry three times daily (*n* = 58); cranberry at breakfast, then placebo at lunch/dinner (*n* = 67); and placebo three times daily (*n* = 63). The dosage was modified to twice daily after trial commencement to improve compliance. Trial results suggest a protective effect from cranberry against UTI recurrence, (Preparation was juice, dose not noted).[21]

The safety of cranberries and their general healthful properties, along with combined empiric evidence of numerous practitioners, suggest that it is reasonable for women with no other significant health problems to use cranberry products for the prevention of recurrent UTI.[22] A recent review article on cranberry summarizes that "recent, randomized controlled trials demonstrate evidence of cranberry's utility in urinary tract infection prophylaxis … Cranberry is a safe, well-tolerated herbal supplement that does not have significant drug interactions."[23] Recommended daily doses of cranberry for the prevention of UTI vary. Based on the available literature, the therapeutic dose of cranberry juice is 300 mL daily, three 8-oz glasses of unsweetened juice daily, or one cranberry extract tablet (300 to 400 mg) twice daily.[8,23]

Echinacea

Echinacea is used as a protocol for women with an acute UTI and for prevention of chronic UTI. Although echinacea is not used to directly address the UTI, it is included as an adjunct for overall immune support.

Uva Ursi

Uva ursi (Fig. 13-2) is one of the most commonly used urinary tract disinfectants in modern herbal medicine.[17] The leaves, taken as a cold or hot infusion, decoction, or tincture, are primarily used as an antiseptic in UTIs.[7] Uva ursi is commonly combined with urinary demulcents, such as marshmallow root or corn silk, and also may be taken with an herbal diuretic, most commonly dandelion leaf, but goldenrod or birch leaf may be used as well. Diuretics are contraindicated in pregnancy. Cold infusion reduces the tannin content of the product, making it easier for the digestive system to handle and reducing the nausea sometimes associated with its use; however, cold preparations might be inadvisable for immunocompromised patients because of the potential for microbial contamination from the herbs. Uva ursi is approved by the German Commission E for the treatment of inflammatory conditions of the urinary tract.[24] It is widely used in the treatment of uncomplicated acute and recurrent UTI based on its astringent and antibacterial actions, and when antibiotics are not deemed essential.[25] Midwives include the herb as an astringent antiinflammatory in sitz baths and perineal rinses for postnatal perineal healing and as part of treatment of vaginitis and urethritis. Unfortunately, there are few clinical trials and pharmacodynamic studies of uva ursi. In vitro studies using crude leaf preparations and extracts of uva ursi leaf have demonstrated mild antimicrobial activity against known UTI–causing organisms, including *C. albicans, E. coli Staphylococcus aureus,* and *Proteus vulgaris*.[26] Several studies have also demonstrated antiinflammatory activity of the herb, particularly enhanced when extracts are used in combination with antiinflammatory pharmaceutical drugs, such as prednisolone, indomethacin, or dexamethazone.[27,28] One double-blind, placebo-controlled, randomized study of 57 women utilized a combination of hydroalcoholic extract of uva ursi leaves (standardized to an unknown amount of arbutin and methylarbutin) and uva ursi with dandelion leaf (*Taraxacum officinalis*) to evaluate the efficacy of this combination for the prevention of recurrent UTI. Inclusion in the study required that otherwise healthy individuals had suffered at least three episodes of cystitis in the past year and at least one episode in the last 6 months before this study. Patients received either the extract ($n = 30$) or placebo ($n = 27$), three tablets three times daily for 1 month, and were then followed for 12 months. At the end of the 12-month monitoring period, significantly more women in the placebo group experienced recurrent cystitis compared with the treatment group ($p < .05$). No adverse effects were reported.[29,30]

> ### 🍃 ANTIMICROBIAL HERBS
>
> Two primary herbs used as antimicrobials in the treatment of lower urinary tract infection (UTI) are cranberry fruit and uva ursi leaf. Some controversy exists in using these two herbs together based on the disputed belief that uva ursi must be used in an alkaline urinary environment for efficacy, and that cranberry products acidify the urine. Modern herbal practice and emerging evidence suggest that there may be no reason to avoid combining these herbs. It appears that, although an alkaline environment may enhance the efficacy of uva ursi, effectiveness as an antimicrobial is not dependant on the urinary pH; in fact, cranberry may not significantly reduce urinary pH. Herbalists have long combined these herbs in UTI treatment protocol with excellent outcomes.

Some amount of disagreement can be found in the literature regarding the requirement of an alkaline pH environment for the efficacy of this herb. Some authors postulate that a reduced urinary pH inhibits the efficacy of the herb; others similarly argue that increasing the alkalinity of the urinary environment enhances the efficacy of the herb; yet others state that activity is not dependent on urinary pH. Given the reliability of this herb generally, it is prudent to conclude that if uva ursi does not seem to be working, the addition of four 00 capsules of the equivalent of 1 tablespoon of sodium or potassium bicarbonate may be taken once or twice daily, divided between uva ursi doses, to alkalinize the urine in such situations before making a final determination about efficacy.[22,25,31,32]

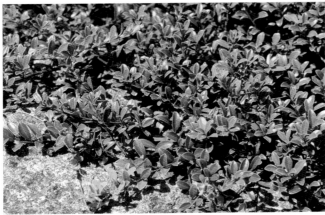

FIGURE 13-2 Uva ursi *(Arctostaphylos uva ursi)*. (Photo by Martin Wall.)

The question of whether this herb is safe for use in pregnancy is difficult to definitely answer based on the available evidence. The *Botanical Safety Handbook* gives this herb a class 2b and 2d rating—not to be used in pregnancy—a caution that is reiterated by many authorities.[24,29,33,34] However, the reasons for contraindication are variable and not well supported, ranging from alleged uterotonic and oxytocic activity to "theoretical fetotoxicity."[29,34] The original source of the concern of oxytocic activity appears to stem from Brinker, who reported that there is "empirical" evidence of oxytocic action, with no further explanation.[35] Low Dog states that the herb has potential fetotoxicity because of its hydroquinone content. Studies using pure hydroquinone (i.e., not the whole herb or whole herb products) have produced microtubulin dysfunction in bone marrow, and exposure of human lymphocytes and cell lines to hydroquinone has been shown to cause genetic damage.[22] However, giving the pure constituent is not the same as giving a whole herb, which is a perennial problem in assessing the safety of herbs with conventional pharmaceutical testing models. Although Upton state that mutagenicity may be associated with this herb, other researchers report on low potential for mutagenicity and negative Ames test.[29] In animals administered 100 and 400 mg/kg per day of arbutin, no signs of fetal toxicity were observed.[29] Uva ursi has been used by midwives as a mainstay treatment of acute symptomatic cystitis in pregnancy for over two decades in the United States with no adverse reports associated with its use.[36] Empiric observation demonstrates less recurrence of UTI with uva ursi versus treatment with antibiotics. The transference to infants of arbutin/hydroquinone from uva ursi use during lactation has not been researched and therefore is not recommended by German authorities; however, the risk remains speculative.[24] McKenna and coworkers recommend using only the lowest doses during lactation, observing the infant for side effects, and using the herb under the guidance of a knowledgeable lactation expert.[7] It is always prudent to avoid the medical use of herbs during the first trimester unless absolutely necessary. In the case of uva ursi, it is advisable to avoid it entirely during the first trimester, and to use it only if it is the best option for treatment of UTI later in pregnancy, using only at a minimal effective dose and for minimal duration. Further research in this area is clearly needed, particularly given the volume and frequency of UTIs among pregnant women.

Yarrow

In vitro studies of the essential oil and methanol extracts of several species of yarrow found *Achillea millefolium* to be active against a number of pathogenic organisms, including *S. aureus*, *K. pneumoniae*, *Pseudomonas aeruginosa*, *Salmonella enteritidis*, *Aspergillus*, and *C. albicans*, and also to possess antioxidant activity.[37,38] Water extracts have also demonstrated antimicrobial activity.[39] Two studies, however, though identifying antimicrobial activity in a number of herbs, did not demonstrate antimicrobial activity of yarrow.[40,41] The German Commission E lists among its actions: antibacterial, astringent, and spasmolytic.[24] No other literature was identified evaluating use of yarrow for UTI. Herbalists typically recommend the tea, 1 cup two to four times daily, for its antimicrobial and mild diuretic effects. Mills and Bone assert that limited use in pregnancy has not been associated with adverse fetal outcomes. Evidence of increased fetal damage in animal studies exists, with unknown relevance to human consumption. Yarrow is generally contraindicated during pregnancy because of its potentially high thujone content and emmenagogic activity.[34,42]

Demulcent and Antiinflammatory Herbs
Calendula, Thyme, and Lavender

Calendula is typically used as a topical antiinflammatory rinse with mild antimicrobial activity, either in the form of an infusion or diluted tincture, 1 Tbsp per 125 mL water. Thyme and lavender are used topically for their antimicrobial activity and mild antiinflammatory activity in the form of peri-rinses for the treatment of urethritis associated with vulvovaginitis, and also for the reduction of rectal to urethral microbial spread. They can be used as infusions or the essential oils can be diluted in tea or warm water. Ingredients for a sample peri-rinse are provided in Topical Treatments for Urethritis (see earlier discussion) Topical use of these herbs is considered safe during pregnancy.

Goldenrod

Goldenrod is an antiinflammatory, diuretic herb and spasmolytic favored for its beneficial effects in the treatment of UTI, which have been successfully demonstrated in both animal and uncontrolled human trials.[25,43] It is described by the German Commission E monographs and European Scientific Cooperative on Phytotherapy (ESCOP) as used for irrigation therapy for diseases of the lower urinary tract, especially for inflammation, as well as for prevention and treatment of urinary calculi and renal gravel. The flavonoid (including quercetin), saponin, caffeic acid derivatives, and glycosides have been described as the active components.[39] Goldenrod is taken as an infusion of 3 to 4 g of dried herb per 150 mL water that is steeped 10 minutes and taken two to three times daily.[25,39] It is suggested to take in conjunction with copious fluids.[24,25,39] ESCOP contraindicates the use of European goldenrod in patients with edema because of impaired cardiac or renal function.[25] Patients with allergies to plants in the *Compositae* family should avoid use of this herb. No data are available on use during pregnancy and lactation.

Marshmallow Root

Marshmallow root is soothing and antiinflammatory to the throat and GI system.[25] It is an excellent addition to water extracted uva ursi infusions and decoctions for its demulcent, soothing effects in the treatment of UTI.[42] The roots are rich in mucilage, which is composed largely of polysaccharides. Lack of studies on the pharmacodynamics of this herb in the urinary system make it impossible to conclude whether there are direct or indirect effects on the urinary epithelium of the urinary tract, but combination with uva ursi certainly reduces the possible irritation to the GI caused by the high-tannin content of that herb. Alcohol is not an effective menstruum for extraction of polysaccharides; therefore only water-based extraction methods are used for marshmallow.

Antispasmodic Herbs

Discussions of specific antispasmodic herbs are found elsewhere in this book. All of the herbs listed in Table 13-2 as antispasmodics are used specifically for their unique ability to relieve spasms in the pelvic organs, mostly through their action on smooth muscle. Yarrow has mild antispasmodic properties, as well as mild antimicrobial activity. Kava kava has a reputation for marked action specifically on the bladder, and is especially valued for treatment of neurogenic bladder pain. Yarrow and kava kava are contraindicated in pregnancy and should be used with caution in lactation. Wild yam has been used historically for its ability to ease spasms in the hollow organs, and is considered a valuable herb for the treatment of cramping associated with lower UTI, as are cramp bark and black haw. Black cohosh is specifically indicated for pelvic discomfort and cramping that are also associated with drawing pains in the lower back and legs. Yarrow may be taken as a tea or infusion, alone or added to other UTI specific herbs; otherwise these types of herbs, including yarrow, generally are included in tincture form with other herbs for UTI, typically as 10% to 50% of the formula.

NUTRITIONAL CONSIDERATIONS/ ADDITIONAL THERAPIES

Probiotics

There is limited research on the influence of diet on UTI. Midwives and herbalists commonly suggest a reduction in dietary sugar consumption and an increase in fluid intake, with the addition of cranberry juice as discussed. Because UTIs are often caused by bowel flora, which are pathogenic in the urinary tract, one train of thought is that modification of bowel flora may lead to a reduction in recurrent UTI.[44-47] The use of probiotics to restore normal vaginal flora and thus provide a competitive bacterial barrier to uropathogens is emerging as an area of research in the prevention of recurrent UTI.[1,13] Proponents of this approach use specific microorganism strains to restore the vaginal lactobacilli microflora such that the indigenous lactobacilli recover, or the patient retains some degree of acidic pH and protection against infection. The basis for use of probiotics emerged from clinical observations in 1973, when a study of healthy women showed an association between lactobacilli presence in the vagina and absence of UTI history. Results from a limited number of studies have demonstrated a significant reduction in recurrence rate of UTI using one or two capsules vaginally per week for 1 year, with no side effects or yeast infections. A two-strain combination is recommended for vaginal use: *Lactobacillus rhamnosus* GR-1 is used for its anti–gram-negative activities and resistance to spermicide, and *L. fermentum* RC-14 is included for anti–gram-positive cocci activities and hydrogen peroxide production. Various protocols have been explored, such as administration postmenses, one or two capsules per week, or one capsule daily for 3 days.[44] Studies are needed to determine whether healthy people and those prone to recurrent urogenital infections benefit from daily ingestion of probiotics, such as *L. rhamnosus* GG, the most clinically documented probiotic strain for gut health. A study using this strain in fermented milk has suggested some reduction in UTI recurrences. The potential for intestinal probiotics to influence bladder and vaginal health through immune modulation has not been fully explored.[6]

L. crispatus is also emerging as a potentially beneficial probiotic strain. A 2011 double-blind phase 2 RCT tested intravaginal *L. crispatus* for UTI prevention ($n = 100$, average age 21). Women with a history of recurrent infection were randomized to receive either the probiotic (10 billion CFUs/mL) or placebo daily for 5 days, then once weekly for a 10-week period. Outcomes were measured by urine analysis, and vaginal swabs were collected at weeks 1 and 10. Results suggest efficacy of this strain for UTI prevention.[48] A phase 1 trial was conducted in Egypt to assess the use of a 5-day treatment of *L. crispatus* vaginal suppository for recurrent UTI prevention in women ($n = 30$) against a placebo suppository. Results pertaining to efficacy are unclear. Seven out of the 15 women receiving the *L. crispatus* suppository developed pyuria (dose and CFU not noted).[49]

Researchers in one study concluded that dietary habits may be an important risk factor in UTI recurrence. One-hundred-thirty-nine women from a health center for university students or from the staff of a university hospital (mean age: 30.5 years) with a diagnosis of an acute UTI were compared with 185 age-matched women with no episodes of UTIs during the past 5 years. Data on the women's dietary and other lifestyle habits were collected by questionnaire. A risk profile for UTI expressed in the form of adjusted odds ratios (ORs) with 95% CIs was modeled in logistic regression analysis for 107 case control pairs with all relevant information. Frequent consumption of fresh juices, especially berry juices, and fermented milk products containing probiotic bacteria (e.g., yogurt, cultured milk, cheese) was associated with a decreased risk of recurrence of UTI. A preference for berry juice over other juices, and consumption of fermented milk products three times weekly were both associated with a reduction in recurrent UTI.[12] The efficacy of probiotics depends on having the proper strains prepared and stored to maintain their activity. According to Low Dog, a recent analysis of 20 probiotic products claiming to contain specific *Lactobacillus* species found 30% of products to be contaminated with other organisms, and 20% of products contained no viable species whatsoever.[22]

Vitamin C

Vitamin C is used as a bacteriostatic and acidifying agent in the treatment of UTIs. Studies have shown, however, that it actually does not significantly acidify the urine. It is likely, therefore, that it has a bacteriostatic action through other mechanisms not yet fully elucidated. It was demonstrated by Carlsson and colleagues that large amounts of a bacteriostatic gas (i.e., nitric oxide [NO]) are formed in mildly acidified nitrite containing human urine and that NO formation is greatly enhanced by the addition of vitamin C. Moreover, mildly acidified nitrite-containing human urine showed antimicrobial activity against three of the most common urinary pathogens; this inhibitory effect was further increased after addition of ascorbic acid.[50]

👤 CASE HISTORY: TREATMENT OF AN UNCOMPLICATED LOWER URINARY TRACT INFECTION IN A NONPREGNANT WOMAN

Lisa, a 32-year-old married mother of four young children, has a history of urinary tract infection (UTI) since her teenage years. Throughout her adult years, infections have recurred regularly, and with more frequency during times of stress. She has always received antibiotic treatment in the past. She is overweight (5'2" and 220 pounds), with no reported health problems, an unremarkable gynecologic history, and no history of pyelonephritis or other renal problems. She has been a regular patient in a midwifery practice through the pregnancy and birth of her fourth child, now 3 months old and breastfeeding. Her pregnancies were uneventful, though likely with undiagnosed gestational diabetes. She had mild transient glucosuria, and large babies (on average, 9 pounds); the most recent birth resulted in a shoulder dystocia that was resolved with no consequences to mother or newborn. She has not been diagnosed with gestational diabetes, but was told that she could be at risk for the later development of adult onset diabetes. She has a family history of marked obesity (i.e., mother, sister).

Lisa presents with an acute, severe UTI; by 10 PM, when she phoned the office on an emergency basis, she had a complete inability to void accompanied by pain (8 on a scale of 1 to 10), nausea, and malaise. She is afebrile on self-reporting, and has no other symptoms, but is extremely anxious and does not want to go on another round of antibiotics, particularly while breastfeeding. Her husband had picked up an over-the-counter medication for her to take to help her void. She does not know the name of it but described it as a "little blue pill" that she has used several times before. It did not help and now she is concerned. She was reassured that her UTI was a solvable problem, but that given the hour we needed a strategy. Her husband agreed to make the 45-minute drive to the office to fill a prescription from the apothecary, and she began an herbal protocol immediately, with a 24-hour observation period. If symptoms improved she would continue with the botanical protocol; if they did not, or at any point worsened, she would obtain medical treatment.

Her protocol is a standard botanical UTI intervention as follows:

Days 1 to 2
Drink:
- One 6- to 8-oz glass of water or diluted, unsweetened cranberry juice, alternating every hour throughout the day.
- ½ cup of uva ursi and marshmallow infusion four times daily (see Table 13-1 for preparation)
- 500 mg vitamin C and 4 mL of echinacea tincture every 4 hours
- If necessary for spasmodic bladder, take 3 mL antispasmodic tincture of equal parts of wild yam, cramp bark, and yarrow

Avoid:
  All sugar, including honey, maple syrup, and other natural sugars, in food products.

Days 3 to 5
Repeat days 1 to 2 protocol but reduce all doses by 50% frequency.

Days 6 to 7
Repeat days 3 to 5, but take only ¼ cup of the decoction.

Lisa began the protocol immediately that night, and given the acute situation, woke repeatedly throughout the night to continue. By 4 AM she voided copiously, and by morning her symptoms had improved mildly but not significantly. She continued the protocol throughout the day with no further improvement. By 4 PM, suggested she take two 00 capsules of baking soda with her next two doses of the uva ursi decoction, after which marked improvement ensued. By the next morning, she was voiding normally and beginning to feel symptom free. By day 3, she was completely symptom free and continued the protocol until completed. She phoned 3 weeks later saying she was thrilled that she had not had her typical relapse and was able to avoid antibiotics. We discussed her tendency to UTI, as well as the possible association with diabetes, and she was encouraged to reduce the sugar consumption that was a regular part of her heavily carbohydrate-based vegetarian diet. She was also reminded of the importance of voiding soon after she felt the urge, rather than waiting until a convenient time when she was not busy with her small children, and to urinate before she sat down to nurse the baby, rather than holding it until the baby was finished.

👤 CASE HISTORY: TREATMENT OF AN UNCOMPLICATED LOWER URINARY TRACT INFECTION IN A PREGNANT WOMAN AT 8 WEEKS' GESTATION

Note: The following case is from the late 1980s, before the publication of contraindications to the use of uva ursi during pregnancy and before the American Congress of Obstetricians and Gynecologists (ACOG) recommendation for antibiotic treatment of all UTI in pregnancy. Should a pregnant woman experience recurrent infection, cranberry juice, increased fluids, and vitamin C, along with lifestyle changes, should be considered, or appropriate antibiotic therapy employed.

Michelle, age 24, phoned early in the morning with presenting symptoms of frequent urination, light, irregular uterine cramping, and blood-tinged vaginal mucus. She was 8 weeks pregnant with her first child and planning a home birth with a midwife. She had no other medical problems. Vaginal examination revealed a closed cervix and speculum inspection revealed no evidence of blood in the vaginal canal or around the cervix. Her past history of frequent UTIs and current symptoms suggested that UTI might be the problem, and a urine dipstick provided preliminary confirmation. She suspected that she might be slightly dehydrated from the intense heat of summer, and she and her partner had also had sex the previous morning. Michelle wanted to avoid antibiotics if at all possible because of a history of vaginal candidal infections occurring after past treatment for UTI, but understood that if symptoms persisted, antibiotics would be necessary. A 24-hour trial was agreed upon with support of her family doctor, with medical intervention to be sought should symptoms worsen or persist, and a prescription for an antibiotic made available.

Michelle immediately began an intensive regimen of cranberry juice concentrate diluted in water every 2 hours, alternated with an 8-oz glass of water every 2 hours; 500 mg vitamin C four times daily; and ¼ cup of uva ursi and marshmallow root infusion every 2 hours, prepared with 7 g each of the herbs steeped in 1 L of boiling water. The herbs were left to sit in the infusion, the liquid being strained off for each dose.

Within 8 hours, symptoms began to improve, and all cramping and spotting had completely ceased by 24 hours. She decreased the dose and frequency of the uva ursi and marshmallow infusion to ½ the original recommendation for the next 24 hours, and after this remained on the cranberry juice preparation for 5 days, drinking three glasses per day, and maintaining a high water intake. She had no further episodes of recurrence and gave birth to a healthy child after a full-term pregnancy, with no complications, at home.

INTERSTITIAL CYSTITIS

The syndrome of chronic urinary bladder inflammation, pelvic pain, and frequent urination was dubbed *interstitial cystitis* (IC) in the nineteenth century. There is no uniform or pathognomonic histopathologic lesion; rather, IC represents part of a spectrum of irritative pelvic syndromes not clearly resulting from infection.[51] Although some patients have ulcerations of the bladder epithelium, these occur in less than 10% of cases. IC generally affects women beginning around 40 years of age, and also affects men.[52] Generally speaking, IC waxes and wanes but does not tend to spontaneously remit except in a minority of patients. Although anxiety, depression, and psychosocial distress (including inability to work owing to pain and frequency of urination) are common accompanying complications, and the condition can cause significant disruption in QOL, the condition itself does not progress and has no known life-threatening complications. A combination of identifying underlying causes and treating inflammation and pain, along with attention to QOL issues, is important.

PATHOPHYSIOLOGY

IC is a multifactorial disorder with no definitively established medical etiology.[51] Connections to allergy or autoimmunity are suspected based on features of the illness and associations with other allergic or autoimmune diseases. In the past decade, research attention has focused on the deterioration of the glycosaminoglycan layer of the bladder epithelium, as well as the role of NO.[53,54]

SYMPTOMS AND SIGNS

Signs and symptoms of IC include:
- History of progressive urinary frequency and nocturia
- No evidence of UTI
- Marked suprapubic pain when the bladder is full
- Pain in the urethra or perineum that is relieved on voiding
- Hematuria, especially when urination has been delayed (e.g., because of bladder over distention)
- Patient often has a history of allergies
- Chronic pelvic pain
- Dyspareunia

Physical examination is usually normal, although there may be some suprapubic tenderness and bladder region–tenderness when palpated transvaginally. Anxiety and stress often accompany the preceding symptoms.

DIAGNOSIS AND DIFFERENTIAL DIAGNOSIS

IC diagnosis is one of exclusion. Other causes of pelvic pain and urinary frequency, including infectious urethritis or cystitis, bladder polyps, bladder cancer, endometriosis, and vaginitis, must be ruled out. Although diagnosis is often presumed based on the clinical picture, cystoscopic examination can help to confirm the diagnosis.[51] The presence of glomerulations or a Hunner's ulcer strongly correlates with IC. Some also consider pain on bladder distention produced by intravesical instillation of water, saline, or potassium solutions to be diagnostically significant.

CONVENTIONAL TREATMENT

One definitive review of IC sums up conventional treatments for the condition thus: "Although the symptoms of IC can be controlled with one of a variety of treatments in the overwhelming majority of patients, there is little evidence that treatment accomplishes anything more than influencing the symptomatic expression of the disease, rather than curing the condition."[51] There are three categories of standard therapy available: oral, intravesicular, and surgical.

Oral Treatment

Amitriptyline, a tricyclic antidepressant, is one of the most commonly prescribed oral medications for patients with IC. Although apparently effective in uncontrolled trials, no controlled trials have been reported.[51] The most common adverse effect of amitriptyline is sedation, and thus it is usually given at bedtime. It is contraindicated in patients with conduction disorders or arrhythmias, unstable angina, congestive heart failure, or orthostatic hypotension.

Hydroxyzine and other H_1 receptor antagonist antihistamines also have been used, although they are not supported by controlled clinical trials.[55] It can take 3 months to see a benefit from these drugs, and they tend to be most effective in patients with allergies.[56] The major adverse effect of these drugs is sedation.

Pentosan sodium polysulfate is a synthetic glycosamino-glycan administered orally. It has been repeatedly shown to induce remission in approximately 30% of patients who take it, particularly if they have milder symptoms of shorter duration.[51,56] It may take many months for benefits to appear, and many more for optimal effects. The most common adverse effects are nausea, rash, diarrhea, and reversible alopecia.[51] Rarely hemorrhage can occur.

The final category of oral medications routinely prescribed for patients with IC are nonsteroidal antiinflammatory drugs (NSAIDs) and opioid analgesics. Nonspecific NSAIDs and cyclooxygenase (COX)-2–specific NSAIDs appear to be equally effective for relief of pain related to IC, although they have not been proved effective for this condition in controlled trials. COX-2 inhibitors are considered safer than nonspecific NSAIDs, but are also dramatically more expensive. Ceiling effects are noted for both types—that is, no added benefit is achieved above a certain dose.[51] Both types can cause GI bleeding, although COX-2 inhibitors are less likely to do so. Both also have significant renal toxicity. Opioid analgesics, with the significant problems of sedation, respiratory depression, dependence, addiction, and other problems, are generally considered a last resort in patients with chronic pain. Unlike NSAIDs, opioids do not have an efficacy ceiling.

Intravesicular Treatment

There are two major intravesicular therapies available: dimethyl sulfoxide (DMSO) and heparin. Less common intravesical therapies that will not be discussed here include silver nitrate, Clorpactin, and hyaluronic acid. DMSO was the first Food and Drug Administration (FDA)–approved treatment for IC—interesting because it is a natural product and because no controlled clinical trial data supported its efficacy. Using a solution of 50% DMSO on an outpatient or self-administration basis, approximately 35% of patients go into remission after one to three cycles of treatment.[56] Unfortunately the treatment tends to lose efficacy over time. The main adverse effects are acute symptom flare-up for 24 hours after instillation (sometimes compensated for by prior instillation of a topical anesthetic or systemic opioid analgesic) and intense sulfurous odor of breath and body after use.

Intravesical heparin requires long-term use (minimum 2 to 6 months) before benefits begin to be noticed, but they can be significant.[51] Benefits do not appear to be sustained unless treatment is continued more or less indefinitely. There is no systemic absorption of heparin administered in this fashion and thus no effect on coagulation or bone density.

Surgical Treatment

Hydrodistention is the most common surgical procedure for treatment of people with IC. It consists of anesthetizing the patient, and then distending the bladder with water and holding it in the enlarged state for a period of 15 or more minutes.[51] Symptoms are usually immediately relieved after hydrodistention and remain in remission for up to 24 months. However, they almost always return. Repeat treatments can be effective. Controlled clinical trials have not been published. This procedure can help in the diagnosis of IC as it often makes glomerulations or Hunner's ulcers obvious. Perhaps surprisingly, there is no indication that this treatment results in long-term bladder dysfunction, although there is a significant risk of bladder rupture. For the fewer than 10% of patients who have severe symptoms not relieved by these therapies, more invasive surgery is contemplated.[51] These procedures include resection of Hunner's ulcers, neurotomies, cystectomies, augmentation cystoplasties, and neo-bladder construction. Results vary considerably and there are many possible adverse effects, necessitating a careful, thorough decision-making process before choosing this method of treatment.

BOTANICAL TREATMENT OF INTERSTITIAL CYSTITIS

The botanical practitioner's approach should include identification of underlying factors. In addition to incorporating botanicals that reduce inflammation and pain, consideration should be given to the potential allergic etiology in this condition. This editor's experience is that utilizing an elimination type of dietary approach along with a low inflammation core diet is very helpful in identifying potential allergic food triggers. In many patients, gluten is a culprit and a 3-month trial of a strictly gluten-free diet can be helpful.

A large number of medicinal plants are utilized clinically in patients with IC based on observed botanical actions (Table 13-3). There is a general absence of clinical trials for botanicals for the treatment of this condition. This parallels the fact that many of the pharmaceuticals prescribed for IC patients also have not been subjected to controlled clinical trials.

The most important categories of herbs for treatment are mucilaginous or reflex demulcent herbs, antiinflammatories, anodynes, pelvic lymphagogues, spasmolytics, astringents, anxiolytics, and bladder tonics. Herbs with these actions are aimed at treating underlying causes and pathophysiologic processes, as well as alleviating symptoms. Immunologic support (e.g., via use of adaptogens; see Chapter 5) is a potentially important means to successful treatment in patients exhibiting this condition in conjunction with a history of allergies or atopy.

Demulcent Herbs

Herbs rich in complex polysaccharides are believed to induce mucus secretion in the urinary tract after oral administration, possibly through neurologic pathways.[57] Marshmallow leaf and root, hollyhock leaf and root, couch grass rhizome, slippery elm bark, and corn silk stigmata are among the many herbs commonly used for this purpose. Many herbal practitioners believe that reflex demulcent herbs such as these may help restore or support the glycosaminoglycan (GAG) layer and/or epithelium of the bladder, although restoration of the GAG layer is not a definitive treatment.[58,59] It is unknown if this action is truly operational in patients with IC, although many patients report at least some symptomatic relief while taking demulcent herbs. The demulcent herbs cited here have

TABLE 13-3 Botanical Treatment Strategies for Interstitial Cystitis

Therapeutic Goal	Therapeutic Activity	Botanical Name	Common Name
Soothe inflammation, relieve pain	Demulcent/Mucilage	*Alcea rosea*	Hollyhock
		Althea officinalis	Marshmallow
		Elymus repens	Couch grass
		Ulmus rubra	Slippery elm
		Verbascum thapsus	Mullein
		Zea mays	Corn silk
Relieve inflammation and pain	Antiinflammatory	*Betula* spp.	Birch
		Echinacea spp.	Echinacea
		Glycyrrhiza glabra	Licorice
		Melilotus officinalis	Sweet clover
		Populus tremuloides	Quaking aspen
		Solidago canadensis	Goldenrod
Relieve pain	Spasmolytic	*Cannabis sativa*	Marijuana
	Anodyne	*Herniaria glabra*	Rupturewort
	Analgesic	*Lobelia inflata*	Lobelia
		Paeonia brownii	Peony
		Piper methysticum	Kava kava
		Pulsatilla vulgaris	Pulsatilla
		Valeriana sitchensis	Pacific valerian
Relieve accompanying stress and anxiety	Anxiolytic	*Cannabis sativa*	Marijuana
		Passiflora incarnata	Passionflower
		Pulsatilla vulgaris	Pulsatilla
		Piper methysticum	Kava kava
		Scutellaria lateriflora	Skullcap
Improve bladder circulation, reduce local inflammation	Lymphagogue	*Fouquieria splendens*	Ocotillo
		Galium aparine	Cleavers
Improve bladder tone	Astringent	*Anemopsis californica*	Yerba mansa
	Tonic	*Chimaphila umbellate*	Pipsissewa
		Ephedra viridis	Mormon tea
		Equisetum arvense	Horsetail
		Rhus aromatica	Sweet sumac
		Zea mays	Corn silk

no known adverse effects. The usual preparation and dose of each is to stir approximately 1 Tbsp of powder into 4 to 8 oz of water, and drink this two to three times daily. This amount of powder also can be taken as capsules. Optionally, 5 to 10 mL of a glycerite can be administered three times daily. These herbs do not work well as tinctures because the polysaccharides are not very soluble in ethanol. These herbs should not be administered simultaneously with other herbs or drugs because the polysaccharides may alter absorption of many agents.[60]

Antiinflammatory Herbs

Antiinflammatory herbs are also likely to be important in any botanical approach for patients with IC. The botanical constituent quercetin is the best example supporting the potential benefit of antiinflammatory herbs. The only botanical medicine that appears to have been studied in a modern clinical IC trial is the antiinflammatory, antioxidant flavonoid, quercetin.

In an open trial, 1 g twice daily for 4 weeks brought symptomatic relief to 20 of 22 male and female volunteers with IC.[61] There were no adverse effects, although two people

dropped out of the study. For acute symptoms, as much as 1 g five times a day of quercetin may be necessary. Freeze-dried stinging nettles may also reduce histamine because it works synergistically in combination with quercetin. It is a combination that many botanical practitioners use with great reported success for seasonal allergies, and may be safely incorporated into a botanical plan for treating IC.

Quercetin is also often combined with bromelain, a plant enzyme complex, on the theory that bromelain enhances absorption of quercetin and because bromelain itself has systemic antiinflammatory activity that clearly affects the lower urinary tract.[62] A typical dose of bromelain is 500 to 1000 mg three times daily between meals. Taking bromelain with food causes it to act as a protease in the digestive tract and may reduce systemic absorption and activity.

Many herbs influence multiple inflammatory pathways and also often have other effects on immune cells, as has been well established for echinacea.[63]

Salicylate-containing herbs are commonly used in countering inflammation, with birch leaf and quaking aspen bark having some specific affinity for the genitourinary tract.[64] These herbs have an additional benefit in that they are analgesic. Any of these antiinflammatory herbs may cause mild digestive upset. Birch and quaking aspen may theoretically inhibit platelet aggregation, although there is no clinical evidence of bleeding with these herbs or interaction with other antiplatelet or anticoagulant agents. Clinical research with the related herb willow cortex shows no significant effect on platelet aggregation in humans.[65]

Two antiinflammatory herbs hold a special place in the treatment of people with IC—*Glycyrrhiza glabra* (licorice) and *Glycyrrhiza uralensis* (gan cao) root. These plants have been studied in depth and found to have several actions that should have a beneficial effect on IC patients. Licorice and gan cao contain compounds that are antiinflammatory, immunomodulating, antioxidant, and inhibit abnormal complement.[66-69] This, coupled with the historical use of these herbs to treat inflammatory diseases and inflammatory autoimmune conditions, makes them well suited as treatment for IC.

Spasmolytic and Anxiolytic Herbs

One herb that seems to be among the most commonly prescribed for people with IC is kava kava *(Piper methysticum)* root. This herb has repeatedly been shown to be an effective anxiolytic in double-blind, placebo-controlled trials.[70]

IC, like so many chronic conditions with an inflammatory component, involves the inseparably linked mind and body. To this end, an anxiolytic herb such as kava might be helpful in a psychoneuroimmunologic way. Indeed, a neurogenic hypothesis of the etiology and pathogenesis of IC has recently gained ground.[71] Many practitioners ascribe kava's benefits to the spasmolytic properties of the herb, a theory that correlates with the fact that the bladder of the IC patient often contracts when it reaches a certain, abnormally low point of fullness.[71]

A typical adult dose of kava tincture for IC treatment is 3 to 5 mL three times daily. Standardized extracts of this herb are not recommended for use because some use acetone as a solvent, and such concentrated extracts differ sufficiently from the natural state of the herb that they cannot be ruled out as a possible cause of the handful of reports of hepatotoxicity. Kava is nonaddictive and nonsedating in small doses. It improved mental function compared with diazepam in a clinical trial.[72] Because of lack of information it should be avoided in pregnancy and lactation. Pending further study, it should be avoided in patients with preexisting liver disease or those concomitantly taking hepatotoxic drugs.

Lymphagogue and Astringent Activity

Astringent herbs may be antiinflammatory. Sweet sumach does have a history of use in treating symptoms of IC. The usual dose of tincture is 1 to 2 mL three times daily. It may cause nausea, in which case it should be taken with food. Mormon tea stem and related native American species in the genus are also used as urinary tract astringents. These species, unlike their Asian cousins (particularly *Ephedra sinica* or ma huang), do not contain ephedrine or pseudoephedrine.[58] They are rich in tannins. Because Mormon tea is also diuretic, it

may be irritating to some patients and should not be taken as a tea in most cases. In cases of acute pain episodes, a sitz bath made by adding a handful of Mormon tea herb to the bath water may help relieve symptoms. Mormon tea may cause nausea when taken internally; taking it with food usually eliminates this problem. Yerba mansa root grows exclusively in the southwest desert of the United States and northern Mexico. It also contains tannins and has a strong reputation in Southwestern herbal traditions as a mucous membrane tonic, mild antimicrobial, and as a mild diuretic.[58] It also has moderate anodyne effects. Although unrelated to goldenseal, it acts similarly to this useful plant.[58] Yerba mansa is considered specific for chronic inflammatory bladder conditions, although it has not been the subject of research.[58] The usual dose of tincture is 3 to 5 mL three times daily. It may cause nausea; taking it with food eliminates this problem. Owing to the limited distribution of this plant in the wild, care should be taken in obtaining it from a sustainable source. All astringent herbs should not be combined with alkaloid-rich herbs or most drugs because tannins interfere with the absorption of these agents.[60]

Ocotillo is an unusual plant native to the southwestern United States and northern Mexico. There is no modern research on this plant, which clinically acts as the most specific pelvic lymphagogue I have encountered. It seems to be helpful in all instances of chronic pelvic conditions characterized in traditional herbalism as being "congested," including IC. Owing primarily to habitat loss and the fact that it is a slow-growing desert plant, ocotillo is potentially threatened in the wild. Therefore it is important to find a source of sustainably harvested herb. The usual dose of tincture is 3 to 5 mL three times daily, or smaller doses when combined with other herbs in formulae. Sweet sumach bark or root belongs to the *Anacardiaceae* family along with its greatly feared cousin, *Rhus toxicodendron* (poison ivy). Sweet sumach does not contain urushiol and does not cause dermatitis. It is high in tannins and has an astringent effect that appears to be specific to the urinary tract.[73]

Bladder Tonics

Several nonastringent herbs traditionally have been considered bladder tonics, meaning that they support the urinary bladder in a very general way. They have not been the subject of modern research to determine the mechanisms involved. Pipsissewa herb, horsetail herb, cleavers herb, and mullein root are four such herbs. All four are completely benign, even at large doses. Because they can be diuretic,[74] high doses may aggravate some patients with IC. Generally, they are used in lower doses for long periods of time combined with other herbs to promote general healing. Investigation of these widely used, gentle herbs is warranted to determine the degree of efficacy and their actions. A typical dose of tincture of any of these is 2 to 4 mL three times daily or less when combined with other herbs in formulae. Although these humble herbs do not conform well to the dominant pharmacologic model, their utilities cannot be overstated.

Anodyne/Analgesic Activity

A wide range of herbs are available to reduce pain associated with IC. Of course, the underlying causative aspects of this condition must be treated foremost to help eliminate the cause of pain, but sometimes it is necessary to suppress pain to make a person's life bearable. The simplest and safest botanical anodynes are herbs normally thought of for relieving insomnia and anxiety—the nervines. These include Pacific valerian root, passionflower leaf, and skullcap leaf and flower. All three are central-acting anodynes and are safe for regular use. There is little research on the analgesic mechanism of these herbs, although preliminary animal studies do support that they are active.[75] A typical dose of tincture of these herbs is 3 to 5 mL three times daily, although taking higher doses more frequently (up to 10 mL five times a day) are indicated for more serious pain. If sleep problems are a distinct element of a patient's case, nervines should be taken at bedtime. Some people may become drowsy when taking nervines during the day, but often there is no problem. Some studies show these herbs actually increase daytime alertness by improving sleep quality at night.[76] These same studies showed no signs of addiction and no interaction with alcohol, facts that are strongly supported by clinical experience. A much more potent, central-acting analgesic is pulsatilla leaf and flower. Although generally active orally, suggesting possible activity in the central nervous system, the widespread use of topical pulsatilla by native peoples for arthritis and related conditions suggests it also may have local anodyne effects.[77] Pulsatilla contains glycosides that, although more toxic when fresh, are also more active. I feel that fresh pulsatilla is superior to dried, and simply recommend a lower dose to avoid adverse effects. A typical dose of fresh-plant tincture is three to five drops three times daily, or more frequently (up to every 2 hours) until the pain is alleviated. Signs of overdose include nausea, weakness, bradycardia, hypotension, mydriasis, paralysis, seizure, or coma. Pulsatilla is contraindicated in pregnancy and lactation.

A more controversial but effective analgesic is marijuana leaf and seed. Clearly, this herb remains illegal in most jurisdictions for political reasons, but some patients still consider using it on their own volition, making it important to understand it. Cannabinoids from marijuana have long been known to have central analgesic effects, probably mediated through cannabinoid receptors.[78,79] Tetrahydrocannabinol is not the most potent cannabinoid in many animal studies, suggesting the whole herb may be more effective or possibly broader in its activity.[80] This concept is supported by other evidence suggesting the whole plant is safer than its constituents in isolation.[81] Substantial evidence also shows that cannabinoids and flavonoid compounds in marijuana are antiinflammatory.[82] Marijuana has not been specifically reported to alleviate pain or other symptoms in people with IC (Table 13-4).

NUTRITIONAL CONSIDERATIONS

Avoidance of various foods in the diet has been suggested as helpful by many sources, although controlled trials are lacking. The mechanism by which food would exacerbate IC pathogenesis or symptoms has not been determined, although food allergy and leakage of irritating food chemicals (e.g., caffeine) excreted in the urine out of the bladder across a damaged bladder wall might explain this phenomenon. Because of the heterogeneity of response among patients, the most reasonable approach would be to have patients eliminate foods that individually seem to bother them and look for effects on symptoms. For patients who are uncertain, an elimination-challenge diet will likely produce better results than avoiding an arbitrary list of possible triggers that might miss what actually has the most damaging influence.

L-Arginine has been advocated as a potential therapy for IC patients because of the possible role of NO in the disease. An initial open trial found that 1.5 g daily was helpful at reducing voiding discomfort and pain over 6 months.[83] A subsequent open study using 3 to 10 g daily found no effect on symptoms or NO production over 5 weeks.[84] A double-blind trial involving 53 patients who took 1.5 g for 3 months found that it decreased pain intensity significantly compared with placebo, and just barely missed statistical significance in reducing pain frequency and urgency.[85] More research is needed, but a trial of 1.5 g arginine daily is worth considering in most IC patients.

ADDITIONAL THERAPIES

Bladder Retraining

Bladder retraining is an important element of any treatment approach because other treatments often do not significantly improve bladder capacity after long-term low-volume voiding.[56] It consists simply of determining the average time between urinations, then gradually having the patient increase the interval by small increments each month, usually by 10 to 15 minutes per month. This approach has resulted in more than doubling the voiding intervals in some patients. It should be noted, however, that it will probably only succeed if pain symptoms have first been alleviated.

Stress Reduction

Stress reduction can take many forms, including regular light exercise, meditation, self-hypnosis, visualization, or regular have been recommended, although their efficacy has not been assessed.[86]

Sitz Baths, Perineal Massage, and Trigger Point Therapy

Warm sitz baths have also been advocated for pain relief without support from clinical trials. Perineal muscle massage and trigger point therapy have been advocated to relieve pain. In one case series involving 52 women and men (10 with IC and the rest with urgency-frequency syndrome), a series of manual trigger release techniques performed per anus and per vagina weekly or biweekly for 8 to 12 weeks resulted in moderate-to-marked improvement in

TABLE 13-4 Condition and Botanical Medicine Summary Table

Botanical	Antimicrobial/Antiseptic	Antispasmodic	Analgesic/Anodyne	Antiinflammatory	Anxiolytic	Astringent/Tonic	Demulcent	Diuretic	Lymphagogue
Achillea millefolium	X	X		X					
Actaea racemosa							X		
Alcea rosea	X			X			X		
Althea officinalis		X					X		
Anemone pulsatilla			X						
Anemopsis californica	X			X					
Arctostaphylos uva ursi	X			X					
Betula spp.				X					
Calendula officinalis		X							
Cannabis sativa			X						
Chimaphila umbellate		X							
Corydalis ambigua			X						
Dioscorea villosa		X							
Echinacea spp.	X								
Elymus repens							X		
Ephedra viridis						X			
Equisetum arvense						X			
Eschscholzia californica		X	X						
Fouquieria splendens									X
Galium aparine									X
Glycyrrhiza spp.	X		X	X					
Herniaria glabra			X						
Lavandula officinalis	X	X			X				
Lobelia inflata		X		X					
Melilotus officinalis									
Paeonia brownii		X	X						
Passiflora incarnata		X	X		X				
Piper methysticum		X	X		X				
Piscidia piscipula			X						
Populus tremuloides				X					
Pulsatilla vulgaris		X							
Quercetin				X					
Rhus aromatica						X			
Scutellaria lateriflora					X				
Solidago canadensis				X					
Solidago virgaurea		X		X					
Thymus vulgaris	X								
Ulmus rubra							X		
Vaccinium macrocarpon	X								
Valeriana sitchensis		X	X						
Verbascum thapsus								X	
Viburnum opulus		X							
Viburnum prunifolium		X							
Zea mays								X	

70% of participants with IC.[87] A similar set of techniques also has been reported to be helpful in a smaller series of four patients with IC.[88]

Acupuncture and Transcutaneous Electrical Nerve Stimulation

Acupuncture and transcutaneous electrical nerve stimulation (TENS) are methods of pain reduction with preliminary support from clinical trials. Needling the spleen 6 point was associated with reduction in frequency, urgency, and dysuria in one case series.[89] A case series found that high or low frequency suprapubic TENS applied daily for 30 to 120 minutes was associated with good pain relief or remission of symptoms in 23% of patients with nonulcerative IC and 54% with ulcerative disease.[90] A combination of acupuncture and TENS resulted in only minor pain relief in an open trial.[91]

🌸 TREATMENT SUMMARY FOR INTERSTITIAL CYSTITIS

- Use mucilaginous or reflex demulcent herbs, antiinflammatories, anodynes, pelvic lymphagogues, spasmolytics, astringents, anxiolytics, and bladder tonics.
- Teach bladder retraining exercises after pain symptoms have first been alleviated.
- Use stress reduction methods, including regular light exercise, meditation, self-hypnosis, visualization, and warm sitz baths.
- Perineal muscle massage and trigger point therapy have been advocated to relieve pain.
- Avoid foods that might exacerbate interstitial cystitis pathogenesis or symptoms on an individual basis.
- Acupuncture and transcutaneous electrical nerve stimulation (TENS) are adjunct methods of pain reduction that can be considered.
- L-Arginine has been advocated as a potential therapy for interstitial cystitis patients.

14

Breast Cancer Prevention and Supportive Therapies

For the majority of women with breast cancer, complementary and alternative medicine (CAM) has become a standard part of their treatment and healing.[1]

THE BREASTS AND THE BREAST EXAMINATION

Anatomy of the Breasts

The breasts of an adult woman are tear-shaped mammary glands (Fig. 14-1), which are technically developmentally modified sweat glands with the potential for milk production. A layer of subcutaneous adipose tissue surrounds the glands and extends throughout the breast itself, composing 80% to 85% of the normal breast. The breasts are supported by and attached to the pectoral muscles of the thorax by ligaments. Each breast contains 12 to 25 circularly arranged lobes radiating around the nipple. Each lobe is made up of numerous lobules containing clusters of alveolar glands that produce milk in a lactating woman. The alveolar glands transport the milk into lactiferous ducts that drain each respective lobe. Each lactiferous duct widens to form an ampulla, and then narrows before termination at openings in the nipple. A band of circular smooth muscle surrounds the base of the nipple; longitudinal smooth muscle fibers extend this ring, encircling the lactiferous ducts as they converge toward the nipple. The adipose tissue and configuration of lobes determine the size and shape of the breast.

The darker-pigmented area around the nipple is called the areola. Its size and color varies from 2 to 6 cm in diameter and from pale pink to deep brown depending on age, parity, and skin pigmentation. The areola contains numerous small oil-producing glands called Montgomery's tubercles, which serve to lubricate the areola; these become more pronounced during pregnancy.[2]

The breasts possess arterial blood supply and venous return, as well as a lymphatic drainage system divided into two main categories: superficial (including cutaneous) drainage and deep parenchymatous drainage. The lymph system serves to filter infection and protect the body from disease. Additionally, the breast has a nerve supply; the nipple is highly innervated, and for many women is a highly sensitive, erogenous area.

Women's breast shape, size, and "tone" are as highly variable as are women themselves. Yet because of a narrow range of acceptable breast appearance in Western culture, many women are dissatisfied with their breasts. According to the American Society for Plastic Surgery, nearly 250,000 breast augmentation procedures were performed in 2005. Breast augmentation for teenagers accounted for 3841 procedures in 2003. The number of breast augmentations increased 7% from 2002 to 2003. When physicians were asked the primary reason their patients offered for wanting a breast augmentation, 91% said it was to improve the way they feel about themselves.[3]

CYCLIC INFLUENCES ON BREAST TISSUE

The breast tissue is highly influenced by the hormonal changes of the menstrual cycle. The three major hormones affecting the breast are estrogen, progesterone, and prolactin. Estrogens cause proliferation of mammary ducts, whereas progesterone causes growth of lobules and alveoli. Many women experience breast swelling, tenderness, and pain in the 10 days preceding menstruation, largely because of distention of the ducts, hyperemia, and edema of the interstitial tissue of the breasts. These changes regress, along with the symptoms, during menstruation and the postmenstrual phase.

During pregnancy, in response to progesterone, breast size and turgidity increase significantly; this is accompanied by deepening nipple and areolar pigmentation, nipple enlargement, areolar widening, and an increase in the number and size of Montgomery's tubercles. In response to hormonal signals, the alveoli enlarge, and their lining cells (i.e., acini), increase in number and size (i.e., hyperplasia and hypertrophy). The breast ductal system branches markedly. In late pregnancy, the fatty tissues of the breasts are almost completely replaced by cellular breast parenchyma. Secretion of colostrum may begin during pregnancy. After birth, the fully mature breasts secrete milk in response to prolactin.

During menopause, because of lack of hormonal stimulation, the breast undergoes a process of involution, eventually regressing to an almost infantile state.

Fibrous Breast Tissue

Many women have fibrous breast tissue, which upon palpation may cause them to think they have abnormal breast tissue or a problematic lump. Fibrocystic breasts are discussed in chapter 11 in Fibrocystic Breasts and Breast Pain. Women with fibrocystic breasts should also learn to perform breast self-examination (BSE). In addition, other normal masses may be present; for example, cysts that are not a cause for

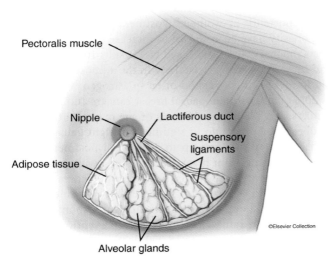

Pectoralis muscle

Nipple

Lactiferous duct

Suspensory ligaments

Adipose tissue

©Elsevier Collection

Alveolar glands

FIGURE 14-1 Anatomy of the female breast. (From Seidel HM: *Mosby's guide to physical examination,* ed 6, St. Louis, 2006, Mosby; © Elsevier Collection.)

concern but that should be regularly evaluated for changes. Women can learn to differentiate the usual pattern of lumps and identify new or unusual lumps. Information on the normal breast pattern from the patient may help her physician to differentiate between a new mass and a stable lump.

BREAST CANCER

Breast cancer is perhaps the single most important medical concern women face today. Although there has been an overall decrease in breast cancer rates in the United States in recent decades, in 2007 there were more than 180,000 new cases of invasive breast cancer and 40,910 breast cancer–related deaths. This is equivalent to a breast cancer diagnosis every 2 minutes.[4] Breast cancer is the leading cause of cancer in women, accounting for one third of all cancer cases.[2] All women are affected by breast cancer—whether by literal diagnosis or a lifetime of worry about whether they will experience this disease.[4] It has been estimated that 50% of all women in the United States at some point in their lives will ask their physicians about a concerning lump or other worrisome breast finding with the anxiety that they have breast cancer. Many have known a friend, relative, or colleague who has gone through a possible or actual breast cancer diagnosis.

Breast cancer, from etiology to treatment, is a vast and complex topic with an enormous amount of literature. There is controversy over screening methods, treatments, and the role of complementary and alternative medicine (CAM) therapies in the care of women with breast cancer. There are still many unknowns in cancer diagnosis, prevention, and treatment. It would be impossible to elucidate the entire topic of breast cancer, or even that of breast cancer and CAM, within the confines of a single chapter. It is hoped that this chapter will help the reader begin to understand the magnitude of breast cancer as a disease that affects all women, whether as a direct clinical reality or a lifelong concern; to understand nonmodifiable and modifiable

breast cancer risk factors; to gain perspective on the complexity of issues women face regarding screening and, if diagnosed, choices regarding their treatment, including whether and how to use CAM therapies. This chapter does not provide guidelines for the botanical treatment of breast cancer, although it does direct readers to additional resources on evidence for botanicals commonly used in cancer treatment protocol.

Risk Factors for Developing Breast Cancer

Breast cancer is the result of the complex interaction of multiple factors—hormonal, genetic, environmental, and lifestyle.[4] Breast cancer risk factors can be divided into nonmodifiable and modifiable risks. The former are heritable or genetic, although it is arguable that genetics can be favorably or negatively influenced by either beneficial or harmful environmental exposures, diet, and therapies that target genetic processes such as transcription and tumor suppression; thus to some extent, they may be modifiable. Modifiable factors include diet, obesity, alcohol intake, and environmental exposures.

Genetics

Germ line mutations are responsible for no greater than 10% of human breast cancers.[2] However, women with specific mutations have a much higher lifetime risk of developing breast cancer, are more likely to experience breast cancer at an earlier age than the average population, and may experience more severe forms of the disease. *BRCA1* and *BRCA2* are known as tumor suppressor genes. Women who have inherited a mutated *BRCA1* allele from either parent have a 60% to 85% lifetime likelihood of developing breast cancer (as well as a 33% chance of developing ovarian cancer). Women with this gene born after 1940 have an even higher risk, attributed to increased exposure to cancer-promoting environmental factors, and Ashkenazi Jewish women have an increased likelihood of carrying this mutation.[2] Mutation of the p53 tumor suppressor gene, such as occurs in the inherited Li-Fraumeni syndrome, is associated with an increased incidence of breast cancer and other cancers, as are phosphatase and tensin homolog (PTEN) tumor suppressor mutations. Heightened oncogene expression is seen in approximately 25% of breast cancer cases. Erb-2 (HER-2 neu), a member of the epidermal growth factor receptor (EGFR) superfamily, is a product of oncogene overexpression, and can contribute to malignant transformation of human breast epithelium.[2] Women with a genetic cancer predisposition are considered high risk for breast cancer and may receive recommendations for prophylactic cancer treatment including oophorectomy, elective mastectomy, and chemotherapy with tamoxifen, raloxifene, and/or aromatase inhibitors (AIs) (see discussion later).[4]

Endogenous Hormone Exposure

Breast cancer is a hormone-dependent disease manifesting as a malignant proliferation of clonal epithelial cells lining the ducts or lobules of the breast.[2] Its hormonal dependence is demonstrated by the fact that women who lack functioning ovaries and who never received hormone replacement therapy (HRT) do not develop breast cancer. Women are 150 times more likely to develop breast cancer than are men because of greater exposure to estrogen and progesterone.[2] Although women may develop breast cancer at any age, there is a slight decline in breast cancer incidence after menopause, accompanying naturally declining levels of estrogen and progesterone; however, as women age they have a statistically increasing likelihood of being diagnosed with breast cancer, likely as a result of a lifetime of accumulated exposures (0.4% chance of diagnosis between 30 and 40 years of age; 4% chance between the ages of 70 and 80 years).[2,3]

Three life cycle events appear to significantly influence a woman's overall risk of developing breast cancer: age at menarche, age at first pregnancy, and age at menopause. Women who begin to menstruate at age 16 have 50% to 60% of the risk of developing breast cancer compared with those who experience menarche at age 12.[2] Having a full-term pregnancy by age 18 confers a 30% to 40% lower risk of developing breast cancer compared with women who have no children. Menopause (natural or surgical) that occurs 10 years before the median age of 52 years old for menopause decreases lifetime breast cancer risk by approximately 35%.[2] Breastfeeding duration has been shown by meta-analysis to also confer substantial protection against breast cancer regardless of age at first pregnancy or number of pregnancies.[2] The risk reduction is directly correlated with a decreased amount of time during which breast tissue is exposed to endogenous estrogens. International variation in breast cancer rates has also supported the role of hormonal exposure as an etiologic factor in breast cancer. Asian women, for example, have been found to have significantly lower serum estrogen and progesterone levels, and have breast cancer rates of 10% to 20% of women in westernized nations (see Phytoestrogens and Breast Cancer).

Alcohol Intake

Even modest amounts of regular alcohol consumption (e.g., one glass of wine daily) has been associated with a 26% increased risk of breast cancer on the basis of multiple cohort studies.[2,4] Folic acid supplementation may modify this risk somewhat.[2] The risk of breast cancer needs to be weighed against the cardioprotective effects of modest alcohol intake.[2]

Dietary Fat Intake and Obesity

Dietary fat intake has been a focus of much research and debate. The dietary fat hypothesis, which proposed a correlation between amount of dietary fat intake and breast cancer incidence, is based on the observation that national per capita fat consumption is highly correlated with breast cancer mortality rates. However, per capita fat intake is also associated with economic prosperity, and this is accompanied by other factors that are also related to breast cancer risk, such as early menarche, low parity, later age at first birth, and lower levels of physical exercise.[5] Studies have failed to show a direct correlation between consumption of specific types of dietary fats or the amount of fat in the diet, and breast cancer.[6] However, excessive caloric intake from any source in adolescent girls has been shown to lead to earlier menarche, whereas in older women can delay the onset of menopause, which as discussed are risk factors for breast cancer development.[2]

Obesity has been correlated with increased risk of all-cause mortality in women.[7] Postmenopausal weight gain and obesity have been shown to increase breast cancer risk by as much as 50%.[4] Increased risk results from prolonged and increased aromatase activity in the adipose tissue leading to increased conversion of fat to estrogen.[2,4,7] As many as 20% of all postmenopausal breast cancers and 27% of all cancers in women over 70 years of age may be attributable to obesity or moderate to significant weight gain after the fifth decade of life, and up to 50% of all postmenopausal deaths resulting from breast cancer may be attributable to obesity.[7] Obesity is also a risk factor for poor breast cancer prognosis with larger tumor size, greater risk of metastases, poorer surgical outcome, and less efficient response to chemotherapy and radiation. The Cancer Prevention Study II concluded that as many as 18,000 deaths of women in the United States older than 50 years of age could be prevented if women maintained a body mass index (BMI) of less than 25 kg/m^2 throughout adulthood.[7] Weight loss and maintenance of weight in the BMI range of 19 to 25 kg/m^2 has been shown to reduce breast cancer risk by about 30%.[4]

Environmental Hormone Exposure

Exogenous hormone exposure may play a significant risk in the etiology of breast cancer. There is well-supported evidence that many commonly used chemicals and widespread environmental pollutants act as hormone disruptors.[8] Polycyclic aromatic hydrocarbons (PAHs) and polychlorinated biphenyls (PCBs), in conjunction with certain genetic polymorphisms involved in carcinogen activation and steroid hormone metabolism, cause mammary gland tumors in animals specifically by mimicking estrogen, or increasing susceptibility of the mammary gland to carcinogenesis.[9] Evidence regarding dioxins and organic solvents is sparse and methodologically limited but also suggestive of an association between breast cancer and exposure.[9] Scientist Rachel Carson suggested the role of environmental contamination in human cancers several decades ago; however, it is only in recent years that the role of exogenous hormones acting as hormone disruptors has begun to be seriously studied, and a great deal is unknown.

Although older studies suggested an association between oral contraceptive (OC) use and breast cancer, more recent meta-analyses imply little to no breast cancer risk from their use.[2,4] The Women's Health Initiative trial found a correlation between risk of breast cancer (and increased cardiovascular risk) and HRT, particularly with conjugated equine estrogens (CEE) plus progestins. Further, women with a prior breast cancer diagnosis have an increased rate of recurrence with HRT.[2] Minimizing unnecessary human exposure to known endocrine disruptors and other carcinogens should be high on our national medical and environmental research budgets.

Prior Radiation Exposure

Women with Hodgkin's lymphoma who were treated with thoracic radiation have a significantly higher risk of developing breast cancer because of radiation exposure.[4]

Lifetime versus Age-Adjusted Risk of Developing Breast Cancer

The figure that one in eight women will develop breast cancer is slightly misleading and may create unnecessary fear in women. Based on statistics from 2002 to 2003 from the National Cancer Institute (NCI), 12.7% will be diagnosed with cancer in their lives, and it is from this figure that the "one in eight" statistic is derived. However, lifetime risk is a cumulative average and does not reflect a woman's risk at different ages. The age-adjusted risk gives women a more realistic, although still generalized, picture of their risk of developing breast cancer. According to the NCI's Surveillance, Epidemiology, and End Results statistics (http://seer.cancer.gov), a woman's chance of being diagnosed with breast cancer is:

- From age 30 through age 39: 0.43% (often expressed as 1 in 233)
- From age 40 through age 49: 1.44% (often expressed as 1 in 69)
- From age 50 through age 59: 2.63% (often expressed as 1 in 38)
- From age 60 through age 69: 3.65% (often expressed as 1 in 27)

Of course, as discussed, many more factors than gender, age, and nationality contribute to breast cancer risk. To adjust for such factors as genetics, weight, and lifestyle, a number of statistical tools have been devised to calculate what might be closer to actual risk for any individual woman. The most widely used scale is the Gail model, which is available as a risk calculator for individuals and practitioners to use via the NCI Web site at www.cancer.gov/bcrisktool.[4,10,11] The tool is not a valid method of calculating breast cancer or recurrence risk in women who have already had a diagnosis of breast cancer, lobular carcinoma in situ (LCIS), or ductal carcinoma in situ (DCIS). One research group suggests that another model, the Rosner and Colditz model, more accurately classifies women according to their risk stratification; however, it is not as widely used as the Gail model.[11]

Race/ethnicity and socioeconomic status have been associated with delayed diagnosis of breast cancer, and therefore may contribute to poorer outcomes. Breast cancer outcomes are also worse for uninsured and Medicaid patients than for privately insured patients.[12]

Breast Cancer in Pregnancy

During pregnancy, breast tissue is stimulated by increased levels of estrogen, progesterone, prolactin, and human placental lactogen (HPL).[2] Breast cancer occurs at a rate of 1 per 3000 to 4000 pregnancies. Pregnant or lactating women should have any persistent breast or axillary lumps evaluated by a gynecologist. Too often breast lumps in this population are dismissed by women or health care professionals as the result of hormonal changes, unfortunately sometimes leading to detection of breast cancer only once it has become advanced.

CONVENTIONAL RISK REDUCTION STRATEGIES

Conventional breast cancer risk reduction strategies include[4]:
- For all women:
  - Lifestyle modification (e.g., maintaining a healthy BMI; exercising; alcohol avoidance)
  - Surveillance (i.e., clinical breast examination [CBE], mammography or other appropriate imaging, BSE)
- For high-risk women:
  - Risk reducing surgery (e.g., oophorectomy, mastectomy)
  - Chemoprevention with tamoxifen, raloxifene, and/or AIs

Surveillance
Breast Self-Examination

A recent review by the Cochrane group, the results of several large randomized trials, and a review by the United States Preventative Services Task Force (USPSTF) all concluded that BSE does not reduce breast cancer specific mortality, and in fact, may increase the number of unnecessary biopsies women receive for benign findings, and it is no longer recommended by the medical community for women to perform BSE as part of health prevention and maintenance.[3] Nonetheless, it is a noninvasive method that some women find self-empowering or reassuring to perform, and which may sometimes lead to the early detection of breast cancer.[2] Women should be informed about the potential risk of BSE findings leading to unnecessarily invasive testing and they should be taught to perform the BSE correctly to maximize the value of the examination.

Breast cancer is a leading cause of death in American women. Overall exposure to circulating and environmental estrogens, lifestyle factors, and genetic predisposition may all contribute to breast cancer development. The clinical practitioner should include a thorough breast examination as part of routine gynecologic care. It is a simple technique, and when done properly, can be an important part of overall cancer screening. In recent years, the value of the BSE has come under scrutiny, and large trials suggest that it is not helpful in reducing cancer mortality and may actually contribute to an overall higher rate of unnecessary breast biopsies. It is clear that if women wish to perform BSE, they should be taught to do so correctly. Numerous Web sites provide invaluable resources on BSE for patients and care providers. The following discussion provides very general guidelines for BSE.

When to Perform a Breast Self-Examination

Hormonal changes associated with the menstrual cycle normally increase breast lumpiness and swelling. These changes are particularly noticeable just before the menstrual period. Therefore it is advisable to perform a BSE a few days to a week after menstruation has ended. Women using OCs are advised to perform their BSE each month on the day they begin a new package of pills.

BOX 14-1   Breast Self-Examination

Breast Changes and Warning Signs
- A new lump or hard knot in the breast or armpit
- A lump or thickening that does not decrease in size after menstruation
- A change in the size, shape, or symmetry of the breast
- Thickening or swelling of the breast
- Dimpling, puckering, or indention in the breast
- Dimpling, skin irritation, or other change in the breast skin or nipple
- Redness or scaliness of the nipple or breast skin
- Nipple discharge, other than breast milk, in a lactating woman, especially if the discharge is bloody, clear and sticky, dark, or occurs without squeezing the nipple
- Nipple tenderness or pain
- Nipple retraction
- Any breast change that appears to be cause for concern

Differentiating Breast Lumps by Palpation
- Normal, noncancerous lumps such as cysts are typically soft, smooth, and moveable. They tend to fluctuate in size with the menstrual cycle. Also, if a lump, knot, or other "difference" is found in one breast, the woman should examine the other breast. If the lump or texture is symmetric between breasts, it is likely to be normal breast tissue.
- Questionable lumps are usually firm, irregular nodules that are fixed in place. They do not typically fluctuate in size with the menstrual cycle.

   WARNING: A physician should evaluate persistent lumps or abnormalities as soon as possible.

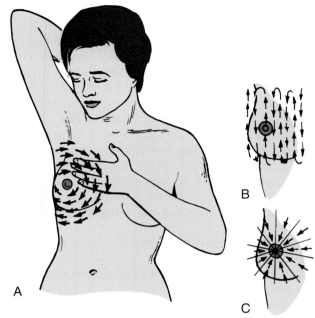

FIGURE 14-2 Comprehensive breast examination illustrations showing directions for three methods of breast self-examination (BSE): **A**, Spiral. **B**, Square. **C**, Wedge. (From Lowdermilk DL, Perry SE: *Maternity & women's health care,* ed 9, St. Louis, 2007, Mosby.)

Unfortunately, too many women do not carry out this simple technique. Selecting 1 day each month is the easiest reminder—encourage patients to circle this date on their calendars or post a reminder to themselves. It is easier to remember once it becomes routine. Pregnant women should continue to perform BSE throughout the pregnancy. An examination should also be performed by the care provider at the onset of pregnancy before the beginning of dramatic pregnancy-induced breast changes, and again later in the pregnancy and postnatally. Pregnancy does not preclude the development of breast cancer. The biggest problem with breast cancer during pregnancy is it going undetected because of lack of regular breast examinations.

In 80% of all cases, breast lumps and changes do not signal breast cancer. However, women should report all unusual changes (Box 14-1) to their health care provider and seek a clinical evaluation. Many women put off telling their doctor out of fear. It can be reassuring for patients to know that at least 50% of all women will seek evaluation for a suspicious lump or breast change at some point in their life.

Performing the Breast Self-Examination

BSE requires examining the entire chest area and both breasts, as well as the axillary area. Although it does not matter in what order the steps of the BSE are performed, it is

essential that all steps be performed so that no area remains overlooked. Therefore women should perform the BSE systematically each time. A log or journal, with an entry after each examination, can help a woman keep track of her findings, and can help her to objectively track any changes she might notice. The instructions that follow are adapted from the American Cancer Society.

General Rules

- BSE should be done in a warm, comfortable, private place free from distractions. This allows women to be mindful of the examination, and the warmth allows the breast tissue to relax, facilitating the examination.
- BSE should be conducted using the pads, not the tips, of the three middle fingers.
- The right hand should be used to examine the left breast, the left hand to examine the right breast.
- The woman should examine all tissue from the midaxillary line to the clavicle and to the sternum. Evidence suggests that a vertical pattern (Fig. 14-2) is most effective for covering the entire breast without missing any breast tissue.
- Three levels of pressure should be applied: light, medium, and firm.
- The breast should be examined in small "massaging" circles when using the patterns shown in Figure 14-2. The fingers should maintain contact with the breast at all times. Lifting the fingers could lead to an area being missed.
- BSE should be performed both lying down and in an upright position. The upright portion of the examination

BOX 14-2 Palpating the Lymph Nodes

Lymph nodes are easily slightly enlarged by noncancerous processes, such as infection. Occasionally, a cancer may cause lymph node enlargement. Lymph node changes or enlargement should be reported to the woman's physician.

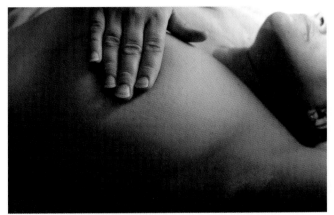

FIGURE 14-3 Patient position for breast examination lying down. (From Seidel HM: *Mosby's guide to physical examination,* ed 6, St. Louis, 2006, Mosby; © Elsevier Collection.)

BOX 14-3 Nipple Discharge

Most suspicious nipple discharges are found to be caused by noncancerous conditions. In approximately 10% of all cases, nipple discharge is caused by cancer. In women younger than 30 years of age, less than 10% of nipple discharge is caused by cancer.
- Green or yellow discharge is usually normal.
- Bloody, dark, or clear and sticky discharge is considered abnormal.

WARNING: A physician should evaluate unusual nipple discharge.

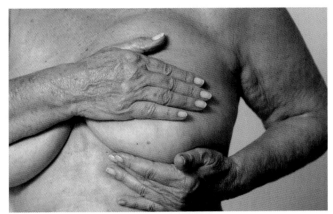

FIGURE 14-4 Patient position for upright breast examination. From (Seidel HM: *Mosby's guide to physical examination,* ed 6, St. Louis, 2006, Mosby; © Elsevier Collection.)

can be done in the shower. Additionally, a visual inspection should be done in front of a mirror.
- A small amount of oil, soap, or powder may be applied to the fingers to reduce friction and allow the fingers to glide more smoothly over the skin.
- The following areas should be examined thoroughly with each BSE:
  - Outside: armpit to collar bone, and below the breast
  - Middle: the breast itself
  - Inside: the nipple area

Although cancerous growths are most likely to be found in the upper, outer breast quadrant or behind the nipple, they can occur in any area of the breast, chest, or lymph network (Box 14-2); therefore a thorough examination is essential.

Step 1: Breast Self-Examination While Lying Down

Lie down with a pillow or folded towel under the right shoulder and place the right arm behind the head (Fig. 14-3). Check the entire breast and armpit area using the pads of the first three middle fingers on the left hand to feel for lumps, changes, or irregularities in the right breast.

1. With the pads of the fingers, use the vertical pattern. Press firmly enough to know how the breast feels. Examine each breast separately and feel for any new lumps, changes, or irregularities. A firm ridge in the lower curve of each breast is normal.
2. The examination should then be repeated on the left breast, using the finger pads of the right hand (the pillow or folded towel should also be moved under the left shoulder at this time).
3. The nipple should also be checked for changes. After making an initial examination, noting changes of

appearance, gently squeeze the nipple to check for discharge of fluid (Box 14-3). Check the color, consistency, and whether the discharge occurs spontaneously or by squeezing. Depress the nipple deep into the hollow beneath it, noting unusual resistance, hardness, or lumps beneath the nipple. Also check the nipple for cracking.

Step 2: Breast Self-Examination Upright and In Front of a Mirror

The upright position (Fig. 14-4) can facilitate examining the upper and outer portions of the breasts and armpit. The lying down portion can either precede or proceed the upright portion. Both a lying down and an upright examination should be performed at each monthly BSE. Examining the breasts in front of a mirror allows women to check for changes in shape, direction, or texture of the breasts. It should be done in a warm area with good lighting. The mirror should allow inspection of the torso from the waist to the neck.

1. Place the arms at the sides. Looking in the mirror, check the breasts for any changes in size, shape or position, dimpling or puckering of the skin, indented or misshapen nipples, other changes in the nipple, redness, swelling, or other irregularities.
2. Repeat this process with the hands on the hips, pressing firmly to flex the chest (i.e., pectoral muscles). Bend

forward with the hands on the hips and note any irregularities.

3. Raise the arms overhead or put the hands behind the head. Turn to each side to check the breasts in profile. Note any changes in symmetry between the right and left breast. Remember, it is often normal for women to have one breast that is larger or a different shape than the other.

Step 3: Breast Self-Examination in the Shower (Optional but Optimal)

Palpating the breasts in the shower is helpful because the skin can be lubricated by soap. Some breast changes can be felt more easily when the skin is wet and soapy. The BSE can be performed in the shower on a monthly basis, or can be used to enhance the previous examinations when trying to more thoroughly feel a lump or other tissue change.

Clinical Breast Examination

The Clinical Breast Examination (CBE) is an important but often overlooked or deferred part of the routine physical examination. The CBE makes a small but important contribution to breast cancer detection, with approximately 5% to 10% of breast cancers identified solely by CBE, independent of mammography.[3] As with BSE, CBE should be properly performed using a vertical technique to maximize the likelihood of finding abnormal breast changes, and the breasts should be visualized with the woman in a variety of designated positions. One study reported that variations in CBE technique led to a 29% variation in sensitivity and a 33% variation in specificity.[3] The most important aspect of the CBE contributing to practitioner sensitivity in detecting abnormalities is the amount of time taken to perform the examination.[3]

Mammography, Magnetic Resonance Imaging, and Ultrasound

There are two basic categories of mammography: screening mammography done in asymptomatic patients with no breast abnormalities and diagnostic mammography done in patients with breast symptoms or abnormalities. Mammography employs a machine that compresses the breast and delivers low-dose radiation to the tissue to allow visualization of breast lesions or abnormalities. In low risk patients with no known breast abnormalities, two images are typically taken per breast at two different angles, although additional compression images or magnifications may be required, particularly if there are breast symptoms. Mammograms are usually done as an outpatient procedure.

Numerous randomized controlled trials (RCTs) performed since the 1960s have demonstrated decreased risk of breast cancer death in women randomized to receive mammography. Although a well-publicized meta-analysis questioned the value of mammography as a breast cancer screening test based on flaws identified in earlier studies, further meta-analysis by the USPSTF concluded that these flaws did not significantly affect outcomes, and recommended screening mammography every 1 to 2 years for women older than 40 years of age

and annually for women over age 70 with no comorbidities that decrease life expectancy.[3,13-21]

Screening mammography is associated with reduced size and stage of breast cancer at diagnosis. Sensitivity is estimated to be between 60% and 90%.[3] Many mammography testing facilities have begun to use computer-aided detection systems designed to assist radiologists in interpreting; however, recent research has found that these tools actually decrease sensitivity and increase false positive results, and since their introduction, breast cancer detection rates have not changed substantially.[3,22] There is no greater benefit to annual mammograms compared with every 2 years in women younger than 70 unless they are at high risk for breast cancer or breast cancer recurrence.[13] High-risk women with a family history of breast cancer should begin screening when they are 10 years younger than the age at which their youngest relative to be diagnosed with breast cancer received a diagnosis. No trials to date have evaluated an age end point for screening mammography. Two trials have enrolled women older than age 65; none have evaluated mammography in women older than age 74 years.[13]

Mammography is the only imaging method that has been demonstrated through RCTs to be effective for breast cancer screening. Current recommendations call for screening mammography every 1 to 2 years beginning at age 40 for low-risk women, and annual screening for women older than 70 in the absence of comorbid disease that lowers life expectancy.[13]

The risk of radiation exposure associated with mammography is of concern to many women. The Biological Effects of Ionizing Radiation (BEIR V) review estimated that the potential total annual added risk of breast cancer mortality resulting from mammography (300 mrad for two-view examination of both breasts) to be 41.9/100,000 for women age 25, 30.9/100,000 for women age 30; 21.4/100,000 for women age 35; 13.8/100,000 for women age 40; and 3.9/100,000 for women age 50, compared with an estimate of greater than 3000 deaths that would occur as a result of naturally occurring breast cancers among women who do not receive screening mammography.[23-25]

Concerns have also been raised about the possible short- and long-term detrimental effects of false positive mammograms on women's psychoemotional well-being. Based on a recent systematic review, a false-positive mammogram does increase anxiety, sometimes substantially, but usually only short-term, and may actually lead women in the United States to increase their diligence about receiving breast screening in the future.[26]

Mammography is less sensitive in younger women, likely a result of greater breast tissue density in younger women as well as faster rate of cancer growth.[3] For women with dense breasts, particularly women younger than 30, screening ultrasound is commonly recommended; however, the European Group for Breast Cancer Screening concluded that there is no evidence to support the use of screening ultrasound at any age.[27] In contrast, in a prospective, uncontrolled study of 11,130 women with dense breasts screened with mammography, clinical examination, and bilateral whole breast ultrasound over approximately 2 years, screening breast ultrasound increased the number of women diagnosed with nonpalpable invasive cancers by 42%.[28] Another option is digital mammography, which may be more sensitive in women younger than 50 with dense breasts; however, it is expensive and not widely available.[22,28]

Recently magnetic resonance imaging (MRI) has been receiving attention as a breast cancer detection tool owing to its greater sensitivity in detecting breast cancer in high-risk women and its ability to increase earlier diagnosis.[3] MRI, however, is also associated with a higher rate of false-positives than is mammography, and it is costly. The latest American Cancer Society recommendations recommend screening MRI in addition to mammograms for women who meet at least one of the following conditions[29]:

- They have a *BRCA1* or *BRCA2* mutation.
- They have a first-degree relative (i.e., parent, sibling, child) with a *BRCA1* or *BRCA2* mutation, even if they have yet to be tested themselves.
- Their lifetime risk of breast cancer has been scored at 20% to 25% or greater, based on one of several accepted risk assessment tools that look at family history and other factors.
- They had radiation to the chest between the ages of 10 and 30.
- They have Li-Fraumeni syndrome, Cowden syndrome, or Bannayan-Riley-Ruvalcaba syndrome, or may have one of these syndromes based on a history in a first-degree relative.

MRI should be considered an adjunct to mammography and CBE in the detection of breast cancer in high-risk women, or when there is a suspicious finding with these other routine screening methods.

Risk-Reducing Surgery

Although this is an aggressive option, risk-reducing surgery may be reasonable for women with a high-risk hereditary predisposition to breast cancer. Prophylactic oophorectomy may be the preferred primary strategy for risk reduction before mastectomy because it is effective and is not associated with visible physical alteration and thus can spare women the struggles with body image that accompany mastectomy.[4] Surgical menopause before age 35 is established as protective against breast cancer; however, it is also a risk factor for osteoporosis and cardiovascular disease.[10]

Chemoprevention

It should be noted that no chemopreventative strategy to date has demonstrated increased health or survival benefits.[4] Tamoxifen and raloxifene will only reduce the incidence of estrogen receptor–positive cancers, and have no effect on estrogen receptor–negative cancer.[10] Side effects can be considerable and often make it difficult to complete the 5-year course of prophylactic treatment. Nonetheless, these drugs have shown significant chemopreventive effects.

Risk of developing breast cancer, and hence the value of preventative therapy, must be weighed against the risks of medication adverse effects.

Tamoxifen

In 1998, the Food and Drug Administration (FDA) approved tamoxifen, a first-generation selective estrogen receptor modulator (SERM) with both estrogenic and antiestrogenic effects, as an effective breast cancer prophylactic agent at a dose of 20 mg/d for 5 years. Its estrogen receptor–blocking effects make it effective against breast cancer.[4] Four prospective randomized trials and one meta-analysis of prophylactic tamoxifen use demonstrated a significant reduction in breast cancer occurrence at rates of 43% to 69% in women across all age groups, and also a reduction in risk of second primary and contralateral breast cancer.[4,10,11] However, there was no mortality benefit in any of the trials, and use of the drug is associated with both mild and serious adverse effects, including hot flashes, vaginal discharge, endometrial cancer (2 per 1000 women per year), stroke (doubled risk), and life-threatening thromboembolic disease (double to triple the risk of deep vein thrombosis and pulmonary embolism).[10] These risks are most prevalent in postmenopausal women and those with comorbidities.[4]

Raloxifene

Raloxifene is a second-generation SERM with mechanisms of action similar to tamoxifen, but which does not produce endometrial proliferation to the extent of tamoxifen and therefore does not carry the same risk of causing endometrial cancer, although otherwise its side effect profile is similar to tamoxifen.[4,10,11] Women taking raloxifene may also experience dyspareunia, weight gain, and musculoskeletal problems compared with those taking tamoxifen; however, those in the latter group are more likely to experience more vasomotor symptoms and leg cramps, although they report improved sexual functioning.[4] Raloxifene increases bone mineral density in postmenopausal women and is FDA–approved for the prevention and treatment of osteoporosis an advantage for those women taking it prophylactically for breast cancer risk. Raloxifene is not recommended for premenopausal women.[4,11]

Aromatase Inhibitors

Conversion of androgens to estrogen in peripheral adipose and muscular tissue is called aromatization. At menopause, when the ovaries cease to produce significant quantities of estrogen, aromatization becomes the primary source of estrogens in postmenopausal women. AIs are used to reduce this process and substantially reduce breast tissue estrogen exposure. At present, they have been studied only as adjuvant therapies for breast cancer treatment; no RCTs have been completed for breast cancer prophylaxis as of the time of this writing.[4]

SIGNS AND SYMPTOMS OF BREAST CANCER

Early findings of breast cancer include a nontender mass that may be firm to hard, and with poorly defined borders; however, there may be abnormal mammography findings in the absence of a palpable mass. In 70% of cases, a painless lump is the presenting complaint. Later, there may be nipple or skin retractions (i.e., peau d'orange), axillary lymphadenopathy, breast enlargement with signs of inflammation, and adherence of a mass to the chest wall or the skin. There can be breast pain; nipple discharge that is watery, serous, or sanguineous; nipple erosion, itching, or enlargement; changes in breast size, shape, and symmetry; and rarely, edema of the axilla or arm. When there is metastatic disease, there may be more generalized symptoms of weight loss and jaundice, and commonly there is back or bone pain, which can have severe consequences if accompanied by spinal cord compression.

Conditions to consider that may present with breast lumps or other breast changes include fibrocystic breasts, intraductal papilloma, lipoma, fat necrosis, mastitis (in lactating women), breast abscess, and phyllodes tumor.

DIAGNOSIS

Diagnosis of breast cancer requires a multidisciplinary team of experts. Initially, suspicion may be raised by the woman herself, who detects a lump on BSE; a lump may be found incidentally upon routine CBE by her midwife, gynecologist, internist, or family doctor; or a lump may be found by a radiologist reading a mammogram. At this point, the woman is referred for screening mammography, also done by a radiologist if she has not had imaging, and if a lump is confirmed by mammography, a biopsy is performed to obtain tissue samples that are analyzed for the presence of cancer cells by a pathologist. If breast cancer is confirmed, additional health professionals are consulted, including but not limited to breast surgeons and oncologists.

Diagnostic Imaging

Abnormal radiographic findings include clustered microcalcifications, densities, or architectural distortions.[2] If a radiologic abnormality is detected, this should be considered contextually. If it is a nonpalpable lesion with a low index of suspicion in a low-risk woman, a follow-up mammogram in 3 to 6 months is considered reasonable.[2] If a probably benign lesion is identified, a stereotactic core or surgical biopsy may be recommended, and if the lesion is clearly suspicious, a surgical biopsy is usually performed.[2]

Diagnostic Procedures

Fine needle aspiration (FNA), open biopsy, and computerized stereotactic or ultrasound-guided needle biopsies are all current methods for obtaining cell and tissue samples that can be sent to a pathology laboratory for analysis, and if cancer cells are present, staging.

Laboratory Testing

Laboratory testing for breast cancer, in addition to examining tissue samples sent for pathology assessment, includes looking for serum markers of breast cancer, especially those that may indicate disease severity, recurrence, or metastases.

Staging

Breast cancer staging is based in the tumor-node-metastasis (TNM) model and guides not only diagnosis, but treatment strategies as well. Within the term, *tumor* refers to the histologic classification of the lesion and determines the type and severity of the tumor (i.e., grading). *Node* refers to the number of lymph nodes involved; sentinel lymph node biopsy is an importance advance in node staging, sparing women invasive lymph surgery when possible. *Metastasis* refers to the number of tumor sites and distance from the primary tumor. Additionally, the presence of hormonally positive or negative receptors is determined. Comprehensive cancer diagnosis and treatment guidelines, including breast cancer staging, are available from the National Comprehensive Cancer Network at https://www.nccn.org/professionals/physician_gls/f_guidelines.asp.

Prognosis

There are numerous prognostic variables in breast cancer. Tumor staging is considered the most important of these. Additional variables include[2]:

- The presence of estrogen and/or progesterone receptors (associated with a lower relapse rate)
- Measures of tumor growth, including S-phase analysis (higher S-phase suggests a greater risk of relapse, but is also associated with a greater response to chemotherapy)
- Histologic classification of the tumor
- Expression of tumor markers (i.e., overexpression of erbβ is associated with a poorer prognosis, as are p53 mutations)
- The presence of neovasculature is associated with a poorer prognosis

Patterns of tumor gene expression are increasingly being recognized as significant in breast cancer prognosis, and certain patterns may reliably predict disease-free internals and survival more accurately than any other prognostic variables.[2]

CONVENTIONAL BREAST CANCER TREATMENT

The mainstays of conventional cancer treatment include surgery, chemotherapy, radiation, and endocrine treatment. Breast cancer treatment is highly complex and well beyond the scope of this chapter to discuss. Readers are referred to the National Comprehensive Cancer Network (Box 14-4) for the 2008 recommended breast cancer treatment guidelines. Women undergoing treatment require a central care coordinator and a strong support network.

BOX 14-4   Resources for Complementary and Alternative Medicine/Herbal Medicine and Cancer

The University of Texas MD Anderson Cancer Center
  www.mdanderson.org/topics/complementary
  www.mdanderson.org/departments/cimer
National Comprehensive Cancer Network
  https://www.nccn.org/professionals/physician_gls/f_guidelines.asp

COMPLEMENTARY AND ALTERNATIVE MEDICINE BREAST CANCER TREATMENT

How Many Women Are Turning to CAM for Breast Cancer Treatment?

Estimates are that between 34% and 60%, but as many as 83%, of cancer patients use some form of CAM, with an estimated out-of-pocket cost of up to $7200/year in the United States.[1,30-33] Women with breast cancer use more CAM than individuals with other types of cancer, and more CAM therapies than women who do not have cancer.[32,34] In one study of CAM use among women with breast cancer, 72% of CAM users used two or more CAM approaches, 49% used three or more, and 15% used seven or more CAM approaches, including prayer/spiritual healing and psychotherapy/support groups.[35] Herbs, vitamins, massage, acupuncture, homeopathy, and mind–body healing are among the therapies frequently used. Most women use complementary therapies in conjunction with conventional medical cancer treatment, although about 2% of women with breast cancer may choose to forego conventional therapy completely and use alternative therapies only.[36]

Why Women Are Choosing CAM Cancer Therapies

The primary reasons women cite for CAM use include desire to enhance their chance of survival, reduction of risk of disease recurrence, relief of disease symptoms, relief from psychological distress, enhancement of immunity, minimization of conventional treatment-related side effects, and improvement of quality of life.[31,34,37] Some women report that CAM use gives them a feeling of hope and a sense of greater control over their lives.[1,34] Increasing interest in CAM may also partially be a result of the limitations of conventional breast cancer treatment.[35]

Desperation can be a motivator toward CAM use, with cancer patients wanting to explore every possible option at their disposal.[38] The fear and confusion wrought by a breast cancer diagnosis and the hope of finding a cure can make women vulnerable to trying therapies that have no basis of safety or efficacy, and which may be ineffective at best and costly or dangerous at worst.

Several studies have found that women who use CAM therapies as part of their breast cancer treatment plan are more likely to have higher levels of psychosocial stress and anxiety and to report poorer quality of life than those who choose conventional treatment alone.[34] This is a perplexing finding with several possible explanations. For example, women who use CAM therapies may be more personally reflective about their stresses because it has been found that CAM users tend to be more spiritually involved in their illnesses and tend to try to gain a deeper holistic view of their illness than non–CAM users.[34] Women who self-medicate with various herbs or nutrients in addition to conventional therapy also may have previously undetected underlying disorders, such as previously undiagnosed depression in women taking St. John's wort. Women who experience more psychological distress associated with their illness may be self-selective for CAM, which is seen as more supportive in nature than conventional care.[34]

The Complexity of Choosing CAM Therapies

In spite of the widespread use of CAM therapies among women with breast cancer, these therapies remain largely marginalized from mainstream cancer care. This appears to result from lack of a strong evidence base for many of the therapies, leading to concern over the risks of therapies and how they might interact or interfere with conventional treatments, and also to differences in how healing is conceptualized and quantified by conventional and CAM practitioners.[1,34] Lack of scientific evidence available on CAM therapies means that patients wishing to incorporate CAM into their care are left to rely on hearsay, Internet information, or anecdotal evidence. An Internet search for cancer and either complementary or alternative medicine yields more than 3.4 million Web sites.[36] Distinguishing accurate from unreliable information is nearly impossible for even the educated patient.[33] Many women ultimately do their own extensive medical literature research, which is difficult and time consuming for a lay person, and even there, the evidence is limited, confusing, and contradictory. This is frequently an exhausting and frustrating process on top of the emotional and physical toll of dealing with breast cancer and treatment, and many women find they have to turn to family or friends to help them with the burden of research. This may compound a sense of helplessness or conflict.

Available information on CAM and breast cancer is often contradictory regarding both its safety and value, causing tremendous confusion. Further, because many oncologists and other physicians remain skeptical about the use of CAM in cancer care, women experience a gap between their conventional care and their desire to use, or their actual use of, CAM that can lead to inner conflict and tension as an added burden in their care, and this stress may not be insignificant.[1] As a result, many women who wish to use CAM therapies to enhance their conventional treatment, support their immunity, or mitigate side effects of conventional therapies often forego CAM therapies while undergoing conventional treatment out of fear of harmful effects, particularly with chemotherapy.[1] Significantly, as many as 64.5% of patients do not disclose CAM use to their health care providers.[31] Reasons for this include fear of disapproval from the practitioner, patient perception that the practitioner lacks knowledge of CAM therapies and therefore there is no reason to discuss them, lack of expressed practitioner interest in the patient's possible use of CAM, and patient perceptions that herbs and supplements are not medications and therefore have no bearing on medical treatment.[39]

Given women's desire to include CAM in their breast cancer treatment plans, it is essential that oncologists and other members of the oncology care team be articulate in CAM options, helping women to navigate the complex and overwhelming array of available options. Some options may be beneficial, and many others may be harmful; the care team should be open to the conversation to honor their patient's desire to incorporate CAM into their care. It has been suggested that because of their widespread use, access to CAM therapies should be part of standard oncology treatment.[31] What is currently needed are models that bridge the gap between CAM and conventional therapies, allowing for an integrated, interdisciplinary model of care that allows women to comfortably and safely access and incorporate a variety of beneficial and safe treatment modalities into their breast cancer care; also important is relieving women with breast cancer of the onus of responsibility for obtaining and deciphering all of their treatment information.[1]

Mistrust Between Conventional and CAM Practitioners

There is generally an enormous gap of mistrust separating oncologists and CAM practitioners. Alternative practitioners base their mistrust of conventional physicians and practices on the historical precedence of the evolution of conventional medicine in the United States and the subsequent marginalization of nonconventional practitioners, combined with a general mistrust of cancer treatments that have historically sometimes proved to be as harmful as they have been helpful.[39] Conventional practitioners maintain a mistrust of CAM practitioners and products because CAM is widely available and unregulated, allowing just about anyone to put up a shingle or market a product offering the hope of a cancer cure.[39] This latter environment is also highly problematic for those CAM practitioners who do possess substantial knowledge and training, but who remain unregulated because of lack of available credentialing pathways in the United States, and are thus categorically lumped into being labeled as quacks or "snake oil salesmen" rather than being integrated into the oncology care team.[39]

Differing conceptual paradigms of healing have only reinforced this gap, with a lack of a common language upon which to converse about the possibility of a cross-disciplinary or integrated model of cancer care. Fortunately, a growing number of oncologists and other physicians are beginning to recognize the important role CAM plays for women in their approach to treating and healing from breast cancer; the potential value of CAM therapies in relieving suffering and improving patient quality of life; and possibly improving medical outcomes. Nonconventional practitioners must recognize that most women with breast cancer want to take an integrated approach to their treatment, and do not wish to forego conventional care altogether. Unfortunately, alternative practitioner attitudes toward conventional cancer care may lead women who wish to take an integrative approach to feel guilty for doing so, or may encourage women to rely on unproved therapies, resulting in a delay in seeking appropriate conventional medical care. A cross-disciplinary, integrated approach would allow women to receive the best of both worlds in the safest and most effective manner, and

requires the cooperation and collaboration of both conventional and nonconventional health care providers to bridge the existing gap.

Incidence of Botanical Medicine Use for Breast Cancer

A survey conducted at eight clinical sites of the University of Texas MD Anderson Cancer Center found that the most frequently used CAM therapies were herbs and/or vitamins, with 62% of women surveyed using them. Less than 53% of women discussed herbal use with their physicians, and less than a third considered herbal products to be medications.[31]

Limitations in Botanical Breast Cancer Treatment Research

Numerous herbs have shown anticancer activity and antitumor properties in vitro. Several herbs have been the source for anticancer compounds currently in use as cancer chemotherapy, such as vincristine and vinblastine from periwinkle (*Vinca* spp.) and taxanes from the Pacific yew tree. Botanicals continue to be a major source of research into novel natural compounds that might hold further promise in cancer treatment.

Although many studies using botanical products have had promising results, none have definitively demonstrated altered disease progression in patients with breast cancer.[37] Because of a bias against unconventional cancer therapies, funding and publishing of studies on CAM cancer therapies, including herbs, has historically been limited. Lack of involvement of nonconventional practitioners in research on herbs, either owing to exclusion by mainstream research institutions or lack of CAM practitioner training in research methodologies, may lead to studies that do not reflect the actual clinical use of herbs; for example, herbal products included in clinical trials may be of inadequate standards or used in inappropriate doses.[31,37] For many botanical products, lack of product characterization, standardization, reproducibility, safety, and basic information on pharmacology remain an obstacle to their use and acceptance by oncologists.[31,40] Several research institutions, such as the NCI and the University of Texas MD Anderson Cancer Center, have placed botanical medicine and cancer among of their research priorities, and have acknowledged the importance of including nonconventional practitioners who use botanicals in establishing study designs.

Herbs Used in the Treatment of Breast Cancer

Based on preliminary in vitro research and the efficacy of botanical products in the treatment of a variety of medical conditions, it is reasonable to expect that herbal medicines may offer numerous possibilities as preventative and therapeutic interventions for patients with cancer (Box 14-5).[41] An extensive body of literature exists documenting the in vitro and in vivo effects of isolated chemical constituents and single botanical entities. Little research is being done, however, in the actual practice of clinical herbal medicine and even less in herbal medicine and cancer. Many herbal practitioners, mindful of their dubious legal position in the United States, do not treat cancer at all, and others who do tend to fulfill a supportive, adjunctive role rather than becoming the primary care provider.[41] As a consequence the records of botanical practitioners are often inaccessible, and lack of a standardized system of record keeping in the profession often leads to inadequate documentation of clinical botanical care. In reviewing the efficacy of herbal medicine in treating breast cancer, there is a dearth of reliable, reproducible evidence.[41]

The following is a brief discussion of the herbs and strategies most commonly cited in popular and medical literature for use in the botanical care of women with breast cancer.

Immunostimulation

One of the most commonly cited reasons women with breast cancer give for using herbs is to stimulate or enhance immune function. A number of herbs have immunostimulatory effects. Conventional cancer therapies are known to have adverse effects on immunity, and low cell counts can interfere with treatment schedules.[37] Therefore, it makes sense that herbal therapies used to boost the immune system might be beneficial to patients undergoing conventional therapies. However, there is concern that these therapies may interfere with the tumor-killing effects of conventional treatments.[37] Further, the immune system is incredibly complex and there are numerous immunostimulatory effects that are irrelevant to cancer treatment. For example, immunologic functions related to inflammation and allergic reaction may have little to do with a beneficial cancer response, although stimulating natural killer (NK) cell functioning is an important response. Therefore it is critically important that research be conducted on the immunologic end points of claims for botanical therapies used to modify immune function and how these relate to

conventional treatment goals and interact with conventional therapies.[37] Herbs commonly used as immunostimulants include maitake and other medicinal mushrooms, astragalus, and many adaptogenic herbs, the latter of which are also used to modulate the stress response (see Chapter 5).

Medicinal Mushrooms

Medicinal mushrooms are among the most commonly prescribed anticancer natural products with data from controlled clinical trials suggesting possible benefit in cancer treatment.[42] Maitake mushroom *(Grifola frondosa)* is among those used. Medicinal mushrooms contain a class of polysaccharides known as beta-glucans that promote antitumor immunity related to antibody–Fc interactions by activating complement receptors. Mouse models have demonstrated that beta-glucans act synergistically with therapeutic antibodies such as trastuzumab or rituximab.[42]

Human data are limited, and at this time there is insufficient evidence to recommend for or against the use of oral maitake for any indication; however, they are commonly ingested as a food and appear safe for general consumption.

Antioxidants and Green Tea

As many as 25% to 84% of patients with cancer use antioxidant supplements. Both in vitro and in vivo research suggest an antitumor role for antioxidants, including inhibition of tumor cell growth, induction of cellular differentiation, alterations in cellular redox, and enhanced effects of cytotoxic therapies. Chemotherapeutic agents such as alkylating agents, antimetabolites, and radiation lower antioxidant status, generating free radicals that have cytotoxic effects.[43] Cancer patients are often told not to take antioxidant herbs and supplements during the course of conventional treatment because of the apprehension that antioxidants will reduce the efficacy of these therapies by eliminating the free radicals. However, adjunctive therapies such as mesna and amifostine, also antioxidants, are commonly given along with other chemotherapeutic agents and do not reduce their efficacy, although antioxidants do appear to reduce the frequency and severity of toxic effects associated with chemotherapy.[43] In 2005, antioxidants were the most popular CAM therapy used for treating breast cancer.[44]

Green tea, prepared from the leaves of *Camellia sinensis*, has been consumed as a beverage for nearly 50 centuries. Next to water, it is the most widely consumed beverage in the world.[45] Multiple lines of evidence, mostly from population-based studies, suggest that green tea consumption is associated with reduced risk of cancer, including breast cancer.[45-48] Epigallocatechin gallate (EGCG), a major polyphenol found in green tea, is a widely studied chemopreventive agent with potential anticancer activity. Green tea polyphenols inhibit angiogenesis and metastasis, and induce growth arrest and apoptosis through regulation of multiple signaling pathways.[45] Apparently, EGCG functions as an antioxidant, preventing oxidative damage in healthy cells, but also as an antiangiogenic agent, preventing tumors from developing a blood supply needed to grow larger. Epidemiologic studies suggest that green tea compounds could protect against cancer, but data are inconsistent, and limitations in study design prevent generalizability of published findings.[49] Some limited evidence suggests that green tea may have down-regulatory effects on circulating estrogen levels, proposed as possibly beneficial in estrogen receptor–positive breast cancers.[50] High consumption of green tea was closely associated with decreased numbers of axillary lymph node metastases among premenopausal stage I and II breast cancer patients, and with increased expression of progesterone and estrogen receptors among postmenopausal patients.[51]

It is recommended that women consume at least four to five cups of green tea per day for chemoprotective effects. Tea is much lower in caffeine than coffee, and is a healthy alternative. Decaffeinated green tea products provide a comparable level of antioxidants to caffeinated green tea and may be substituted by caffeine-sensitive individuals.[52]

Phytoestrogens and Breast Cancer

Phytoestrogens are plant-derived nonsteroidal estrogens that are structurally or functionally similar to endogenous estradiol.[53] The major classes of phytoestrogens discussed here are the isoflavones (i.e., daidzein, genistein) and the lignins (i.e., enterodiol, enterolactone). Phytoestrogens are able to bind to the estrogen receptor, and although stimulating it, do so at only a minimal fraction of the strength of endogenous 17-β-estradiol. It is believed that this weaker binding actually acts as an antiestrogenic effect in the presence of a high endogenous amount of estrogen, preventing the stronger endogenous estrogen from binding to estrogen receptors.[52,54]

Soy is the richest dietary source of isoflavones, whereas flax is a major dietary source of lignins. Findings of low rates of breast cancer among Asian women who regularly consume soy products in their diets, and the fact that breast cancer rates begin to approximate those of US women when Asian women consume a Western diet, has stimulated a significant amount of research into the possible protective role of dietary phytoestrogens against breast cancer.[54,55] Conversely, trends in increased consumption of phytoestrogens as a dietary supplement as a result of the popularity of phytoestrogens based on these findings has raised serious concerns that their estrogenic effects may actually increase the risk or recurrence of breast cancer; thus in spite of a great deal of research, the topic of phytoestrogens and breast cancer remains highly controversial.[54]

Research on the health benefits of soy foods and soy extracts and isolates is contradictory and confusing. Twenty-two case control and cohort studies examined the incidence of breast cancer among women with and without a diet high in phytoestrogens. A meta-analysis of 21 studies found a significantly reduced incidence of breast cancer among past phytoestrogen users. Increased radiologic density has been associated with a four- to sixfold increased risk of breast cancer.[56] Three clinical trials have demonstrated an inverse association between dietary phytoestrogen intake and breast density, two using similar isoflavones and one reporting on lignins.[57-59]

None of the available RCTs documents a protective effect of phytoestrogens on the clinical end points of breast cancer.[60] Women who were high soy consumers during adolescence demonstrate a 23% risk reduction compared with matched controls, and consuming soy in adult life and adolescence increases the risk reduction to 47%. Phytoestrogens may induce differentiation of breast epithelium during early childhood and puberty, thus making the breast epithelium less sensitive to noxious agents such as chemical carcinogens. Breast epithelia may no longer be sensitive to phytoestrogens after pregnancy.[60] Eating little soy in adolescence but more in adult life does not confer any advantage.[61] This is clinically significant because it promotes the use of soy as an early preventative but it challenges the usefulness of soy products to treat breast cancer in women who have not grown up eating such foods. The value of soy supplementation postadolescence is of dubious value, and one study actually demonstrated increased breast density in women who consumed large amounts of soy as adults.

Controversy exists as to the clinical significance of all these findings, and there is as yet no consensus of scientific opinion. The variability in outcomes of studies looking at the protective effects of phytoestrogens may result from individual variability in phytoestrogen metabolism and bioavailability and content of isoflavones in supplements. Both isoflavone and lignin metabolism are dependent on gut flora. Individual differences in gut flora, bowel transit time, and genetic polymorphisms comprise variations that may encourage or inhibit the conversion of phytoestrogens into beneficial metabolites. A study by Setchell and colleagues analyzed 33 different phytoestrogen supplements for isoflavone content and found that there were considerable differences between the amount the manufacturer claimed to be in the product and the actual content.[62] Dietary fiber content affects the absorption, reabsorption, and excretion of estrogens and phytoestrogens.[63-65] Additionally, because phytoestrogen metabolism is dependent on availability of specific gut flora, antibiotic use may interfere with metabolism of phytoestrogens.[54]

In summary, the relationship between phytoestrogens and breast cancer appears to be dependent on a number of variables, including age at exposure, individual variability in metabolism, endogenous hormone levels, form in which phytoestrogens are consumed (i.e., as foods or supplements), and whether soy products are fermented, which may increase bioavailability.[54,62,66] Adolescent exposure to soy foods appears to be one key to its protective effects against breast cancer.[67] Although it cannot be stated without a doubt that there is no increased breast cancer risk from a diet high in phytoestrogen-containing foods, there are no data indicating that prolonged use of a phytoestrogen-rich diet induces malignant growth of hormone-dependent tissue.[60] Including phytoestrogen-rich foods such as tofu, tempeh, soy milk, and flax seeds as part of an overall balanced diet is considered likely to be safe, and possibly even health promoting; however, supplemental intake of phytoestrogen products is not advisable, particularly for women with a history of breast cancer or breast cancer risk.[54]

Reduction of Side Effects of Conventional Therapies and Disease Symptoms

Patients commonly turn to CAM therapies for the reduction of side effects of conventional therapies and disease symptoms.[68] Acupuncture relieves nausea and vomiting associated with chemotherapy, postmastectomy massage reduces lymphedema, and mind–body therapies help relieve the stress and pain associated with breast cancer treatment.[37,68] A number of herbs may be considered for the reduction of nausea, pain, and anxiety associated with treatment.

Ginger (*Zingiber officinalis*) has been shown to be effective in several trials in reducing nausea associated with chemotherapy and surgery. Its mechanism of action, although not entirely known, appears to be a possible anti-serotonin (5-HT) action, possible reduction of gastrointestinal (GI) motility, and reduction of feedback to central chemoreceptors.[52] Although not all trials have demonstrated efficacy, given generally positive findings, a high level of safety, and a low side effects profile, it may be considered safe for use in patients experiencing nausea and vomiting during cancer treatment. High doses may theoretically inhibit platelet function.[52]

St. John's wort (*Hypericum perforatum*) is used to treat mild to moderate depression. Its mechanisms of action include inhibition of the reuptake of 5-hydroxytryptamine (5-HT), dopamine (DA), norepinephrine (NE), and gamma (γ)-aminobutyric acid (GABA), and L-glutamine in vitro.[68] Because of its interaction with cytochrome P450 (CYP) 3A4, it has been shown to lower the efficacy of irinotecan and tamoxifen.[68]

Kava kava (*Piper methysticum*) and passionflower (*Passiflora incarnata*) can be considered for patients with anxiety. The former has been associated with hepatotoxicity. The latter is also used for insomnia and neuralgias, and has a very good safety profile, although it may potentiate centrally acting sedative drugs.

Black Cohosh

Women undergoing chemotherapy for breast cancer experience increased intensity of menopausal symptoms, particularly hot flashes. Black cohosh has commonly been recommended for reduction of this troublesome symptom, and although many women report it effective, research evidence suggests that it is no more effective than placebo for women undergoing chemotherapy-induced menopausal vasomotor symptoms.[69]

The Hoxsey Formulae and Essiac

The Hoxsey formulae are a combination of an externally applied yellow or red salve, respectively containing arsenic sulfide, sulfur, and talc or antimony trisulfide, zinc chloride, and bloodroot; and a cathartic, immune-stimulating liquid tonic to be taken internally consisting of a mixture of licorice, red clover, burdock root, stillingia root, barberry, cascara, prickly ash bark, buckthorn bark, and potassium iodide. A similar formula intended for oral use, without the buckthorn bark and with more cascara sagrada and prickly ash, was listed in the 1926 United States *National Formulary* (ed 5) and the 1936 sixth edition

as an official remedy known as "Compound Fluidextract of Trifolium," and was first described in 1898 in the *King's American Dispensatory*. A 2002 survey of naturopathic physicians in the United States and Canada treating patients with breast cancer reported that the Hoxsey formula was used by 29% of the 161 responders treating localized breast cancer and 24% of the 72 responders treating metastatic breast cancer.[70] No toxicity associated with the Hoxsey tonic has been reported, but the potential of toxicity exists from some of its components. No peer-reviewed scientific studies have been published regarding the effectiveness of the treatment.[71] The topical applications are potentially caustic and damaging to the breast tissue.

Essiac—typically a combination of burdock root (*Arctium lappa*), Indian rhubarb (*Rheum palmatum*), sheep sorrel (*Rumex acetosella*), and the inner bark of slippery elm (*Ulmus fulva* or *U. rubra*)—has become one of the more popular herbal remedies for breast cancer treatment, secondary prevention, improving quality of life, and controlling negative side effects of conventional breast cancer treatment.[72] The formula may also variably include blessed thistle (*Cnicus benedictus*), red clover (*Trifolium pratense*), kelp (*Laminaria digitata*), and watercress (*Rorippa nasturtium aquaticum*).[71] In vivo and animal studies have reported antioxidant effects, competitive estrogen receptor binding, immune stimulation, inhibition of cell proliferation including human cancer cells, and laxative and bile-stimulating activities. Results have been inconsistent and have required doses greater than recommended for general consumption to achieve. A phase 2 trial in collaboration with the British Columbia Cancer Agency was discontinued apparently because of difficulties in enrolling patients.

A cohort study ($n = 510$) by Zick and coworkers was done to determine the effects of Essiac on health-related quality of life (HR-QOL) between women who are new Essiac users (since breast cancer diagnosis) and those who have never used Essiac; secondary end points were differences in depression, anxiety, fatigue, rate of adverse events, and prevalence of complications or benefits associated with Essiac during standard breast cancer treatment. The study found that Essiac does not appear to improve HR-QOL or mood states and seemed to have a negative effect, with Essiac users doing worse than the non-Essiac users.[72] This might be attributed to the fact that the group of users comprised younger women with more advanced stages of breast cancer, and both of these subgroups of patients have been shown to be at a significantly increased risk for negative mood states and/or a decreased sense of well-being. The women were taking low doses (total daily dose 43.6 ±30.8 mL) of Essiac that corresponded to the label directions found on most Essiac products. Friends were the most common source of information, and most women were taking Essiac to boost their immune systems or increase their chances of survival. Only two women reported minor adverse events, whereas numerous women reported beneficial effects of Essiac.[72]

In another study, researchers evaluated the effects of Essiac and another popular herbal product, Flor-Essence, on a line of human breast cancer cells. Exposure to the tonics produced a dose-dependent increase in estrogen-receptor activity but did not affect cell proliferation. The authors concluded that Flor-Essence and Essiac herbal tonics can stimulate the growth of human breast cancer cells through estrogen receptor–mediated as well as estrogen receptor–independent mechanisms of action.[73] According to Low Dog,[52] there is no compelling evidence that these products reduce tumor size, prolong survival, or improve quality of life.

Escharotic Salves

Escharotic treatments have been used historically as topical applications, commonly called "black salves" intended to draw out the tumor from the underlying tissue. They frequently include bloodroot *(Sanguinaria canadensis)*, an herb traditionally used as a blood purifier, and zinc chloride, a caustic agent, although ingredients vary widely. Escharotic treatments are commonly used by patients wishing to avoid surgical lumpectomy, with the promise that they are effective and safe. However, they are more commonly neither. The damage done to breast tissue from the topical use of these salves can be significant and permanently disfiguring. Use of escharotic treatments sometimes has resulted in much more radical breast surgery than simple lumpectomy would have, both owing to the damaging effects of the salves, and also to delay in obtaining appropriate medical care. I recommend that their use be entirely avoided in the treatment of breast cancer.

AFTER BREAST CANCER

Only recently have the emotional, social, and even medical complexities of life after breast cancer begun to be recognized. Even the terminology remains uncertain—do women think of themselves as breast cancer survivors? Do they move on, or spend their lives worrying about recurrence? Are there preventative strategies they can use to reduce their risk of recurrence? Currently there are probably more questions than answers. From a medical standpoint, the following follow-up guidelines are recommended[2]:

- History, symptom review, and physical examination (including CBE) should be performed every 3 to 6 months for 3 years; every 6 to 12 months for 2 years, and then annually
- BSE can be performed monthly
- Mammogram should be done annually
- Pelvic examination should be performed annually
- Patient should receive ongoing education about recurrence symptoms and ongoing care coordination

Many women continue to use herbal and nutritional supplements, along with a healthy lifestyle, throughout their lives to maintain health and prevent breast cancer recurrence.

15

Pregnancy and Botanical Medicine Use and Safety

So 8 days late, huh, you must be getting a little uncomfortable? ... If you're anxious there are a few ways to help things along ... actually there are things you can do ... just some home remedies .... I've found that some of them are very effective ... there's an herbal tea you can drink ....

Obstetrician in Friends, *The One Where Rachel Is Late*

The charge that herbal medications are not well tested in pregnancy is true, but it is just as true that conventional medications are not well tested in pregnancy. The medication-related embryopathies with which we are familiar are nearly all associated with conventional prescription drugs: thalidomide, anticonvulsants, ACE inhibitors, misoprostol, lithium, and isotretinoin. The most common embryopathy affecting humans is fetal alcohol syndrome, which is not associated with an herbal medication. This observation does not mean that herbal medications are safe, but only underscores the need to be well informed when prescribing in pregnancy. Let's recommend medications in pregnancy that have been adequately studied, without assuming that all conventional medications are on one side of a divide and all herbal medications are on the other side.[1]

PREVALENCE OF HERB USE DURING PREGNANCY

Herbs have been applied in the treatment of difficulties arising during pregnancy and childbirth since time immemorial, with texts and treatises on the uses of herbs for childbearing problems dating at least back to ancient Egypt. Childbearing women commonly experience minor complaints for which the use of natural remedies may be preferable to the woman, who perceives them as gentler and safer than over-the-counter (OTC) and prescription pharmaceuticals. The appropriate use of herbs medicinally during pregnancy requires specialized knowledge and a healthy dose of caution. This chapter presents a discussion of the prevalence of herb use during pregnancy and childbearing, possible risks, and general guidelines for responsible use. Subsequent chapters discuss the use of herbs for specific pregnancy concerns.

Herbal medicines are commonly used by pregnant women for a variety of complaints, as well as for nutritive and tonic purposes, such as the use of ginger to treat nausea and vomiting of pregnancy (NVP) or the traditional use of raspberry leaf as a uterine tonic. There is considerable evidence of increasing herb prescribing by obstetric health professionals, particularly certified nurse-midwives (CNMs).[2] The introductory quote to this chapter suggests a mainstreaming of herb use even by obstetricians—enough so that it would be mentioned by an obstetrician-gynecologist (OB-GYN) on the popular television sitcom *Friends* when one of the characters is seeking advice for her postdates pregnancy.

Epidemiologic studies and surveys from the United States, United Kingdom, and Australia estimate a range of approximately 7% to 45% of women using herbs during pregnancy.[2-5] A recent survey of 587 pregnant women by Glover and colleagues revealed that a total of 45.2% of participants in a rural obstetric population had used herbal medications (95.8% had used prescription and 92.6% had self-prescribed OTCs).[6] In another study, a one-page questionnaire examining the use of all prescription and nonprescription medications, including herbal remedies, was sent to parturients expected to deliver within 20 weeks who had preregistered with the hospital's admissions office. Sixty-one percent of the women responded to the survey, with 7.1% reporting the use of herbal remedies. Only 14.6% of users considered herbs to be medications. Herbal medicine use was most prevalent (17.1%) in parturients in the 41- to 50-year age range (5.6% of parturients). In another study, approximately one third of 463 postpartum women surveyed in the United States reported having used complementary and alternative medicine (CAM) therapies during pregnancy.[7] Of 734 pregnant women that responded to one survey, 46% used herbal remedies at the recommendation of their health care provider; 54% did so at the recommendation of a friend or family member.[2]

Botanical medicine use is likely even higher in communities observing traditional practices, for example, among Hispanic Americans or Asian Americans, where herb use is an inherent cultural practice. Internationally, traditional herb use during pregnancy is common. For example, a report from the King Edward VIII Hospital in South Africa demonstrated use of a specific traditional herbal formula among 55% of 229 patients randomly selected for interview upon admission in early labor.[8]

Articles and studies published in prominent nurse-midwifery and obstetric journals (i.e., *Journal of Nurse-Midwifery, Obstetrics and Gynecology,* and *Clinical Obstetrics and Gynecology*) indicate that a large number of CNMs use herbal medicines clinically or are interested in learning to do so.[9-12] A study of CNMs in North Carolina indicated that 90% of midwives recommend CAM therapies to patients, with 80% of respondents suggesting herbal therapies for labor stimulation.[9] A survey of 596 health care professionals in Leicestershire, United Kingdom, found that 34% of midwives and 18% of nurses used complementary therapies in their practices.[13] According to Jeanne Raisler, former associate editor of the *Journal of Nurse-Midwifery*, "Herbal healing is probably the complementary therapy most widely used by midwives."[12]

WHY ARE HERBS BEING USED DURING PREGNANCY?

One of the primary reasons women cite for stopping conventional medication during pregnancy is concern for risks to the fetus.[2] A recent report by Lo and Friedman indicates that more than 90% of all conventional medications prescribed for pregnant women have not been proved safe for use during pregnancy.[14] The specter of the thalidomide and DES (diethylstilbestrol) disasters are sufficiently recent to remind us of the hazards of "safe" pharmaceutical use during pregnancy. Many pregnant women turn to botanical therapies over pharmaceutical medications, believing them to be safer and gentler. Women planning natural birth also may feel that the use of herbs is more philosophically harmonious with their overall belief that childbearing is a natural experience and are more likely to use herbal preparations than those who are not preparing for natural birth.[2] Thus the use of herbal medicines represents both a philosophic and medical choice.

Midwives recommend herbal medicines for a variety of reasons, including support of patient choice, a shared belief in the naturalness of birth and the use of herbs as a natural extension of this belief, and as a way to help pregnant and postpartum women avoid more invasive and costly medical interventions that may be perceived as overly aggressive or unnecessary.[15] For example, Tiran suggests that the possibility of cephalic version of breech presentation through the use of moxibustion (see Breech Presentation and Version) may avoid the costs (and risks) of cesarean section, and

adequate management of NVP may reduce hospital admission for hyperemesis gravidarum.[16]

Midwives are in a key position to interface with pregnant clients about the use of botanical therapies. The philosophic compatibility between herbal medicine, midwifery, and nursing care philosophies reinforces a perceived "rightness" of botanical medicine use.[11,17,18] Unfortunately, few midwives are adequately trained in the use of botanical medicines during pregnancy. Education on the use—or at least safety and risks—of botanicals in the childbearing cycle should be a requisite part of training for all midwifery and obstetric care providers.

LACK OF TRAINING IN OBSTETRIC BOTANICAL MEDICINE USE

The medical and alternative literature on botanicals for pregnancy and birth often contains erroneous or inadequate information on the use of herbs during childbearing.[15,19,20] Herbs may be recommended, for example, with insufficient explanation of possible risks, without specified dosage ranges, and may be based on theoretic or academic knowledge rather than training or clinical experience. In one well-cited survey conducted by McFarlin and coworkers of nurse-midwives on their use of herbal remedies during pregnancy, most midwives who responded reported that they had learned about the use of herbs by word of mouth.[21] Several articles report on the need for further training in botanicals for nurse-midwives, citing its absence from curricula.[12,16,22]

Lack of practitioner training in botanical medicines for pregnancy might mean that practitioners are inappropriately recommending botanical therapies to their patients, either by recommending herbs that might be contraindicated, recommending inappropriate doses, not identifying safe and high-quality botanical products for patients, or recommending inappropriate durations of use. Further, practitioners with limited knowledge cannot accurately evaluate advice patients might receive from other sources, such as the Internet, a common source of misleading information on herbs and pregnancy.[23] There is clearly a need to include education on obstetric botanical medicine use in the growing number of CAM education programs in medical and nursing programs. Adequate practitioner knowledge is critical to the well-being of both patients involved in the prenatal and lactation dyad.

HERBS MOST COMMONLY USED DURING PREGNANCY

The herbs cited in the medical literature as those most frequently used for pregnancy complaints varies slightly among studies, but includes echinacea, St. John's wort, ephedra, peppermint, spearmint, ginger root, raspberry leaf, fennel, wild yam, meadowsweet, blue cohosh, black cohosh, castor oil, evening primrose, garlic, aloe, chamomile, pumpkin seeds, and ginseng. In one study, patients cited lower gastrointestinal (GI) problems, anxiety, nausea and vomiting, and urinary tract problems as the most common reasons for using complementary therapies in pregnancy.*

Midwives most frequently recommend herbs for nausea and vomiting, labor stimulation, perineal discomfort, lactation disorders, postpartum depression, preterm labor, postpartum hemorrhage, labor analgesia, and malpresentation.[9] Most of the herbs cited as commonly used are generally considered safe and gentle, even for use during pregnancy; however, several, including blue cohosh, ephedra, aloe (internally), and St. John's wort (internally) are not appropriate and may even be harmful (see further discussions on blue cohosh throughout this and subsequent sections of this chapter).

SAFETY, EVIDENCE, AND POTENTIAL ADVERSE EFFECTS OF BOTANICAL USE DURING PREGNANCY

Little is known scientifically about the risk of using herbs during pregnancy because most have not been formally evaluated and ethical considerations severely limit human clinical investigation during pregnancy.[†]

Much the same can be said for the use of many pharmaceuticals during pregnancy. Bone identifies five primary risks associated with the use of herbs during pregnancy[26]:

1. Toxicity to the mother, which might indirectly affect the fetus
2. Toxicity to the fetus
3. Teratogenesis
4. Increased miscarriage risk
5. Poor neonatal health

An additional potential risk is the consequences of delayed administration of necessary medical therapy in favor of herbs, regardless of their safety.[27] Most of what is currently known about botanical use during pregnancy is based on a significant body of historical, empirical, and observational evidence, and limited pharmacologic and animal studies. There has been little evidence of harm from the use of botanicals during pregnancy. When apparent adverse events have occurred, cause and effect have been difficult to establish because of a range of confounding factors.[23] Also, adverse events reports typically have involved the consumption of known toxic herbs, adulterations, or inappropriate use or dosage of botanical therapies. In general, there have also been relatively few case reports of adverse drug interactions involving herbal medicines.[28] Overall, most herbs have a high safety profile. Many practitioners take this as proof of safety, believing that whole herbs are inherently safer than concentrated pharmaceutical drugs.[10,11] However, lack of proof of harm is not synonymous with proof of safety. Some of the harmful effects of herbs may not be readily apparent until long after use has been discontinued, or may only occur with cumulative use.

There is a paucity of human clinical trials on the safety and efficacy of Western botanical therapies during pregnancy. Two human clinical trials evaluated raspberry leaf for its effects on labor outcome with positive findings; a study conducted on echinacea safety after varying lengths of pregnancy use found no harmful effects; and several studies have evaluated the safety and efficacy of ginger root for the reduction of NVP, finding it safe and effective.[29-31] Most often, the results of clinical trials are positive.[3] Nonetheless, many researchers feel that in the absence of proof of safety, herbs should be entirely avoided during pregnancy.[3] However, many midwives and pregnant women continue to use herbs based on satisfaction with their safety, efficacy, and outcomes, and on the knowledge that many pharmaceutical preparations recommended during pregnancy also carry unknown risks.

Controls over the manufacturing of herbs do not entirely protect consumers from the accidental or deliberate adulteration, sophistication, or contamination of herbal products, all of which can pose problems during pregnancy. In one study of 200 different herbal products, 83% were found to be contaminated with undeclared pharmaceuticals or heavy metals, including lead, arsenic, and mercury.[5] Adulteration occurs when one herb is accidentally or deliberately substituted for another. Rarely, toxic herbs have been found as adulterants in otherwise completely benign herbal products, for example, adulteration of skullcap (*Scutellaria lateriflora*) with the toxic *Teucrium*, or common plantain (*Plantago* spp.) with *Digitalis* spp. (foxglove). One case in the literature reports on the substitution of the herb *Periploca sepium* for *Eleutherococcus senticosus*.[26,32] This substitution resulted in a case of hyperandrogenization of the fetus ("hairy baby syndrome") as a result of the mother mistakenly taking the adulterated product throughout her pregnancy. Chinese patent products and imported Asian herbal formulae should be viewed with utmost caution during pregnancy because they are well known to contain adulterants, heavy metals, and added pharmaceutical medications frequently not listed on the label, all of which can pose a threat to the safety of the pregnant woman and her fetus.

Negative outcomes have been reported for a limited number of herbal products used by parturient women. Ernst provides a thorough review of these in *Herbal Medicinal Products During Pregnancy: Are They Safe?*[3] Causality remains uncertain. Adverse reports cited by Ernst and others include[8,10,33]:

- One case of ovarian hyperstimulation in a woman undergoing in vitro fertilization and taking *Vitex agnus-castus*
- One case of fetal alcohol syndrome in a 29-year-old Chinese woman taking an herbal product containing 19% alcohol regularly throughout pregnancy, with negative report of other alcohol consumption
- One case of hypertension in a 3-week postpartum mother and neonate associated with maternal consumption of dong quai; hypertension disappeared within 48 hours of discontinuation of the herbal product
- Case report of a 15-month-old Chinese female with congenital deformity of an accessory phallic urethra arising in the vicinity of the anus

---

*References 2, 4, 7, 10, 23.
†References 2, 5, 9, 24, 25.

- Possible association between maternal consumption of blue cohosh as a partus preparator and neonatal cardiac arrest, neonatal congestive heart failure, and neonatal stroke in three respective cases
- Maternal hepatotoxicity allegedly from a Chinese herbal product called Shou-Wu-Pian
- Neonatal hepatotoxicity and death caused by liver failure in a female Swiss infant associated with maternal consumption of an herbal tea known to be high in pyrrolizidine alkaloids (PAs)
- Congenital meningoencephalocele and cerebellar agenesis in a baby born to a woman who had consumed a known toxic herb, *Tripterygium wilfordii*, for rheumatoid arthritis throughout her pregnancy

Other herbal products that have been associated with increased complications include a possible correlation between a German sinus preparation (i.e., Sinupret) and increased rates of miscarriage, stillbirth, and malformations; increased rate of meconium-stained amniotic fluid with maternal use of castor oil; and increased meconium staining and possibly related fetal distress with use of a traditional South African herbal pregnancy formula called isihlambezo; and a case of a baby born with veno-occlusive disease (VOD) after the mother consumed a coltsfoot-containing cough syrup throughout her pregnancy.[3,8]

USING HERBS DURING PREGNANCY

The most prudent approach to the use of herbs during pregnancy is to avoid all herbs during the first trimester unless medically indicated (i.e., severe NVP preventing adequate nutritional intake, threatened miscarriage) and used with proper guidance, and to otherwise only use herbs during the remainder of pregnancy if there is a compelling reason for their therapeutic use, greater safety in a botanical option than a pharmaceutical one, or lack of a suitable pharmaceutical alternative. Beverage and nutritive teas that are known to be safe in moderate amounts (e.g., red raspberry, spearmint, chamomile, lemon balm, nettles), and ingestion of normal amounts of cooking spices are excepted from these restrictions; however, practitioners and pregnant women should be aware that herbs may be contaminated with heavy metals or adulterated. For example, an industry recall of the nutritive tonic herb nettles occurred some years ago owing to high lead content of a batch that had been released to the market. It is therefore best for pregnant women to use only organically grown and carefully cultivated herbs, and to avoid all products with a high likelihood of contamination or adulteration.

The following key points are essential to remember when using botanical medicines during pregnancy:
- Natural is not synonymous with safe.
- Many botanical medicines contain potent pharmacologic constituents.
- Many constituents consumed by the mother can pass through the placenta and reach the fetus.
- Physiologic and metabolic changes during pregnancy may influence the pharmacokinetics of herbs, thus changing expected actions or safety; for example decreased bowel transit time may affect dosing, and renal and hepatic changes may affect the metabolism and excretion of herbal constituents.
- Actions that may be acceptable in the mother may be inappropriate, or even harmful, for the baby.
- Herbs can have unknown and idiosyncratic effects in the pregnant woman or her baby.
- Herbs with known teratogenic, mutagenic, or abortifacient properties should be avoided.
- Highly concentrated herbal products should be avoided.
- Long-term use and high doses of alcohol-based products (i.e., tinctures), especially during the first trimester, should be avoided.
- Herbs may affect the developing fetal endocrine and/or nervous system.
- Herbs can disrupt pregnancy and lead to miscarriage or premature labor.

CONTRAINDICATED HERBS FOR PREGNANCY AND LACTATION

There are several specific categories of herbs that are historically avoided during pregnancy to minimize risks to the maternal–embryonal/fetal dyad (Table 15-1). A discussion follows, as well as an extensive list of contraindicated herbs for pregnancy and lactation.

Abortifacients and Emmenagogues

Abortifacients are those herbs that may induce miscarriage/abortion (Table 15-2). The amounts required to induce an abortion may pose toxicity risks to the mother, including kidney and liver damage. Because the risks of maternal intake of these herbs to the fetus are unknown, women who have attempted to abort unsuccessfully may require a follow-up clinical abortion. Abortifacients should be entirely avoided during pregnancy and herbal abortion is not a recommended method of intentional pregnancy termination.

Emmenagogues are defined in herbal medicine as herbs capable of stimulating the menstrual flow even when it is not due, and are also to be avoided during pregnancy. For centuries, they have been colloquially defined as "herbs for delayed menses," sometimes a euphemism for eliminating an unwanted pregnancy. Many emmenagogic herbs are therefore also abortifacients. There is disagreement in the literature as to what actually constitutes an emmenagogue. Certain herbs such as chamomile are frequently and erroneously listed as emmenagogic. Other herbs, such as dong quai and peony, are considered emmenagogic, and in fact do have uterine stimulatory activity, but are nonetheless used extensively in the Chinese and Japanese formulary for the prevention of miscarriage. Finally, the recorded data on other herbs are contradictory; for example, ashwagandha has been described as an abortifacient yet was used historically to prevent miscarriage. Many herbs that are high in essential oil content are undisputed emmenagogues, although the presence of essential oils in an herb does not

TABLE 15-1   Herb Categories to Avoid During Pregnancy

Category	Examples
Abortifacients and emmenagogues	Angelica (Angelica archangelica) Mugwort (Artemesia vulgaris) Pennyroyal essential oil Rue (Ruta graveolens) Safflower (Carthamus tinctorius) Scotch broom (Cytisus scoparius) Tansy (Tanacetum vulgare) Thuja (Thuja occidentalis) Wormwood (Artemesia absinthium) Yarrow (Achillea millefolium)
Alkaloids*	Barberry (Berberis vulgaris) Borage (Borago officinalis) Coltsfoot (Tussilago farfara) Comfrey (Symphytum officinale) Goldenseal (Hydrastis Canadensis) Oregon grape (Mahonia aquifolium)
Essential oils and volatile oils*	Pennyroyal (Mentha pulegium) Peppermint (Mentha piperita) Oregano (Origanum vulgare) Sage (Salvia officinalis) Tansy (Tanacetum vulgare) Thuja (Thuja occidentalis) Thyme (Thymus vulgaris)
Nervous system stimulants/depressants	Coffee (Coffea arabica) Ephedra sinica Guarana (Paullinia cupana) Kava kava (Piper methysticum)
Phytoestrogens	Hops (Humulus lupulus) Isoflavone extracts Red clover (Trifolium pratense)
Stimulating laxatives	Aloe vera (Aloe barbadensis) Buckthorn (Rhamnus cathartica) Cascara sagrada (Rhamnus purshiana) Castor oil (Ricinus communis) Rhubarb (Rheum rhabarbarum)
Teratogens	Cherry bark (Prunus spp.) Galbanum (Ferula spp.) Hellebore (Veratrum spp.) Jimson Weed or Angel's Trumpet (Datura spp.) Lupine (Lupinus spp.) Nightshade (Solanum spp.) Parsnip (Trachymene spp.) Poison hemlock (Conium spp.) Ragwort (Senecio spp.) Tobacco (Nicotiana spp.)

Note: The herbs listed under each category are representative examples and are not exhaustive. Additional herbs may fall into any of these categories.
*Avoid internal use; external use may be acceptable under the guidance of an experienced botanical medicine practitioner.

mean it acts as an emmenagogue.[26] Commonly accepted abortifacients and emmenagogic herbs include (but are not limited to) tansy, thuja, safflower, scotch broom, rue, angelica, mugwort, wormwood, yarrow, and essential oil of pennyroyal.[26]

TABLE 15-2   Commonly Used Botanicals with Possible Abortifacient, Emmenagogue, or Oxytocic Activity

Common Name	Botanical Name
Blue cohosh	Caulophyllum thalictroides
Coleus	Coleus forskohlii
Cotton root bark	Gossypium spp.
Eucalyptus	Eucalyptus spp.
Goldenseal	Hydrastis canadensis
Motherwort	Leonurus cardiaca
Mugwort	Artemisia spp.
Pennyroyal	Mentha pulegium
Tansy	Tanacetum vulgare
Yarrow	Achillea millefolium

Essential Oils and Volatile Oils

Essential oils and volatile oils are capable of crossing the placenta and reaching the fetus, and may have effects on the developing fetal nervous system. In significant doses, essential oils can be emmenagogic. Concentrated essential oils should never be taken internally during pregnancy and should not be used neat (i.e., undiluted) topically. Oils known to be specifically emmenagogic because of their essential oil content (e.g., thuja, pennyroyal, tansy) should be entirely avoided during pregnancy. Common herbs with high volatile oil content such as chamomile, lavender, spearmint, and peppermint, but which are considered generally safe during pregnancy, should be used in moderation; however, they have not been associated with adverse clinical outcomes.

Teratogens and Mutagens

The word *teratogen* has its origins in the Greek *terato*, meaning "monster." Teratogens are substances that cause structural abnormalities in the fetus. The drug thalidomide was a powerful example of a teratogen, and its legacy has left an imprint on those who prescribe medications to pregnant women. There is extremely limited knowledge about which herbs are teratogenic. Most of what is known is derived primarily from animal studies, observation of teratogenesis in grazing cattle, and suspected teratogenicity in humans from ingestion of suspected harmful herbal products. Known teratogens include those plants in the *Lupinus*, *Veratrum*, *Conium*, and *Solanum* genera; and suspected teratogenic substances can be found in *Astragalus*, *Nicotiana*, *Ferula*, and *Trachymene* genera. Plants in the *Datura*, *Prunus*, *Sorghum*, and *Senecio* genera may also contain teratogenic substances.[26] The primary means for identifying the propensity for this type of reaction is through general toxicologic screenings or through pharmacovigilance programs. Birth defects that occur between conception and birth are caused by teratogenic agents, whereas mutagens cause direct changes in the nucleus of cells.

The potential for mutagenicity is discerned through in vitro assays, most notably Salmonella microsome test (i.e., Ames assay) or rodent tests, and then followed by animal studies. In both types of tests, isolated compounds rather than complete

TABLE 15-3 Botanicals Containing Pyrrolizidine Alkaloids

Common Name	Botanical Nomenclature
Borage*	*Borago officinalis*
Butterbur	*Petasites hybridus*
Coltsfoot	*Tussilago farfara*
Comfrey	*Symphytum officinale*
Eyebright	*Euphrasia officinalis*
Life root	*Senecio aureus*

*Borage oil does not contain pyrrolizidine alkaloids.

herbal products are most often investigated. Unfortunately, simple in vitro toxicity screenings do not reveal much useful data because they often cannot be extrapolated to human use. The presence of a mutagen in a product does not automatically contraindicate the use of the substance in pregnancy. There are many commonly consumed substances such as basil, black pepper, coffee, tomatoes, and potatoes that contain toxic compounds, including those with mutagenic or teratogenic potential. However, consumption of these in pregnancy is not contraindicated when consumed as a normal part of the diet.

Alkaloids

Alkaloids are a highly bioactive category of plant compounds, many of which may have adverse effects on the developing embryo/fetus. One such group is the PAs, known to cause VOD, an adverse outcome that has been observed in fetuses when the herb has been ingested regularly by their pregnant mothers (Table 15-3). Comfrey, coltsfoot, and borage herb (not borage oil) are the main herbs that have been implicated, containing varying amounts of PAs. They should therefore be avoided for internal use and should be used only short term topically when there is broken skin because there is a minimal risk of transdermal absorption into the bloodstream. Germany has established limits for external application of toxic PAs to no more than 100 µg daily. In addition to causing VOD, PAs are carcinogenic and mutagenic. Botanicals containing toxic PAs should not be used in pregnancy or lactation. PAs have been reported to be secreted into the milk of nursing animals. Also, new mothers should be cautioned against excessive or frequent use of salves, oils, and balms made from herbs known to contain toxic PAs, such as comfrey (*Symphytum officinale*) for sore breasts associated with breastfeeding.

Oral consumption of berberine alkaloid–containing herbs is also typically best avoided during pregnancy. Although there are no documented reports of adverse events in pregnancy associated with their use, they have been implicated in neonatal jaundice when used in pregnancy.[34] Herbs in this category include goldenseal, goldthread, barberry, and Oregon grape root. Topical and vaginal applications appear to be safe for use during pregnancy.

Laxatives

Stimulating laxatives, including Cascara sagrada, castor oil, buckthorn, aloes, and rhubarb, are to be avoided. Senna is generally contraindicated by midwives and herbalists for use during pregnancy, though Mills and Bone state that is has not been associated with adverse effects and therefore should not be contraindicated in pregnancy.[26] Constipation is best addressed with gentle, nonstimulating bulk laxatives (e.g., flax, psyllium) and lifestyle approaches such as dietary changes and exercise.[26] Laxatives containing anthraquinone glycosides are considered overly stimulating during pregnancy because their effects of increasing intestinal peristalsis can lead to sympathetic uterine stimulation. Yellow dock, however, is one anthraquinone-containing laxative that herbalists and midwives frequently except from this rule; it is much gentler in effects and is commonly added to formulae for treating anemia because of its purported iron-fortifying actions.

Phytoestrogens

Numerous plants, including food plants, such as legumes, contain phytoestrogens, which are an integral part of a healthy diet. Asian diets, which include large amounts of tofu and other soy products, are particularly high in phytoestrogens, and abnormal levels of fetal and neonatal problems have not been observed compared with other populations. Nonetheless, there is concern that high consumption of phytoestrogens during pregnancy may exert abnormal hormonal effects on the developing embryo or fetus, particularly in female embryogenesis, as occurred with the drug DES. Although phytoestrogens are dramatically weaker than DES, because of unknown effects, it is best to avoid specifically supplementing the diet with concentrated phytoestrogen supplements. Additionally, herbs with known hormonal activity, including hops, red clover, and isoflavone extract supplements, are best avoided for long-term use or in large doses during pregnancy.

Nervous System Stimulants/Depressants

Herbs that strongly affect the nervous system, including stimulants such as ephedra, guarana, and large amounts of caffeine-containing herbs, including coffee and green and black teas, may have adverse effects on pregnancy and the developing embryonic and fetal nervous system, and should be avoided during pregnancy. Kava kava, a strong anxiolytic and sedative herb, has recently been implicated in cases of hepatotoxicity. Although many of the cases appear not to be causally related to the herb, the herb does appear to have idiosyncratic hepatotoxic effects, and should be avoided during pregnancy and lactation in favor of other, safer botanical options.

A WORD ABOUT PARTUS PREPARATORS

Partus preparators are herbs used during the last weeks of pregnancy to tone and prepare the uterus for labor. Historically, they have been used to facilitate a rapid and easy delivery. Herbs commonly used as partus preparators include blue cohosh (*Caulophyllum thalictroides*), black cohosh (*Actaea racemosa*), partridge berry (*Mitchella repens*), and spikenard (*Aralia racemosa*), among others. The use of such herbs to prepare women for labor begs the question of why one would use an herbal preparation to prepare the body for something it naturally knows how to do. Furthermore, the safety of these herbs before the onset of labor is questionable. Case reports have appeared in the literature suggesting an association between blue cohosh and profound cerebral ischemic episodes or myocardial infarction in the neonate.[35,36] Blue cohosh contains a number of potent alkaloids, including methylcysteine and anagyrine, the latter of which is known to have an effect on cardiac muscle activity. Other side effects of blue cohosh include maternal headache and nausea. Yet as previously stated, the use of blue cohosh represents one of the widely applied botanical medicines by midwives, and one of those most commonly included in late pregnancy formulae self-prescribed by pregnant mothers. The risks associated with extended third trimester ingestion of blue cohosh specifically suggest that it should be avoided as a partus preparator. It seems that it would be preferable, unless otherwise indicated for the health of the mother and baby, to focus attention on nonpharmacologic methods of preparing for labor.

CONTRAINDICATED HERB LISTS AND BOTANICAL SAFETY CLASSIFICATIONS

The herbal literature is rife with lists of herbs contraindicated in pregnancy and lactation. Limitations are inherent in most of these lists, particularly in their lack of specifics as to how and when each herb is contraindicated. Herbs may sometimes be broadly contraindicated in pregnancy yet in actuality be only contextually contraindicated; for example, they are absolutely contraindicated during the first and second trimesters but may be reasonably used during labor, or they may be safe in small doses for a very limited duration. Culinary herbs, appearing on many contraindicated lists, when used in moderation as food seasonings, pose no harm to the fetus or mother. Herbs such as aloe vera, calendula, and even comfrey may be used topically with no risk but are to be avoided for internal use, yet are contraindicated on such lists with no differentiation, leading to confusion about safety. Certain contraindications have become pervasive myths, for example, the frequent contraindication of chamomile in pregnancy owing to its alleged action as an abortifacient.[37] In fact, chamomile provides an excellent example of how misapplication of a scientific finding can lead to unjustified contraindication of a safe herb. A study conducted in 1979 found teratogenic effects using a concentrated extract of alpha (α)-bisabolol at high doses. No teratogenic effects were seen at lower doses and the dose of the oil constituent required to cause teratogenicity are far greater than it would ever be possible for someone drinking the tea to ever approximate. However, based on this single study, chamomile was erroneously contraindicated for consumption during pregnancy.[38]

Finally, herbs may be contraindicated based on theoretical reasons; for example, ashwagandha, which in traditional Ayurvedic medicine was used to prevent miscarriage, is contraindicated on the basis that it might cause uterine contractions, predicated on a single anecdotal report with no details

on duration, mode of use, nor dose that has been reiterated several times in the scientific literature. To complicate matters, certain herbs that are contraindicated by Western herbalists and Western scientific research for use during pregnancy are regularly used in traditional medicine from non-Western cultures; for example, dong quai (Angelica sinensis) is prescribed as a blood tonic for pregnant women in China, and listed in China and Japan in official formulae for the prevention of miscarriage, yet is considered contraindicated in Western herbal medicine.

The *Botanical Safety Handbook* has categorized herbs for use in pregnancy and lactation as follows[39]:

- Category 2b: "Not to be used during pregnancy unless otherwise directed by an expert qualified in the appropriate use of this substance"
- Category 2c: "Not to be used while nursing unless otherwise directed by an expert qualified in the appropriate use of this substance"

Table 15-4 is an amalgamation of contraindicated herb lists from *The Botanical Safety Handbook, The Natural Pregnancy Book,* and *Women's Health in Complementary and Integrative Medicine,* all compiled by authors with significant knowledge of botanical safety and obstetric botanical use. It is not exhaustive, leaving out many obscure herbs, and focusing on those herbs the clinician is likely to encounter, consider, or question. It also does not cover many herbs from traditional Chinese medicine or the Ayurvedic materia medica. Table 15-4 also includes categoric designations of caution and contraindication according to Mills and Bone, which are subsequently discussed.

Mills and Bone suggest that a descriptive classification scheme for the risk of herbs during pregnancy, similar to that used for drugs in pregnancy, would be more useful than contraindicated lists in helping practitioners sort through the inconsistencies in the literature.[26] They recommend the use of the Australian Therapeutic Goods Administration (TGA) Prescribing medicines in pregnancy http://www.tga.gov.au/prescribing-medicines-pregnancy-database (Table 15-5) as the guideline for a similar classification of herb use and safety during pregnancy and lactation, which they have begun to outline based on available evidence. They suggest that practitioners might use these guidelines to choose at which level(s) they are comfortable prescribing botanical medicines for pregnant women. For example, only those herbs that are considered benign or have been demonstrated to be safe would meet the criteria for category A (e.g., red raspberry leaf, ginger, echinacea); those herbs definitively contraindicated, such as the internal use of comfrey or other PA–containing herbs, would be relegated to categories D or below. More conservative practitioners would have the option of recommending only those herbs in category A; others might prescribe from categories A to B3, herbs from categories C would primarily be avoided throughout pregnancy and would be contraindicated during first trimester, and those from D to X would be contraindicated entirely throughout pregnancy. Much work is still needed to classify herbs according to this scheme, and classifications may shift as new data become available.

TABLE 15-4 Herbs Contraindicated in Pregnancy with American Herbal Products Association and Mills and Bone Safety Classifications

Common Name	Botanical Name	Botanical Safety Handbook Classification	Mills and Bone Classification*	Exceptions
Achyranthes	Achyranthes bidentata	2b	NC	
Albizzia	Albizia julibrissin	2b	NC	
Alder buckthorn	Rhamnus frangula	2b, 2c	NC	
Aloe (dried juice)	Aloe spp.	2b, 2c	B3	Safe for topical use
Andrographis	Andrographis paniculata	2b	B3	
Angelica	Angelica archangelica	2b	NC	
Arnica	Arnica montana	2b	X	Safe for topical use; unbroken skin only
Ashwagandha	Withania somnifera	2b	B1	Used in Ayurveda to prevent miscarriage
Barberry	Berberis vulgaris	2b	P/C	
Basil leaf	Ocimum basilicum	2b, 2c	NC	Safe for normal culinary use
Bethroot	Trillium spp.	2b	NC	
Birthwort	Aristolochia clematitis	NC	NC	
Black cohosh	Actaea racemosa	2b, 2c	B2	Classically used to prevent miscarriage
Bladderwrack	Fucus vesiculosus	2b, 2c	B2	
Blessed thistle	Carbenia benedicta	2b	NC	
Blood root	Sanguinaria canadensis	2b	NC	
Blue cohosh	Caulophyllum thalictroides	2b	D	Possibly safe for short-term use during labor only, and with proper monitoring of fetal heart tones
Blue flag	Iris versicolor	2b	B1	
Blue vervain	Verbena hastata	2b	NC	
Borage	Borago officinalis	2a	NC	
Broom	Sarothamnus scoparius	NC	NC	
Buchu	Barosma betulina	2b	B2	
Buckthorn	Rhamnus cathartica	2b, 2c	NC	
Bugleweed	Lycopus spp.	2b, 2c	P/C L/X	
Butterbur	Petasites hybridus	NC	NC	
Butternut	Juglans cinerea	NC	NC	
California poppy	Eschscholzia californica	2b	B2	
Cascara sagrada	Rhamnus purshiana	2b, 2c	B2	
Celandine	Chelidonium majus	2b	C	
Chaparral	Larrea tridentata	2b	C	
Coltsfoot	Tussilago farfara	2b, 2c	NC	
Comfrey	Symphytum officinale	2a, 2c	NC	Safe for topical application for short duration but avoid on large areas of broken skin
Corydalis	Corydalis yanhusuo	2b	NC	
Cotton root	Gossypium herbaceum	2b	NC	
Cowslip	Primula veris	2b	NC	
Elecampane	Inula helenium	2b, 2c	B2	
Ephedra (Ma Huang)	Ephedra vulgaris	2b, 2c	B3	
Fenugreek	Trigonella foenum-graecum	2b	B3	
Feverfew	Tanacetum parthenium	2b	B3	
Gelsemium	Gelsemium sempervirens	NC	NC	
Ginseng	Panax quinquefolius	NC	A	Used during pregnancy in Traditional Chinese Medicine
Goldenseal	Hydrastis canadensis	2b	C	Safe for topical and suppository use

TABLE 15-4 Herbs Contraindicated in Pregnancy with AHPA and Mills and Bone Safety Classifications—cont'd

Common Name	Botanical Name	Botanical Safety Handbook Classification	Mills and Bone Classification*	Exceptions
Gotu kola	Hydrocotyle asiatica	NC	B1	
Goat's rue	Galega officinalis	NC	B3	
Guggul	Commiphora mukul	2b	C	
Horsetail	Equisetum spp.	2d	B2	
Ipecac	Ipecac ipecacuanha	2b	NC	
Juniper berries	Juniperus communis	2b	NC	
Kava	Piper methysticum	2b, 2c	B1	
Licorice	Glycyrrhiza glabra	2b	A	Possibly safe for medically indicated uses for short duration
Lily of the valley	Convallaria majalis	NC	NC	
Lobelia	Lobelia inflata	2b	NC	
Male fern	Dryopteris filix-mas	2a, 2c	NC	
Mistletoe	Viscum album	2b	NC	
Motherwort	Leonurus cardiaca	2b	B3	
Mugwort	Artemisia vulgaris	2b	NC	
Nutmeg	Myristica officinalis	NC	NC	Safe for normal culinary use
Oregon grape root	Mahonia aquifolium	2b	C	Safe for topical use
Osha	Ligusticum porteri	2b	NC	
Parsley	Carum petroselinum	2b	NC	Safe for normal culinary use
Pasqueflower	Pulsatilla vulgaris	NC	C	
Pennyroyal	Mentha pulegium	2a, 2b	NC	
Periwinkle	Vinca spp.	NC	NC	
Peruvian bark	Cinchona spp.	2b	NC	
Pleurisy root	Asclepias tuberosa	2b	NC	
Pokeweed	Phytolacca decandra	2b	D	
Prickly ash	Zanthoxylum americanum	2b	B2	
Red clover	Trifolium pratense	2b	NC	
Rosemary	Rosmarinus officinalis	2b	B1	Safe for culinary use
Rue	Ruta graveolens	2b	NC	
Rhubarb	Rheum palmatum	NC	NC	
Sage	Salvia officinalis	2b	C	
Sarsaparilla	Smilax officinale	NC	NC	
Senna	Cassia senna	2b, 2c	A	
Shepherd's purse	Capsella bursa-pastoris	2b	B3	
Spikenard	Aralia racemosa	2b	NC	
Stillingia	Stillingia sylvatica	3	NC	
Sweet flag	Acorus calamus	2b	NC	
Tansy	Tanacetum vulgare	2b, 2c	D	
Thuja	Thuja occidentalis	2b	D	
Tumeric	Curcuma longa	2b	A	Safe for normal culinary use
Wild indigo	Baptisia tinctoria	2b	NC	
Wormwood	Artemisia absinthium	2b, 2c	D	
Yarrow	Achillea millefolium	2b	B3	Safe for topical application

L, Lactation category; *NC,* not categorized; *P*, pregnancy category.
*Only for those herbs appearing on this list. Mills S., Bone K: The Essential Guide to Herbal Safety, St. Louis, Churchill Livingstone, 2005.

Based on their review of the literature using sources similar to those accepted in this text, they have developed the categorization that appears in Table 15-6. Mills and Bone clearly take the approach that with proper use and knowledge of risks and contraindications, herbs can be safely applied therapeutically during pregnancy and lactation. Their classification itself, however, introduces further inconsistencies and sometimes contradicts other recognized lists of herbs contraindicated during pregnancy. For example, Mills and Bone include licorice in Category A, "Drugs which have been taken by a large number of pregnant women and women of childbearing age without any proven increase in the frequency of malformations

TABLE 15-5 The Australian Therapeutic Goods Association Classification for Drugs in Pregnancy

Category	Definition
Category A	Drugs that have been taken by a large number of pregnant women and women of childbearing age without any proven increase in the frequency of malformations or other direct or indirect harmful effects on the fetus having been observed.
Category B1	Drugs that have been taken by only a limited number of pregnant women and women of childbearing age, without an increase in the frequency of malformations or other direct or indirect harmful effects on the human fetus having been observed. Studies in animals have not shown evidence of an increased occurrence of fetal damage.
Category B2	Drugs that have been taken by only a limited number of pregnant women and women of childbearing age, without an increase in the frequency of malformations or other direct or indirect harmful effects on the human fetus having been observed. Studies in animals are inadequate or may be lacking, but available data show no evidence of an increased occurrence of fetal damage.
Category B3	Drugs that have been taken by only a limited number of pregnant women and women of childbearing age, without an increase in the frequency of malformations or other direct or indirect harmful effects on the human fetus having been observed. Studies in animals have shown evidence of an increased occurrence of fetal damage, the significance of which is considered uncertain in humans.
Category C	Drugs that, owing to their pharmacologic effects, have caused or may be suspected of causing harmful effects in the human fetus or neonate without causing malformations. These effects may be reversible.
Category D	Drugs that have caused, are suspected to have caused, or may be expected to cause, an increased incidence of human fetal malformations or irreversible damage. These drugs also have adverse pharmacologic effects.
Category X	Drugs that have such a high risk of causing permanent damage to the fetus that they should not be used in pregnancy or when there is a possibility of pregnancy.

Note: For drugs in B1, B2, or B3 categories, human data are lacking or inadequate and subcategorization is therefore based on available animal data. The allocation of a B category does NOT imply greater safety than the C category. Drugs in category D are NOT absolutely contraindicated in pregnancy (e.g., anticonvulsants). Moreover, in some cases the D category has been assigned on the basis of suspicion.

TABLE 15-6 Mills and Bone Classification for Herbs in Pregnancy

Category	Examples
Category A	Bilberry fruit, Chamomile (German), Cranberry, Echinacea, Garlic, Ginger, Ginseng,* Licorice,* Raspberry leaf, Senna,* Turmeric
Category B1	Astragalus, Blue flag, Boswellia, Bupleurum, Burdock, Butcher's broom, Chaste tree, Codonopsis, Evening primrose oil, Ginkgo, Goat's rue, Gotu kola, Hawthorn, Kava, Myrrh, Passionflower, Rosemary, Schisandra, Siberian ginseng, St. John's wort, St. Mary's thistle, Valerian, Willow bark, Withania
Category B2	Bacopa, Black cohosh, Black haw, Black walnut, Bladderwrack, Buchu, Calendula, California poppy, Cascara, Celery seed, Chickweed, Cleavers, Corn silk, Couch grass, Cramp bark, Cranesbill root, Damiana, Dandelion, Devil's claw, Elder flowers, Elecampane, Euphorbia, Eyebright, False unicorn, Fringe tree, Gentian, Globe artichoke, Goldenrod, Grindelia, Gymnema, Hops, Horsetail, Hydrangea, Lavender, Lemon balm, Lime flowers, Marshmallow, Mullein, Nettle, Peppermint, Prickly ash, Pygeum, Saw palmetto, Shatavari, Skullcap, Thyme, Wild lettuce, Willow herb, Yellow dock, Ziziphus seed
Category B3	Aloe, Andrographis, Bittersweet, Crataeva, Ephedra, Fennel, Fenugreek, Feverfew, Horse chestnut, Meadowsweet, Motherwort, Rehmannia, Shepherd's purse, Tribulus, White horehound, Wild cherry, Yarrow
Category C	Barberry and Indian barberry, Bearberry, Bugleweed, Chaparral, Dong quai, Goldenseal, Greater celandine, Guggul, Oregon grape, Pasque flower, Sage, Tylophora
Category D	Blue cohosh, Cat's claw, Jamaican dogwood, Pau d'Arco, Poke root, Tansy, Thuja, Wormwood
Category X	Arnica, Boldo

*Recent literature suggests that the regular use of large amounts of licorice in pregnancy, including licorice candy containing real licorice extract (not just licorice or anise flavor) may lead to preterm birth. These other herbs are also contraindicated for use during pregnancy on other lists. Strandberg T, Andersson S, Jarvenpaa A, et al: Preterm birth and licorice consumption during pregnancy, *Am J Epidemiol* 156(9):803–805, 2002; Mills S, Bone K. *The essential guide to herbal safety.* St Louis: Elsevier, 2005.

or other direct or indirect harmful effects on the fetus having been observed"; licorice is contraindicated for use during pregnancy in lists provided by Low Dog and McGuffin and colleagues, among others, and which has recently been associated with premature delivery after regular consumption of licorice candy during pregnancy.[38-40] Their support of the use of senna as a category A herb is another example.

What becomes clear is that there is still a tremendous amount to be learned about the effects of herbs used during pregnancy. Given the inconsistencies, it is best for practitioners and patients to use only those herbs with a proven safety record or to use herbs during pregnancy only when the risks of a conventional medical therapy clearly outweighs theoretical but unproven risks of an herb.

FORMS OF ADMINISTRATION APPROPRIATE DURING PREGNANCY

The forms in which herbs are administered (e.g., tincture, tea) can affect their strength and efficacy. During pregnancy, various forms can be chosen to maximize or minimize the volume and availability of more or less desirable constituents in a preparation, as well as exposure to other unwanted substances; for example, using water-based extracts to minimize extraction of bioactive compounds, or avoiding excessive consumption of alcohol by minimizing alcohol-based preparations. Chapter 3 provides a full discussion of forms of administration. The following brief discussion addresses the specific nuances of administration of herbs during pregnancy.

Internal Forms of Herbal Medicines

Internally used preparations that might be considered during pregnancy include teas and infusions, decoctions, syrups, tinctures (alcohol- and glycerin-based), capsules, and rarely, enemas. Each of the internal forms offers specific advantages and disadvantages. For example, infusions are water-based extracts and are less effective at extracting many of the bioactive compounds that are more readily extracted when alcohol, which is hydroethanolic, is used as a solvent. Thus water-based preparations are considered by many herbalists to be gentler and safer. Further, because water-based preparations are more dilute than, for example, concentrated alcohol extracts, one must consume a larger volume of the preparation to approximate a comparable dose of a more concentrated form of preparation; thus this is a limiting factor for excessive dosing.

The sheer unpalatability of many herbs, particularly those that are considered very strong medicinally or even toxic, frequently serves as an inherent mechanism to prevent excessive consumption of a harmful herb. The heightened taste sensitivity frequently accompanying pregnancy further reinforces this—many pregnant women find excessive consumption of liquids nauseating and thus they are only able to consume limited amounts of strong-tasting medicinal teas during the gestational period. Water-based preparations also allow ease in evaporating off strong essential oils even from teas that are considered safe for general use (e.g., chamomile, mint), but that do contain essential oil fractions.

A clear disadvantage of water-based preparations is that the volume of liquid (e.g., tea, infusion) one must consume for an effective dose may be difficult to achieve for the aforementioned reasons. Decoctions are concentrated water-based preparations made by simmering or long steeping of a larger ratio of herbs to water than is used for tea. They can be further reduced by simmering down to a concentrate, to which

a sweetener is added for flavor, thickening, and as a preservative; this allows for tablespoon-sized doses rather than cup-sized doses. This can be an effective solution; however, for women who must limit their sugar intake because of gestational or true diabetes, the added sugar must be taken into account.

Tinctures, which are hydroethanolic extractions, offer the advantage of being highly concentrated and are self-preserved, allowing the patient to take small dose sizes. They eliminate the effort of preparation inherent in using teas. Thus they are easy to consume and convenient. Taste often can be masked either by the addition of vegetable glycerin or a flavoring extract, or by "hiding" the dose in a small quantity of fruit juice. These factors often lead to increased compliance with a botanical protocol. However, there are disadvantages to tinctures. Because the water–alcohol combination is such an effective solvent, the medicines contain a full array of plant compounds, some of which might be undesirable for consumption during pregnancy. Additionally, there are concerns regarding the use of alcohol during pregnancy, although the volume of alcohol per dose is typically very small (e.g., in a 5-mL dose of a 40% alcohol tincture, the patient is receiving 2 mL of alcohol; even at three doses per day, this is one fifth of an ounce of alcohol per day). However, in the first trimester, it may be advisable to avoid alcohol entirely. The practitioner and the patient need to determine the risks and benefits of using tinctures during pregnancy on an individual basis. Many naturopathic physicians, herbalists, and midwives are quite comfortable with their use on a limited, as-needed basis.

Capsules and pills, unless made from liquid extracts of freshly milled herb, are notoriously not fresh, and many herbalists consider them less-than-reliable medicines, preferring the use of water- and alcohol-based extracts. A number of companies, however, do make high-quality pills and capsules using plant extracts rather than dried herbs bound with fillers. Understanding of manufacturing practices is essential in determining the quality and reliability of any herbal product.

Because of the high level of absorption that occurs through the intestinal mucosa, enemas may be classified as a form of internal administration. Although they are rarely given during pregnancy (there is some risk that the use of an enema during pregnancy can stimulate uterine contractions through stimulation of bowel evacuation), they can be extremely useful in limited conditions, such as hyperemesis gravidarum, when the pregnant mother is unable to take or retain anything orally. The herbal enema can be a well-tolerated route of administration to provide and retain both fluids and medicine.

External Forms of Herbal Medicines

Externally administered forms of herbal preparations include medicated and extracted oils, baths, compresses, washes, periwashes, vaginal suppositories, creams, salves, and ointments. There is little risk from the topical use of botanical extracts, whether water-, oil-, or alcohol-based during pregnancy, when applied primarily to unbroken skin. One exception is the topical use of concentrated, undiluted (i.e., neat) essential oils, which should be avoided. Extracted nonessential oils, for example calendula oil, and many highly diluted essential oils can be safely used topically for the treatment of skin infections (e.g., fungal infections), for massage to promote relaxation (e.g., three to five drops of lavender and rose essential oils diluted in 2 tablespoons of a carrier oil such as almond oil), or for muscle spasms and aches (e.g., three to five drops each of wintergreen oil and cinnamon oil in 4 tablespoons of almond oil). Certain essential oils, however, are contraindicated for use during pregnancy.

Certain constituents, such as the hepatotoxic PAs present in comfrey, are capable of passing into the bloodstream through the skin. Although the risk is minimal from this small amount of potential exposure, it may be wise to avoid prolonged use of comfrey-containing products on large areas of broken skin during pregnancy.

Vaginal suppositories (see Chapter 3) often may be used safely during pregnancy for the treatment of vaginal infections, providing the herbs they contain are safe for such use during pregnancy. Herbs with suspected or known teratogenicity or mutagenicity, such as thuja, should be avoided, as well as those that might cause uterine stimulation. However, herbs that are typically contraindicated for oral consumption often may be used vaginally in late pregnancy for the treatment of vaginal infection. This should be done with knowledge of the individual herbs in the preparation, or in consultation with a qualified herbalist. Douches should be avoided during pregnancy because of risk of embolism; peri-washes may be used for a vulvar and perineal rinse.

SUMMARY

Herbs can provide substantial relief of common complaints and concerns that arise during pregnancy and childbirth. The power of herbs should be respected during pregnancy, and therefore they should be used with caution. However, many herbs may be contraindicated on the basis of very limited findings, erroneous reports, or by association with a problem rather than a proven causal effect. Many herbs that have not been evaluated may, nonetheless, offer simple, safe, gentle, and effective solutions for many common pregnancy problems ranging from anemia to vaginitis. Practitioners need to be better educated about patients' choices when it comes to herbal medicines; further research needs to be conducted into the safety and efficacy of herbs for both the mother and her baby. In addition, a comparative safety analysis should be done with the herbs and pharmaceuticals commonly used during pregnancy, which are often used without proper proof of safety during the childbearing cycle.

Fertility Challenges

Infertility is defined as the inability to conceive after 12 months of unprotected intercourse in a couple of reproductive age attempting to conceive. Approximately 90% of couples achieve conception within this time, and a further 15% of normally fertile couples take longer than 12 months to become pregnant. Research has shown that even couples in their late thirties have a 91% chance of conceiving naturally within 2 years, and recent studies estimate that an average of 25% to 40% of women have a live birth without treatment during the 3 years after the first infertility consultation, even without treatment.[1-3] Nevertheless, of the approximately 60 million women of reproductive age in the United States in 2002, about 1.2 million, or 2%, had had an infertility-related medical appointment within the previous year and an additional 13% had received infertility services at some time in their lives.[4] This number has increased in recent decades because of societal demographic changes, particularly the aging of the baby boom generation, leading to an increased size of the reproductive age population, and more couples delaying fertility for the sake of careers.[1]

Infertility is not synonymous with sterility and it is important to differentiate these terms. Sterility is defined as the inability to achieve pregnancy and affects only 1% to 2% of couples.[2] Primary infertility refers to those who have never before conceived and secondary infertility to those who have achieved conception at some time in the past (regardless of pregnancy outcome) and thereafter became infertile.[5]

FEMALE FACTORS AFFECTING FERTILITY

The main types of female infertility include ovulatory disorders (25%) and tubal diseases (20% to 25%), including endometriosis (5%). Ovulatory factors are suspected when menstrual abnormalities are reported. Male infertility is the primary cause in approximately 25% of cases and contributes to an additional 15% to 25% of cases.[1] Thorough evaluation of the couple will point to a probable cause in 85% to 90% of cases.[2] Ovarian factors are primarily associated with follicular phase disruptions. An inadequate luteal phase is said to account for only 3% to 4% of fertility failure. Examples of all of the factors that account for fertility challenges are listed in Table 16-1.

Unexplained and coexisting factors account for approximately 10%-20% of infertility cases and can be a result of

The Editor wishes to thank *Botanical Medicine for Women's Health*, ed 1 contributor to this chapter Angela J. Hywood.

environmental and/or occupational exposure to toxicity such as heavy metals, radiation, solvents, DES (diethylstilbestrol), smoking, and exogenous androgens and/or estrogens from environmental and food sources. Nutritional deficiency, stress, and age can all contribute to fertility problems. Abnormal body mass index (BMI), including being underweight or overweight, can cause amenorrhea and infertility. The fertility of a woman begins to significantly decline between the ages of 35 to 38 and sharply declines after the age of 40.

MALE FACTORS AFFECTING FERTILITY

Male factors affecting fertility include:
- Endocrine disorders of the hypothalamus, pituitary, adrenal glands, thyroid
- Anatomic disorders of the male reproductive tract
- Sperm abnormalities
- Abnormal spermatogenesis resulting from chromosomal abnormalities, infection, radiation, or chemical exposure
- Abnormal motility resulting from Kartagener's syndrome (i.e., the absence of cilia), testicular varicoceles, or antibody production (i.e., male immune-mediated infertility)
- Sexual dysfunction, including erectile and ejaculatory dysfunction or decreased libido
- Unexplained factors
- Environmental and occupational toxicity such as exposure to heavy metal, DES, radiation, and exogenous androgens and estrogens
- Nutritional deficiency, particularly zinc and selenium
- Psychological stressors

DIAGNOSIS

Initial evaluation of infertility must include a thorough workup of both partners for male and female factors that might cause fertility problems.

Evaluation of Male Factors
Primary evaluation includes:
- A thorough medical history and physical examination
- Semen analysis

A secondary evaluation is recommended and usually includes more holistic measures:
- Genitourinary infection screening
- Heavy metal screening

TABLE 16-1   Causes of Fertility Challenges

Factor	Examples
Ovulatory	Defects of the ovaries
	Anovulatory cycles
	Hyperprolactinemia
	Hypothalamic dysfunction
	Pituitary dysfunction
	Gonadal dysgenesis
	Premature ovarian failure
	Ovarian resistance
Metabolic	Thyroid disorders
	Adrenal disorders
	Liver disease
	Renal disease
	Androgen excess (i.e., adrenal or neoplastic causes)
Pelvic	Common infection (e.g., genitourinary infections such as *Chlamydia trachomatis, Ureaplasma urealyticum, Mycoplasma hominis,* and *Neisseria gonorrhoeae* causing inflammation, infections, and scar tissue)
	Chronic inflammation manifesting as pelvic inflammatory disease
	Uterine or fallopian adhesions
	Endometriosis (attributed to 5% of cases of infertility)
	Fibroids
	Structural abnormalities
Cervical (evident in only about 3% of cases)	Hostile mucus (e.g., sperm antibodies; abnormal viscosity or pH)
	Cervicitis and infections
	Acquired surgical damage to the mucus-producing endocervical glands (e.g., cone biopsy, laser ablation, cryotherapy) associated with cervical dysplasia or neoplasia
Immune mediated	Lack of blocking antibodies
	Autoimmune disease such as systemic lupus erythematosus
	Immunophenotypes
	Antithyroid antibodies
	Antiphospholipid syndrome

Data from Kaider A, Kaider B, Janowicz P, et al: Immunodiagnostic evaluation in women with reproductive failure, *Am J Reprod Immunol* 42(6):335–346, 1999.

- Male hormone panel
- Adrenal stress index (ASI)

Semen analysis can rule out the most likely abnormalities in male factors. Sperm count, motility, morphology, pH, and white blood cell count need to be reviewed. If the male has not had a semen analysis within the past 3 months before the initial visit to the practitioner, it is suggested that this test be recommended. Spermatogenesis takes approximately 74 days; hence, the viability of the sperm will depend on the environment over the 74-day time frame in which the sperm were developing. If, for example, the man was exposed to dangerous solvents, toxic heavy metals, or radiation, his sperm parameters may reflect abnormalities. The morphology is the most relevant parameter to review because this indicates the most likely chance of that sperm resulting in conception and hence the actual sperm viability. The percentage morphology reflects the number of normally shaped sperm within the sample.

Several genitourinary infections are known to significantly affect both male and female fertility, including *Chlamydia trachomatis, Ureaplasma urealyticum, Mycoplasma hominis,* and *Neisseria gonorrhoeae.* Subclinical infection can contribute to unexplained infertility. Not only can these genitourinary tract infections adversely affect fertility, but they also can potentially cause miscarriage and birth defects.

Evaluation of Female Factors

Primary evaluation should include:
- Thorough medical history and physical examination
- Expanded female hormonal panel
- Evaluation for thyroid disorders
- Evaluation for immunologic disorders, including autoimmune conditions
- Genitourinary infection screening as described earlier for male evaluation
- Cervical cytology

A secondary evaluation is recommended, especially for unidentified infertility:
- Heavy metal screening
- Salivary ASI

In a tertiary evaluation for pelvic factors, minor surgery is often required. These tests require referral to a reproductive medical specialist. These tests and procedures, although sometimes necessary, are invasive, painful, and expensive:
- Hysterosalpingogram for investigation of tubal patency, congenital malformations, polyps, and distal and proximal occlusions
- Transvaginal ultrasound for detection and monitoring of the developing follicle on the ovary
- Endometrial biopsy sampling to determine the maturation of the endometria
- Laparoscopy for detection of tubal abnormalities such as agglutinated fimbria or adhesions, tubal cysts, and endometriosis
- Serum tests for immune-mediated infertility

Mutual Fertility Testing

The postcoital test (i.e., Sims-Huhner test) is an evaluation of the sperm's interaction within cervical mucus postcoitally. This test is designed to evaluate the number of sperm that survive within the mucus and their duration of survival. This test can rule out parameters such as inadequate quantity and clarity of cervical mucus, spinnbarkeit (fibrosity, or stringiness of mucus) of greater than 8 cm, and nonforward progressive sperm in the mucus. When the quality and quantity of mucus is good, yet the test results are abnormal, then further evaluation for cervical mucus antisperm antibodies is warranted. It is a debatable test for efficacy but is used to assess cervical hostility to sperm. Hostile mucus can result from the presence of sperm antibodies and/or an unfavorable pH of cervical mucus.

Noninvasive Home Evaluation and Patient Participation: Thermo-Symptal Monitoring, and Mucus and Cervical Evaluation for Detection of Ovulation

As fertility evaluation can be physically invasive, traumatic, and cost prohibitive, there are some useful tests women can do themselves at home. One easy technique is thermo-symptal monitoring, which involves the monitoring and recording of the basal body temperature (BBT) and recording of cervical mucus secretions on a daily basis throughout the cycle. Although convenient and cost-effective, thermo-symptal monitoring requires consistent commitment and a learned awareness of the body's subtle signs of fertility. This awareness can help the couple refine conception timing and allow the woman a sense of participation in her own program toward achieving pregnancy.

Basal Body Temperature Monitoring

The luteal phase of the cycle is characterized by the production of progesterone from the corpus luteum. Progesterone is a thermogenic hormone that elevates the core body temperature in the luteal phase of the cycle. When adequate progesterone is produced as a result of ovulation having occurred, the BBT elevates and remains elevated for approximately 10 days after ovulation; at this point either menses occurs, in which the temperature will drop, or pregnancy is established, in which the temperature will continue to elevate to a third phase as the progesterone continues to be produced into the pregnancy. This elevation in temperature usually occurs 1 to 2 days after ovulation.

Interpretation of the Basal Body Temperature

In the follicular, preovulatory phase of the menstrual cycle in a healthy woman, the temperature reading is approximately 97° F. An increase in temperature greater than 97° F in the luteal phase, after day 13 or 14, is indicative of a normal ovulation in 90% of cases. If the temperature maintains above this temperature after 16 days, this is suggestive of pregnancy. The BBT is measured orally first thing upon waking in the morning, before any activity, with a specific fertility thermometer (i.e., thermocrystal basal thermometer). The temperature is best taken at the same time each day, after at least 6 hours of sleep. The routine should commence on the first day of the cycle, which corresponds to the first day of menstrual flow. Sleeping with an electric blanket, heated waterbeds, or other heating or cooling devices near the body may disrupt the BBT and adversely affect the reading; hence they need to be avoided when monitoring BBT. BBT cannot be used by the couple to predict ovulation; it only confirms ovulation retrospectively by indicating the event of luteinization but is considered a relatively reliable assessment of the preovulatory phase. Used as a single tool, it proves to be of limited value.

When BBT is monitored concurrently with cervical mucus observations, it can be a very informative and valuable tool for the couple.

Monitoring Cervical Mucus Changes

Daily monitoring of the texture, quality, and quantity of cervical mucus secretions can be useful to predict ovulation. Cervical mucus secretions change throughout the cycle under the influence of estrogen and progesterone. Approximately 2 or 3 days before ovulation occurs, the estrogen levels peak and the nature of the mucus changes from a pasty thick or milky consistency to a distinctive spinnbarkeit: stretchy mucus (usually 6 to 10 cm) of wet consistency and opaque color. It resembles a similar texture and nature to raw egg white. At this stage of the cycle, the mucus is an optimal reservoir to nourish sperm and encourage their survival for conception. When seen under a microscope, fertile spinnbarkeit mucus dries into a distinctive crystalline fernlike pattern. Small, inexpensive ovulation predictor microscopes for home use are available to assist couples in predicting ovulation. Saliva is usually used on the microscope as an alternative to cervical mucus because saliva mimics the ferning pattern of the spinnbarkeit at ovulation. When estrogen levels are lower in the early follicular phase and midluteal phase of the cycle, the mucus secretions are thin, milky, and sparse in nature. When a woman is monitoring cervical mucus, it is recommended she feel the texture of the mucus at the vaginal opening between the forefinger and thumb. Do not use toilet tissue to collect the sample; it absorbs moisture and may lead to misinterpretation of the mucus viscosity. Home test kits that measure urinary LH levels are available for ovulation prediction. These are single use tests and their disadvantage is the expense when used regularly.

The Texture and Shape of the Cervix

Some women experiencing infertility may produce inadequate quantities of cervical mucus or experience difficulty feeling the texture of the mucus. In this case she can be taught to feel the texture of the cervix itself. When cervical tissue is not under the influence of peak estrogen levels it feels hard, cartilaginous (imagine feeling the end of the nose; this is a similar texture), and the cervical os is closed. At the time of the LH surge and estrogen peak, the cervix becomes soft, "ripe," and palpable (imagine feeling the texture of the cheeks; this is a similar texture) and the cervical os is slightly open.

CONVENTIONAL TREATMENT APPROACHES

Despite developments in fertility knowledge and technologies, the overall prognosis for achieving childbirth with reproductive technologies is approximately 50%, and declines as women age. Each treatment option has overt and hidden costs, including emotional, physical, and financial burdens, often without justification because of lack of success. Couples entering fertility treatment need to be fully cognizant of the potential price of treatment in all of these areas, and the benefit versus costs must be evaluated. Patients must also consider the high frequency and implications of a multiple pregnancy, a common outcome with assisted reproductive technologies. Psychological support should be available to all couples considering reproductive technologies, with no blame laid upon either partner, and a realistic appraisal of the chances for success and failure of treatment honestly provided. Reproductive expert Marcelle Cedars advises, "The option of child-free living should also be included in any discussion. At times couples must be advised to stop treatment if the likelihood for success is quite low. Frequently this is a very difficult time for both the patient and the physician, but fruitless treatment should be avoided."[1]

Ovulatory Factors

The conventional treatment of ovulatory factors is determined by the conclusive diagnosis made after clinical investigation. With conventional infertility therapy, the chances of conception are said to be 15% to 25% per cycle, depending on the degree of drug-induced ovarian stimulation. If failure to conceive after a maximum of 12 cycles persists, then assisted reproductive technology (ART) is recommended as the next option by allopathic medical reproductive specialists.

Ovarian Stimulation Therapy

Induction of ovulation is said to be successful in 90% to 95% of cases with administration of particular pharmaceutical drugs in a given scenario. Each given scenario depends on a specific set of circumstances, such as hormonal imbalances or failure of a prior drug approach.

In cases of elevated follicle-stimulating hormone (FSH), indicating ovarian failure, postmenopause, or ovarian resistance, fertility cannot be restored using drugs. Options for these women include adoption, or embryo or egg donation. Success of pregnancy with embryo or egg donation is reported to be approximately 40%, but this does not reflect live birth statistics for the given scenario. This scenario also gives rise to multifactorial ethical, legal, financial, and psychosocial issues.

In the case of chronic anovulation with normal FSH and normal prolactin levels, first line therapy is clomiphene citrate, a nonsteroidal, antiestrogen drug. This drug is prescribed for women with oligomenorrhea, amenorrhea (including polycystic ovarian syndrome [PCOS] and psychogenic amenorrhea), and women who have insufficient estradiol levels or luteal phase deficiency (progesterone failure). This is administered orally at 50 to 250 mg daily on days 5 to 10 of the cycle. It is often combined with corticosteroids, estrogen, and midcycle human chorionic gonadotropin (hCG), and followed up with monthly hormonal testing or ultrasound to establish the drug's efficacy in stimulating the follicle and ovulation. Clomiphene citrate is reported to be successful in stimulating ovulation in 70% of cases. The pregnancy rate from use of this drug is only 35%. In 50% of women who use clomiphene citrate, it stimulates more than one follicle, and the incidence of multiple births is 8%. It is recommended that it not be used for longer than six cycles. Use for longer than 12 months may

increase the risk of ovarian cancer. Side effects of clomiphene citrate include hot flashes, breast tenderness, mood swings, visual problems, thick cervical mucus, luteal phase deficiency (although it is routinely prescribed for this problem), ovarian enlargement, abdominal-pelvis bloating, and discomfort. Ovarian hyperstimulation syndrome has been associated with this drug therapy.

Where there is failure to respond to clomiphene citrate, or in patients with pituitary insufficiency and/or hypothalamic insufficiency, unexplained infertility, or endometriosis, a second line of treatment is used to induce ovarian stimulation: human menopausal gonadotropin (hMG), a pituitary peptide hormone. This is a combination of FSH and luteinizing hormone (LH) derived from the urine of menopausal women. Administration is by intramuscular injection one to two times per day at a dose of 75 to 600 IU/day. This drug regimen is also used to stimulate the ovaries in preparation for ART procedures such as in vitro fertilization (IVF), gamete intrafallopian transfer (GIFT), or zygote intrafallopian transfer (ZIFT). hMG is said to be successful in stimulating ovulation in 85% to 90% of cases. It increases the multiple pregnancy rates up to 20% and increases the risk of both ovarian hyperstimulation syndrome and ovarian cancer. Side effects include mood swings and ovarian hyperstimulation.

When the diagnosis of hypothalamic dysfunction has been established and ovarian stimulation using clomiphene citrate fails, gonadotrophin-releasing hormone (GnRH), a hormone produced by the hypothalamus, is administered. This step is said to restore ovulation in nearly all cases. Restoring ovulation does not necessarily result in a successful pregnancy.

When elevated prolactin levels are causing amenorrhea or luteal phase defects are confirmed (e.g., in PCOS), bromocriptine is used. In this circumstance, thyroid function is also evaluated, as primary hypothyroidism can cause elevated prolactin levels. Many pharmaceutical drugs can also cause hyperprolactinemia as a side effect. This needs to be considered and ruled out. Hyperprolactinemia is treated using bromocriptine, a dopamine agonist. Administration is either oral or vaginally at doses of 2.5 mg twice daily or 0.5 mg twice a week. Bromocriptine does not increase the risk of inducing multiple pregnancies. Side effects include weakness, nausea, and nasal congestion.

Pelvic Factors

Endometriosis and the effects of salpingitis are the most common problems causing infertility related to pelvic factors. These affect the structural health of the fallopian tubes, as well as uterine and endometrial tissue. Salpingitis is usually caused by infections with microorganisms such as *N. gonorrhea* and *C. trichomatosis;* other infective organisms include *Escherichia coli, M. hominis,* and *U. urealyticum.*[6] Bacterial vaginosis is common among these women. Antibiotic drugs are the usual treatment for these infections.[7] The treatment option for moderate and advanced endometriosis is usually surgical; at the time of a laparoscopy, resection and ablation is performed. Fibroids are usually left untouched and are only addressed if multiple miscarriages have been a problem. ART is available for those who are unable to conceive after surgery for common pelvic factors.

Cervical Factors

Inadequate midcycle cervical mucus is treated in one of two ways. Either low-dose estrogen or hMG is given mid to late in the follicular phase, or hMG is given, to stimulate ovarian production of estrogen. If this fails, the couples are recommended to use artificial insemination (AI), one of the oldest fertility treatments still used. If cervicitis is a possible causal factor, the antibiotic doxycycline is administered. If surgery (commonly cone biopsy or laser ablation) or congenital issues render the endocervical glands absent or damaged, intrauterine insemination (IUI) procedures can result in pregnancy in 20% to 30% of cases within three cycles of treatment. Those who fail to have a positive outcome are offered the possibility of IVF, GIFT, or ZIFT.

Unexplained Infertility

When both partners' evaluations yield negative results, this is defined as unexplained infertility. This is found in only 10%-20% of cases.[7] The main courses of treatment for couples with unexplained fertility include observation of the cycle and refining of timing techniques for intercourse, ovarian stimulation, IUI, GIFT, and IVF.

THE BOTANICAL PRACTITIONER'S PERSPECTIVE

Botanical treatment of infertility cannot address overt physical impediments to fertility; however, it can provide treatment and support for numerous fertility-related problems, such as hormonal dysregulation, thyroid and adrenal disorders, genitourinary infections, immune dysregulation, and stress-related problems (Table 16-2). The herbal consultation also takes into account factors such as nutritional deficiency and occupational/environmental exposures. Most importantly, a holistic practitioner reviews the case as a totality of contributing factors, not simply a reproductive issue.

Fertility challenges should be approached as an opportunity for the couple to engage in an active treatment plan to improve their overall health, rather than just a quest for reproduction. Couples should be encouraged to participate in a 3- to 4-month period of preconception care, in which their

TABLE 16-2 Botanical Treatment Strategies for Female Infertility			
Therapeutic Goal	**Therapeutic Activity**	**Botanical Name**	**Common Name**
Hormonal regulation	Hormonal regulation	*Actaea racemosa*	Black cohosh
Fertility tonic	Fertility tonic	*Angelica sinensis*	Dong quai
	Proestrogenic	*Asparagus racemosa*	Shatavari
	Proprogesterogenic	*Chamaelirium luteum*	False unicorn
	Reproductive tonic	*Dioscorea villosa*	Wild yam
	Regulate prolactin	*Paeonia lactiflora*	White peony
	Unknown activities	*Serenoa repens*	Saw palmetto
		Tribulus terrestris	Tribulus
		Vitex agnus-castus	Chaste berry
Support immune response	Antimicrobial	*Albizia lebbeck*	Albizia
Treat vaginal infection	Immunotonic	*Echinacea* spp.	Echinacea
Reduce inflammation	Antiinflammatory	*Glycyrrhiza glabra*	Licorice
		Hydrastis canadensis	Goldenseal
Detoxification of environmental toxins	Promote phase 1 and phase 2 detoxification	*Bupleurum falcatum*	Bupleurum
		Picrorhiza kurroa	Picrorrhiza
	Support hepatic function	*Schisandra chinensis*	Schisandra
		Silybum marianum	Milk thistle
	Antioxidant activity	*Camellia sinensis*	Green tea
		Curcuma longa	Tumeric
		Ginkgo biloba	Ginkgo
		Rosmarinus officinalis	Rosemary
		Silybum marianum	Milk thistle
		Vitis vinifera	Grape seed
Relieve stress	Nervines	*Avena sativa*	Milky oats
		Leonurus cardiaca	Motherwort
		Matricaria recutita	Chamomile
		Melissa officinalis	Lemon balm
		Scutellaria lateriflora	Skullcap
		Stachys betonica	Wood betony
			(Also see index for references to nervines throughout the text)
Relieve stress	Adaptogens	See Chapter 5	

overall health can be improved with the use of herbs, nutrition, and dietary and lifestyle modification. Thus not only will they then improve their chance of natural conception, but they will be more likely to have a healthy, complication-free pregnancy and a healthy child. Additionally, for many couples, the attempt to conceive can become mechanical, lacking in passion, and plagued by a repeating cycle of expectation and disappointment. Ideally, botanical treatments for infertility attend to this problem, offering common sense and herbal strategies for restoring sensuality and passion to conception.

Herbal therapy requires a minimum commitment of 3 to 4 months to improve the fertility of a couple before conception, and in general, is ideally done when the couple is not concurrently taking any pharmaceutical fertility drug. Herbal medicines and nutritional supplements are prescribed for each individual situation, with appropriate dietary and lifestyle modification, stress management, and detoxification measures, if necessary (e.g., caused by environmental toxin exposure). The protocol should be revised on a regular basis (e.g., monthly) until conception occurs. If conception has not resulted after 12 months of holistic therapy, then other medical options may be considered. The treatment protocol in the remainder of this chapter focuses on botanical treatments for female fertility.

Herbs that enhance fertility might be divided into categories, and although they may overlap, they serve different purposes in nurturing reproductive health and general wellness. These categories include nutritive herbs that build the blood (e.g., rehmannia, dong quai) and support hepatic function (e.g., milk thistle); herbs that restore hormonal balance (e.g., chaste berry) and impart pelvic tone (e.g., shatavari); herbs that improve pelvic circulation (e.g., dong quai); and adaptogenic (e.g., ashwagandha) and nervine herbs (e.g., vervain), which help to reduce stress and improve the stress response.

Herbs can also be used externally in the form of essential oils to stimulate sexual desire (i.e., aphrodisiacs), and include amber, sandalwood, rose, jasmine, and ylang-ylang. A few drops can be carefully placed on the body (i.e., slightly diluted in a carrier oil such as almond oil), used in an atomizer to scent the air, sprinkled onto linens, or placed in a bath.

DISCUSSION OF BOTANICAL PROTOCOL

Black Cohosh

Black cohosh was thought to have estrogen-modulating activity and is used for both ovarian insufficiency affecting fertility and estrogen dominance affecting infertility (e.g., one factor in PCOS). It has been described as a selective estrogen receptor modulator (SERM). It was a favorite herb of the native North American Indians and Eclectic physicians for amenorrhea, as a uterine tonic, and for a number of other gynecologic applications.[8-10] Black cohosh has been subjected to extensive clinical trials, demonstrating some estrogen-modulating activity and ability to reduce elevated LH levels, but not affecting FSH and prolactin in any way. In modern herbal applications, black cohosh is indicated for infertility associated with anovulation, PCOS, ovulatory pain, and secondary amenorrhea. Some common side effects have been noted, including a frontal headache

with a dull, full, or bursting feeling, and a low frequency of stomach complaints, including nausea and vomiting. These side effects are most likely with the high end of a therapeutic daily dose. Recent concerns have arisen that black cohosh may be associated with liver disease, including liver failure; therefore caution should be observed with its use. It is recommended that this herb be avoided in pregnancy.

Chaste Berry

Chaste berry has a long history of use for regulating menstrual cycles, which may result from its ability to regulate prolactin levels, enhance corpus luteum development, and correct relative progesterone deficiency. *Vitex agnus-castus* is beneficial for ovulatory factors associated with infertility, in particular modulating the anterior pituitary's production of LH and mildly inhibiting FSH. *V. agnus-castus* has been shown to downregulate the production of excess prolactin in hyperprolactinemia via dopaminergic activity.[8,11] In an uncontrolled study, chaste berry reduced elevated prolactin levels in 80% of 34 women with hyperprolactinemia at a dosage of 30 to 40 mg per day for 1 month and improved symptoms of a variety of menstrual disorders, including secondary amenorrhea, cystic hyperplasia of the endometrium, deficient corpus luteum function, metrorrhagia, polymenorrhea, and oligomenorrhea.[8] Chaste berry reduces thyrotropin-releasing hormone (TRH)–induced prolactin release (essentially a pituitary–thyroid axis problem), normalizes shortened luteal phases, corrects luteal phase progesterone deficiencies, and reduces premenstrual syndrome (PMS) symptoms in women with luteal phase defects caused by latent hyperprolactinemia. In two uncontrolled studies involving 45 infertile women with normal prolactin and pathologically low progesterone, 39 of the women achieved pregnancy after 3 months on chaste berry. In a second study involving 31 women with infertility, after 3 months 15 of these women were pregnant. Of these women who became pregnant using chaste berry, seven previously had amenorrhea, four had luteal insufficiency, and four had been diagnosed with unexplained infertility. A 2006 double-blind randomized controlled trial (RCT) tested the use of the polyherbal supplement Fertilityblend (FB; containing chaste berry, green tea, L-arginine, vitamins [e.g., zinc folate], and minerals) for the improvement of fertility in women. A group of 93 women met eligibility criteria (i.e., unable to conceive for 6 to 36 months) and were randomized to receive the supplement or placebo for 3 months. Outcomes measured included BBT, progesterone, menstrual cycle length, and rates of conception. The FB group ($n = 53$) experienced more days with BBT higher than 98° F, high midluteal serum progesterone, normalization of menstrual cycle length, and 26% of women were pregnant after 3 months. In contrast, the control group ($n = 40$) did not experience changes among these parameters, and a 10% pregnancy rate was observed. The treatment was well tolerated (Dose information not available).[12]

Chaste berry should be considered a first-line botanical therapy for infertility associated with secondary amenorrhea, hyperprolactinemia, and luteal insufficiency, and should be given for a duration of at least 3 to 6 months. Chaste berry is particularly effective in restoring the menstrual cycle in a woman after years of taking oral contraceptive pills, and improving low LH levels. The daily dose of chaste berry needed to improve ovulatory factors affecting fertility is 1 to 4 mL of tincture or 500 to 1000 mg of dried berries daily. It is best taken as a single dose in the morning. Chaste berry is preferably not taken with other progesterone drugs and may interact antagonistically with pharmaceutical dopamine receptor antagonist drugs.

Dong Quai

Dong quai has been used in Traditional Chinese Medicine (TCM) as a female reproductive tonic, menstrual regulator, and remedy for amenorrhea for at least 20 centuries. Dong quai is regarded as a tonic for women with fatigue and low vitality. Traditional prescribing indicated dong quai for conditions of what is referred to as congealed blood, evidenced by clots in the menstrual blood, endometriosis, and dark, sluggish menstrual flow, and is typically used in formulae to harmonize the blood. In one uncontrolled trial involving infertility resulting from tubal occlusion, a dong quai extract was administered via vaginal irrigation (i.e., douche) for up to 9 months. Approximately 80% of the women regained tubal patency and 53% became pregnant. The known constituents of dong quai include coumarins, essential oils, ferulic acids, psoralens, vitamin B_{12}, and folinic acid, the active form of folic acid. Dong quai does not have estrogenic activity.

Dong quai is contraindicated for women with heavy bleeding and those with a history of spontaneous miscarriage. This herb is contraindicated for use with warfarin and anticoagulant medications because it may increase bleeding time.

False Unicorn

False unicorn has been used historically as a female reproductive tonic, particularly for infertility and atony of the female reproductive organs. It was used by the Eclectic physicians as a uterine tonic to promote tone and vigor of the reproductive organs. For infertility, false unicorn is used when there is insufficient cervical mucus and amenorrhea. It was considered useful for congestion or stagnation of the uterus and ovaries, in which the menstrual blood is dark, sluggish, and clotted. Although not well characterized phytochemically, the steroidal saponins chamaelirin and diosgenin have been identified in false unicorn, and are postulated to exert an estrogen-modulating activity via interaction with estrogen receptor sites of the hypothalamus. There is no known toxicity or contraindication to use of false unicorn; however, this plant is a threatened species because of excessive wild harvesting and may soon be endangered. Therefore this herb should only be used if other steroidal saponin–containing herbs such as tribulus and wild yam do not deliver a desired result and only when absolutely indicated.

Goldenseal

Goldenseal was the chief herb used by the Eclectics as a mucous membrane tonic. It was used for acute and subacute inflammation of the mucous membranes, especially when accompanied by discharge or mucus catarrh. It is valuable for the treatment for inflammation and infection of the genitourinary tract. The constituents include isoquinoline alkaloids, hydrastine, berberine, hydrastinine, and canadine. Goldenseal is a valuable remedy for ulceration, inflammation, and erosion of the cervix, affecting both quality and quantity of the cervical mucus. It can be used in both topical and internal applications.

Saw Palmetto

The Eclectic physicians used saw palmetto as a urinary and reproductive tract remedy for inflammation. It was widely used for ovarian pain, pelvic congestion, and atrophy of the ovaries. It proves to be a useful herb to include for infertility in cases of pelvic factors associated with infertility and infertility caused by PCOS. It is known to inhibit the production of prolactin from the pituitary.[13] If there is a history of genitourinary infection or pelvic inflammatory disease (PID), Saw palmetto is a valuable herb. The daily dose is 2 to 4 mL of a dried plant extract.

Shatavari

Shatavari is a traditional Ayurvedic herb. The root is used medicinally. In the Indian medicine system, shatavari is said to "give her capacity to have a hundred husbands."[14] In traditional Ayurvedic gynecologic prescribing, shatavari has been used as a nutritive tonic, general female reproductive tonic, fertility tonic, treatment for sexual debility, and as an aphrodisiac. It has also been used traditionally as a tonic for lactating women to improve the quality and quantity of breast milk. Pharmacologic research has found the key constituents of shatavari are steroidal saponins, including shatavarin-I, alkaloids, and mucilage. The presence of the steroidal saponins suggest shatavari's activity as an estrogen modulator and a menstrual cycle regulator. Shatavari has adaptogenic and immunomodulating properties and is a very useful tonic herb for women with stress-induced and immune-mediated infertility. It has antibacterial action; hence it should be considered a general reproductive tonic for any woman who has a history of genitourinary infections. There are no known contraindications to the use of shatavari. The daily dose is 4.5 to 8.5 mL of a dried plant extract.

Tribulus

There is little information on the traditional use of tribulus leaf. In Ayurvedic medicine, the fruit has been used for improving male fertility and male erectile function, uterine disorders, urinary disorders, kidney stones, gout, and gonorrhea. As a result of Bulgarian research, tribulus has become a popular herb for the treatment of infertility, menopause, and low libido. It acts as a general tonic and aphrodisiac, and is used to restore vitality, reduce the physiologic effects of stress, and is a powerful fertility tonic for both men and women.[8]

Open-label clinical trials have demonstrated improvements in both male and female infertility.[15] Bulgarian research has identified a unique steroidal saponin known as a furostanol saponin, calculated to be no less than 45% protodioscin. The leaf is noted to be higher in the unique saponin than the fruit. Other active constituents include phytosterols and spirostanol glycosides. The results of studies and clinical trials with tribulus have been remarkable, both in animal and human models. When given at a dose of 750 mg per day for 5 days it increased serum FSH and estradiol compared with baseline in females, and increased LH and testosterone in males, demonstrating an increase in sex hormone production for both men and women.[8] The steroidal saponins are thought to bind and weakly stimulate the hypothalamic estrogen receptor sites. The tonic activities of tribulus have been shown to act by intensifying protein synthesis and enhancing the activity of enzymes associated with energy metabolism. It increases iron absorption from the small intestines and inhibits lipid peroxidation during stress. This leads to more muscle strength and improved endurance and stamina.[8]

Another stunning study showed that tribulus increased serum growth hormone, insulin, and aldosterone without exceeding normal values. Protodioscin, the steroidal saponin in tribulus, has been shown to improve sexual desire via the conversion of protodioscin to dehydroepiandrosterone (DHEA).[16] It has been observed that tribulus grown in different soils does not consistently produce the important active fucosterol, protodioscin. To ensure the desired clinical results, it is recommended to use only Bulgarian-grown tribulus standardized to 40% furosterol saponins by ultraviolet (UV) analysis. It is not interchangeable with Chinese or Indian tribulus. When samples of these were analyzed, they were shown to contain only 3% steroidal saponins by UV analysis, and none of these steroidal saponins are the unique and desirable furosterols. Specific female fertility studies have been conducted with tribulus. In an open study with 36 infertile women who were given tribulus on days 5 to 14 of the menstrual cycle for 2 to 3 months, 6% became pregnant as a result of normalized ovulation, 61% demonstrated normalized ovulation and no pregnancy, and 33% demonstrated no effect from tribulus within the 2- to 3-month time frame of the study.[17] In this same study, another subgroup of women used tribulus concurrently with pharmaceutical ovarian stimulation via the drug epimestrol. Of the 62 women in this group, within 2 to 3 months 39% had normalized ovulation and resultant pregnancy, 35% had normalized ovulation with no pregnancy, and the remaining 26% had no effect from the combined therapy. The results obtained from using tribulus concurrently with epimestrol were better than using the drug alone.

Although no increased frequency of fetal malformation or other harm has been observed in limited use by women during pregnancy, tribulus is considered contraindicated in pregnancy according to TCM; in at least one animal study, decreased survival was observed in the offspring of penned pregnant ewes fed the herb.[15] In dogs, an alcoholic extract of the whole plant produced a sharp vasodepression through a cholinergic mechanism.[17] Ingestion of tribulus by sheep produced outbreaks of a locomotor disorder known as staggers, an asymmetric locomotor disorder in sheep produced by a central functional abnormality.[18] Ingestion of tribulus

caused photosensitivity in animals. No human or animal teratogenicity data are available, and scientific evidence for the safe use of tribulus during pregnancy is not available. The daily dose of tribulus is equivalent to 40 g per day of dried leaf or a concentrated extract standardized to contain a minimum of furostanol saponins like protodioscin at 300 to 400 mg per day. It is best used on days 5 to 14 of the menstrual cycle for enhanced fertility. It is essential to ensure phytoequivalence for optimal therapeutic outcomes. It is advisable to discontinue tribulus use during the luteal phase of the menstrual cycle, and to absolutely not resume use if pregnancy is suspected.

White Peony

White peony is commonly used in traditional Chinese and Japanese medicine for gynecologic conditions. It is generally used for infertility associated with PCOS, hyperprolactinemia, endometriosis, ovarian failure, and androgen excess. *Paeonia lactiflora* has been shown to positively influence low progesterone, reduce elevated androgens (e.g., testosterone), and modulate estrogen and prolactin. In vitro, the active constituent paeoniflorin has been shown to affect the ovarian follicle by its action on the aromatase enzyme. Aromatase is important for follicular maturation, ovulation and corpus luteum function, steroid hormone synthesis, and the regulation of conversion of androgens to estrogens. The biofeedback in the pituitary and hypothalamus rely on aromatase to regulate prolactin and GnRH. Excess levels of prolactin and GnRH inhibit the activity of aromatase. In TCM, *P. lactiflora* is always used in combination with other herbs. A TCM formula that contains *P. lactiflora* and used in application for infertility is Keishi-Bukuryo-Gan (TJ-25) or Cinnamon and Hoelen Formula. One study with TJ-25 demonstrated, when used for 14 consecutive days in rats, increased plasma levels of LH by 94%, FSH by 67%, and estradiol by 50%. This formula is thought to be a GnRH antagonist and mildly antiestrogenic. When combined with *Glycyrrhiza glabra*, *P. lactiflora* is effective at promoting fertility and improving pregnancy rates in cases of androgen excess, as learned from the TCM Licorice and Peony Formula.[19] This combination regulates LH to FSH ratios.

Wild Yam

Wild yam has been used traditionally for uterine and ovarian spasm, including dysmenorrhea. When used for infertility it is employed to optimize estrogen levels and improve the quality and quantity of cervical mucus, if the cervical mucus is too viscous or too sparse. The active constituents of wild yam include the steroidal saponins dioscin and gracilin, and quinuclidine alkaloids such as dioscorine and tannins. It is useful as an antispasmodic to sooth oviductal and fallopian tube spasm, which can interfere with conception and implantation. For optimal bioavailability, the herb relies on adequate gut flora to enable conversion of the steroidal saponin aglycone diosin to diosgenin. It is currently speculated that the bowel flora consumes a glycoside molecule from diosin, liberating diosgenin. Diosgenin is absorbed through the mucous membranes of the bowel into the bloodstream. Diosgenin may exert its effect by interaction at the hypothalamic estrogen receptor sites, regulating the production of estrogen by encouraging an increased production of FSH from the pituitary. Wild yam has demonstrated an estrogenic activity in vitro, and was shown to enhance estradiol by binding to estrogen receptor cites. Wild yam has no known side effects, interactions, or contraindications.

Immune Support

Immunologic factors affecting fertility are prevalent. Most cases result in recurrent spontaneous miscarriage; however, in some cases immunologic concerns prevent conception. The development of antisperm antibodies is one such circumstance. In a study of 1020 female patients with primary or secondary infertility, serum antisperm antibody, antiovarian antibody, antiendometrial antibody, and antihCG antibody levels were tested. Patients were treated with dexamethasone, vitamin E, and vitamin C for three cycles consecutively as one course. After one course of treatment with corticosteroids, the disappearance rates of the antibodies mentioned were over 90%, and the average pregnancy rate was up to 30%. Corticosteroid use is associated with significant side effects.[7] Herbs can be used either as an alternative first-line therapy or concurrently. An example of herb–drug synergy was seen when *Glycyrrhiza glabra* and cortisone were successfully used together to minimize the dose dependence of the corticosteroid drug.[8] *Glycyrrhiza glabra* has a cortisol-sparing action, as well as antiinflammatory and adrenal restorative actions. It is contraindicated in hypertension, and steroid doses need to be modulated.

Rehmannia glutinosa is also of benefit in immune-mediated infertility and subfertility. Constituents in cured (i.e., cooked in wine) rehmannia, known as di huang, have been shown to inhibit antibody formation and reduce allergic reaction. Rehmannia has been shown to reduce the suppressive side effects of corticosteroid drugs on endogenous levels of corticosteroids. It would be a valuable adjunctive therapy for a woman with immune-mediated infertility if using this drug therapy. It is sweet and warm in property and has been used to regulate menstruation and promote blood production, and is preferred in this application over the raw rehmannia.

Echinacea is a well-known traditional immune-enhancing herb. It was widely used by Native Americans and then adopted by the Eclectic physicians for general immune support and infections. It is beneficial in the preconception stage of an infertility protocol to help immune surveillance. Echinacea can be aptly described as an immune modulator, assisting in enhanced phagocytosis and immune recognition. This may just be the key factor needed to regulate or prevent the onset of an autoimmune issue preventing conception or continued pregnancy. This action of echinacea is thought to be as a result of the presence of alkyl amides within the Echinacea root.[20]

Albizia is a traditional Ayurvedic herb with antiallergenic properties. It has been shown to stabilize mast cells, reducing levels of allergy-inducing antibodies.[13] Although not phytochemically well defined, albizia is a useful herb to support women who are producing antisperm antibodies.

NUTRITIONAL CONSIDERATIONS

Diet can play a significant role in fertility. Specific nutrients enhance normal reproductive function and fertility, thus assisting in resolving conception problems when these are insufficient in the diet. These include zinc (found in pumpkin and sunflower seeds, brewer's yeast, wheat germ, soybeans, eggs, seafoods, and meats), calcium (found in dairy products, leafy green vegetables, seaweeds, almonds, and blackstrap molasses), magnesium (found in whole grains, dark-green veggies, blackstrap molasses, nuts, and seafoods), vitamin C (found in citrus fruits, rose hips, cherries, currants, alfalfa sprouts, cantaloupe, strawberries, broccoli, peppers, and tomatoes), and folic acid (found in dark-green leafy vegetables, root vegetables, whole grains, milk, salmon, and brewer's yeast). Women who are very thin, with scanty or irregular periods or anovulation, may be able to achieve cycle regularity, ovulation, and conception by gaining enough weight to bring them into a normal weight for height range.

Between 1990 and 1993, Foresight, a British medical association for the promotion of preconception, conducted a study using a nutritional and lifestyle modification preconception care program. The results were nothing less than remarkable. There was a tenfold reduction in the expected incidence of miscarriage and birth defects and over 80% success rate with unexplained infertility. It was evaluated that before the study was started, 60% of the women drank alcohol regularly and 57% of the women involved were previously smokers. Out of the 367 couples in the study, 327 (89%) of them successfully became pregnant and 327 children were born. All of these babies were born healthy. Among the 204 couples with infertility problems, 175 (86%) were able to achieve a healthy pregnancy.[21] One of the most significant aspects of these results was the involvement of both partners in the program—both female and male factors were concurrently addressed. In addition to nutritional supplementation, the study included lifestyle and social modifications, including the cessation of both smoking and coffee and alcohol consumption. Smoking cigarettes and coffee consumption have been linked to subfertility and delayed conception.[22-24] Based on the Foresight study, the suggested preconception care nutritional program is outlined in Table 16-3.[21]

Antioxidants

A secondary analysis of RCT data aimed to determine whether antioxidant intake in women was associated with shorter time to pregnancy (TTP) among couples undergoing treatment for infertility. The authors concluded that shorter TTP was observed among women with BMI <25 kg/m² with higher vitamin C intake, women with BMI ≥25 kg/m² with

TABLE 16-3   Preconception Care Nutritional Supplementation

Nutrient	Daily Dose
Beta carotene	6 mg
Vitamin E	500 IU
Vitamin D	200 IU
B_1, B_2, B_3, B_5	50 mg each
B_{12}	400 µg
B_6	Up to 250 mg
Biotin	200 µg
Choline	25 mg
Inositol	25 mg
Para-aminobenzoic Acid (PABA)	25 mg
Folic acid	500 mg
Vitamin C	2000-3000 mg
Bioflavonoid	300 mg
Calcium	800 mg
Magnesium	400 mg
Potassium	15 mg
Iron	15 mg
Iodine	75 µg
Selenium	100-200 µg
Zinc	20-60 mg
Chromium	100-200 µg
Omega-3 essential fatty acids (e.g., evening primrose oil)	500-1000 mg
Omega-6 essential fatty acids (e.g., fish oil, flaxseed oil)	500-1000 mg

increased β-carotene, women <35 y with higher β-carotene and vitamin C, and women ≥35 y with higher vitamin E. There were no differences in mean intake of any of the antioxidants between women who delivered a live infant during the study period versus those who did not.[25]

Omega-3/Polyunsaturated Fatty Acids

Essential fatty acids, found in wild cold-water fish, most vegetable oils, flaxseed oil, evening primrose oil, borage oil, and black current oil, are important for conception. A prospective study on the effects of preconception omega-3 polyunsaturated fatty acids (PUFA) intake, estradiol levels, and IVF and sperm injection outcome found that high α-linolenic acid (ALA) increased baseline estradiol, and high docosahexaenoic acid (DHA) and eicosapentaenoic acid (EPA) decreased estradiol as well as the number of follicles after ovarian stimulation.[26]

Vitamin D

A prospective cross-sectional study was conducted to investigate IVF outcome in women with 25-hydroxy-vitamin D ($25OH-D_3$) deficiency (i.e., serum levels <20 ng/mL). The women had normal body weight and were of reproductive age with adequate ovarian follicles. A group of 335 women participated, but 154 had low serum vitamin D levels. Women with higher serum vitamin D levels demonstrated more high-quality embryos and higher pregnancy rates than women who were deficient.[27] A 2011 cohort study ($n = 82$) elucidated the predictive capacity of follicular $25OH-D_3$ on

the outcome of ART. Both serum and follicular vitamin D were measured along with clinical pregnancy rates. It was observed that most of the women were vitamin D deficient, but this did not appear to be a factor in ART outcomes. The researchers observed serum and follicular vitamin D levels to be highly correlated.[28] A cohort study ($n = 173$) investigated vitamin D status and clinical pregnancy rates after IVF. Patients were classified as having vitamin D sufficiency (≥75 nmol/L) or deficiency (<75 nmol/L); the clinical pregnancy rates of each group were monitored. Women who had sufficient vitamin D levels were also observed to have significantly higher pregnancy rates, and (statistically nonsignificant) higher rates of implantation.[29] A 2010 cohort study ($n = 84$) similarly aimed to determine whether follicular $25OH-D_3$ levels in women undergoing IVF correlated with vitamin repletion status. Unlike the previous study, the researchers found that women with higher serum and follicular $25OH-D_3$ were more likely to become clinically pregnant.[30] Several additional reviews expound on the role of vitamin D in fertility and conception.[31-33]

ADDITIONAL THERAPIES

Stress Management and the Mind–Body Approach

There is a direct relationship between fertility and stress; it is as much an endocrine experience as an emotional reality. The Longitudinal Investigation of Fertility and the Environment (LIFE) study was a 2014 couple-based prospective cohort study ($n = 501$ couples) investigating whether women's stress levels were associated with fecundity and infertility. Using markers of salivary cortisol and α-amylase, women with higher α-amylase exhibited a 29% reduction in fecundity; according to researchers, that equaled a greater than twofold increased risk of infertility.[34] The human body has extensive hormonal responses to the environment, especially stress, which occur at the hypothalamic and pituitary levels. The anterior pituitary is responsible for regulation of the female menstrual cycle. In response to stress, the adrenals release the hormone cortisol, known to adversely affect the menstrual cycle. The effects of stress are mostly associated with long menstrual cycles and delayed ovulation. Stress and elevated cortisol have also been linked to elevated prolactin levels. Stress management strategies should include lifestyle modifications, including exercise, yoga, and emotional release techniques. Physiologically, the hypothalamic-pituitary-adrenal (HPA) axis can be supported with adrenal tonic herbs such as licorice and rehmannia, in combination with adaptogenic herbs such as eleuthero (*Eleutherococcus senticosus*) and ashwagandha. These herbs act to regulate the HPA axis and assist in general adaptation. There is also increasing evidence that a behavioral approach might be effective in infertility treatment. A study of 54 women who completed a behavioral treatment program based on ability to elicit a relaxation response demonstrated decreased anxiety, depression, and fatigue. Additionally, 34% of the women became pregnant within months of completing the program. Behavioral therapy should be considered as therapy itself, or in conjunction with other treatments, including ART.[35]

Addressing Environmental and Occupational Toxicity Associated with Infertility

Environmental and occupational toxicity has been linked to infertility, subfertility, spontaneous miscarriage, intrauterine growth retardation, and various birth defects, and is currently blamed for declining fertility. The particular toxins linked to infertility include heavy metals, pesticides, environmental estrogens, volatile organic solvents, and radiation.[36,37] Heavy metals most often linked to subfertility are lead, mercury, and cadmium.[36,38]

🌿 FORMULAE FOR INFERTILITY: VARIOUS ASSOCIATED CONTRIBUTING FACTORS

Estrogen Balancing and Ovarian Tonic Formula (for Follicular Phase Problems)

Chaste berry	(Vitex agnus-castus)	30 mL
Shatavari	(Asparagus racemosa)	30 mL
Schisandra	(Schisandra chinensis)	20 mL
Black cohosh	(Actaea racemosa)	10 mL
Wild yam	(Dioscorea villosa)	10 mL
		Total: 100 mL

Dose: 5 mL three times daily

Luteal Insufficiency Formula

White peony	(Paeonia lactiflora)	50 mL
Licorice	(Glycyrrhiza glabra)	25 mL
Chaste berry	(Vitex agnus-castus)	15 mL
Blue cohosh	(Caulophyllum thalictroides)	10 mL
		Total: 100 mL

Dose: 15 mL per day in the morning

Formula for Hyperprolactinemia

White peony	(Paeonia lactiflora)	30 mL
Ashwagandha	(Withania somnifera)	30 mL
Gymnema	(Gymnema sylvestris)	15 mL
Chaste berry	(Vitex agnus-castus)	12.5 mL
Licorice	(Glycyrrhiza glabra)	12.5 mL
		Total: 100 mL

Dose: 5 mL three times daily

Formula for Elevated Luteinizing Hormone

White peony	(Paeonia lactiflora)	65 mL
Black cohosh	(Actaea racemosa)	35 mL
		Total: 100 mL

Dose: 2 mL twice daily

Formula for Low Levels of Luteinizing Hormone

Tribulus*	(Tribulus terrestris)	60 mL
Chaste berry	(Vitex agnus-castus)	40 mL
		Total: 100 mL

Dose: 20 mL twice daily

Formula for Elevated Follicle-Stimulating Hormone

Tribulus*	(Tribulus terrestris)	80 mL
Shatavari	(Asparagus racemosus)	10 mL
Chaste berry	(Vitex agnus-castus)	5 mL
Wild yam	(Dioscorea villosa)	5 mL
		Total: 100 mL

Dose: 10 mL three times daily

Formula for Elevated Testosterone/Androgens

Tribulus*	(Tribulus terrestris)	75 mL
Schisandra	(Schisandra chinensis)	10 mL
White peony	(Paeonia lactiflora)	10 mL
Licorice	(Glycyrrhiza glabra)	5 mL
		Total: 100 mL

Dose: 10 mL three times daily

Formula for Pelvic Factors/Uterine Tonic

White peony	(Paeonia lactiflora)	25 mL
Shatavari	(Asparagus racemosus)	25 mL
Saw palmetto	(Serenoa repens)	20 mL
False unicorn	(Chamaelirium luteum)	15 mL
Goldenseal	(Hydrastis canadensis)	15 mL
		Total: 100 mL

Dose: 5 mL three times daily

Formula for Cervical Factors (Sperm Antibodies, Mucous Membrane Integrity)

Saw palmetto	(Serenoa repens)	30 mL
Echinacea	(Echinacea spp.)	25 mL
Wild yam	(Dioscorea villosa)	20 mL
Rehmannia	(Rehmannia glutinosa)	25 mL
		Total: 100 mL

Dose: 5 mL three times daily

---

*Because of the high dose requirements of tribulus, a concentrated extract in a tablet preparation is often more desirable for optimal patient adherence.

One study examined the association between occupational chemicals and radiation exposure in 281 infertile women compared with 216 fertile women. The study concluded there was an increased risk of infertility among women exposed to volatile organic solvents, chemical dust, pesticides, and video display terminals (i.e., radiation). The women exposed to volatile organic solvents and chemical dust had an increased incidence of ovulatory problems. Tubal factors and endometriosis were also associated with solvents and chemical dusts. Endometriosis and cervical factor infertility were associated with exposure to video display terminals (i.e., radiation).[39]

Environmental contamination is widespread; therefore exposure to toxins is virtually ubiquitous. Research suggests that oxidative stress and electron transfer are the underlying causes of drastic health concerns such as infertility. The treatment framework should include multifaceted preventative measures, such as botanical and nutritional antioxidant therapy and liver support.[40] Herbal therapy with a focus on liver support and improvement of phase 1 and 2 liver detoxification are helpful in the preconception period and during the infertility treatment to aid effective conjugation of sex hormones and toxins. Herbs such as *Silybum marianum*, *Schisandra chinensis*, *Picrorhiza kurroa*, and *Bupleurum falcatum* have demonstrated hepatoprotective and hepatorestorative activity, and assist with improvement of liver function and the detoxification processes in the body.[41] To protect against the damaging effects of radiation exposure, foods and herbs rich in antioxidants have been shown to protect and regulate gene activity. Herbs that exhibit antioxidant activity include *Ginkgo biloba*, *Vitis vinifera*, *S. marianum*, *Rosmarinus officinalis*, *Camellia sinensis*, and *Curcuma longa*.

Acupuncture and Traditional Chinese Medicine

Acupuncture can be considered for women suffering from infertility and has been shown to be of benefit in those with luteal phase defects. In TCM, the diagnosis of kidney insufficiency is said to relate to luteal phase defects. Using acupuncture to regulate the kidney may help regulate the hypothalamus pituitary ovarian axis.[42,43]

CASE HISTORY

A young couple had been trying to conceive for 28 months before seeking holistic therapy. They had been through one failed in vitro fertilization (IVF) attempt 6 months earlier, which motivated them to explore other options. The female was 30 years old, and from medical evaluation, the fertility complications resulted from female factors. The menstrual history has been normal with menarche at age 14 and a regular 34-day cycle. She was aware of texture changes to her cervical mucus and noted that she experienced fertile mucus on days 16 or 17 of the cycle each month and experienced cramps on the first day of her menses. Her general medical history included anxiety, depression, insomnia, and hypoglycemia.

Drug and Supplement History

She has been taking a prenatal folic acid B$_{12}$ supplement but was never advised by her medical doctor to take any other supplements. A few years prior, she took Prozac but discontinued this therapy because of side effects. She managed her depression and anxiety with counseling and regular yoga.

Reproductive History

Her reproductive medical history was complex and included hyperprolactinemia, a moderate degree of pelvic endometriosis, and mild cervical erosion with chronic inflammatory changes. She had a history of pelvic inflammatory disease associated with a *Chlamydia trachomatis* infection that had been treated with doxycycline. Blood tests indicated progesterone failure with a late luteinizing hormone (LH) surge and elevated prolactin levels. She experienced premenstrual breast tenderness and mood changes on a monthly basis.

A previous laparoscopy, performed before the initial IVF attempt, revealed endometriosis and endometrial adhesions; her left ovary was tethered to the left broad ligament. During this procedure, the endometriosis was excised and ablated. A hysterosalpingogram before the IVF attempt revealed inflammation and edema in the fallopian tubes and some fallopian blockage. High-pressure oil perturbation was performed and bilateral tubal patency was then established; her fallopian tubes were clear and apparently functional at 18 months.

A previous postcoital test indicted she had been diagnosed with "hostile mucus," with very few sperm moving in the mucus upon postcoital evaluation. Antisperm antibodies were detected in her mucus.

Additional Assessment

The client had regular lifestyle exposure to significant levels of radiation, including interstate and overseas flights five to six times per year, daily use of a cellular phone, recent spinal x-rays because of lower back pain, and daily exposure to video display terminals from working on a computer. She drank alcohol moderately (two glasses two to three times per week) and consumed 16 oz of coffee on a daily basis. Her diet was high in animal protein.

Treatment Protocol

Black cohosh	(*Actaea racemosa*)	15 mL
Ginger	(*Zingiber officinale*)	15 mL
White peony	(*Paeonia lactiflora*)	15 mL
Chaste berry	(*Vitex agnus-castus*)	15 mL
Goldenseal	(*Hydrastis canadensis*)	15 mL
Albizia	(*Albizia julibrissin*)	15 mL
Rehmannia	(*Rehmannia glutinosa*)	10 mL
		Total: 100 mL

Dose: 10 mL twice daily, before food, through the cycle

Additionally:
- *Tribulus terrestris,* standardized to 100 mg furostanol saponins such as protodioscin: two tablets twice daily on days 5 to 14 of the cycle
- Tablet formula of *Vitis vinifera* extract standardized to contain procyanidins 42.5 mg per tablet; *Camellia sinensis* extract standardized to contain catechins 83.35 mg per tablet; *Curcuma longa* extract standardized to contain curcuminoids 70.4 mg per tablet; *Rosmarinus officinalis* extract 1000 mg per tablet. Dose of three tablets per day was given.
- Tablet formula of *Echinacea angustifolia* extract containing alkyl amides 2.5 mg per tablet and *Echinacea purpurea* extract containing alkyl amides 2.65 mg per tablet. Dose of four tablets per day was given.
- Full preconception nutritional program, as per Foresight studies, including lifestyle modifications.
- Diet: High in fish protein. High in *Brassicae* and green leafy vegetables. Low starch, dairy, and refined carbohydrates. Organic produce was advised when possible. Coffee, caffeine, and alcohol were eliminated.

Rationale

The primary clinical concern was a past history of pelvic and fallopian inflammation, endometriosis, and hormonal imbalance. Considering her history of chlamydia and endometriosis, the use of immune tonics and antiinflammatories was essential.

Black cohosh was included for hormonal modulation. Ginger was included for its antiinflammatory and circulatory tonic action. White peony was included to regulate the LH surge and reduce the elevated prolactin in conjunction with chaste berry. Goldenseal was included for mucous membrane trophorestorative and antiinflammatory action. Rehmannia was included as an antiinflammatory, adrenal tonic, and immune support. Albizia was included as an antiallergenic herb to address the immunologic complications with the antisperm antibodies. The couple was also advised to use barrier contraception (e.g., condom) to reduce her exposure to her partner's sperm during the preconception period of 4 months. Echinacea was used as a general immune modulator because her case demonstrated a need for nonspecific immune support. A combination of turmeric, rosemary, green tea, and grape seed was prescribed for antioxidant and antiinflammatory activity. These herbs also aid the microvascular circulation to the uterus, ovaries, and fallopian tubes to promote healing. Tribulus was added as a general tonic; one known to promote fertility.

Follow-Up Appointments
Second Consultation (8 Weeks Later)
During the weeks between consultations, an ordered test showed no heavy metal toxicity and no active genitourinary infection. The patient commented that her cycle had become shorter and was now 32 days, with no premenstrual breast tenderness, improved mood stability, and increased sense of relaxedness. Overall, she remarked on improvements in energy and sleep quality, increased ability to focus, and she was positive and relaxed. Her treatment protocol remained unchanged.

Third Consultation (8 Weeks Later)
On a second postcoital test, there was no evidence of antisperm antibodies. Her mucus was now healthy; she could support a natural conception. There was no abdominal tenderness and no pain at menses. Hormonal reevaluation was conducted and prolactin, estrogen, progesterone, LH, and FSH were within normal ranges. She continued on her protocol.

Conclusion of Care
She remained on the protocol for 3 more months, at the end of which the couple successfully conceived. The total duration of treatment was 18 weeks, of which 12 weeks was focused on preconception care. During that time, the couple was advised not to try to conceive and instead focus on resolving health concerns and preparing for a healthy, conscious conception. She went on to have a complication-free, healthy pregnancy and a natural, drug- and surgery-free home birth. She gave birth to a 7 lb 8 oz baby girl after 39.5 weeks of gestation. The mother commented that she was healthier during her pregnancy than she had ever been and the experience of using a holistic approach to resolve her fertility challenges had taught them the fundamental principles of diet, health, and the subtle signs of her body's fertility. She now uses natural thermo-symptal charting as an awareness technique for natural contraception.

Pregnancy: First Trimester

The state of a woman's health is indeed completely tied up with the culture in which she lives and her position in it, as well as in the way she lives her life as an individual. We cannot hope to reclaim our bodily wisdom and inherent ability to create health without first understanding the influence of our society on how we think and care for our bodies.[1]

Dr. Christiane Northrup, obstetrician/gynecologist

PREGNANCY CARE AND PRENATAL WELLNESS

The past decades have tremendously improved the outcomes of high-risk pregnancies and birth, yet with these improvements have come the ubiquitous presence of technological intervention in nearly all aspects of normal childbearing as well. Yet the safety and efficacy of the routine use of many interventions is not clear, with a striking lack of an evidence base for many.[2,3] Nonetheless, the number and frequency of interventions has risen steadily since the 1950s. Since 2003, cesarean section has been the most common hospital surgical procedure performed in the United States, with 1.2 million of these major abdominal surgeries each year, accounting for more than 25% of all US births at a national cost of $14.6 billion in total charges. In spite of spending more money and using more technologies on obstetric care than any other country in the world, the United States ranks only 25th in birth outcome and infant mortality worldwide. Dr. Marsden Wagner, former Director of the World Health Organization's (WHO) European Regional Office, remarked at an international medical conference that hospital births "endanger mothers and babies—primarily because of the impersonal procedures and overuse of technology and drugs."[4]

The desire to avoid excessive technology and an inclination toward natural approaches to health, combined with many women's perceptions that obstetric care is grossly impersonal, has led women to seek alternatives to conventional obstetric care. Homebirth has become an increasingly popular option because of its astounding safety record and the intimate prenatal, birth, and postnatal care experience it offers women.[5-9] Many women choose to self-medicate with alternative therapies, such as herbs, and turn to sources that may not be reliable for information. Although the treatment of common pregnancy complaints with gentle herbs and simple home remedies has generally proved safe, women are increasingly seeking advice through the Internet, books, and alternative practitioners for potentially serious problems than can arise during the childbearing cycle. Thus it is essential for practitioners to become knowledgeable about natural therapies and be willing to have an open dialog with their clients about their concerns and preferences. This is to help pregnant women access intelligent and accurate information about the safety and efficacy of such therapies during the childbearing cycle, and to avoid harmful therapies and obtain appropriate medical care as needed.

DIET, NUTRITION, EXERCISE, LIFESTYLE, AND PSYCHOEMOTIONAL HEALTH: CENTRAL TO OPTIMAL CHILDBEARING HEALTH

Health education and preventative care through diet and nutrition, exercise, and healthful lifestyle are the cornerstones of an optimal childbearing experience that may play the most pivotal roles, outside of genetics, in shaping pregnancy health; as a result, they significantly influence the health of the baby. In addition to routine prenatal care, attention should be given to the psychoemotional wellness of the emerging mother, her changing identity as a woman, and her changing family status. Although a presentation of diet, nutrition, exercise, and lifestyle approaches to prenatal health is beyond the scope of this edition, as is a discussion of the psychological and emotional factors that support a healthy pregnancy, the importance of these factors cannot be overstated.

HERBS AS PART OF PREGNANCY WELLNESS

Schools of thought differ on whether herbs should be used routinely—or at all—during pregnancy. Some ascribe to the belief that because most herbs have not been proven safe for use during pregnancy, they should be entirely avoided, whereas others see certain herbs more as foods that can provide an additional source of nutrition during pregnancy, or as tonics that can encourage and support optimal pregnancy health and uterine function.[10,11] Many consider the choice of whether herbs are appropriate for use during pregnancy to be circumstantial; for example, dependent on the nature of the condition being treated and the risk benefit of herbs compared with medical intervention for that particular condition. Certain conditions are beyond the scope of herbal treatment, and practitioners should be keenly aware of the symptoms that herald such conditions and indicate the absolute need for medical care.

> **WARNING/DANGER SIGNS DURING PREGNANCY:** The following signs at any stage of pregnancy suggest that there may be a problem requiring medical treatment. These are beyond the scope of what botanical care can treat. A patient with any of these signs should be referred immediately to an obstetrician or midwife for assessment and appropriate medical intervention.
>
> **Warning Signs**
> - Vaginal bleeding
> - Initial outbreak of herpes blisters during the pregnancy
> - Severe pelvic or abdominal pain
> - Persistent, severe midback pain
> - Edema of the hands and face
> - Severe headaches, blurry vision, or epigastric pain
> - Rupture of membranes before 37 weeks of pregnancy
> - Regular uterine contractions before 37 weeks of pregnancy
> - Cessation of fetal movement

It can be useful to see herbs on a continuum between food and medicine. There are many herbs whose constituents are mostly benign, nutritive substances such as carbohydrates, vitamins, and minerals (Table 17-1).[12-17] Herbs such as nettles *(Urtica dioica)*, milky oats *(Avena sativa)*, and red raspberry leaf *(Rubus idaeus)* are examples. On the other hand, there are numerous herbs whose use in pregnancy is entirely contraindicated for safety reasons (see Chapter 15). Somewhere between these categories are herbs not appropriate for daily, routine intake, but which can be used if necessary for brief or more extended periods of time for specific conditions. In addition to common complaints of pregnancy, pregnant and lactating women are also subject to the run of the mill complaints and illnesses we all face—colds, indigestion, headache—for which they may seek herbal care. Many of these problems can be addressed safely and gently with the herbs listed in the following or discussed in subsections of this chapter.

Table 17-1 provides an overview of a number of herbs that are generally considered safe for general use during pregnancy, reasons for use, and doses. The remainder of this chapter is dedicated to common pregnancy complaints and problems, and the herbs that are often used in their treatment.

THE ROLE OF HERBS IN THE PREVENTION AND TREATMENT OF MISCARRIAGE

Miscarriage, medically referred to as spontaneous abortion (SAb), is the spontaneous, unexpected, and often unexplained loss of a pregnancy before 20 weeks' gestation. Miscarriage is the most common pregnancy complication; however, the exact incidence is unknown because the actual incidence of conception in the population is uncertain. One in seven clinically recognized pregnancies will miscarry, and in studies of women attempting to conceive, SAb occurs in 10% to 15% of conceptions.[18-20] Based on studies of pregnancies achieved through assisted reproductive technologies, 50% of conceptions result in miscarriage. Miscarriage rate is related to maternal age, with rates under 2% for women younger than 30 years of age, and between 5% and 10% for women older than 40 years old. Miscarriage rates decline to less than 3% if there is a healthy fetus present at 8 weeks of gestation (as visible upon ultrasonogram) in healthy women. *Note:* The term *fetus* is used throughout this chapter; however, the term *embryo* is the technically correct developmental term for any baby less than or equal to 8 weeks of gestation.

Although miscarriage may occasionally be welcome in the case of an undesired pregnancy, it is generally accompanied by a sense of loss, grief, or sadness, and a woman may experience self-doubt or self-reproach (e.g., "Maybe I miscarried because of that glass of wine I had last week, or maybe it was because I was ambiguous about being pregnant."). In addition to supportive physical care, women need emotionally sensitive care providers who can understand and empathize that the loss of a pregnancy may matter a great deal to the mother.

CAUSES OF MISCARRIAGE

Numerous factors contribute to miscarriage; however, the etiology of most individual miscarriages is never determined. Causes of miscarriage can originate with either parent or the conceptus (all structures that develop from the zygote). Investigation into specific causes of miscarriage in individual women is generally not pursued unless the woman miscarries recurrently. Causes include:
- Fetal factors
- Maternal factors
- Age
- Environmental exposure
- Infection
- Physical and congenital abnormalities
- Endocrine disorders
- Immunologic factors
- Coagulation disorders
- Nutritional deficiencies
- Psychological factors
- Paternal factors

SIGNS AND SYMPTOMS OF MISCARRIAGE

Signs and symptoms of miscarriage include:
- Vaginal bleeding (i.e., brown or bright red "spotting" or bleeding)
- Abdominal cramping, pain, or contractions that become increasingly regular
- Passing of clots, tissue, or a gush of fluid
- Diminished subjective signs of pregnancy (e.g., nausea and vomiting of pregnancy [NVP], breast tenderness)
- Cervical dilatation

TABLE 17-1 **Herbs Demonstrated as Safe for General Use in Pregnancy Based on Clinical Studies**

Common Name	Botanical Name	Reason for Use	Clinical Trials in Pregnancy	Typical Daily Dose	Comments
Red raspberry leaf	Rubus idaeus	Mineral-rich nutritive tonic; uterine tonic to promote an expedient labor with minimal bleeding; can also be used as an astringent in diarrhea	Positive[12,13]	1.5-5 g/day in tea or infusion	Highly astringent herbs can theoretically interfere with intestinal nutrient absorption
Echinacea	Echinacea spp.	Reduce duration and recurrence of colds and URI	Positive[14]	5-20 mL tincture	The dose listed here and considered safe by herbalists is higher than that used in the study by Gallo et al[14]
Ginger	Zingiber officinale	Antinauseant and antiemetic for NVP, hyperemesis gravidarum, and general nausea	Positive[15,16]	Up to 1 g dried powder/day	Higher doses of ginger are traditionally considered emmenagogic Untreated hyperemesis gravidarum in pregnancy can cause serious adverse outcomes
Cranberry	Vaccinium macrocarpon	Prevent and relieve UTI	None identified	16-32 fl oz of juice/day	Untreated UTI in pregnancy can cause serious adverse outcomes
Chamomile	Matricaria recutita	Promote general relaxation; treat insomnia; treat flatulence	None identified	1-5 g/day in tea	No reasonable contraindications[17]

URI, Upper respiratory infection; NVP, nausea and vomiting of pregnancy; UTI, urinary tract infection.

DIAGNOSIS

Diagnosis and staging of miscarriage is made primarily upon ultrasound findings and the presence of cervical dilatation. Ultrasonography is considered the most important and useful diagnostic tool for SAb. Passage of complete embryonic or fetal tissue, cessation of pregnancy symptoms, and negative hCG levels for pregnancy are indicative of miscarriage; however, self-diagnosis on the basis of passage of large amounts of "tissue," abatement of pregnancy symptoms, and a negative home pregnancy test are not proof of miscarriage. What appears to be embryonic or fetal tissue can actually be clots, pregnancy symptoms can fluctuate, and home pregnancy tests can give false negative results.

DIFFERENTIAL DIAGNOSIS

Bleeding in early pregnancy can be a sign of serious problems. Major causes of early pregnancy bleeding, other than miscarriage, that must be ruled out include ectopic pregnancy and cervical, vaginal, or uterine pathology (e.g., trauma, polyp, cervicitis, neoplasia). Molar pregnancy (i.e., hydatidiform mole) also should be ruled out. Some women experience a small amount of bleeding on implantation, known as physiologic bleeding, which typically is not of concern.

CATEGORIES OF MISCARRIAGE

Miscarriage is divided into six primary categories. Which category a woman fits into dictates the care she will need to receive. If miscarriage is threatened, then measures to prevent miscarriage are appropriate and may be effective, whereas if miscarriage is inevitable, preventative measures will not be effective and supportive care and appropriate medical care for safely completing the miscarriage are warranted.

Threatened Abortion

The term *threatened abortion* is used when there is vaginal bleeding before 20 weeks of gestation. This may be accompanied by abdominal aching or cramping. Upon vaginal examination, the cervix is found undilated. Incidence is 25% of pregnant women experiencing some quantity of vaginal bleeding; of these, 50% ultimately miscarry. When there is threatened abortion caused by a number of factors, including hormonal dysregulation or vaginal infection, for example, preventative strategies sometimes may avert a miscarriage; however, in the case of a nonviable fetus, miscarriage eventually progresses to inevitable abortion.

Inevitable Abortion

In inevitable abortion, there is both bleeding and lower abdominal cramping, accompanied by some degree of cervical dilatation.

Bleeding may range from minimal to severe and even life threatening. Inevitable miscarriage should not be treated with strategies to prevent miscarriage; rather, confirmation that the baby is no longer alive should be obtained and support for miscarriage completion should be provided. Most women miscarry spontaneously without complications or need for physical support, although emotional support may still be needed.

Incomplete Abortion

An incomplete abortion involves vaginal bleeding, cramping (i.e., contractions), cervical dilatation, and incomplete passage of the products of conception. A woman experiencing incomplete abortion frequently describes passage of clots or pieces of tissue and reports vaginal bleeding. The cramping may be rhythmic or laborlike, although less intense than a full-term labor. At this point, the baby has already died and has either been passed or is part of the retained tissue. Treatment focuses on helping the woman to complete the miscarriage process by expelling any retained tissue, and facilitating emotional and physical healing.

Complete Abortion

With complete abortion, all of the uterine contents of pregnancy are expelled, after which cramping and bleeding subside, the cervix returns to an undilated state, and the uterus begins to involute. Other symptoms of pregnancy disappear, and a pregnancy test will yield a negative result. Only emotional support is generally required.

Missed Abortion

Missed abortion refers to a fetus that has died but is retained in the uterus, often with no signs of ensuing miscarriage. This condition may persist for several weeks before miscarriage spontaneously commences. In some cases, it will not commence without assistance. Left untreated beyond approximately 4 weeks, missed abortion can lead to serious maternal infection and rarely, disseminated intravascular coagulopathy (DIC) in the mother, which can be fatal. Medical care must be obtained.

Habitual (or Recurrent) Abortion

Habitual (or recurrent) abortion refers to a history of repeated miscarriage, defined as three or more successive pregnancy losses. Habitual miscarriage suggests the need for medical evaluation of a couple and ongoing care for what may be chronic problems (e.g., hormonal dysregulation, infection). Of women who experience a first miscarriage, only 1% experiences a second miscarriage; however, for women who have never had a live birth and who have had two or more miscarriages, the risk of subsequent miscarriage is in excess of 40%.

CONVENTIONAL TREATMENT APPROACHES

Initially, an ultrasound should be performed to determine whether a live fetus is present. A live baby is born in 94% of pregnancies in which there was a threatened miscarriage. Conventional treatment of threatened miscarriage includes a "wait and watch" (i.e., expectant) approach with reassurance to the use of bed rest, administration of progesterone, use of uterine muscle relaxant drugs (i.e., tocolytics), or other therapies when appropriate, such as specific treatments for systemic lupus erythematosus (SLE) or antiphospholipid syndrome (APS):

- Expectant approach
- Bed rest
- Progesterone therapy
- Uterine muscle relaxants (i.e., tocolytics)

Conventional treatment of inevitable miscarriage includes hospital admission for pain medication if needed, and ultrasound to determine whether the fetus is alive or whether miscarriage is incomplete. In incomplete abortion where there has been substantial blood loss, appropriate emergency procedures are followed, including resuscitation if needed, administration of intravenous (IV) fluids, blood work, and treatment of shock and infection if present. A dilatation and evacuation is performed to empty the uterus of any remaining products of conception, and medication for pain and infection prophylaxis is administered as appropriate. Missed abortion is typically first identified during routine ultrasound examination, or because of a discrepancy between maternal growth, or subjective or objective pregnancy signs, and time elapsed since the missed period. In these cases, a "wait and see" attitude may be adopted for up to several days to 2 weeks (depending on the time elapsed since the missed abortion first occurred) to see if completion of the abortion ensues spontaneously; surgical removal of the conception products may be scheduled to prevent the risk of hemorrhage and infection.

Women presenting with a history of miscarriage should be evaluated for the presence of any of the factors named earlier that are associated with miscarriage. Diabetes mellitus, thyroid diseases, and immunologic factors should be ruled out. Chromosomal evaluation of both partners should be performed, and an evaluation of the woman's reproductive anatomy should be performed. Presence of infection and infectious organisms should be ruled out, and if present, treated. Cervical incompetence often can be treated successfully with cervical cerclage—a suture placed in the cervical os in the first trimester of pregnancy.

Rho(D) immune globulin human (RhoGAM) should be administered within 72 hours of miscarriage to all women who are Rh− to prevent maternal sensitization and possible Rhesus isoimmunization of a fetus in a subsequent pregnancy.

Support and counseling should be provided because miscarriage is frequently accompanied by feelings of guilt, shame, and grief. Practitioners should reassure couples that it is unlikely that anything either parent did caused the pregnancy loss. Women with a history of repeated miscarriage may need significantly more counseling than women experiencing a first miscarriage.

BOTANICAL TREATMENT FOR MISCARRIAGE: THREATENED AND HABITUAL

This section provides botanical strategies for miscarriage prevention in the event of threatened miscarriage (Table 17-2), and basic support for habitual abortion when resulting from

TABLE 17-2	Botanical Treatment Strategies for Miscarriage Prevention in the Event of Threatened Miscarriage and Habitual Abortion		
Therapeutic Goal	**Therapeutic Activity**	**Botanical Name**	**Common Name**
Relieve uterine contractions	Uterine antispasmodic	*Dioscorea villosa*	Wild yam
		Viburnum opulus	Cramp bark
		Viburnum prunifolium	Black haw*
Increase progesterone	Progestogenic	*Vitex agnus-castus*	Chaste berry
Improve uterine tone	Uterine tonics	*Chamaelirium luteum*	False unicorn
		Mitchella repens	Partridge berry

*Black haw *(Viburnum prunifolium)* may be used interchangeably with cramp bark.

progesterone insufficiency. See Case history. When there is incomplete or missed abortion, special attention needs to be given to the risk of infection and subsequent coagulopathy. Women who miscarry are at some increased risk for postmiscarriage anxiety and depression. Emotional support during and after a miscarriage, as well as during a subsequent pregnancy, is often necessary. Botanical treatments for postpartum depression (see Chapter 21) can be extrapolated for use when needed.

> **WARNING:** Appropriate treatment/prevention of miscarriage requires specialized obstetric knowledge and may require hospitalization, particularly if there is cervical length shortening or cervical dilatation when the fetus is close to a viable age, or if there is excessive bleeding. Miscarriage can lead to maternal hemorrhage, and if left incomplete, maternal infection. The care of an obstetrician or midwife should be sought in conjunction with botanical care for the treatment or prevention of miscarriage.

Whenever possible in the prevention of habitual miscarriage, the practitioner will want to try to establish a cause. When this is not possible, a thorough personal and medical history often provides clues to the direction the practitioner can take in establishing an herbal protocol. Both the etiology and botanical treatment of habitual miscarriage are often complex. Unfortunately, emerging theories and understanding of the immunologic, endocrine, and thrombopathic bases of miscarriage are often more advanced than can be matched by current research on botanicals. Most current botanical protocol for miscarriage are based on traditional uses. This section highlights miscarriage prevention for uterine irritability and progesterone insufficiency, which is treated with long-term use of chaste berry (*Vitex agnus-castus*), begun several months before conception and continued until several weeks past the time of prior miscarriage; cramp bark or black haw are also included during this time, and wild yam once pregnancy is established, to prevent cramping. Uterine tonic herbs, particularly partridge berry (*Mitchella repens*) and false unicorn root (*Chamaelirium luteum*), are commonly included in formulae as well. False unicorn is an endangered herb; therefore it is recommended

to use only cultivated sources. Traditional Chinese Medicine (TCM) can play an important role in miscarriage prevention when there is habitual abortion; its constitutional diagnostic model and corresponding herbal and dietary protocol can be specifically tailored to a woman's constitution and imbalances.

HERBALIST/MIDWIFE PROTOCOL FOR HABITUAL MISCARRIAGE

Begin formula 3 months before conception and continued until at least 2 weeks past the latest week's gestation of previous miscarriages (e.g., if a previous miscarriage occurred at 8 weeks, continue the formula until at least 10 weeks).

Chaste berry	(*Vitex agnus castus*)	50 mL
Cramp bark	(*Viburnum opulus*)	30 mL
Partridge berry	(*Mitchella repens*)	20 mL
		Total: 100 mL

Dose: 5 mL twice daily

HERBALIST/MIDWIFE PROTOCOL FOR THREATENED MISCARRIAGE WITH CRAMPING AS THE PRIMARY SYMPTOM

Cramp bark*	(*Viburnum opulus*)	70 mL
Wild yam	(*Dioscorea villosa*)	30 mL
		Total: 100 mL

Dose: 3 to 5 mL every 30 to 60 minutes for up to 4 hours, depending on severity and regularity of cramping. This protocol can be repeated up to twice daily for 3 consecutive days.

*Black haw *(Viburnum prunifolium)* may be used interchangeably with cramp bark.

In case of threatened miscarriage, the Western herbal practitioner will need to address commonly overlooked factors, such as overwhelming stress, dehydration, or malnutrition. Urinary tract infection (or other infection) should be ruled out, and if present, treated (see Chapter 13). Women should attempt to achieve an optimal body weight before conception; underweight women in particular should bring their weight to within a normal body mass index to

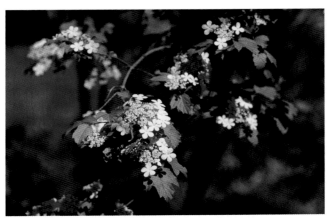

FIGURE 17-1 Cramp bark *(Viburnum opulus).* (Photo by Martin Wall.)

ensure adequate hormone production. Herbs can be used to reduce uterine contractions associated with threatened miscarriage. The most commonly used herbs include cramp bark (Fig. 17-1), black haw, and wild yam, either alone or in combination.

Black Haw, Cramp Bark, and Wild Yam

When there is uterine cramping in the absence of cervical dilatation, cramp bark *(Viburnum opulus)* and black haw *(Viburnum prunifolium)* are used to arrest uterine spasm.[21,22] These herbs, which can be used interchangeably or together for this purpose, have a long history of use as spasmolytics during pregnancy, especially for miscarriage, dating back well over a hundred years by Western herbalists, and even longer by Native American tribes.[21,22] Black haw was official in the *United States Pharmacopoeia* in 1882, its uses as an antispasmodic and preventative for miscarriage popularized by the Eclectic physicians. Cramp bark is included in the *British Herbal Pharmacopoeia* and is used by herbalists in the United Kingdom for miscarriage prevention.[17,21] The active principles are unknown; however, it is thought that at least four active substances that have been identified, including scopoletin and aesculetin, have uterine spasmolytic activity.[23]

Another herb with a long history of use for relieving uterine contractions is wild yam *(Dioscorea villosa).* Although this herb has developed the erroneous reputation for use as a progesterone supplement, wild yam contains no progesterone, nor can it be converted by the body into progestogenic substances. This does not preclude its efficacy and reliability as a uterine antispasmodic that combines well with both cramp bark and black haw; however, no research was identified that either supports or refutes its traditional uses.[17]

Chaste Tree

Chaste tree or berry *(Vitex agnus-castus)* is used by midwives and herbalists to prevent miscarriage associated with low progesterone, where it may exert its effects via enhancing corpus luteum function.[24,25] Although researchers

are still uncertain as to the exact mechanism of action of *V. agnus-castus,* it appears to have a regulatory effect on luteinizing hormone (LH), follicle-stimulating hormone (FSH), and progesterone, as well as the ability to reduce elevated prolactin levels via dopaminergic activity, and has shown positive effects in improving premenstrual syndrome (PMS) symptoms and luteal phase defects.[25-30] It is used alone and in conjunction with topical United States Pharmacopeia (USP) progesterone when the latter is prescribed by an obstetrician or midwife for miscarriage prevention. Placebo-controlled studies for teratogenicity and mutagenicity were conducted in rats, and even when the animals were administered 74 times the dose typically consumed by humans, no toxicity nor aberrations in fetal development were seen.[25] Although it is sometimes given acutely, for the herb to have efficacy as a miscarriage preventative it is ideally given for at least 3 months before conception and continued well into the first trimester to maintain stable progesterone levels. The most recent edition of the *Botanical Safety Handbook* provides no contraindications to continued use during pregnancy.

 CASE HISTORY

> This case history illustrates the versatility of herbs for treating miscarriage-related problems. The patient initially presented with a missed abortion, which she went on to complete with herbal support, and then she desired to maintain pregnancy after a history of several miscarriages.
>
> **Initial Appointment**
> Jan is a 30-year-old woman in dire emotional distress having been informed that day by her nurse-midwife that her 10-week-old fetus had died and that her pregnancy was no longer viable. The certified nurse-midwife (CNM) and obstetrician told her it appeared that the baby had been dead for about 3 weeks, and recommended dilatation and curettage (D&C). Jan was concerned about the procedure; this was her third miscarriage and she was afraid that the D&Cs might contribute to uterine scarring and cause problems in a future pregnancy, and she desperately wanted to have another child. Jan requested assistance in completing the miscarriage herbally and wanted help, should she become pregnant again, to prevent miscarriage.
>
> **Past Medical History**
> Jan had twins 4 years ago after an uneventful pregnancy, and has been unable to carry a pregnancy to completion since then, having had three miscarriages. In the year after the birth of the twins, Jan gained 30 pounds (height is 5'8" and current weight is 210 pounds) and had a serious bout of depression for which she took antidepressants for about 1 year, and then discontinued. After a year of not understanding what was wrong with her, she went to an endocrinologist and was diagnosed with hypothyroidism, for which she was taking Synthroid. Her thyroid condition is well managed and her thyroid tests are normal. Though she has not been experiencing chronic depression, the miscarriages have really caused her to feel down.

Continued

👤 CASE HISTORY—cont'd

Treatment Protocol: Missed Abortion

The goal is to stimulate uterine contractions and promote the expulsion of the fetus from the uterus. Jan's cervix was closed and firm at the initial appointment. We discussed giving the protocol a strict time limit of 5 days, after which she agreed to have a D&C if the protocol was not effective. Her CNM and obstetrician agreed to support her in this choice.

1. To initiate cervical ripening, *Oenothera biennis,* in the form of evening primrose oil (EPO), was given orally as follows: two 500 mg capsules, twice daily, for a total of 2000 mg per day, for 2 days. Also, Jan was instructed to digitally apply 1500 mg EPO to the cervix. (The woman can do this herself, her partner can do it, or she can go to a midwife for the treatment; however, the efficacy of this practice has not been demonstrated by clinical trials.)

2. After 24 hours of EPO, Jan began taking an oral administration of the following tincture:

Cotton root bark	*(Gossypium herbaceum)*	40 mL
Black cohosh	*(Actaea racemosa)*	40 mL
Blue cohosh	*(Caulophyllum thalictroides)*	20 mL
	Total: 100 mL	

Instructions: Beginning in the morning, take 2.5 mL every hour for 4 hours, and then discontinue. She was instructed that if no contractions commenced, she was to repeat the next day. If no contractions ensued on day 2, she was to discontinue on the third day, and resume for two more days on days 4 and 5.

3. The client was instructed to keep on hand *Angelica archangelica, Hamamelis virginiana,* and hemostatic herbs should bleeding be heavy, and was given strict instructions on when to seek medical care.

Contractions began after the first 24 hours of the herbal protocol, and she continued the herbs until miscarriage seemed inevitable. She miscarried within the next 24 hours and was pleased with the results, and relieved to be through this part of her ordeal.

Treatment Protocol: Miscarriage Prevention

Eight months later, the client, who has a history of progesterone insufficiency, depression, and irritability, became pregnant again. At this point she was placed on the following herbal protocol to prevent miscarriage:

Tinctures of:

Chaste berry	*(Vitex agnus-castus)*	60 mL
Cramp bark	*(Viburnum opulus)*	25 mL
Wild yam	*(Dioscorea villosa)*	15 mL
	Total: 100 mL	

Dose: 5 mL three times per day

Jan continued this protocol throughout the first trimester of her pregnancy. Late in her pregnancy, she sent a note saying, "I have had a great pregnancy so far." The client carried this pregnancy to term and gave birth to a healthy baby boy.

NAUSEA AND VOMITING OF PREGNANCY AND HYPEREMESIS GRAVIDARUM

NVP, generally referred to as "morning sickness," is a common pregnancy discomfort. Its association with pregnancy was documented on papyrus dating as far back as 2000 BCE. The earliest reference is in Soranus' *Gynecology* from the second century CE.[31] Some degree of nausea, with or without vomiting, occurs in 50% to 90% of all pregnancies. It generally begins at about 5 to 6 weeks of gestation and usually abates by 16 to 18 weeks of gestation. As many as 15% to 20% of pregnant women will continue to experience some degree of NVP into the third trimester, and approximately 5% will continue to experience it until birth.[32,33] The socioeconomic effect of NVP on time lost from either paid employment or household work is substantial, with one study reporting as many as 8.6 million hours of paid employment and 5.8 million hours of household work lost each year because of NVP.[34] Additionally, women experiencing more extreme versions of NVP or hyperemesis gravidarum are vulnerable to social isolation, and possibly depression, as a result of their symptoms—they are simply too ill to engage in their normal social activities, or they isolate themselves to avoid the embarrassment of being caught vomiting publicly.[35]

Morning sickness is actually a misnomer for this condition; the symptoms are not limited to the morning, and may occur at any time of day. In fact, in 80% of women, symptoms persist throughout the day. It has been jokingly said the condition is called morning sickness because it starts in the morning and lasts all day. Both the etiologies and role of NVP in pregnancy remain uncertain. Several physiologic etiologies have been proposed. It has been suggested that NVP actually serves a protective function for the pregnancy. Flaxman and Sherman proposed, for example, that morning sickness causes women to avoid foods that might be dangerous to themselves or their embryos, especially foods that, before widespread refrigeration, were likely to be heavily laden with microorganisms and their toxins.[36] Studies have demonstrated that women who experience some degree of NVP are less likely to miscarry or experience stillbirth.[36,37]

SYMPTOMS OF NVP AND HYPEREMESIS GRAVIDARUM

The spectrum of symptoms and severity of NVP range from mild to severe nausea to gagging, retching, and vomiting, and from mild discomfort with minimal food and smell aversions to severe aversions and discomfort. Extreme NVP with unrelenting vomiting is called hyperemesis gravidarum, and is a medical condition, as opposed to NVP, which in its milder forms is actually considered normal.

Symptoms of hyperemesis gravidarum include persistent vomiting (and often dry heaving as well), weight loss exceeding 5% of prepregnancy body weight, and ketonuria unrelated to other causes.[38] It is generally incapacitating. It is estimated that hyperemesis occurs in 0.3% to 2% of pregnancies.[39] Hyperemesis typically persists into the second trimester, and may continue until the time of birth. Hospitalization for hyperemesis is common, peaking at approximately 9 weeks of gestation and leveling off at around 20 weeks. The pathogenesis of hyperemesis is unknown. Symptoms generally resolve by midpregnancy regardless of treatment. When properly treated, hyperemesis gravidarum is associated with a very low morbidity and mortality rate. Without adequate treatment, the mother may experience micronutrient deficiency, Wernicke's encephalopathy caused by vitamin B_1 deficiency, and consequences of malnutrition, for example, propensity toward infection or slow-healing wounds. There does not appear to be an increased risk of birth defects in babies born to mothers with hyperemesis gravidarum, and although women with hyperemesis gravidarum may experience substantial weight loss in early pregnancy, as long as overall pregnancy weight gain is normal, there does not appear to be any difference in birth weight.[40-43] Low birth weight is likely to occur in babies born to mothers who do not make up their pregnancy weight later in pregnancy.[39,40,44-46]

RISK FACTORS FOR NVP AND HYPEREMESIS GRAVIDARUM

In a study of the risk factors for NVP and hyperemesis, hyperthyroid disorders, psychiatric illness, previous molar pregnancy, preexisting diabetes, gastrointestinal (GI) disorders, and asthma were all statistically significant risks, whereas maternal smoking and maternal age older than 30 were associated with decreased risk. Singleton (one child) pregnancies, as well as multiple pregnancies, were associated with statistically significant increased risk of hyperemesis.[47] Women with gastroesophageal reflux disease (GERD) are more likely to experience NVP and hyperemesis.

During pregnancy, esophageal, gastric, and small bowel motility are impaired as a result of smooth muscle relaxation fostered by increased levels of female sex hormones. This dysmotility could contribute to NVP. Hormonal changes leading to changes in lower esophageal tone may also provoke NVP, in addition to heartburn.[48,49] Psychological factors, particularly feelings of ambivalence about the pregnancy, have been suggested as part of the etiology; however, this theory has not been borne out by psychological evaluation of women with this condition, and studies are confounded by the fact that the experience of hyperemesis can lead to feelings of ambivalence.[50] Elevated serum concentrations of estrogen and progesterone have been implicated as pathogenic factors, as have decreased prolactin levels and elevated human chorionic gonadotropin (hCG); however, none of these associations has been definitely demonstrated.[51] Other proposed pathogenic factors include abnormal gastric motility, nutrient deficiencies, alterations in lipid levels, changes in the autonomic nervous system, genetic factors, and infection with *Helicobacter pylori*.[52-55]

DIAGNOSIS

There is no specific diagnosis for NVP. Nausea, accompanied by a missed menstrual period or other confirmation of pregnancy, is usually adequate. Hyperemesis gravidarum, likewise, is a clinical diagnosis. There is not a definitive point of demarcation separating a diagnosis of NVP from hyperemesis. The sheer persistence of the vomiting accompanied, as mentioned, by weight loss exceeding 5% of prepregnancy body weight and ketonuria unrelated to other causes is considered diagnostic.[38] Although NVP can cause significant inconvenience and changes in daily activities, hyperemesis is usually markedly debilitating, and many practitioners consider persistent vomiting and marked debility diagnostic of hyperemesis. Women with persistent vomiting are evaluated by ultrasound for the presence of trophoblastic disease (e.g., hydatidiform mole) and multiple pregnancy. Serum electrolyte levels, as well as free thyroxine (FT_4), are also checked. Differential diagnosis for nausea and vomiting is extensive; other pathologic causes ranging from endocrine disorders to neoplastic conditions should be ruled out, particularly for nausea and vomiting that commence after 10 weeks of gestation. Concurrent signs such as abdominal pain, fever, headache, goiter, abnormal neurologic findings, diarrhea, constipation, or hypertension suggest a problem other than NVP or hyperemesis gravidarum. Nausea and vomiting that occur in the latter half of pregnancy could be associated with preeclampsia, HELLP syndrome (hemolysis, elevated liver function tests, low platelets), and fatty liver of pregnancy, and should be ruled out.

CONVENTIONAL TREATMENT OF NVP AND HYPEREMESIS GRAVIDARUM

Conventional treatment for both NVP and hyperemesis gravidarum includes supportive therapy and nonpharmacologic and pharmacologic interventions. Nausea that is mild and self-limiting is considered normal and does not require treatment.[35] The supportive and nonpharmacologic therapies used in conventional care are the same as those used in conjunction with botanical care, and are described under Nonpharmacologic Treatment of Nausea and Vomiting of Pregnancy and Hyperemesis Gravidarum. Pharmacologic treatment may be necessary in severe or refractory cases, and after nonpharmacologic interventions have failed to bring relief or improvement, in order for women to function in their daily lives and gain nutrition without IV or enteral feeding methods.

The mainstay of pharmacologic treatment for these conditions is the use of antiemetic drugs.[40,56,57] Antiemetics have been shown to be more effective than placebo, and do not appear to increase birth defect risk; however, evidence of safety from well-designed trials is not substantial.[58] Thus many women and doctors remain wary of their use, especially in the first trimester. Most women are content to wait out the normal, mild to moderate first trimester nausea without significant intervention as long as it does not interfere with their ability to function.

When pharmacologic intervention is required, it is advisable to start with drugs with minimal known side effects, and progress to other drugs only if these are ineffective and antiemetic therapy is necessary.[59] Antihistamines are also successfully used as antiemetics to control NVP.[58] A meta-analysis reviewed 24 controlled studies including over 200,000 first trimester exposures and found that these medications had a protective effect, with a reduction in birth defects.[57] A number of other antiemetic medications are used including several of the dopamine antagonists; these appear to be helpful and are not associated with teratogenicity.[58]

Corticosteroids have been used for women with severe, unresponsive hyperemesis. The mechanisms of action are poorly understood, and the results of controlled trials have been contradictory.[58,60-64] Prolonged use of oral corticosteroids in pregnancy may increase the risk of preterm premature rupture of membranes (PPROM) and the risk of cleft palate, the latter when administered before 10 weeks of gestation.[65,66] Given the potential risks and undetermined benefits, the American Congress of Obstetricians and Gynecologists (ACOG) advises against the use of corticosteroids for treatment of hyperemesis unless as a last resort.[67]

NONPHARMACOLOGIC TREATMENT OF NVP AND HYPEREMESIS GRAVIDARUM

Mazotta, Magee and colleagues conducted an extensive review of MEDLINE, the Cochrane Database of Systematic Reviews, and bibliographies and texts for the effectiveness of maternal therapies for NVP (including randomized controlled trials [RCTs] of drug treatment versus placebo, no therapy, or another drug therapy). The researchers focused on observational, controlled studies for adverse fetal effects, specifically the incidence of major malformations, because treatment of NVP usually involves administration of medication during the first trimester. Physical outcome measures were evaluated. The findings indicated that some women prefer more "natural," nonpharmacologic therapies for NVP, such as dietary and lifestyle changes, pyridoxine, ginger, and/or stimulation of the pericardium 6 (P6) Neiguan point (e.g., Sea-Bands). Theoretically, these therapies are not considered harmful to the fetus.[68] The goals of nonpharmacologic treatment for both NVP and hyperemesis gravidarum include reducing the symptoms and enabling the mother to obtain nutrition from foods and fluids. Malnutrition and dehydration are both significant concerns when there is a near complete inability to eat or drink, or when there is persistent vomiting.

Nutrition: Food and Fluids
Trigger Avoidance
Women with hyperolfaction are especially prone to NVP and hyperemesis. Avoiding triggers of nausea and/or vomiting, for example, offending smells or tastes, can be helpful. This can be difficult to effectively achieve as preferences and aversions are continually changing for the pregnant woman, and are highly individual. It is for this reason that simple comfort measures, such as dry crackers, ginger ale, and so forth, may only yield fleeting results. Many women with NVP find that most measures only work for a limited time, often for a few consecutive days, and that the very substance that led to some improvement may often then join the ranks of the offending agents. For some

women, tooth brushing is a major trigger that stimulates gagging or vomiting. Avoiding brushing when nauseated can help, and using a toothpaste that is low-foaming and with a mild minty flavor can help minimize an adverse response. Some women find foregoing the toothpaste altogether for a time can be helpful. Using a child's size toothbrush, and avoiding getting the brush, toothpaste, or "spit" in the back of the mouth, can be helpful. Many women find the sight of certain foods distasteful enough to trigger nausea or vomiting; for example, the meat or fish department of the market. Avoiding these departments, or having someone else do the grocery shopping until intolerable nausea has passed, can reduce trigger exposure. Iron-containing supplements cause gastric irritation, and thus should be avoided until NVP or hyperemesis is overcome. Women with very severe NVP or hyperemesis may be triggered by even the thought or the mention of food. In such cases, avoiding exposure to all food images may be necessary. Additional triggers include stuffy rooms, odors (e.g., perfume, chemicals, smoke), heat, humidity, noise, visual or physical motion (e.g., flickering lights, driving), and inadequate rest.[69,70]

Protein and Carbohydrates

Avoid hypoglycemia by eating small, regular meals or snacks, including immediately upon waking in the morning, before bed, and even during the night, if necessary. Women with mild to moderate nausea, with or without minimal vomiting, often respond to intake of dry, slightly salty foods, such as crackers, toast, and pretzels, as well as high-protein foods.[71] Many women find that eating simple, carbohydrate-based meals, for example, a baked potato or plain pasta with a small amount of butter and salt, can be easily digested and allay nausea. A small amount of slightly sweetened yogurt is often a tolerable snack, and can easily be eaten at any time of day or night.

Fluids

Fluids that pregnant women commonly find tolerable include cold water with a squeeze of lemon or lime; sparkling water with lemon, lime, or orange flavor; ginger ale; and small amounts of grapefruit juice, lemonade, or purple grape juice. Clear broth, bouillon, or miso broth may also be tolerated by some women. Although it is critical that women with hyperemesis adequately replace lost fluids, drinking large amounts of fluids is, in itself, often a trigger for nausea and vomiting. Therefore drinking very small amounts at a time, as little as several tablespoons of liquid every 15 minutes or so, is frequently more effective than trying to drink larger amounts of fluids. Women should also be encouraged to drink a couple of tablespoons of fluid after each episode or vomiting.

Nutritive Enemas

In severe cases, an enema containing Pedialyte can dramatically and quickly improve the mother's status, and preempt the need to hospitalize her for IV nutrition. This can be repeated up to several times daily for a few days as a supplement to the woman's nutritional intake. Quite often this is enough to raise her energy and fluid level so that appetite is restored and she is able to eat and drink on her own. Many women find this an option they prefer to try before a more invasive trip to the hospital becomes necessary.

Intravenous Fluid and Nutrient Replacement

Should oral fluid or food intake be impossible to achieve, and a nutritive enema either ineffective or an undesirable treatment to the mother, IV nutrition will be necessary. Infusion of IV lactated Ringer's solution supplemented with electrolytes and vitamins can relieve symptoms of dehydration in 1 to 2 days.[33] Minerals including magnesium, phosphorus, and potassium need to be supplemented, and 100 mg IV thiamine for 2 to 3 days is recommended for women who have vomited for longer than 3 weeks.[33] Plasma sodium should be corrected at a careful rate to avoid osmotic demyelination syndrome, which can occur with too quick a replacement.

Nutrient Supplements

Pyridoxine (i.e., vitamin B_6), 10 to 25 mg by mouth, three to four times daily, has been demonstrated to improve mild to moderate nausea in women with NVP, although it does not seem to be effective in the treatment of vomiting.[56,72,73]

Acupuncture/Acupressure

A number of studies have been published demonstrating the effectiveness of acupuncture and acupressure for the suppression and relief of nausea and vomiting, including NVP.[74-78] Treatment has focused on what is referred to in TCM as the Neiguan point, pericardium 6 (P6), an acupuncture point on the underside of the wrist. Acupuncture has been systemically tested in a limited number of trials. A single-blind, randomized, controlled trial in which 593 women less than 14 weeks pregnant with nausea and vomiting were treated weekly for 4 weeks found no difference in vomiting but less nausea and dry retching in treatment women versus controls. Although acupuncture clearly seems to be effective, it requires administration by a trained acupuncturist, regular access to which is a limitation for many women, and shows no apparently greater benefit than acupressure, which women can self-administer. Further, acupuncture treatment requires ongoing visits, which incur a much greater cost than the one-time purchase of acupressure bands, which can be used repeatedly.[79]

In one study, researchers randomly assigned 33 women with hyperemesis gravidarum to acupuncture treatments on P6 or to mock treatments at a different location. After 2 days, all treatments were stopped for an additional 2 days to allow any effects to dissipate. The groups were then reversed for 2 additional days of treatment. Before treatment, all women were vomiting. On day 3, only 7 out of 17 women (41%) receiving active acupuncture were still vomiting compared with 12 out of 16 (75%) receiving mock treatment. After the active and mock treatment groups were switched, more of the women in the active treatment group ceased vomiting. The women in the active treatment group also reported decreased nausea.[80] In another study, reported in the *Journal of Reproductive Medicine*, 41 patients had P6 treated with an acustimulation device at the Department of Maternal-Fetal Medicine at Eastern Virginia Medical School.[81] Before treatment, patients averaged a score of 4.2 on a nausea severity scale, with five being completely debilitating nausea. Posttreatment device effectiveness averaged 4.2, with significant or complete relief rated 5. All neonates were evaluated for congenital abnormalities and all neonates were found to be normal. The researchers concluded that because current pharmacologic treatments for nausea in early pregnancy are not consistent, efficacious, or without unwanted side effects or increased teratogenic risks, acustimulation of P6 in pregnancy may prove to be a significant therapeutic alternative.

Stimulation of the P6 Neiguan point, three fingers above the wrist on the palmar aspect of the forearm, has been shown to alleviate NVP by at least 50%. (P6 stimulation for 5 minutes four times daily, or as continuously as possible, may be administered by acupuncture, acupressure, manual pressure, Sea-Bands, or by a small transcutaneous electrical nerve stimulation [TENS] unit [e.g., ReliefBand].) The small sample sizes and the failure of most trials to blind outcome assessment complicate interpretation of results. However, the acupuncture principles and practices for the treatment of nausea and vomiting using P6 and for the alleviation of pain have been effectively and successfully extended to the treatment of postsurgical nausea and postsurgical pain relief.[82] Because acupressure stimulation is safe and inexpensive as well as simple for women to achieve on their own at home with the use of wrist bands (e.g., Sea-Bands), it is a reasonable part of a protocol for the treatment of NVP and hyperemesis. For nausea and vomiting, pressure is applied to the P6 point on the inside of the wrist, about 2 to 3 finger widths proximal to the wrist crease, between the tendons, about 1 cm deep. Manually, the woman or someone else applies pressure for 5 minutes every 4 hours. Alternately, pressure can be applied by wearing an elasticized band with a 1-cm round plastic protruding button that is centered over the acupuncture point.[79] The Food and Drug Administration (FDA) has recently approved a wristband-type, miniaturized, battery-operated TENS unit designed to stimulate the P6 acupuncture site. Called the ReliefBand, it has been found to be helpful for mild to moderate nausea and vomiting but not for severe symptoms.[78] It is available over the Internet for a relatively cheaper price, and clients with NVP may want to pursue this option.[79]

🌾 **TREATMENT SUMMARY FOR NAUSEA AND VOMITING OF PREGNANCY AND HYPEREMESIS GRAVIDARUM**

The following treatments may be tried individually or in combination, according to the woman's needs, preferences, and severity of her condition.

Nonpharmacologic/Nutritional Treatments
- Avoid triggers
- Avoid hypoglycemia with small, frequent intake of foods and beverages
  - High-protein, low-fat snacks
  - Dry crackers, pretzels, pasta, baked potatoes, or other bland, slightly salty foods
  - Carbonated beverages, beverages with lemon or lime, ginger ale, slightly salty clear broth or bouillon

Continued

TREATMENT SUMMARY FOR NAUSEA AND VOMITING OF PREGNANCY AND HYPEREMESIS GRAVIDARUM—cont'd

- Supplementation with vitamin B_6 (10 or 25 mg three times per day)
- Acupuncture/acupressure at P6, or an individually designed professional acupuncture program
- Hypnosis or psychotherapy
- Nutritive enemas or parenteral nutrition in severe cases

Pharmacologic Treatments

- Antiemetics
  There are NO drugs that are Food and Drug Administration (FDA)–approved for the treatment of morning sickness. However, drugs such as dimenhydrinate, diphenhydramine, and melamine have been used. Prescription medications used include prochlorperazine (Compazine), ondansetron (Zofran), meclizine (Antivert), promethazine (Phenergan), and metoclopramide (Reglan).
- Hospitalization when there is complete inability to eat or drink, or if there is persistent weight loss

Botanical Treatments

- Ginger root has demonstrated efficacy and safety, up to 1 g/day, for the treatment of nausea and vomiting of pregnancy (NVP) and hyperemesis
- Other effective herbs include peppermint, wild yam, dandelion root, chamomile, and black horehound. These have a traditional basis of safe and effective use and can be taken regularly throughout the day.
- Peppermint oil can be used as aromatherapy as needed.
- Marijuana is commonly used as self-medication for nausea, vomiting, and loss of appetite. Results of safety studies in pregnancy are contradictory and the legal status makes use controversial; nonetheless, practitioners should inquire about patient's use and advise safe use if the patient is likely to continue to use regardless of practitioner's recommendations (i.e., avoid potentially adulterated "street" products).

Aromatherapy

A double-blind clinical trial tested the effect of lemon essential oil scent inhalation on NVP. One-hundred pregnant women experiencing NVP were randomized to inhale lemon essential oil or placebo control as needed for nausea. Effects on emesis were measured using 24-hour Pregnancy-Unique Quantification of Emesis, and statistically significant improvements were observed on mean scores in the lemon group compared with controls.[83]

Hypnosis and Psychotherapy

A limited number of studies have demonstrated the efficacy of hypnosis in reducing NVP in some patients.[84] Psychotherapy is more likely to be beneficial if anxiety is playing a role in the etiology of the condition.[85] Because it is a safe intervention and because many women become anxious, depressed, or isolated when dealing with protracted vomiting, some form of counseling is a reasonable part of a treatment plan if it can be afforded.

BOTANICAL TREATMENT OF NVP AND HYPEREMESIS GRAVIDARUM

According to Borrelli and colleagues, the potential teratogenic effects of drugs administered during the critical embryogenic period of pregnancy drastically limit their use.[86] Because of this, many pregnant women turn to complementary and alternative therapies including vitamins, herbal products, homeopathic preparation, acupressure, and acupuncture.[86-88] A recent literature survey reports that the most commonly used botanicals for the treatment of morning sickness are ginger, chamomile, peppermint, and raspberry leaf.[89] Only ginger has been subjected to investigation of its safety and efficacy for NVP.

The botanical approach to treatment of NVP and hyperemesis gravidarum, like conventional therapy, includes supportive, nonpharmacologic, and pharmacologic therapies, the latter in the form of antinauseant/antiemetic and antispasmodic herbs, and the use of gentle herbs that support digestion (Table 17-3). The supportive and nonpharmacologic therapies used with herbal interventions are the same as those used with conventional therapies, and are described under Nonpharmacologic Treatment of Nausea and Vomiting of Pregnancy and Hyperemesis Gravidarum. NVP can be challenging to treat with consistent effectiveness in any individual woman because it is difficult to find a single remedy that works consistently, especially over a prolonged time period. Typically, women find relief from a specific protocol for a short duration, only to find themselves nauseated by the remedy that helped in the first place. Therefore it is preferable to have a "repertoire" or options a woman can try, and suggest she rotate these to create some variety and not become resistant to any single approach.

The literature is unclear and contradictory regarding the safety of the herbs used for NVP during pregnancy, which is especially concerning because they are used most extensively during the first and early second trimesters when embryonic/fetal development is critical. Historical and anecdotal use suggests a high degree of safety, but as with as substances taken during pregnancy, care should be exercised. Specific safety data are presented with individual herbs.

Ginger

The best studied herb for NVP is *Zingiber officinale* (Fig. 17-2)[90-94] A recent systematic literature search by Borrelli and colleagues identified six double-blind RCTs with a total of 675 participants and a prospective observational cohort study that met the inclusion criteria for the review. The methodological quality of 4 of 5 of the RCTs was high according to the Jadad scale. The six studies are outlined in Table 17-4.[86]

Four of the six RCTs (*n* = 246) showed superiority of ginger over placebo; the other two RCTs (*n* = 429) indicated that ginger was as effective as the reference drug (i.e., vitamin B_6) in relieving the severity of nausea and vomiting episodes, including one study by Fischer-Rasmussen and coworkers that demonstrated efficacy and was superior to placebo for

TABLE 17-3 Botanical Treatment Strategies for Nausea and Vomiting of Pregnancy and Hyperemesis Gravidarum

Therapeutic Goal	Therapeutic Activity	Botanical Name	Common Name
Reduce nausea and vomiting	Antinauseant Antiemetic	*Cannabis* spp. *Mentha piperita* *Zingiber officinale*	Marijuana Peppermint Ginger
Relieve stomach cramps	Antispasmodic	*Dioscorea villosa* *Matricaria recutita*	Wild yam Chamomile
Support digestion/appetite	Digestive bitters	*Ballota nigra* *Taraxacum officinale*	Black horehound Dandelion root

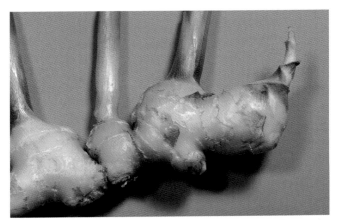

FIGURE 17-2 Ginger root *(Zingiber officinale)*. (Photo by Martin Wall.)

the treatment of hyperemesis gravidarum.[96] The observational study and RCTs showed the absence of significant side effects or adverse effects on pregnancy outcomes. There were no spontaneous or case reports of adverse events during ginger treatment in pregnancy.[86] A 2009 single blind RCT ($n = 67$) tested the use of ginger to alleviate nausea and vomiting in pregnant women. Women were randomized to receive ginger treatment (250 mg capsules four times daily) or placebo for 4 days. Mean gestational age of participants was 13 weeks. The women were evaluated using a questionnaire before and after treatment, twice daily. Compared with controls, the women treated with ginger experienced significant improvement.[97] Two additional studies suggest that ginger is either comparable to or superior to vitamin B_6. A 2009 double-blind study compared the efficacy of ginger to B_6 for reducing nausea and vomiting in pregnant women. Seventy women (who attended prenatal clinics at or before 17 weeks) were randomized to receive either 1000 mg ginger or 40 mg B_6 daily for 4 days. Women tracked the number of vomiting episodes and graded nausea severity using visual analog scale (VAS) starting 24 hours before treatment (i.e., baseline) and through the four consecutive days of treatment. Compared with baseline, women treated with ginger experienced a greater reduction in nausea and vomiting (29/35) compared with the B_6 group (23/34) ($p = .52$) (Preparation not disclosed).[98] An earlier comparative study (2007) also tested ginger against B_6 for NVP. The 126 women (gestational age less than or equal to

16 weeks) included in the trial were currently experiencing nausea and vomiting and required antiemetics (with no medical complications or hospitalization requirement). The women were randomized to receive either 650 mg of ginger or 25 mg of B_6 three times daily for 4 days. Symptom severity was measured by three aspects of Rhode's Index (i.e., episodes of nausea, duration of nausea, number of vomits) starting 24 hours before treatment (i.e., baseline) and through the four consecutive days of treatment. Results suggested that both interventions were effective in reducing NVP. However, the mean score reduction posttreatment with ginger was greater than with B_6. Mild side effects were recorded in both groups (in about a quarter of the women): sedation, heartburn, and arrhythmia (Preparation not disclosed).[99]

The evidence, both scientific and traditional, is that ginger is safe and effective for some women with mild or moderate NVP.[79] It can be taken in the form of ginger ale (i.e., with real ginger), ginger tea sipped in small doses (to avoid nausea that may occur from drinking large amounts of any fluid), ginger capsules, or even candied ginger or spiced ginger cookies. It is generally recommended that women take up to 1 g daily because this is the largest amount that has been studied in clinical trials and been demonstrated as safe. Ginger ale must have real ginger in it, not just ginger flavoring, to be effective. The use of ginger is affordable and many women find this an acceptable approach, preferring to try this before resorting to conventional medications. The various routes of administration allow women to change how they are taking it regularly, which can help them avoid becoming sensitized to and nauseated from the ginger flavor. Occasionally, some women find the flavor unpleasant; adding peppermint leaf to the tea may improve the flavor for these women. Capsules allow women to avoid the smell and taste; however, some may find that eructation is unpleasant. As with all NVP remedies, there will be a great deal of individual variety determining what is palatable and tolerable.

Peppermint

Peppermint has a long history of use as a digestive aid, for improving digestion after meals, and calming nausea, flatulence, and abdominal spasms. The role of peppermint in the treatment of NVP has not been investigated; however, some benefit has been shown for the treatment of postoperative nausea, and also for the treatment of esophageal dysmotility, a physiologic finding that is also postulated as part

TABLE 17-4   Clinical Trials Demonstrating Efficacy of Ginger for Nausea and Vomiting of Pregnancy

Author	Study Design	Weeks of Gestation	Dose	Control	Treatment Duration	Main Outcome
Fischer-Rasmussen et al, 1990[15]	Randomized, double-blind, cross-over	<20	250 mg, 4 times/day	Placebo	4 days	Based on a 4-point subjective scoring system for severity and relief of nausea and vomiting and weight loss measurement, ginger was better than placebo in alleviating or eliminating NVP.
Vutyavanich et al, 2001[16]	Randomized, double-blind	<17	250 mg, 4 times/day	Placebo	4 days	Based on severity of nausea and vomiting (subjective reporting); number of vomiting episodes; and occurrence of side and adverse effects on pregnancy, ginger was more effective than placebo in reducing the severity of nausea and vomiting.
Keating and Chez, 2002[92]	Randomized, double-blind	<12	250 mg, 4 times/day	Placebo	2 weeks	Using a 10-point scale to evaluate the duration and severity of nausea and vomiting, ginger was more effective than placebo in reducing nausea and stopping vomiting.
Sripramote and Lekhyananda, 2003[93]	Randomized, double-blind	<17	500 mg, 3 times/day	Vitamin B_6	3 days	Using a visual analog scale to evaluate severity of nausea, number of vomiting episodes, and occurrence of adverse effects, ginger was found to significantly reduce nausea score, and fewer vomiting episodes were noted.
Willetts et al, 2003[94]	Randomized, double-blind	<20	125 mg, 3 times/day	Placebo	4 days	Ginger was observed to be more effective than placebo in reducing nausea and retching. No effects on vomiting symptoms were reported.
Smith et al, 2004[95]	Randomized, double-blind	>8, <16	350 mg, 3 times/day	Vitamin B_6	3 weeks	Ginger was found to be as effective as vitamin B_6 at days 7, 14, and 21 in reducing nausea, dry retching, and vomiting compared with baseline.

NVP, Nausea and vomiting of pregnancy.
Data from Borrelli F, Capasso R, Aviello G, et al: Effectiveness and safety of ginger in the treatment of pregnancy-induced nausea and vomiting, *Obstet Gynecol* 105(4):849–856, 2005.

of the etiology of NVP.[48,100] Anecdotally, peppermint has a calmative effect on the stomach, in addition to reducing nausea, in women with NVP.[101] It is taken as a tea in small sips (often combined with ginger for a pleasant-tasting tea), in the form of peppermint-flavored candies, or peppermint oil scent indirectly inhaled as aromatherapy. For the latter, many pregnant women have found it effective to douse a small piece of cotton wool with peppermint oil and place this in a small glass vial that can be carried around in the pocket, opened, and whiffed as needed; for example, during car travel.[102] It is considered a safe and gentle remedy; however, peppermint herb is rich in volatile oils that can cross the placenta; thus care should be taken to use only if necessary and in small amounts as a tea only, and not as a tincture or essential oil for ingestion. Neither the *Botanical Safety Handbook* nor the German Commission E contradict the use of peppermint during pregnancy.[103,104]

Black Horehound

British trained herbalists commonly use black horehound in the treatment of motion sickness and NVP with reports of great effects.[96] The safety of this herb during pregnancy has not been evaluated. It is typically taken in small doses (e.g., 1 to 2 mL tincture three times/day) in combination with ginger, chamomile, or peppermint. It may also be added to a small amount of ginger ale or carbonated water (see Dandelion Root).

Wild Yam

Wild yam has been used in herbal medicine as an antispasmodic for not only the uterus and bladder, but for the stomach and intestines as well. The Eclectic physicians reported its use for the treatment of NVP, a use which has found its way into contemporary midwifery-botanical practice.[102,105,106] Steroidal saponins in the plant may exert estrogenic effects by binding with endogenous estrogen receptors in the hypothalamus; however, this has only been demonstrated in vitro. There is no evidence to contraindicate the use of this herb during pregnancy, nor research on its safety or efficacy during pregnancy. There are no reports in the literature of wild yam having emmenagogic effects.[107] It is typically taken in repeated doses of small amounts (e.g., 20 to 30 drops) in tincture form, sometimes combined with dandelion root tincture (see the following) or added to ginger tea, when other remedies alone have failed.

Dandelion Root

Dandelion root is traditionally used as a gentle digestive bitter to improve digestion, increase bile flow choleretic, relieve nausea and vomiting, and improve appetite. The bitter constituents in dandelion increase bile flow and act as an appetite stimulant.[107,108] There are no reports in the literature of dandelion being either safe or contraindicated during pregnancy.[107] Herbalist-midwives may recommend it taken alone in small doses (e.g., 1 to 15 drops) as a tincture in water, or this same dose added to half a glass of ginger ale or lemon-flavored carbonated water. It has a mildly bitter taste, but diluted is not typically offensive to pregnant women.

Cannabis

Cannabis (i.e., marijuana) has at least a 4000-year history of use as a medicinal plant, including extensive use for the treatment of gynecologic and obstetric conditions in many cultures throughout the world.[109-111] It was first described in Western medical literature by a physician in Ohio who used an extract of *Cannabis indica* to successfully remedy a near-fatal case of hyperemesis gravidarum.[112] Cannabinoids, delivered in the form of pharmaceutical preparations (e.g., nabilone, delta-9-tetrahydrocannabinol) or directly smoked by the patient, are effective in reducing chemotherapy-induced nausea, vomiting, and anorexia, and may significantly improve appetite and ability to eat and drink.[113-117] It is used extensively by patients undergoing treatment for cancer and human immunodeficiency virus (HIV), and may provide novel therapies for other GI disorders including gastric ulcers, irritable bowel syndrome, Crohn's disease, secretory diarrhea, paralytic ileus, and GERD.[113-117] The 5-HT$_3$–receptor antagonists, including cannabinoids, offer enhanced control of emesis and cause few side effects.[118] Marijuana use may improve treatment adherence in patients undergoing treatments with protocol that have a high rate of side effects, such as HIV and cancer chemotherapy.[119] Clinical trials that have looked at the efficacy of cannabis as an antiemetic have found it better than conventional antiemetics.[120] Not only does cannabis reduce nausea and vomiting, but it has a significant effect on improving appetite and caloric intake.[115,121-123] Patients with multiple sclerosis (MS) symptoms report reductions in nausea and improved ability to eat and drink among improvement in other

MS–related symptoms.[124,125] In addition to its effects on central nervous system receptors, new research suggests the role of cannabinoids in the treatment of esophageal dysfunction as one of its mechanisms of action.[126] There are strong indications that cannabis is better tolerated than tetrahydrocannabinol (THC) alone because cannabis contains several additional cannabinoids, like cannabidiol (CBD), which antagonize the psychotropic actions of THC, but do not inhibit the appetite-stimulating effect.[127]

Cannabis is reported to be the most widely used recreational drug in pregnancy, with use during pregnancy in developed nations estimated to be approximately 10% to 20%.[128,129] Not uncommonly, it is self-prescribed for NVP.[79,130] A 2003 to 2004 survey of 84 female users of medicinal cannabis recruited through two compassion societies in British Columbia, Canada, found that of the 79 respondents who had experienced pregnancy, 51 (65%) reported using cannabis during their pregnancies. Although 59 (77%) of the respondents who had been pregnant had experienced nausea and/or vomiting of pregnancy, 40 (68%) had used cannabis to treat the condition, and of these respondents, 37 (over 92%) rated cannabis as "extremely effective" or "effective."[130] It is widely used by Rastafarian women in Jamaica and elsewhere to treat NVP, as well as other complaints; for example, labor pain.[130] Because of its status as an illegal drug, as well as the general ethical issues that arise regarding conducting clinical studies during pregnancy, no formal clinical trials that examine the efficacy of this herb for use during pregnancy have been conducted.[129,130] Because of its widespread use, its safety during pregnancy has been the subject of significant investigation; however, according to Westfall and colleagues, it is important to be cognizant when evaluating marijuana and pregnancy safety data that data derived from recreational use may not be equivalent to that which might be derived from therapeutic use in terms of adverse effects.[130] The influence of cannabis use during human pregnancy, and indeed, the medical use of marijuana generally, has been fraught with contradictions and controversies.[129]

A recent MEDLINE database search by Karila and coworkers conducted for articles indexed from 1970 to 2005 using the terms *cannabis/marijuana, pregnancy, fetal development, newborn, prenatal exposure, neurobehavioral deficits, cognitive deficits, executive functions, cannabinoids,* and *reproduction* suggested that cannabis use during pregnancy is related to diverse neurobehavioral and cognitive outcomes, including symptoms of inattention, impulsivity, deficits in learning and memory, and a deficiency in aspects of executive functions in the child.[129] However, composite learning scores in these studies were not lower than controls, and adverse effects on learning were not significant when home factors were included.[131] It is therefore difficult to ascribe direct effects on learning and behavior to maternal cannabis consumption during pregnancy.[130] A report by Park and associates states that few studies have been conclusive regarding the effects of cannabis use during pregnancy.[130] Cannabis use has been correlated with low birth weight, prematurity, intrauterine growth retardation, presence of congenital abnormalities, perinatal death, and delayed time to commencement of respiration. Increased evidence of increased meconium staining was observed in newborns of heavy marijuana users who were from low-risk pregnancy and socioeconomic categories.[129] Studies evaluating the use of cannabis during pregnancy have been confounded by the failure to separate the effects of alcohol versus marijuana on the newborn.[128,132] A large survey ($n = 12,060$) of British women showed no significant different in growth of the babies among women who did versus did not use cannabis during pregnancy, based on self-report. Another large survey ($n = 12,885$) of women in Copenhagen, which controlled for both alcohol and tobacco use, showed similar findings. A multisite study in the United States ($n = 7470$ women) showed no correlation between maternal cannabis intake and adverse pregnancy outcome, including premature birth, low birth weight, or placental abruption. A study of Jamaican births ($n = 9919$) showed no correlation between maternal cannabis use and perinatal morbidity or mortality.

Side effects of use reported in the HIV community and general population include more side effects, feeling high, sedation, euphoria, dizziness, dysphoria or depression, hallucinations, paranoia, and arterial hypotension.[120] Chronic cannabis use has been reported to affect memory in patients using it to treat HIV chemotherapy-induced symptoms, and a study found that acutely, cannabis can impair driving response.[117,133] Clearly, cannabis has effects on brain activity, cognition, perception, and function. Herbalists consider cannabis to be a reliable antiemetic, antinauseant, antianorexic, and analgesic. It is also considered to have mild oxytocic effects.[101]

What remains unknown is the effect of small amounts of marijuana intake during pregnancy for the specific treatment of NVP, anorexia, and weight loss, both independently and compared with no treatment or the use of conventional antiemetics. As it can be expected that some population of pregnant women entering the clinic with NVP will be self-medicating with cannabis, it is important to elicit honest communication from the patient, using a nonjudgmental approach, to ascertain how much cannabis the woman is using and what effects she feels it is having. Drug adulterants such as ketamine and others are common in street products, and can pose serious and dangerous consequences to the mother and fetus.

Pregnancy: Second Trimester

HEARTBURN (GASTROESOPHAGEAL REFLUX) IN PREGNANCY

Heartburn is caused by a reflux of gastric acids into the lower esophagus, usually occurring after meals or when lying down.[1] The gastric acids irritate the esophagus, causing a burning sensation behind the sternum that may extend into the neck and face, and may be accompanied by regurgitation, nausea, and hypersalivation. Inflammation and ulceration of the esophagus may result.[2] Up to two thirds of women experience heartburn during pregnancy.[3] Rarely, it is an exacerbation of preexisting disease. Symptoms may begin as early as the first trimester and cease soon after birth. Most women first experience reflux symptoms after 5 months of gestation; however, many women report the onset of symptoms only when they become very bothersome, long after the symptoms actually began.[3] The prevalence and severity of heartburn progressively increases during pregnancy.[4]

The exact causes of reflux during pregnancy include relaxed lower esophageal tone; secondary effects from hormonal changes during pregnancy, particularly the influence of progesterone; and mechanical pressure of the growing uterus on the stomach.[3] However, some studies have demonstrated that, in spite of increased intraabdominal pressure as the uterus expands during pregnancy, the high abdominal pressure and the low pressure in the esophagus are maintained by a compensatory increase in lower esophageal sphincter (LES) pressure, supporting the finding by Lind and colleagues (http://www.ncbi.nlm.nih.gov/pmc/articles/PMC1923974/pdf/canmedaj01259-0003.pdf) that the LES pressure rose in response to abdominal compression in pregnant women without heartburn.[5] Other possible contributing factors include an alteration in gastrointestinal (GI) transit time. For example, some studies have suggested that ineffective esophageal motility (i.e., decreased amplitude of distal esophageal contractions) is the most common motility abnormality in gastroesophageal reflux disease (GERD).[6]

DIAGNOSIS

A diagnosis of heartburn in pregnancy is generally based on clinical picture. The association of other signs and symptoms is important in ruling out underlying causes. Anorexia, hiatus hernia, and gastric ulcers are the more common causes in pregnancy. Other systemic illnesses of the respiratory, cardiac, or GI tract that are associated with GI irritation or substernal pain need to be taken into account when forming a diagnosis. Preeclampsia must be ruled out on a pregnant woman in her third trimester complaining of epigastric or right upper quadrant abdominal discomfort.

CONVENTIONAL TREATMENT APPROACHES

Medical treatment in pregnancy focuses on symptomatic relief. Complications caused by reflux in pregnancy are rare because of its short duration, and thus upper endoscopy and other diagnostic tests are not typically indicated.[3] Complications, however, can include esophagitis, bleeding, and stricture formation. Care should follow a "step-up algorithm" (i.e., start with simple and noninterventional strategies and add on as needed) beginning with lifestyle modifications and dietary changes. Antacids or sucralfate are considered the first-line drug therapies. If symptoms persist, histamine-2 (H_2)–receptor antagonists can be used. Proton pump inhibitors (PPIs) are reserved for women with intractable symptoms or complicated reflux disease. Promotility drugs (agents that enhance the emptying of the stomach) may also be used. All but omeprazole are Food and Drug Administration (FDA) category B drugs during pregnancy. Most drugs are excreted in breast milk. Of systemic agents, only the H_2–receptor antagonists, with the exception of nizatidine, are safe to use during lactation.[3]

There are limited data regarding the safety of antacids during pregnancy, and teratogenicity is a significant concern.[3] One retrospective case-controlled study in the 1960s reported a significant increase in major and minor congenital abnormalities in infants exposed to antacids during the first trimester of pregnancy.[3] Analysis of individual antacids has shown no such associations, and most aluminum-, magnesium-, and calcium-containing antacids are considered acceptable in normal therapeutic doses during pregnancy.[3] One study "found a higher rate of congenital anomalies in children of women who took an antacid in the first trimester."[7] Side effects of antacids are diarrhea, constipation, headaches, and nausea. Compounds containing magnesium trisilicate can lead to fetal nephrolithiasis, hypotonia, respiratory distress, and cardiovascular impairment if used long-term and in high doses. Magnesium sulfate can slow or arrest labor and may cause convulsions. Magnesium-containing antacids should be avoided during the last few weeks of pregnancy. Antacids containing sodium bicarbonate should not be used during

The editor wishes to thank *Botanical Medicine for Women's Health*, ed 1 contributors to this chapter: Elizabeth Mazanec and Mary Bove.

pregnancy because they can cause maternal or fetal metabolic alkalosis and fluid overload. Pregnant women receiving iron for iron deficiency anemia should be monitored carefully when antacids are used because normal gastric acid secretions facilitate the absorption of iron, and iron and antacids should be taken at different times during the day to avoid problems.[3] There are also little data to support the efficacy of antacids during pregnancy.[7]

According to Richter:

Medications for treating GERD are not routinely or rigorously tested in randomized, controlled trials in pregnant women because of ethical and medicolegal concerns. Most recommendations arise from case reports and cohort studies by physicians, pharmaceutical companies, or the FDA. Voluntary reporting by the manufacturers suffers from an unknown duration of follow up, absence of appropriate controls, and possible reporting bias.[3]

Some believe that over-the-counter (OTC) antacids should be avoided in pregnancy because they can lead to an excess intake of aluminum and salt and interfere with absorption of potassium, phosphorus, calcium, and drugs such as anticoagulants, salicylates, and vitamin E.[8] One small double-blind randomized control trial in pregnancy was identified for H_2–blockers. It found that 150 mg of ranitidine taken twice daily improved symptoms over a placebo by 44% and supposedly demonstrated no risk. However, the results were equal in the antacid alone group, who experienced reduced symptoms of 44%.[9]

BOTANICAL TREATMENT

Herbal treatment for heartburn during pregnancy focuses on simple lifestyle and dietary modification, and the use of gentle herbs to soothe and protect the esophageal epithelium (Table 18-1). A mild antacid herb may also be included in more bothersome cases. Nervines (e.g., chamomile, skullcap, passionflower) can be added to a protocol if heartburn is causing sleeping problems or if stress is contributing to digestive difficulties. Herbs for treating heartburn are best taken as teas or lozenges (e.g., slippery elm bark lozenges) rather than as tinctures, both to bathe the alimentary canal as they are

ingested and avoid the potentially irritating effects of alcohol in the tinctures. Further, demulcent herbs are best extracted in water for maximum efficacy (see Chapter 3).

General Recommendations for Preventing/ Relieving Heartburn

A number of foods have been associated with an increase in reflux, either by increasing gastric acid or relaxing LES pressure. Individuals with GERD may wish to experiment with avoiding all, or some, of these possibly offending items or practices:

- Fatty or spicy foods
- Coffee (decaffeinated or caffeinated), chocolate, and alcohol[10,11]
- Eating within 2 hours before lying down
- Tomato products; for example, tomato sauce, pizza
- Peppermint and ginger[12]
- Drinking more than one cup of fluids with a meal

Other practices may help to improve symptoms:

- Eat small frequent meals (i.e., six to eight a day)
- Elevate the head of the bed 6 inches
- Chew gum

Interestingly, few clinical trials have been conducted demonstrating beneficial effects of eliminating offending foods or practices, including those listed in the preceding, with the exception of elevation of the head of the bed.[13] One pilot study found benefit of a very low (<20 g/daily) carbohydrate diet on distal esophageal pH and GERD symptoms patterns.[14] Nonetheless, many women report improvement with a combination of these changes.

Discussion of Botanicals

Almonds

Chewing raw almonds is a treatment relied on by many midwives for the reduction of heartburn. Instruct clients to thoroughly chew 8 to 10 raw almonds and swallow. This may be repeated several times daily. Almonds are nutritive and there are no expected side effects or contraindications to the use of this food.

Marshmallow Root

Marshmallow root has similar properties to slippery elm—it is mucilaginous, soothing, and antiinflammatory to epithelial surfaces. Evidence for the use of this herb stems largely from traditional use. Though this herb has been used for centuries, there are remarkably few clinical trials evaluating its safety or efficacy. It has no known expected toxic effects; caution should be observed when using this herb in combination with blood sugar–lowering medications, though the risk is theoretical. It has been suggested that this herb might interfere with drug absorption. Although this has never been demonstrated clinically, it may be prudent to avoid taking this herb at the same time as taking other medicinal agents, and instead take marshmallow root and other medications several hours apart.[15] Herbalists, however, commonly combine marshmallow with other herbs for the digestive tract. Unlike slippery elm, marshmallow is not available in convenient lozenges;

TABLE 18-1	Botanical Treatment Strategies for Heartburn		
Therapeutic Goal	Therapeutic Activity	Botanical Name	Common Name
Relieve esophageal irritation and inflammation	Demulcents	*Althea officinalis*	Marshmallow root
		Ulmus fulva	Slippery elm bark
Improve esophageal sphincter tone	Unknown	*Amygdalis communis*	Almonds

therefore it must be prepared as an infusion, and sipped as needed throughout the day or during an acute episode of heartburn.

Slippery Elm

Ulmus rubra is a nutritive demulcent, rich in mucilaginous polysaccharides. Slippery elm's emollient actions have led to its traditional use for centuries for soothing irritated tissue and coating and protecting the digestive tract.[15] Its high calcium content may have some antacid effects. The herb may be taken as a tea; however, it has a thick, mucuslike consistency that can be unpleasant to women with NVP. To avoid this, one to two teaspoons of slippery elm can be added to oatmeal instead; it is has a pleasant, slight maple syrup–like flavor and is easy to take this way. The easiest and most effective way to use the herb is in the form of slippery elm lozenges, which may be purchased in a conveniently prepared form (e.g., Thayer Slippery Elm Lozenges), are quite palatable, and may sucked on as needed up to 8 to 12 per day. Supporting evidence for the herb's benefits is drawn from traditional use, and extrapolation from effects of the mucilaginous constituent of the herb. There is no known toxicity, and in fact slippery elm has been used in some baby foods and adult nutritional foods.[15]

IRON DEFICIENCY ANEMIA

Iron is essential to multiple metabolic processes, including oxygen transport (critical to muscle and brain functioning), DNA synthesis, and electron transport. Iron balance in the body is carefully regulated to guarantee that sufficient iron is absorbed to compensate for body losses of iron. Either inadequate intake of absorbable dietary iron or excessive loss of iron from the body can cause iron deficiency. Menstrual losses are highly variable, ranging from 10 to 250 mL (4 to 100 mg of iron) per menses. Women require twice the iron intake of men to maintain normal stores, and can expect to lose approximately 500 mg of iron with each pregnancy without careful attention to adequate dietary intake and supplementation.[16] Iron deficiency anemia occurs when all of the body's iron stores have been entirely depleted. This section focuses on the iron needs of the pregnant and lactating woman.

Iron deficiency is the most common nutritional deficiency worldwide, affecting 20% of the world's population. It is considered the most common health problem faced by women worldwide, adjusted for all ages and economic groups, and is a marker of overall poor nutritional status.[17] Poor socioeconomic status does, however, further increase the risk of iron deficiency anemia.[18] It is estimated that worldwide, 20% to 50% of all maternal deaths are related to iron deficiency anemia.[19]

During pregnancy the blood volume expands by about 35% to 50%, with additional iron required to meet the needs of the fetus, placenta, and increased maternal tissue. In the second and third trimesters, iron requirements increase to three times the nonpregnant needs. Women who do not supplement iron during pregnancy are usually unable to maintain adequate iron stores throughout and are at increased risk for developing iron deficiency anemia. Women who have a history of iron deficiency anemia before pregnancy, low iron stores at the onset of pregnancy, or those with heavy menstrual blood loss, are at further risk for anemia during pregnancy.[16,20] Iron deficiency anemia decreases quality of life because of symptoms of fatigue, weakness, loss of appetite, and increased susceptibility to infection (see Symptoms), and increases the risk of a number of problems including severe anemia from normal blood loss during labor, requiring blood transfusions. Fetal iron stores in the first 6 months of life are dependent on maternal stores during pregnancy.[20] Postpartum anemia is a contributing factor to postpartum depression.[20]

SYMPTOMS

Symptoms of iron deficiency anemia include:
- Easy fatigability
- Tachycardia
- Palpitations
- Tachypnea on exertion
- Pica (e.g., craving for nonfood items, e.g., ice chips, laundry starch, dirt)
- Muscle dysfunction
- Appetite loss
- Constipation
- Poor scholastic performance
- Altered resistance to infection
- Altered behavior
- Smooth tongue*
- Brittle nails*
- Cheilosis (i.e., fissures at the corners of the mouth)*

Improving iron status noticeably and rapidly improves most of these symptoms.

DIAGNOSIS

Iron deficiency anemia is diagnosed on the basis of simple, inexpensive screening tests. Hematocrit (Hct) and hemoglobin (Hb), both of which can often be done in-office by an obstetrician or midwife, are the most commonly ascertained values. The mean cell volume (MCV) is done to assess red blood cell (RBC) size to rule out anemia caused by nutritional deficiencies other than iron; for example, vitamin B_{12} deficiency, which causes macrocytic anemia. Hct is a measure of the percentage of whole blood occupied by RBCs, the oxygen and iron-carrying portions of the blood; Hb is the concentration of iron-containing protein in the RBCs. The normal Hct in nonpregnant women ranges from 36% to 45%. However, in pregnant women, because of normally increased blood volume (i.e., physiologic hemodilution of pregnancy), values can be as low as 34% in singleton and 30% in twin or multiple pregnancy, even with normal iron stores, and does not necessarily indicate a true anemia. Normal Hb for women

---

*In severe iron deficiency.

ranges between 12 to 16 g/dL, with a drop down to 10.5 possibly normal in midpregnancy (i.e., weeks 16 to 28) owing to physiologic hemodilution.[16] Diagnosis also may be made on the basis of an increase in Hb levels after supplementation has begun. Additional tests, including serum ferritin concentration and transferrin levels can also be used to differentiate iron deficiency anemia from other forms of anemia. This is usually only necessary during pregnancy when anemia is refractory to treatment.

DIFFERENTIAL DIAGNOSIS

Iron deficiency anemia can be a result of chronic internal bleeding that can occur, for example, in the case of GI disease (e.g., inflammatory bowel disease, celiac disease, peptic ulcer disease). Causes of microcytic anemia that must be ruled out include thalassemia, anemia of chronic disease, sideroblastic anemia, and lead poisoning.

CONVENTIONAL TREATMENT

Conventional treatment of iron deficiency anemia relies primarily on diet and iron supplements.

Diet

Red meat, poultry, and fish are good sources of heme iron, the most absorbable form. Iron deficiency anemia is lowest in areas where red meat is a dietary staple. Dietary sources of nonheme iron include blackstrap molasses, dried apricots, raisins, dark green leafy vegetables (e.g., kale, collards), kidney beans, lentils, mussels, oysters, pine nuts, pumpkin seeds, quinoa, tempeh, tofu, and wheat germ. Nonheme sources of iron are also an important part of the diet, though not as readily absorbable. A carefully planned diet rich in a variety of iron sources can allow vegetarians to meet their dietary iron needs.

Iron Supplements

Oral iron supplements are an inexpensive, generally safe, and simple way to treat iron deficiency. Because iron is best absorbed from the duodenum and proximal jejunum, time-released and enteric-coated preparations are not very effective, and they are also much more costly. Ascorbic acid increases the absorbability of nonheme iron. Taking 250 mg of vitamin C with iron supplement is therefore advisable. Phytates, oxalates, carbonates, calcium, and tannins, found in foods such as cereals, dietary fiber, tea, coffee, eggs, and milk, interfere with iron absorption; therefore iron supplements should not be taken with food. Antacids also interfere with iron absorption, and should be given several hours before or after taking iron supplements. Antibiotics also interfere with iron absorption. GI side effects are common (10% to 20% of patients report GI side effects) with conventional iron supplements (see Botanical Treatment for herbal alternatives). Constipation is a common complaint, as are nausea, vomiting, abdominal discomfort, and diarrhea. Elemental iron in the forms of ferrous sulfate, ferrous fumarate, or ferrous gluconate may be substituted with ferrous sulfate elixir, a liquid preparation that may cause fewer GI symptoms. Improvement can usually be observed starting approximately 7 days after the onset of iron supplementation. Also, though a less effective therapy, iron supplements may be taken with meals to avoid discomfort. The various forms of iron commonly used therapeutically appear to be equally effective. In severe cases where oral iron is unable to be tolerated, parenteral iron may be given. It is considered optimal to remain on iron supplements for approximately 6 months after iron levels return to normal to adequately replenish depleted iron stores. Low-dose iron supplementation (e.g., 30 mg/day) throughout pregnancy is as effective as higher dose supplementation (e.g., 60 mg day) and less likely to cause side effects.[17] If a patient does not respond to iron therapy, the possibility of an underlying disorder or coexisting disease (e.g., GI bleeding, thalassemia) must be addressed. Malabsorption is also a common problem leading to refractory anemia.

BOTANICAL TREATMENT

The use of various forms of elemental iron have been a part of both folk and Western medical herbal tradition for at least the past few hundred years, whether in the form of iron nails stuck in apples to infuse the apples with iron for consumption by pioneer women, or the use of ferrum supplements by the Eclectic physicians. As stated earlier, side effects from iron supplements are common. For pregnant women who may be experiencing GI symptoms caused by the pregnancy itself, such as nausea, vomiting, or constipation, regular elemental iron supplements may be intolerable. Although there is almost no evidence in the literature evaluating the efficacy or safety of herbs used as "iron tonics," their use is popular among herbalists, midwives, and pregnant women (Table 18-2). Clinical observation has demonstrated a high level of efficacy and minimal side effects (Case History) with a limited number of botanical supplements. The herbs in this section are those most commonly used in contemporary midwifery and herbal practice.

TABLE 18-2 **Botanical Treatment Strategies for Iron Deficiency Anemia**			
Therapeutic Goal	Therapeutic Activity	Botanical Name	Common Name
Provide dietary/ supplemental iron	Iron tonic	*Medicago sativa*	Alfalfa
		Rumex crispus	Yellow dock
		Taraxacum officinale	Dandelion root
		Urtica dioica	Nettles
			Floradix Iron + Herbs
			Liquid chlorophyll
Treat blood and yin deficiency		*Angelica sinensis*	Dong quai
		Paeonia lactiflora	White peony

Floradix Iron + Herbs

This product is a popular, easily assimilable source of elemental iron and iron-rich herbs, including aqueous extracts of carrot, nettle wort, spinach, kelp, blackberry, cherry, and beet root concentrates, among other herbal and food ingredients. A 2-tsp (10-mL) daily dose provides 100% of the daily dose of pyridoxine (i.e., vitamin B6), 125% of cyanocobalamin (i.e., vitamin B12), and 10 mg (56%) of iron. Many of the herbs in the product have not been evaluated for use during pregnancy; however, no adverse outcomes from use of the product have been identified. Most women find Floradix palatable and easy to digest.

Nettles

The leaf of the nettle plant, prepared as a strong infusion, is a popular tonic used by many herbalists for treating iron deficiency anemia; many herbalists stand by it as one of their primary anemia treatments. The fresh leaves, which lose their sting when cooked, can also be eaten as an iron-rich green leafy vegetable, if one has access to them. The leaves are also rich in chlorophyll, for which they are commonly a commercial source, and a rich source of vitamin C.[21] As with other herbs used for the treatment of iron deficiency anemia, the amount of iron in any given dose has not been quantified; however, pregnant women and midwives report good results with symptoms of anemia, particularly fatigue. It is rarely used as a singular treatment but rather as part of a protocol for anemia. It has been suggested, although not demonstrated, that the astringency of this herb might interfere with iron absorption. A 1975 review article by Farnsworth and coworkers reported that stinging nettle was a potential abortifacient, and that its constituent, 5-hydroxytryptamine was a uterine stimulant; however, frequent use of large doses of this herbal infusion in midwifery practice has demonstrated no evidence of such activity.[22]

Yellow Dock and Dandelion Root Iron Tonic

The use of yellow dock root, in combination with dandelion root, is perhaps one of the most popular Western herb tonics used by midwives.[23,24] It is typically prepared as a syrup with blackstrap molasses (see recipe), itself rich in iron (and calcium), to be taken daily, usually in a 1- to 2-Tbsp dose. In this form it is easily digestible, though some women report mild nausea if taken on an empty stomach. Yellow dock is listed in Dr. Duke's Phytochemical and Ethnobotanical Databases (www.ars-grin.gov/duke) as an iron-containing herb; however, the amount of iron per any single dose of this herb is difficult to quantify and has not been evaluated in regard to its use as an iron supplement. The herb is touted by traditional herbalists, as is dandelion, not only for its iron content but also for its actions on the liver. It is believed to increase uptake of dietary iron. Neither the veracity of this claim nor possible mechanisms have been evaluated. The use of yellow dock as an iron tonic is presented in the 1918 edition of Remington's *Dispensatory of the United States of America*:

The roots of this plant are said to possess the power to take up the iron present in the soil, and fix it in the form of organic compounds of iron. By watering the plants with a solution of iron carbonate, roots are said to be obtained that contain 1.5% of iron. Rumex is said to give good results in the treatment of chlorosis and anemia. The authors gave the dried and powdered root during meals in doses of 15 to 45 grains (1 to 3 g), in view of their good results they regard it as a valuable iron medicine. Dock root is given in powder or in decoction.[25]

Note that yellow dock is sometimes considered contraindicated in pregnancy because it is a mild anthraquinone laxative; however, clinically it has not been observed to be associated with increased uterine activity. The gentle laxative (i.e., aperient) effects relieve anemia-associated constipation and build iron.

DANDELION–YELLOW DOCK SYRUP FOR IRON DEFICIENCY ANEMIA

Yellow dock root *(Rumex crispus)*: ½ ounce (14 g)
Dandelion root *(Taraxacum officinale)*: ½ ounce (14 g)
Directions: Prepare a decoction by simmering both herbs (1 oz/28 g total) in 4 cups of water, uncovered, until reduced to 1 cup. Strain the liquid thoroughly, discard the herb material), and add ½ cup blackstrap molasses, mixing until blended. Cool to room temperature. Keep refrigerated. The product will keep for up to 2 weeks refrigerated.
Dose: 1 to 2 Tbsp, up to twice daily, depending on the severity of the anemia.

Alfalfa

In 1915, Dr. Richard Willstätter, a German chemist, was awarded the Nobel Prize in chemistry for elucidating the structure of chlorophyll. Willstätter observed that the chlorophyll molecule bears a striking resemblance to Hb, except that its centerpiece is a single atom of magnesium rather than iron. Today, commercial liquid chlorophyll is derived mostly from alfalfa, and is popularly used to improve iron levels in iron deficiency anemia. No data evaluating the efficacy or safety of chlorophyll use during pregnancy have been identified. In fact, little data exist on the safety or efficacy of alfalfa, though some preliminary studies have suggested possible beneficial effects in lowering cholesterol.[15] The herb may also have some hypoglycemic and antifungal effects.[15] Alfalfa is considered to have minimal risk when used as a food source (e.g., a normal serving of alfalfa sprouts) during pregnancy and lactation.[21] Animal studies (nonpregnant and lactating) have demonstrated no toxicity when alfalfa seeds or saponins are ingested in large quantities over an extended period of time (up to 6 weeks of consumption of seeds and 8 weeks for saponins).[15] However, the herb, particularly the seeds and seed products (e.g., alfalfa sprouts) are contraindicated in patients with systemic lupus erythematosus (SLE), in whom it has been reported to cause exacerbations and pancytopenia.[15] The constituent thought to be responsible for this effect, L-canavanine, is not present in the leaf; however, lupuslike syndrome has been reported with consumption of leaf-containing tablets. This may be caused by adulteration of leaf products with L-canavanine–containing plant parts. Alfalfa contains the phytoestrogen coumestrol, which may have estrogenic properties. A 1975 paper by Farnsworth and coworkers on the antifertility effects of herbs stated that alfalfa has uterine stimulant activity; however, no other such findings have been reported in the literature or observed by clinical herbalists.[22] Alfalfa is rich in vitamin K, and thus is contraindicated with anticoagulant therapies (e.g., warfarin) with which it may interfere. It may also interact with hypoglycemic drugs, lower blood glucose levels, interfere with lipid-lowering medications, and should not be taken with chlorpromazine. Clinically, liquid chlorophyll, combined with other iron-raising protocols, has been observed to rapidly improve Hb more quickly than the protocol used alone, and without adverse effects (see Case History).

👤 CASE HISTORY

> Celeste is a 28-year-old woman who is 29 weeks pregnant with her second baby. She has a history of iron deficiency anemia for which she has been under the care of her obstetrician. In spite of 6 weeks of treatment, her hematocrit (Hct), which is 29, has not increased. Her physician doubled her iron supplement to 60 mg/day, and she has been experiencing side effects, including severe constipation for 2 weeks, nausea, and abdominal cramps. Her skin color has a slightly greenish tint around her mouth and under her eyes. She is deeply fatigued and has a poor appetite, as well as daily headaches.
>
> Recommendations:
> - Discontinue the prescription iron supplement
> - Take Floradix Iron + Herbs as instructed on the bottle
>
> After 1 week, Celeste was still constipated, so she was instructed to add the following to her plan:
>
> For constipation:
> - Take yellow dock dandelion root syrup (1 Tbsp each morning)
> - Soak four dried prunes and 1 tablespoon of bran in ½ cup warm, unfiltered apple juice until prunes are soft. Eat/drink entire portion once each morning.
>
> Three weeks after the initial visit (31 weeks pregnant), Celeste's Hct had risen to 30, and she was having regular bowel movements—one soft, formed stool per day or every other day. It was recommended that she continue taking the preparations for constipation each morning for a couple of additional weeks. It was also recommended that she add 1 Tbsp liquid chlorophyll to her protocol daily, and take 250 mg vitamin C with each dose of Floradix. It was somewhat urgent to quickly raise her Hct because her due date was only 9 weeks away.
>
> At 34 weeks of pregnancy, Celeste's Hct was 32, and now that her bowels were regular, she was instructed to start eating beef stew three times per week (i.e., organic beef). At 36 weeks, Celeste's Hct was 34, and by 37 weeks it had risen to 35. Celeste gave birth at home at 38 weeks, with the midwife who had assisted her in treating her anemia, to a healthy baby boy.

PRETERM LABOR AND UTERINE IRRITABILITY

Preterm labor occurs before the end of the pregnancy week 37. Preterm birth is one of the leading causes of infant mortality and also long-term disability in the United States.[26-28] In spite of improvements in the outcome of prematurely born infants, the rate of premature delivery has continued to rise, largely as a result of assisted reproductive technologies (ARTs) and multiple pregnancies, although poor nutrition and lower socioeconomic status continue to play a major role. In 2004, 12.5% of all births in the United States occurred before 32 weeks of gestation. Rates of preterm birth are highest among African American women, adolescents, women older than 40, unmarried women, and women with lower socioeconomic status. Additional factors that contribute to premature labor include prior preterm birth, history of second trimester pregnancy loss, preterm premature rupture of the membranes (PPROM), multiple gestation, concurrent obstetric or medical complications, uteroplacental insufficiency, cigarette smoking, drug use, alcohol intake, lack of prenatal care, uterine abnormalities, infections, loop electrosurgical excision procedure (LEEP), and fetal congenital abnormalities.[28,29] Stress, dehydration, domestic violence, emotional abuse, closely spaced pregnancies, and jobs that require long periods of standing are also thought to be contributory to premature labor.[29,30]

The following specific conditions are associated with premature labor: urinary tract infections, vaginal infections, sexually transmitted infections and possibly other infections, diabetes, hypertension, preeclampsia, and clotting disorders (i.e., thrombophilia).[30] Dietary patterns also play a role. Decreased frequency of eating is associated with an increased risk of premature labor. Women who consume three meals and two snacks daily throughout pregnancy appear less likely to experience premature onset of labor.[31] Low or no fish consumption, associated with inadequate intake of omega-3 fatty acids, is also associated with an increased risk of premature labor.[32] Other nutritional deficiencies, notably vitamin C, may also be related to increased risk of premature labor.[33]

Uterine irritability is a stressful and annoying pregnancy problem in which the pregnant woman experiences frequent uterine contractions, ranging from mild to painful, that generally come in an irregular pattern, although they may appear to mimic early labor. Women with uterine irritability have an increased risk of premature labor; however, the presence of an irritable uterus is not indicative of labor, and may simply be a source of ongoing concern to the mother, her family, and care providers, and a bother to the mother.

SIGNS AND SYMPTOMS

Women should be advised to contact their health care providers or go to the hospital immediately if they are experiencing the following:
- Contractions every 10 minutes or more frequently
- Rupture of membranes (ROM)

- Vaginal bleeding
- Pelvic pressure
- Dull lower backache
- Menstrual-like cramps
- Abdominal cramps with or without diarrhea

Unfortunately, diagnosis of early preterm labor is difficult and has a high false positive rate, which may lead to possibly harmful interventions for thousands of women. Screening methods for preterm labor such as routine cervical assessment, transvaginal ultrasonography, fetal fibronectin (fFN) detection, and home uterine activity monitoring have not been shown to be beneficial at actually preventing preterm labor, although some of these methods may detect risk or early symptoms, and fFN testing can provide information on the likelihood of a woman entering labor in the 2 weeks after the test.[28]

Medical evaluation for the presence of premature labor includes assessment for the following signs:

- Uterine activity that is suggestive of a labor pattern (i.e., increasingly regular contractions coming with increasing frequency)
- ROM
- Vaginal bleeding
- Cervical dilatation, effacement, and station

MEDICAL TREATMENT

Strategies to prevent preterm delivery have focused on early diagnosis of preterm labor symptoms and on clinical markers such as cervical change, uterine contractions, vaginal bleeding, and changes in fetal behavior. Bed rest and home uterine monitoring have not led to a reduction in preterm birth rates. Because bed rest can lead to potential adverse effects on women and their families, clinicians should not routinely advise women to rest in bed to prevent preterm birth.[34] The medical priority is to halt the progression to premature birth whenever possible and also treat underlying medical contributing causes, and assure fetal lung maturity and the availability of proper neonatal care if preterm birth becomes inevitable. Medical treatments used to arrest premature labor include the use of tocolytic agents (e.g., terbutaline, magnesium sulfate, ritodrine, and nifedipine); corticosteroid therapy to stimulate fetal lung maturity; and treatment of underlying causes of premature labor, for example, antibiotics for specific infections. Complications of the use of these medications vary according to the drug, and include but are not limited to pulmonary edema, profound hypotension, muscular paralysis, cardiac arrest, respiratory depression, hypokalemia, hyperglycemia, arrhythmias, myocardial ischemia, and maternal death. A

risk–harm evaluation is done based on the week's gestation of the pregnancy, status of the fetus, and reason for premature labor when determining whether to arrest labor medically or to allow labor to proceed. If premature labor is diagnosed and is progressing, the pregnant woman is transferred to a care facility equipped to care for the premature newborn.

BOTANICAL TREATMENT

Women in active, progressing, premature labor require hospitalization for birth to guarantee the neonate access to appropriate medical care necessary for survival after birth. The use of botanicals is not adequate treatment if a woman has premature cervical dilatation, ruptured membranes, or regular contractions with signs of labor progress. However, women experiencing uterine irritability or threatened premature labor with mild irregular contractions only may respond effectively to botanical uterine spasmolytics. Active labor must be ruled out by a qualified obstetric care provider and the situation carefully and appropriately monitored.

Uterine spasmolytics such as cramp bark (*Viburnum opulus*) and black haw (*Viburnum prunifolium*) can be given in repeated doses every 15 minutes with 2 to 3 mL of these herbs over a 2- to 3-hour period. This should yield a demonstrable reduction in uterine irritability. Other herbs that may be combined with the aforementioned to create an additive musculoskeletal relaxant effect include wild yam (*Dioscorea villosa*) and Jamaican dogwood (*Piscidia piscipula*). The latter two herbs are considered appropriate for acute use only during pregnancy; long-term effects are unknown and possibly unsafe. However, no adverse effects are expected from acute use over a few hours within recommended doses (i.e., Jamaican dogwood up to 2 mL every 30 minutes for 2 hours, combined with an equal amount of either cramp bark or black haw at each dose). These herbs are not recommended for use during the first trimester, and should not be used for more than three consecutive days as described. Midwives may also recommend warm baths to which have been added 5 to 7 drops of lavender oil for relaxation, visualization, and other mind–body techniques for stress reduction. Bathing is contraindicated if there has been ROM. Emotional support of the mother is essential, and herbs for anxiety may be given short term in small doses if necessary.

Premature labor can progress to birth in a short time; thus these herbs should not be relied on if premature labor is occurring unless in an appropriate medical setting and in conjunction with medical observation and care; no studies have been conducted to examine the safety or efficacy of botanical treatments to arrest premature labor contractions.

Pregnancy: Third Trimester

CONSTIPATION DURING PREGNANCY

Constipation is defined as having bowel movements fewer than three times per week. The stools are typically hard, dry, small in size, and difficult to eliminate. Constipation may be accompanied by straining, pain, bloating, cramping, and the sensation of a full bowel. It is a bothersome common complaint of pregnancy, particularly in the second and third trimesters. Women who are habitually constipated may become more so during pregnancy. The prevalence of constipation in pregnancy is reported to be 11% to 38%.[1] It has been generally accepted that decreased gastric motility in pregnancy is a result of increased circulating progesterone levels. More recent experimental evidence suggests that elevated estrogen concentrations are involved in delayed motility through an enhancement of nitric oxide release.[1,2] Slow transit time of food through the intestinal tract leads to increased water absorption and thereby to constipation. Dietary factors, particularly inadequate fiber intake and lack of exercise, contribute to constipation, as does increased pressure of the growing uterus on the rectum as pregnancy becomes advanced.[3] Ignoring the urge to have a bowel movement can also contribute to the problem. Iron deficiency anemia can contribute to constipation, as can elemental iron supplements.

DIAGNOSIS

Constipation first presenting in pregnancy does not require an extensive evaluation, and is considered a normal pregnancy complaint.[4] Constipation accompanied by other symptoms, for example, blood in the stools, or that is unresponsive to treatments, requires further investigation to rule out possible pathology.

CONVENTIONAL TREATMENT OF CONSTIPATION

Most patients respond to simple dietary and lifestyle measures. Treatment during pregnancy is similar to that for the general population; however, special care must be taken to avoid medications that may be harmful to the fetus or disrupt the pregnancy.[4]

The first line of treatments for constipation include:
- Increasing water consumption to eight glasses per day: Avoiding dehydration will keep the stools softer and make them easier to pass; liquids that contain caffeine (e.g., coffee, tea, cola) increase dehydration.
- Increasing dietary fiber to 20 to 35 g/day: High-fiber foods increase stool bulk and facilitate bowel evacuation; high-fiber food sources include fruits, vegetables, whole grains and bran cereals, and beans.
- Minimizing consumption of constipating food items: For example, ice cream, meats, cheese, and high-fat foods can increase constipation, especially in a low-fiber diet.
- Increasing daily activity: Even increased daily walking, as well as other forms of exercise, will prevent constipation.
- Encouraging use of the bathroom as soon as there is the urge to eliminate: Putting off the need to have a bowel movement can actually blunt the sensation over time, leading to constipation.
- Trying to have a bowel movement at a regular time each day: Sit on the toilet and try to relax each morning shortly after awakening. Some women, particularly in advanced pregnancy, find that putting their feet up on a step-stool (or a Squatty Potty) while sitting on the toilet relieves pressure of the uterus on the lower intestines, facilitating a bowel movement.

Should these measures not be adequate to treat the problem, bulk laxative fiber supplements, or, if necessary, osmotic or stimulating laxatives can be used.

Fiber Supplementation: Bulk-Forming Laxatives

Fiber supplements, which are bulk-forming laxatives, are effective, safe, and without side effects when used in appropriate doses; however, limited studies are available on the use of laxatives in pregnancy.[1] In addition to softening the stool by keeping more fluid in the bowel lumen, the presence of the increased bulk is thought to stimulate intestinal peristalsis.[5] Examples include wheat fiber (e.g., wheat bran), psyllium, flax seed, and pectin; it is recommended to consume up to 25 g per day.[6] Laxative effects may take 3 to 7 days to be noticeable. If side effects occur, switching to a different bulk laxative may help. Taken in excessive qualities they can lead to cramping, gas, diarrhea, and bloating.[4,6] Bulk laxatives have a pregnancy B category (Table 19-1).[4,6] Stool softeners are not recommended for use during pregnancy.

The editor wishes to thank *Botanical Medicine for Women's Health*, ed 1 contributors to this chapter: Laurel Lee and Christopher Hobbs.

TREATMENT SUMMARY FOR CONSTIPATION

- Increase fluid intake, especially water and noncaffeinated beverages.
- Increase consumption of high-fiber foods such as fruits, vegetables, whole grains, and beans.
- Decrease consumption of constipating foods, particularly those high in fat, such as cheese, milk, and ice cream.
- Increase exercise, even a brisk walk once daily.
- Do not ignore or delay the urge to have a bowel movement—when you've got to go, you've got to go!
- *Herbs are not a substitute for dietary and lifestyle changes!*

TABLE 19-1 Food and Drug Administration Categories for Drug Use During Pregnancy

Category	Description
A	Adequate, well-controlled studies in pregnant women have not shown an increased risk of fetal abnormalities.
B	Either: Animal studies have revealed no evidence of harm to the fetus; however, there are no adequate and well-controlled studies in pregnant women. Or: Animal studies have shown an adverse effect, but adequate and well-controlled studies in pregnant women have failed to demonstrate a risk to the fetus.
C	Either: Animal studies have shown an adverse effect and there are no adequate and well-controlled studies in pregnant women. Or: No animal studies have been conducted and there are no adequate and well-controlled studies in pregnant women.
D	Adequate well-controlled or observational studies in pregnant women have demonstrated a risk to the fetus. However, the benefits of therapy may outweigh the potential risk.
X	Adequate well-controlled or observational studies in animals or pregnant women have demonstrated positive evidence of fetal abnormalities. The use of the product is contraindicated in women who are or may become pregnant.

Adapted from Meadows M: Pregnancy and the drug dilemma, *FDA Consum* 35(3):16–20, 2001.

Osmotic Laxatives

Osmotic laxatives are indigestible sugars that work by increasing the amount of fluid that is retained in the bowel. Sorbitol, lactulose, and glycerin appear to be safe sources for use during pregnancy. Saline, phosphorus, and magnesium salt laxatives, including many prepackaged enemas, are not advisable during pregnancy because they can cause salt retention in the mother.[7]

Stimulant Laxatives

Stimulant laxatives are best used in pregnancy only after other measures have failed to relieve constipation. Examples of stimulant laxatives include senna, cascara sagrada, and aloes. Of these, only senna is considered safe for use during pregnancy (see later senna discussion). Approved as an over-the-counter (OTC) medication, senna is an herb and is thus discussed in the following section with other botanicals. Stimulants are more likely to cause side effects of diarrhea and abdominal pain than are bulk laxatives.[8]

BOTANICAL TREATMENT FOR CONSTIPATION

Botanical treatment for constipation relies on a combination of the practical dietary and lifestyle changes presented in the preceding, and gentle herbs that either increase bulk and moisture in the bowel or gently stimulate bowel activity. These herbs may be used singly, or in combination, and are combined with a carminative herb—one that relieves gas and griping—to prevent side effects sometimes associated with laxatives. Examples of carminatives that can be safely used for short durations during pregnancy include ginger root and anise seed. Stimulant laxatives are used only for short durations (up to 2 weeks) to avoid dependence. When using herbal bulk-forming laxatives, it is important to make sure the patient is drinking plenty of water because the bulk laxative will absorb large amounts of water from the colon. There have been few studies evaluating the safety or efficacy of natural laxatives in pregnancy. A number of herbal preparations available in health food and grocery stores contain herbs that are not appropriate or safe for use in pregnancy, including cascara sagrada, aloe, and buckthorn (see Box 19-1). Aloe may be teratogenic, whereas the other herbs are associated with increased uterine activity. Practitioners should inquire of their pregnant patients whether they are using preparations containing these herbs if constipation is a problem and direct them to safer food-based, lifestyle, and herbal alternatives.

Foods and food agents commonly used to relieve constipation include wheat bran, which is a high-fiber source, prunes (soaked in water or apple juice until soft and plump), and fruits high in sorbitol, including apples, pears, apricots, and cherries. Molasses is both high in iron and is a gentle laxative, and therefore excellent for constipation associated with anemia.[9] Commonly used herbs are listed in Table 19-2. In Traditional Chinese Medicine (TCM), constipation is considered a symptom of blood deficiency, and may be treated with dong quai and peony formula, discussed in Iron Deficiency Anemia (see Chapter 18).

Discussion of Botanicals for Constipation During Pregnancy

Prunes (Dried Plum)

Prunes are a well-known "home remedy" for the treatment of constipation, particularly in the form of prune juice. They are considered safe and effective. A 2011 single-blind crossover randomized controlled trial (RCT) ($n = 40$; 3 men and 37 women, mean age 38 years) tested psyllium fiber (11 g) against dried plums (50 g) for the treatment of constipation. The dietary fiber content of psyllium fiber and dried plums both equaled 6 g. Patients were enrolled into one of the experimental groups for 3 weeks and tracked daily symptoms and

TABLE 19-2　Botanical Treatment Strategies for Constipation

Therapeutic Activity	Botanical Name	Common Name
Bulk laxatives	*Linum usitatissimum*	Flax (i.e., linseed)
	Plantago psyllium; P. ovata	Psyllium
Lubricating laxatives	*Glycyrrhiza glabra*	Licorice
Stimulating laxatives (i.e., aperients)	*Cassia senna; C. angustifolia*	Senna
	Rumex crispus	Yellow dock root

BOX 19-1　Commonly Used Botanical Laxatives That Are Contraindicated During Pregnancy

Aloe *(Aloe vera)*
Cascara *(Frangula purshiana)*
Buckthorn *(Rhamnus cathartica)*
Chinese rhubarb *(Rheum palmatum)*
Castor oil *(Ricinus communis)*

bowel movements in a diary. After the conclusion of the first leg, a 1-week washout period was granted. Then the experimental groups crossed over. The dried plum treatment was more successful than the psyllium in treating constipation ($p < .05$), but both were rated as equally palatable.[10]

Psyllium Seed and Husk

Psyllium seeds, as well as ispaghula seeds, which have comparable activity, are bulk laxative agents.[11] Psyllium seeds shorten bowel transit time by increasing the intestinal contents and stimulating stretch receptors and thereby peristalsis. The whole seeds or husks are soaked in water or apple juice for several hours and then they are taken with a large amount of liquid. Bowel movements are usually achieved within 6 to 12 hours after taking the preparation.[5] Rarely, allergic reactions have occurred.[5] The preparation should not be taken by patients with swallowing difficulties because choking can occur.

Senna Leaf and Pod

Senna, a quick-acting, generally reliable stimulating laxative, is taken as a tea. The tea formula Smooth Move utilizes senna as a primary ingredient and was tested for constipation management in nursing home residents. A group of 86 patients was assigned to receive Smooth Move or placebo daily for 28 days, along with standard treatment. The total number of bowel movements was the primary outcome. Using intent to treat analysis, the Smooth Move group experienced more bowel movements than the placebo group (1 cup of SmootheMove tea daily).[12] The mechanism of action of senna leaf is primarily via anthracoids (i.e., sennoside A and B), or anthraquinone glycosides. Senna is considered appropriate for use in acute cases, though is not ideal for chronic use—it is preferable to make dietary changes, including increasing dietary fiber, and to use bulk laxatives. When used alone senna can elicit loose stool with significant griping, and is therefore traditionally combined with a small amount of ginger root, anise seed, fennel seed, spearmint, or peppermint for their carminative action (see Formula 1 in Box 19-2). Though modern herbalists have tended to consider senna contraindicated for use during pregnancy, with the supposition

that the markedly increased bowel peristalsis stimulated by the herb might lead to reflex uterine activity and thus may have indirect emmenagogic effects, it is considered safe for use during pregnancy by obstetricians, and is recommended regularly for constipation in pregnancy. According to the European Scientific Cooperative on Phytotherapy (ESCOP) there are no reports of undesirable or damaging effects during pregnancy or on the fetus when senna is used in accordance with the recommended dosing and use schedule. However, because of experimental data concerning a genotoxic risk from several anthracoids (i.e., emodin, aloe-emodin), the herb should be avoided during the first trimester or taken only under medical supervision.[13] Two studies reported that human and animal data do not support concerns that senna laxatives pose a genotoxic risk to humans when taken properly.[14-16] A 2010 case-control study evaluated the association between severe constipation, accompanying laxative treatment in pregnant women, and congenital abnormalities (CA) in children. Cases were selected from the data set of the population-based Hungarian Case-Control Surveillance System of Congenital Abnormalities (HCCSCA) 1980 to 1996. Data from 22,843 cases with CA and 38,151 matched controls without CA were utilized. Pregnant women (i.e., 78 cases, 144 controls) with prospective and medically recorded constipation were included for the analysis. Senna was not observed to have teratogenic effects.[17] A review article reported that senna appears to be the most appropriate stimulant laxative to use during pregnancy.[18] Small amounts of active metabolites are excreted in the breast milk, and though these do not appear to have a laxative effect in the newborn, its use is not recommended during lactation.[13] The dose recommended by ESCOP is individualized to the smallest possible dose that produces a comfortable, soft, formed stool. Weiss and Fintelmann stated that small doses of 1 to 2 g soften the stools within 5 to 7 hours.[11] It is recommended that the herb be used only short-term for occasional constipation. Senna preparations are typically taken at bed time to produce a bowel movement the next morning.

Yellow Dock Root

Yellow dock is sometimes contraindicated during pregnancy because of its anthraquinone glycoside contents. Clinically, it is widely used by midwives as a gentle stimulating laxative because it is effective yet much milder than senna, which is generally avoided when possible. According to the *Botanical Safety Handbook,* this herb contains only a small amount of anthraquinone glycosides and has a mild laxative effect.[19]

BOX 19-2 Formulae for Constipation

Formula 1: Laxative Tea (adapted from the German Standard Registration)[5]

Senna leaf	(Cassia senna)	15 g
Anise seed	(Pimpinella anisum)	3 g
Chamomile blossoms	(Matricaria recutita)	5 g
Spearmint leaf	(Mentha spicata)	5 g
	Total: 28 g (1 oz)	

Directions: Prepare 1 to 2 teaspoons as an infusion. Steep for 10 minutes. Take 1 cup each evening.

Formula 2: Dandelion–Yellow Dock Syrup

Yellow dock root	(Rumex crispus)	14 g
Dandelion root	(Taraxacum officinale)	14 g
	Total: 28 g (1 oz)	

Directions: Prepare a decoction by simmering both herbs in 4 cups of water, uncovered, until reduced to 1 cup. Strain the liquid thoroughly, discard the herb material, and add ½ cup blackstrap molasses, mixing until blended. Cool to room temperature. Keep refrigerated. The product will keep for up to 2 weeks refrigerated.

Dose: 1 to 2 tablespoons, up to twice daily.

Limited maternal use has not been observed to cause any increase in fetal malformation or other harmful effects to the fetus.[20] The use of yellow dock for constipation is illustrated in Dandelion–Yellow Dock Root Syrup (see Formula 2 in Box 19-2), and in the case history in iron deficiency anemia.

Licorice Root

Herbalists favor the use of licorice root for its intestinal moistening abilities. According to Wichtl, licorice root is included in laxative herbal tea formulae because it potentiates the activity of anthraquinone-containing herbs (e.g., senna), lowering the required dose of the anthraquinone laxative.[21] A 2010 two-arm, open-label, uncontrolled pilot study ($n = 31$ patients who met Rome II criteria, 10 afflicted with constipation) tested two herbal formulae in the treatment of irritable bowel syndrome (IBS). The first formula (i.e., DA-IBS) was formulated to treat diarrhea-predominant IBS and consisted of bilberry fruit powder, slippery elm bark, agrimony aerial parts, and cinnamon quills. The second formula (i.e., C-IBS) was designed to ameliorate constipation-predominant IBS and included slippery elm bark, lactulose, oat bran, and licorice root. DA-IBS administration was associated with a small yet still significant increase in a few IBS symptoms. But C-IBS performed significantly in alleviating constipation-predominant symptoms. The C-IBS group experienced a 20% increase in bowel movement frequency and significant reductions in straining, abdominal pain, bloating, and global IBS symptom severity ($p = .0005$), as well as improvements in stool consistency ($p < .0001$) (Dose information not available).[22]

Because of its effects on glucocorticoids, excessive doses (>50 g per day) over a prolonged period can result in hypokalemia, hypernatremia, edema, hypertension, and cardiac disorders, and in extreme cases, pseudoaldosteronism. Symptoms disappear within days of discontinuation of the herb.[21] Two recent reports on high-dose licorice consumption, in the form of licorice candy containing actual glycyrrhizin-containing licorice, during pregnancy, demonstrated no increase in maternal hypertension or low birth weight; however, both studies demonstrated a significant increase in preterm (<37 weeks) delivery. In one study, the risk of preterm delivery was greater than double the risk of women not consuming licorice.[23,24] No studies demonstrate harm or adverse outcomes with short-term use of modest doses of licorice. It is recommended that licorice not be used in excessive doses or for prolonged periods during pregnancy; as with senna, it should be used for acute use for up to several days at a time.

CASE HISTORY

Sara, a nurse, was pregnant with her second baby. Her husband, Jeff, is a physician. In addition to these pregnancies, Sara had experienced two miscarriages, one before her first live birth, and the second between the two pregnancies. At 10 weeks of gestation, Sara was experiencing moderate constipation, so she decided to go to the local health food store and try a natural laxative. She purchased a prepackaged mix containing a number of herbs including senna, cascara sagrada, and buckthorn. Concerned about the safety of these herbs she called her obstetrician for information. He told her that herbs do not do anything, and that it was fine to take them. Sara took the herbs for 5 days, after which time she began having cramping and spotting. She miscarried 3 days later. Although the miscarriage may have been entirely unrelated to the use of these herbs, this case illustrates a serious lack of knowledge on the part of the obstetrician and the need for medical education to include training at least in the herbs contraindicated in various circumstances, for example, pregnancy.

See also iron deficiency anemia case history box in Chapter 18.

HYPERTENSION IN PREGNANCY

Hypertension is the most common medical problem of pregnancy, affecting 10% of all pregnant women.[25] The condition can lead to devastating outcomes with significantly increased risks of placental abruption, disseminated intravascular coagulation (DIC), cerebral hemorrhage, hepatic failure, and acute renal failure.[26] Hypertensive disorders of pregnancy are a significant cause of maternal and perinatal morbidity and mortality, and therefore require accurate diagnosis and proper medical management. Complementary and alternative medicine (CAM) treatments for hypertensive disorders during pregnancy should *always* accompany proper medical management *in conjunction* with the care of an obstetrician.

Hypertensive disorders of pregnancy are divided into four categories according to the National High Blood Pressure Education Program (NHBPEP) 2000 Working Group:

1. Preeclampsia–eclampsia
2. Chronic hypertension
3. Preeclampsia superimposed on chronic hypertension
4. Gestational (transient) hypertension[26]

Hypertension itself is defined as a sustained increase in blood pressure greater than 140/90. Elevated blood pressure should be documented on at least two consecutive occasions more than 6 hours apart, using the appropriate-size blood pressure cuff, to make a diagnosis of hypertension. Diastolic pressure should be considered the number at which the phase V Korotkoff sound is auscultated. Patients should be told to avoid tobacco and caffeine for at least 30 minutes before a blood pressure reading, and should be encouraged to relax for 10 minutes before evaluation.[26] The definition of hypertension as a 30 mmHg systolic and/or 15 mmHg rise over baseline is now considered invalid because it is recognized that up to 73% of all women in their first pregnancies experience a diastolic rise of this magnitude at some point in the pregnancy with no subsequent development of pathology.[27] Nonetheless, close observation of these women is recommended.[25] Each type of hypertensive disorder of pregnancy has specific diagnostic criteria (Box 19-3).

DESCRIPTIONS OF HYPERTENSIVE DISORDERS OF PREGNANCY BY CLASSIFICATION AND GENERAL CONVENTIONAL TREATMENT APPROACHES

A great deal of debate and uncertainty surrounds the etiology, classification, and medical treatment of pregnancy hypertensive disorders. The following discussion provides a brief overview of the salient points of each of the pregnancy hypertensive disorders and their specific medical treatments based on current recommendations.

Preeclampsia

Preeclampsia is a disease specific to pregnancy, with "cure" occurring only upon delivery of the placenta. The etiology of preeclampsia remains unknown, although there are numerous theories. It appears that it is a complex, multifactorial condition with genetic factors, immunologic factors, altered inflammatory pathways, insulin resistance (e.g., obesity, hyperlipidemia, glucose intolerance), endothelial dysfunction, macronutrient and micronutrient deficiencies, altered placental angiogenesis, and subclinical infections possibly participating in the risk of developing this condition.[25,28] Advanced maternal age, first pregnancy, poor nutrition, residence at high altitudes, and lack of adequate prenatal care have also been associated with increased risk.[28] There is a common thread in all cases: poor placental perfusion associated with maternal vasoconstriction and subsequent maternal multiorgan failure.[25]

Early identification of preeclampsia increases the likelihood of proper early management and reduction of poor prenatal outcome. Unfortunately, in spite of a great deal of investigation into serum markers that might help to identify women at risk of developing preeclampsia, no reliable markers have been found, nor is there a consistent standard for clinical identification of this potentially devastating condition.[25] Similarly, no preventative measures for preeclampsia have been identified with any certainty. Current pharmacotherapy is able to reduce

---

BOX 19-3   Diagnosis of Hypertensive Disorders Complicating Pregnancy

Preeclampsia
Minimum criteria:
- Blood pressure (BP) = 140/90 mmHg after 20 weeks of gestation
- Proteinuria = 300 mg/24 hours or = 1 + dipstick

Increased certainty of preeclampsia:
- BP = 160/110 mmHg
- Proteinuria 2.0 g/24 hours
- Serum creatinine >1.2 mg/dL unless known to be previously elevated
- Platelets <100,000 mm
- Microangiopathic hemolysis (increased LDH (lactate dehydrogenase))
- Elevated alanine transaminase (ALT) or aspartate transaminase (AST)
- Persistent headache or other cerebral or visual disturbance
- Persistent epigastric pain

Eclampsia
- Seizures that cannot be attributed to other causes in a woman with preeclampsia. *This is a medical emergency!*

Chronic Hypertension
- BP = 140/90 mmHg before pregnancy or diagnosed before 20 weeks of gestation *Or*
- Hypertension first diagnosed after 20 weeks of gestation and persistent after 12 weeks postpartum

Preeclampsia Superimposed on Chronic Hypertension
- New-onset proteinuria = 300 mg/24 hours in hypertensive women but no proteinuria before 20 weeks of gestation
- Sudden increase in proteinuria or blood pressure or platelet count <100.000 mm in women with hypertension and proteinuria before 20 weeks of gestation

Gestational Hypertension (Transient Hypertension)
- BP = 140/90 mmHg for first time during pregnancy
- No proteinuria
- BP return to normal <12 weeks postpartum
- Final diagnosis made only postpartum
- May have other signs of preeclampsia, for example, epigastric discomfort or thrombocytopenia
- 15% to 25% of women will go on to develop preeclampsia; gestational age at diagnosis of transient hypertension is inversely related to likelihood of developing preeclampsia

Note that edema is no longer considered a diagnostic criterion of preeclampsia because it is found in many normal pregnancies and is not a reliable indicator.

blood pressure and prevent the development of eclampsia (i.e., preeclampsia with seizures), but it cannot stop the progression of the condition once it is established. Fetal intrauterine growth restriction is a major consequence of this disease. Initial ultrasound at 18 to 20 weeks of gestation documents baseline fetal growth. When a woman is diagnosed with preeclampsia, serial ultrasounds at 28 to 32 weeks of gestation and then monthly until term are suggested for objective measurement. Fetal well-being tests such as nonstress tests (NST) and biophysical profile (BPP) are ordered in the third trimester. Fetal movement counts are helpful as a subjective measurement the woman can do at home. A variety of therapeutic strategies have been evaluated for the prevention and treatment of preeclampsia. These are discussed in the following.

Diuretics

Diuretics were once assumed to be a beneficial part of treatment of preeclampsia with its attendant hypertension and edema. However, women with preeclampsia are actually hypovolemic and hemoconcentrated; therefore the use of diuretics may exacerbate the condition, and thus their use for this condition has been abandoned.[25]

Salt Restriction

There is no evidence that salt restriction is of any benefit in the prevention or treatment of preeclampsia.[29,30]

Antihypertensive Medication

Antihypertensive therapy for women with preeclampsia does not affect the underlying disease process or improve mother–baby outcome.[30] Further, antihypertensive medications have been associated with adverse side effects, including total placental hypoperfusion; thus their use is reserved for the treatment of chronic and severe hypertension.[30]

Aspirin

Data from randomized trials and meta-analyses have been conflicting on the prophylactic and therapeutic effects of low-dose aspirin for preeclampsia. The use of aspirin is predicated on the fact that widely disseminated endothelial dysfunction and platelet disturbances are associated with the etiology of this condition. Low-dose aspirin is thought to be effective because of its thromboxane synthesis inhibition, with consequent reduction in platelet aggregation, as well as its ability to inhibit free radical formation (i.e., lipid peroxides) and support of resistance to angiotensin II in pregnant women with increased susceptibility to this vasoconstriction substance.[25,31,32] The most recent systematic review of all randomized trials to meet the reviewer's inclusion criteria (39 trials with a total of 30,563 women) showed a positive safety profile with a moderate, but significant, reduction in the risk of preeclampsia regardless of weeks gestation at trial entry or dose of aspirin. A 15% reduction in incidence of preeclampsia was observed, with an 8% reduction in preterm birth and a 14% reduction in risk of perinatal death.[33] In spite of disagreement of the value of aspirin for preeclampsia in earlier studies, all studies have demonstrated that aspirin use in recommended doses during pregnancy appears safe.[25] Recent evidence suggests that the earlier in pregnancy that the aspirin is started, the greater the benefit. The recommended dosage range for optimal effects is between 80 and 150 mg per day, specifically to be taken at bedtime.[34,35]

Calcium

Studies on the efficacy of calcium supplementation for prophylaxis and treatment of preeclampsia have been equivocal. A recent, large, multicenter, randomized prospective trial of 2 g of elemental calcium versus placebo given to healthy, nulliparous pregnant women beginning in their second trimester showed no differences in the incidence or severity of hypertensive disorders.[36] However, a more recent trial demonstrated benefit for women who were at very high risk for developing preeclampsia.[37] A proposed mechanism is via prevention of a compensatory rise in parathyroid hormone associated with low serum calcium, and consequently, smooth muscle contraction; however, this remains theoretical.[25]

Vitamins C and E

Oxidative stress has been proposed as a mechanism associated with the development of preeclampsia. Further, studies have demonstrated decreased levels of antioxidant levels in women with preeclampsia. This has prompted evaluation into the use of vitamin C and E supplements as possible prophylaxis and therapy. The risk of developing preeclampsia was seen to be lower in high-risk women begun on supplementation at 16 to 20 weeks of gestation compared with placebo.[25] At this point, the role of antioxidants in this condition remains unclear. For women wishing to supplement vitamin C during pregnancy, it is recommended not to exceed 2000 mg per day to avoid the risk of sensitivity or neonatal rebound scurvy.

Chronic Hypertension

Chronic hypertension is defined as hypertension that predated pregnancy, or hypertension beginning before 20 weeks of gestation. This diagnosis is not easy to establish in women who have not had care before pregnancy and because hypertension before 20 weeks of gestation can also be indicative of preeclampsia that can occur early in pregnancy in a limited number of conditions.[25] Blood pressure levels are less suggestive of poor maternal or fetal outcomes, including fetal growth retardation, prematurity, preeclampsia, placental abruption, and maternal or perinatal morbidity and mortality than are the onset of proteinuria and symptoms of preeclampsia.[38,39] The health care professional may order electrocardiography, echocardiogram, ophthalmologic examination, and renal ultrasound. Women with mild hypertension (i.e., 140 to 159 mmHg systolic or 90 to 105 mmHg diastolic) generally do well in pregnancy and, overall, do not need antihypertensive medication. In fact, women already taking antihypertensive medications may need to decrease the dose because some studies have shown decreased uteroplacental blood flow and fetal growth with medication.[40] Tapering or stopping antihypertensive medications is done under close observation. Antihypertensive therapies are given to reduce the risk of maternal stroke and cardiovascular complication in women with a diastolic blood pressure of greater than 105 mmHg. Recommendation of antihypertensive treatment is done when blood pressure levels reach or exceed 160 mmHg systolic or 100 to 106 mmHg diastolic, when abnormal laboratory values are found, and certainly with a combination of both abnormal factors. Oral antihypertensive medication with methyldopa or labetalol is typically recommended. Methyldopa does not appear to have negative effects on uteroplacental blood flow.[41] Some women, however, do not tolerate it well because of drowsiness. Labetalol, a combined alpha- and beta-blocker, is another choice and can also be prescribed postpartum when breastfeeding. Ideally, women with chronic hypertension need to be evaluated before pregnancy for severity of the hypertension, modification of lifestyle habits, and target organ damage (i.e., heart, kidney). Women with significant renal impairment (i.e., serum creatinine 71.4 mg/dL) may have further deterioration in pregnancy. Women with cardiac abnormalities may have underlying diseases in addition to chronic hypertension. Most women with mild chronic hypertension (i.e., 140/90 mmHg) have no end organ involvement and can have uncomplicated pregnancies.

Gestational (Transient) Hypertension

Elevated blood pressure appearing after 20 weeks without proteinuria and with normal laboratory values in a previously normotensive woman generally results in a good outcome.[25] However, gestational hypertension is considered a provisional term. Although most women will not develop subsequent problems, up to 25% will go on to develop symptoms of preeclampsia.[42] Women with gestational hypertension appear to be at significantly increased risk of maternal and perinatal morbidity, with elevated rates of preterm delivery, infants that are small for gestational age, and abruptio placenta occurrence significantly increased compared with the general obstetric population, and similar to rates reported for women with severe preeclampsia.[42] Thus women with a diagnosis of gestational hypertension should be monitored closely, with weekly prenatal visits optimal. Ultrasound and fetal well-being tests are appropriate in the third trimester. If symptoms of preeclampsia develop, women are treated as is appropriate for that condition. If elevated blood pressure readings persist 12 weeks postpartum, a diagnosis of chronic hypertension is made retrospectively.

BOTANICAL TREATMENT OF HYPERTENSION IN PREGNANCY

Improperly treated pregnancy hypertensive disorders can have dire consequences for the mother and baby. It is not recommended that pregnant women attempt self-medication for pregnancy hypertension, nor that this be done by inexperienced practitioners. The best treatment is obstetric medical care accompanied, when appropriate, by prudent use of herbal medicines as adjunct therapy, under the guidance of an herbalist, naturopath, or midwife trained in the use of botanical medicines in pregnancy. Although popular for the treatment of hypertension in the nonpregnant population, herbal diuretics such as dandelion leaf (*Taraxacum officinale*) are not appropriate for the treatment of pregnancy hypertensive disorders, and may potentially cause exacerbation. The herbs discussed in the following are those commonly used for treating gestational and chronic hypertension that are considered generally safe for use during pregnancy. Botanical treatment for preeclampsia is not recommended and has not been investigated.

Cramp Bark and Black Haw

Cramp bark and black haw have been used by midwives as part of herbal antihypertensive protocol for gestational hypertension. Traditionally, they have been used as musculoskeletal relaxants during pregnancy, and to treat irritable uterus, prevent premature labor, and relieve incoordinate uterine contractions.[43,44] They are taken in tincture form for this purpose, either alone or more typically with relaxing nervines and hawthorn (Table 19-3).

Garlic

Garlic has mild antihypertensive properties and inhibits platelet aggregation and inflammation. No studies have evaluated the efficacy or safety of garlic use for pregnancy hypertension. Garlic is a common food used during pregnancy worldwide, and in modest doses is not expected to cause any adverse effects. The German Commission E gives no contraindication to its use during pregnancy, nor does the *Botanical Safety Handbook*, which does however provide a caution about use during lactation because of active constituents passing through the breast milk.[45-47] (McKenna and colleagues note that the dose of constituents received through breast milk is actually quite small.[46]) A randomized

TABLE 19-3	Botanical Treatment Strategies for Hypertension in Pregnancy		
Therapeutic Goal	**Therapeutic Activity**	**Botanical Name**	**Common Name**
Reduce blood pressure	Antihypertensives	*Allium sativum*	Garlic
		Crataegus spp.	Hawthorn
		Ganoderma lucidum	Reishi
		Viburnum spp.	Cramp bark, black haw
Stress reduction, relaxation	Nervines	*Lavandula officinalis*	Lavender
		Passiflora incarnata	Passionflower
		Viburnum spp.	Cramp bark, black haw

control study of 100 primigravid women given either 800 mg/day of garlic tablets or placebo during third trimester pregnancy to evaluate the effect of garlic supplementation on preeclampsia found that pregnancy outcomes were comparable in both groups. There were no reports of side effects in the garlic group other than garlic body odor and nausea, nor reports of an incidence of adverse fetal outcomes or spontaneous abortion.[48] Garlic odor was identifiable in the amniotic fluid of a small group of pregnant women taking garlic supplements.[49] It is commonly recommended that because of its antithrombotic effects, garlic use should be discounted 7 days before surgery.[46] A recent Cochrane review evaluating the effects of garlic on preeclampsia and its related complications concluded that there is insufficient evidence to recommend increased garlic intake for preventing preeclampsia and its complications, and that side effects have not been reported with its use in pregnancy.[50] Although the actual risk of bleeding is uncertain, it is prudent to discontinue the medicinal use of garlic 3 weeks before the due date to minimize any increased risk of bleeding because women with hypertensive disorders during pregnancy are more likely to enter labor early.

Hawthorn

Hawthorn has been used for treating a variety of cardiovascular conditions, and has noted antioxidant effects and antiplatelet aggregating effects, which may be of benefit in preventing pregnancy hypertension.[45,46,51] Other noted actions are an increase in the integrity of the blood vessel wall, improvement in coronary blood flow, and positive effects on oxygen use.[46] There are no known contraindications or restrictions to the use of this herb during pregnancy or lactation.[45-47]

Reishi

Although not classically used for the treatment of hypertension in pregnancy, it is worth mentioning that the medicinal mushroom *Ganoderma lucidum* has demonstrated positive results in research looking at its antihypertensive effects, as well as effects against diabetes and hyperlipidemia.[52-54] One interesting study looked at the effects of reishi on glomerular function, and found that it was able to improve hemodynamic flow in glomerular disease and reduce proteinuria. The beneficial effect of *G. lucidum* appears to be multifactorial, including the modulation of immunocirculatory balance; antilipid, vasodilator, and antiplatelet effects; and improved hemodynamics. Together with vitamins C and E, this herb helped to neutralize oxidative stress and suppress the toxic effect to the glomerular endothelial function.[55] Extracts of reishi polysaccharides have demonstrated significantly improved basal nitrous oxide (NO) release and endothelium-dependent relaxation but without affecting endogenous nitrous oxide synthase (NOS) activity. These results suggest that this herb has the potential to improve endothelium-dependent relaxation in mineralocorticoid hypertension.[56] In a study evaluating the clinical effects of lyophilized *G. lucidum* extract, 53 patients were divided into two groups: group I consisted

of essential hypertensive patients, and group II consisted of mild hypertensive or normotensive patients. The patients were instructed to take six tablets containing 240 mg of the extract per day. Biochemical and hematologic examination were performed for 21 test items, and the following results were obtained.[1] In regard to hypertension, blood pressure significantly decreased in group I, but did not in group II, thus showing that *G. lucidum* has an ameliorating effect on hypertension.[2] In regard to biochemical and hematologic effects, the oral intake did not result in any change in the values of any of the 21 test items beyond the normal range, except that total cholesterol decreased slightly and fibrinogen increased slightly. It was therefore concluded that *G. lucidum* has blood pressure lowering effects on patients with essential hypertension and will not have any side effects on patients with essential or border line hypertension during 6 months of oral intake.[57] In one study, however, reishi did not demonstrate any observable differences in body mass index (BMI), blood pressure, urine catecholamines, cortisol, plasma antioxidant status, or blood lymphocyte subsets between groups. There were, however, decreases in triacylglycerol, plasma insulin, and homeostasis model assessment insulin resistance, and increases in high-density lipoprotein (HDL) cholesterol.[58] No safety data on use during pregnancy were identified.[59] Reishi may be taken alone or in combination with other herbs, and may be taken as a liquid extract or in solid (i.e., pill) form (Box 19-4).

BOX 19-4 Protocol for Chronic or Gestational Hypertension

Tincture Formula for Cardiovascular Support

Hawthorn	*Crataegus oxyacantha*	40 mL
Cramp bark or black haw	*Viburnum* spp.	30 mL
Passionflower	*Passiflora incarnata*	30 mL
		Total: 100 mL

Dose: 5 mL twice daily

Also:
Garlic: One clove of fresh garlic daily or garlic capsules (dose according to specific product)
Reishi: 2 mL tincture twice daily
Daily supplementation:
- 2 g calcium citrate with 500 mg magnesium citrate
- 1000 mg vitamin C
- 400 IU vitamin E

Diet: Emphasize a heart-healthy diet of fresh fruits, especially dark-colored berries rich in the vascular-protective antioxidant anthocyanidin; vegetables, whole grains, legumes, nuts, fresh fish, and poultry. Avoid high fat, fried, and processed foods.
Exercise: 30 minutes walking daily (unless otherwise prohibited).
Relaxation: Daily yoga, meditation, or biofeedback exercises.
Warm (not hot) baths: 2 to 3 times/week with ½ cup Epsom salts and 5 to 10 drops lavender essential oil added to the bath.

ADDITIONAL THERAPIES

Nutritional Considerations

A diet rich in calcium, magnesium, and potassium may lessen cardiovascular risk. A diet rich in fruits, vegetables, whole grains, legumes, nuts, good-quality oils, and low-fat foods is associated with decreased hypertension and may be especially beneficial for women with chronic hypertension. A 2013 RCT tested early pregnancy phytonutrient supplementation against placebo for the prevention of preeclampsia. Out of 684 enrolled women, 39% ($n = 267$) completed the trial. The women were randomized to receive treatment or placebo according to risk status, and primary outcome was preeclampsia. The investigators did not find a difference between groups on this outcome. However, nonsignificant trends toward placenta-related complications were noted in the supplement group. They also reported slightly decreased rates of respiratory distress syndrome in infants born to mothers in the supplement group (Dose and preparation information not available).[60] Essential fatty acids (EFAs) may also be beneficial in the prevention of pregnancy hypertension. Vascular sensitivity to angiotensin II was determined in the midtrimester of pregnancy in women after taking a diet with supplemented EFAs and vitamins. The EFAs linoleic and dihomo-gamma-linolenic acid were administered as evening primrose oil capsules (i.e., Efamol) for 1 week before the study. Vascular sensitivity was then determined in response to 4, 8, and 16 ng kg-1 min-1 angiotensin II. Vitamin supplements (i.e., Elevit) were given with the Efamol capsules. Seven women were studied, and their vascular sensitivity compared with controls on normal diet. The vascular sensitivity was significantly reduced in all the patients on essential fatty acid supplements, and all values fell below the mean of the control group.[61]

Exercise and Stress Management

Exercise and relaxation practices have generally been shown to be beneficial in the reduction of hypertension as part of therapeutic lifestyle choices. Although the role of exercise and stress management in the prevention of preeclampsia is not established, it is certainly beneficial in the management of chronic hypertension. Regular walking, yoga, meditation, biofeedback, and other gentle techniques are safe during normal pregnancy.

GROUP B STREPTOCOCCUS INFECTION IN PREGNANCY

Group B streptococcus (GBS) is a normal inhabitant of the intestinal tract and colonizes the vaginal tracts of many women; it can be demonstrated by culture of combined rectal and vaginal swabs in 15% to 30% of pregnant women on random sampling.[62]

In the 1970s, GBS, or infection with *Streptococcus agalactiae*, emerged as a leading cause of pneumonia, sepsis, and meningitis in newborns.[63] Most bacterial transmission to the neonate occurs during birth via passage of the baby through the birth canal, or via ascendant bacteria during labor with ruptured membranes. Premature babies and babies of mothers with prolonged or preterm premature rupture of membranes (PPROM) are at higher risk of infection. GBS can also cross the membranes, so cesarean section is not protective and carries additional surgical risks to the mother. Infection is categorized as either early or late onset.

Early onset disease symptoms manifest within a few hours, and up to a week after birth. In a study of 148,000 infants born between 2000 and 2008, nearly all of the 94 infants who developed early GBS infection were diagnosed within an hour after birth—suggesting that early GBS infection probably begins *before* birth.[64] Antibiotic prophylaxis administered to the mother during labor, as is discussed in the following, is used to prevent early-onset infection in the neonate.

Late-onset disease develops through contact with hospital nursery personnel and usually manifests in the first 3 months after birth. Up to 45% of health care workers carry the bacteria on their skin, and may transmit the infection to newborns.[65] Meticulous hand-washing practices in the hospital are essential for reduction of nosocomial disease transmission.

Women with these factors may be more likely to carry GBS:

- African American women
- Multiple sexual partners
- Male-to-female oral sex
- Frequent or recent sex
- Tampon use
- Infrequent hand-washing
- Younger than 20 years old[66]

Though GBS transmission rates are high, the rate of neonatal sepsis is surprisingly low. The mortality rate from early onset GBS infection is 2% to 3% for full-term infants and as high as 20% to 30% for premature infants born before 33 weeks of gestation.[67]

Over 1600 cases of early-onset infections occur in newborns annually, with as many as 80 deaths per year.[63] Although the mortality rate of GBS is relatively low, morbidity can be significant. In addition to extensive stays in the neonatal intensive care unit, which is costly and emotionally demanding for families, it is estimated that up to 44% of infants who survive GBS with meningitis end up with long-term health problems, including developmental disabilities, paralysis, seizure disorder, hearing loss, vision loss, and small brains.[68]

If a pregnant woman carrying GBS is not treated with antibiotics during labor, the baby's risk of becoming colonized with GBS is approximately 50%. Note that most colonized babies do not develop GBS infection. The risk of developing a *serious, life-threatening GBS infection,* according to the Centers for Disease Control and Prevention (CDC), is 1% to 2% (2010).[67] If a GBS–positive woman is treated with antibiotics during labor, chances of her infant developing an early GBS infection declines by 80%, or from 1% to 0.2%.[69]

Note that GBS can also cause maternal bladder and uterine infections, and increases the risk of premature labor, PPROM, and stillbirth.

DIAGNOSIS

The gold standard test used in screening is a bacterial culture of a sample collection from a simultaneous vaginal and rectal swab. The best time to test for the presence of the organism is between weeks 35 and 37.[63] Testing at this time is as much as 50% more effective at predicting and preventing perinatal disease than screening earlier in pregnancy, although the numbers of organisms in any individual might fluctuate, making detectable levels variable. CDC guidelines published in 2002 recommend universal screening for pregnant mothers between 35 and 37 weeks of gestation.[63] The FDA has recently approved a new "quick" test that can diagnose GBS in pregnant women in about an hour. Some studies have shown the test to be up to 94% sensitive, whereas other studies show less consistent results. Because GBS resistance to specific antibiotics has developed, especially to those used for penicillin-allergic women, culture and sensitivity testing is recommended. Urine testing in the first trimester that reveals the presence of urinary GBS infection suggests an increased risk for GBS infection in late pregnancy, and is also a method of diagnosis.

- The United Kingdom National Screening Committee states that pregnant women in the UK should not be screened for GBS. The UK follows the risk-based approach. This includes giving antibiotics in-labor to all women who have fever, prolonged rupture of membranes longer than 18 hours, GBS in urine at any time during pregnancy, preterm labor, or a prior infant with GBS. This means that many women who are actually GBS negative receive antibiotics directed at GBS, just based on their risk factors. In the UK, the rate of early GBS infections is 0.5 per 1000 births, which is slightly higher than the rate of 0.2 per 1000 births in the U.S. In the UK, it is not considered cost effective to screen the whole population of pregnant women to lower the early GBS infection rate by 0.2 to 0.3 cases per 1000.
- The Royal College of Obstetricians does not recommend routine screening for GBS during pregnancy. However, they do state that in-labor antibiotics could be considered if GBS was detected in passing or if women have any of the risk factors listed earlier. Many women are already receiving antibiotics for these reasons.

There is controversy in the UK over the lack of access to GBS testing within the National Health Service. Group B Strep Support is a consumer-based charity that advocates for women to have access to GBS screening in the UK. The Society of Obstetricians and Gynaecologists of Canada (SOGC) recommends offering GBS screening to all pregnant women and treating those who are positive with intravenous (IV) antibiotics.

CONVENTIONAL TREATMENT APPROACHES

The American College of Obstetricians and Gynecologists (ACOG), the American Academy of Pediatrics, and the CDC published guidelines in 1996 recommending a risk-based (i.e., screening) approach to determine when to recommend IV antibiotic prophylaxis during labor.[70,71] It was determined that women with the following risk factors should be offered IV antibiotics during labor and delivery, not before labor:

- Fever during labor
- Rupture of membranes 18 hours or more before delivery
- Labor or rupture of membranes before 37 weeks

As of 2002, the CDC revised the 1996 guidelines, recommending routine screening for all pregnant women between 35 and 37 weeks of gestation, and universal treatment for women who test positive for GBS during pregnancy (Box 19-5).

> **WARNING:** Women with negative vaginal and rectal GBS screening cultures within 5 weeks of delivery do not require intrapartum antimicrobial prophylaxis for GBS even if obstetric risk factors develop (i.e., delivery at <37 weeks' gestation, duration of membrane rupture >18 hours, or temperature >100.4° F [>38.0° C]).

The use of prophylactic perinatal IV antibiotics is attributed with a 70% reduction in the incidence of GBS disease during the last 10 years. In spite of this reduction in incidence, early-onset GBS-related diseases such as pneumonia and meningitis remain a cause of illness and death in newborns in the United States, with a rate of approximately 80 deaths annually.

An alternative conventional treatment to IV antibiotic prophylaxis that has been investigated in Europe but is not employed in the United States other than by midwives is the use of chlorhexidine vaginal flushing. A randomized controlled study was conducted to investigate the efficacy of intrapartum vaginal flushing with chlorhexidine compared with ampicillin in preventing GBS transmission to neonates. The study evaluated outcomes of singleton pregnancies delivering vaginally. Rupture of membranes, when present, must not have occurred more than 6 hours prior. Women with any gestational complication, with a newborn previously affected by GBS sepsis, or whose cervical dilatation was greater than 5 cm were excluded. A total of 244 GBS–colonized mothers at term (screened at 36 to 38 weeks) were randomized to receive either 140 mL chlorhexidine 0.2% by vaginal flushing every 6 hours or ampicillin 2 g IV every 6 hours until delivery. Neonatal swabs were taken at birth at three different sites (i.e., nose, ear, and gastric juice). A total of 108 women were treated with ampicillin and 109 with chlorhexidine. Ages and gestational weeks at delivery were similar in the two groups. Nulliparous women were equally distributed between the two groups (ampicillin, 87%; chlorhexidine, 89%). Clinical data such as birth weight (ampicillin, 3365 ± 390 g; chlorhexidine, 3440 ± 452 g) and Apgar scores at 1 minute (ampicillin, 8.4 ± 0.9; chlorhexidine, 8.2 ± 1.4) and at 5 minutes (ampicillin, 9.7 ± 0.6; chlorhexidine, 9.6 ± 1.1) were similar for the two groups, as was the rate of neonatal GBS colonization (chlorhexidine, 15.6%; ampicillin, 12%). *Escherichia coli*, on the other hand, was significantly more prevalent in the ampicillin (7.4%) than in the chlorhexidine group (1.8%, $p < .05$). Six

BOX 19-5   Centers for Disease Control and Prevention 2002 Group B Streptococcus Treatment Guidelines[63]

- All pregnant women should be screened at 35 to 37 weeks of gestation for vaginal and rectal group B streptococcus (GBS) colonization. At the time of labor or rupture of membranes, intrapartum chemoprophylaxis should be given to all pregnant women identified as GBS carriers. Colonization during a previous pregnancy is not an indication for intrapartum prophylaxis in subsequent deliveries. Screening to detect GBS colonization in each pregnancy will determine the need for prophylaxis in that pregnancy.
- Women with GBS isolated from the urine in any concentration during their current pregnancy should receive intrapartum chemoprophylaxis because such women usually are heavily colonized with GBS and are at increased risk of delivering an infant with early-onset GBS disease. Prenatal culture-based screening at 35 to 37 weeks of gestation is not necessary for women with GBS bacteriuria. Women with symptomatic or asymptomatic GBS urinary tract infection (UTI) detected during pregnancy should be treated according to current standards of care for UTI during pregnancy.
- Women who have previously given birth to an infant with invasive GBS disease should receive intrapartum chemoprophylaxis; prenatal culture-based screening is not necessary for these women.
- If the result of GBS culture is not known at the onset of labor, intrapartum chemoprophylaxis should be administered to women with any of the following risk factors: gestation less than 37 weeks, duration of membrane rupture longer than 18 hours, or a temperature higher than 100.4° F (>38.0° C). Women with known negative results from vaginal and rectal GBS screening cultures within 5 weeks of delivery do not require prophylaxis to prevent GBS disease even if any of the intrapartum risk factors develop.
- Women with threatened preterm (<37 weeks of gestation) delivery should be assessed for need for intrapartum prophylaxis to prevent perinatal GBS disease.
- In the absence of GBS UTI, antimicrobial agents should not be used before the intrapartum period to treat GBS colonization. Such treatment is not effective in eliminating carriage or preventing neonatal disease and may cause adverse consequences.

- GBS–colonized women who have a planned cesarean delivery performed before rupture of membranes and onset of labor are at low risk for having an infant with early-onset GBS disease. These women should not routinely receive intrapartum chemoprophylaxis for perinatal GBS disease prevention.
- For intrapartum chemoprophylaxis, the following regimen is recommended for women without penicillin allergy: penicillin G, 5 million units intravenously (IV) initial dose, then 2.5 million units IV every 4 hours until delivery. Because of its narrow spectrum of activity, penicillin is the preferred agent. An alternative regimen is ampicillin; 2 g IV initial dose, then 1 g IV every 4 hours until delivery (AI).
- Intrapartum chemoprophylaxis for penicillin-allergic women takes into account increasing resistance to clindamycin and erythromycin among GBS isolates. During prenatal care, history of penicillin allergy should be assessed to determine whether a patient is at high risk for anaphylaxis, that is, has a history of immediate hypersensitivity reactions to penicillin (e.g., anaphylaxis, angioedema, urticaria) or history of asthma or other conditions that would make anaphylaxis more dangerous. Women who are not at high risk for anaphylaxis should be given cefazolin; 2 g IV initial dose, then 1 g IV every 8 hours until delivery. For women at high risk for anaphylaxis, clindamycin and erythromycin susceptibility testing, if available, should be performed on isolates obtained during GBS prenatal carriage screening. Women with clindamycin- and erythromycin-susceptible isolates should be given either clindamycin, 900 mg IV every 8 hours until delivery; or erythromycin, 500 mg IV every 6 hours until delivery. If susceptibility testing is not possible, susceptibility results are not known, or isolates are resistant to erythromycin or clindamycin, the following regimen can be used for women with immediate penicillin hypersensitivity: vancomycin, 1 g IV every 12 hours until delivery.
- Routine use of antimicrobial prophylaxis for newborns whose mothers received intrapartum chemoprophylaxis for GBS infection is not recommended. However, therapeutic use of these agents is appropriate for infants with clinically suspected sepsis.

neonates were transferred to the neonatal intensive care unit, including two cases of early-onset sepsis (one in each group). In this carefully screened target population, intrapartum vaginal flushing with chlorhexidine in colonized mothers displayed the same efficacy as ampicillin in preventing vertical transmission of GBS. Moreover, the rate of neonatal *E. coli* colonization was reduced by chlorhexidine.[72]

This is an option that many midwives in the United States are beginning to employ in home birth settings; clearly more investigation of this option should be conducted to determine whether it is a safe and effective alternative to routine intranatal IV prophylaxis for neonatal GBS infection. Until then, IV antibiotic prophylaxis remains the recommended standard.

BOTANICAL TREATMENT OF GROUP B STREPTOCOCCUS

Choosing to Use Botanical Therapies for Reducing Group B Streptococcus Infection During Pregnancy

Despite the 2002 revised protocol, many pregnant women prefer to avoid routine antibiotic prophylaxis for a variety of reasons including:

- Philosophic reasons (i.e., they prefer to minimize medical intervention or want a "natural" approach)
- Concern about sequelae (i.e., effect on neonatal microbiome, increased risk of atopic disease and diabetes

later in life because of antibiotic exposure prenatally or at the time of birth, development of resistant infections, increased likelihood of neonatal Candida infection [i.e., thrush])

- Choice of birth setting (i.e., home birth, making it difficult if not impossible to access antibiotic prophylaxis in labor)

For women choosing to birth naturally at home, the use of prophylactic IV antibiotics in labor is sometimes not a realistic option—in most states, home birth midwives are unable to administer IV medications. Home birth midwifery protocol therefore continues to follow the risk-assessment model, transporting to the hospital for IV antibiotic prophylaxis should indications arise, including rupture of membranes longer than 18 to 24 hours (length of time varies with the protocol of different medical and midwifery communities) or any signs of infection. GBS–positive women planning home births commonly seek herbal options prenatally for reducing their microbial load, hoping to avoid PPROM, thus prolonging the length of time before the need to transport to the hospital during delivery.

Herbal treatment has been empirically demonstrated to be effective in reducing GBS colonization if it is started 2 to 3 weeks before the onset of labor. Note that herbal prophylaxis is done during pregnancy and not as a substitute for intranatal antibiotic prophylaxis. It is common for women in this situation to also use herbs to augment labor in the event of PPROM to encourage birth to occur within the allotted 18- to 24-hour window. PPROM is discussed elsewhere in this book.

Should women choose to follow an herbal protocol for reducing GBS colonization, it is imperative that the protocol be accompanied by retesting as close to the expected due date as possible but with enough time to receive results before labor. GBS–positive pregnant women should be made fully aware of the risks of GBS before laboring without antibiotic prophylaxis. Women should also be informed that, in cases in which antibiotics are declined intranatally for the mother, they might then be routinely administered to the baby if she transports to the hospital and if at any time during the pregnancy she had a positive GBS test. Faced with these choices, a woman may prefer to receive antibiotic prophylaxis herself rather than have it directly administered to the baby. Yet other facilities and practitioners will allow antibiotics to be deferred unless there is ROM for more than 24 hours, allowing a period of observation of the baby for signs of infection rather than routinely administering antibiotics intranatally or postnatally. Women who test GBS positive during pregnancy should discuss their concerns and options with their obstetric and pediatric care providers prenatally. There is no substitute for antibiotics in women with signs of infection and prolonged rupture of membranes (i.e., >24 hours since rupture), and all newborns exhibiting signs of GBS infection *must* receive immediate and aggressive antibiotic therapy.

Given the potential narrow time frame between a positive GBS test at 35 to 37 weeks and the time of birth, especially considering the possible need for antibiotic follow-up and the increased risk of premature rupture of membranes and premature labor associated with GBS, midwives may consider an initial culture during pregnancy earlier than the recommended 35 to 37 weeks of gestation, particularly in women with a history of chronic urinary tract infection (UTI) or vaginal yeast infection. Although a positive result earlier in pregnancy is not predictive of risk of neonatal infection, earlier testing allows time to address the potential problem using botanical strategies, with a reculture during the predictive period. This approach is consistent with the preventative philosophies of both herbal medicine and midwifery care, and also allows adequate time for more aggressive medical intervention with antibiotics should this be optimal.

Botanical Protocol for Group B Streptococcus

Botanical treatment for GBS infection relies on the vaginal application of antimicrobial herbs, and the internal (i.e., oral) use of probiotics to normalize intestinal flora and reduce *S. agalactiae* colonization. When women have had a protracted history of GBS infection, with repeated urogenital infections or other signs of decreased immune response, for example, frequent colds, or sore throats, an internal herbal protocol to enhance immunity is sometimes recommended; however, options during pregnancy are somewhat limited.

Many herbs are known in Western herbalism for their antibacterial actions. These include garlic, oregano, myrrh, thyme, and tea tree oil, to name a few. After an exhaustive search of a number of key medical and chemical databases, however, no clinical trials looking at the clinical treatment or prevention of GBS infection with herbal medicine are available in the world literature. In vitro tests show *S. agalactiae* to be inhibited by a number of herbs; however, many of these are not safe for use during pregnancy.

> ### 🖋 TREATMENT OF GROUP B STREPTOCOCCUS
>
> There is absolutely no substitute for antibiotics in women with a history of a positive group B streptococcus (GBS) test and prolonged rupture of membranes (>24 hours since rupture). All newborns exhibiting signs of GBS infection *must* receive immediate and aggressive antibiotic therapy.

Given the paucity of research available directly on this topic, and the long history of clinical efficacy of many botanicals in reducing a variety of infections, including vaginal infections, contemporary herbal practitioners tend to rely on traditional indications of herbs enhanced by contemporary understanding of disease pathology and herbal pharmacology for developing modern clinical applications. Those herbs most commonly used by herbalists, midwives, and naturopathic physicians for the treatment of GBS are listed in Table 19-4. Information on specific categories of herbal actions and exemplary herbs follows.

The basic approach for treating GBS is the nightly insertion of either vaginal suppositories or capsules of

TABLE 19-4	Summary of Botanical Treatment Strategies for Group B Streptococcus		
Therapeutic Goal	**Therapeutic Activity**	**Botanical Name**	**Common Name**
Reduce microbial infection	Antibacterial	*Allium sativum*	Garlic
		Baptisia tinctoria	Wild indigo
		*Berberis vulgaris**	Barberry
		Chrysanthemum morifolium	Chrysanthemum
		*Coptis chinensis**	Goldthread
		Commiphora molmol	Myrrh
		Echinacea purpurea	Echinacea
		Ganoderma lucidum	Reishi
		Gardenia augusta	Gardenia
		*Hydrastis canadensis**	Goldenseal
		Ligustrum lucidum	Ligustrum
		*Mahonia aquifolium**	Oregon grape root
		Melaleuca alternifolia	Tea tree
		Origanum vulgare	Oregano
		Thymus vulgaris	Thyme
		Usnea spp.	Usnea
Reduce local inflammation, support tissue integrity	Antiinflammatory Vulnerary	*Althea officinalis*	Marshmallow
		Calendula officinalis	Calendula
		Glycyrrhiza glabra	Licorice
		Hypericum perforatum	St. John's wort
		Symphytum officinale	Comfrey root
	Astringent	*Achillea millefolium*	Yarrow
		Hamamelis virginiana	Witch hazel
		Quercus spp.	Oak bark

*Coptis, goldenseal, barberry, and Oregon grape root all contain berberine, which may theoretically increase the risk of neonatal jaundice; thus they are contraindicated for oral use during pregnancy. These herbs may be used safely in vaginal preparations in the last 4 weeks of pregnancy.

antimicrobial, antiinflammatory, and vulnerary herbs for a minimum of 3 weeks before the onset of labor. The suppositories, which are the most effective delivery model, are typically inserted in the evening before bed, and the woman instructed to wear a panty liner to prevent damage to bedding and underclothes from leakage as the suppository melts in the vaginal canal. This melting allows the vaginal and cervical tissue to be slowly bathed in the herbs and emollient. This is repeated nightly for 14 days, a 2-day break allowed, and reculturing done. Some practitioners choose to alternate nightly between the use of a suppository and an inserted capsule or garlic clove. A single 00-sized capsule can be filled with goldenseal powder and the woman instructed to insert these into the vaginal fornix (the superior portions of the vagina, extending into the recesses created by the vaginal portion of cervix) every other night for the same duration as the suppository protocol. Again, a panty liner is worn. Perianal rinses are also sometimes used if there is heavy colonization or history of repeated urogenital infection. Astringent herbs may be included in topical preparations if there is a great deal of tissue irritation because they also help to improve tissue integrity and make the tissue less permeable to infection. *Douching should be avoided* because it is not an optimally safe practice during pregnancy and may also drive microorganisms upward toward the uterus. The combination of actions of herbs reduces microbial load

and reinforces the integrity of the vaginal tissue, reducing the ability of organisms to colonize in fissures and irritated areas. Probiotics are used concurrently on a daily basis to maximize the body's ability to produce flora that prevents overgrowth of GBS and enhances the presence of normal vaginal flora. Satisfactorily low levels of the organism should be achieved at least 1 to 2 weeks before the onset of labor. Should GBS bacteriuria persist later than this, an antibiotic protocol can be offered, according to CDC guidelines.

Discussion of Botanical Protocol for Group B Streptococcus
Immunomodulators

This is an important therapeutic category for women with a history of repeated or intractable vaginal or UTIs. These herbs are taken as decoctions or tinctures with the goal of strengthening the immune response. Herbs with low toxicity that can be given in therapeutic doses include medicinal mushrooms such as *Lentinus edodes* (shiitake), *Trametes versicolor* (turkey tails), and *G. lucidum* (reishi). They can be safely employed for extended use throughout the pregnancy and are taken at a dose of 6 to 12 g for decoction, 1 to 4 g of a 5:1 powdered extract as an instant tea, or in capsules, 1 to 4 twice daily.

Echinacea is the only antimicrobial, immune-enhancing botanical to have a study specifically validating its safe use during pregnancy, and is the herb most confidently relied upon by most midwives for this purpose. Inefficacy of echinacea products in treating infections is most likely owing to poor-quality product or inadequate dosing. Liquid extracts of fresh echinacea, rather than dried, powdered, or encapsulated products should be used; strong infusions can also be made from high-quality dried plant material. The dose should be approximately 5 mL daily for general prophylactic use and up to two to three times that quantity for aggressive reduction of GBS colonies.

Garlic can also be used during pregnancy safely. Although it may be more of a theoretical than an actual concern, because of concerns of increased bleeding with high levels of garlic consumption, the practitioner may wish to discontinue its oral administration 2 weeks before the due date.

Topical Antimicrobial Treatment

Antimicrobial herbs most commonly included in suppositories for GBS treatment include goldenseal, thyme, oregano, calendula, tea tree, and usnea. They are used in combination in forms most appropriate to each herb, for example, powder, tincture, or essential oil. An example of a suppository recipe, designating proper forms, can be found in the case history for GBS, and a discussion of suppository preparation can be found in Chapter 3. Garlic cloves have a long history of use as suppositories for the treatment of vaginal infections. A single garlic clove (*not* a full bulb!) is carefully peeled to avoid nicking of the garlic flesh, dipped in a small amount of olive oil, inserted into the vaginal fornix, and left overnight. Whereas the suppositories and capsule will melt and do not require removal, the clove may fall out on its own when the woman urinates in the morning, or it may need to be manually removed by the woman if it does not spontaneously drop out. The woman can be instructed to remove the clove with a clean finger; some patients may find this offensive, and can be directed to the previous strategies. Capsules are usually filled with only one or two herbs, usually stronger antimicrobials, in powder form. Perhaps most commonly applied is goldenseal root powder, which is inserted on alternate nights to the suppository, as described in the preceding.

NUTRITIONAL CONSIDERATIONS

Probiotics

Lactobacillus spp. have been shown to strongly inhibit the growth of GBS in vitro by increasing the acidity of the environment.[73] One small placebo-controlled clinical trial of healthy, fertile, nonpregnant women compared the effects of wearing a probiotic saturated panty liner to a placebo panty liner. Transfer of the probiotic to the vagina was found, and the women who had higher levels of *Lactobacillus* spp. in the vagina had lower levels of GBS.[74] No such study has been conducted in pregnant women, but would be of great interest. Nonetheless, given its safety, and also benefits in protecting against

atopic disease in the newborn when a probiotic is taken by pregnant women in the third trimester, a high-quality probiotic blend containing *Lactobacillus* spp. is highly recommended. Two capsules can be taken with the morning meal, and one or two with the evening meal. The active dose is from 9 to 12 billion organisms per day. *L. reuteri* and *L. rhamnosus* may be especially useful in the recolonization of healthy vaginal flora.

ADDITIONAL THERAPIES

Improper toilet hygiene (i.e., wiping back-to-front after a bowel movement) and anovaginal sexual contact, both of which can increase transmission of GBS to the vaginal canal, should be avoided.

CASE HISTORY

Lisa, a 22-year-old woman, 36 weeks pregnant, tested positive for vaginal group B streptococcal (GBS) infection with routine screening. She was asymptomatic with no accompanying history of vaginal infection or urinary tract infection (UTI). She was planning a home birth and did not have ready access to intranatal antibiotics because of the political climate of home birth midwifery in her community. Home birth midwifery protocol with GBS is quite strict, and thus her midwife would require her to transport to the hospital for IV antibiotics within 18 hours of rupture of membranes (ROM), regardless of her stage of labor. Her midwife supported her choice to reduce GBS infection prenatally in the hopes of achieving a negative culture and keeping her birth options open. The following treatment protocol was maintained for 2 weeks, and then Lisa was recultured for GBS.

Group B Streptococcal Treatment Protocol
Nightly insertion of the following vaginal suppository blend for at least 5 nights per week, for 3 weeks (see Chapter 3):
  To ½ cup each of melted coconut oil and cocoa butter add:
    1 Tbsp calendula oil
    ½ tsp each of rosemary, lavender, and rosemary essential oils
    2 tsp tincture of *Usnea barbata*
    2 tsp tincture of *Thymus vulgaris*
    2 Tbsp *Hydrastis canadensis* powder
    1 Tbsp *Ulmus rubra* powder
    1 Tbsp *Commiphora molmol* powder
  Instructions: Begin at 36 weeks. Wear a light menstrual pad each night to protect underwear and bedding because the oil and goldenseal powders can stain as the suppository melts.

Lisa continued protocol for 2 weeks at which time a vaginal culture for GBS was performed. Culture came back negative 3 days later. She continued the protocol for an additional week (3 weeks total). A final culture several days before she went into labor also yielded a negative GBS finding. She continued the protocol until 40 weeks, at which time she gave birth to a healthy 7 lb 7 oz boy, at home, after 18 hours of labor with no preterm premature rupture of membranes (PPROM). The baby was closely observed in the neonatal period, and showed no signs of infection.

TREATMENT SUMMARY FOR GROUP B STREPTOCOCCUS BEFORE LABOR ONSET

- If group B streptococcus (GBS) is detected before 36 weeks and woman has history of GBS, chronic vaginal candidiasis, or recurrent urinary tract infection (UTI), begin treatment with nutritional and botanical strategies to improve immunity.
- Zinc, vitamin A, folate, and vitamin C to adequate pregnancy amounts
  - Assess hemoglobin and hematocrit to determine whether anemia is present and supplement iron if needed.
  - Use echinacea or other immunity-enhancing herbs daily, 2 to 5 mL tid for up to 6 weeks.
- Reduce stress through stress reduction exercises, modifying stressful situations, and use of nervines and adaptogens as needed.
- Treat accompanying conditions such as UTI or vaginal infection.
- If greater than 36 weeks gestation, use oral and topical antimicrobial agents to reduce colonization, heal vaginal tissue, and improve resistance to infection. Orally, consider echinacea, garlic extracts, and medicinal mushrooms as immunomodulators.
- Apply suppositories nightly for 2 weeks consecutively, and reculture. Specific herbs to consider for suppositories are presented in Table 19-4 and discussed in this section.
- In all cases, include a high-dose active probiotic daily.

PRURITIC URTICARIAL PAPULES AND PLAQUES OF PREGNANCY

Pruritic urticarial papules and plaques of pregnancy (PUPPP) is the most common specific dermatologic condition affecting pregnant women, with an incidence of 1 per 120 to 1 per 300 pregnancies.[75] Seventy-five percent of women who develop PUPPP are pregnant for the first time, and it is 8 to 12 times more likely to occur in women with multiple gestations.[76] PUPPP usually develops in the third trimester, although the condition may have its onset in the postpartum, and rarely earlier in pregnancy.[75] PUPPP is referred to as polymorphic eruption of pregnancy (in the United Kingdom), toxemic rash of pregnancy, and late-onset prurigo of pregnancy, although PUPPP is the name most commonly used in the United States.[77]

The condition presents as erythematous papules within the striae, usually of the abdomen and thighs, which eventually spread to the extremities and become hives (i.e., urticarial plaques). The periumbilical area, breasts, face, palms, and soles usually remain unaffected. The hallmark of this condition is pruritus (i.e., itching), which can be extreme, disturbing sleep and preventing normal daily activities. The pruritus of PUPPP can be so uncomfortable as to cause women to feel quite desperate. Pruritus may worsen immediately after delivery, but generally resolves by 10 to 15 days postpartum. Rarely, the condition may resolve before birth. Most women do not experience a recurrence with subsequent pregnancies; however, when a recurrence does occur, it is almost always much milder than the original case.[75] The condition

is not associated with any adverse maternal, fetal, or neonatal outcomes.[75]

The exact etiology of PUPPP is unknown. One popular theory, supported by the fact that women with larger babies, multiples, or greater maternal weight gain are more likely to develop PUPPP, is that the abdominal stretching of pregnancy leads to an inflammatory response in the connective tissue.[75,77] More recently, a maternal response to fetal circulating antigens has been proposed as an etiologic theory, based on the fact that fetal skin tissue has been found in maternal lesions.[75,78,79]

DIAGNOSIS

There are no specific laboratory diagnostic methods for PUPPP. Diagnosis is made clinically and on the basis of exclusion of other conditions (see Differential Diagnosis). Histopathology and immunochemistry are noncontributory to the diagnosis.

DIFFERENTIAL DIAGNOSIS

Differential diagnosis includes all conditions that may cause hives, and specifically, pemphigoid gestationis, adverse cutaneous drug reaction, allergic contact dermatitis, metabolic pruritus, and atopic dermatitis.

CONVENTIONAL MEDICAL TREATMENT FOR PUPPP

Treatment for PUPPP consists of high-potency topical steroids, ideally tapering these off after 7 days of therapy. Oral prednisone in doses of 10 to 40 mg/day has been used for severe cases when the pruritus is unbearable to the woman. Symptoms are often relieved after 24 hours of oral treatment. Oral antihistamines are generally ineffective. Early delivery is sometimes discussed when the symptoms are unbearable and treatment is ineffective; however, early delivery does not usually give relief of symptoms.[77] Fortunately, symptoms are usually greatly improved with several days of steroid treatment.[75] The safety of antenatal steroid use remains controversial; short-term or single course use is advisable, and the safety of use is greater in the third trimester than in the first trimester.

BOTANICAL TREATMENT OF PUPPP

Many women, either unable to achieve adequate relief with conventional therapies, or concerned about the safety of steroid use during pregnancy, prefer to try natural alternatives for treating PUPPP. Treatment strategies include:
- Use of topical and oral antiinflammatories
- Nervines to improve sleep, which is often seriously impaired owing to physical discomfort
- Nervines to relieve irritability from itching
- Traditional hepatic alterative herbs, which have been empirically shown to improve a number of skin conditions
- Use of adaptogens as immunomodulators

BOX 19-6   Herbal Protocol for Pruritic Urticarial Papules and Plaques of Pregnancy

Topical Treatment

As needed daily, shower and apply the extracted milky liquid of rolled oats (*Avena sativa*). Pat dry and then rinse affected areas with witch hazel extract. Then apply the following cream daily, *repeated as needed* to maintain symptom relief:

Mix

3 oz cream base
10 mL each of the following tinctures:

St. John's wort	(*Hypericum perforatum*)
Skullcap	(*Scutellaria baicalensis*)
Licorice	(*Glycyrrhiza glabra*)

Internal Treatment

Tincture for relief of pruritic urticarial papules and plaques of pregnancy
  Combine:

Nettle leaf tincture	(*Urtica dioica*)	30 mL
Licorice root	(*Glycyrrhiza glabra*)	30 mL
Dandelion root	(*Taraxacum officinale*)	20 mL
Passionflower	(*Passiflora incarnata*)	20 mL
		Total: 100 mL

Dose: Take 3 to 4 mL repeated up to four times daily

Also: Take an herbal nervine tea or tincture as needed.

In botanical therapy, the health of the skin is believed to reflect the health of the other eliminatory and detoxification organs (i.e., bowels, lymph system, liver). When these are not functioning optimally or are overtaxed, as may be a natural consequence of the increased burden of pregnancy on the body, it is believed this will manifest in skin problems, including inflammatory disorders. Topical treatments are therefore almost universally accompanied by systemic treatments (Box 19-6).

Although the use of conventional antihistamines has not demonstrated efficacy in the treatment of PUPPP, nettle leaf, which appears to have antihistaminic activity, has been empirically observed to be helpful in the treatment of conditions with hives as a key feature, including PUPPP.

Herbs used to promote sleep are discussed later in Insomnia in Pregnancy.

Treatments are divided into those for topical and internal use, and are recommended to be used in combination. Effects may be expected after 2 to 3 days of regular use, although some women gain relief more quickly and for some it may take up to a week to notice results. Many women report that herbal treatments provide only temporary relief, requiring them to reapply topical remedies often; however, they find this an acceptable alternative to steroid use during pregnancy.

The effects of using oral corticosteroids and herbs internally simultaneously during pregnancy has not been studied; therefore owing to unknown safety, is not recommended. However, the use of oral steroids and topical herbal treatments, or conversely, oral herbal treatments and topical steroids, may be acceptable. Women using oral medications for the treatment of PUPPP should inform their medical providers about their use of herbs before beginning an herbal protocol (Table 19-5).

Topical Applications

The vehicle via which topical applications are delivered in the case of PUPPP will depend entirely on the mother's response to any given preparation. PUPPP presents as itchy, irritating, and inflamed. The urticaric lesions may be discrete, but often, as the condition progresses, become contiguous, requiring application of medicine to a large area. Salves may not be the best delivery mode because they may actually feel as if they are "sealing in" the hot, inflamed sensation. Similarly, applying tinctures directly to the skin is not advisable, although tinctures may be highly diluted in water or witch hazel extract and used as compresses. Washes made of herbal teas can be used as compresses as well, although they are inconvenient to prepare daily. Similarly, herbal extracts can be added to aloe vera gel and applied this way. A highly absorbent cream base to which herbal extracts are added is perhaps the optimal delivery mode; the cream is soothing and allows broad application of herbs, and the preparations are easy to make in large batches, store well, and are highly portable should travel or application at work be necessary. Topical applications will need to be reapplied multiple times per day, or as needed, for symptomatic relief. Women should be advised that products containing oil may stain clothing or bedding.

🌿 PUPP TREATMENT SUMMARY

- Conventional therapy includes the use of topical and oral corticosteroids, usually taken high dose (10 to 40 mg) for up to 1 week, and then tapering down as symptoms subside.
- Botanical therapy primarily consists of the use of topical and oral antiinflammatory and nervine herbs.
- An antiinflammatory diet supplemented with essential fatty acids may be helpful.

Baking Soda Paste

Baking soda paste is reported by women on "mother blogs" (Internet) to relieve itching from PUPPP. Enough water is mixed with baking soda to form a paste and this is applied directly to affected areas.

Chamomile

Chamomile has been approved by the German Commission E for the treatment of inflammatory skin conditions.[80] Although there appear to be no contraindications to its use topically or internally (with the exception of rare allergy),

TABLE 19-5   **Botanical Treatment Strategies for Pruritic Urticarial Papules and Plaques of Pregnancy**

Therapeutic Goal	Therapeutic Activity	Botanical Name	Common Name
Relieve inflammation	Antiinflammatory	*Aloe vera*	Aloe vera
		Avena sativa	Oatmeal
		Glycyrrhiza glabra	Licorice
		Hamamelis virginiana	Witch hazel
		Matricaria recutita	Chamomile
		Scutellaria baicalensis	Chinese skullcap
	Antihistaminic	*Urtica dioica*	Nettle leaf
	Hepatic Alternatives/Aperients	*Rumex crispus*	Yellow dock
		Taraxacum officinale	Dandelion root
Prevent striae gravidarum		*Centella asiatica*	Gotu kola
Promote relaxation and sleep as needed	Nervine	*Avena sativa*	Milky oats
	Sedative	*Eschscholzia californica*	California poppy
		Passiflora incarnata	Passionflower
Immunomodulation	Adaptogen	*Ganoderma lucidum*	Reishi
		Schisandra chinensis	Schisandra
		Withania somnifera	Ashwagandha

herbalists have noted that with some conditions, for example, pediatric eczema, chamomile oil extracts may actually exacerbate irritation. For patients wishing to use chamomile for topical treatment of PUPPP, a cream preparation is advised. Chamomile tea may also be taken internally as a relaxing, mild sleep-promoting tea or tincture.

Chinese Skullcap

Chinese skullcap, or "scute," is used in TCM to clear heat and drain dampness, which, from a modern medical perspective, might be interpreted as treating inflammation.[81] The antiinflammatory effects are attributed to the herb's flavonoids, and antioxidant and antihistamine activity.[81,82] Only recently is this herb finding its way into Western herbal medicine practice. Little published data were identified specifically on the use of Chinese skullcap for skin conditions; however, clinical evidence from herbal practice suggests a high degree of efficacy and safety in the treatment of inflammatory skin conditions, including eczema and dermatitis. Tincture may be added to a cream base and applied topically, either alone or mixed with herbs, for example, licorice root and St. John's wort extracts. Internal use of Chinese skullcap is not recommended during pregnancy because of teratogenicity in animal studies. It may be used internally, short term, during the postpartum should PUPPP arise during that period or persist past the time of birth.[83]

Gotu Kola

Because one of the theories on the etiology of PUPPP is connective tissue damage as a result of abdominal stretching, with manifestation in the striae, it seems a reasonable consideration to minimize striae development if at all possible. A Cochrane Collaboration review of topical agents for stretch mark prevention identified two randomized trials involving a total of 130 women. One study involving 80 women indicated that, compared with placebo, massage with a cream (i.e., Trofolastin)

containing *Centella asiatica* extract, alpha-tocopherol, and collagen-elastin hydrolysates was associated with less women developing stretch marks. A second study of 50 women compared massage using an ointment (i.e., Verum) containing tocopherol, panthenol, hyaluronic acid, elastin, and menthol with no treatment. Massage with the ointment was associated with fewer women developing stretch marks. The two papers reviewed may show that any cream massaged onto the abdomen, thighs, and breasts (i.e., areas most affected by stretch marks) may be of some benefit. There may be additional benefit from certain ingredients in the cream and the ointment described, but it is unknown which constituent(s) is beneficial. Neither preparation is widely available.[84] Gotu kola is widely used by herbalists for the treatment of connective tissue damage. Practitioners should be aware that a number of cases of contact dermatitis from topical use were identified in the literature (nonpregnant patients); therefore caution is advised and patch testing recommended before general use.[85-87]

Oatmeal Baths

To apply oats topically, the rolled oats are moistened and the milk extracted and added to bath water or rubbed on the body in a bath or shower.[88] Two handfuls (about 1 cup) of rolled oats are placed into a large clean sock or rolled in a towel or bandana that can be tied at the top. The sac is taken into the bath or the shower, and as the oats soak up the water the cloth is squeezed firmly in the palm of the hand. A milky liquid will begin to be exuded, and it is this liquid that is allowed to fill the tub or rubbed over the body in the shower, and then rinsed off. This oat milk is very soothing and emollient. This can be repeated as needed even several times daily.

St. John's Wort

St. John's wort oil is a classic topical burn treatment.[89] Both St. John's wort extract and hyperforin have demonstrated inhibitory effects in epidermal immune response when applied topically, and suggest a role for this soothing application in the treatment of inflammatory skin conditions. It is popularly used by herbalists for inflammatory and microbial skin conditions. St. John's wort demonstrates good cosmetic skin tolerance.[90,91]

Witch Hazel, Aloe Vera

Witch hazel extract, applied as a compress, has long been used as a topical agent for reducing inflammatory and pruritic skin conditions. It is recognized by ESCOP and approved by the German Commission E as a treatment for skin irritations and minor inflammatory dermatologic and mucosal conditions.[80,92] A comparative study looking at witch hazel versus cortisone for the treatment of erythema found it to be slightly less effective than cortisone but still noteworthy in its effects, whereas a study on the outcome of treatment of sunburn with witch hazel versus no treatment found that it led to a significant reduction in erythema and visible skin damage. It has demonstrated a mild antiinflammatory effect in patients suffering from atopic neurodermatitis and psoriasis.[92]

Aloe vera gel is a soothing topical liquid from the aloe vera plant. Popular for pain relief and healing from burns and other skin conditions for thousands of years, some women find temporary relief from the itching of PUPPP with topical application of the gel. Promising preliminary research suggests that aloe has immunostimulatory properties that may improve wound healing and dermatologic inflammation.[93] There is no contraindication to liberal topical use during pregnancy; aloe should not be used internally during pregnancy.

Internal Use
California Poppy, Passionflower

See Insomnia in Pregnancy for discussion of the safety and efficacy of these herbs that are commonly used to treat sleep difficulties in pregnancy.

Dandelion Root, Yellow Dock

An entire category of herbs, known historically and to this day as "alteratives," and referred to colloquially as "blood cleansers," are included in the treatment of many skin conditions. Dandelion root is perhaps one of the most commonly used, and is popularly cited on "mother blogs" on the Internet as prescribed by midwives in the treatment of PUPPP. No human clinical trials have been conducted to support the use of dandelion root for skin conditions and there are no data in the scientific literature of dandelion either being safe or contraindicated during pregnancy.[94-96] Yellow dock is used similarly to dandelion root. Note that yellow dock is sometimes considered contraindicated in pregnancy because it is a mild anthraquinone laxative; however, clinically it has not been observed to be associated with increased uterine activity or other adverse outcomes.

Licorice

Glycyrrhizin has exhibited a range of corticosteroid-like activities when injected in animals and humans, including inhibition of prostaglandin synthesis similar to cortisone. Compounds in the root inhibit 5-lipoxygenase formation and leukotriene biosynthesis in vitro.[97] It is commonly used by herbalists for a wide variety of inflammatory complaints ranging from gastrointestinal (GI) disorders, for which it is best studied, to inflammatory skin conditions such as eczema. Its use for PUPPP is empirically based. Two recent reports on high-dose licorice consumption throughout pregnancy, in the form of licorice candy containing actual licorice extract rather than licorice flavor, demonstrated no increase in maternal hypertension or low birth weight; however, both studies demonstrated a significant increase in preterm (<37 weeks) delivery. In one study, the risk of preterm delivery was greater than double the risk of women not consuming licorice.[98,99] No studies demonstrate harm or adverse outcomes with short-term use of modest doses of licorice, including a study of 110 case reports on the use of glycyrrhizin injections for treating viral hepatitis during pregnancy that showed no adverse effects.[94] It is recommended that licorice not be used in excessive doses or for prolonged periods during pregnancy; however, use for up to a week at a time appears to be safe. A comparative study of the safety and efficacy of licorice versus cortisone use during pregnancy for the treatment of PUPPP would be informative. Women with hypertension should not take licorice during pregnancy.

Milky Oats

The tincture of milky oats is considered a reliable nerve tonic, especially for use when there is nervous exhaustion or general debility. The medicinal use of oats during pregnancy has not been studied; however, taken as food, no adverse effects have been noted in pregnancy.[88] The tincture may be used alone, but it is more commonly taken in combination with other nervine or sedating herbs; for example, chamomile, St. John's wort, California poppy, passionflower, and lavender.

Nettle Leaf

Stinging nettle leaf has demonstrated significant antiinflammatory activity; it is used for the treatment of rheumatoid arthritis and allergic rhinitis.[92] Herbalists have found nettle to be a reliable herb in the treatment of numerous systemic and dermatologic inflammatory conditions. It may be taken as tea or in freeze-dried capsules. No serious adverse effects were reported in five clinical studies with a total of 10,368 patients using hydroethanolic extracts corresponding to an equivalence of 9.7 g of dried leaf daily for periods ranging from 3 weeks to 12 months. Minor side effects included GI upset and allergic reaction (1.2% to 2.7% of cases).[92] Nettle leaf is one of the most commonly used herbs by midwives who commonly recommend it to help build iron levels. It has been suggested, although not demonstrated, that the astringency of this herb might interfere with iron absorption. A 1975 review article by Farnsworth and colleagues reported that stinging nettle was a potential abortifacient, and that its constituent 5-hydroxytryptamine was a uterine stimulant; however, frequent use of large doses of this herbal infusion in midwifery practice has demonstrated no evidence of such activity.

NUTRITIONAL CONSIDERATIONS

Essential Fatty Acids

Some women report finding relief from the daily addition of EFAs to their diets. A high-quality combination EFA product containing plant-source oils and fish oils is recommended. Women supplementing with fish oils during pregnancy should not exceed daily recommended allowances for vitamins A and D and should only take products that exclude the presence of heavy metal contaminants.

VARICOSITIES IN PREGNANCY

Varicosities are exceedingly common during pregnancy, when they often appear for the first time. Forty percent of all pregnant women are affected.[100] They most commonly appear on the lower legs and rectum (i.e., hemorrhoids), although vulvar varicosities may also occur. The physiologic changes of pregnancy are responsible for the development of varicosities. These include hormonal changes that cause increased fragility of the blood vessel walls, along with increased iliac venous pressure owing to the enlarging uterus, leading to reflux of blood in the vessels, subsequent rupture of valves, and the appearance of varicosities.[100] More recently, the "weak-wall hypothesis" proposed that varicosities arising in pregnancy are actually the result of an inherited predisposition to weakness in the vein wall that allows progressive venous dilation even at normal venous pressures, with valve failure occurring as a consequence.[101] Further, it is now recognized that the saphenous veins contain estrogen and progesterone receptors that may play a role in pregnancy-mediated varicose vein development, although the role of these receptors is not entirely known.[101,102]

Varicosities may be accompanied by throbbing, a feeling of heaviness, aching, heat, and pain, and with leg varicosities there may be ankle edema and phlebitis. Varicosities frequently regress in intensity during the postpartum; however, they may also persist, with continued symptoms and worsening of venous distention.[103] Hemorrhoids are predisposed to bleed and are further aggravated by constipation, which also commonly increases in pregnancy. Venous thrombosis is a complication that occurs in less than 10% of pregnancies, and which requires immediate medical management. In severe cases, and especially in the postpartum and as women age, chronic venous insufficiency and venous ulceration can become problematic. These conditions, too, require medical care in conjunction with complementary therapies.

This section focuses on the treatment of uncomplicated superficial leg varicosities and hemorrhoids during pregnancy; thus the range of herbs is limited to those herbs and supplements considered safe for use by pregnant women; these treatments, however, can be applied to anyone with varicosities.

TREATMENT OF VARICOSITIES IN PREGNANCY

Supportive therapy for leg varicosities includes leg elevation, compression with support hose, sleeping in a left lateral decubitus (i.e., side-lying) position, regular exercise, and avoidance of long periods of standing or sitting.[101,103] Anticoagulant therapy is used when needed to prevent thromboses. Hemorrhoids are treated with topical antihemorrhoid preparations and avoidance of straining when having a bowel movement. Surgical treatment for hemorrhoids is rarely required during pregnancy; when surgery is required for either hemorrhoids or leg varicosities, it is preferably done between pregnancies.[101] Most often, vulvar varicosities also require only supportive treatment; severe vulvar varicosities may require attention during vaginal birth to prevent them from rupturing and bleeding extensively.

BOTANICAL TREATMENT OF VARICOSITIES IN PREGNANCY

There is very little published evidence in either the herbal or scientific literature on the use of botanicals for the prevention or treatment of varicosities in pregnancy. Topical treatments that include horse chestnut and witch hazel extracts are commonly recommended. Black tea (in tea bags) are commonly used by midwives as a highly astringent "home remedy" used topically for the treatment of hemorrhoids, both during pregnancy and postnatally. Other herbs that may be used topically include witch hazel, yarrow, and white oak bark. Arnica may sometimes be recommended for external use, but should not be used on broken or open skin. The use of nettle leaf infusion, taken regularly as a tea, is often recommended for its reputed hemostatic and venotonic actions. Horse chestnut is a popular herb in Europe, taken internally for the treatment of venous insufficiency. Bilberry is an important venotonic herb used internally with a good safety for pregnancy. Foods high in rutin and bioflavonoids are commonly used to improve vascular tone and integrity. The herbal approach to the treatment of hemorrhoids includes gentle measures to alleviate constipation if this is a concurrent problem, and thus minimize straining during bowel movements. Gotu kola, which is sometimes used for varicosities and venous disorders, is not safe for internal use during pregnancy, and has been associated with contact dermatitis with topical use, so it is recommended that patch testing be done before applying liberally (Table 19-5).[104-107]

Arnica

Topical arnica applications are sometimes included in treatment protocol for varicosities. According to Schulz and coworkers, it is uncertain whether arnica extracts are active topically and if so, by what mechanism.[108] Clinical herbalists, however, report on the remarkable and rapid ability of arnica flowers to reduce bruises and swellings when applied topically

TABLE 19-6   Botanical Treatment Strategies for Varicosities

Therapeutic Activity	Botanical Name	Common Name
Astringent	Aesculus hippocastanum	Horse chestnut
Venotonic	Arnica montana	Arnica
Hemostatic	Camellia sinensis	Green tea
	Hamamelis virginiana	Witch hazel
	Quercus alba	White oak bark
	Urtica dioica	Nettle leaf
	Vaccinium myrtillus	Bilberry

to the affected areas. No studies were identified on the use of arnica for the treatment of varicosities. The herb is most commonly applied as an oil or gel, is not applied to broken skin, and should not be used internally. The oil may be applied two to three times daily, either alone or in combination with other herbal preparations. As the rectal mucosa is highly vascular and absorptive, it is recommended that arnica be used for leg varicosities only, and that other herbs (e.g., witch hazel, black tea) be used to reduce hemorrhoids (see Table 19-6).

Bilberry

Bilberry, a relative of the blueberry, is used as a vasoprotective herb, one of its many virtues. It has demonstrated potent effects on vascular permeability in animal and in vitro models, and a number of positive human trials have been done, though their methodological quality was not strong.[104] Bilberry has been reported to be safe for internal use during pregnancy and efficacious in the treatment of gestational hemorrhoids and venous insufficiency of pregnancy.[109] It is taken in two or three divided doses of 160 to 340 mg per day, depending on the severity of the condition.[109] It may also be taken in liquid extract form. Bilberry can be taken prophylactically in women with a predisposition to varicosities or a family history of gestational varicosities.

Horse Chestnut

Horse chestnut seed extract (HCSE) preparations are widely prescribed in Europe for the treatment of venous insufficiency and vascular fragility. They are taken orally. A review of the scientific literature yields seven well-designed studies that support the superiority of HCSE over placebo and suggest that the herbal product may be equal to compression stockings in efficacy.[104] A 2012 Cochrane review examined the efficacy and safety of HCSE versus placebo or reference therapy for CVI (chronic venous insufficiency) treatment. For the meta-analysis, reviewers searched CENTRAL, AMED, and Phytobase for RCTs related to HCSE. Product manufacturers were also consulted for unpublished trial data. Trials that examined combination products were excluded. The reviewers concluded that there is an improvement in CVI–related signs and symptoms with HCSE compared with placebo, and adverse events were mild and infrequent.[110] Although the herb is generally not recommended for use in pregnancy, this is

owing to lack of data rather than contraindication based on known adverse effects. No teratogenic effects have been observed in animals given very high doses of extract by oral route, although fetal body weights were reduced compared with controls.[111] Steiner conducted a double-blind, placebo-controlled study of HSCE use during pregnancy. Fifty-two women with leg edema owing to pregnancy-induced venous insufficiency received 300 mg of Venostasin (i.e., 240 to 290 mg of HSCE standardized to 50 mg escin) twice daily for 2 weeks. No adverse effects were observed (Fig. 19-1).[112]

🌿 TREATMENT SUMMARY FOR VARICOSITIES AND HEMORRHOIDS DURING PREGNANCY

- Women with leg varicosities should be encouraged to take a brisk walk each day. This can also be beneficial for women with hemorrhoids accompanied by constipation because regular exercise reduces constipation.
- When constipation accompanies hemorrhoids, dietary changes and gentle herbal and nutritional approaches should be taken to relieve constipation to avoid unnecessary rectal pressure and straining to pass stools.
- Compression stockings can be used in the event of extensive, painful, or swollen leg varicosities.
- Leg elevation for 30 minutes twice daily temporarily relieves ankle edema and discomfort associated with varicosities.
- Topical applications can be used two to four times daily to relieve swelling associated with varicosities.
  - For leg varicosities, compresses of witch hazel extract or arnica ointment can be applied.
  - For hemorrhoids, black tea bag compresses or other herbal extract compresses (e.g., witch hazel) can be applied as needed. A convenient way to apply witch hazel to hemorrhoids is with medication-saturated cosmetic pads. Women can take a stack of cosmetic pads, place them in a 4-oz wide mouth jar with a screw top, and fill the jar to cover the pads with witch hazel extract purchased from the pharmacy. A few drops of lavender essential oil can be added as well for its pleasant scent and soothing action when applied topically. A pad can be tucked in next to the hemorrhoids and changed several times daily. This can be used in conjunction with, alternated with, or in lieu of the tea bags. Both are quite effective as reducing the hemorrhoids and relieving itching and irritation. The black tea is more effective.

Continued

TREATMENT SUMMARY FOR VARICOSITIES AND HEMORRHOIDS DURING PREGNANCY—cont'd

- An herbal suppository can be inserted nightly to shrink hemorrhoids and relieve itching, burning, and irritation. Use 4 oz of cocoa butter and 2 Tbsp each of marshmallow root, white oak bark, and goldenseal powders, as well as 2 Tbsp of calendula oil, which is vulnerary. See Chapter 3 for instructions on making suppositories. These can be made in batches that can be stored in the refrigerator for several weeks and used as needed. Women should be informed that the oil can stain clothing and bedding, and therefore a menstrual pad should be worn with nightly insertion of the suppository.
- Internally:
  - 120 to 360 mg bilberry extract two to three times daily, depending on the severity of the varicosities or hemorrhoids
  - Nettle infusion: 2 Tbsp dried organic nettle leaf steeped 30 minutes in 1 cup of boiling water. Strain and drink the liquid. Take 2 cups daily.
  - 2 to 5 mL horse chestnut seed extract (HSCE) twice daily, depending on severity of varicosities
  - 500 mg vitamin C with bioflavonoids twice daily

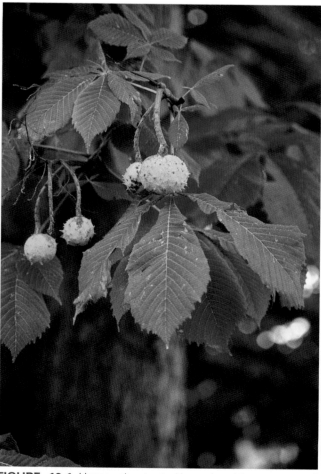

FIGURE 19-1 Horse chestnut *(Aesculus hippocastanum).* (Photo by Martin Wall.)

Nettle Leaf

Nettle leaf is highly valued by herbalists for its purported venotonic actions, and is used by herbalists and midwives for the treatment of varicosities.[113] It is taken internally as a strong daily nutritive infusion. Its use is empirically based. No herbal or scientific studies were identified on the use of nettle leaf for the treatment of varicosities. Animal studies are lacking on the use of this herb in pregnancy. No harmful effects to the fetus have been identified. The lignins in nettle, as well as their intestinal transformation products, have been shown to bind sex hormone–binding globulin (SHBG) in vitro; however, ethanol extract of the aerial parts of nettle did not demonstrate significant antiimplantation activity when given to female rats.[111]

Pine Bark Extract

A clinical trial tested Pycnogenol for *postpartum* symptomatic hemorrhoids.[114] Forty-nine women with hemorrhoids after their second pregnancy were enrolled within the third month after pregnancy. They were randomized to receive either Pycnogenol 150 mg/day or placebo control. After 6 months, 75% in the Pycnogenol group with third-degree hemorrhoids were symptom-free in comparison to 56% of controls. In the fourth-degree hemorrhoid group, 70% of women in the treatment group were symptom-free in comparison with 36% of the controls. Another earlier RCT tested 150 mg Pycnogenol for treatment of severe CVI. Ninety-eight women were randomized into three groups: 150 mg Pycnogenol, elastic stockings, or 150 mg Pycnogenol plus elastic stockings. Outcomes were assessed using ambulatory venous pressure (AVP) and refilling time (which were comparable between groups at baseline). After 8 weeks of treatment, a decrease was seen in ankle swelling rate, resting flux, transcutaneous pO(2), and clinical symptom scores in all groups. The combination group exhibited greater improvement over single treatment groups. The results indicated that Pycnogenol performed better than compression in attenuating CVI signs and symptoms.[115] Safety data on the use of pine bark extract in pregnancy is lacking, and therefore cannot be recommended.

Witch Hazel, Black Tea, White Oak, Yarrow

Witch hazel bark, black tea, and white oak bark are tannin-rich, highly astringent herbs commonly used as topical remedies for the treatment of hemorrhoids (Fig. 19-2). Yarrow is also quite astringent, and although more commonly used for bleeding, may sometimes be included in topical preparations. These herbs are not intended for internal use in pregnancy (with the exception of small amounts of black tea as a beverage). They can be used in a variety of forms, including as strong washes or diluted extracts applied with a cotton ball, or in herbal suppositories (see the following discussion) to be inserted nightly to reduce local swelling and inflammation. Black tea bags are a very convenient and acceptable remedy because they are easily accessible, affordable, and simple to prepare. Women can be instructed to purchase commercial tea bags and steep 1 per application in ¼ cup of boiling water (as if making a cup of tea with a very small amount of water). When the tea has cooled, the liquid can be discarded, the tea

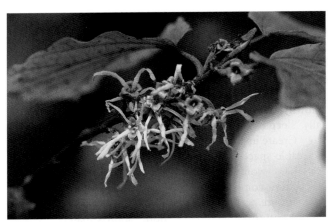

FIGURE 19-2 Witch hazel *(Hamamelis virginiana).* (Photo by Martin Wall.)

bag slightly wrung out, and the bag applied to the hemorrhoids. Women must be warned that the tea will permanently stain fabrics and bedding. Putting a menstrual pad in an old pair of underwear to hold the tea bag in place for up to 30 minutes at a time is effective, or the woman can simply apply the tea bag manually for several minutes, sitting over the toilet or in the shower, two to three times daily.

Food Sources of Rutin

Rutin is a naturally occurring flavonoid in many foods, especially buckwheat, apricots, cherries, grapes, grapefruit, plums, and oranges. It is often used in patients with capillary fragility, varicose veins, bruising, or hemorrhoids.[116] Most clinical studies have used hydroxyethylrutoside (HER), a standardized mixture of rutinosides. In a study of 37 pregnant women given 300 mg of rutoside three times daily for 8 weeks versus placebo, rutoside reduced symptom scores for pain, feelings of leg heaviness and tiredness, nocturnal cramps, and paraesthesias associated with varicosities compared with placebo in women with visible varicosities and these symptoms after 28 weeks of gestation. Rutosides also have led to reduction of ankle size compared with placebo; ankle size increased in the placebo group. Adverse effects are rare and transient. The most commonly reported adverse effects include dizziness, headache, dry mouth, tiredness, nausea, dyspepsia, diarrhea, constipation, and skin rash. Rutin appears to be safe during pregnancy. Its safety after 28 weeks of gestation has been confirmed in two human trials. Scientific evidence for the safe use of rutin during lactation is not available. Given the uncertainty of the safety of rutoside preparations, it is recommended that pregnant women consume foods rich in rutin and take a complete vitamin supplement with bioflavonoids, including rutin, rather than a rutoside product.[116]

❙ INSOMNIA IN PREGNANCY

The International Classification of Sleep Disorders has proposed that the occurrence of either insomnia or excessive sleepiness that develops during pregnancy be called *pregnancy-associated sleep disorder* in recognition of the association of sleep disturbance with pregnancy and the self-limited nature of these problems.[117] In nonpregnant populations, sleeping less than 5 hours per night has been observed to adversely affect both mood and performance, and places individuals at increased risk of adverse events such as motor vehicle accidents.[117] Postpartum sleep deprivation may increase the risk for mood disorders ranging from postpartum depression to overt psychosis.[117] Disrupted sleep during pregnancy is associated with poorer obstetric outcomes, in particular length of labor and type of delivery. In a prospective, longitudinal follow-up of 131 pregnant women, Lee and Gay demonstrated that women who slept less than 6 hours at night had longer labors and were 4.5 times more likely to have cesarean deliveries.[118] Given the potential magnitude of adverse events associated with sleep disturbances, serious attention should be given to this complaint during pregnancy and its effects on a woman's quality of life and health.

Physiologic, hormonal, and physical changes of pregnancy are responsible for a variety of sleep disorders. Women may experience insomnia, night waking, parasomnias (e.g., restless leg syndrome [RLS]), leg cramps, hypersomnia, or snoring.[118-120] The growing uterus and the pressure it places on the lower back, diaphragm and stomach, and simply its weight, require pregnant women to adopt a variety of positions to sleep comfortably and avoid associated discomforts; for example, heartburn, or pressure on the inferior vena cava, leading to paresthesias of the distal extremities and shortness of breath. Increased need to urinate during the night, exaggerated dreams, worries over the increased responsibilities of pregnancy and parenthood, anxieties over the birth, and many other concerns also can interfere with sleep and severely decrease its quantity and quality. The effects of estrogen and progesterone in pregnancy also alter the quality of sleep, although the extent to which this occurs as a result of hormones is not clear. However, indirectly, hormonal effects such as increased nasal congestion can dramatically affect sleep.[118,121] Pregnancy may also exacerbate existing sleep disorders, or exacerbate medical conditions (e.g., acid reflux, asthma) that affect sleep. Chronic pain is a common cause of sleep disturbances, and may also be exacerbated during pregnancy (see Case History).

Sleep disorders of pregnancy have a predictable pattern relative to the trimesters. During the first trimester, sleep duration and quality at night are often decreased, although women require more and report that they are apt to fall asleep much more easily than usual during the day, commonly with an increased desire to nap. The second trimester usually leads to a return of a woman's normal sleep patterns. In the third trimester, women show increased wake after sleep onset and decreased sleep quality, and frequently complain of restless sleep, leg cramps, and frightening dreams.[118-120] Some amount of night waking during pregnancy may be the body's natural and intrinsic way of preparing the mother for the inevitable night waking that accompanies having a breastfeeding newborn and infant; therefore regardless of treatment, this may be unavoidable.

Lack of sleep or poor sleep quality can affect a woman's sense of well-being during her waking hours, increase irritability, lead to depression, decrease appetite, affect memory, and may affect concentration and functioning at normal daily tasks. As discussed earlier, significantly diminished sleep during pregnancy may also have a deleterious effect on the birth experience.[118]

MEDICAL TREATMENT OF INSOMNIA IN PREGNANCY

The exact incidence of sleep disorders in pregnancy is unknown, but it is estimated that as many as 90% of women experience them during the third trimester.[117,118] There are no clinical trials of various treatment modalities in this group of patients.[119] It is important to identify etiologic factors and to treat any associated or underlying medical conditions. RLS may represent folate or iron deficiency, hormonal changes of pregnancy, or more rarely, may be a sign of end-stage renal disease or peripheral neuropathy.[122] It is usually transient in pregnancy, occurring most commonly in the third trimester and disappearing by the time of birth.[122] Insomnia associated with a more serious psychiatric disorder, for example, severe depression, anxiety disorders, or bipolar disorder, may require specific pharmaceutical treatment. Risks associated with the use of pharmaceutical medications during pregnancy must be seriously considered.

The medical treatment of RLS in pregnant women is difficult; most of the drugs commonly used for this problem are not safe for use during pregnancy. Nonpharmacologic treatments are recommended, such as leg stretching before sleep and support hose if varicosities are prominent. Iron supplementation is suggested because this condition is associated with iron deficiency. Opioids are used sometimes in the second or third trimester in severe cases.[123]

GENERAL TREATMENT OF SLEEP DIFFICULTIES IN PREGNANCY

Sleep quality in pregnancy is often greatly improved by improving the sleep environment—both internally and externally—through simple, common sense measures. For example, during growth spurts, the fetus places significantly increased nutritional demands on the mother—night waking may simply be a result of hunger, but this frequently goes unrecognized by the mother, or hunger is ignored in the effort to avoid getting out of bed—with sleep nonetheless compromised. Placing a snack near the bed and having the mother eat freely during the night may, in itself, remedy sleep disturbances. Nutritional deficiencies may also affect sleep quality. This is discussed under Nutritional Considerations. It is common for people to use stimulants during the day, for example, increased caffeine (e.g., coffee, chocolate, tea, soda) intake, when they are not getting adequate restful sleep at night. Unfortunately, such behavior can further exacerbate sleep difficulties, making it difficult to finally unwind when one is ready for sleep. Encourage pregnant patients to engage in healthful activities to increase wakefulness during the day, for example, taking a refreshing walk, using aromatherapy (e.g., peppermint oil in an infuser) in their work area to increase concentration, eating well, drinking plenty of water, and avoiding stimulant use as much as possible; this can be beneficial in promoting sleep and at least will not make sleep efforts more difficult.

Pregnant women can be encouraged to incorporate the following simple suggestions for encouraging sleep into their daily "sleep hygiene" practices:

- Create an environment conducive to sleep: a comfortable space with adequate pillows to support the pregnant woman comfortably; the ability to darken the room completely and block out extraneous disturbing sound.
- A gentle yoga session done approximately an hour before bed, followed by a warm bath, can promote relaxation before sleep.
- Take a warm bath about an hour before bed. Add 5 to 7 drops of relaxing essential oils to the tub, for example, lavender and rose oils.
- Get into bed 30 minutes before intended sleep and read, or take some time to write in a journal.
- Play quiet, relaxing music in the room, especially if other noises prevent sleep, or if troublesome thoughts are keeping the woman awake.
- Use aromatherapy to create a relaxing ambience.
- If possible, have a partner give the pregnant woman a foot and leg massage as she is trying to go to sleep.
- Encourage the woman to identify hunger as a possible cause of sleep disturbance. Eating a light snack just before sleep, and having a snack at the bedside or readily available in the kitchen to eat during the night if hunger awakens her can make a huge difference. Tell women that even if they do not feel hungry, if they wake in the middle of the night and cannot fall back to sleep, try eating something light—this will often help even if hunger was not obvious. Snack suggestions include low fat organic yogurt, toast with nut butter, crackers, cereal with a small amount of milk, hard cheese, or a banana.
- Use cognitive behavioral therapy to help a woman cope with troublesome thoughts if these are the prime culprit preventing sleep, and have the woman develop strategies for dealing with her primary concerns.
- Although napping is not an alternative to a good night's sleep, it is essential, whenever possible, for pregnant women to nap when they are unable to get adequate sleep at night.
- Avoid caffeine after late afternoon, disturbing television programs, watching television close to bed time and in bed, spicy meals in the evening, eating heavy foods within 2 hours of sleep, and tension in the bedroom.

BOTANICAL TREATMENT OF INSOMNIA IN PREGNANCY

There is a limited range of safe conventional pharmaceutical options for treating insomnia during pregnancy, and

TABLE 19-7 Herbs for Treating Sleep Disturbances During Pregnancy

Therapeutic Goal	Therapeutic Activity	Botanical Name	Common Name
Promote sleep, relieve anxiety (generally considered safe during pregnancy)	Nervine Sedative Spasmolytic	*Lavandula officinalis* *Matricaria recutita* *Melissa officinalis*	Lavender Chamomile Lemon balm
Promote sleep, relieve anxiety (stronger herbs, see Chapter 6)	Nervine Sedative Spasmolytic	*Eschscholzia californica* *Passiflora incarnata* *Scutellaria lateriflora* *Valeriana officinalis*	California poppy Passionflower Skullcap Valerian
Relieve restless legs	Spasmolytic	*Viburnum* spp.	Cramp bark, black haw

interestingly, most pregnant women do not report sleep disorders to their physicians.[117] It is nonetheless a problem for which women commonly seek relief, and therefore frequently turn to natural products. It is essential that the normalcy of symptoms, for example, RLS, be established before treating. However, once it is determined that the sleep disturbance is a simple pregnancy discomfort, gentle herbal therapies may be tried. Several herbal medicines appear to be safe during pregnancy and provide modest improvement in sleep quality; however, experimental and clinical data on the use of these during pregnancy is, with minimal exception, lacking. General recommendations should be incorporated before or in conjunction with botanical use. For women with severe sleep disorders but who are not willing to use pharmaceutical drugs, stronger herbs may be considered; however, because studies evaluating their safety during pregnancy are largely lacking, their use should be limited to short term, and first-trimester use should be avoided. Examples of such herbs include passionflower (*Passiflora incarnata*), skullcap (*Scutellaria lateriflora*), California poppy (*Eschscholzia californica*), and valerian (*Valeriana officinalis*). Herbs commonly used during pregnancy for difficulty falling asleep or poor sleep quality, and which have a good safety profile, are presented in the following; further discussion of the evidence for these herbs, as well as additional herbs for insomnia, is presented in Chapter 6. Readers are also directed to Chapter 6 for insomnia secondary to anxiety.

Teas are an excellent form for using sleep-promoting aromatic herbs such as chamomile, lavender, and lemon balm; unfortunately, drinking tea close to bedtime often causes the pregnant woman to awaken within a couple of hours after falling asleep with the need to urinate, thus defeating the benefits of the herbs. Therefore it is recommended that tea not be taken closer than 2 hours before bed, and that frequent small amounts of tincture be taken instead to build an effective dose over a period of 1 to 2 hours, with a dose of 2 mL of any single herb or a combination of any two or three taken every 15 to 30 minutes for 1 to 2 hours before attempting to sleep (Table 19-7).

Chamomile

Chamomile is commonly taken as a tea, although it may also be included in tincture formulae, as a gentle calming and sleep-inducing herb.[124] Clinical trials are generally lacking, and the only one identified did not show a statistically significant improvement in primary insomnia.[125] Studies in mice and rats have shown anticonvulsant and central nervous system depressant effects, respectively.[124,126] Chamomile is erroneously placed on lists of herbs contraindicated during pregnancy; however, this is based on a single 1979 study that found teratogenic effects using a concentrated extract of α-bisoprolol at high doses. No teratogenic effects were seen at lower doses, and the dose of the oil constituent required to cause teratogenicity is far greater than it would ever be possible for someone drinking the tea to ever approximate.[127] No harmful effects have been reported from the use of chamomile during pregnancy or lactation.

Cramp Bark/Black Haw

Considered generally safe for use during pregnancy, these closely related herbs have a long history of use for the treatment of spasmodic muscle discomforts.[128] Although they have not been studied for the treatment of RLS during pregnancy, they have been used traditionally for spasmodic pain in the legs and back, and particularly in the calf.[128-130] Today, midwives and herbalists consider these herbs in the treatment of back pain, leg discomfort associated with RLS, and leg cramps, which may interfere with sleep, used in conjunction with appropriate relaxation techniques and nutritional supplementation.

Lavender

Lavender oil's effects on sleep have been evaluated in murine models. Mice exposed to repeated dosing have demonstrated a more rapid sleep onset with longer duration of sleep, and exposure of mice to a lavender scented atmosphere in a dark cage resulted in depression of motor activity.[131,132] Lavender oil has also been shown to inhibit the stimulant effects of caffeine.[131] In a clinical study on four benzodiazepine-dependent geriatric patients on stopping this treatment, there was a significant decrease in sleep duration, which was restored to previous levels by substitution of aromatherapy with lavender oil.[133] In a study comparing single 3-minute inhalations of the scents of lavender and rosemary (mental-stimulating effects) in 40 subjects, the lavender group showed increased beta power (via electroencephalogram [EEG]), suggesting drowsiness; less depressed mood; and reported feeling more relaxed and performed the math computations faster and more accurately.[134] A 2014 controlled pilot study ($n = 50$) of intermediate care unit patients tested lavender aromatherapy for sleep quality improvement. Control groups received standard care for insomnia, and treated patients received 3 mL of 100% lavender oil in a glass jar at bedside. Sleep quality was monitored through the Richards-Campbell Sleep Questionnaire and vital sign data points taken throughout the night. The treated group exhibited lower blood pressure than the control group ($p = .03$). The mean sleep scores were higher in the intervention than control groups (48.25 versus 40.10), but the difference was insignificant.[135] In another study, researchers tested lavender fragrance on insomnia and depression in 42 female college students. Participants self-reported improvements in sleep latency and sleep satisfaction at lower concentrations, and improvements in depressive moods during treatment weeks at higher concentrations of lavender fragrance.[136]

Although data in pregnancy are lacking, lavender appears to be a safe and gentle herb for sleep promotion. The herb may be taken as a tea or tincture; the oil should never be taken internally but can be added to a warm bath (5 to 7 drops per tub of water) and the woman encouraged to soak for 20 minutes each night before sleep, or the oil can be placed in an aromatherapy infuser near the bed. A recent article in the *New England Journal of Medicine* suggested a possible estrogenic effect in young boys regularly exposed to topical products containing lavender oils. Although the products were not characterized, and the case reports do not clearly implicate lavender use, practitioners should be aware that this is an emerging concern and that other essential oils have been associated with estrogenic effects. Short-term use may be preferable until further research in this area has been conducted; however, no adverse effects have been previously reported with the external use of lavender oil or lavender oil–containing products in spite of widespread use (Fig. 19-3).[137]

Lemon Balm

Lemon balm is approved by the German Commission E for the treatment of insomnia of nervous origin.[138] Lemon balm is beneficial in moderating subjective mood in response to mild psychological stress and may be capable of inducing a mood-state compatible with inducing sleep.[124,139] No mutagenic or genotoxic effects have been observed in experimental models.[9] Patients with thyroid disorders or taking thyroid medications should avoid the use of lemon balm during pregnancy owing to theoretical risk of reduction of thyroid function from this herb (see Chapter 5).[127]

ADDITIONAL THERAPIES

Nutritional Considerations

In addition to addressing hunger as a possible cause of sleep disturbances (see the general recommendations), certain nutritional deficiencies may be associated with insomnia and other sleep disorders, for example, leg cramps and RLS. Adequate intake of iron, folate, B vitamins, calcium, and magnesium are essential for optimal sleep during pregnancy and appropriate supplementation should be introduced when there are sleep disorders.

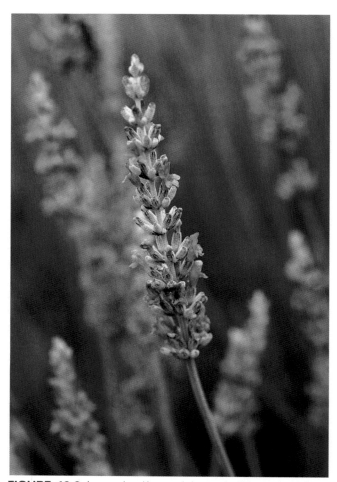

FIGURE 19-3 Lavender (*Lavandula* spp.). (Photo by Martin Wall.)

 CASE HISTORY

Perri had experienced chronic insomnia and back pain for years, which had been severely exacerbated by her first pregnancy 5 years ago. The back pain began after a car accident about 7 years ago, and is believed by her doctors to be caused by muscle spasm. Perri is a school teacher in otherwise good health with a stable home life. Now in week 14 of her second pregnancy, she is anxious that her growing uterus will worsen both her back pain and insomnia. She did not want to use pain killers or the antidepressants she had previously been prescribed and had taken until she became pregnant with this baby. She consulted with an herbalist about alternatives that might be safe and effective for sleep promotion. After taking a careful history, the herbalist determined that the back pain was really the underlying cause of the sleep disorder, and decided to begin treatment by addressing the chronic pain; however, because of pregnancy, herbal options were limited to mild herbs. Perri was instructed to do the following daily:
- 15 minutes of gentle yoga stretches upon waking.
- 15 minutes of gentle yoga 1 hour before bed.
- Warm bath 30 minutes before sleep each night. Seven drops of lavender essential oil are to be added to each tub.
- Perri was provided with an herbal ointment containing cramp bark (*Viburnum opulus*) capsicum (*Capsicum*

Continued

officinalis), and lobelia (*Lobelia inflata*) to be rubbed into the tight areas of her back twice daily (she will need to get her partner to apply this).
- Cramp bark (*Viburnum opulus*) tincture to be taken as follows:
  - 2 mL in warm water four times daily, including one dose 30 minutes before sleep
  - 5 mL of the following tincture to be taken in two divided doses (2.5 mL each) 1 hour and again 30 minutes before bed;
  - Equal parts of tinctures of passionflower (*Passiflora incarnata*), skullcap (*Scutellaria lateriflora*), chamomile (*Matricaria recutita*), and lavender (*Lavandula officinalis*)

Perri followed this protocol for 3 weeks and came in for a subsequent appointment. She subjectively reported that her back pain had improved by about 80%, and that for the first time she was getting a full night's sleep. She could not be more pleased. She reported that the improved sleep made a huge difference in the experience of her back pain, and vice versa, the decreased pain allowed her to sleep more comfortably. No subsequent prescriptions were necessary, and Perri gave birth to a healthy, full-term baby boy after an uneventful pregnancy and birth.

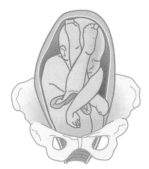

Frank breech

FIGURE 19-4 Frank breech. (Redrawn from Lowdermilk DL, Perry SE: *Maternity & women's health care,* ed 9, St. Louis, 2007, Mosby.)

BREECH PRESENTATION AND VERSION

Breech presentation is when the fetus presents with the buttocks, knees, or feet, rather than the head, toward the vaginal canal during pregnancy. It is common in early pregnancy when the fetus has ample room to move around. As the pregnancy progresses, the baby has less space to move around. The fetal head will tend to gravitate toward the pelvis and the baby will assume a position it often maintains until labor. By 32 weeks of pregnancy, the prevalence of breech presentation is reduced to 16%, and by term it is 3% to 4%. The likelihood that a baby in the breech position at 36 weeks will remain so until the time of birth is 25%; however, spontaneous version to a cephalic (i.e., head first) presentation may occur at any time. Preterm babies are more likely to present breech than those born at full term.

There are three classifications of breech presentation:
1. Frank breech, which is when the fetus has both hips flexed and both knees extended so its feet are near its head (Fig. 19-4). This occurs in 50% to 70% of breech presentations.
2. Footling or incomplete breech, in which the fetus has one or both hips or one or both knees not flexed. As a result, one or both feet present before the buttocks (Fig. 19-5). This occurs in 10% to 40% of breech presentations.
3. Complete breech refers to a fetus with both hips and both knees flexed. The feet are opposite the fetal trunk rather than the head, but do not present in advance of the buttocks (Fig. 19-6). This occurs in 5% to 10% of breech presentations.

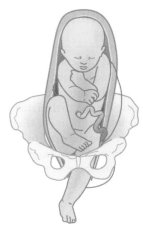

Single footling breech

FIGURE 19-5 Footling (incomplete) breech. (Redrawn from Lowdermilk DL, Perry SE: *Maternity & women's health care,* ed 9, St. Louis, 2007, Mosby.)

REASONS FOR BREECH PRESENTATION

In most cases a persistent breech position is nonpathologic in origin, being a random occurrence or a combination of the dynamics between the maternal pelvic and fetal head shapes.

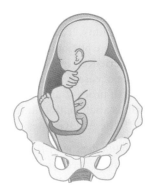

Full breech

FIGURE 19-6 Complete breech. (Redrawn from Lowdermilk DL, Perry SE: *Maternity & women's health care,* ed 9, St. Louis, 2007, Mosby.)

Breech presentation itself presents little risk to the fetus. In some cases, however, persistent breech position is the result of a maternal, fetal, or placental problem. Maternal factors that may contribute to breech presentation include uterine abnormalities that change the normal shape of the uterus, for example, bicornate uterus or uterine fibroids; multiparity that leads to uterine and abdominal wall laxity, changing the shape of the uterus; and a deformed or contracted maternal pelvis. Placental abnormalities, for example, placenta previa, which prevent the fetal head from properly entering the pelvis can contribute to breech position, as can amniotic fluid volume abnormalities (e.g., polyhydramnios, oligohydramnios). Any factors that alter either the normal fetal shape or normal fetal mobility can contribute to breech presentation, and include fetal anomalies (e.g., anencephaly, hydrocephaly), multiple pregnancy (e.g., twins), short umbilical cord, and fetal demise. Previous breech birth is considered a risk factor for breech presentation in subsequent pregnancies.

RISKS OF BREECH PRESENTATION AND BREECH BIRTH

Breech presentation itself presents little risk to the fetus. Risk occurs when there are predisposing maternal, fetal, or placental factors that cause the baby to present breech. Breech birth does appear to increase the risk to the fetus.[140] The exact extent to which this is so is uncertain, as are the reasons. Before the 1950s, vaginal delivery was the preferred method for breech presentation in the United States. In 1970, cesarean rates for breech were 12%. By 2002, this rate had risen to 86.9%.[141] The ACOG Committee on Obstetric Practice currently recommends use of external cephalic version (ECV) and planned cesarean delivery for persistent singleton breech presentation at term. This recommendation was amended to allow vaginal delivery of a term singleton breech if there is detailed patient informed consent, under hospital-specific protocol guidelines for eligibility and labor management, and by a health care provider experienced in vaginal breech delivery.[141]

There is significant controversy regarding whether cesarean section is necessary or improves outcome, and just how great a risk there is with vaginal breech birth.[142] Several studies demonstrate decreased morbidity and mortality to the fetus with elective cesarean; however, this is accompanied by increased maternal morbidity. It has been suggested that the risk of breech birth is more attributable to the fact that most obstetricians are inexperienced in breech birth management because of the high use of cesarean delivery, than to inherent risks in the breech birth process, and that with skilled management, breech birth is a safe option in the absence of complicating factors.[143-146] The ACOG states:

> The number of practitioners with the skills and experience to perform vaginal breech delivery has decreased. Even in academic medical centers where faculty support for teaching vaginal breech delivery to residents remains high, there may be insufficient volume of vaginal breech deliveries to adequately teach this procedure.[141]

To avoid the need for unnecessary cesarean section, obstetric and midwifery care providers recommend that attempts be made to turn the baby to a cephalic presentation before the onset of labor. This section focuses on the use of ECV and moxibustion as two techniques that may be attempted with potential for success. Although this section addresses breech presentation as something to be changed, I wish to emphasize that breech presentation is most often a variation of normal rather than a pathologic condition, and that a discussion on changing the breech to a cephalic presentation is in no way meant to disparage vaginal breech birth.

SIGNS, SYMPTOMS, AND DIAGNOSIS OF BREECH PRESENTATION

With breech presentation, the mother is likely to report more upper abdominal discomfort, indigestion, and greater fetal movement in the upper, rather than lower, abdomen. The care provider may identity the breech presentation upon abdominal palpation. Ultrasound visualization is used as confirmation. Breech presentation is sometimes first diagnosed upon vaginal examination in labor.

CONVENTIONAL TREATMENT OPTIONS FOR TURNING A BREECH PRESENTATION: EXTERNAL CEPHALIC VERSION

The primary method used to turn a breech baby to a cephalic presentation is ECV. ECV is the manual transabdominal rotation of the fetus into a cephalic presentation. The practice was popular in the 1960s and 1970s but fell out of favor because of fetal deaths associated with the procedure. However, the practice was revived in the 1980s and is now considered a safe and effective means for avoiding cesarean section caused by breech presentation.[147-150] ACOG recommends ECV as a standard procedure for turning a breech to avoid cesarean section when the maternal–fetal dyad meets eligibility criteria.[141,151] ECV is performed in the hospital with a surgical room set up should emergency cesarean be necessitated as a result of complications, which occasionally occur as a result of the procedure, including cord entanglement, fetal hypoxia, premature rupture of the membranes, separation of the placenta, and even fetal death.[152] The procedure may be performed with or without tocolysis (i.e., medications to relax the uterus) or anesthetic administered to the mother. Use of tocolysis or anesthetic may facilitate the procedure and reduces pain to the mother.[153,154] Rho(D) immune globulin should be given to RH–negative mothers before attempting a version. The average success rate for the procedure is 58%. Efficacy is greater when the procedure is performed between 34 and 37 weeks, compared with later in pregnancy, although the fetus may revert to its previous position, thus requiring that the procedure be repeated.

BOTANICAL TREATMENT OPTIONS FOR TURNING A BREECH PRESENTATION

Moxibustion for Breech Presentation

Moxibustion is a TCM technique that involves the use of a cigar-shaped stick of compressed *Artemisia vulgaris* herb, lit and indirectly applied as a heat source over the acupuncture point Bladder 67 (BL67) (i.e., zhi yin) on the outer edge of the fifth (pinky) toenail, on each foot (the moxa is *not* applied directly to the skin) (Fig. 19-7). The technique is repeated twice daily for 15 minutes on each foot for 7 to 10 days, and is discontinued when the fetus has felt to have turned. Fetal activity is observed to increase during the treatment period, followed by movement of the baby into a cephalic presentation. In a study by Cardini and colleagues published in *JAMA* in 1998, the authors reported that of 130 women with breech babies who received moxibustion beginning at 33 weeks of gestation, 75.4% of babies were cephalic by 35 weeks of gestation versus 47.7% in the control group. Because no studies had previously been carried out on Western populations, pregnant Italian women at 33 to 35 weeks of gestational age carrying a fetus in breech presentation were enrolled in a randomized controlled trial involving BL67 point stimulation and an observation group. A total of 240 were randomized to receive active treatment (acupuncture plus moxibustion) or be assigned to the observation group. Bilateral acupuncture plus moxibustion was applied at the BL67 acupoint. The primary outcome of the study was fetal presentation at delivery. Fourteen cases dropped out. The final analysis thus was made on 226 cases, 114 randomized to observation and 112 to acupuncture plus moxibustion. At delivery, the proportion of cephalic version was lower in the observation group (36.7%) than in the active-treatment group (53.6%). Hence, the proportion of cesarean sections indicated for breech presentation was significantly lower in the treatment group than in the observation group (52.3% versus 66.7%).[155] Ewies and Olah report that moxa is a safe, painless, inexpensive, and easily administered option, but emphasize the small sample sizes of most studies, with lack of randomization.[156] The Cochrane Review reports no side effects associated with use of moxibustion in pregnancy.[157] Patients should be advised that the smell of burning moxibustion is similar to the smell of marijuana. I have had several patients who had house guests or business associates who thought they were smoking cannabis. It may be suggested that clients use moxa outside or away from an area of business. One funny anecdote with moxa use is of a real estate agent who told a patient that if she wanted to sell her house, which was on the market during the time the patient was using moxibustion for breech version, she might want to smoke her marijuana somewhere else. The patient explained and demonstrated the moxa use to the realtor, and afterward completed her treatments outside, in spite of it being late autumn! She had had a cesarean for a breech baby with her first pregnancy, and was delighted when, after 4 days of treatment at 37 weeks of gestation, her baby changed to a cephalic presentation and she gave birth vaginally at 39 weeks to a vertex baby.

Although from a Western medical perspective, the mechanism of action is entirely unknown, the treatment appears to be entirely safe, is inexpensive, and is applied externally only. It is certainly a preferable alternative to ECV or cesarean section for the management of persistent breech presentation. Because it is advised to be done from 34 weeks onward, treatment does not preclude the decision to perform external version or surgical delivery.

ADDITIONAL TECHNIQUES

Postural Management of Breech Presentation

Five studies involving a total of 392 women were included in a Cochrane review on the efficacy of postural management for changing a breech to a cephalic presentation. Postural management includes the use of slant boards upon which the mother lies on her back at a 45-degree angle with her head down, and other similar techniques that are thought to coax the baby to change position. The authors of the review concluded that there is insufficient evidence from well-controlled trials to support the use of postural management for breech presentation. The numbers of women studied to date, however, remains relatively small.[158]

Hypnosis

In a study by Mehl, 100 women with breech presentation between 37 weeks and term were compared with a similarly matched control group and achieved a version rate of 81% compared with 48% in the nonintervention group. It is thought that because psychophysiologic factors may influence breech presentation, relaxing the mother's abdominal musculature or preparing her mentally and emotionally for delivery through the use of hypnotism or other techniques may assist

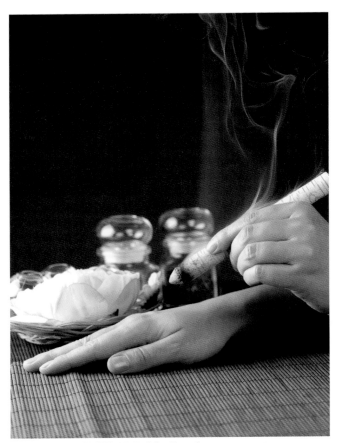

FIGURE 19-7 Moxibustion treatment.

in achieving cephalic version.[152] There are no studies in the literature on the use of hypnosis for breech version.[152]

Other

Small nonrandomized, noncontrolled studies and case reports suggest that there may be some small benefit to a variety of techniques for changing breech position. These include yoga, chiropractic, and homeopathic methods, as well as the use of ginger paste applied in place of moxibustion to stimulate heat to BL67.[152] One of these methods has been systemically evaluated. Use of music applied to the mother's abdomen, a popular technique promoted on the Internet, has only been minimally studied in conjunction with the use of ECV with tocolytic drugs, making it difficult to evaluate the usefulness of the studies.[152]

Labor and Birth

FACILITATING LABOR: INDUCTION, AUGMENTATION, AND DYSFUNCTIONAL LABOR

Labor induction refers to the medical stimulation of contractions before the onset of spontaneous labor to cause labor to commence.[1] One of the most commonly performed obstetric procedures in the United States, rates of labor induction more than doubled between 1990 and 1998 from approximately 9.5% to 21%.[2,3] Reasons cited for this increase include widespread availability of cervical ripening agents, convenience to physicians, pressure from patients, and medicolegal constraints.[4] In spite of obstetric recognition that normal human gestation is 40 to 42 weeks (i.e., postterm pregnancy is defined as pregnancy past 42 weeks of gestation), conservative obstetric practice frequently results in the suggestion, admonition—or insistence—by medical practitioners that their pregnant patients begin labor at, or close to, 40 weeks of gestation. Data to support or refute the benefits of elective inductions are limited.[4] Risks to the mother and fetus include those related to the medications used, risks of iatrogenically induced prematurity, and the increased risk of operative delivery, which is more likely to occur as a consequence of labor induction.[5] According to a Cochrane review of outcomes of labor induction of fetal/neonatal death that compared awaiting spontaneous labor versus a policy of induction after 41 weeks of gestation, including a total of 19 trials and over 8000 women, it was reported that there were intranatal and neonatal deaths when a labor induction policy was implemented after 41 completed weeks or later. However, such deaths were rare with either policy.[6] In a matched cohort study from 1996 through 1997, 7683 women with elective induced labor were compared with 7683 women with spontaneous labor; results in all categories were significantly higher when labor was induced electively: cesarean section rates (9.9% versus 6.5%), instrumental delivery (31.6% versus 29.1%), epidural analgesia (80% versus 58%), and transfer of the baby to the neonatal ward (10.7% versus 9.4%).[5] Studies from the United States have reported similar findings, with a doubling of operative delivery with induction.[7-10] Nulliparous women are especially at risk of cesarean section as a result of induction, and an unfavorable cervix at the time of induction appears to be the greatest contributing cause to need for operative delivery.[1,7] Elective induction leads to an estimated 12,000 excess cesarean sections per annum at a cost of over $100 million.[1] Overall, it is advisable to avoid elective induction unless medically indicated.[10]

Labor induction should only be undertaken when the benefits to either the mother or fetus outweigh the risks of maintaining the pregnancy.[1] Accepted indications for labor induction include[1]:

- Preeclampsia/eclampsia and hypertensive disorders
- Maternal diabetes mellitus with a macrosomic infant ≥4000 g
- Prelabor/premature rupture of membranes (P/PROM)
- Chorioamnionitis
- Intrauterine fetal growth restriction (IUGR)
- Isoimmunization
- Fetal death
- Postterm pregnancy

Contraindications to labor induction include[1]:

- Prior classical uterine incision
- Active genital herpes infection
- Placenta or vasa previa
- Umbilical cord prolapse
- Certain fetal malpresentations (e.g., transverse lie)

Labor augmentation refers to the use of medications to stimulate contractions in an already commenced labor when contraction rate or intensity is inadequate to accomplish birth of the baby, or labor has slowed or stopped. Methods of augmenting labor commonly employed by medical professionals include administration of Pitocin via intravenous (IV) drip and artificial rupture of the membranes (AROM). Dysfunctional labor is failure to progress in the presence of a normal labor pattern, or the contraction pattern itself may be uncoordinated, leading to ineffectual labor. The results are protracted, stalled, or obstructed labor. Factors contributing to dysfunctional labor include but are not limited to pelvic abnormalities, fetal malpresentation, macrosomic fetus, and maternal sedation.

MEDICAL APPROACHES TO LABOR INDUCTION AND AUGMENTATION

The literature on the use of medical interventions for the induction and augmentation of labor is extensive, and far beyond the scope of this textbook to fully present. This section provides a brief synopsis of the most commonly used methods for induction and augmentation, and their safety and efficacy. Readers are encouraged to search the Cochrane

Database, which has an extensive collection of articles (more than 400) reviewing methods of labor induction.

Oxytocin Induction

Synthetic oxytocin (Pitocin) is one of the most commonly used and most potent uterotonic agents available. It is given IV for purposes of induction (as an antihemorrhagic, it may be given intramuscularly) via an infusion pump that allows exact dosing with various dosing protocols. Dosing is done incrementally, starting with small amounts and increasing until contractions come at 2- to 3-minute intervals, and typically not exceeding 40 mU/min. Oxytocin is more effective when administered in the presence of a ripened cervix (i.e., it is softening and has the ability to stretch); thus methods to induce ripening (e.g., prostaglandins via suppositories or oral administration, cervical manipulation, amniotomy) may be used just before or in conjunction with oxytocin administration. Oxytocin use alone is less effective than prostaglandins for inducing labor. Labor induction with oxytocin is associated with an increased rate of cesarean section.[11] Any agent that increases uterine contractions can lead to hypercontractility of the uterus, and can interfere with blood flow to the uterus, and consequently the fetus, with ensuing fetal distress.[12] This is a less frequent complication with oxytocin than with misoprostol. There is some evidence to suggest that use of oxytocin may be associated with an increased incidence of fetal hyperbilirubinemia; however, it is unclear whether this is a direct result of oxytocin use, or associated with other pregnancy factors, such as preterm labor.[12]

High-dose oxytocin (i.e., 40 mU) given over a prolonged period in hypotonic solution (>3 L), or in rapid infusion, can lead to hyponatremia and hypotension, respectively, with resultant serious consequences.

Stripping the Membranes

Stripping the membranes, also called "sweeping the membranes," is thought to release prostaglandin F2-alpha (PGF2α) from the decidua and membranes, or prostaglandin E2 (PGE2) from the cervix, causing cervical ripening and instigating contractions. It is widely used by obstetricians and midwives, often done as a routine part of vaginal and cervical examinations in women who are close to or past term, but often undocumented—possibly because it is not generally thought of as an invasive technique by many practitioners (although many midwives do consider it invasive, especially when done without the mother's permission).[1] In a meta-analysis of 24 trials, (n = 2797) 20 comparing sweeping of membranes with no treatment, three comparing sweeping with prostaglandins, and one comparing sweeping with oxytocin, risk of cesarean section was similar between groups. Sweeping of the membranes, performed as a general policy in women at term, was associated with reduced duration of pregnancy and reduced frequency of pregnancy continuing beyond 41 weeks and 42 weeks. It was effective at preventing the need for formal induction in one out of eight women. No evidence of a difference in the risk of maternal or neonatal

infection was observed. Discomfort during vaginal examination and other adverse effects (e.g., bleeding, irregular contractions) were more frequently reported by women allocated to sweeping. Studies comparing sweeping with prostaglandin administration were of limited sample size and did not provide evidence of benefit. The authors of the meta-analysis concluded that sweeping the membranes is effective in some women at inducing labor, is generally safe in the absence of other complications, and reduces the need for other forms of induction; however, its rate of effectiveness seems limited.[13] Weekly membrane stripping appears to shorten the interval of time to spontaneous labor at term, although improvement in pregnancy outcome has not been demonstrated by large, randomized trials.[1] Risks of membrane stripping include premature rupture of membranes (PROM), infection, disruptions of occult placenta previa, and rupture of vasa previa, though these are rare outcomes of this procedure.

Artificial Rupture of Membranes

AROM, or amniotomy, is performed when the cervix is partially dilated and effaced, and with the fetus in a vertex presentation with the head well applied to the cervix to avoid prolapse of the umbilical cord (or other presenting part). Fetal monitoring accompanies the procedure, as does evaluation of the color of the amniotic fluid to detect for the presence of meconium staining—a possible indication of fetal distress. A Cochrane review identified two trials comprising 50 and 260 women, respectively, that were considered eligible for inclusion in the review of amniotomy alone for labor induction. Conclusions were unable to be drawn on the use of amniotomy alone versus no intervention, nor amniotomy alone versus oxytocin alone. Compared with single-dose application of vaginal prostaglandins in women with a favorable cervix in a single center trial, a higher rate of oxytocin augmentation was required in the amniotomy alone group (44% compared with 15%). Combined use of amniotomy and IV oxytocin is more effective than amniotomy alone. Limited data suggest that the efficacy of oxytocin plus amniotomy is similar to that of prostaglandins alone.[14] Amniotomy is associated with an increase in cesarean section rate. With regard to neonatal outcomes, fewer babies are born with Apgar scores of less than seven, but no statistically or clinically significant differences have been observed in other measures of neonatal morbidity, such as umbilical artery acid-base disturbances and admission to intensive care units.[15] Risks of amniotomy include intrauterine infection, umbilical cord prolapse, and disruption of an occult placenta previa or vasa previa with subsequent maternal hemorrhage. Serious complications, however, are rare.[12]

Prostaglandins

Although the exact mechanisms triggering the onset of labor remain unknown, the production of prostaglandins by the body is implicated in the commencement of cervical ripening and stimulation of uterine contractions. Administration of prostaglandins for labor induction is considered preferable to oxytocin use because the latter does not lead to cervical ripening but only contractions. The use of prostaglandins for labor stimulation appears to decrease the need for obstetric analgesia, and increases the likelihood of birth without operative delivery within 12 to 24 hours of onset of treatment. These advantages, however, are accompanied by increased risk of uterine hyperstimulation with its increased risk of fetal distress and maternal uterine rupture—a surgical emergency. Prostaglandins used include PGE2 and PGF2α; PGE2 is considered safer and equally effective and therefore is the prostaglandin of choice.[12] The optimal route, frequency, and dose of prostaglandins have not been determined.[16-18] Dinoprostone, either in the form of Cervidil or Prepidil, both Food and Drug Administration (FDA)–approved drugs for this purpose, is the agent of choice, and is most commonly administered by direct cervical application via vaginal route; this has proved to be effective with the fewest side effects. Introduction of IV oxytocin approximately 12 hours after administration of dinoprostone is common practice to facilitate labor onset.

Misoprostol (Cytotec) is a synthetic prostaglandin E1 (PGE1) analog available as 100- and 200-μg tablets, which can be broken to provide 25- or 50-μg aliquots and can be administered orally or intravaginally. Misoprostol is approved by the FDA for the prevention and treatment of gastric ulcer disease related to chronic nonsteroidal antiinflammatory drug use.[1] In most countries, it has not been licensed for use in pregnancy; however, off-label use is common because the drug is inexpensive, stable at room temperature (unlike other prostaglandin drugs), and effective in causing cervical ripening and uterine contractions. Misoprostol is highly effective at initiating labor; reduces the need for oxytocin administration, epidurals, and cesarean section; and shortens time to delivery by as much as 8.7 hours.[19] The use of misoprostol has been associated with uterine hyperstimulation, tetanic contractions, precipitous labor, and possibly an increased incidence of uterine rupture, which can be fatal for both mother and fetus.[19] Uterine hyperstimulation with fetal heart rate changes and meconium staining of the amniotic fluid—indicative of fetal distress—are increased with misoprostol use. The optimal dose and timing of misoprostol use remain unknown.

Oral misoprostol appears to be more effective than placebo and is at least as effective as vaginal dinoprostone. However, because of increased risk of uterine hyperstimulation and lack of certainty in dosing, vaginal administration, which is also effective, and associated with a slightly decreased risk of hyperstimulation and other side effects compared with the oral route, is considered preferable.[19] If misoprostol is used orally, the dose should not exceed 50 mcg.[19] In countries where misoprostol remains unlicensed for the induction of labor, practitioners may prefer to use a licensed product, for example, dinoprostone, for legal reasons.[19] Studies to date have not been large enough to determine the actual risk of uterine rupture, which has been anecdotally associated with misoprostol use.[20] Misoprostol, however, is contraindicated for women with a history of prior cesarean delivery or other previous major uterine surgery owing to increased risk of uterine rupture. Of particular concern also is the use of misoprostol in the home birth setting, where equipment for adequate measurement of uterine contractions is unavailable, as is rapid access to emergency surgery in the event of fetal distress or uterine rupture.

Mechanical Stimulation Methods

Mechanical methods of labor induction include use of a Foley balloon catheter and hygroscopic dilators. In the former method, a Foley balloon catheter is passed, uninflated, into the undilated cervix and then inflated; it may be used alone or in combination with pharmacologic methods of induction. The combination of balloon catheterization and prostaglandin administration appears to significantly increase the likelihood that a woman will deliver within 24 hours of the procedure; however, the benefit of the two methods combined has not been shown to be more effective than use of oral misoprostol alone. Hygroscopic dilators are inserted into the vaginal canal after application of a topical anesthetic, and gradually swell as they absorb moisture. The swelling, in addition to mechanical effects on the cervix leading to dilatation, may serve to disrupt the chorioamnionic decidual interface, causing lysosomal destruction that results in prostaglandin release. Laminaria, made from seaweed, is a typical hygroscopic dilator; synthetic agents are also available. Hygroscopic dilators do not appear to be as clinically effective as PGE2 gels and are associated with an increased risk of maternal postpartum infection and neonatal infection.[1]

MEDICAL APPROACHES TO DYSFUNCTIONAL LABOR

The causes of and medical treatments for dysfunctional labor (i.e., dystocia) are extensive. This section provides only a brief overview of the pathophysiology and medical interventions. Labor is considered dysfunctional when any of the stages of labor is protracted with no progress made in cervical dilatation and fetal descent. During the latent phase of labor, it is recommended that women alternate rest or sleep with periods of activity (e.g., walking). Cervical effacement, uterine activity, and fetal status are periodically evaluated. Eight-five percent of women progress to the active phase of labor, 10% cease uterine activity, and approximately 5% require oxytocin induction if it is necessary to expedite labor. If labor dysfunction arises during active phases, the underlying reason for arrest is ideally determined; for example, obstruction resulting from a macrosomic baby or contracted pelvis, or fetal head malposition (e.g., persistent asynclitism). Various methods may be used to facilitate labor, including amniotomy, oxytocin infusion, and epidural or other agents to relax pelvic musculature and allow the mother to rest. The fetus is monitored throughout. If fetal status remains normal and there is minimal risk of cord prolapse, ambulation may be allowed or encouraged. If labor does not progress normally with these, and possibly other interventions, or if fetal status becomes compromised, surgical delivery (i.e., cesarean section) ultimately must be performed.

TABLE 20-1 Botanical Treatment Strategies for Labor Induction, Augmentation, and Dysfunction

Therapeutic Goal	Therapeutic Activity	Botanical Name	Common Name
Stimulate contractions	Uterine stimulant	Caulophyllum thalictroides	Blue cohosh
		Gossypium herbaceum	Cotton root
		Ricinus communis	Castor oil
		Rubus idaeus	Red raspberry leaf
Stimulate cervical ripening	Prostaglandin	Oenothera biennis	Evening primrose oil
Coordinate uterine activity	Uterine spasmolytic	Actaea racemosa	Black cohosh
		Leonurus cardiaca	Motherwort
		Viburnum spp.	Cramp bark/black haw
Promote smooth muscle relaxation	Uterine spasmolytic	Actaea racemosa	Black cohosh
		Leonurus cardiaca	Motherwort
		Viburnum spp.	Cramp bark/black haw
Relieve labor pain	Analgesic/sedative	Corydalis ambigua	Corydalis
		Eschscholzia californica	California poppy
		Piscidia piscipula	Jamaican dogwood
Relieve maternal anxiety and tension	Anxiolytic Nervine	Eschscholzia californica	California poppy
		Humulus lupulus	Hops
		Leonurus cardiaca	Motherwort
		Matricaria recutita	Chamomile
		Passiflora incarnata	Passionflower
		Valeriana officinalis	Valerian

BOTANICAL APPROACHES TO FACILITATING LABOR

Midwives use a wide variety of approaches to facilitate the onset and progress of labor when these are not occurring spontaneously or when otherwise indicated (Table 20-1). Although midwives honor the fact that the timing and pace of labor and birth are highly individual, there are times when legal or medical restrictions require that women birth within certain time parameters; for example, by 41 weeks of gestation or within 18 hours of ROM for women to birth at home in certain states where home birth midwifery is licensed. These constraints require that midwives and their pregnant clients work creatively with a breadth of options to expedite labor and birth. Also, birth does not always progress smoothly, obstructed by any number of sometimes benign but nonetheless problematic factors such as malpresentation of the fetal head (i.e., persistent asynclitism), and maternal fear, anxiety, pain, or pelvic tension. A combination of these factors is very common; asynclitism can lead to uncoordinated contractions and maternal fatigue, which increase pain, tension, and anxiety—thus creating a vicious cycle that ultimately leads to medical intervention. Often, a combination of agents to alter the maternal response via uterine stimulation or maternal relaxation and noninvasive measures such as nipple stimulation, changes of maternal position, and relaxation techniques, can facilitate labor. Rarely is any single technique used in isolation; rather, several techniques are more commonly employed, ideally in an orderly and rhythmic fashion to initiate a healthy, active labor pattern. Botanical choices are selected according to the individual needs and either physiologic or pathophysiologic response to labor, and are used in conjunction with options presented in **Additional Methods** Table 20-2.

The role of a knowledgeable and supportive care provider serving as a labor facilitator—a midwife, understanding obstetrician, or doula—cannot be underestimated in its effects on facilitating a healthy labor and birth process. Further, to effectively intervene with natural, noninvasive strategies, it is essential that the care provider adequately understand the mechanics, physiology, and psychology of birth. For example, although many think that it is adequate to stimulate contractions in a stalled or dysfunctional labor using uterine stimulants, effective labor requires a delicate balance between contraction and relaxation—this yields coordinated uterine contractions, cervical dilatation, and fetal descent. Therefore it is often more effective to use both uterine stimulant and uterine antispasmodic herbs in combination to achieve an effective labor pattern. Similarly, if a woman is exhausted and contractions are faltering, promoting sleep may actually achieve a better and faster outcome than stimulating contractions. Table 20-2 will help the reader to identify a combination strategy that might be applied to the individual woman. Practitioners must be knowledgeable about when medical intervention becomes required, and of course it is essential that the mother and fetus be adequately and properly monitored during labor and efforts to stimulate labor. As discussed in the following, blue cohosh, for example, has been associated with rare adverse cardiovascular effects on the fetus, and more commonly with milder side effects as a result of maternal use.

The following section discusses herbs specifically used to stimulate contractions or used as spasmolytics specifically for

TABLE 20-2 General Approaches to Labor Problems

Labor Problem	General Strategy	Botanical Strategy	Additional Methods
Postdates pregnancy (>41 weeks and 6 days)	Stimulate labor	Uterine stimulants Prostaglandins	Nipple stimulation Sexual intercourse (if possible); orgasm Maternal activity (e.g., walking)
Obstetric pressure to induce (e.g., legal, hospital, or obstetric practice policy)	Stimulate labor	Uterine stimulants Prostaglandins	Nipple stimulation Sexual intercourse (if possible); orgasm Maternal activity (e.g., walking)
PROM	Stimulate labor	Uterine stimulants Prostaglandins	Nipple stimulation Sexual intercourse (if possible); orgasm Maternal activity (e.g., walking)
Labor stalled or ceased Prolonged labor Dysfunctional labor	If maternal exhaustion predominates	Uterine spasmolytic sedatives	Hot baths if no ROM or hot showers if ROM Promote sleep with massage, visualization, music
	If fetal malposition is present (i.e., asynclitism)	Uterine spasmolytics	Maternal pelvic relaxation with hot baths if no ROM or a hot shower if ROM Maternal position changes and movement
	If maternal anxiety or fear predominates	Anxiolytics Nervines	Verbal/emotional support
	If maternal pain predominates	Uterine spasmolytics Analgesics/sedatives	Verbal/emotional support Maternal pelvic relaxation with hot baths if no ROM or a hot shower if ROM Maternal position changes and movement

PROM, Premature rupture of membranes; *ROM*, rupture of membranes.

labor. Analgesics, sedatives, and nervine herbs are discussed throughout this book.

Castor Oil

Castor oil is a potent cathartic extracted from the castor bean (Fig. 20-1). Use of this herb to stimulate labor appears to date back to ancient Egypt.[21] It remains a commonly used folk method to induce labor, and has made its way into obstetric practice, with its use commonly suggested by midwives. There are scant data evaluating its clinical efficacy. In a clinical trial, a single dose of castor oil was compared with no treatment. There was no evidence of a difference between cesarean section rates, meconium staining of the amniotic fluid, or Apgar score. No data were presented on neonatal or maternal mortality or morbidity. Nausea was a side effect in all women who ingested castor oil.[21] Overall, the trial was of poor methodological quality and no determination can be made regarding efficacy for labor induction.

Blue Cohosh

Caulophyllum thalictroides (blue cohosh) (Fig. 20-2), a native of the eastern and central woodlands of the United States, has been used traditionally and historically as an anticonvulsant, antirheumatic, febrifuge, emetic, sedative, and most notably, a gynecologic aid.[22,23] It has been used for labor induction, amenorrhea, dysmenorrhea, menorrhagia, and to induce abortion.[22] Blue cohosh was official in the *United States Pharmacopoeia (USP)* from 1882 to 1905 for labor induction, and in the *National Formulary* from 1916 to 1950.[24] It was a

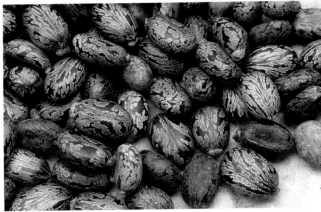

FIGURE 20-1 Castor plant beans *(Ricinus communis)*. (Photo by Martin Wall.)

major ingredient in the popular Eclectic preparation Mother's Cordial, which also included *Mitchella repens, Rubus idaeus, Actaea racemosa,* and *Chamaelirium luteum*. At least one company (Herbalist & Alchemist, New Jersey) still makes this preparation; however, the blue cohosh has been removed as an ingredient in the product because of safety concerns. The practice of labor induction with blue cohosh remains a popular choice both among self-prescribers and obstetric professionals in the United States and abroad, with one large survey indicating widespread use among nurse-midwives.[25]

Blue cohosh is listed in the *British Herbal Pharmacopoeia* (1983) as a spasmolytic and emmenagogue.[26] It may also be used

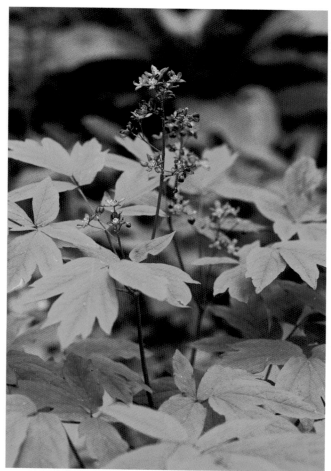

FIGURE 20-2 Blue cohosh *(Caulophyllum thalictroides)*. (Photo by Martin Wall.)

as a uterine and ovarian tonic, and for the treatment of a variety of menstrual complaints, including menorrhagia, amenorrhea, dysmenorrhea, and pelvic congestion syndrome.[27,28] It is commonly used as a partus preparator to ease parturition, and for labor induction and augmentation.[27] It has also been used as an abortifacient.[27] Use of blue cohosh during pregnancy is a widespread practice among midwives and pregnant women.[25] Maternal ingestion has been associated with a range of fetal and neonatal side effects and adverse outcomes, including fetal tachycardia, increased meconium, profound neonatal congestive heart failure, and perinatal stroke.[25,29-31] There is one case report of a neonate born with complications including myocardial infarction and profound congestive heart failure to a mother who ingested blue cohosh as a partus preparator. The newborn remained critically ill for several weeks but eventually recovered. All other causes of myocardial infarction were excluded.[30] In another case report, a child was born with severe multiorgan failure associated with the use of a blue and black cohosh combination. The child required significant resuscitation at birth and sustained permanent central nervous system (CNS) damage.[32] Neither the amount and duration nor preparation used were disclosed. The effects in both cases have been attributed to vasoactive glycosides in the herb. A 21-year-old woman developed

symptoms of nicotinic toxicity, including tachycardia, diaphoresis, abdominal pain, vomiting, and muscle weakness and fasciculations after using blue cohosh in an attempt to induce an abortion. These symptoms likely resulted from methylcytosine known to be present in blue cohosh. The patient's symptoms resolved over 24 hours and she was discharged.[33]

Alkaloid and glycoside components in blue cohosh suggest possible mechanisms for these effects, as well as teratogenicity and mutagenicity.[33,34] Methylcysteine exhibited teratogenic activity in rat embryo culture (REC), an in vitro method to detect potential teratogens. Taspine showed high embryotoxicity but no teratogenic activity in the REC.[34] Toxic effects of the plant's constituents include coronary vasoconstriction, tachycardia, hypotension, and respiratory distress.[24] However, Low Dog cautions that the quality of the case reports to date and the value of some of the testing methods used to establish toxicity may be questionable. For example, although REC tests have shown teratogenicity and embryotoxicity, "neither the National Institute of Environmental Health Sciences nor the Environmental Protection Agency recognizes these tests as an appropriate screen for human reproductive risk."[24] Similarly, it has been speculated that anagyrine, which produces known malformations in ruminant livestock, may do so only after metabolism by microflora in the ruminant gut.[24]

The *Botanical Safety Handbook* classifies this herb as 2b, not to be used during pregnancy; however, it states that *Caulophyllum* may be used as a parturient near term to induce childbirth under the supervision of a qualified practitioner.[35] Canadian regulations require that any products containing this herb be labeled as not for use in pregnancy.[35] Given the volume of blue cohosh use in the United States alone, and the general paucity of reports of its side effects, as well as a lack of comparison of side effects with conventional medications for labor augmentation (e.g., Pitocin, misoprostol), it remains uncertain how great a risk is posed by the use of blue cohosh, particularly for short-term labor augmentation as opposed to long-term use as a partus preparator. Low Dog states, "The human case reports, flawed as they are, paint a picture that is consistent with the evidence provided by the in vitro and animal studies."[24] The most conservative route is to avoid its use entirely as a partus preparator, and possibly at all during pregnancy, until safety information is established. Midwives and mothers choosing to use blue cohosh to augment labor should observe assiduous fetal heart monitoring during use and should discontinue use promptly if deviations are observed. No discussion on the safety of blue cohosh during lactation is reported in the literature.[27] One case report in the literature describes an infant born to a mother who had consumed anagyrine-containing goat milk; however, as stated, it is not known whether activation of this compound requires metabolism in the ruminant gut.[24] Many direct-entry midwives have discontinued use of the herb because of safety concerns.[36]

The Use of Herbs as Partus Preparators and for Labor Induction

The use of herbs for labor stimulation is popular, both with self-prescription among pregnant women and prescription by midwives.[25,37-39] The pressure to give birth by a certain date to avoid artificial induction is the primary incentive behind such use, followed by the desire of pregnant women to avoid protracted pregnancy for personal comfort. In a study by Westfall and Benoit, a panel of 27 women was interviewed in the third trimester of pregnancy, and 23 of the same participants were reinterviewed postpartum (50 interviews total). Many of the women said they favored a natural birth and were opposed to labor induction at the time of the first interview. However, all but 1 of the 10 women who went beyond 40 weeks of gestation used self-help measures to stimulate labor. These women did not perceive prolonged pregnancy as a medical problem. Instead, they considered it an inconvenience, a worry to their friends, families, and maternity care providers, and a prolongation of physical discomfort.[40]

A national survey of 500 members of the American College of Nurse-Midwives and 48 nurse-midwifery programs was conducted by McFarlin and colleagues to determine whether they were formally or informally educating students in the use of herbal preparations for cervical ripening, induction, or augmentation of labor.[25] Ninety surveys were returned from certified nurse-midwives (CNMs) who used herbal preparations to stimulate labor and 82 were returned from CNMs who did not. Of the CNMs who used herbal preparations to stimulate labor, 93% used castor oil, 64% used blue cohosh, 63% used red raspberry leaf, 60% used evening primrose oil (EPO), and 45% used black cohosh. The most cited reason for using herbal preparations to stimulate labor was that they are "natural," whereas the most common reason for not using herbal preparations was the lack of research or experience with the safety of these substances. Although 78% of the CNMs who used herbal preparations to stimulate labor directly prescribed them and 70% indirectly suggested them to clients, only 22% had included them within their written practice protocols. Seventy-five percent of the CNMs who used herbal preparations to stimulate labor used them first or instead of Pitocin. Twenty-one percent reported complications including precipitous labor, tetanic uterine contractions, nausea, and vomiting. CNMs who used herbal preparations to stimulate labor were more likely to deliver at home or in an in-hospital or out-of-hospital birthing center than CNMs who never used herbal preparations to stimulate labor.[25]

Initiation of labor may be medically necessitated in some cases of postdatism or in the advent of PROM. Labor augmentation is required when contractions in a previously active labor cease or become ineffective. The use of a variety of herbs and approaches, including some of those used to induce or augment labor, are commonly a part of the protocol for prolonged or dysfunctional labors. The herbs most commonly used for labor induction are blue cohosh (*Caulophyllum thalictroides*) and black cohosh (*Actaea racemosa*).

The use of herbs to prepare women for labor begs the question of why one would use an herbal preparation to prepare the body for something it naturally knows how to do, and seems antithetical to the principles upon which herbal medicine philosophy is built—to trust the body's innate wisdom. Although a small percentage of women truly need pharmacologic help with induction, most women can enter labor naturally, and given proper support, experience labor and birth without the use of drugs for augmentation. The widespread use of blue cohosh to stimulate labor may be a problem in itself, but more importantly, it is symptomatic of a greater medicosociologic problem. Health practitioners in the position to do so must help to educate their colleagues about the natural process of labor and a woman's (and baby's) ability to accomplish it successfully and safely, thus mitigating the need for unnecessary pharmacologic intervention.

Cotton Root

The historical use of cotton root bark as an emmenagogue and abortifacient is discussed in Chapter 15. Ellingwood considered cotton root specifically for uterine inertia, to increase uterine contractions, and also prevent postpartum hemorrhage.[41] The plant was marketed by Lloyd Pharmaceuticals and Eli Lilly as an oxytocic, emmenagogic agent. The *USP* listed cotton root as a parturient from 1860 to 1880.[42] Cardiotoxic and hepatotoxic effects have been reported in animals and in vitro with gossypol, an isolated chemical constituent used medically. Altered hormone levels and other metabolic effects have been mainly reported in animals and in vitro, but are reported in human studies as well.[43] Gossypol is present in the seed in 0.5% concentration, and in lesser concentrations throughout the plant.

The root bark extract (not gossypol) is currently used by Western herbalists as an emmenagogue in cases of amenorrhea and as a uterine antihemorrhagic. It is increasingly used by midwives as an alternative or adjunct to blue cohosh as a labor stimulant in postterm pregnancies, for PROM, or for stalled labor. No studies were identified in the literature on use of whole plant extracts, nor the use of this herb for labor stimulation; thus the safety and efficacy of this herb as a labor stimulant cannot be determined. This herb may have teratogenic effects if taken during early pregnancy, and may induce abortion, so it should not be used earlier in pregnancy than at the intended onset of labor. It is generally given in tincture form, usually in combination with other uterine stimulants, and often antispasmodic herbs. Repeated doses of 2 to 3 mL every 2 hours often result in contractions after four to six doses.

Red Raspberry

Red raspberry leaf is perhaps one of the most historically venerated herbal uterine tonics. It is used during pregnancy to strengthen the uterus, improve labor outcome, and prevent excessive bleeding after birth. Its use continues to be highly popular. One study indicates that approximately 63% of US midwives use this herb to stimulate labor.[25] Although it does not appear that raspberry leaf is very effective for labor stimulation or shortening the duration of labor, recent research has found that the consumption of raspberry leaf tea during pregnancy may in fact improve labor outcome and reduce the need for medical intervention at birth. The results of a double-blind, randomized, placebo-controlled trial consisting of 192 low-risk, nulliparous women who birthed their babies between May 1999 and February 2000 at a large tertiary-level hospital in Sydney, Australia found that raspberry leaf, taken in tablet form from 32 weeks' gestation until labor, caused no adverse effects for mother or baby, and although it did not shorten labor, a lower rate of forceps deliveries between the treatment group and the control group (19.3% versus 30.4%) was observed.[44] Another study consisted of 108 mothers; 57 (52.8%) consumed raspberry leaf products, whereas 51 (47.2%) were in the control group. The findings suggested that raspberry leaf can be taken safely during pregnancy to shorten labor with no expected side effects for women or their babies. The study also reported a decreased likelihood of preterm and postterm gestation, and fewer obstetric interventions, including decreased amniotomy, cesarean section, forceps delivery, and vacuum extraction in the group that had taken raspberry leaf compared with the control group.[45] Herbalists and midwives consider raspberry leaf to be a gentle, effective nutritive medicament, and recommend it be taken in the form of an infusion, 1 to 3 cups daily. Of all the herbs that might be considered for labor preparation, raspberry leaf products appear to be the safest.[24]

Evening Primrose Oil

EPO is a rich source of essential fatty acids, especially gamma (γ)-linolenic acid (GLA), which function as precursors for prostaglandin synthesis. EPO is widely used by many midwives, both applied topically to the cervix and taken orally, to encourage cervical ripening in an effort to shorten labor and decrease the incidence of postterm pregnancies. Sparse data are available to support this use, although many midwives report it to be effective based on observational reports and anecdotes (Case History). One study was identified that investigated the effect of oral EPO on the length of pregnancy and selected intrapartum outcomes in low-risk nulliparous women. A two-group retrospective quasi-experimental design conducted on a sample of women who received care in a birth center compared selected outcomes of 54 women taking EPO in their pregnancy with a control group of 54 women who did not. Findings suggested that the oral administration of EPO from week 37 until birth did not shorten gestation or decrease the overall length of labor. Further, in this study, the use of orally administered EPO may have been associated with an increase in the incidence of prolonged rupture of membranes, oxytocin augmentation, arrest of descent, and vacuum extraction.[46] Numerous studies of EPO have found no toxicity. Rare side effects include headache and gastrointestinal upset.[47]

Black Cohosh

Black cohosh was considered an excellent remedy to treat both "false pains in the pregnant uterus, and aid true pains" making "labor easier and quicker and give a better getting up."[48] One Eclectic physician gave a report to the Chicago Gynecologic Society of a study of 160 primiparous and multiparous women to whom he gave a combination of black cohosh and sarsaparilla during the last 4 weeks of pregnancy. By his account, the women experienced decreased length of labor, with minimal neuralgic cramping and irregular pain in the first stage, greater relaxation of the "soft parts," energetic and rhythmic contractions throughout the remainder of labor, and decreased incidence of lacerations and good maintenance of contractions after delivery (he compared the effects with those of ergot).[49]

Black cohosh was an ingredient in the popular Eclectic preparation Mother's Cordial, which was used as a labor preparatory blend in the late nineteenth and early twentieth centuries. It continues to be popular today, with one survey indicating that as many as 45% of nurse-midwives responding used it to stimulate labor. It is frequently combined with blue cohosh as a popular labor stimulant formula. It is spasmolytic and antiinflammatory to the smooth and skeletal muscles, making it effective in the treatment of dysmenorrhea, and perhaps suggesting a mechanism for its observed efficacy in treating spasmodic pain in labor and incoordinate uterine contractions.[50,51] Black cohosh is approved by the German Commission E for the treatment of premenstrual complaints and dysmenorrhea.[52,53] It is indicated for muscular pains, nervous tension, and has been noted to have antiinflammatory and analgesic effects.[54,55] It is often used by midwives to relax spasmodic contractions and help coordinate uterine smooth muscle activity to promote effective contractions in combination with a more stimulating uterine tonic, for example, blue cohosh or cotton root bark (see Blue Cohosh for warnings regarding its use during pregnancy and labor). Several case reports have suggested a possible hepatotoxic effect of black cohosh. As of 2006, several Western nations, including Canada, have issued requirements that all black cohosh products be labeled with a warning about the risk of hepatotoxicity from consumption. The United States has not issued such a warning, based on prior findings that the herb appears reasonably safe. At this time, the safety of the herb for use during pregnancy and lactation is uncertain; long-term use (>2 days) is not advisable. Some herbalists report that patients sometimes experience a frontal headache with use of this herb. If this occurs, discontinue use; this side effect resolves with discontinuation.

Motherwort

Motherwort is considered a uterine spasmolytic and tonic, exerting both actions for the result of easing spastic uterine contractions, for example, in a protracted first stage of labor, and improving the resting tone of the uterine tissue. It is also a favored nervine and anxiolytic, including for panic disorders and to promote sleep. It is widely used by herbalists and midwives during labor, the puerperium, and for **Premenstrual syndrome** with dysmenorrhea (**PMS-D**). Its common name, motherwort, literally means "healing herb for mothers," suggesting a long history of use for these purposes. Most evidence for the use of motherwort is based on traditional medicine and clinical observation.[23,53] No side effects are expected from appropriate use during labor; the herb is considered contraindicated earlier in pregnancy because of its history of use as an emmenegogue.[24] It is typically taken in tincture form.

Cramp Bark/Black Haw

Cramp bark, in small doses, was considered by the Eclectics to be an excellent partus preparator, easing irregular uterine contractions and "greatly facilitating a speedy and uncomplicated normal labor."[41] It was also used for after pains and prevention of postpartum hemorrhage because of its tonifying effects exerted on uterine smooth muscle. It was considered specific for erratic uterine cramping and pain.[41,56] These herbs are still widely used by contemporary midwives and herbalists for uterine cramping, with many finding it effective for spasmodic contractions and a protracted early labor. Either may be used in tincture form, alone or combined with other herbs as appropriate, for example, with nervines or sedatives to promote rest during the first stage. There are no adverse effects or side effects expected with use of this herb.

ADDITIONAL METHODS OF FACILITATING LABOR

Nipple Stimulation

Nipple stimulation is commonly recommended by midwives as part of a protocol to stimulate labor. The mother is instructed to apply traction and a pulling, rolling motion to the nipples either simultaneously or separately but sequentially, for 15 to 30 minutes at a time, and repeat this up to two or three times daily for several days if needed. It is more effective to have a partner apply the nipple stimulation because it is difficult to achieve the required force on oneself. A 2005 Cochrane review of the effects of breast stimulation on onset of labor identified six trials with a total of 719 women. Analysis of trials comparing nipple stimulation with no intervention found a significant reduction in the number of women not in labor at 72 hours. However, this result was only seen in women with a favorable cervix at the onset of stimulation. Interestingly, a major reduction in the rate of postpartum hemorrhage was reported (0.7% versus 6%). There was no significant difference in the cesarean section rate (9% versus 10%), nor in rates of meconium staining. There were no instances of uterine hyperstimulation. Three perinatal deaths were reported.[57] Chayen and Kim, in a clinical trial of 317 patients taking contraction stress tests using stimulation with an automatic breast pump, found that contractions were successfully achieved in 84.2% of cases, with uterine hyperstimulation observed in 4.1% of tests performed. They reported that side effects and complications were minimal.[58] In another study by Chayen and colleagues, nipple stimulation with an electric breast pump was compared with oxytocin infusion as a means of labor induction. The time from stimulation to the onset of regular uterine activity, to 200 Montevideo units of uterine activity, and the time until entrance into the active phase of labor were significantly shorter in the

nipple stimulation group. Once the women were in active labor, there was no difference between the groups in the length of labor or mode of birth. Although nipple stimulation is not as effective as oxytocin induction, it appears to be effective for many women, and may be considered a safe, effective alternative to try before turning to pharmaceutical or mechanical labor stimulation.[59]

Sexual Intercourse

Prostaglandins have been extensively studied for their role in stimulating the onset of labor, particularly ripening the cervix. Human semen is a rich biological source of prostaglandins, with a high prostaglandin concentration. The use of intercourse to stimulate labor has become a modern "folk" tradition, and it is widely recommended among midwives when labor stimulation is required. The typical recommendation is intercourse two to three times daily, for 2 to 3 days in a row. Of course, this assumes the mother is in a heterosexual, sexually active relationship. The recommendation is generally made in conjunction with additional techniques for labor stimulation (e.g., nipple stimulation, herbs). It is uncertain whether any stimulating effects resulting from sexual intercourse result from the mechanical stimulation of the lower uterine segment, the endogenous release of oxytocin as a result of orgasm, or the direct action of prostaglandins in semen. Furthermore, nipple stimulation may be part of the process of initiation if this occurs in the context of sexual activity. These various factors are very difficult to standardize for clinical studies in comparison with other interventions for labor induction.[60] A Cochrane review identified one study of 28 women, from which the authors determined that no meaningful conclusions could be derived.[60] As long as the membranes are intact, there is not placenta previa, and the mother is comfortable with this approach, there is no harm in incorporating intercourse into efforts to stimulate labor.

Acupuncture

Acupuncture has been used in Asia and Europe to decrease the pain of labor, effect cervical ripening, and stimulate the onset of labor. It has been suggested that acupuncture neuronal stimulation may increase uterine contractility either by central oxytocin release or parasympathetic stimulation of the uterus. A Cochrane review on the effects of acupuncture on labor stimulation found that although there are a number of studies looking at acupuncture labor effects, few are of high quality. Induction of labor using electroacupuncture was reported by Yip and coworkers[61] in 1976 with a success rate of 67% of women ($n = 31$), with pregnancy duration ranging from 38 to 42 weeks. Another study ($n = 12$) using acupuncture with and without electrical stimulation had a success rate of 83% with an average time between induction and delivery of 13.1 hours. In a third study, 34 term and postterm women and seven women with intrauterine fetal deaths were induced using electroacupuncture. Labor was successfully induced in 32 (78%) women.[62] These and a limited number of additional observational studies to date suggest that acupuncture for induction of labor appears safe, has no known teratogenic effects, and may be effective.[62] The evidence regarding the clinical effectiveness of this technique is limited.

Homeopathy

Homeopathy is popularly used for labor induction. The homeopathic extract of *Caulophyllum thalictroides* is proposed to be useful in establishing labor, or when uterine contractions are short and irregular or there is an arrest of uterine contractions.[63] It is commonly recommended that pregnant women ingest one tablet daily for the last few days before the due date or desired onset of labor, or alternatively to dissolve a tablet in a glass of water and sip from the glass from time to time, or whenever a contraction is imminent. A double-blind placebo-controlled matched cohort study by Beer and Heiliger compared *Caulophyllum* with placebo in 40 women at term with PROM and no onset of contractions. Women were administered *Caulophyllum* or a placebo hourly for 7 hours. Each active tablet consisted of 250 mg *Caulophyllum* (trituration D4) and inert binders.[64]

A study by Dorfman and associates compared five homeopathic therapies with placebo in 93 women from 36 weeks pregnant; 53 women were randomized to the treatment group and 40 to the placebo group. The trial examined the effect of the homeopathic therapy on length of labor and difficulty of labor. The information on any side effects arising from *Caulophyllum* was unclear and it was unclear as to how women assessed the tolerability of *Caulophyllum*. No data were provided on side effects.[65] The Cochrane Collaboration concluded that both trials were of weak methodological quality and no meaningful conclusions could be drawn on the efficacy of *Caulophyllum* for inducing labor or improving labor-related outcomes.[66] Additionally, they commented that the use of *Caulophyllum* may not represent common homeopathic practice, in which the prescribing of a therapy is typically individualized.[66] However, it may represent common over-the-counter self-prescribing that is based on more common generic prescriptions, of which it should be noted that the adverse effects that may be associated with the use of the herb blue cohosh (*Caulophyllum thalictroides*), discussed in the preceding, are not expected with the homeopathic preparation, in which no identifiable chemical compounds remain.

Walking and Positional Changes

Controversy exists regarding the relationship between maternal position in labor and outcome, such as labor duration, subjective discomfort, and fetal outcome.[67] In cultures not influenced by Western society, women progress through the first stage of labor in upright positions and change position as they wish with no evidence of adverse effects to either the mother or fetus.[12,68,69] The technologic approach to birth endemic to Western culture with nearly ubiquitous reliance on interventions such as continuous fetal monitoring, epidural use, and continuous IV infusion, relegates women to a supine position during labor. Numerous studies have demonstrated that this position may increase the risk of

adverse effects to both the mother and her passenger, as well as impinging on the effective progress of labor.[70] Effective contractions, and therefore effective fetal descent and prevention of dystocia, are essential to labor progress and can be facilitated with ambulation and positional changes in labor.[12] Further, moving around can increase a woman's sense of control in labor by providing a self-regulated distraction from the challenge of labor and also may decrease her need for analgesia.[70] The use of a variety of positions, changes of position throughout labor as needed, and maternal ambulation in labor are considered by midwives to be fundamental to the prevention and management of labor dystocia, particularly when associated with remediable fetal malpresentation, such as asynclitism. Further, changes in maternal position, such as from supine to left lateral or hands-and-knees, can be effective in relieving fetal cord compression and therefore fetal distress associated with the supine position.[71-74] Midwives frequently encourage positions that are not only physiologic for the mother, her maximal comfort and labor effectiveness, and the position of the fetus, but also positions that facilitate optimal maternal support, such as access to massaging her lower back to relieve the pain of labor in the lower back (Fig. 20-3).

A limited number of studies have evaluated the effects of maternal position on labor outcome, and most of these evaluated positions prescribed by obstetric care providers rather than those chosen by laboring women for themselves.[67] In a study by Carlson and colleagues, it was observed that left to select their own positions, a total of 80 laboring patients selected from no less than 59 different positions during the course of labor, with a greater variety of positions chosen in early labor, but more positional changes occurring during second stage. The most commonly selected position for labor was lateral recumbent.[67] Outcome measures were not evaluated in this study. The hands-and-knees position during labor has been recommended on the theory that gravity and buoyancy may promote fetal head rotation to the anterior position and reduce persistent back pain. A Cochrane review based on two studies found that the use of hands-and-knees position for 10 minutes twice daily to correct occipitoposterior position of the fetus in late pregnancy does not affect this change; however, it did not evaluate the use of this position during labor or for more extended lengths of time.[75] A study by Stremler and coworkers was conducted to evaluate the effect of maternal hands-and-knees positioning on fetal head rotation from occipitoposterior to occipitoanterior position, persistent back pain, and other perinatal outcomes. Thirteen labor units in university-affiliated hospitals participated in this multicenter randomized controlled trial. Study participants were 147 women laboring with a fetus at 37 weeks of gestation and confirmed by ultrasound to be in occipitoposterior position. Seventy women were randomized to the intervention group (hands-and-knees positioning for at least 30 minutes over a 1-hour period during labor) and 77 to the control group (no hands-and-knees positioning). The primary outcome

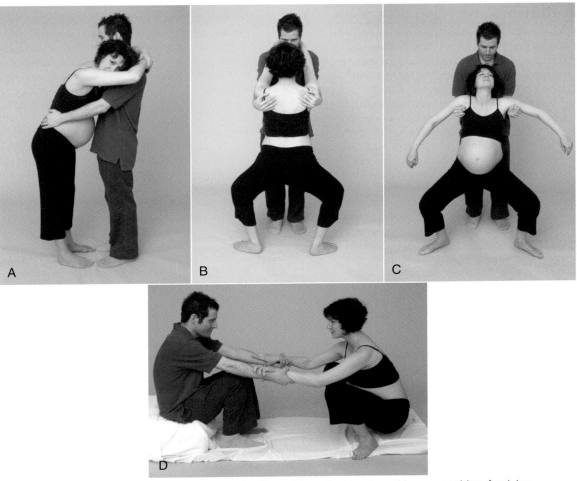

FIGURE 20-3 Positional changes to facilitate labor. **A,** Hands-and-knees position for labor. **B,** Left lateral recumbent position. **C,** Standing position with massage. **D,** Supported squat. (From Stillerman E: *Prenatal massage: a textbook of pregnancy, labor, and postpartum bodywork,* St. Louis, 2008, Mosby.)

was occipitoanterior position determined by ultrasound after the 1-hour study period, and the secondary outcome was persistent back pain. Other outcomes included operative delivery, fetal head position at delivery, perineal trauma, Apgar scores, length of labor, and women's views with respect to positioning. Women randomized to the intervention group had significant reductions in persistent back pain. Eleven women (16%) allocated to use hands-and-knees positioning had fetal heads in occipitoanterior position after the 1-hour study period compared with five (7%) in the control group. Trends toward benefit for the intervention group were seen for several other outcomes, including operative delivery, fetal head position at delivery, 1-minute Apgar scores, and time to delivery. The authors concluded that maternal hands-and-knees positioning during labor with a fetus in occipitoposterior position reduces persistent back pain and is acceptable to laboring women, and this option of a position for labor should be made available to women laboring with a fetus in occipitoposterior position.[76]

LABOR STIMULATION PROTOCOL

Midwives use a variety of protocol to stimulate labor. They are applied in a supportive atmosphere conducive to labor, with the primary labor support person(s) present, and ideally, appropriate monitoring available for mother and fetuses (e.g., maternal blood pressure and labor progress, fetal heart tones). A typical protocol for initiating labor is presented in the Case History. Other herbs may be added to the protocol, such as nervines if there is anxiety. Women are not encouraged to attempt to stimulate labor before 40 weeks, unless otherwise medically instructed, because of the risk of inducing premature labor. The labor initiation protocol is typically applied over an 8-hour time course, and if not effective on the first attempt, it may be repeated the next day. It is not recommended to repeat this for more than two consecutive days. Some mothers find the castor oil intolerably nauseating; if so, repeat the abdominal massage and skip castor intake; some mothers may experience a frontal headache. This is most likely a result of the black cohosh. If this occurs, discontinue the tincture for the next dose and thereafter substitute cramp bark or black haw for the black cohosh.

👤 CASE HISTORY

Alison, a 38-year-old mother of two, was 34 weeks pregnant with her third baby when her midwives told her that her baby was getting too big and she should prepare herself for an early induction at 38 weeks or a cesarean delivery. Her previous baby, now age 8, was born by cesarean section at term after 30 hours of labor because of the baby's large size (9 lb 8 oz) and an ineffectual labor. She was not pleased about the idea of another cesarean, and therefore was excited to be preparing for a VBAC (vaginal birth after cesarean) in the hospital with a midwife and obstetrician practice. She had no medical risk factors and was not diabetic. With her midwife's support, she found a direct entry midwife in the community who practiced herbal medicine, and contacted her to discuss possible alternative methods of initiating labor as early as 36 weeks. The midwife told Alison that 36 weeks is too early, but to discuss a reasonable goal with her primary care midwife and then they could discuss options. Alison came back to the herbalist-midwife with a reasonable due date of the beginning of week 38. The herbalist midwife gave Alison a protocol, and agreed to help if all of the care providers involved in Alison's prenatal and delivery care supported the use of the herbs. All agreed. Alison's protocol was as follows:

- Beginning at 37 weeks of gestation, for 1 week, apply 1500 mg of EPO to the cervix daily and take 1000 mg EPO orally. Alison was instructed that the cervical application could be accomplished by digital application or by using the oil as a lubricant during intercourse, which was also recommended several times weekly.
- On the first day of week 38, or in this case, the intended due date, Alison was to follow a specific protocol for 8 hours and then discontinue.

8 AM

1.5 mL each blue and black cohosh (*Caulophyllum thalictroides* and *Actaea racemosa*) and 0.5 mL ginger root (*Zingiber officinale*) in a combined tincture

30 minutes nipple stimulation

8:30 AM

Long walk (i.e., 30 minutes)

9 AM

1.5 mL each blue and black cohosh (*Caulophyllum thalictroides* and *Actaea racemosa*) and 0.5 mL ginger root (*Zingiber officinale*) in a combined tincture

9:30 AM

Massage of selective acupressure points or acupuncture treatment for mother

10 AM

1.5 mL each blue and black cohosh (*Caulophyllum thalictroides* and *Actaea racemosa*) and 0.5 mL ginger root (*Zingiber officinale*) in a combined tincture

Castor oil abdominal massage: Warm castor oil by running bottle under hot water or putting in a basin of hot water. Apply with effleurage-style massage for 20 to 30 minutes.

10:30 AM

Hot shower or bath (the latter if membranes are intact)

11 AM

1.5 mL each blue and black cohosh (*Caulophyllum thalictroides* and *Actaea racemosa*) and 0.5 mL ginger root (*Zingiber officinale*) in a combined tincture

Dose 1 Castor oil: 2 oz castor oil in blender with 4 oz orange juice; blend on high speed with pinch of baking soda to emulsify, and have mother drink down quickly. Have mother sit and rest quietly, and if needed, suck a piece of candied ginger or a mint lozenge to quell nausea.

11:30 AM

Have mother rest.

12 PM

Light lunch

1.5 mL each blue and black cohosh (*Caulophyllum thalictroides* and *Actaea racemosa*) and 0.5 mL ginger root (*Zingiber officinale*) in a combined tincture

12:30 PM

Long walk if mother is not limited to "bathroom range" from castor oil

1 PM

1.5 mL each blue and black cohosh (*Caulophyllum thalictroides* and *Actaea racemosa*) and 0.5 mL ginger root (*Zingiber officinale*) in a combined tincture

30 minutes nipple stimulation

1:30 PM

Dose 2 Castor oil: 2 oz castor oil in blender with 4 oz orange juice; blend on high speed with pinch of baking soda to emulsify and have mother drink down quickly. Have mother sit and rest quietly, and if needed, suck a piece of candied ginger or a mint lozenge to quell nausea.

2 PM

1.5 mL each blue and black cohosh (*Caulophyllum thalictroides* and *Actaea racemosa*) and 0.5 mL ginger root (*Zingiber officinale*) in a combined tincture

3 PM

1.5 mL each blue and black cohosh (*Caulophyllum thalictroides* and *Actaea racemosa*) and 0.5 mL ginger root (*Zingiber officinale*) in a combined tincture

4 PM

1.5 mL each blue and black cohosh (*Caulophyllum thalictroides* and *Actaea racemosa*) and 0.5 mL ginger root (*Zingiber officinale*) in a combined tincture

Alison was told that she should start the protocol after a good breakfast as early in the morning as possible, to absolutely discontinue the protocol at the end (do NOT take additional doses of the herbs) and then to try to have a good dinner, do something relaxing, and get to bed early; labor rarely starts immediately with the protocol, but often starts as long as 8 to 12 hours after.

At 37 weeks, Alison went to her nurse-midwife who checked her cervix and found it to be uneffaced and undilated. By ultrasound, the baby's weight was estimated at approximately 8 lbs. Alison followed the instructions for using the EPO and went to her midwife for a follow-up appointment to determine whether any progress occurred with this treatment; she was found to be 50% effaced and 1 cm dilated. At the onset of 38 weeks, Alison followed the 8-hour protocol, ending at about 6 PM. She had dinner with her family and then she and her husband went to a movie. She got to bed at about 11:30 PM and was awakened at about 2 AM with strong contractions. These persisted and by about 6 AM she could no longer tolerate the discomfort and felt the need to go to the hospital. In her mind, she was disappointed because with her previous labor she had labored for 30 hours and only progressed to 6 cm; now she felt she was giving up already and assumed she would have another cesarean. She arrived at the hospital about 45 minutes later, and was found to be 9 cm dilated. She birthed a healthy 8.5-lb baby boy within the hour, vaginally, and with no complications for the mother or baby. The family was entirely pleased and the nurse-midwife amazed at the efficacy of the herbal protocol. The herbalist-midwife saw the mother and child when he was 7 years old; both were in excellent health, and the mother still ecstatic over the birth experience.

PAIN IN LABOR

Knowledge is the most powerful thing as far as pain.[77]

The experience of pain in labor is a complex individual experience, and perhaps one of the greatest areas of anticipatory anxiety for pregnant women. Epidural anesthesia is currently used in almost two thirds of all labors in the United States, a reflection of the immense desire of women to avoid the pain normally associated with labor.[78,79] Although epidural anesthesia can be an invaluable tool in the management of difficult labors and births, and many women report that epidural analgesia is very helpful, it is not without potential risks, including increased length of labor, need for operative vaginal delivery, likelihood of perineal laceration, increased incidence of maternal fever leading to increased use of neonatal antibiotics and sepsis evaluations, increased use of oxytocin augmentation, and possible increase in need for cesarean section.[77,79] There are little data evaluating the effects of epidural anesthesia on breastfeeding and mother–infant bonding; however, it has been observed that women who experience operative deliveries are more likely to experience postpartum depression, which can significantly affect mother–child interaction. Women are poorly informed about the potential side effects of epidural (and other) anesthesia, and what little information they are given is commonly provided in active labor, even at the height of a contraction, when it is impossible for a woman to make an informed choice.[79] Further, women are rarely offered nonpharmacologic alternatives for pain relief, in spite of the fact that numerous studies show that the use of doulas, continuous labor support, using various positions for labor, massage during labor, sterile water injections, acupuncture, and other modalities lessen labor pain.[79-81]

This chapter casts no judgment on the choice of women to receive epidural anesthesia for pain relief, and endorses its judicious use in difficult labors. It is every woman's right to choose how to birth, and to have access to all of the tools available for her to do so safely and with as much support, comfort, and confidence as possible. However, this chapter does encourage practitioners to give women the ability to make fully informed decisions by apprising them of nonpharmacologic and pharmacologic interventions equally, ideally before or during labor, with adequate information to make a realistic appraisal of risks and benefits. It also encourages birthing centers and hospitals to see alternative methods of pain management as safe, cost-effective means of caring for laboring patients rather than resorting to the routine use of interventions that can lead to unnecessary additional interventions and complications.

Unlike other chapters in this book, which emphasize the use of botanical therapies, this section provides an overview of the many possible options for pain management in labor that are commonly used by midwives and other practitioners, of which herbs are only a small part.

The nonpharmacologic approach to pain includes a wide variety of techniques to address not only the physical sensations of pain but also to prevent suffering by enhancing the psycho emotional and spiritual components of care. Pain is perceived as a side effect of a normal process, not a sign of damage, injury, or abnormality. Rather than making the pain disappear, the midwife and other caregivers assist the woman to cope with it, build her self-confidence, and maintain a sense of mastery and well-being.[82]

Penny Simkin and April Bolding

ASSUMPTIONS ABOUT LABOR AND BIRTH: OBSTETRIC VERSUS MIDWIFERY BELIEFS

According to childbirth sociologist Carol Sakala, a prevalent assumption of the biomedical approach to labor pain is that many or most women require pain medication during labor.[77] In direct contrast, midwives assume that women intrinsically know how to birth, and that with adequate prenatal preparation and support during the birthing process, pain medication is often unnecessary.[77,83] Midwives recognize that a routine, homogenous approach to pain management in labor, even using nonpharmacologic methods, is inherently ineffective, and that care providers must be able to respond to the unique needs of individual laboring women with a variety of tools in their repertoire, and be creative and responsive in the moment.

Midwives believe that not only is education about the process of labor and birth essential, but so is a close and trusting relationship with the care provider, or in the least, a doula who can be both a support person and an advocate for the mother. Midwifery wisdom appears to be consistent with what women actually report as the most important factors leading to a feeling of satisfaction with birth, none of which include pain relief as important. A recent systematic review concluded that the four factors associated with satisfaction with the childbirth experience are[79]:

- Amount of support received
- Quality of relationship with care provider
- Involvement in decision making
- Personal expectations

Midwives, whose professional care is based on a mother-centered empowerment approach, and caregivers that include complementary and alternative medicine (CAM) as part of the repertoire they offer mothers for labor support, are more likely to be perceived by patients as consistent with these factors.[84]

Hospital-based preparation (e.g., childbirth classes) commonly spends more time preparing women for the interventions they can expect as part of routine hospital practices than building their sense of personal empowerment and choice. Childbirth classes designed by midwives (e.g., Birthing from Within), in contrast, are more likely to emphasize skills and tools that can be used by the mother/couple to achieve as natural a birth as possible. Changing medical attitudes to embrace the possibility of natural birth as a routine childbirth practice will be necessary to expand the repertoire of non-pharmacologic interventions available to women birthing in medical institutions. It has been demonstrated in European hospitals that such attitude changes can lead to changes in practice that translate into reductions in unnecessary medical and surgical interventions, improving outcomes for both mother and baby.[85] "Hospitals with low cesarean section rates have achieved this goal by embracing the belief that supportive labor care and the least intervention create the best opportunity for a good birth experience."[85]

PSYCHOLOGICAL PREPARATION FOR LABOR

Every birth experience is unique and unpredictable. Preparing for labor is not dissimilar to preparing for a hiking trip. You train in advance; know the terrain; pack your gear, your trail mix, and other provisions; stock your first aid kit; check the weather; and set out, prepared and expecting the best. Hopefully, you have good weather and a clear trail. But sometimes the unforeseen happens—the trails are closed because of rock slides, there is an unexpected thunder storm, or you slip and sprain your ankle. In the event of these problems, one takes an alternate route, breaks out the rain gear and seeks shelter, or abandons the trip and gets medical attention. So it is with birth. We make our plans, but sometimes the best-laid plans are not what birth has in store—so we have to choose an alternate route. Empowerment and self-determination, tempered by flexibility, are perhaps the most important attributes with which women can enter labor.

Rarely does a woman give birth and later say "that was easy." Even with quick and seemingly (to the observer) easy births, the mother goes through enormous physiologic, psychological, emotional, and perhaps even spiritual changes. At the least, a woman usually remarks that it was work. For most women labor is hard work, and a lot of it, perhaps for hours, perhaps protracted over days. Sometimes resources are available to help a woman cope with the intensity of it—a comforting partner, midwife, doula, or obstetrician who can give reassurance, massage, or herbs if needed to relieve anxiety, fear, or pain—enabling the mother to endure a great deal of work to birth her baby. Other times, in the absence of such resources, or in spite of the best resources, medical intervention is needed in the form of pharmacologic pain relief or operative delivery.

Women led to believe that labor can be painless, fast, and easy, whether by using herbs, hypnotherapy, or the power of positive thinking are often sorely disappointed and ill-prepared as they get past the initial contractions. Although any of these tools may be useful adjuncts to a well-prepared woman, in the absence of preparation for a broad range of possible experiences, and acceptance that labor cannot entirely be controlled or planned, they may set a woman up for a sense of failure if things do not go according to plans, hopes, and expectations. Further, women who approach their prenatal preparation "arming" themselves with techniques to avoid pain in labor are probably not preparing effectively. The point of pain relief techniques is not necessarily to make labor "pain free," but to give women tools to help them cope as they find their inner resources to get through labor. As practitioners, we can best help women and couples to prepare for labor and birth by honestly discussing the range of realities and possibilities inherent in the experience, and the options for maximizing coping skills. Helping women to become more comfortable and trusting in their bodies, more self-aware, more empowered to express their needs and preferences, and helping to create a safe place in which pregnant and laboring women can express their fears and pain are all powerful parts of labor preparation.

CONTINUOUS LABOR SUPPORT

The word "continuous," as it relates to labor support, has been defined in various ways. In one study, in which staff nurses were the support providers, "continuous" was defined as "a minimum of 80% of the time from randomization to delivery." In a meta-analysis of trials of labor support, "continuous" was defined as "without interruption, except for toileting, from shortly after admission to the hospital or entry into the study, and during the birth of the child." Labor support with a midwife or doula usually includes continuous presence, emotional support (e.g., reassurance, encouragement, guidance); physical comforting (e.g., assistance in carrying out coping techniques; use of touch, massage, heat and cold, hydrotherapy, positioning, and movement); information and guidance for the woman and her partner; facilitation of communication (e.g., assisting the woman to express her needs and wishes); and nonmedical information and advice, anticipatory guidance, and explanations of procedures.[82] Continuous support provided by another woman with birth experience consistently has been demonstrated to reduce labor pain and improve labor outcomes—a fact long known by traditional midwives worldwide. The perhaps seminal studies on this were reported by Kennell and colleagues, who found that the continuous presence of a supportive companion (i.e., doula) during labor and delivery in two studies in Guatemala shortened labor and reduced the need for cesarean section and other interventions. In a US hospital with modern obstetric practices, 412 healthy nulliparous women in labor were randomly assigned to a supported group ($n = 212$) that received the continuous support of a doula, or an observed group ($n = 200$) that was monitored by an inconspicuous observer. A control group was formed of 204 women after delivery. Continuous labor support significantly reduced the rate of cesarean section deliveries (supported group, 8%; observed group, 13%; control group, 18%) and forceps deliveries. Epidural anesthesia for spontaneous vaginal deliveries varied across the three groups (supported group, 7.8%; observed group, 22.6%; control group, 55.3%). Oxytocin use, duration of labor, prolonged infant hospitalization, and maternal fever followed a similar pattern. The authors concluded that the beneficial effects of labor support underscore the need for a review of current obstetric practices.[86] A Cochrane meta-analysis found a decrease in operative vaginal deliveries, cesarean section, fewer requests for pain medication, and increased birth satisfaction when continuous labor support was given.[87] Interestingly, fear of labor in itself has been shown to decrease pain tolerance.[88] The support of a caring woman during pregnancy and in labor, herself educated and experienced in matters of birth, can be instrumental in dispelling and alleviating fear. Prenatally, midwives are aware that they can have a dual role in becoming both a trusted support person and someone who can help a woman to reframe or reprogram her misapprehensions and misconceptions about childbirth, so that the mother might enter labor with reduced anxiety.[77]

VARIOUS POSITIONS

Unrestricted, women will assume a variety of positions that they find conducive to labor and birth. Possible positions for labor and birth include semiseated, squatting, hands-and-knees, kneeling, side-lying, and standing. Women may birth in a shower, birthing tub, on a bed, a birthing stool, or on the floor. Midwives have long assisted women in labor by having them change positions to facilitate rotation of the baby's head and downward descent of the baby, or having the mother shift positions to relieve discomfort when possible, such as laboring on the hands-and-knees to relieve lower back pressure and to rotate a baby from a posterior position, or rocking the hips during contractions to accomplish the same. Fourteen studies have been conducted in which women were randomized to various positions in labor; of these, two have shown a decrease in the use of analgesia. Randomizing women to specific birthing positions is not the same as individualizing birthing positions to optimize the mother's comfort, nor is it comparable with the mother intrinsically identifying the positions in which she is most comfortable laboring.

MASSAGE

Massage is a tool used almost ubiquitously by midwives throughout labor, whether of the lower back, or gentle effleurage of the abdomen, legs, neck and shoulders, or forehead (Fig. 20-4). Massage is tailored to the specific physical needs of the mother and her stage in labor; for example, during early labor, a deep foot massage can help a mother to sleep through contractions and get needed rest; in more advanced labor,

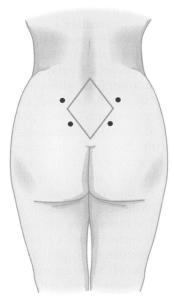

FIGURE 20-4 Sites for firm acupressure massage or sterile water injections. (From Stillerman E: *Prenatal massage: a textbook of pregnancy, labor, and postpartum bodywork,* St. Louis, 2008, Mosby.)

firm lower back pressure might be welcomed; and during transition, light touch across the forehead can relieve tension. Even just simple touch can be a great comfort.[79] Massage can be used throughout labor, with women in a variety of positions from side-lying to standing, and requires no special equipment (although massage oil or hand cream can be used to prevent chaffing or irritation to the mother's skin). Training in specific massage techniques can be beneficial for optimal relief of discomfort, and is easy for the labor partner, doula, or midwife to learn; however, it is not necessary to have special training to be effective and comforting.

A number of studies have explored the effects of massage on labor pain. In a study by Chang and colleagues, 60 primiparas in labor were randomly assigned to either a massage or control group and tested using the self-reported Short-Form McGill Pain Questionnaire (SF-MPQ) at three phases of cervical dilation: phase 1 dilation (3 to 4 cm), phase 2 dilation (5 to 7 cm), and phase 3 dilation (8 to 10 cm). The massage group received standard nursing care and massage intervention, whereas the control group received standard nursing care only. The results of this study showed that in both groups, as cervical dilation increased, there were significant increases in pain intensity as measured by SF-MPQ; massage lessened pain intensity at phases 1 and 2, but there were no significant differences between the groups at phase 3. The results of this study indicate that, although massage cannot change the characteristics of pain experienced by women in labor, it can effectively decrease labor pain intensity at phases 1 and 2 of cervical dilation during labor.[89] Another study evaluated a program of massage, controlled breathing, and visualization performed regularly by birth partners from 36 weeks of gestation and assisted by a trained professional; this occurred after hospital admission during labor and birth. The intervention was designed in light of experimental findings that repeated massage sessions over 14 days increased the pain threshold by an interaction between oxytocin and opioid neurons.[90] A 4-week time frame was selected to coincide with a physiologic increase in maternal pain threshold. To detect the effects of massage during labor on maternal cortisol and catecholamines, cord venous blood was taken to measure plasma concentrations after birth. Twenty-five nulliparous and 10 multiparous women participated in the study. Cortisol values were similar to published studies after labor without massage, but pain scores on a visual analog scale (VAS) done at 90 minutes after birth were significantly lower than scores recorded 2 days. The mean score was 6.6. Previous studies suggested that a reduction from 8.5 to 7.5 would significantly reduce pharmacologic analgesia in labor.[90-92] A study by Field and associates of 28 average socioeconomic women from diverse ethnic backgrounds (Hispanic, 57%; Anglo-American, 34%; African American, 9%) were randomized to receive massage in addition to coaching or breathing, or to receive coaching and breathing in the absence of massage. Based on self-reporting using a Likert scale, women in the massage group reported a pain reduction from 5.0 to 3.5, whereas the women in the control group actually reported an increase from 4.3 to 5.0.[1-5,93]

A 2012 randomized controlled trial (RCT) tested the effects of massage intervention compared with attendant presence and control for reduction of labor pain. A group of 120 primiparous women was allocated to receive either massage (administered in 30-minute intervals), the presence of an attendant, or standard care control. Pain scores were self-reported, and anxiety and overall satisfaction were assessed with VAS. The women who received massage experienced less anxiety and pain than controls, and lower pain compared with the attendant group. The women who received an attendant experienced less anxiety than the massage group.[94] Another study tested the effects of massage against music therapy for labor pain reduction. A group of 100 primiparous women was randomized to receive either massage or music therapy. Using VAS, the massage group experienced a statistically significant decrease in pain scores over the music group ($p = .009$).[95] Further studies suggest that massage may reduce the intensity but not the qualitative character of pain. A clinical trial tested massage against standard care control for labor pain reduction ($n = 60$ primiparous women). The primary outcome was measured using the self-reported McGill Pain Questionnaire at three phases of cervical dilation: 3 to 4 cm, 5 to 7 cm, and 8 to 10 cm. Results suggest that massage benefited pain intensity at the first and second phases, but not the third. Interestingly, the most commonly used words to describe the pain were similar between the experimental and control groups: sore, sharp, heavy, throbbing, and cramping.[96] Even more studies concluded there was a benefit of massage intervention and breathing on labor pain;[97] reflexology was also found to be beneficial.[98,99]

HYDROTHERAPY

Maternal anxiety and pain may prolong labor and contribute to fetal distress.[100] Hydrotherapy during labor can promote relaxation and decrease pain without the risks caused by other treatments. Hydrotherapy can include warm baths, birthing pools, or a hot shower, ideally with an adjustable flow spray nozzle with a firm massage setting. A pilot study by Benfield and coworkers on the psychophysiologic effects of hydrotherapy on maternal anxiety and pain during labor was conducted. Using a randomized, pretest-posttest control group design with repeated measures, 18 term parturients were assigned to a control or an experimental group. Experimental subjects were placed in a tub of 37° C (98.6° F) water for 1 hour during early labor. The Wilcoxon two-sample test revealed statistically significant effects. At 15 minutes, bathers' anxiety and pain scores were decreased compared with nonbathers. At 60 minutes, bathers' pain scores were decreased compared with nonbathers. After 15 minutes of immersion, bathers had a significantly greater increase in plasma volume than nonbathers. No significant differences were found in urine catecholamines or maternal–fetal complications. The small sample limits conclusions, but the findings offer preliminary support for the therapeutic effects of bathing in labor for acute, short-term anxiety and pain reduction.[100] A 2013 RCT tested 20-minute warm shower interventions on first labor stage pain ($n = 92$, 80 completed). Using VAS and the Labour Agentry Scale, women who received the warm showers reportedly experienced less pain.[101] But there may be limitations to the effects of hydrotherapy. A 2010 pilot study ($n = 11$) aimed to determine the effects of hydrotherapy on anxiety, contraction responses, and neuroendocrine changes during labor. Eleven term women took body temperature baths for 1 hour. Outcomes were measured by taking blood samples and applying pain and anxiety questionnaires at baseline, and 15 and 45 minutes into bathing. The investigators concluded statistically significant decreases in anxiety, vasopressin, and oxytocin at 15 and 45 minutes, as well as decreased contraction frequency. Significant decreases in pain and cortisol were not observed. However, women with higher baseline pain and cortisol responded to the hydrotherapy.[102]

A review of the literature suggests that a primary effect of immersion is a central blood volume bolus, which occurs almost immediately after bathing begins. Subjective maternal responses to bathing in labor have been favorable. No maternal or infant infections have been attributed to bathing by parturients with either intact or ruptured membranes. Maternal bathing in labor does not appear to affect infant Apgar scores or stress hormones at birth. No clear evidence exists to indicate that hydrotherapy increases cervical dilation, increases fetal descent, reduces uterine dyskinesia, shortens labor, decreases use of epidurals or analgesia, or decreases rates of operative delivery or hemorrhage. Study findings indicate support for using hydrotherapy for rapid relief of pain and anxiety in labor.[103] Midwives have observed that the overuse of water, especially full immersion in warm tubs for extended durations during labor, actually can lead to maternal exhaustion and delays in labor. Although there is no way to individualize the amount of time a woman spends in water during labor, personal midwifery experience suggests emphasizing the use of short baths or showers and massage in early labor, and using warm tubs and full immersion at longer lengths in later stages of active labor. Women may enter the water at any point in labor, but when there is cervical dilatation less than 5 cm, bathing may diminish the frequency or intensity of contractions, as may staying in the water for greater than 2 hours continuously.[104] Having the mother get out of the tub and walk around and cool off periodically may prevent prolonged labor. To prevent maternal dehydration during long immersions, fluid intake should be encouraged. Immersion in baths is contraindicated in labor when there is evidence of maternal infection, excessive vaginal bleeding, conditions requiring continuous fetal monitoring, with continuous oxytocin infusion, or a nonreassuring fetal heart rate pattern.

AROMATHERAPY

Many midwives and mothers report that soothing scents can enhance a sense of comfort and well-being in the laboring mother's environment. Scents may be chosen for their relaxing effects (e.g., lavender), soothing effects (e.g., lavender, vanilla), or stimulating effects (e.g., peppermint). Essential oils, distributed via diffuser or spray bottle, may be mixed into massage oil, added to a warm bath, or placed on a washcloth in the bottom of a hot shower. One extensive observation study of 8058 mothers in childbirth was the largest research initiative in the use of aromatherapy within a health care setting. The study involved a range of participants, from mothers who experienced a low-risk, spontaneous labor and birth to those whose labor was induced and those who had vaginal operative delivery and cesarean section. The study took place over a period of 8 years, which enabled a more challenging test of the effect of aromatherapy on intrapartum midwifery practice and outcomes. In the study, a total of 10 essential oils were used, plus a carrier oil, which were administered to the participants via skin absorption and inhalation. The study found little direct evidence that the practice of aromatherapy per se reduced the need for pain relief during labor, or the incidence of operative delivery. But a key finding of this study suggested that two essential oils, clary sage and chamomile, were effective in alleviating pain. The evidence from this study suggested that aromatherapy can be effective in reducing maternal anxiety, fear, and/or pain during labor. The use of aromatherapy appeared to facilitate a further reduction in the use of systemic opioids in the study center, from 6% in 1990 to 0.4% in 1997 (measured per woman).

Bitter orange has been tested for labor pain reduction, and has demonstrated positive results. A 2014 RCT tested bitter orange hydrosol fragrance inhalation for pain reduction in the first stage of labor. A group of 126 primiparous women was randomized to inhale a spray of 4 mL of hydrosol or saline control every 30 minutes. Pain measurements were taken at baseline and at cervical dilations of 3 to 4 cm, 5 to 7 cm, and 8 to 10 cm. The researchers reported equivalent pain scores in the control and experimental group at baseline, but a noted reduction in pain perception in the experimental group.[11,105] The same group of researchers (2014) tested bitter orange oil fragrance inhalation for anxiety reduction in the first stage of labor. The study also consisted of 126 women, so it is likely that the same group was utilized. The women were randomized to inhale the fragrance of 4 mL of oil or saline control every 30 minutes. Anxiety levels were measured at baseline (method not noted) and at cervical dilations of 3 to 4 cm, 5 to 7 cm, and 8 to 10 cm. Though precise data and methods of assessing outcomes were not provided, the authors claim that the experimental group experienced less anxiety than the control group.[106] Aromatherapy is an inexpensive care option. The study reports a minimal incidence of associated symptoms. Out of 8058 mothers in the extensive study, 1% recorded an associated symptom, all of which were mild in nature.[107,108]

HERBS FOR PAIN RELIEF

Independent midwives commonly use herbs for pain relief in labor when other, nonpharmacologic methods have not produced adequate results and the mother appears to be suffering. Although the analgesic and sedative actions of herbs are not as quick-acting or powerful as pharmaceuticals, their actions can be gently effective, most with minimal risk of serious side effects, and their use does not preclude subsequent administration of pharmaceutical intervention should it eventually be required. It is not usually expected that herbal medicines will entirely relieve the pain associated with labor; rather they are used to "take the edge off," promote sleep when needed, and relax incoordinate uterine contractions that may be leading to ineffective and thereby unnecessarily painful labor. The herbs discussed in the following are those that are purely analgesic or sedating in action, and that are most commonly used by midwives for labor pain. These herbs are typically combined into formulae and given repeatedly over a short period of time (e.g., every 15 minutes for 1 hour until desired effect [e.g., sleep, pain relief] is achieved) and repeated as necessary. Maximum daily doses are provided in Table 20-3.

STERILE WATER INJECTIONS

Intracutaneous sterile water (ISW) injections made adjacent to the posterior superior iliac spines are believed to cause distention of the skin, which leads to stimulation of nociceptors and mechanoreceptors, creating a localized sensation that may act as a counterirritation to uterine contraction pain (see Fig. 20-4). A randomized controlled trial ($n = 134$) was conducted comparing the effectiveness of three nonpharmacologic approaches for relief of back pain: (1) ISW; (2) transcutaneous electrical nerve stimulation (TENS); and (3) standard care, including back massage, whirlpool bath, and liberal mobilization. Women self-evaluated both intensity and affective dimensions of pain using VAS. Their evaluations of control and satisfaction were assessed using

TABLE 20-3 Herbs for Pain Relief in Labor

Herb	Use in Labor/Effect	Cautions	Form/Dose for Labor
Black cohosh (Actaea racemosa)	Relieve spastic uterine contractions; relieve lower back pain; relieve leg pain; general musculoskeletal relaxant	Concerns have recently been raised about the hepatotoxicity of black cohosh; the actual risk has not been determined	Tincture 2 mL repeated every 15-60 minutes, up to 6 doses total in 24 hours, not to exceed 2 days' use
California poppy (Eschscholzia californica)	Promote sleep	Sedating at excessively high doses	Tincture 1-2 mL repeated every 30-60 minutes, up to 6 doses total in 24 hours
Cannabis* (Cannabis spp.)	Relieve sensation of uterine pain; promote deep relaxation; relieve anxiety; general musculoskeletal relaxant; promote appetite	Not legally available; risk of positive drug test; risk of adulteration or contamination of product with harmful drugs; paranoia or increased anxiety in mother	Tincture; smoked in "pin joint" (i.e., very thin marijuana cigarette), 1-2 puffs as needed
Cramp bark (Viburnum opulus)	Relieve spastic uterine contractions; relieve lower back pain; general musculoskeletal relaxant	No expected adverse effects; possible mild hypotensive effects with large or repeated doses	Tincture 2-3 mL repeated every 15-60 minutes, up to 15 in 24 hours; not to exceed 2 consecutive days
Hops (Humulus lupulus)	Sedating; promotes sleep	Can be strongly sedating at higher doses; not recommended in patients with severe depression	Tincture 1-2 mL every 1-2 hours, up to 8 mL in 24 hours
Motherwort (Leonurus cardiaca)	Relieve spastic uterine contractions; relieve anxiety	No expected adverse effects	Tincture 1-3 mL repeated every 30-60 minutes, up to 15 mL in 24 hours
Passionflower (Passiflora incarnata)	Relieve anxiety; promote rest/sleep	No expected adverse effects	Tincture 1-3 mL repeated every 30-60 minutes, up to 15 mL in 24 hours

*Because of illegality, this herb is not recommended for use unless under medical prescription.

adapted versions of the Labour Agentry Scale and the Labour and Delivery Satisfaction Index. The results indicated that women in the ISW group rated the intensity and unpleasantness of pain during the experimental period significantly lower than women in the standard care group or the TENS group. Mean pain intensity at 15 and 60 minutes after randomization was significantly reduced in the ISW group compared with the two other groups.[109]

In another study, 45 pregnant women in the first stage of labor presenting with lower back pain were randomized into two groups. One group received ISW in the lumbosacral region, whereas the other group was given corresponding subcutaneous (in comparison to intracutaneous) injections of isotonic saline, regarded as a placebo treatment. In the group that received ISW injections the mean pain score was significantly more reduced compared with the placebo group at 10, 45, and 90 minutes after the treatment. The midwives' blind estimation of the effectiveness of treatment was consistent with the subjective patient assessment. However, the requirement of meperidine was similar in the two groups. The analgesic method presented was found to be an effective treatment against lower back pain during the first stage of labor.[110]

BIOFEEDBACK

Biofeedback is a noninvasive system that utilizes monitoring instruments to provide visual or auditory feedback to patients based on physiologic responses of which they are usually unaware, for example, pulse or respiratory rate, allowing the patient to gain a sense of self-reliance in their ability to alter these parameters. In a study of 55 first-time mothers randomly assigned to either childbirth classes or childbirth classes plus biofeedback training, women who used biofeedback during labor reported significantly lower pain than women in the control group. Seventy percent of women in the control group requested epidural anesthesia, versus only 40% in the biofeedback group.[111]

ACUPUNCTURE

Although the mechanisms of action remain unknown, findings from three randomized controlled trials (Western-based) have concluded that acupuncture during labor can reduce the use of pain medication in labor.[112,113] Numerous trials have been done in China with similar conclusions; however, the quality of these trials has not always met standards for inclusion in meta-analyses. According to the results of a systematic review by Lee and Ernst, three RCTs were identified, and their methodological quality was generally good.[114] Two RCTs compared adjunctive acupuncture with usual care only and reported a reduction of meperidine and/or epidural analgesia. One acupuncture placebo-controlled trial showed a statistically significant difference in both subjective and objective outcome measures of pain. No adverse events were reported in any of the trials. The LI4 and SP6 points have demonstrated particular benefit for labor-associated pain.[115,116] The reviews concluded that the evidence for acupuncture as an adjunct to conventional pain control during labor is promising; however, they commented on the paucity of research upon which to assert definitive conclusions.[114] Whether acupuncture in combination with other forms of nonpharmacologic support (e.g., continuous labor support, massage, and positional changes) would be more effective than acupuncture used alone has not been evaluated.

HYPNOSIS

A 2012 Cochrane review examined the evidence for hypnosis in labor pain management settings. Seven RCTs met the inclusion criteria, involving 1213 women. The reviewers noted that all but one trial had a moderate to high risk of bias. Six of the trials tested antenatal hypnosis, and one tested hypnosis during labor. No differences were seen in the experimental versus control groups regarding use of pharmacologic pain relief, spontaneous vaginal birth, satisfaction with pain relief, satisfaction with the childbirth experience, admissions to the neonatal intensive care unit, or breastfeeding at discharge from hospital. The reviewers found some evidence of benefit on measures of pain intensity, length of labor, and maternal hospital stay.[117]

Two studies on the effects of hypnosis on pain in labor were identified. In one study, 82 first-time low-risk mothers were randomized to attend routine weekly prenatal classes plus individual hypnosis sessions focusing on relaxation and pain relief, or prenatal classes alone. Based on a linear analog scale, no significant difference in subjective reporting of pain relief was reported between the groups and there was no difference in rate of pharmacologic pain medication used in labor.[107] In a 1975 study, 60 primiparous women were randomly assigned to either hypnosis induction classes or relaxation and breathing exercise during childbirth classes. Ischemic pain thresholds were measured before labor and during labor with a standardized pain questionnaire. Women in the hypnosis group received less pain medication in labor than the control group.[111] Hypnotherapy is not widely used by midwives unless women have specific deep-seated fears about labor or past experiences that block effective preparation.

YOGA

Yoga and movement therapy may ease the discomforts associated with labor. A 2008 trial ($n = 74$) tested the efficacy of a yoga program during pregnancy for maternal comfort, labor pain, and birth outcomes. Participants enrolled in six 1-hour yoga sessions at specific gestational intervals. The yoga therapy was associated with higher maternal comfort during labor (as well as comfort at 2 hours postpartum) and shorter labor time. There were no differences seen in pethidine use, labor augmentation, or infant Apgar scores at minutes 1 and 5 between the experimental and control groups. The type of yoga therapy was not disclosed, nor were the methods by which the outcomes were measured, limiting the interpretation of the results.[118] Other types of movement therapy may be helpful. A recent RCT tested a dance-based movement therapy on labor pain scores ($n = 60$ primiparous women). Pain outcomes were assessed with VAS, and results were analyzed using the T-test and Chi-square. Using VAS, the mean pain scores were decreased in women using dance labor ($p < .05$) compared with standard care controls.[119]

The Postpartum

POSTPARTUM CARE OF THE MOTHER

On Crete, right after a baby is born, it is given chamomile tea. The mother's breasts and nipples are washed with chamomile tea before she nurses. When visitors come to the hospital to see the new baby, the first question they ask is "has she/he drunk the chamomile yet?" The tea is considered the perfect thing for both mother and child after the excitement of labor. Once the baby has had its first chamomile, it is a huge relief to everyone because it is a sign that they are healthy and now part of the clan. In the hospital near the village I live in part of the year, there is a special room for brewing chamomile for the new mothers and babies.[1]

Patricia Kyritsi Howell, Herbalist

WHAT IS THE POSTPARTUM?

The postpartum (i.e., *puerperium*) is defined as the 6-week period of time beginning immediately after birth, during which the reproductive organs and maternal physiology return toward the prepregnant state. Catabolic processes cause the uterus to rapidly return from a weight of approximately 1000 g at the time of birth to approximately 50 g by the third postpartum week through a process called *involution*. Although the vagina does not return entirely to its prepregnancy state, vaginal and pelvic tissue normally regains most of its prepregnant tone. The cardiovascular system likewise returns to its prepregnant level of vascular resistance and volume. Because of all of these changes in tissue size and fluid levels, women in the immediate week after birth experience marked diaphoresis and diuresis, accompanied by dramatic weight loss. In addition to these changes, women normally experience vaginal bleeding; the lochia, which begins as a menstrual-like discharge in the hours after birth, tapers to a pale, thin, or mucuslike fluid by 3 weeks after birth. Many women normally experience some lochial flow for up to 6 weeks or so postpartum. During the puerperium, women who choose to breastfeed also experience the physical changes (e.g., breast changes) that accompany lactation, whereas those who do not experience gradual drying of their milk supply with diminished breast engorgement over the first few postpartum days. Most women experience disturbance of sleep rhythm and regularity as a result of tending to their newborn, and emotional fluctuations as a result of hormonal and psychoemotional adjustments (see Postpartum Depression).

REDEFINING POSTPARTUM IN A WOMAN-CENTERED WAY

Many consider 6 weeks to be an arbitrary and terribly limited definition of time allocated for the postpartum, recognizing that it takes much longer than 6 weeks to fully physically and emotionally recover from the demands placed on a woman by pregnancy and birth, and much longer than this to adjust to the demands of motherhood. The postpartum is a time of enormous physical, emotional, psychological, and social change, whether associated with the birth of a first child or subsequent children. The adjustments are potentially much more difficult if there have been complications or loss associated with the birth. Each passage through birth and into motherhood is a journey into the unknown, with new hopes, fears, expectations, and demands. Although newborns are doted upon with kisses, praise, and gifts, most women receive little special attention and nurturing during this time, leaving many new mothers stressed, exhausted, or overwhelmed. The fact that women are no longer considered obstetric patients after 6 weeks also reflects the belief that women are expected to be physically recovered enough to resume their previous responsibilities. Defining the postpartum as a finite period of 6 weeks leads many new mothers to feel as if they are taking too long to "get it together," or that they are overwhelmed by something that just should not be such a big deal.

Societal expectations also revolve around this arbitrarily allotted 6-week period. Many employers expect women to be back to work after 6 weeks; obstetricians' and midwives care packages end at 6 weeks; and even husbands, other relatives, and friends expect mom to be able to cope on her own by then. Yet most women, when given the opportunity to express their feelings about their postpartum experience, say that they needed more help, support, care, guidance, and understanding than they received, and for much longer than 6 weeks after birth (Box 21-1). Most mothers say that they do not really begin to feel like their old selves for at least 6 to 8 months after birth, and many never feel quite like their old selves again. Most admit that they had feelings of profound joy as well as stress, anxiety, and confusion during those early days, weeks, and months of becoming a mother.

Postpartum women experience a significant rate of physical health problems; however, little attention has been given

---

BOX 21-1   **Basic Needs of the New Mother**

- Time to focus on the newborn and older children
- A good, confidential, listener
- To feel protected, honored, and nurtured
- Reassurance that they are doing a good job
- Noncritical support and advice
- Praise and encouragement
- To have complaints and concerns taken seriously by family and care providers
- Time-out now and then for a bath, a shower, or a quiet moment
- Ample, healthy food
- Adequate rest
- Respect for their emotions

---

to research in this area beyond recent research into postpartum depression (PPD).[1,2] Substantial postpartum morbidity is known to exist and this is not routinely assessed as the postnatal assessment.[3] In a study of 11,701 postpartum women, nearly half had health problems within 3 months after the birth that continued for more than 6 weeks, and that they had never experienced before. The symptoms of ill health that they confronted sometimes lasted for months or years afterward, and many of them never told their doctors about their problems.[2] In general, the cursory nature of postnatal care does not facilitate the intimacy required for women to express the nature of their physical complaints, and thus most obstetricians have not recognized the extent to which postpartum women experience health complaints. Interestingly, recent studies have questioned the effectiveness of postpartum medical visits in meeting the postpartum health needs of mothers, and have concluded that "the present 6-week postnatal examination does not appear to meet the health needs of women after childbirth: its content and timing should be reviewed."[3]

Postpartum visits should focus on the challenges women face during this time, and should provide women with the opportunity to express their concerns and expectations, both physically and emotionally. In *Reactions to Motherhood: The Role of Post-Natal Care*, midwife Jean A. Ball states:

> *The main focus of postnatal care has traditionally been that of ensuring the physical recovery of the mother from the effects of pregnancy and labor and establishing infant feeding patterns ... The emotional and psychological needs of mothers have not received much attention until recently and there has been an assumption that these needs will automatically be met if the first two aspects of care are satisfied. The organization of postnatal care has accordingly been based upon this premise.[4]*

According to a study by Buchart et al, "Listening to women is an essential element in the provision of flexible and responsive postnatal care that meets the felt needs of women and their families."[5] By developing an open dialogue with women during pregnancy, care providers can help women to realistically prepare for the postpartum before birth, and overcome

difficulties that might be inhibiting their recovery as well as their experience of motherhood. This chapter highlights the need for extensive family and social support for the mother after birth in the prevention of this potentially devastating problem. It must be recognized, however, that the need for such support is not limited to the prevention of PPD, but for the promotion of the overall wellness of the new mother, and by extension, her child and family. Indeed, many postpartum difficulties can be averted with adequate postpartum support of the mother, both from her immediate personal community (e.g., family, friends, co-workers) and from her health care providers.

Increasingly, the postpartum doula is becoming an important figure in the postpartum care of new mothers. In the United States, doula services are privately hired; however, in many European countries, postpartum visiting nurses are a common part of routine obstetric care. Beginning in the mid 1980s in the United States, postpartum mother care services, which now routinely employ certified doulas, began cropping up in major cities around the United States, providing in-home help and giving new mothers non-medical assistance and advice on such matters as breastfeeding and newborn care.

Unfortunately, the cost of such services is prohibitive to most. Optimally, doula care should be incorporated into maternal care services because postpartum support has definitely been demonstrated to reduce postpartum morbidity, especially associated with depression (see Postpartum Depression).

THE USE OF HERBS FOR POSTPARTUM CARE

The use of medicinal herbs has been an intrinsic part of postpartum care in cultures throughout the world. Herbal teas and other preparations are given for a variety of reasons, including preventing infection, treating colic, and nourishing the mother and child. Herbs have been used both internally and topically to reduce bleeding, ease pain from cramping, increase breast milk production, heal and soothe the perineal area, and relax the mother.[6-10] References to traditional herb use after birth abound in historical and sociologic references, although the ethnobotany is often not specific. For example, women in Thailand have been known to drink a mixture of tamarind, salt, and water to "strengthen the womb," whereas women of the Seri Indian tribe of Mexico drank "seep willow tea" to "stop bleeding after birth."[11] The Jicarilla women chewed the root of wild geranium to assist in "expelling uterine blood."[11] Herb use was common in Colombia and Jamaica, as it was in Southeast Asia.[12] In Burma, a paste of tumeric is rubbed onto the body to prevent blood stasis and encourage good circulation while expelling the afterbirth blood.[12] In Micronesia, women are given baths of tumeric paste after birth.[1] In both Ayurvedic and Traditional Chinese Medicine (TCM), herbs are a routine aspect of postpartum care, and have been for thousands of years.

There is little evidence on the number of women in the United States using herbs for postpartum complaints;

however, it is likely consistent with the volume of herb use during pregnancy, or slightly higher; the use of herbal teas for increasing lactation is very popular, and women and care providers are often less hesitant to use herbs outside of pregnancy. Numerous articles appearing in nursing, medical, and midwifery journals describe the use of herbs for postpartum care.[6-10] Chapters 15 and 22 discuss the safety of herb use during lactation. The remainder of this chapter presents information on treatments for common postpartum problems.

COMMON POSTPARTUM COMPLAINTS

After birth, women experience a number of common physiologic changes that can lead to discomfort (e.g., sweating, engorged breasts, after birth pains), problems resulting from pregnancy or birth (e.g., hemorrhoids), and discomforts associated with breastfeeding (e.g., engorgement, sore nipples). Hemorrhoids are discussed in Chapter 17, and problems associated with lactation in Chapter 22.

After Pains

After pains are associated with the normal process of uterine involution—the return of the uterus to its prepregnant size. Involution involves the clamping down of the uterine myometrium, a process that is accompanied by menstrual cramp–like pain that varies from mild to very severe. Many women turn to nonsteroidal antiinflammatory medications (NSAIDs) such as ibuprofen to relieve the discomfort, whereas others, preferring not to use pharmaceuticals while breastfeeding, turn to herbs. Herbs such as cramp bark (*Viburnum opulus*), black haw (*Viburnum prunifolium*), and motherwort (*Leonurus cardiaca*) are excellent choices as they are both antispasmodic and uterotonic.[13,14] This is important because uterine laxity might actually exacerbate the contractions as the uterus tries to involute. The herbs facilitate the physiologic process and provide relief of cramping and possibly, with the viburnums, mild analgesia. Simple teas such as catnip (*Nepeta cataria*) and chamomile (*Matricaria recutita*) have empirically been shown to be effective, providing an apparently synergistic effect when used together for mild cramping, and with tinctures of cramp bark, black haw, and/or motherwort added for severe discomfort.[15]

A popular treatment among independent midwives for the relief of after pains, and for supporting recovery of the pelvic organs and "qi" of the body after childbirth, is the use of the TCM practice of moxibustion (Box 21-2). This technique, previously discussed for turning a breech baby when applied to acupuncture points on the small toe, is applied to the lower back and abdominal area over the uterus to warm the mother, reduce pain, and support involution. It is repeated once or twice daily, for 30 minutes, for the first week after birth, usually starting on day 2 or 3 postpartum.

Note that abdominal pain, especially if accompanied by fever or foul-smelling vaginal discharge, can be symptomatic of endometritis, a potentially life-threatening uterine infection requiring immediate antibiotics.

POSTPARTUM DEPRESSION

Postpartum depression is a crippling mood disorder, historically neglected in health care, leaving mothers to suffer in fear, confusion, and silence. Undiagnosed it can adversely affect the mother–infant relationship and lead to long-term emotional problems for the child. I have described it as 'a thief that steals motherhood.'[16]

Cheryl Tatano Beck

PPD is a potentially devastating mood disorder thought to affect approximately 15% but as many as 28% of new mothers, with an estimated 400,000 women suffering from this condition annually. Twenty-five percent of these women are likely to develop PPD in the first 3 months postpartum and 25% of these women are at increased risk of developing severe, chronic depression.[1] PPD generally has a slow and insidious onset, beginning at 2 to 3 weeks postpartum; however, it can occur anytime in the first year postpartum, and may last up to a year or longer. Symptoms of PPD include irritability, depression, guilt, hopelessness, chronic exhaustion, despair, feelings of inadequacy, insomnia, agitation, loss of normal interests, joylessness, difficulty relaxing or concentrating, memory loss, confusion, inability to function, emotional numbness, inability to cope, irrational concern with baby's well-being, and thoughts of hurting oneself or baby (Box 21-3). Women with postpartum depression may become obsessed by the terrifying feeling that their depression and anxiety are interminable. They may feel extremely detached from their family, including husband, baby, and other children. They may be plagued by fear of hurting the baby, causing them panic and anxiety, leading them to distance themselves from the baby, and exacerbating feelings of inadequacy as a mother; thus it has been described as "a thief that steals motherhood."[16,17]

Despite multiple visits to care providers in the postpartum period, postpartum depression often goes unrecognized by the obstetrician or midwife, with symptoms of depression commonly dismissed as "just the baby blues," leaving women in need of treatment and care with none, and prolonging the terrible desperation they feel without an explanation.[16,18-20] Undiagnosed PPD can adversely affect the mother–infant relationship and lead to long-term emotional consequences for both.[16] For most women, a diagnosis of PPD comes as a welcome relief—putting their experience into the context of an explainable illness for which there is treatment. It can provide a framework that helps them, as well as their family, begin to make sense of what is happening. It is essential that care providers learn to recognize the many symptoms and manifestations of PPD to ensure that it is recognized and that women receive adequate support and treatment.[21]

ETIOLOGY AND RISK FACTORS FOR PPD

Despite its prevalence, the etiology of PPD remains unknown.[22] Smokers are at increased risk for PPD.[23] In a survey of 574 women in Ontario, of whom 9.9% were diagnosed with PPD, there was a higher rate of PPD among women with

BOX 21-2   Moxibustion for Essential Postpartum Care

In Traditional Chinese Medicine (TCM), heat is a significant part of healing for the woman who has recently given birth. One of the three major factors considered important for the health of postpartum women is "sparing the exterior," which means protecting against wind and avoiding cold drafts. Childbirth is thought to deplete what is called the *wei chi*. The wei chi is the body's protective immune capacity, specifically found on the surface of the body and in the lungs. Special herbs are given to protect the woman and nourish the wei chi, and the woman is expected to remain indoors for 1 month after birth.

There is an area of the body known as the *Ming Men*. This literally translates as Life Gate, or Life Gate Fire, and correlates to the TCM concept of the kidneys, which are said to govern the functions of reproduction, sexuality, growth, and decline. It also controls the relaxation of the pelvis, which allows the baby to be born. Rest and heat are the two cardinal factors that facilitate proper closure of the Life Gate. Incomplete recovery is believed to lead to later chronic health problems and general weakness, which may become worse with each successive birth. Heat treatments, in the form of moxibustion, may be added to the postpartum care routine to ensure optimal recovery.

Moxa is Chinese mugwort *(Folium Artemisia* spp.*)*, traditionally used internally for the treatment of gynecologic problems. For external use, it comes in the form of a rolled stick, much like a cigar, but completely covered by a fine linen paper. The end of this stick, when lit and held close to the skin, sends a deep, penetrating warmth into area. The technique of moxibustion was featured in an article in the *Journal of the American Medical Association* (November 11, 1998), in which researchers concluded that the technique is reliable for turning babies from the breech to the head down position. No research has yet been published on its use for postpartum care, but midwives who incorporate this technique into their clinical practices, and mothers who have received this technique, can attest to its value.

To Give a Moxibustion Treatment

1. Have the mother lie in a comfortable position on her side or belly. Use pillows to support her if her breasts are sore or enlarged from breast feeding. Make sure the room is warm.
2. Provide some ventilation, but do not allow the mother to receive a chill or draft. A window may be slightly open on the opposite side of the room, or use "little smoke" moxa in cold weather. It is more difficult to light but does not emit as much smoke.
3. Peel the outer paper wrapper off the moxa stick. Light the moxa stick with the inner paper left on it. Blow on the end until it is a burning ember. Roll off any excess ash in an ashtray or dish until the tip of the moxa becomes slightly cone shaped.
4. The area on the body you want to treat extends over the sacrum on the back, and the area from just above the pubic bone on the front to about an inch below the navel to 3 inches on either side of the midline of the lower abdomen.
5. Holding the moxa stick 1 to 2 inches over the correct area, begin to move the stick in tiny circles about 2 inches in diameter, until the area becomes warm and slightly pink. Then move to an adjacent spot until the whole area has been treated. Do not touch the mother with the moxa, and periodically knock ashes off into your ashtray or dish to prevent them from falling on her. Do not treat to the point of burning or stinging pain, and instruct the mother to tell you if any area is becoming too hot.
6. Continue treating the back for 15 minutes, then "massage the heat inward" for several minutes before proceeding to treat the abdomen.
7. A woman may give herself a moxa treatment on the abdomen if no one is available to do the treatment on her back.
8. To extinguish the moxa, place it upside down into a small dish of sand, run the tip until water until not lit, or use a specially made moxa extinguisher. Use fire safety precautions when treating with moxa.
9. Begin treatments the first day after birth, and continue daily for 1 to 2 weeks.

---

a prior history of depression, among women whose pregnancy was unplanned, among those who described the course of pregnancy as "difficult," and among women who described their general health as "not good."[24] Women with a history of premenstrual dysphoric disorder (PMDD) may also be at increased risk.[25] Breastfeeding mothers may be significantly less likely to develop PPD than nonbreastfeeding mothers, and breastfeeding may have unknown protective biological factors against PPD.[23,26,27] A recent revision of the predictive factors for PPD lists prenatal depression, child care stress, life stress, lack of social/marital support, prenatal anxiety, low marital satisfaction/poor relationship, history of depression, a difficult infant temperament, maternity blues, low self-esteem, low socioeconomic status, single motherhood, and unplanned/unwanted pregnancy as the most important risk factors for PPD.[28-33]

Many hormones have been investigated for their possible causative roles, and PPD is commonly attributed to the rapid change in hormones in the postpartum period; however, the role of hormones in PPD remains inconclusive.[22,34] PPD has also been attributed to thyroid insufficiency (i.e., hypothyroidism), which is commonly found in the 2 to 5 months after birth. Recent research suggests that the abrupt physiologic drop in insulin levels that occurs during the postpartum period after the slow rise throughout pregnancy may induce mood disorders by affecting serotonin secretion in the brain. Low blood sugar can also have a dramatic effect on mood; therefore postpartum women must ensure adequate caloric intake through a well-balanced diet to minimize the risk of depression resulting from hypoglycemia. It has been suggested that a carbohydrate-rich diet in the postpartum period may be a preventative or adjunctive treatment of postpartum mood disorders.[22] Inadequate intake of essential fatty acids, protein, B vitamins, zinc, and iron also have been associated with PPD. Women who have experienced significant blood loss at birth may be predisposed to depression

BOX 21-3 Symptoms of Postpartum Depression

Agitation
Anxiety or panic attacks
Chronic exhaustion
Clumsiness
Confusion
Decreased appetite or extreme cravings
Depression
Despair
Difficulty relaxing or concentrating
Emotional numbness
Fear
Feelings of inadequacy
Frequent crying or inability to cry
Guilt
Hopelessness
Inability to cope
Inability to function
Insomnia
Irrational overconcern with baby's well-being
Irritability
Joylessness
Lack of attention to appearance
Loneliness
Loss of normal interests
Memory loss
Mood swings
Nightmares
Thoughts of hurting oneself or baby
Withdrawal from social contacts

caused by anemia and its accompanying increased fatigue and tendency to infection. Fatigue also appears to be highly correlated with PPD, especially persistent fatigue occurring by day 14 postpartum.[35]

Lack of social and emotional support during pregnancy, labor, birth, and in the postpartum period have all been associated with an increased risk of developing PPD. One PPD study found that poor support with newborn care showed a positive correlation with PPD, whereas affiliation with a secular group was a positive preventative factor.[36] A study looking at the effect of a supportive partner in the treatment of PPD found a significant decrease in depressive symptoms in the group where the partner provided the mother with significant support, whereas another discovered that women with PPD "reported less practical and emotional support from their partners and saw themselves as having less social support overall."[37] Clearly, adequate social support is an important variable in preventing PPD. Even a therapist can lead to significant improvement in PPD. In one study, interpersonal psychotherapy was demonstrated to reduce depressive symptoms, improve adjustment, and was shown to be an alternative to drug therapy, especially for breastfeeding mothers.[38] It is important for women who are experiencing extreme or prolonged symptoms to seek help.

A study conducted in Switzerland found that among the most significant risk factors for PPD are social or professional difficulties, deleterious life events, early mother–child separation, and negative birth experience.[39] Birth experience may have a dramatic effect on a woman's self-perception as she enters motherhood, yet is generally overlooked. Assisted delivery (e.g., cesarean, forceps, and vacuum extraction) may be associated with higher rates of postnatal depression, as are bottle-feeding, dissatisfaction with prenatal care, having unwanted people present at the birth, and lacking confidence to care for the baby after leaving the hospital.[40,41] A study by Edwards et al indicated that there is an increase in rates of PPD among women who have had cesarean sections, a finding that women themselves report.[42,43] Although this finding has been debated, clinical experience suggests that disappointment in the birth experience affects a new mother's self-confidence. Considering that 25% to 40% of American women now deliver by cesarean section, this certainly illuminates the need to both reduce cesarean rates and provide counseling and support for those women who have birthed operatively. Furthermore, one study indicates that women who were cared for by midwives had lower rates of depression in the postnatal period; another study revealed a significantly lower rate of depression among women who had given birth at home compared with hospital vaginal delivery. Women reported that a sense of control and being informed about choices in their health care greatly improved their psychological state.[44]

Few women experience all of the symptoms of PPD; some may exhibit only a few, some many. It is the duration, severity, and complexity of the symptoms that distinguishes PPD from the common and normally occurring "baby blues," which occurs in 50% to 70% of new mothers. Baby blues is thought to be a result of normal postnatal hormonal and other physiologic adjustments, and is self-limiting, usually beginning at about day 3 or 4 postpartum and lasting only up to about 14 days.[45] Symptoms include crying, irritability, fatigue, anxiety, and emotional lability.[16] Further, the baby blues tends to be punctuated by periods of elation, whereas PPD lacks the elation and the periods of depression are more intense and prolonged. Women with baby blues require support and reassurance but no treatment is necessary, although attention to nutrition, sleep, and support are essential. If symptoms persist past 2 weeks, depression should be ruled out.

Postpartum psychosis is an extreme postpartum mood disorder, occurring in 1 to 2 per 1000 new mothers, usually having its onset a few weeks after birth, but up to 3 months after, occurring most often in primiparas, and being more likely to require hospitalization for treatment. Other mood disorders than can occur in the postpartum period include panic attacks, postpartum obsessive-compulsive disorder, postpartum traumatic stress disorder, and postpartum bipolar disorder.[16]

Any woman experiencing extreme depression, suicidal thoughts, or thoughts of harming her baby requires immediate professional help through her physician, an emergency hotline, or the local emergency room. Early identification and treatment of PPD can decrease the duration and consequences of the condition for a woman and her family.

PREVENTION OF POSTPARTUM DEPRESSION

Many care providers are afraid to talk to women prenatally about PPD, thinking it might frighten them. In fact, a woman will be better prepared to recognize the need for help and get it if she is informed that this could happen ahead of time. According to Jane Honikman, founder of Postpartum Support International, "Ignorance and denial are the two greatest barriers to this problem."[1] Many women enter pregnancy and become mothers with an unrealistic and romanticized picture of motherhood. There are also tremendous social pressures on women to conform to the image of being happy and grateful. Yet new motherhood can also bring fatigue, feelings of being overwhelmed and inadequate, a sense of social isolation for women who have abandoned previous social or work activities to be home with the baby, and body image issues as a result of changes that occurred during pregnancy and accompanying lactation. Social pressures on mothers strongly contribute to many mothers' sense of inadequacy—leaving them feeling that "everyone else does it better than I do, and is happy, why can't I?" Single mothers face additional burdens, concerns, and fears unique to the task of raising a baby alone.

Talking about PPD before birth can actually have a positive effect on reducing depression because it can help a mother develop realistic goals and expectations for herself for after the birth, and recognize the need to establish a support network for herself if she is not part of an actively supportive family or community. The need for family and community support, especially for women at risk for PPD, but for all new mothers, cannot be overestimated, and should be planned before the birth. The new mother's ability to get adequate rest, proper and ample nourishment, social interaction, time for self-care, support with breastfeeding, and access to a woman skilled in newborn care and the needs of the new mother (e.g., a doula) who can answer questions and reassure her should be established before birth. For women with a history of PMDD, depression, or previous episodes of PPD after prior births, special care should be taken to assure support and even postpartum psychological or psychiatric care; preventative measures should be taken during pregnancy to optimize nutrition, as this may help to allay symptoms (see Nutritional Considerations).

CONVENTIONAL TREATMENT APPROACHES

If a woman develops depression during pregnancy or is at risk for this problem, the most important thing she can be encouraged to do is to seek support. She needs to stay connected with other women who understand what she is going through. She can do this by participating in counseling and support groups. Support groups during pregnancy can help reduce both depression and anxiety. Cognitive behavioral therapy and even just talking about depression with friends can decrease a woman's shame around that diagnosis. Decreasing that shame can allow light through the gaps in the darkness for her. Discovering that other women are also experiencing similar symptoms decreases the woman's sense of loneliness and isolation and sometimes can have an uplifting effect on her mood.

Family and group therapy can be important if there are relationship stressors or domestic problems. This kind of therapy can help the woman and her partner and/or family to cope better with pregnancy challenges, which can ease the burden of depression for the woman.

Avoiding changes in medication during pregnancy, if possible, is optimal. For example, a woman may enter pregnancy while taking an antidepressant. During her first trimester, she may then either stop taking the medication abruptly because of safety concerns for her baby, or she may need to change her antidepressant because of safety issues that can affect her. As a result, she may tend to have more significant depression during her pregnancy than a woman who just takes a stable dose of an antidepressant throughout the pregnancy. Even if a woman stops taking the medication for the first trimester and then returns to her prior dose afterward, she is less likely to have optimized mental health than if she had continued taking a stable dose of her original medication.

The biggest problem with treatment for PPD is the uncertainty about causative factors. There is no consensus on the use of hormonal therapy in the treatment of PPD.[34] The safety of maternal use of psychotropic medications while breastfeeding is controversial. In 2001, expert consensus guidelines for the treatment of depression in women were published. The expert panel concluded that few studies published evaluate pharmacologic or nonpharmacologic treatments for PPD. Antidepressant medications and psychosocial interventions were recommended as first-line treatments regardless of the mother's breastfeeding status, with the exception of treatment of minor depression, for which the use of antidepressants was considered warranted only if the woman was not breastfeeding. A 2001 comprehensive review by Burt and colleagues that looked at the use of psychotropic medication in breastfeeding women since 1955 found no controlled studies evaluating safety.[46] In contrast, Hale suggests that many of these drugs are well-studied and safe, although demonstrates that most do enter breast milk in varying quantities and may cause side effects in the infant, including sedation, somnolence, respiratory arrest, colic, jitteriness, and withdrawal.[47]

There is emerging data suggesting risk of antidepressants to the infants of nursing mothers using selective serotonin reuptake inhibitors (SSRIs); therefore it is essential that a careful plan of treatment be considered for mothers committed to breastfeeding. Chambers et al identified an association between maternal SSRI use in late pregnancy and persistent pulmonary hypertension (PPH) in the newborn. The authors stated, "Although our study cannot establish causality, several possible mechanisms suggest a casual association is possible."[48] Another physician writes:

> Any drug that affects infant growth, in or ex utero, should be regarded with suspicion and should not be written up as a recommendable solution for postpartum depression, comparable with innocuous and effective methods such as psychotherapy, nurse home visits, and group therapy. The

available evidence indicates that even when infant serum levels are low or undetectable, side effects may occur. There is an ample body of evidence that SSRIs taken during pregnancy cause neonates to suffer withdrawal symptoms, which all by itself is a matter for concern. Postpartum depression is an issue that should not be taken lightly, but, as history shows, the short-term benefits of drugs that have not been sufficiently studied do not weigh up against the tragic long-term disasters they might provoke.[49]

Unfortunately, because untreated PPD can have significant and long-term consequences for mother, child, and family, a careful risk–benefit comparison must be done for use of medication versus nonpharmacologic treatment. In cases of severe PPD, medication may be unavoidable.

Nonpharmacologic treatments for PPD can be effective primary treatments depending on the severity of symptoms and the woman's ability to comply, and can be used in conjunction with pharmacotherapy. Nonpharmacologic treatments include psychosocial supports, psychotherapy (individual and/or couple), group therapy, and medications. Attention to nutrition, fluid, sleep, and social support status are essential.[34] Many women turn to alternative therapies for PPD, concerned about the risk of pharmacotherapy while nursing. Alternative therapies can constitute part of effective adjunct treatment for PPD.[50] Therapies to consider include nutritional and herbal supplements, aromatherapy, acupuncture, and both maternal and infant massage. These are discussed under Nutritional Considerations and Additional Therapies.

THE BOTANICAL PRACTITIONER'S PERSPECTIVE

PPD is complex to treat because of multifactorial causes, so addressing the big picture and the details is important. Optimal nutrition and blood-sugar balance are cornerstones of a healthy mood. Blood-sugar fluctuations, particularly hypoglycemia, can exacerbate depression. In addition, when a person's blood sugar fluctuates, that person develops inflammatory processes, which, through inflammatory mediators, can exacerbate depression. New mothers should be encouraged to "graze" by eating something healthy with good-quality protein and fat every 2 to 3 hours.

Adequate rest is incredibly important, but easy to overlook. Lack of sleep can cause depression and decrease the ability to cope, and may also increase inflammatory processes, causing a burden on the adrenal system and the hypothalamic-pituitary-adrenal (HPA) axis, which adds further to depression.

Another important action that clinicians need to tell women about is to get ample and regular exercise during pregnancy. We know that physical activity on a regular basis decreases depression. An interesting study, from researchers at the University of Michigan, found that pregnant women who participated in a 10-week program combining mindfulness with specific yoga āsanās had significantly reduced depressive symptoms. Exercise and movement can make a difference in a woman's mood.[51]

Although herbs can be tremendously beneficial, effective treatment depends on a holistic approach that includes the most appropriate choice of herbs in conjunction with nutritional, social, and psychological interventions. The effect of PPD on the mother, infant, and family should not be minimized, and medical interventions should be sought in severe cases, and even in milder cases if botanical therapies are not effective. It is difficult to know how much time to allot to determine whether herbs are bringing adequate improvement because they can take several weeks to make a noticeable effect. However, this is also the case with psychotropic drugs. It is essential that the practitioner remain in regular contact with the patient, and continually evaluate her status and progress to ascertain whether treatment is effective or it is necessary to use other interventions.

Herbal remedies are the primary pharmacologic therapy for the treatment of depression in many European countries, and are increasingly being recognized in the United States as safe and effective alternatives to many psychotherapeutic medications for mild to moderate depression and anxiety (Table 21-1). Herbs such as St. John's wort, kava kava, lavender, lemon balm, passionflower, and valerian have been used in the treatment of a number of mood disorders including depression, anxiety, restlessness, insomnia, and irritability.[52,53] Herbs, such as many adaptogens, can also be used to treat fatigue, nervous exhaustion, hormonal dysregulation, and blood sugar dysregulation. Unfortunately, almost no studies have been conducted on the safety and efficacy of herbs for the treatment of PPD, or the safe use of herbs during lactation.

The application of herbs for the treatment of PPD is largely extrapolated from traditional herbal treatments for general depression. The use of adaptogens in this context is predicated on their marked ability to improve the stress response, and via the HPA axis, to regulate cortisol and blood sugar levels, an important adaptation during times of increased and prolonged stress, as new motherhood is for many, and especially so for those at risk of PPD. Safety is an important concern when herbs are to be applied prophylactically during pregnancy for women with a history of PPD, and during lactation, especially for a prolonged period as is often necessary with PPD. Table 21-2 ranks these herbs according to the scale developed by Hale (Table 21-3) for the evaluation of drugs for the treatment of PPD during lactation; I modified this for relevance to herbal medicine. When there is a history of previous PPD, it is best to focus on preventive nutritional strategies during pregnancy, as well as ensuring that proper social supports are in place, and reserving the use of herbs to the postpartum period for optimal safety to the fetus. Nutritional and social/psychological strategies can be continued postnatally, and herbal interventions begun immediately after birth with a history of PPD, or even prophylactically for a woman with significant risk factors for developing PPD. In women with no history or risk factors, or who present at their first appointment with symptoms, herbs can be started as needed.

Adaptogens

The role of adaptogens in improving stress resistance and response is extensively discussed in Chapter 5. No studies

TABLE 21-1	Botanical Treatment Strategies for Postpartum Depression		
Therapeutic Goal	**Therapeutic Activity**	**Botanical Name**	**Common Name**
Improve the stress response	Adaptogen See Table 5-4		
Support and nourish the nervous system	Nervine tonic	*Withania somnifera*	Ashwagandha
		Panax quinquefolius	American ginseng
		Verbena officinalis	Blue vervain
		Eleutherococcus senticosus	Eleuthero
		Panax ginseng	Ginseng
		Avena sativa	Milky oats
		Hypericum perforatum	St. John's wort
Improve general relaxation and relieve stress	Nervine relaxant	*Verbena officinalis*	Blue vervain
		Matricaria recutita	Chamomile
		Lavandula officinalis	Lavender
		Melissa officinalis	Lemon balm
		Tilia spp.	Linden
		Avena sativa	Milky oats
		Leonurus cardiaca	Motherwort
		Passiflora incarnata	Passionflower
		Scutellaria lateriflora	Skullcap
Reduce anxiety	Anxiolytic	*Matricaria recutita*	Chamomile
		Piper methysticum	Kava kava
		Leonurus cardiaca	Motherwort
		Passiflora incarnata	Passionflower
		Hypericum perforatum	St. John's wort
		Valeriana officinalis	Valerian
		Ziziphus spinosa	Ziziphus
Alleviate depression	Antidepressant	*Eleutherococcus senticosus*	Eleuthero
		Panax ginseng	Ginseng
		Piper methysticum	Kava kava
		Rosmarinus officinalis	Rosemary
		Hypericum perforatum	St. John's wort
Promote sleep, relieve insomnia	Sedative	*Withania somnifera*	Ashwagandha
		Eschscholzia californica	California poppy
		Matricaria recutita	Chamomile
		Lavandula officinalis	Lavender
		Melissa officinalis	Lemon balm
		Passiflora incarnata	Passionflower
		Scutellaria lateriflora	Skullcap
		Valeriana officinalis	Valerian
Support steady hormonal states	Hormonal regulator	*Angelica sinensis*	Dong quai
		Paeonia lactiflora	Peony
		Vitex agnus-castus	Chaste berry
Build energy and stamina	Blood tonic	*Angelica sinensis*	Dong quai
		Polygonum multiflorum	Fo Ti
		Panax ginseng	Ginseng
		Urtica dioica	Nettle
		Peony lactiflora	Peony
		Rehmannia glutinosa	Rehmannia
		Schisandra chinensis	Schisandra

have been conducted on the use of these herbs for PPD; however, they are widely used by herbalists for the treatment of general depression and no adverse effects are expected from their use during lactation. Use during pregnancy is generally not recommended. Women at high risk for developing PPD can begin the use of adaptogens in the days or weeks after birth to improve the ability to handle stress, withstand sleep deprivation, and also to improve

nonspecific resistance. Ashwagandha may have anxiolytic activity.[54] Schisandra is used to calm the spirit, for insomnia, palpitations, and poor memory. Contradictory information exists on its safety in pregnancy. It is generally contraindicated in pregnancy owing to its potential for increasing uterine contractions. However, no adverse effects on the fetus have been observed with maternal use, and in fact, some studies have demonstrated increased fetal

TABLE 21-2   Safety of Herbs for Postpartum Depression During Pregnancy and Lactation

Herb	Risk Category During Lactation*	Risk During Pregnancy†
American ginseng (*Panax quinquefolius*)	See Ginseng	
Ashwagandha (*Withania somnifera*)	L1	B1
Blue vervain (*Verbena officinalis*)	No data	Unknown
California poppy (*Eschscholzia californica*)	L2/L3	B2
Chamomile (*Matricaria recutita*)	L1/L2	A
Chaste berry (*Vitex agnus-castus*)	L2	B1
Dong quai (*Angelica sinensis*)	L2/L3	C
Eleuthero (*Eleutherococcus senticosus*)	See Ginseng	
Ginseng (*Panax ginseng*)	L1/L2	A
Kava kava (*Piper methysticum*)	L3-L5	B1
Lavender (*Lavandula officinalis*)	L1/L2	B2
Lemon balm (*Melissa officinalis*)	L1/L2	B2
Milky oats (*Avena sativa*)	L1/L2	B1
Motherwort (*Leonurus cardiaca*)	L1/L2	B3
Nettle (*Urtica dioica*)	L1/L2	B2
Passionflower (*Passiflora incarnata*)	L1/L2	B1
Peony (*Paeonia lactiflora*)	L2/L3	B1
Rosemary (*Rosmarinus officinalis*)	L2	B1
Schisandra (*Schisandra chinensis*)	No data	B1
Skullcap (*Scutellaria lateriflora*)	L1/L2	B2
St. John's wort (*Hypericum perforatum*)	L2/L3	B1

*See Table 21-3 for ranking scheme.
†See Chapter 15 for Mills and Bone/ Australian Therapeutic Goods Association (TGA) classification scheme for herb safety during pregnancy.
Data from Blumenthal M: *The complete German Commission E monographs: therapeutic guide to herbal medicines*, Austin, 1998, American Botanical Council; Mills E, Duguoa J, Perri D, et al: *Herbal medicines in pregnancy and lactation: an evidence-based approach*, Boca Raton, 2006, Taylor and Francis; Mills S, Bone K: *The essential guide to herbal safety*, St. Louis, 2005, Churchill Livingstone; Basch E, Ulbricht C: *Natural standard herb and supplement reference: evidence-based clinical reviews*, St. Louis, 2005, Mosby.

TABLE 21-3   Lactation Risk Categories

Risk Category		Description
L1	Safest	No adverse effects observed in infants of lactating mothers. Controlled studies demonstrate no increased risk
L2	Safer	Limited studies demonstrate no increased risk. Known constituent profile suggests no increased risk. Extensive historical/traditional use profile suggests no evidence of risk
L3	Moderately safe	No controlled studies in breastfeeding women or controlled studies demonstrate minimal adverse effects
L4	Possible risk	Positive evidence of risk, but benefits may make risk acceptable
L5	Contraindicated	Significant documented risk. Significant potential for risk based on known constituent profile

Adapted from Hale T: *Medications and mother's milk: a manual of lactation pharmacology*, ed 10, Amarillo, 2002, Pharmasoft Publishing.

weight and improved birth outcome with use of adaptogens see Chapter 5. Although these herbs are considered compatible with lactation, it is best to avoid their use during pregnancy owing to inconclusive evidence of safety.[55]

Nervine Relaxants, Sedatives, Tonics, and Anxiolytics

St. John's wort (SJW) is the most thoroughly studied herb for the treatment of depression. It is the primary medication used for depression in several European countries and it has become a popular alternative to pharmaceutical antidepressant medications in the United States. A 2008 Cochrane review evaluated the evidence base for SJW in the treatment of depression. The reviewers included 29 trials (5489 patients) with 18 comparisons with placebo and 17 comparisons with standard antidepressants. After review, the following conclusions were drawn: SJW is superior to placebo in patients with major depression; SJW is as effective as antidepressants for depression; SJW has fewer side effects than standard antidepressants.[56] As of 2002, 34 controlled clinical trials of more than 3000 patients have demonstrated the efficacy of this herb for treating mild to moderate depression.[57] No studies have evaluated the herb for either efficacy or safety in the treatment of PPD.[50] The herb is not contraindicated for use during pregnancy; however, safety studies are lacking. There is one published case report in which low levels of hyperforin were detected in the breast milk of a woman consuming 300 mg/day; however, no constituents of the herb were detectable in the baby's plasma and no adverse effects were observed in either.[58] In another study, researchers tested breast milk samples of five mothers taking 300 mg of SJW three times daily and found traces of hyperforin using tandem mass spectrometry.[59] Lactation and medication expert Hale states that recent data suggest transfer to milk is minimal and that SJW appears to be safe for use during lactation.[47] Because of its potent ability to induce cytochrome P450 3A4, a major drug-metabolizing enzyme in the liver, SJW is contraindicated with the use of other drugs, including monoamine oxidase inhibitors (MAOIs) and SSRIs.[60]

Kava kava is traditionally used to promote a calm, relaxed mood and as a ceremonial and social drink by Pacific Islanders.[61] It used extensively in Europe and the United States as a treatment for anxiety and insomnia, both of which are associated with PPD.[62] The 2009 Kava Anxiety Depression Spectrum Study (KADSS) was a 3-week placebo-controlled, double-blind, crossover trial ($n = 60$) that used an aqueous standardized extract of kava to evaluate its efficacy in the treatment of anxiety and depression. Using the Hamilton Anxiety scale, as well as the Beck Anxiety Inventory and Montgomery-Asberg Depression scales, the kava extract was found to be significantly more efficacious ($p < 0.0001$) compared with controls. It was also well tolerated, with no serious adverse or hepatotoxic effects observed (Kava extract dose not noted).[63] Kava has been shown to improve general relaxation response time.[64] Studies have demonstrated kava to be a highly effective treatment for anxiety.[65] Kava has been shown to be significantly more effective than placebo in clinical trial participants with moderately severe, nonpsychotic anxiety disorder, perhaps even more effective than benzodiazepines.[66] It has been generally well tolerated at recommended doses, although individuals taking higher doses of kava may experience fatigue, unsteadiness, appearance of intoxication, and skin changes.[66] As of 2000, however, approximately 60 adverse case reports suggesting a link between kava use and liver failure have led to the governments of at least eight countries to remove kava from the general market. The German Commission E contraindicates the use of kava during pregnancy and lactation; however, no specific data on pregnancy and lactation exists. Ethnobotanical information suggests that the herb is avoided to maintain fertility and during pregnancy, but information on use during lactation is not reported.[61] Insufficient information on the use of kava during lactation makes it difficult to predict safety. The risk of hepatotoxicity from the herb versus risks of conventional drugs for anxiety treatment, including addiction and infant sedation or toxicity, must be investigated and evaluated.[61] However, until then and in light of recent concerns raised about kava and hepatotoxicity, it is prudent to avoid this herb during lactation. The herb is definitely contraindicated during pregnancy because of possible risk.

Motherwort is perhaps the classic historical herb for PPD, anxiety with palpitations, and stress. The name of the herb itself, *mother wort*—a healing herb for mothers—and its botanical name *Leonurus cardiaca*—heart of a lion—are evocative of its traditional healing uses. Today, the herb finds its way into many gynecologic formulae. It is used as a uterine tonic and antispasmodic, as a bitter to stimulate the liver, as a nervine and sedative, and in the treatment of stress, anxiety, and palpitations, including the latter in the treatment of hyperthyroidism. It is very popular for its perceived ability to modulate irritability and emotional lability. It may possess some hormonal activity, although this has not been thoroughly evaluated. Most of the evidence for this herb remains largely anecdotal.[67] It is approved by the German Commission E for nervous cardiac conditions and as an adjuvant for thyroid hyperfunction.[53] Motherwort is contraindicated in pregnancy but is safe during lactation.

Blue vervain has been used historically as a galactagogue and to treat nervous exhaustion; however, no studies have been done to confirm its efficacy.[53] Limited studies have demonstrated some effects on the endocrine system where it appears to stimulate follicle-stimulating hormone (FSH) and luteinizing hormone (LH). It may also have antithyrotropic effects and synergistic effects with prostaglandin E2, although the significance of these effects is unknown beyond possibly contributing to the herb's traditional use as an emmenagogue.[67] The herb is used by herbalists similarly to motherwort for its perceived ability to modulate irritability and emotional lability. It is contraindicated in pregnancy but is safe during lactation.

California poppy is used by herbalists as a mild sedative to promote sleep and reduce nervousness and anxiety; it is calming but not heavily sedating. It has demonstrated anxiolytic, mild sedative, and hypnotic effects. It should be considered when there is disturbed sleep (see Insomnia) or anxiety (see Anxiety). It was a popular drug in the late 1800s, when it was sold as a pharmaceutical product by Parke-Davis as a soporific (i.e., sleep-inducing) and analgesic agent. Extracts of California poppy inhibit catecholamine degradation and epinephrine synthesis. The former activity may be especially responsible for the herb's sedative and antidepressant activities. Sedative, anxiolytic, and muscle relaxant effects have been observed experimentally in animals injected with California poppy extracts. Two controlled clinical trials demonstrated normalization of sleep without carryover effects when combined with corydalis (*Corydalis cava*).[68]

Passionflower is approved by the German Commission E for the treatment of nervous restlessness, and recommended by the European Scientific Cooperative on Phytotherapy (ESCOP) for the treatment of tenseness, restlessness, irritability, and difficulty with falling asleep, indications for which herbalists generally prescribe this herb.[53,69] Pharmacodynamic studies and a limited number of clinical trials that have been conducted appear to support its empirical uses as an anxiolytic and sedative herb.[69] Safety during pregnancy is not established; the herb is compatible with lactation.

Skullcap has been used traditionally as a relaxing nervine to support and calm the nervous system, for nervous exhaustion, excitability, overwork, sleep disorders, depression, and exhaustion from mental strain.[68] A recent clinical trial tested the mood effects of skullcap on 43 healthy volunteers. Participants were randomized to receive 350 mg of skullcap or placebo three times daily for 2 weeks. The group was characterized as nonanxious using the Beck Anxiety Inventory. The authors observed a significant group effect and posited a carryover effect between skullcap and placebo groups. Mood disturbance was assessed by Profile of Mood

States and the skullcap group exhibited significant decreases from baseline scores compared with controls (Specific preparation was not mentioned).[70] There is little pharmacologic or clinical research on this widely used herb, and there has been some controversy in the literature regarding its efficacy. A double-blind, placebo-controlled study of healthy subjects by Wolfson and Hoffmann demonstrated noteworthy anxiolytic effects.[71] Because of potential of adulteration with the hepatotoxic herb germander (*Teucrium chamaedrys*) it is best to avoid this herb during pregnancy; notwithstanding this concern, its use is safe during lactation. Obtaining the herb from a reliable source should largely mitigate the concern of adulteration.

Milky oats, chamomile, lavender, and lemon balm are all pleasant tasting, gentle nervines with a long history of use for the nursing mother to promote relaxation, ensure ample breast milk, and as treatment both through the mother and directly to the baby for a fussy or colicky baby. They remain common ingredients in many "mother's milk" (i.e., galactagogue) formulae and are considered safe for use during both pregnancy and lactation.

FORMULAE FOR POSTPARTUM DEPRESSION

The following examples of formulae for the treatment of various PPD symptoms can be used both by nursing and non-nursing mothers. Formulae can be modified for the individual needs of specific patients as required. Additionally, drinking herbal tea is a relaxing ritual for new mothers—a few minutes to sip a cup of hot tea can not only be medicinal but a needed moment for quiet and calm. A cup of hot tea can be taken while nursing or holding the baby even if mom cannot get a moment to herself. Mother's milk tea is a relaxing and delicious favorite of many women.

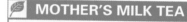

MOTHER'S MILK TEA

Combine the following herbs:

1 oz dried chamomile flowers	(*Matricaria recutita*)
1 oz dried catnip	(*Nepeta cataria*)
¼ oz fennel seeds	(*Foeniculum vulgare*)
⅛ oz dried lavender blossoms	(*Lavandula officinalis*)

Place 1 tablespoon of the dried herbs in a cup or teapot and cover with 1 cup of boiling water. Cover the cup or pot and steep the herbs for 10 minutes. Strain and sweeten if desired.
Dose: 1 to 3 cups/day

FOR IRRITABILITY AND WEEPINESS

For an irritable nervous system, jumpiness and anxiety, quick angering, or frequent weepiness.

Blue vervain	(*Verbena officinalis*)	25 mL
Motherwort	(*Leonurus cardiaca*)	25 mL
Skullcap	(*Scutellaria lateriflora*)	25 mL
Nettle	(*Urtica dioica*)	25 mL
	Total: 100 mL

Dose: 3 to 4 mL with water, 2 to 5 times daily

FOR GENERAL DEPRESSION WITH IRRITABILITY

Recommended by Simon Mill and Kerry Bone in *Principles and Practice of Phytotherapy* specifically for the treatment of postpartum depression caused by hormonal effects and adrenal depletion. They also recommend an addition of 2 mL of *Vitex agnes-castus* upon rising each day.

Ashwagandha	(*Withania somnifera*)	30 mL
St. John's wort	(*Hypericum perforatum*)	25 mL
Blue vervain	(*Verbena officinalis*)	20 mL
Licorice	(*Glycyrrhiza glabra*)	15 mL
Ginseng	(*Panax ginseng*)	10 mL
	Total: 100 mL

Dose: 5 mL in water, three times daily

NUTRITIONAL CONSIDERATIONS

Important nutritional/dietary strategies include improving overall caloric intake through a well-balanced diet, ensuring adequate consumption of complex carbohydrates, and ensuring adequate intake of vitamins and minerals through foods, supplemented with a multivitamin mineral supplement for lactating women. Ample fluid intake is very important, especially for the lactating mother, who needs approximately 2 L per day. B-complex supplementation has been anecdotally reported to improve symptoms of depression and anxiety. Avoiding caffeine, chocolate, coffee, and caffeinated sodas, and keeping sugar consumption to a minimum may help erratic shifts in blood sugar, energy levels, and thus emotions.

Essential Fatty Acids

Essential fatty acids are critically important to a healthy functioning nervous system.[72,73] Evidence indicates an association between omega-3 polyunsaturated fatty acids (PUFAs) and depression.[74,75] The relationship between omega-3 PUFAs and depression is biologically plausible and is consistent across study designs, study groups, and diverse populations, which increases likelihood of a causal relationship.[76] Recently, *The Mothers, Omega-3, and Mental Health Study* tested the efficacy of omega-3 supplementation in perinatal major depressive disorder. A group of 126 pregnant women (108 completed) who were deemed at risk for depression were randomly assigned to receive either eicosapentaenoic acid (EPA)–rich fish oil (1060 mg EPA plus 274 mg docosahexaenoic acid [DHA]), DHA–rich fish oil (900 mg DHA plus 180 mg EPA), or soy oil placebo. Outcomes were measured using Beck Depression Inventory (BDI) and Mini-International Neuropsychiatric Interview at baseline, 26 to 28 weeks, 34 to 36 weeks, and 6 to 8 weeks postdelivery. Serum fatty acids were assessed at baseline 34 to 36 weeks. BDI scores did not significantly differ between groups, but serum EPA and DHA concentrations were elevated in the experimental groups. Serum concentrations of DHA at 34 to 36 weeks were inversely related to BDI scores in late pregnancy.[77] A 2011 systematic review evaluated available evidence for the association between omega-3 supplementation and perinatal depression risk. Ten studies met the inclusion criteria, and results were mixed. Six studies found no association between omega-3 supplementation and reduction of perinatal depression risk, two had a positive association, and two studies yielded mixed results. The reviewers acknowledged heterogenous study designs. Furthermore, it was noted that higher omega-3 dose ranges were associated with positive outcomes.[78] Some trials have reported negative results. A 2010 double-blind multicenter randomized controlled trial (RCT) on the effects of maternal DHA supplementation in pregnancy on perinatal depression and neurodevelopment of offspring did not find significant effects. A group of 2399 women at five hospitals was recruited to participate (if they were at <21 weeks of gestation) and were randomized to receive 800 mg/d of DHA or vegetable oil control. Depressive outcomes were measured via Edinburgh Postnatal Depression Scale at 6 weeks and 6 months postpartum. There was also a follow-up on cognitive and language development for the children ($n = 726$) assessed by the Bayley Scales of Infant and Toddler Development at 18 months. Significant changes in depressive scores were not observed in the DHA group compared with controls. Cognitive and language development scores in children were also nonsignificant between groups.[79]

The evidence to date supports the adjunctive use of omega-3 fatty acids in the management of unresponsive depression.[80] Several studies suggest that DHA fatty acid supplements given to nursing mothers may reduce the incidence of PPD and also improve early infant development. High EFA intake and high fish consumption have been inversely correlated with incidence of depression.[81,82] In fact, higher intake of DHA by nursing mothers is related to a lower reported incidence of PPD, with women in Singapore consuming 81 lb per year per woman and reporting 0.5% incidence of PPD compared with women in South Africa who consume on average 8.6 lb of fish per year per woman, and reporting an incidence of 24.5% PPD per year. Women in the US fall about halfway between these extremes in both fish consumption and PPD incidence.[75] The DHA content of mother's milk in the United States is among the lowest in the world—about 40 to 50 mg in US women, 200 mg in European women, and about 600 mg in Japanese women. Women who want to increase their DHA levels can take dietary supplements or eat more tuna, salmon, and other foods rich in DHA. To avoid mercury contamination, however, current guidelines suggest limiting fish to 12 oz of cooked fish per week during pregnancy and breastfeeding, and avoiding shark, swordfish, king mackerel, and tilefish. The dose of omega-3 PUFAs required for supplementation to prevent or treat PPD is still not entirely clear. The recommended daily dose of 200 mg DHA has not been consistently sufficient in trials, whereas 1 g/day of EPA has shown more consistent benefits, and has been demonstrated to be superior in relieving symptoms such as delusion, hallucinations, and bizarre behavior in major depression. It is recommended that women supplement with 1 to 3 g/day of a fish oil supplement containing both DHA and EPA.[57] Twenty

fish oil supplements tested for mercury levels by an independent laboratory were found to be free of detectable levels of mercury.[57] Many reputable fish oil companies will offer product information that addresses this concern for professionals and consumers.

🌿 FOR DEPRESSION WITH ANXIETY

When anxiety is the predominant symptom accompanying depression.

Kava kava	*(Piper methysticum)*	20 mL
Ashwagandha	*(Withania somnifera)*	20 mL
St. John's wort	*(Hypericum perforatum)*	20 mL
Motherwort	*(Leonurus cardiaca)*	15 mL
Schisandra	*(Schisandra chinensis)*	15 mL
Licorice	*(Glycyrrhiza glabra)*	10 mL
		Total: 100 mL

Dose: 3 mL in water, two to four times daily

🌿 FOR DEPRESSION WITH MILD SLEEP DIFFICULTY

Primarily for insomnia and exhaustion related to insomnia.

Passionflower	*(Passiflora incarnata)*	30 mL
Skullcap	*(Scutellaria lateriflora)*	20 mL
Chamomile	*(Matricaria recutita)*	20 mL
Linden	*(Tilia* spp.)	20 mL
Lavender	*(Lavandula officinalis)*	10 mL
		Total: 100 mL

Dose: 3 to 4 mL in water, three to five times daily, to promote a relaxed state throughout the day

Can be taken 2 to 4 mL every 30 minutes for 2 hours before bed to promote sleep.

ADDITIONAL THERAPIES

Massage for Mom and Baby

Therapeutic massage for the mother can provide an important opportunity for stress release and time to self-nourish on a regular basis, and can impart of feeling of being cared for.[50] A study by Field et al found that depressed teenage mothers receiving massage (10 sessions reported) experienced decreased depression and anxiety, had statistically significant behavior changes, and decreased salivary cortisol levels after a session.[83] Infant massage, which mothers can easily be trained to do, may also have benefits not only for the infant of the depressed mother via insuring contact and bonding that may become neglected with PPD, but also for the mother. Infants who receive massage regularly may sleep better and be less fussy, reducing potential stress, anxiety, and depression triggers for the mother, but also the act of giving infant massage can improve the mother's sense of connection and attachment to her baby and helping her to feel confident handling the baby and validated as a "good mother" for the effort she is making. A study by Onozawa et al found that depression scores were reduced for both mothers with PPD and their infants as a result of regularly attending infant massage classes, and mother–infant inter-actions were improved.[84]

Aromatherapy

Scent can uplift the spirit, and its connection to memory and emotion has been well-documented. Several scents have been traditionally used to relieve depression; most notable among these is lavender oil. A 2012 pilot study tested aromatherapy for anxiety and depression in postpartum women. A group of 28 women (0 to 18 months postpartum) was randomly assigned to receive aromatherapy (essential oil blend of *Rose otto* and *Lavandula angustifolia* at 2% dilution) or inhala-tion controls. Treatments were 15 minutes twice weekly for 4 weeks. Baseline scores did not differ between the two groups, but endpoint scores suggest favorable mental health outcomes for the aromatherapy group.[85]

Although there is not data on the use of herbs to treat PPD, some evidence suggests the positive effects of laven-der oil for the treatment of general depression.[50] The dilute oil may be used in a massage oil, or may be diffused in the room with an oil diffuser, sprinkled onto a pillow, or added to a bath. Massage may be a particularly beneficial way of utilizing aromatherapy. A 1-day pilot study tested the acute psychological effects of aromatherapy massage in healthy postpartum women. Thirty-six healthy primiparous moth-ers participated on day 2 postdelivery. Sixteen women received aromatherapy massage, and 20 were in the con-trol group. The women in the massage group had decreased posttreatment scores compared with controls.[86] Care should be taken when oils are applied to the skin; they should be diluted enough not to cause irritation. Usually several drops of essential oil to several tablespoons of carrier oil (e.g., almond oil), and 3 to 7 drops of undiluted essential oil added to a full bath, are adequate.

👤 CASE HISTORY: POSTPARTUM DEPRESSION

Anne began her prenatal care with a midwife at 9 weeks pregnant with her second child. At age 39, she had post-poned this second pregnancy for 6 years largely out of fear of reexperiencing the postpartum depression (PPD) that had debilitated her after the birth of her first child. Her first preg-nancy had been uneventful, although she recalled losing a large amount of blood at birth. In the weeks and months post-partum, she reported symptoms of depression to her mid-wife, but these were dismissed as normal for the adjustment to motherhood. She tried St. John's wort with no noticeable improvement. At 1 year postpartum, the symptoms became severe, with suicidal thoughts. She had gained a significant amount of weight (50 lbs) over her prenatal and pregnancy weights, which added to her depression, and she was expe-riencing serious marital discord, so she sought the help of a psychiatrist. Anne spent over a year trying different prescrip-tion medications singly and in combinations. Finally, with a combination of three antidepressant drugs and a synthetic form of T3 hormone, she was symptom-free and remained so for several years. With the help of a prenatal psychiatry

specialist, she was able to eventually wean off most of the drugs, which she did so she could become pregnant. She remained on a single antidepressant medication for the first couple of weeks of pregnancy and then discontinued this as well. She did not like the idea of being on pharmaceuticals at all, as this did not fit with her "natural philosophies" about medicine, and felt entirely uncomfortable using the drugs during pregnancy.

Upon beginning her relationship with a new midwife for this pregnancy, she had a tremendous amount of anxiety about the potential for repeated PPD. Her midwife worked with her to develop a plan that included postnatal support, about which her husband was educated during the course of the pregnancy, nutritional supplementation with an emphasis on essential fatty acid intake, a plan to begin using appro-priate herbs immediately postpartum, and a back-up plan to access medical care if needed. She talked a great deal with her midwife about feelings of abandonment after her first pregnancy, and anger that her practitioner had not recognized the PPD. Her new midwife agreed to be available by pager for an extended postnatal period of time so that Anne would have the assurance that she was not going to feel isolated or alone, and that she could reach her midwife should she feel panicked. This was very reassuring to her throughout the pregnancy.

Anne's diet was revised to include fewer simple carbohy-drates (she ate a good deal of refined and natural sugars) and more whole grains and ample protein. She was encouraged to get in the habit of eating often to prevent hypoglycemia. Her pregnancy was mostly uneventful with the exception of occasional migraines and severe itching, which were treated botanically. She gave birth to a healthy baby but again had a significant blood loss after the birth and was instructed in boosting her iron nutritionally and with Floradix Iron + Herbs for 6 weeks postnatally. Her midwife was in frequent con-tact with her, specifically inquiring about social and emotional aspects of her adjustment. Her husband was much more supportive. She took 3 g of a combination of docosahexae-noic acid (DHA) and eicosapentaenoic acid (EPA) in the form of fish oil, and also 1500 mg of evening primrose oil daily. Immediately postpartum she also began taking the following tincture:

Motherwort	(*Leonurus cardiaca*)	25 mL
Eleuthero	(*Eleutherococcus senticosus*)	25 mL
Blue vervain	(*Verbena officinalis*)	20 mL
Passionflower	(*Passiflora incarnata*)	20 mL
Lavender	(*Lavandula officinalis*)	10 mL
		Total: 100 mL

Dose: 5 mL twice daily

Anne remained on this protocol for 6 months postnatally and had no depression. She went off the formula at this point, but kept a 200 mL bottle on hand "for emergencies." She resumed taking the formula at 8 months postpartum because of feeling "overwhelmed," and remained on it for several more months, after which time she discontinued the formula and remained symptom free. She used no pharma-ceutical drugs at any time in the postpartum period with her second child.

TREATMENT SUMMARY FOR POSTPARTUM DEPRESSION

- Postpartum depression (PPD) is a multifactorial problem requiring attention on many levels, including social, psychological and emotional, nutritional, and biochemical. There is no single magic solution.
- Proper identification of women at risk and diagnosis of PPD is essential to the wellness of the mother, child, and family.
- Preventative strategies such as securing maternal parenting education and support for the postpartum period, and ensuring proper parental nutrition, are essential.
- Essential fatty acid supplementation (i.e., 1 to 3 g/day combined eicosapentaenoic acid [EPA] and docosahexaenoic acid [DHA]) and adequate cold-water fish consumption (i.e., up to 12 oz/week; avoid excess owing to potential for mercury toxicity) during pregnancy and in the postpartum may prevent or alleviate PPD.
- Ample complex carbohydrate intake in the postnatal period may be beneficial in preventing drastic drops in insulin level and thus maintain adequate levels of serotonin, preventing PPD.
- Botanical therapies include the use of adaptogens, nervine tonics, antidepressant herbs, and nervine relaxants and sedatives (see Table 21-1).
- Additional therapies such as maternal massage, infant massage, and the use of lavender oil aromatherapy can be beneficial.

POSTPARTUM PERINEAL HEALING

Episiotomy is one of the most commonly performed procedures in obstetrics. In 2000 approximately 33% of women giving birth vaginally had an episiotomy. Historically, the purpose of this procedure was to facilitate completion of the second stage of labor to improve both maternal and neonatal outcomes. Maternal benefits were thought to include a reduced risk of perineal trauma, subsequent pelvic floor dysfunction and prolapse, urinary incontinence, fecal incontinence, and sexual dysfunction. Potential benefits to the fetus were thought to include a shortened second stage of labor resulting from more rapid spontaneous delivery or from instrumented vaginal delivery. Despite limited data, this procedure became virtually routine resulting in an underestimation of the potential adverse consequences of episiotomy, including extension to a third- or fourth-degree tear, anal sphincter dysfunction, and dyspareunia.[87]

American College of Obstetricians and Gynecologists

The perineum is a muscular body at the inferior boundary of the pelvis, bordered superiorly by the muscles of the levator ani, and inferiorly by fascia. It is bordered by the vaginal introitus anteriorly and the rectal sphincter muscles and rectum posteriorly (Fig. 21-1). Because of the mechanical stresses of the baby's presenting part, particularly the head, on the perineum during birth, the perineum is subject to tearing during the second stage of labor (i.e., pushing). In the 1920s, episiotomy, the surgical cutting of the perineum, became a routine procedure for second stage labor, predicated on the belief that the normal mechanical stresses of birth posed the risk of considerable overstretching of the pelvic floor muscles, predisposing women to long-term or permanent damage and risk of pelvic organ prolapse and incontinence. The final stitch placed in a repair job has often been referred to as the "husband's knot," and it was not uncommon for an obstetrician to inform the new mother or her partner that she would be "better than new" after the repair! Medically, it is considered easier to repair a smooth surgical incision than a possibly jagged laceration that occurs naturally.

By the 1980s, episiotomy was being performed in rates in excess of 60% of all vaginal births.[88] More recently, emerging evidence of the lack of benefit of episiotomy, and associated risks, along with increased demand from maternal consumers that this procedure be avoided, has led to a significant decline in episiotomy rates to as low as 30% to 35% of all vaginal deliveries (against a backdrop of 27.5% of hospital deliveries now occurring by cesarean section).[89] As stated in the introductory quote, limited data supported the efficacy or safety of this procedure in preventing maternal damage as a result of normal vaginal childbirth, and the procedure itself has resulted in deleterious consequences for innumerable women, with soreness, itching, thickening, and scarring of the perineal tissue leading to lack of pliability and dyspareunia as common complaints.

Ironically, not only does routine episiotomy not reduce perineal trauma in most instances, episiotomy incisions frequently extend from first-degree lacerations to third- and fourth-degree lacerations, involving the pelvic floor musculature, rectum, and anal sphincter, with the emergence of the baby over the perineum. In fact, episiotomy is the overriding factor in the length of perineal tearing.[90] Bleeding is a common complication, and infection and permanent sphincter dysfunction not rare. Infection has led to anovaginal fistula, and rarely, infection has resulted in maternal mortality.[87]

It has a common obstetric myth that episiotomy is necessary in cases where expediting delivery in the second stage of labor is warranted for the safety of the fetus, or where the likelihood of spontaneous laceration to the mother seems high. Examples of these indications include ominous fetal heart rate, operative vaginal delivery such as forceps, shoulder dystocia, or a "short" perineal body. However, several trials suggest evidence supporting these claims is lacking. Two recent trials also failed to show evidence that episiotomy improved neonatal outcome, provided better protection of the perineum, or facilitated operative vaginal delivery.[91,92] Current evidence-based medicine does not support liberal or routine use of episiotomy. Although there is a role for episiotomy for a limited number maternal or fetal indications, such as avoiding severe maternal lacerations or facilitating or expediting emergency deliveries, a recent systematic evidence review found that prophylactic use of episiotomy does not appear to result in maternal or fetal benefit.[89] In fact, it

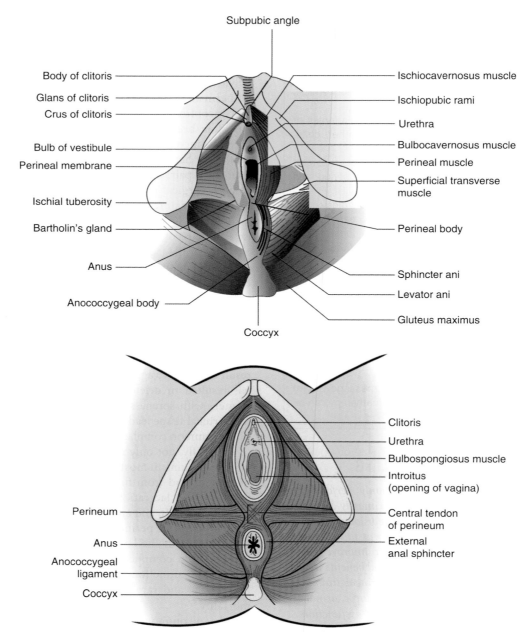

Subpubic angle

Body of clitoris

Glans of clitoris

Crus of clitoris

Bulb of vestibule

Perineal membrane

Ischial tuberosity

Bartholin's gland

Anus

Anococcygeal body

Coccyx

Ischiocavernosus muscle

Ischiopubic rami

Urethra

Bulbocavernosus muscle

Perineal muscle

Superficial transverse muscle

Perineal body

Sphincter ani

Levator ani

Gluteus maximus

Clitoris

Urethra

Bulbospongiosus muscle

Introitus (opening of vagina)

Central tendon of perineum

External anal sphincter

Perineum

Anus

Anococcygeal ligament

Coccyx

FIGURE 21-1 The female perineum and pelvic floor muscles. (From Padubidri VG, Daftary SN: Shaw's Textbook of Gynecology, ed 16, India, 2015, Elsevier (top image), Pfenninger JL, et al: Pfenninger & Fowler's Procedures for Primary Care, ed 3, 2011, St. Louis, Saunders.) (bottom image).

appears to confer more harm than benefit.[88] Nonetheless, of those women who prefer elective cesarean section rather than vaginal delivery, 80% do so because of the fear of perineal damages.[93]

PREVENTION OF PERINEAL TEARS

Perineal tearing, even in the absence of episiotomy, is a common occurrence accompanying vaginal childbirth. Tears are generally first- or second-degree tears, with third- or fourth-degree tears involving the musculature and rectum

more likely to occur as a result of a tear that extends an episiotomy. Repair of natural tearing, as well as episiotomy, can lead to noticeable and prolonged discomfort and mild to moderate dysfunction for many women, depending on the extent of the damage and the quality of the repair. A systematic review of the English language literature was conducted in 1998 to describe the current state of knowledge on reduction of genital tract trauma. A total of 77 papers and chapters were identified and placed into four categories after critical review: 25 randomized trials, 4 meta-analyses, 4 prospective studies, 36 retrospective studies, and 8 descriptions of practice from textbooks.[94] The case for restricting episiotomy is conclusive—what remains uncertain is which techniques for preventing tears are effective. Midwives have consistently demonstrated reduced rates of perineal damage, with lower episiotomy rates, lower tear rates, and less damage to the perineum.[95,96] Techniques commonly employed include prenatal perineal massage, intranatal perineal massage, and application of hot compresses to the perineum during second state, as well as use of alternative positions to the lithotomy position, including standing, squatting, semirecumbent, and lateral positions. The contribution of maternal characteristics and attitudes to intact perineum has not been investigated to date.[94] Achieving an intact perineum, whether through avoidance of tearing or use of episiotomy, can have significant effects on a woman's long-term health after birth. For example, a study by Signorello et al reported that at 6 months postpartum about one fourth of all primiparous women reported lessened sexual sensation, worsened sexual satisfaction, and less ability to achieve orgasm, compared with these parameters before they gave birth. At 3 and 6 months postpartum, 41% and 22%, respectively, reported dyspareunia. Relative to women with an intact perineum, women with second-degree perineal trauma were 80% more likely and those with third- or fourth-degree perineal trauma were 270% more likely to report dyspareunia at 3 months postpartum.[97]

Prenatal Perineal Massage

Three trials (2434 women) comparing digital perineal massage with control were included in a review of antenatal massage and birth outcome by the Cochrane Collaboration. Antenatal perineal massage was associated with an overall reduction in the incidence of trauma requiring suturing, as well as a reduction in episiotomy. This reduction was statistically significant for women without previous vaginal birth only. No differences were seen in the incidence of first- or second-degree perineal tears or third- or fourth-degree perineal trauma. Only women who had previously birthed vaginally reported a statistically significant reduction in the incidence of pain at 3 months postpartum. No significant differences were observed in the incidence of instrumental deliveries, sexual satisfaction, or incontinence of urine, feces, or flatus for any women who practiced perineal massage compared with those who did not. The authors concluded that antenatal perineal massage reduces the likelihood of perineal trauma (mainly episiotomies) and the reporting of ongoing perineal pain, and is generally well accepted by women. As such, women should be made aware of the likely benefit of perineal massage and provided with information on how to massage.[98] Another study evaluating the associations between perineal lacerations and 13 variables associated with the incidence of perineal lacerations concluded that perineal massage was beneficial not only to primiparous women but also to multipara who had episiotomies with their previous births.[99] Additional studies have demonstrated that women find prenatal perineal massage an acceptable practice.[100]

Birth Position, Practitioner Type, and Prevention of Perineal Trauma

In a study evaluating birth position and midwife versus obstetric outcomes in relation to intact perineum at birth, retrospective data from 2891 normal vaginal births were analyzed using multiple regression. A statistically significant association was found between birth position and perineal outcome, with a lateral position associated with the highest rate of intact perineum (intact rate 66.6%) and squatting for primiparas associated with the least favorable perineal outcome (intact rate 42%). Semirecumbent, standing, and "all-fours" positions led to outcomes of 36.3%, 42.7%, and 44.4%, respectively. The obstetrician group had an episiotomy rate greater than five times that of midwives, and generated tears requiring suturing 42.1% of the time, an average of 5 to 7 percentage points higher than midwives. In midwife-supported births, an intact perineum was achieved 56% to 61% of the time, compared with 31.9% for obstetricians.[95] Additional studies have demonstrated improved perineal outcomes with birth in an upright position.[101] Midwives use a variety of techniques to support the perineum during birth. This study was an attempt to begin to understand which of these factors contribute to improved outcomes, and to what extent. However, it should be remembered that it may be the gestalt of factors together that is ultimately responsible for improved perineal outcome at birth.

Intranatal Perineal Massage and/or Hot Compresses during Birth

In one clinical trial done to evaluate these methods, neither intranatal perineal massage nor hot compresses during second stage of labor reduced the incidence of spontaneous perineal tearing as independent techniques. However, as these measures are not harmful and they provide comfort to many women, their use should not be excluded but should be based on whether they provide maternal comfort.[88]

"Easing the Baby Out" and "No Touching" until Crowning of the Head

Techniques not used by the medical community, but widely reported by midwives, include easing the baby out gently rather than bearing down to push, and not touching the perineum until the baby's head is crowning.[102] The former practice encourages the mother to breathe with urges to push rather than using a Valsalva method; based on observation, this appears to minimize pressure against the perineum as the head begins to emerge, and allows a slow emergence of the head, which may optimize perineal stretching versus a fast delivery with the added force of maternal pushing behind it. Many midwives practice "no touching" rather than aggressive second-stage intranatal perineal massage or the practice of "ironing" the perineum, to thin and stretch it, as is commonly practiced in obstetrics. These techniques have not been studied systematically but may contribute to the improved perineal outcomes associated with midwifery care.

TABLE 21-4 Botanical Treatment Strategies for Perineal Healing

Therapeutic Goal	Therapeutic Activity	Botanical Name	Common Name
Restore tone to tissue; promote healing, protect tissue from infection	Astringent	Achillea millefolium	Yarrow
		Arctostaphylos uva ursi	Uva ursi
		Hamamelis virginiana	Witch hazel
		Myrica cerifera	Bayberry bark
		Quercus spp.	Oak bark
Prevent infection	Antiseptic	Allium sativum	Garlic
		Commiphora molmol	Myrrh
		Lavandula officinalis	Lavender
		Rosmarinus officinalis	Rosemary
		Salvia officinalis	Sage
		Thymus vulgaris	Thyme
Heal tissue	Vulnerary	Calendula officinalis	Calendula
		Symphytum officinale	Comfrey leaf

BOTANICAL TREATMENT FOR PERINEAL HEALING

For women who have experienced perineal trauma with birth, perineal healing is a concern (Table 21-4). Whether as a result of nonsurgical laceration or routine or medically necessitated episiotomy, if a surgical repair was done (i.e., stitches), postpartum perineal discomfort can be significant, with itching, soreness, tenderness, and even pain. Discomfort can sometimes persist for months after childbirth, interfering with normal activities, exercise, and sex. For some women, this has serious implications in their work life and marriage/sexual relationships. Severe perineal trauma at birth, even in the absence of episiotomy, can also lead to delayed return of sexual activity and perineal discomfort.

Astringent herbs such as yarrow, witch hazel, and white oak bark, vulnerary herbs such as calendula and comfrey, antiseptic herbs such as sage and myrrh, and a mild topical analgesic such as lavender can be made into strong decoctions, which can be applied to the perineum via a peri-wash or sitz bath. Alternatively, tinctures of these herbs can be diluted in water and similarly applied. These herbs can accelerate healing from perineal tears and episiotomy, reduce swelling and bruising, and alleviate pain and soreness. Peri-rinses can be used after each use of the toilet, and sitz baths can be taken one to two times daily as needed. These techniques are repeated up to 5 days postnatally. Sample recipes that are popular for use among midwives are described later. See Chapter 3 for instructions on preparing herbal baths, sitz baths, and peri-rinses. With the exception of lavender, which has been studied minimally for this purpose, few studies have been conducted on the use of herbs specifically for postnatal perineal healing. Anecdotally, women report these to be soothing, and look forward to repeating the baths and rinses. These applications are also effective in reducing hemorrhoids postnatally, and for this purpose, may additionally be used directly on the hemorrhoids in the form of compresses of the teas. When using compresses, omit the garlic, which is too irritating to be applied directly, and omit the sea salt, which is unnecessary.

PERINEAL HERBAL BATH I

A blend of beautiful and fragrant blossoms that is soothing, healing, and antiseptic.
Mix these herbs:

Comfrey leaves	(Symphytum officinale)	2 oz
Calendula flowers	(Calendula officinalis)	1 oz
Lavender flowers	(Lavandula officinalis)	1 oz
Sage leaf	(Salvia officinalis)	½ oz
Myrrh powder	(Commiphora molmol)	½ oz
		Total: 5 oz

Also: ½ cup sea salt
Directions: Bring 4 quarts of water to a boil. Turn off heat, and place 1 oz of the mix (not the salt) into the pot. Steep, covered, for 30 minutes. Strain the liquid thoroughly through a fine mesh strainer, and discard the herb material. Add 2 quarts of liquid to the tub, along with the 3½ cups of salt. Reserve the remaining liquid for another bath or alternatively, use the tea in a 4-oz peri-bottle, adding 1 Tbsp of salt per bottle.

PERINEAL HERBAL BATH II

Strongly antiseptic and astringent, this bath, or similar variations of it, is a popular postpartum treatment among home birth midwives. It can be used when there is tearing, bruising, abrasions ("skid marks"), or soreness.
Mix the following dried herbs:

Comfrey leaf	(Symphytum officinale)	1 oz
Yarrow blossoms	(Achillea millefolium)	1 oz
Sage leaf	(Salvia officinalis)	1 oz
Rosemary leaf	(Rosmarinus officinalis)	1 oz
		Total: 4 oz

Also: Peel 1 large fresh bulb of garlic (Allium sativum) and obtain ½ cup of sea salt.
Directions: Peel all of the garlic cloves and place them in a blender with 2 cups of lukewarm water. Blend at high speed until a milky liquid is obtained and the garlic is completely pulverized. Strain through a fine mesh strainer. Bring 6 cups of water to a boil and turn off heat. Add 1 ounce total of the dried herb blend to the pot and steep for 30 minutes, covered.

Strain the liquid thoroughly through a fine mesh strainer or cheesecloth and discard the herb material. Add 1 cup of the garlic "milk" and 4 cups of herb tea to the bath, along with ½ cup of salt. Reserve the remaining liquids for a subsequent bath. Do not use the garlic milk directly or in a peri-bottle—it is too irritating. However, the tea made be used as such, with the addition of 1 Tbsp sea salt per 4-oz peri-bottle.

ASTRINGENT AND ANTISEPTIC TINCTURE

Mix all tinctures and add ½ fl oz of the mix to 4 oz of warm water in a peri-bottle.

Witch hazel bark	*(Hamamelis virginiana)*	½ fl oz
Calendula	*(Calendula officinalis)*	½ fl oz
Lavender	*(Lavandula officinalis)*	½ fl oz
Myrrh	*(Commiphora molmol)*	½ fl oz
		Total: 2 fl oz

Lavender

Lavender herb and oil are traditionally used by herbalists for their antiseptic and mild analgesic properties when applied topically. It is commonly recommended by midwives and herbalists as an ingredient in postpartum sitz baths. Researchers at the Hinchingbrooke Hospital, Huntingdon, Cambridgeshire, undertook a blind randomized clinical trial using a total of 635 postnatal women to test these claims. The women were divided into three groups: the first group was given pure lavender oil, the second group synthetic lavender oil, and the third group an inert substance, each to be used as bath additives daily for 10 days after normal childbirth. Analysis of the total daily discomfort scores revealed no statistically significant difference between the three groups. However, on closer inspection, the outcomes showed that those women using lavender oil recorded lower mean discomfort scores on the third and fifth days than the two control groups, which is a time when the mother usually finds herself discharged home and perineal discomfort is high.[103] As another example, 60 primiparous women participated in a 2012 RCT investigating the efficacy of lavender oil for episiotomy recovery. Women were randomized to receive lavender oil treatment or standard care control. Pain outcomes were assessed with the visual analog scale (VAS), and the REEDA scale (Redness, Edema, Ecchymosis, Discharge, Approximation) quantified wound healing. The women were examined 4 hours, 12 hours, and 5 days postepisiotomy. Researchers observed significant differences in pain measures 4 hours and 5 days after in the experimental group (12 hour measures were not significant). Statistically significant lower scores for REEDA were observed in the experimental group at 5 days after episiotomy.[104] Another recent RCT tested lavender oil in episiotomy recovery. One-hundred-twenty women (primiparous, no comorbidities, spontaneous vaginal delivery with episiotomy) were randomized into equal groups receiving topical lavender oil treatment or povidone iodine control. The women were examined 10 days postpartum. In the lavender oil group 25/60 women reported no pain, and 17/60 women in the control group reported the same ($p = 0.06$). Researchers observed reduced redness in the lavender oil group, but no differences in surgical complications between the two groups.[105]

Breastfeeding and Botanical Medicine

BREASTFEEDING AND HERBS: A COMPREHENSIVE REVIEW OF SAFETY CONSIDERATIONS AND BREASTFEEDING CONCERNS FOR THE MOTHER–INFANT DYAD

Lactation is a healthy function of a woman's body; it benefits the woman and provides the child with the only known perfect food for humans—human milk.[1] The breast and breast milk are what the human baby is evolutionarily adapted to "expect" after birth. Breastfeeding is what the woman's body also "expects" after birth. Although a full description of benefits of breastfeeding is well beyond the scope of this chapter, the American Academy of Pediatrics' (AAP) statement on breastfeeding provides a succinct summary (Box 22-1).[1]

As a society, encouraging breastfeeding of our young is one of the most important health measures we can take. The established risks of not breastfeeding include increased incidence of otitis media, gastrointestinal (GI) infections, respiratory infections, juvenile diabetes, lymphoma, and lowered cognitive function for the baby; the mother is at increased risk for breast cancer, ovarian cancer, and osteoporosis. The beneficial effects of breastfeeding are generally dose related: Exclusive breastfeeding in the first 6 months, followed by significant breastfeeding for at least the first year and beyond is recognized as optimal.[1,2] This "dose" provides the gold standard of nutrition, with which all else must be compared. Benefits to both mother and child are now considered so extensive that the protection, promotion, and support of breastfeeding is a recognized global health activity in all countries; the World Health Organization (WHO) and United Nations Children's Fund (UNICEF) are but two global organizations that have consistently worked toward the goal of increasing breastfeeding rates and duration. Chemical risk to the breastfeeding dyad must be considered relative to the importance of breastfeeding in the optimal manner for the optimal duration.

HERBS AND BREASTFEEDING

Concerns involving herbs and breastfeeding have become commonplace among health care providers. Written information to date is often inadequate for counseling clients/patients: herbal product label information provides insufficient safety information, and reference texts generally present extremely limited data focused only on infant risk.[3-6] Few authors explain the rationale behind contraindications, nor do they provide documentation of adverse reactions, and the criteria for determining risk is typically not defined. Exceptions are McKenna and colleagues,[7] which features an introductory essay on the parameters of herb risk during lactation as well as more detailed discussion of lactation use for each monographed herb, and Mills and Bone,[8] with an extensive chapter on the safety of herbs during pregnancy and lactation. Some texts discourage or contraindicate all herb use during lactation, rendering such books particularly useless.[9] In sharp contrast, the herbal *Physicians' Desk Reference (PDR)* only rarely mentions that use of an herb may require caution during lactation, even when perhaps when it is merited. The German Commission E[3] as well as the American Herbal Products Association (AHPA)'s *Botanical Safety Handbook*[10] provide generally reliable guidelines for the safe use of herbs during lactation.

Breastfeeding mothers, like all other women, have health needs that may at times require treatment, and breastfeeding mothers may choose botanical medicines as their treatment choice. Risk assessment must include those risks to the infant, the mother, and lactation itself. The risk analysis of the herbal medicine must be extended to include the comparison risk of using the relevant pharmaceutical drug.

Detailed information is now available on pharmaceutical drug use during lactation, providing the health care practitioner with sufficient information to counsel breastfeeding mothers. Most prescription drugs have been demonstrated to carry some degree of compatibility with breastfeeding.[11,12] Lactation pharmacology generally has shown limited drug entry into breast milk and few adverse reactions in the infant for most chemical entities. Weaning to use a medication is only rarely considered necessary.[11] Given this, herb safety cannot be evaluated in isolation from drug safety, and the relative safety of most herbs during lactation may be taken as an extension because of the relatively limited side effects and adverse events from herbs compared with pharmaceutical drugs.

Each mother–child nursing pair, or dyad, is considered a unit. Dyads are as unique as any individual, requiring information fitted to their own situation. Just as with drugs, categorical recommendations cannot be made about herbs. Ruth Lawrence, an internationally recognized expert in lactation,

The editor wishes to thank *Botanical Medicine for Women's Health*, ed 1 contributor Sheila Humphrey for her original contributions to this chapter.

BOX 22-1 American Academy of Pediatrics' Policy Statement on Breastfeeding

The American Academy of Pediatrics (AAP) identifies breastfeeding as the ideal method of feeding and nurturing infants and recognizes breastfeeding as primary in achieving optimal infant and child health, growth, and development. The following are excerpts from the extensive AAP policy statement on breastfeeding: Breastfeeding and the use of human milk, *Pediatrics* 115(2):496–506, 2005. The full text is available at www.pediatrics.org/cgi/content/full/115/2/496. Many of these recommendations are identical for high-risk infants, and a section devoted to the nursing of these babies is included in the AAP statement.

It should be noted that midwives and breastfeeding advocates have been recommending many of these policies for at least three decades.

Recommendations on Breastfeeding for Healthy Term Infants

1. Pediatricians and other health care professionals should recommend human milk for all infants in whom breastfeeding is not specifically contraindicated (for significant health reasons, i.e., infectious disease) and provide parents with complete, current information on the benefits and techniques of breastfeeding to ensure that their feeding decision is a fully informed one.
   - When direct breastfeeding is not possible, expressed human milk should be provided. Before advising against breastfeeding or recommending premature weaning, weigh the benefits of breastfeeding against the risks of not receiving human milk.
2. Peripartum policies and practices that optimize breastfeeding initiation and maintenance should be encouraged.
   - Education of both parents before and after delivery of the infant is an essential component of successful breastfeeding. Support and encouragement by the father can greatly assist the mother during the initiation process and subsequent periods when problems arise. Consistent with appropriate care for the mother, minimize or modify the course of maternal medications that have the potential for altering the infant's alertness and feeding behavior. Avoid procedures that may interfere with breastfeeding or that may traumatize the infant, including unnecessary, excessive, and overvigorous suctioning of the oral cavity, esophagus, and airways to avoid oropharyngeal mucosal injury that may lead to aversive feeding behavior.
3. Healthy infants should be placed and remain in direct skin-to-skin contact with their mothers immediately after delivery until the first feeding is accomplished.
   - The alert, healthy newborn infant is capable of latching on to a breast without specific assistance within the first hour after birth. The mother is an optimal heat source for the infant. Delay weighing, measuring, bathing, needle-sticks, and eye prophylaxis until after the first feeding is completed. Infants affected by maternal medications may require assistance for effective latch-on. Except under unusual circumstances, the newborn infant should remain with the mother throughout the recovery period.
4. Supplements (water, glucose water, formula, and other fluids) should not be given to breastfeeding newborn infants unless ordered by a physician when a medical indication exists.

5. Pacifier use is best avoided during the initiation of breastfeeding and used only after breastfeeding is well established.
6. Pediatricians and parents should be aware that exclusive breastfeeding is sufficient to support optimal growth and development for approximately the first 6 months of life and provides continuing protection against diarrhea and respiratory tract infection. Breastfeeding should be continued for at least the first year of life and beyond for as long as mutually desired by mother and child.
   - Introduction of complementary feedings before 6 months of age generally does not increase total caloric intake or rate of growth and only substitutes foods that lack the protective components of human milk.
   - During the first 6 months of age, even in hot climates, water and juice are unnecessary for breastfed infants and may introduce contaminants or allergens.
   - Increased duration of breastfeeding confers significant health and developmental benefits for the child and the mother, especially in delaying return of fertility (thereby promoting optimal intervals between births).
   - There is no upper limit to the duration of breastfeeding and no evidence of psychological or developmental harm from breastfeeding into the third year of life or longer.
7. Mother and infant should sleep in proximity to each other to facilitate breastfeeding.

Role of Pediatricians and Other Health Care Professionals in Protecting, Promoting, and Supporting Breastfeeding
General
   - Promote, support, and protect breastfeeding enthusiastically. In consideration of the extensively published evidence for improved health and developmental outcomes in breastfed infants and their mothers, a strong position on behalf of breastfeeding is warranted.
   - Promote breastfeeding as a cultural norm and encourage family and societal support for breastfeeding.
   - Recognize the effect of cultural diversity on breastfeeding attitudes and practices and encourage variations, if appropriate, that effectively promote and support breastfeeding in different cultures.

Education
   - Become knowledgeable and skilled in the physiology and current clinical management of breastfeeding.
   - Encourage development of formal training in breastfeeding and lactation in medical schools, in residency and fellowship training programs, and for practicing pediatricians.
   - Use every opportunity to provide age-appropriate breastfeeding education to children and adults in the medical setting and in outreach programs for student and parent groups.

Clinical Practice
   - Work collaboratively with the obstetric community to ensure that women receive accurate and sufficient information throughout the perinatal period to make a fully informed decision about infant feeding.
   - Work collaboratively with the dental community to ensure that women are encouraged to continue to breastfeed and use good oral health practices.

Continued

BOX 22-1   American Academy of Pediatrics' Policy Statement on Breastfeeding—cont'd

Clinical Practice—cont'd

- Promote hospital policies and procedures that facilitate breastfeeding. Work actively toward eliminating hospital policies and practices that discourage breastfeeding (e.g., promotion of infant formula in hospitals including infant formula discharge packs and formula discount coupons, separation of mother and infant, inappropriate infant feeding images, and lack of adequate encouragement and support of breastfeeding by all health care staff). Encourage hospitals to provide in-depth training in breastfeeding for all health care staff (including physicians) and have lactation experts available at all times.
- Provide effective breast pumps and private lactation areas for all breastfeeding mothers (patients and staff) in ambulatory and inpatient areas of the hospital.
- Become familiar with local breastfeeding resources (e.g., Women, Infants, and Children [WIC] clinics, breastfeeding medical and nursing specialists, lactation educators and consultants, lay support groups, and breast-pump rental stations).

- Encourage adequate, routine insurance coverage for necessary breastfeeding services and supplies, including the time required by pediatricians and other licensed health care professionals to assess and manage breastfeeding and the cost for the rental of breast pumps.
- Develop and maintain effective communication and coordination with other health care professionals to ensure optimal breastfeeding education, support, and counseling.

Society

- Encourage the media to portray breastfeeding as positive and normative.
- Encourage employers to provide appropriate facilities and adequate time in the workplace for breastfeeding and/or milk expression.
- Encourage child care providers to support breastfeeding and the use of expressed human milk provided by the parent.
- Encourage development and approval of governmental policies and legislation that are supportive of a mother's choice to breastfeed.

Adapted from American Academy of Pediatrics, Policy Statement Section on Breastfeeding, Breastfeeding and the use of human milk, *Pediatrics* 115:496-506, 2005.

---

ended her discussion on herbs in a US government publication about risk with a simple summary statement: "The medicinal use of herbs per se is not a contraindication to breastfeeding."[13] Assessment of risk is possible but must be individualized using basic principles. This first requires an understanding of both lactation and lactation pharmacology.

HOW CHEMICALS ENTER BREAST MILK: WHAT WE KNOW

The science of lactation pharmacology and toxicology has greatly advanced over the last 20 years so that recognized principles of chemical entry into breast milk can be used to determine drug and environmental contaminant risk, even when some information is lacking.[12] Recognition of these principles has greatly advanced the knowledge base and clinical practice of drug prescribing with breastfeeding women.

Almost any chemical a breastfeeding mother ingests that gains entry to her bloodstream will enter her milk to some degree; however, it appears that most substances will only gain entry in minute doses. The oft-quoted rule is 1% of the maternal dose of any medication will enter the milk, and with some exceptions, up to about 10%.[12,14] Pharmaceuticals, especially single-chemical preparations noted for their "magic bullet" effect on target systems, can have profound effects on the mother, yet it is the exception when the infant-received dose is large enough to elicit any pharmacologic effect. In general, no adverse effects are noted when the milk dose of a substance is less than 10% of the mother's ingested dose. Such a dose is typically too small to elicit a pharmaceutical response. From ingestion to milk entry, the same pharmacologic principles for drugs apply to herbs, and there is no a priori reason to think that phytochemicals would be exceptional regarding milk entry.

The blood–breast barrier possesses unique permeability and selectivity regarding passage of any one chemical. Chemicals on the blood side must pass through the cell lining of the breast's alveoli to reach the milk. The amount of any chemical's entry into milk is determined by a number of pharmacokinetic factors: bioavailability, maternal serum levels, degree of protein binding in maternal serum, lipid solubility and the fat content of the milk, degree of ionization and milk pH, molecular size and weight, and the half-life in the maternal plasma compartment.

Bioavailability is an important first determinant of maternal serum levels and has proved useful in predicting the infant serum levels after milk ingestion. If a chemical is not absorbed into the bloodstream from the GI tract, then it cannot reach the breast. The most important factor affecting milk entry after oral availability is the mother's serum level, with breast milk levels almost always directly correlating to maternal serum levels. Chemical entry is primarily by diffusion through the alveolar cells, driven by equilibrium forces between the maternal plasma compartment and the maternal milk compartment. Chemicals do not usually "get stuck" in breast milk, though a few chemicals do sequester or concentrate in breast milk, most notably iodine and alkaloids. Unlike most minerals, iodine is actively transported into breast milk. Nonionized chemicals will more readily enter and leave the milk compartment than ionized chemicals. Because of a shift in pH, weakly basic chemicals such as alkaloids tend to concentrate in the slightly more acidic breast milk, resulting in "trapping" and higher milk to plasma ratios than is typical. The degree of protein binding is also a primary determinant of milk entry. Chemicals must be free in the plasma to diffuse into breast milk. Thus Coumadin, 99% bound to serum proteins, only enters milk in miniscule amounts (0.08 μmole/L), which have been shown to be of no pharmacologic consequence to the infant. Very large molecules, such as insulin and heparin, do not enter breast milk at all. Very small molecules, including ethanol and other volatiles, tend to diffuse more rapidly into and out of milk, with milk levels closely reflecting maternal serum levels. Lipid-soluble chemicals, such as most central nervous system (CNS) drugs, also tend to enter into milk more readily, and can exhibit higher than expected levels. The blood–breast barrier somewhat resembles the blood–brain barrier in this regard.[12]

 FACTORS AFFECTING THE IMPACT OF SUBSTANCES TAKEN BY THE MOTHER ON A CHILD DURING LACTATION

1. Dose present in the milk (i.e., degree of entry)
2. Dose or volume of breast milk received by the child
3. Serum levels attained in the child depend on:
   a. Oral availability in the child
   b. Metabolism of that chemical by the infant
4. Age and health of the child determines elimination capabilities
5. Weight of the child will also determine the effect of the substance (a pediatric dose is always expressed in terms of weight)

Chemical entry into milk is restricted by a secretory epithelium with tight junctures between the alveolar cells of the mammary structure. However, colostrum, produced in the first 3 to 10 days postpartum, is produced before these tight junctures close. Until the alveolar cells swell with high-volume milk production, maternal proteins such as immunoglobulins and most chemicals in the serum have enhanced access to the milk compartment, passing freely between the alveolar cells. Lactation experts agree that relatively larger doses of chemicals enter milk during this time.[12,15] After this time, chemicals can only gain access to the milk compartment through the two-cell membranes of the alveolar cells, usually by diffusion.

The amount of breast milk ingested by the child (i.e., nursing pattern) is probably the most important determinant of risk, and the most variable. The exclusively breastfeeding infant is ingesting a maximal volume of breast milk per body weight. An older infant may also be ingesting a similar volume of milk, but because the child now weighs considerably more at 6 months, possesses a GI tract ready to handle foods other than breast milk, and has a matured elimination capacity, the dose effect will be lessened. At the other end of the spectrum is the token-nursed infant receiving only one to two feedings at the breast per day, or the nursing toddler, who may nurse only occasionally.

Asking the mother the age of the child and about the nursing pattern will quickly place the dyad on the relative risk continuum. The age and weight of the child are largely predictive of the effect of any given herb/medication dose. Another important factor is the maturity of the child's metabolic and eliminative functions. The newborn is the most vulnerable to chemicals ingested by the mother, being born with immature gut, liver, and kidney function. By about the age of 2 weeks, however, the liver is able to effectively metabolize ingested chemicals competently.[15] Kidney clearance capacity increases and becomes fully functional by 4 to 5 months of age. The adult half-life of a chemical is commonly used to give some measure of whether a drug is likely to accumulate in an infant, even though pediatric half-life is not known for most drugs. Chemicals with half-lives of longer than 24 hours are of greatest concern because they will accumulate in the infant.[12] For neonates with immature metabolic capacity and small body size, serum levels can rise to pharmacologically significant levels more quickly, even with drugs of shorter half-lives. Thus great caution is required with premature and low birth-weight infants.[15]

Lactation pharmacology has developed to the point where generalizations about chemicals, synthetic or naturally occurring, are possible, and where a prediction of risk can be made for a particular mother–child pair. Because the dose of breast milk as well as the size and health of a nursing child are highly variable, blanket statements of risk during breastfeeding are gross simplifications that cannot guide clinical practice, although a cautionary statement on an herbal or drug product label helps mothers in determining self-use.

RISKS

Risks of Medications

The AAP, in 1994, 1997, and 2001, reviewed research and clinical information about drug use in lactation, with the latest statement supporting the safety of the use of the vast majority of drugs during breastfeeding. Generally, only the most toxic drugs, such as cancer chemotherapeutics and long half-life radioactive iodine compounds, are absolutely contraindicated. Known adverse events are usually associated with premature babies or those that are small for gestational age, and such effects often reflect the known side effects in adults. Prediction of risk includes the nature and degree of adverse effects. Certain categories of drugs, such as antidepressants, may be of concern. Although clinical use of many of these substances is widespread, despite the AAP's concerns, most lack significant adverse effects.[12] The safety of antidepressant medications during lactation was discussed in Chapter 21.

Interestingly, synthetic hormonal substances such as the progestins are considered compatible with breastfeeding. Some experts are concerned about potential long-term effects on the infant, yet no evidence of this has been found. Other hormonal preparations, such as synthetic thyroid preparations, are noncontroversial and have been used for decades. Synthetic estrogens are an exception; most practitioners report a decrease in milk supply with use of any amount of estrogen in birth control agents.

Measurement of the degree of milk entry of many types of pharmaceutical substances has led to the realization that few drugs can be expected to cause toxic effects in the infant. Animal lactation studies have been done for some, but not all drugs. Newer prescription drugs often lack studies. Yet, lack of specific lactation studies is not considered reason enough to contraindicate a drug. Indeed, many drugs lack even preliminary study of milk entry in animals or humans. The pharmacokinetic characterization of almost all pharmaceuticals does allow more precise prediction of milk entry, although few fall outside of the 1% to 10% milk entry rule predicted simply from maternal oral ingestion. The clinical evidence for use of most drugs has accumulated through publication of case studies, anecdotes, and experimental study of individuals or very small groups made up of a few mother–baby pairs (often fewer than 10). Typically, milk entry is only characterized for one stage of lactation. Very few drugs have been studied over long-term use, where the child has been exposed to the drug over weeks or months, though some drugs are indeed administered in this way. Despite this narrow basis of experimental evidence or quantitative data on drugs during lactation, the increased prescription of medications during lactation has resulted in the documentation of few adverse reactions in children. It is worthy to note here that even drugs such as digoxin, a cardioactive alkaloid with a narrow therapeutic index, is considered compatible with breastfeeding, although close monitoring of mother and baby is necessary to ensure dose limitation.[11] As reassuring as this is to lactation experts, it is clear that the actual evidence for safety is quite limited compared with the evidence for safety in adults. Thus we know a lot about how a pharmaceutical is metabolized in the mother (pharmacokinetics), allowing tolerably accurate prediction of milk dose, yet have an almost nonexistent experimental base of information regarding actual milk entry or effects in large numbers of infants or over all stages of lactation. Quantification of milk entry and infant serum levels for most drugs is surprisingly limited.

In the Absence of Lactation Studies: Herbs versus Medications

The powerful nature of pharmaceuticals that inherently generates side effects and drug interactions, as well as their use in complex medical situations, results in a relatively high rate of adverse events associated with their use compared with herbal medicines.[16] When comparing the merits of medications versus herbs, the relatively narrow basis of evidence for safe use of medications during lactation must still be balanced by the fact that most medications are more completely studied, particularly regarding their metabolism, and that more elaborate pharmacovigilance systems are in place to monitor their use.[17] However, information gained from traditional use cannot be ignored or discarded; traditional information is the basic study material for the scientific discipline of ethnopharmacology, after all. Nor can drug data provided by the pharmaceutical industry be entirely trusted to always provide an objective measure of safety. Indeed, the *PDR*'s statements regarding safety during lactation are singularly useless to guide clinical practice.[12,15] Regarding efficacy, the principle of proportionality should not be overlooked.[18] Are we talking about the mother having cancer or a cold? How important is efficacy in the risk–benefit analysis? The advantages of an herbal treatment that may not work as

quickly or as well compared with a pharmaceutical must be balanced against the need for efficacy.

Herb Risks: Herbs with Pharmacokinetic Information

De Smet and Brouwers provide a systematic review of the state of herbal pharmacokinetics, evaluating the complexities of phytoconstituent bioavailability and pharmacokinetics, and providing a short list of plant constituents where serum levels have been measured.[18] The authors advocate pharmacokinetic study of herbs with narrow safety margins or those commonly used for life-threatening disorders, but point out that for herbs with wide safety margins, available in high-quality preparations and used for minor health disorders, the need for such characterization is unnecessary. Yet bioavailability and serum levels are two measures that are of great utility in assessing herb safety during lactation, if for no other reason than to reassure the doubtful health practitioner. Assessment of herb risk during lactation is hindered by the fact that useful information such as serum levels, half-life, and protein binding are not yet characterized for many phytochemicals. Dose information for any one constituent, usually the "active" constituent, is often available for most controversial or well-researched herbs, and the simple application of the 1% rule to estimate maternal serum levels from oral dose will yield a ballpark estimate of milk entry for the chemical of toxicologic interest. Even if you assume a worse-case scenario and use 10% as the rule, this number is still likely to be very small. Hypericin and soy isoflavones are two examples where serum levels have been measured. Hypericin is a constituent of St. John's wort (*Hypericum perforatum*) that has been considered active, even though more recent studies indicate a number of other constituents may actually be responsible for the antidepressant activity. In any event, hypericin serum levels have been measured at 8.5 ng/mL after a dose of 900 mg/day of the dried herb.[19] This amount represents a very small dose available to diffuse into the milk. The soy isoflavone, genistein, was recently measured in breast milk at concentrations of 0.2 μmol/L in breast milk after ingestion of soy nuts containing 20 mg of genistein.[20] Genistein entry into breast milk appears extremely limited in this study; serum levels were measured at 2.0 μmol/L plasma, representing a 1:10 milk to plasma ratio. This amount is tiny compared with what babies receive when fed soy formula.[21]

Another class of relatively well-studied herbs is the stimulant laxatives that breastfeeding women are cautioned about for good reason; diarrhea can result from local activity of constituents within the GI tract (i.e., compartmental effect). In a study described in Hale, sennosides A and B could not be detected in milk in one study of 20 breastfeeding women using Senokot tablets containing a dose of 8.6 mg sennosides/day.[12] Most (15/23) women in the study reported loose stool; of these, two had babies who also had loose stools. In another study, rhein, an active laxative metabolite of sennosides, was measured in 100 milk samples drawn from 20 women.[22] A daily dose of 15 mg of sennosides was consumed for 3 days before sampling; 0 to 27 ng/mL was found, with over 90%

of the milk samples containing less than 10 ng/mL of rhein. None of the infants had loose stools. However, the senna was combined with the bulking agent, *Plantago ovata,* which may have slowed or lowered absorption of the laxative constituents into the mothers' bloodstreams. In contrast to the German Commission E, senna and cascara are considered compatible with breastfeeding; this statement assumes the necessary short-term use of a standardized product in appropriate doses; occasional diarrhea has been noted in neonates but not older children.[3]

Herb Risk to the Child

Herbs that present a well-documented risk to adults (i.e., those containing aristolochic acid [AA] or toxic pyrrolizidine alkaloids [PAs]) logically can be expected to present some degree of risk to the breastfeeding child. However, most herbs of commerce lack serious side effects when used appropriately, and thus would not be expected to be able to produce them in infants in the tiny doses of phytoconstituents received in breast milk. Synthetic hormones such as progesterones, estrogens, thyroid replacements, and insulins are compatible with breastfeeding, at least regarding infant safety.[11] Thus the proportional risk posed to the child by the relatively much weaker phytohormones would seem slight. This is not to say that adverse effects cannot occur. Herbs that do have adverse side effects when used appropriately or with narrow therapeutic safety range would be predicted to be much more likely to cause similar problems in the breastfeeding child. These herbs must be used with caution when breastfeeding, even in standardized or over-the-counter (OTC) forms. Yet documented infant effects are rarely seen even in the more vulnerable neonates. And, in those instances where the infant has received the plant chemicals through breast milk alone, the adverse effects have been reversible. Appropriate use of herbs by mothers of nursing toddlers is not expected to pose a risk to the child. Still, the mother needs counseling on what appropriate use is, and what potential side effects should be watched for in the child. The strategy of using the medicine and watching the child for expected side effects is advocated by lactation experts.[12,14] If side effects should appear in the infant, the dose is lowered or a different medicinal is used. Obviously, use of questionable herbs during lactation always needs a close look. Alternative approaches that may or may not include the use of other herbs need to be explored or recommended to the mother. A questionable herbal product should not be used by the nursing mother, regardless of the herb. This pragmatic aspect of herb safety cannot be ignored. Education on product selection should be part of any guidance provided to a mother.

The Pregnancy and Lactation Confusion

When reading herbal literature, it is important to determine whether precautions distinguish between pregnancy and lactation. Numerous authors do not make this distinction. To further complicate matters, many authors do not differentiate between self-directed use and supervised use of herbs; thus it is not at all clear under what use conditions such contraindications are thought necessary.

A prime example of confusing pregnancy and lactation precautions is seen in herbs where many authors contraindicate their use during "pregnancy and lactation due to hormonal influences."[6] For oxytocic or uterotonic herbs, this confounding of pregnancy and lactation is unfortunate, as the following discussion shows. Note that "oxytocic" describes an agent capable of causing uterine contractions leading to the delivery of the fetus or placenta. Not all uterotonics are oxytocic or capable of inducing true labor. Oxytocin is the hormone mainly responsible for labor resulting in birth; it is absolutely required for the milk ejection reflex (MER) to occur. Without oxytocin, there is no milk production. (It is worth noting here that women with a healthy pregnancy who continue to nurse their child do not run an increased risk of premature labor.) Agents that are called oxytocic do not necessarily replace oxytocin, although many probably interact in some way at the oxytocin receptor. A synthetic form (i.e., Pitocin) is used to promote labor as well as trigger the MER after birth; it can act at peripheral receptor sites but cannot access the receptor sites within the CNS.

At present, there is no information available on plant constituent interactions with oxytocin or its receptors in the brain or at peripheral sites. Although oxytocic herbs are properly contraindicated for self-use during pregnancy, there is a wealth of data on their usefulness in lactation. Galactagogues are herbs used with the intent of increasing milk production. Most herbal galactagogues common in clinical practice in Western countries have some degree of uterotonic or even oxytocin activity. Indeed, many of the hundreds of herbs traditionally used as oxytocics (i.e., speeding labor and delivery of both infant and placenta) are also traditionally used as galactogogues.[23-25] Recent lactation research has verified that frequent adequate milk removal is the primary mechanism by which milk production can be increased or maintained.[26] Adequate removal of milk immediately increases the rate of milk synthesis in that breast for the next several hours. Oxytocin is needed to remove milk and it is known that increasing the activity of the oxytocin system results in an increased milk flow from the breast; an immediate galactogogue effect. This boost in milk production can stimulate a flagging synthesis rate for a sustained galactogogue effect. Herbs with noted oxytocic effects have been noted to help trigger the MER, as well as to increase milk flow. Both these actions can indeed aid lactation. However, a mother needing help with milk production is best served by consulting with a lactation specialist; judicious use of oxytocic herbs can play an important but complementary role.

Oxytocic activity is but one of many hormonal influences in which pregnancy cautions do not apply during lactation; indeed, hormonal activity risks during pregnancy may be what makes that herb helpful as a galactogogue. Although consumers should be able to easily identify such herbs, and thus avoid their unintentional use during lactation, health care providers should not mistake general consumer warnings as indicative of the need for all breastfeeding women to avoid supervised use when warranted.

Maternal Plant Use and Risks to the Infant

A study done in Minnesota examined the dietary habits of experienced breastfeeding mothers to determine what foods might be associated with colic symptoms in infants.[27] Researchers found a strong association between the consumption of cruciferous vegetables and the degree of crying and other colic symptoms. Clearly, constituents from the mother's diet are able to enter breast milk in sufficient quantity to cause the baby discomfort. It is worth noting that vegetables (i.e., as foods) are consumed in much larger doses than most medicinal plants. No other systematic studies looking at food and adverse reactions in babies have apparently been done, although mothers are routinely told to avoid hot peppers, garlic, and onions by their doctors and others.

Capsaicin, the "hot" constituent in hot peppers, has been noted to cause problems with episodic consumption by the mother, including fussiness, diarrhea, and a red bottom in the baby. However, many mothers who eat hot peppers daily report no such problems. Additionally, infants accustomed to drinking "spicy" milk will readily eat spicy foods when introduced later in the first year. In the *Botanical Safety Handbook,* the authors classify garlic as an herb to use with caution, and cite references where infant ingestion of garlic resulted in death.[10] Clearly, the authors underestimated the dose difference between direct ingestion of a substance, and indirect ingestion of phytochemical constituents through breast milk. Although direct exposure of infants to large quantities of raw garlic may be potentially dangerous, the daily diet of many countries contains medicinal quantities of garlic, yet there are no documented adverse effects of garlic on nursing infants. Garlic is even used as a galactogogue in India. In one human trial, neither efficacy nor harm was demonstrated.[25] New lactation studies of garlic have been done, yielding no adverse effects.[28] Hale inferred it is not known whether garlic constituents enter milk, which overlooks the pioneering work of Mennella and Beauchamp who studied the effect of garlic on breastfeeding infants.[28] In an earlier study, these authors demonstrated greater interest and longer nursing times in infants whose mothers had ingested a dose of garlic. In a 1993 follow-up study in which mothers ingested garlic daily, the novelty wore off, and the infants went back to their usual nursing patterns. None of the infants suffered adverse effects during these tests. Given the widespread use of garlic as a food, and the existence of studies of garlic and breastfeeding infants, the maternal use of garlic to prevent or treat maternal breast candidiasis (i.e., thrush) should be considered a relatively safe and inexpensive alternative to certain medications, such as fluconazole, a powerful antifungal with potential serious adverse effects on the liver.

Allergy and Associated Risks of Direct Feeding on the Baby and Breastfeeding

The risk of allergic reaction to plant chemicals is real and most likely in the first months of life, yet significantly reduced when exposure is restricted through breastfeeding. Not only are the range of plant chemicals reaching the bloodstream reduced but the dose received by the child is very small. Mothers with allergies or atopic and autoimmune diseases will need guidance with allergenic plants, for both her and the baby's protection. It is also important to determine the father's allergy history. When possible, initial use of simple rather than combination remedies will assist identification of the culprit if an allergy should occur in a mother or baby. Allergy, atopic, and autoimmune diseases are rampant in modern society, now in this third generation of widespread formula feeding experimentation. In addition to being proved as a major preventative of allergenic and atopic disease,[15] exclusive breastfeeding in the first 6 months of life is also preventative against an enormous range of diseases of both childhood and adulthood[1]; direct feeding of substances (whether these are considered food, herbs, or drugs) other than breast milk is clearly an introduced risk.[1,29]

The young baby's GI tract is not mature and is still quite "leaky" or permeable to ingested substances, even proteins. Early exposure of the GI tract and flora to foreign substances is thought to set the child up for subtle and frank infections as well as allergies. These effects may have permanent consequences.[14] Associated risks go hand in hand with premature direct feeding. It is possible to confuse a baby with bottle or pacifier nipples when used to administer a remedy or drug; replacing breast milk with other fluids will lessen his desire to nurse. (Young babies may only take 2 ounces at a time, an amount easily undermined with frequent "tonic" feeds.) For mothers already experiencing latching or other breastfeeding difficulties, these risks can become considerable, a fact that is not yet recognized in much of herbalist literature. Alternative treatment methods should be sought first. In some instances (e.g., colic), the mother can pass beneficial plant constituents through the milk without risking disruption of baby's pristine GI tract or throwing her breastfeeding relationship off-track. This wise and much safer method has been long known and is still used by mothers all over the world.

Herbs That Commonly Cause Adverse Effects in Infants: Coffee and Chocolate

Cases of adverse reactions to chemicals, whether drugs or herbs, usually involve newborns. Lawrence and Lawrence stated that adverse drug reactions often can be traced to accumulation of the chemical in the infant, leading to adverse effects with increasing serum levels.[15] Just about the only herbs that are clearly and consistently able to cause adverse effects seen in infants are CNS–stimulant herbs, most commonly those that contain caffeine and other stimulant xanthine alkaloids: coffee, tea, chocolate, yerba mate, cola, and guarana. Even with its strongly alkaloidal nature, caffeine enters into milk in only tiny amounts. However, it tends to accumulate in the neonate, and can cause fussiness and hyperalertness. This effect is used with premature infants in whom tiny controlled doses of caffeine are given directly to prevent apnea. Despite the fact that mild adverse reactions have been documented in some newborns, caffeine is considered safe for use by breastfeeding mothers. Many mothers can ingest one to two cups of coffee per day without incident, even when breastfeeding neonates, although some babies, like some adults, are acutely sensitive to caffeine and react to any amount of caffeine even as they grow older. Mothers soon find out to what degree coffee, tea, or other caffeine-containing herbs are the cause of their baby's irritability and adjust their dose accordingly.[30]

Other Documented Adverse Reactions of Herbs During Breastfeeding

There is a body of literature describing adverse effects when young infants are directly fed herbal preparations or milk substitutes.[1,29] Yet, very few cases of adverse reactions are documented involving infants ingesting medicinal phytochemicals through breastfeeding, and those that do exist usually involve herb ingestion during pregnancy as well. Farnsworth noted one case involving infant death attributed to the mother having used coltsfoot (*Tussilago farfara*) and butterbur (*Petasites officinalis*) during pregnancy as well as after birth while breastfeeding.[16] Both these plants contain hepatotoxic PAs. Without suggesting that the use of such herbs is hazard-free during breastfeeding, it is reasonable to suggest that use during pregnancy alone could have produced significant liver damage before any amount was received through the milk. This case involved toxins that cause irreversible liver damage and death in adults, and underscores the need for contraindication of such substances in plant medicine more than that herbs per se are dangerous during breastfeeding. However, it remains entirely possible that the developing fetus as well as the newborn may be particularly susceptible to the toxic forms of PAs; there are other incidents of children being harmed through direct ingestion of these chemicals. There is no safe dose level established for children and a very stringent one set for adults in Germany. Because the liver can sustain damage without immediate symptoms, it remains necessary to encourage nursing mothers to avoid consuming herbs with any amounts of these toxic substances that can cause irreversible adverse effects. Comfrey and borage are commonly used herbs known to contain various amounts of toxic PAs. The other widely recognized dangerous plant toxin is AA, which is present in essentially all members of the *Aristolochiaceae* family. This toxin is associated with permanent and sometimes fatal kidney failure.[16,18] The limited elimination capacity of infants may place them at greater risk to this toxin.

The "hairy baby" story has entered the lactation textbooks, even though the original report has subsequently been shown to be incorrect.[15,16,31-33] A woman who thought she was ingesting ginseng throughout pregnancy was using twice the dose suggested by the label. She developed signs of androgenization during pregnancy, and the baby was born with significant hirsutism and other signs of androgenization. This incident reported ginseng as the likely culprit. A more thorough investigation showed that the package was actually labeled Siberian ginseng (*Eleutherococcus senticosus*), and that the product was adulterated with the potentially toxic plant, *Periploca sepium*, although Farnsworth noted that in vitro hormonal studies of the adulterant did not show androgenic activity.[16] It was concluded that no likely

cause of the hirsutism could be determined. This case has limited application in evaluating the risk of properly prepared herbal medicines during pregnancy or lactation. The "hairy baby story," however, illustrates the number one deficiency in anecdotal reporting of adverse events involving herbs in medical literature: lack of verified identification of the actual substance consumed.

The first case identified in the literature that involves breastfeeding only was reported by Rosti and colleagues.[34] In a letter published in the *Journal of the American Medical Association (JAMA)*, the authors tell how two mothers were taking high doses (2 L/day) of an herbal tea with the intention of stimulating lactation, twice the usual dosage of galactogogue teas considered appropriate. Assuming a typical tea, prepared in a standard infusion form, a more typical dose would be 1 L/day total at most. Both of their newborns presented with symptoms that included "reduced growth, poor feeding and sucking, restlessness, emesis, hypotonia, lethargy, and weak cry." It is not clear how the babies could be both lethargic and restless at the same time. Poor breast milk intake alone could soon cause symptoms involving poor growth, suck and feeding, lethargy, low muscle tone, and a weak cry but would not explain restlessness or emesis. Obviously something was going on with these babies. The tea was reported to contain "a variety of active ingredients" that the authors listed as "licorice, fennel, anise, and goat's rue." Symptoms resolved in both infants after the mothers discontinued the herbal teas.[34]

Although it is common for mothers to ingest teas made from any or all of these ingredients without precipitating a visit to the emergency room (ER), licorice (*Glycyrrhiza* spp.) and goat's rue (*Galega officinalis*) may be worth examining more closely, simply because of their capacities to induce side effects with excessive or prolonged use. Fennel (*Foeniculum vulgare*) and anise (*Pimpinella anisum*) both contain (trans-anethole), a sweet-tasting compound thought capable of altering CNS activity (at least in high doses). It is quite possible that these babies may have simply been consuming breast milk containing too high a concentration of constituents, too early in the neonatal period, although a distinct lack of other similar adverse events points to other factors. First is the widespread use of such herbs where these mothers come from. In Italy, new mothers as a matter of course go out to buy galactogogue teas in pharmacies, whether they need them or not. Fennel and anise, in particular, are favored there, as they have been for thousands of years. Goat's rue is very commonly used in France, a practice that dates back to antiquity as well. However, plant materials were not positively identified in the article, and adulteration of the presumed plant material is always a possibility, as occurred with the *Periploca* case. Given that fennel and anise both bear striking resemblance to a number of very toxic relatives (i.e., anise and the potentially toxic star anise have similar flavor), the question of plant identity must be raised. The letter does not indicate whether these women presented independently or were somehow connected. Since the letter's publication, no further corroborating cases involving any of these herbs have been published. Very little actual knowledge can be gained from such a letter because the information was not scrutinized by plant or lactation experts and thus is incomplete and unverified.

A report involving the use of dong quai (*Angelica sinensis*) was published as a letter.[35] In this instance, a Chinese American woman, 3 weeks postpartum, developed an acute onset of headache, weakness, lightheadedness, and vomiting and came to the ER for evaluation. In the ER she was found to be hypertensive (195/85). She had no history of hypertension, as verified from her medical record at birth. Blood chemistry and other studies were normal. Earlier that day, she had twice eaten a traditional postpartum soup made by her mother. The soup was reported as being made from *Angelica sinensis* rhizome that the grandmother had purchased in Malaysia before visiting her daughter. Within 12 hours of arrival at the ER, her blood pressure was once again within normal limits and other symptoms had disappeared. The next day, the baby was evaluated by a pediatrician and found to also have elevated blood pressure, which was treated by withholding breast milk. Within 48 hours, his blood pressure was normal. The authors clearly state that as they could not obtain a sample of the actual soup ingested, they could confirm neither the identity of the actual substance ingested, nor its dose. Use of other herbals or other medicines was denied by the mother. The authors did do the next best thing though, and obtained samples of the same product the mother purchased in Malaysia for analysis by a Chinese medicinal expert (unnamed) who said it was indistinguishable from *Angelica sinensis*. What is not mentioned in this article is the lack of any other cases in which ingestion of *Angelica sinensis* has led to high blood pressure. Indeed, the herb is known to be, if anything, hypotensive in studies. Thus the development of hypertension must be considered atypical. This is especially so given that it is a very widespread ancient tradition to use dong quai in postpartum soups for new mothers in Asia. A traditional Chinese medical practitioner in North America has commented that although most ordinary people would know when a new mother is already too "hot" and would not give the soup, it is entirely possible for such a mistake to be made. Further, botanicals imported from China are notorious for being contaminated—it is possible that it was not the herb, per se, but contaminants that, if at all, were associated with this episode.

External Use of Herbs on the Breast and Nipple

Products used to treat thrush or bacterial infections need to be nontoxic and nonallergenic to best ensure safety to the infant, who will be ingesting some share of such products.[31] The taste of an external substance can sometimes cause problems. Some babies refuse the breast upon tasting bitter substances and can quickly develop an aversion to the breast. To avoid this, babies must be nursed before external applications and the nipples rinsed before nursing if there are still obvious residues on the nipple. It is possible that many substances in the cream may be absorbed into the breast tissue and thus enter the nearby milk ducts in relatively large amounts; wiping may not avert all potential problems with a questionable product. The use of potentially toxic herbs such as comfrey (which contains

PAs) should clearly be seen as being an unnecessary risk to an infant, despite the herb's excellent healing properties. Safer alternatives, such as *Calendula officinalis*, should be selected.

The use of essential oils on the breast and nipple is in general riskier than use of less-concentrated water-based herb preparations. Yet tea tree oil is often suggested to treat nipple thrush, a practice that not only lacks evidence of efficacy but may be particularly unwise. First, babies exposed to tea tree oil near their faces and mouths may gag, or in a worst-case scenario, suffer respiratory collapse. This is a well-known phenomenon also known to occur with essential oils of peppermint, camphor, neroli, and cajeput, the last two being from close relatives of tea tree.[3] Tea tree oil can be irritating and sensitizing, leading to contact dermatitis, and there are two cases of toxicity associated with its use.[3] In one case, an adult developed petechiae and leukocytosis after ingesting about 7 cc of the essential oil; in another, a 17-month-old toddler developed ataxia and drowsiness after swallowing less than 10 cc of the essential oil.[12] Taken altogether, tea tree oil should not be used or suggested for nipple thrush, and safer alternatives should be sought.

Risks to the Mother

The lactating breast is metabolically extremely active. All components of the milk are brought through the bloodstream and incorporated directly or assembled in the secretory cells. The breast has dermatologically unique areas—the areola and nipple. The nipples mark the boundary between mucous membranes of the internal ducts and external skin of the areola. The skin of the areola is very thin compared with other skin; both areas are extremely sensitive. It is known that breast sensitivity increases during lactation; this facilitates oxytocin release that is triggered in the brain by suckling. There is reason to believe that the lactating breast may be more unusually sensitive to externally applied substances, perhaps because of increased permeability of the skin.[25,36] It is known that very sensitive mothers can develop eczema from food residues in their babies' mouths. The permeability of the breast has not been directly studied, however. Care should be taken for the mother's safety when applying external products to the breast and nipple.

There are a number of reports of allergic reaction to herbs applied to the nipple, most often in an effort to heal sore nipples. One short communication gives two case histories that involved Roman chamomile (*Chamaemelum nobile*). The herbal cream was applied to sore nipples and resulted in severe exudative eczema on the nipples and the areola.[37] In both cases, the mothers used a product marketed for sore nipples. One mother had used the product with her previous child without difficulty. Roman chamomile is much more frequently reported as a cause of allergic reactions than its relatively innocent cousin, German chamomile (*Matricaria recutita*).

Another case described the use of garlic on the breast, which resulted in skin burns.[36] Although the letter did not include this fact, garlic is a known allergen.[3] The mother was self-treating a rash on her breast that she thought was "thrush," in and of itself a likely misdiagnosis. She placed fresh garlic on the rash and left the area covered for 4 days. The baby had access to the nipple and continued to nurse uninterrupted. The mother immediately experienced pain at the site, which continued for the entire time, but she did not remove the garlic plaster. When she presented to the ER, she was found to have third-degree burns to the site. Through the whole ordeal, the baby was not deterred from breastfeeding, and suffered no consequences. The authors do a first-rate job of differentiating between the risks and benefits of garlic ingestion versus external application, clearly saying that this case has nothing to do with internal garlic use and cannot be used as an argument against it. They also do a good job of finding the rather numerous reports of fresh garlic having caused burns when used externally, and correctly point out that the mother's persistence of use contributed greatly to the event.

Risks and Benefits of Lactation-Modulating Herbs

The risk of herbs during lactation is, in the minds of most practitioners, limited to risk to the infant. Until very recently, both the herbal and pharmaceutical literature restricted consideration of risk to the infant and completely ignored the effect of a medicinal substance on milk supply or fertility.[3,10-12] There are some signs of this changing, perhaps related to the widespread successful use of herbal and pharmaceutical lactation modulators.

Hundreds of plants from all cultures are used as galactogogues.[25] Only a few of these are known and commonly used in the United States and Europe. Fenugreek *(Trigonella foenum-graecum)* (Fig. 22-1), blessed thistle *(Carduus marianum)*, fennel, anise, nettle *(Urtica dioica)*, alfalfa *(Medicago sativa)*, marshmallow *(Althea officinalis)*, and goat's rue have gained acceptance and see widespread, if mostly undocumented, use by lactation specialists. A well-recognized lactation consultant, Kathleen Huggins, wrote of her extensive use of fenugreek in helping hundreds of women increase milk supply.[38] Few side effects were experienced by either mother or baby, although isolated cases of diarrhea or allergic reaction in the mother were noted. Very rarely, an infant may experience diarrhea. Since that report, fenugreek use has become increasingly common and accepted. Combinations of fenugreek and blessed thistle have been recognized to help if taken in sufficient amounts; doses of up to 3 g/day of each have been found efficacious.[14] Mothers need to divide the doses and may find that gradual introduction over a few days avoids side effects. Fears of lowering blood sugar, an effect of fenugreek when consumed at 15 to 100 g/day, are unfounded at this dose range.[39]

Formal studies are rare, however. One pilot study of fenugreek showed a positive effect on pumped milk volume in women.[40] The most commonly used alternative pharmaceutical, metoclopramide, enters the blood–brain barrier and can cause maternal depression after extended use; domperidone does not enter the CNS and is relatively free of side effects, but because of its orphan status in the United States, it has limited availability.

This is truly a situation in which herbs can be viewed as preferable. Galactagogues are useful only when a true low supply issue exists; their role is secondary to basic lactation techniques to building milk supply. General marketing of herbal galactagogues to breastfeeding women is considered unethical because

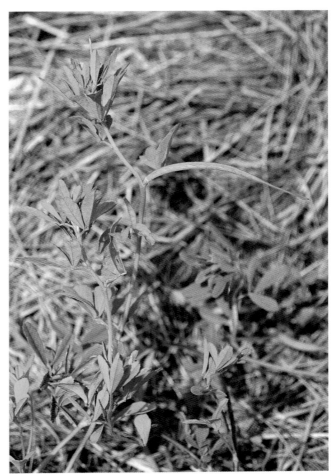

FIGURE   22-1 Fenugreek *(Trigonella foenum-graecum)*. (Photo by Martin Wall.)

it preys upon new mothers' often unfounded fears of inadequate milk. If a real problem exists, sole reliance on an herb may delay effective assistance without fixing the basic problem. It is critical to point out here that failure to establish a good supply in the first week or two of breastfeeding often results in a permanently reduced supply or weaning. Both herbs and pharmaceuticals can be very helpful in inducing and reestablishing lactation and are sometimes used in combination.[14]

It has become better known and accepted that many herbs and a few pharmaceuticals can modulate the process of lactation, affecting milk supply as well as the lactation amenorrhea state. Although herbalists may consider anything that increases milk to be a boon to nursing mothers, this is by no means a safe assumption.

Risks to Lactation

Herbal risks to milk production are not well discussed in the herbal literature. Most reference texts seem to focus entirely on the toxicity risk to the infant, and are not very consistent in identifying which herbs are traditionally used to increase or decrease milk. For example, the German Commission E entries for fennel make no mention of the herb's widespread use as a galactogogue, nor does it mention the use of sage for weaning.[3] The AHPA's comprehensive review of a large number of herbs is to be commended for considering lactation separately from pregnancy, but likewise neglects to consider an herb's potential to increase or decrease milk production.[10] Feltrow and Avila, although contraindicating just about every other herb in their book, did not contraindicate dill, citing its traditional use as a galactogogue.[9] However, the idea that increasing supply is safe, that is always beneficial during breastfeeding, is simply not true. Some mothers may have an overactive MER and produce more milk than their babies can handle; the reasons for this development are unknown. But negative consequences are widely recognized by lactation specialists.[30] Unintentional use of weaning herbs can also cause problems. "Green drinks" that contain parsley juice have been noted to lower supply. Use for oversupply, weaning, or unintentional lowering of milk supply has not been formally studied. These effects are reported in anecdotes gathered by lactation specialists but are in agreement with the traditional lactation use of these herbs. The mechanisms by which herbs may modulate synthesis or supply are far from understood, although for the galactagogues many potential mechanisms, and possibly active constituents, have been summarized in Bingel and Farnsworth's review of galactogogues.[25]

Herbs That Influence Prolactin

Endocrine stimulation of the breasts after birth drives the initial production of milk. In this stage, serum prolactin is high with even higher pulses released in response to a nursing session.[15] Later, autocrine control mechanisms prevail and each breast independently produces milk in response to milk removal.[26] Prolactin levels in later lactation are near normal between nursing sessions but spike after each feeding. Frequent and high prolactin spikes are associated with good milk supply as well as the maintenance of lactation amenorrhea.[15] Nonlactating women do not normally show elevated prolactin levels; indeed, hyperprolactinemia is generally seen as a stress response, and is associated with premenstrual syndrome (PMS) symptoms and some associated infertility states.[7]

Herbal influences on prolactin levels during human lactation have not been studied; studies done in this area have used men or nonlactating women, with the exception of chaste berry *(Vitex agnus-castus)*, which has been studied in lactating women.[41] Although the studies were done before the discovery of prolactin, and suffer from serious lactation study methodology flaws, the findings consistently indicated a galactogogue effect, in line with the herb's ancient and traditional use in Germany. Recent in vitro and in vivo animal studies found an antiprolactin and antigalactogogue effect after intraperitoneal injection with rats.[42-44] However, the question of dose has been raised. In one tantalizing study in men, low doses of a chaste berry extract raised prolactin, whereas high doses lowered prolactin.[45] It is far from clear just what effect chaste berry truly has on human lactation. It is well known, however, that it can be used to induce or reestablish normal ovulation in women with high prolactin

levels. Mohr related that those lactating women who were instructed to continue using chaste berry tincture for more than 2 weeks reported an unexpectedly early return of the menstrual cycle.[41] This return of the menses and fertility after only a few weeks after birth needs to be seen as a loss of benefit to breastfeeding mothers; decreased risk of breast and ovarian cancer is related to the lower estrogen states that are especially prevalent during lactation amenorrhea. On the other hand, other breastfeeding mothers may find this same property of chaste berry of great benefit. Mothers of nursing toddlers may find their fertility is impaired but do not wish to actively wean their children. Chaste berry could restore fertility without the need for stressful mother-led weaning or the use of powerful fertility drugs.

Bugleweed (*Lycopus* spp.) and prolactin have a complex relationship in which at least some studies have found an antiprolactin effect mediated to some degree through its antithyroid actions.[46] Thus it is generally contraindicated during breastfeeding. Given the many unknowns about bugleweed as well as prolactin, and the necessity of seeking expert medical guidance for situations involving the very complex but critical thyroid gland, general avoidance of this herb during lactation unless under the guidance of a qualified practitioner seems sensible.

HEALTH ISSUES AS SEEN IN THE CULTURAL CONTEXT OF THE BREASTFEEDING WOMAN

Herbal literature has shown little understanding of some health issues pertinent to breastfeeding women. Advice on herbs is generally presented in a vacuum, without consideration of larger cultural issues that are pressuring a breastfeeding mother. These may need to be countered first to ensure the best protection and support for breastfeeding. Fatigue, depression, anxiety, and weight loss are common health concerns for women in Western cultures. Breastfeeding mothers are like other women and are afflicted with these health concerns. A breastfeeding mother is often isolated and overwhelmed in her role as mother and exclusive source of food for her baby. She often experiences great challenges in taking on her new role as mother, and can easily feel that breastfeeding is to blame for the fatigue, anxiety, and being over her usual weight. Modern Western culture places great importance to a mother getting back to "normal" quickly, even though this is not really possible. The fact is, children change everything. Many mothers seek pharmacologic assistance to make these adjustments, and true to our culture's fondest beliefs, feel that the answer to their problems lies in a pill, whether it is a prescription or an herb capsule. And herein lies the dilemma: Mothers feel they must take "something" to fix problems that are better addressed through finding a network of supporters, sharing in discussions of parenting and breastfeeding with other mothers, or, for some, seeking counseling. Often, great improvement is experienced once improved communication of the mother's needs is achieved with those closest to her. For example, cognitive therapy is proved to be as helpful as pharmaceutical antidepressants in the treatment of postpartum depression and may be more beneficial in the long term in preventing recurrence with the next child.[30]

Breastfeeding mothers are terribly sensitive to any information that suggests a risk in using any medicinal agent yet are culturally conditioned to greatly underestimate the risks inherent in formula use. Thus she is easily led to wean if it is even hinted that this would be "safer" than using a medicine or more typically, weaning to use a drug. Although few women wean to use an herb (other than tobacco), they may very easily be led to believe that the herbal option is always more dangerous than the pharmaceutical, given the current state of written information. On the other hand, some mothers will not consider anything but the herbal option, thus making it necessary for a rational decision to be made about a particular herb (Box 22-2). It is with these conditions in mind that the following discussion on controversial herbs is offered.

BOX 22-2 Considerations for Herb Use During Lactation

- Have you positively identified the herb(s) in the product to be taken? (The botanical Latin name should be on the package.)
- Have you ascertained the quality and reliability of the herbal product company being considered?
- What is the general nature of this herb? Does it have a wide margin of safety with no suggestion of toxicity? Are expected side effects mild and reversible? Is there any documented adverse effect of the herb on the breastfed child? Again, most herbs are not noted to cause problems in infants, nor expected to, although there are exceptions.
- How old is the baby and how much is she or he nursing? Is this a very young baby or a toddler? Is the baby exclusively breastfeeding or have other food plants already been introduced into the diet? Was this child born small-for-gestational-age or premature? Does this child have health conditions, atopic disease, or allergies? Is the baby taking medications?
- What is the mother's medical history? Is this a safe herb for her? Does she use medications or dietary supplements that will require consideration of potential interactions? Does she or the father of the child have any relevant allergies?
- Is the mother intending to ingest it or use it externally? External use that does not involve the breast is mostly noncontroversial. Essential oils require more caution. Their use on the breast may not be appropriate.
- What are the risks and benefits of the herbs compared with the risks and benefits of the pharmaceutical alternative? And, does she run the risk of being told to wean to use the pharmaceutical alternative?
- Is the reason for taking the herb serious or chronic, or is it minor and self-limiting? In other words, what degree of harm is possible if the therapy does not work? If this is a breastfeeding problem, has she received help and guidance from a lactation specialist? For the sake of her breastfeeding relationship, this last question always should be answered, Yes!

A Note About Alcohol and Tinctures

Tinctures are sometimes contraindicated during lactation out of concern for the infant receiving some alcohol through the milk. In pregnancy, any amount of alcohol can have negative consequences to the fetus; exposure comes at a much more sensitive time in development. However, an occasional drink or regular light drinking (one or fewer drinks per day) is considered compatible with breastfeeding.[11,30] Heavier drinking (two or more drinks every day) may inhibit the MER.[30] Of course, heavy drinking renders the mother unfit for parenting, regardless of how the baby is fed.[14] Appropriate use of tinctures, on the other hand, would not be expected to represent this level of alcohol consumption. Tincture use during breastfeeding would seem to be a nonissue because there is no evidence of harm from a mother enjoying a beer with dinner or a glass of wine or two at a party.[30]

Unsafe Compared with What? Psychoactive Herbs

Depression and anxiety are two issues that often lead a mother to the doctor's office. Antidepressants and anxiolytics have commonly been prescribed during lactation, although their use is not entirely accepted given the potential for alteration of brain chemistry in the infant.[11] However, some antidepressants enter the milk supply to such a small extent that they cannot be detected in the baby's serum at all. These drugs are not absolutely contraindicated in lactation because the risks of formula are greater than any observed effects in the baby and untreated depression in the mother also has been shown to affect the baby's normal development.[14] Of course, such agents are not ever to be used lightly, and should be used at the lowest dose and shortest time possible. When needed, they should not be withheld or weaning forced.

St. John's wort (*Hypericum perforatum*) is an example of a well-studied herb for which considerable evidence has accumulated suggesting it is efficacious for the treatment of mild to moderate depression.[3,7,47] It is expected to be no more of a risk for infant health than any other antidepressant, and perhaps a better risk because it causes fewer side effects in the mother. Few if any effects would be expected in the baby. In a recent study, St. John's wort has been shown to have an acute negative effect on prolactin levels; within hours of ingestion, prolactin levels drop. However, after 2 weeks extending the same animal model, the herb has been found to increase prolactin levels well above those of the control group; selective serotonin reuptake inhibitors (SSRIs) have been found to elicit the same drop in prolactin, with levels later returning to baseline.[48] However, no study of prolactin response in breastfeeding women exists, and the German Commission E report indicated no known problems with milk supply in this widely used herb.[3] If there are no other contraindications to the use of this herb (i.e., concomitant contraindicated medication use), there seems little reason to contraindicate it as a possible therapy for postpartum depression (see Postpartum Depression). There are also a number of other noncontroversial herbal alternatives for many nervous conditions. Valerian, passionflower, and oat straw are just a few of the psychoactive herbs that can be expected to be safe to use during breastfeeding. It is known that anxiolytics such as benzodiazepine can cause sedation in very young infants; necessary use is compatible with breastfeeding when the baby is closely monitored.[11] Nervine and sedative herbs are very mild compared with their pharmaceutical counterparts, and the amount of constituents entering breast milk is unlikely to be sufficient to sedate a baby. Even though these would be expected to readily enter milk, no adverse events are known. Skullcap has been known to be contaminated with the toxic plant germander, so its use should be limited to reliable sources.

Weight Loss and the Infamous Ephedra Dilemma

Weight loss becomes an obsession that sets in with many mothers immediately after birth or within just a few weeks. Despite the biologically important gain of fat during pregnancy that prepares her body to feed the baby for many months, women are culturally guided to quickly return to a nonmaternal state of appearance. Herbal weight loss products abound in our culture, and mothers cannot help but encounter them. Breastfeeding mothers often approach breastfeeding counselors with questions about herbal weight loss products. Although recent bans on ephedra (Ephedra sinica) in dietary supplements has limited access to this herb, more obscure CNS–stimulant plants such as Sida cordifolia or Citrus aurantium are being substituted for ephedra.

Ephedra alkaloids are stimulants that are known to cause overstimulation and sleeplessness in breastfeeding babies.[30,49] As well, pseudoephedrine has recently been confirmed to lower milk supply by lowering prolactin levels at least on an acute basis.[12] In fact, some practitioners use pseudoephedrine in small doses to lower an overactive milk supply. It is interesting to note that the German Commission E did not contraindicate ephedra in doses of up to 300 mg ephedrine per day during lactation, recognizing its utility for asthma and apparently finding little evidence for risk during lactation when used in a traditional episodic manner.[3] Given the stimulant nature of ephedra alkaloids and caffeine, combination products would be expected to yield an additive stimulant effect. Indeed, incidents of serious harm associated with the use of ephedra products typically involve such combination products.

I have known mothers so desperate to lose weight that they said they would wean if they could not use a certain product. Many mothers have a very limited understanding of the risks of formula feeding or the benefits of breastfeeding. They may not know that breastfeeding will provide weight loss in a slow but permanent fashion; indeed, she can expect to lose more weight and keep it off by simply breastfeeding for a year compared with bottle-feeding mothers who dieted. Honest counsel on the risks and benefits of weight loss products, the benefits of breastfeeding for permanent weight loss, and the risks of weaning are essential. As of this time, ephedra–containing weight loss products are no longer commercially available in the U.S.

COMMON LACTATION CONCERNS: CRACKED NIPPLES, ENGORGEMENT, MASTITIS, AND INSUFFICIENT BREAST MILK

Breastfeeding is, undoubtedly, the best nutritional option for the human infant. No substitute provides the essential nutrients needed by the baby, along with the immunologic protection and emotional nourishment provided by breastfeeding. Although not all women are able to breastfeed because of medical reasons, economic limitations, or lack of social support, many women quit breastfeeding because of common breastfeeding problems. Breast and nipple problems can detract terribly from the mother's experience of breastfeeding. Nipple pain can make breastfeeding nearly unbearable; both engorgement and mastitis can be extremely painful and worrisome, and mastitis presents acute illness that is debilitating; insufficient breast milk (or fear that the baby is not getting adequate nourishment) is tremendously anxiety provoking. It is the responsibility of women's health care providers to supply education and support should breastfeeding problems arise, and provide options for treatment that are safe and simple, enabling breastfeeding to continue whenever possible.

Herbal treatments for problems associated with breastfeeding can be identified in botanical writings as far back as ancient Egypt. Arabian physician Avicenna described massaging the breast to improve insufficient milk production, and giving the mother black cumin, carrot, clover, dill, fennel, fenugreek, and leek mixed with fennel water, honey, and clarified butter. Herbs to induce lactation used by seventeenth-century midwives and physicians included aniseed, barley, cumin, dill, fennel, and flax—as well as the traditional well-known treatment, ale. Herbs such as St. John's wort, poppy oil, and red rose water, usually mixed in some form of oil or fat, were applied directly to the nipples for the treatment of sore, cracked nipples.[50] The medieval compendium of women's medicine, the Trotula, mentions applying plasters of vinegar and clay to the breasts for the pain of breast engorgement and mastitis.

Modern midwives have evolved a number of successful strategies for treating breastfeeding problems, and have a track record for long-term breastfeeding among their clients/patients. A number of the aforementioned herbs remain in use today.

SORE, CRACKED NIPPLES

Some amount of nipple soreness in the initial week of breastfeeding, especially with a first baby or with a long time span between pregnancies, is normal. The increased nipple sensitivity common to pregnancy usually begins to subside in the first week postpartum, but until then can lead to heightened discomfort. Normal sensitivity usually persists for 30 to 60 seconds once the baby latches on; pain caused by nipple trauma persists or worsens throughout a feeding. Prenatal nipple preparation has not been shown to be effective in the prevention of nipple pain or irritation after birth.

Nipples may become sore, cracked, and may even bleed because of a variety of reasons, including improper positioning of the breastfeeding baby on the nipple, thrush (*Candida albicans*) infection from the baby's mouth, or use of breast pads, which keep the nipple moist and can aggravate irritation or thrush. *Staphylococcus aureus* and other organisms are less commonly involved in nipple infection. Prevention is the best treatment. A midwife or lactation consultant should be contacted to assist in helping the mother position the baby properly on the breast if there is difficulty with nipple pain or trauma.

General Prevention and Treatment

- Ensure proper position of the baby at the breast; consult with a midwife or lactation consultant if needed.
- If nipples are sore or cracked, gently rinse and pat dry them after each feeding, and let air dry if possible for 10 minutes after each nursing.
- Avoid the use of breast pads, and whenever possible, spend time without a bra. This allows the nipple to remain dry between feedings and eliminates an otherwise friendly environment for microbial growth, especially in the breast pad.
- Treat oral thrush in the newborn to prevent spread to the nipples.
- Plastic breast shells can be worn to prevent irritation from clothing rubbing against the nipples.
- Wash nursing bras regularly if there is infection to avoid recontamination.

Medical Treatment

The medical treatment of breastfeeding-related nipple problems includes the general strategies listed in the preceding, as well as the addition of antibiotic ointments in the treatment of fungal or bacterial infection. Such preparations are applied after each nursing, for 2 to 5 days, and are considered safe for use during breastfeeding. A lanolin ointment may be recommended in the absence of infection, though some women report sensitivity to lanolin and cannot use it. One report recommended that concentrated vitamin E oil preparations be avoided because they can be toxic to the baby in high doses.[51]

Herbal Treatment

In addition to the general treatment strategies described earlier, a number of topical herbal preparations are used to assist in the healing of irritated tissue, and are also used as topical antiinflammatory and antimicrobial agents (Table 22-1). Herbal applications for dry, cracked, painful nipples are usually applied as extracted oil or salve, carefully rubbed on the nipple several times daily after nursing. Excess remaining on the nipple can be wiped off before subsequent feeding. When there is infection, antimicrobial herbs may be used as tincture diluted in water (1:4), also after feeding, repeated throughout the day.

Discussion of Botanicals

Calendula

Calendula has a long history of use as a vulnerary herb. It is approved by the European Scientific Cooperative on Phytotherapy (ESCOP) and the German Commission E for the treatment of minor inflammations of the skin and mucosa, and as an aid in the healing of minor wounds.[52] It is used as an oil extract and in salve for the treatment of inflamed, irritated, sore, or cracked nipples. Hydroethanolic extracts have exhibited antimicrobial and antifungal activity, and may be used as a topical rinse when there is infection.[52] There are no data in the scientific literature that supports or refutes the safety of use during lactation. There are no known or expected risks from minimal ingestion by via short-term maternal use on the nipple.

TABLE 22-1   Herbs Commonly Used to Treat Sore Nipples

Therapeutic Goal	Therapeutic Activity	Botanical Name	Common Name
Heal cracks, fissures	Vulnerary	*Calendula officinalis* *Hypericum perforatum* *Symphytum officinale*	Calendula St. John's wort Comfrey*
Moisten dry, cracked tissue	Emollient		Almond oil Cocoa butter Coconut oil Beeswax
Reduce irritation and inflammation	Antiinflammatory	*Calendula officinalis* *Hypericum perforatum* *Symphytum officinale*	Calendula St. John's wort Comfrey*
Treat fungal and bacterial infection	Antimicrobial	*Camellia sinensis* *Commiphora molmol* *Hydrastis canadensis* *Matricaria recutita* *Melaleuca alternifolia*	Green tea Myrrh Goldenseal Chamomile Tea tree

*See comfrey discussion earlier for safety considerations.

Chamomile

The use of chamomile is supported by the German Commission E and ESCOP for the treatment of skin inflammations and bacterial skin diseases.[3,52] There are no expected contraindications or side effects. Rarely, allergic sensitization has occurred from prolonged use of the herb; however, the risk appears very low, especially when *Matricaria* spp. is used.[52,53] The oil of *Matricaria* has demonstrated activity against *Candida albicans* at a concentration of 0.7%.[52] Several studies evaluating the efficacy of chamomile ointments and hydroethanolic extract in the treatment of topical inflammation and dermatitis have demonstrated improvement, either comparable or superior to cortisone.[52] It is frequently included in herbal salves for the nipples, in combination with other herbs discussed in this chapter.

Comfrey

Comfrey, also a traditional vulnerary, is generally considered safe for topical use in small amounts and for short durations on open skin. However, because of the potential for hepatotoxicity from PAs via ingestion by babies from the mother applying it to the nipples, this herb is NOT considered optimal for topical use on the nipples of breastfeeding mothers other than acutely. Residues should be thoroughly wiped off before nursing, and use should be limited to several days.

Goldenseal

Goldenseal is positively regarded by herbalists for its efficacy as a topical antimicrobial. There are no human clinical trials studying the antimicrobial effects of goldenseal. Goldenseal extract has shown in vitro and in vivo efficacy in the treatment of *Candida* infection on the mucous membranes.[7] It is commonly used in herbal salve to treat nipple infection and promote tissue healing. Berberine is sometimes listed as contraindicated during lactation. This is based on evidence from animal studies that goldenseal has bilirubin-displacing effects and may lead to neonatal jaundice, as well as on the observation that after ingestion of berberine-containing herbs, babies with glucose-6-phosphate dehydrogenase deficiency (G6PD) developed hemolytic anemia and jaundice.[7] After these herbal products were banned for use by the Singapore government, the incidences of neonatal jaundice dropped; yet, they remained high among infants in southern China and Hong Kong, where they were not banned.[7] The issue of safety of goldenseal use during lactation remains inconclusive. Blumenthal states that there are no known contraindications during lactation, but its use should be avoided during lactation until further research has been conducted.[54] No research has been conducted on the minimal amount that might be ingested by an infant from the use of goldenseal in salve on the mother's nipples. No adverse effects, nor neonatal jaundice, has been observed or reported from such use in midwifery practice.

Green Tea

A prospective, randomized trial was conducted of 65 primiparas with sore nipples who were breastfeeding after a vaginal delivery at 37 or more weeks of gestation, who were 36 hours or less postpartum, and had combined mother–infant care. Participants were assigned randomly to one of six treatment groups with one of three regimens (i.e., tea bag compress, water compress, or no compress) randomly assigned to right or left sides. Participants applied the treatments at least four times a day, from days 1 to 5 postpartum. Tea bag and water compresses were more effective than no treatment, with no statistically significant difference between the two types of compresses. The authors concluded that tea bag compresses are an inexpensive, effective treatment for sore nipples during the early postpartum period.[55] Additionally, green tea has demonstrated efficacy against methicillin-resistant *S. aureus*.[56] Water extracts of green tea or green tea bags may be applied directly to the nipple. There are no known adverse effects or contraindications to use.

Myrrh

Local anesthetic, antibacterial, and antifungal effects have been reported with use of the sesquiterpene fractions of myrrh.[57] It is almost always used as an ethanol extract because it is not highly water soluble; it is also used in powdered form in ointments and directly on weeping, sore tissue. The German Commission E monographs support its use for the topical treatment of mild inflammations of the oral and pharyngeal mucosa. The diluted tincture (1:4 with water) is dabbed on the affected area two to three times daily, or the mouth is rinsed with 5 to 10 drops of tincture diluted in a glass of water.[3] It may be used diluted and applied to the nipples several times daily, and is sometimes used as a rinse in the baby's mouth if this is the source of the thrush. Hans Schilcher, a German pediatrician, recommends its use as a treatment for oral thrush in *Phytotherapy in Paediatrics: Handbook for Physicians and Pharmacists*.[58] There are no known safety contraindications to its use for mother or baby in this manner, with oral doses of up to 3 g/kg showing no major side effects.[56]

St. John's Wort

St. John's wort traditionally was used as a topical aid in the healing of cracked and dry nipples, and thrush. Both oil and ointment have demonstrated effectiveness in the treatment of burns and for the healing of skin injuries. Hypericum ointment standardized to 1.5% hyperforin reduced skin colonization of *S. aureus* better than placebo in a prospective, randomized, placebo-controlled, double-blind study of the treatment of subacute atopic dermatitis. There are no known contraindications to use in this manner.[59]

Tea Tree

Current research, presented in a thorough review by Carson and colleagues, supports the use of tea tree oil (TTO) as an antibacterial and antifungal, as well as an antiinflammatory.[60] Limited studies have been done on TTO's use as an antiviral, but a few trials have indicated possible activity against enveloped and nonenveloped viruses.[60] Several studies have demonstrated efficacy against *C. albicans*; however, to date, no clinical trials have been done. A rat model of vulvovaginal candidiasis (VVC) supports the use of TTO for VVC.[60] The mechanisms of antimicrobial action are similar for bacteria and fungi and appear to involve cell membrane disruption with increased permeability to sodium-chloride and loss of intracellular material, inhibition of glucose-dependent respiration, mitochondrial membrane disruption, and inability to maintain homeostasis.[61-64] Perhaps what has attracted the most interest in this herb is that it has demonstrated activity against antibiotic-resistant bacteria. Further, its use in Australia since the 1920s has not led to the development of resistant strains of microorganisms, nor have studies that have attempted to induce resistance, with the exception of one case of induced in vitro resistance in *S. aureus*.[65,66] TTO applied directly to the nipple can be caustic and irritating, and should only be used highly diluted (1:10 with a carrier oil such as almond oil). Further, there is no established safe dose for babies. There are several reported cases of ataxia and drowsiness in young children who consumed 10 mL or less of the oil; therefore TTO is not recommended for use as an oral rinse for babies with thrush, and if it is used to treat nipple thrush, the nipple should be rinsed off thoroughly before nursing.[56]

BREAST ENGORGEMENT

National surveys in the United Kingdom have shown that painful breasts are the second most common reason for giving up breastfeeding in the first 2 weeks postpartum.[67] One factor contributing to pain is breast engorgement. Views differ as to how engorgement arises, although restrictive feeding patterns may be contributory.[67] Engorgement refers to swelling of the breast associated with breastfeeding. Engorgement is classified as early or late in onset, depending on when in the postpartum period it arises. Early engorgement occurs because of edema, inflammation, and accumulated milk, whereas late engorgement is caused by accumulated milk only. Early engorgement typically occurs between 24 and 72 hours postpartum but may occur any time in the first postpartum week. Even a significant amount of engorgement may occur after birth, with a sense of fullness, warmth, and heaviness in the breasts, a normal physiologic change owing to an increase in the vascular supply.[67] In some women, milk production exceeds the baby's demand and excess milk builds up, leading to distention of the alveolar sacs, and consequently hot, tender, swollen, and painful breasts. Edema may occur, if untreated, because of pressure of the surrounding tissue on lymph nodes, preventing their draining.

Early engorgement typically resolves over the first couple of weeks postpartum as the production of breast milk regulates to the breastfeeding demands of the baby. Engorgement can be extremely uncomfortable; the breasts become markedly distended, hard, and hot to the touch. It can also make breastfeeding difficult because nipple protractility is reduced and latching on of the baby to the nipple can be challenging. The mother should be taught strategies to reduce engorgement, make the nipple more accessible to the newborn, reduce discomfort, and nurse regularly to establish the appropriate amount of milk production. Late engorgement occurs anytime during the breastfeeding period, but is most likely to occur in the first year. It commonly occurs if a feeding is missed, allowing milk to build up. It may lead to mastitis, in which there is a blocked milk duct preventing adequate emptying of the breast (see the following) and subsequent local or systemic inflammatory response and local infection. Treatment of early and late engorgement is the same.

General Prevention and Treatment

- The breast should be emptied regularly to prevent and treat engorgement. To facilitate latching on if the nipple is not protracted, the mother can reduce swelling of the areola by initially hand-expressing or pumping a small amount of milk and then putting the baby to the breast.
- Engorgement can be avoided by:
  - Allowing breast milk to freely flow out of the breast not being nursed while nursing on the other side (use a cloth diaper, receiving blanket, or towel to catch the running milk)
  - Avoiding tight-fitting bras
  - Nursing the baby often, on demand, and allowing the breasts to be emptied as much as possible at each feeding
- Hot water running over the breasts can stimulate release of breast milk. Mothers can take a hot shower and let the water spray over the breasts, and let milk run freely out of the breasts; a hot bath will often also stimulate this reflex.
- Hot packs and cold packs both bring relief of discomfort. Women may try each and use the method that brings the greatest relief.
- Pumping the breasts other than to facilitate latching on during engorgement should be avoided because it increases breast milk production beyond the baby's demand, and can increase engorgement.
- Massage appears to play a role in relieving discomfort. This was suggested by a randomized masked trial in 39 women in which application by massage of cabbage leaf extract (not otherwise effective) and placebo provided equivalent symptomatic relief.[68]

Medical Treatment

In addition to the practical strategies described in the preceding, analgesics may be considered for severe pain. The AAP considers acetaminophen and ibuprofen safe and effective for pain relief during breastfeeding.[69] Serrapeptase, a proteolytic enzyme product, is commonly used throughout Europe for the treatment of inflammatory and traumatic swelling as an alternative to salicylates, ibuprofen, and other nonsteroidal antiinflammatory drugs (NSAIDs). Serrapeptase has been used in the treatment of fibrocystic breast disease and breast engorgement. In a double-blind, randomized, placebo-controlled study, 70 patients complaining of breast engorgement were randomly divided into a treatment group and a placebo group. Serrapeptase was superior to placebo in improving breast pain, breast swelling, and induration, with 85.7% of the patients receiving serrapeptase reporting moderate to marked improvement.[70] A review by the Cochrane database found that serrapeptase (Danzen) and bromelain/trypsin complex (OR 8.02, 95% CI 2.8 to 23.3) improved symptoms of engorgement, compared with placebo. Serrapeptase is available as an over the counter (OTC) nutritional supplement.

No data are available regarding its entry into milk or potential side effects in breastfeeding infants.[67]

Herbal Treatment

Midwives routinely use the common sense strategies described under General Prevention and Treatment. These are usually adequate to prevent or relieve engorgement. If there is mastitis, botanical treatment strategies are added (see the following). A popular folk remedy for the treatment of breast engorgement is the application of cabbage leaves to the swollen breasts. Fresh, refrigerated leaves are slightly crushed, for example, by rolling under a rolling pin, and are applied to the breast to draw out heat and inflammation. The leaves are left on until they become warm, and then are changed. This is repeated several times daily. According to a Cochrane review, cabbage leaves were no more effective than the use of gel packs for relieving discomfort.[67]

PLUGGED DUCTS AND MASTITIS

Milk ducts can become plugged, distended, inflamed, and tender owing to localized milk stasis. In mastitis, the plugged ducts are accompanied by infection. The differential diagnosis between plugged ducts and mastitis is the absence of signs of systemic infection including fever, local redness, and myalgia. Plugged ducts are most often easily treated by applying heat and gently expressing the blocked milk. Rarely, a galactocele may form in which the milk congeals into a thick consistency and requires aspiration. Factors contributing to plugged ducts are similar to those for breast engorgement (see the preceding), and similar prevention strategies should be employed, including ensuring proper position of the baby on the nipple during feedings, and using gentle massage and heat to facilitate milk release from the duct. It may take several days to completely empty the duct and for residual soreness to resolve.

Mastitis is a breast infection affecting at least 1% to 3% of lactating women. Symptoms include a hard, tender, inflamed area of one breast, accompanied by fever that can become quite elevated (as high as 104° F). Women almost invariably complain of chills, achiness, and malaise. Infection is commonly caused by *S. aureus*, *Streptococcus agalactiae*, and *Escherichia coli*. Fungal mastitis may also occur, typically owing to *Candida* infection, with sharp, shooting pains a common symptom. Risk factors for developing mastitis include cracked nipples or nipple sores, recent antibiotic use, use of antifungal nipple preparations within 3 weeks, and use of a manual breast pump. Diabetes, steroid use, and oral contraceptive use also increase the risk of *Candida* mastitis. Women who had mastitis with a previous child have an increased likelihood of a repeated episode.[71] Breast abscess may occur in 5% to 11% of women with mastitis.[72] Relapse is common with mastitis; therefore care must be taken to treat completely, and ensure adequate rest and nutrition, as well as avoiding contributing factors (e.g., tight brassieres, improper emptying of the breast).

General Prevention and Treatment

- Encourage bed rest; minimize visitors and social activities to allow adequate rest.
- Drink copious amounts of fluids, especially water, up to 8 ounces every 2 hours.
- The breast should be emptied as completely as possible on the affected side. Breastfeeding on the affected side is encouraged. A breast pump may be used if needed for complete emptying.
- Avoid tight-fitting brassieres and sleeping in positions that lead to compression of the breast.
- Apply hot compresses to the breast to relieve pain and allow a hot shower to run over the breast to encourage draining of blocked ducts.
- Maintain adequate nourishment with grain and vegetable soups.

Medical Treatment

Medical treatment of mastitis includes regular complete emptying of the affected breast (e.g., breastfeeding, pumping), bed rest, pain management with antiinflammatory medications (e.g., ibuprofen), and a 10- to 14-day course of antibiotics. The WHO protocol suggests that breast milk be cultured and antibiotics prescribed according to sensitivity testing in cases in which there is no response to antibiotics in 48 hours, the infection is hospital acquired, there is relapse, or the case is severe.[73] Nystatin treatment is given to the mother and infant for *Candida* mastitis. Should abscess occur, draining may be accomplished with needle aspiration.[74] Women with unresponsive and intractable mastitis should also have other causes ruled out, such as breast cancer.

Herbal Treatment

Herbal treatment for mastitis consists of herbs to treat local inflammation and infection, and those to relieve systemic symptoms associated with fever such as myalgia and chills (Table 22-2). Improvements are usually seen within 12 to 24 hours, and complete recovery usually occurs in 48 hours. Should symptoms worsen, abscesses form, or treatment not lead to adequate results within 72 hours, medical treatment should be sought. Following the general instructions for plugged ducts and mastitis (see the preceding), along with herbal treatment, is essential for good results. As mastitis commonly recurs, general recommendations such as consuming adequate fluids, avoiding tight-fitting bras, and regularly emptying the breasts by breastfeeding are recommended beyond the duration of the infection as a general practice. Women with recurrent mastitis should be evaluated for adequate nutritional intake, particularly iron, protein, vitamin C, and zinc, because deficiencies of these nutrients can lead to susceptibility to infection. Adaptogens should be considered to enhance immunity, particularly if there is fatigue accompanying relapsing mastitis. Herbs to consider when breastfeeding include ashwagandha (*Withania somnifera*) and reishi mushroom (*Ganoderma lucidum*). Additional adaptogens are discussed in Chapter 5.

- Use compresses and tub soaks to apply moist heat to the breasts. Ginger root or chamomile infusion can be used as a compress. Hot water will suffice if nothing else is available.

TABLE 22-2   Herbs Commonly Used to Treat Mastitis

Therapeutic Goal	Therapeutic Activity	Botanical Name	Common Name
Relieve local inflammation	Antiinflammatory	*Matricaria recutita*	Chamomile
		Zingiber officinale	Ginger
Relieve inflammation and treat infection	Antimicrobial	*Echinacea* spp.	Echinacea
Reduce fever	Febrifuge	*Mentha piperita*	Spearmint
		Sambucus nigra	Elder
Relieve flulike symptoms	Antispasmodic	*Humulus lupulus*	Hops
	Analgesic	*Matricaria recutita*	Chamomile
		Melissa officinalis	Lemon balm
		Nepeta cataria	Catnip
		Passiflora incarnata	Passionflower
		Viburnum opulus	Cramp bark
Promote relaxation and sleep	Sedative	*Humulus lupulus*	Hops
		Matricaria recutita	Chamomile
		Melissa officinalis	Lemon balm
		Nepeta cataria	Catnip
		Passiflora incarnata	Passionflower
		Viburnum opulus	Cramp bark
Improve immunity; decrease susceptibility to infection	Adaptogens	*Ganoderma lucidum*	Reishi mushroom
		Withania somnifera	Ashwagandha

- Apply a poultice of freshly grated raw white potato two to three times a day. This is a wonderful remedy because nearly everyone has a potato, and it is remarkably effective in reducing pain, blockage, and inflammation. Remove the poultice when it becomes warm, usually after about 20 minutes, and repeat with fresh grated potato several times daily.
- Take ½ to 1 teaspoon of echinacea tincture every 2 to 4 hours depending on the severity of the problem. Continue for at least 24 hours after all signs of illness are past. There are no known harmful effects related to echinacea use during lactation.
- For high fever, hot elder blossom and spearmint infusion (5 g of each herb steeped for 20 minutes in a quart of boiling water, covered while steeping) can be taken, 2 cups consecutively, to help break a fever. The mother should stay warm under covers to avoid worsening of chill. These herbs are considered safe for short duration during lactation.
- Gentle antispasmodics such as lemon balm, chamomile, and catnip teas may be sipped to relieve muscle tension associated with fever. Cramp bark, passionflower, and hops tinctures may be used safely to relieve myalgia and promote sleep. There are no known harmful effects related to short-term use of these herbs during lactation.

INSUFFICIENT BREAST MILK

Concern over the adequacy of the mother's milk supply is the primary reason that women discontinue breastfeeding in the first few months. Most often the woman is actually producing adequate quantities of milk—the baby's proper growth and development, as well as voiding patterns (i.e., urinary and stool frequency), are important indicators of adequate milk production and intake. Maternal concern over breast milk adequacy usually arises in response to the baby being fussy and wanting to nurse frequently—often because of a growth spurt in which the baby will nurse more to stimulate more milk production—and this is misinterpreted by the mother, her relatives or friends, or a physician who is not knowledgeable about breastfeeding trends and patterns—any of whom might recommend the mother give the baby supplemental feeding of formula or solids, and cause her to feel anxiety.

More rarely, milk supply truly is inadequate, with the baby demonstrating failure to thrive—either slow weight gain or weight loss. As maternal and infant factors other than inadequate milk supply can contribute to poor infant growth and development (e.g., maternal illness, significant stress, cigarette smoking, alcohol consumption, thyroid disorders and other hormonal problems, and certain medications; and infant neurologic disorders, reflux, congenital heart disease, and other conditions), a thorough examination of mother and infant should be performed, and a social history of the mother should be obtained to identify the cause. Proper positioning and sucking by the baby is essential for both adequate milk production, and the baby actually receiving the milk. A baby with a short frenulum, for example, will not be able to suck properly, and a baby with a congenital heart disease may fatigue easily while nursing, and may be unable to suck vigorously enough to maintain milk production. A lactation consultant can help to determine whether the baby is latching on properly; a pediatrician should be consulted immediately if the baby appears to fatigue or develops cyanosis or apnea while nursing.

General Prevention and Treatment

In a healthy woman, the following general strategies will often contribute to an increased milk supply:

- Increased sucking activity, either directly by the baby, or through use of a breast pump. Breast milk production works by demand and supply—the more demand, the greater the supply.
- Adequate food and fluid intake are essential for optimal milk production. Mothers should be directed to one of the many books (e.g., *What to Eat When You're Expecting*) that provide both guidelines and recipes for breastfeeding nutrition. Specific foods commonly recommended for increasing milk supply include oatmeal (cooked from rolled oats, not instant oatmeal) and barley soups and stews.
- Ensure that the baby is latching on properly while nursing.
- Several studies have suggested that increased skin-to-skin contact between mother and baby may prolong the duration and success of breastfeeding and should be considered when there are breastfeeding difficulties.[75,76]
- Adequate delivery of milk to the baby requires not only sufficient production but also an intact let-down reflex. Stress and inhibition can significantly interfere with milk let-down. A lactation consultant or midwife can help the mother to learn to relax during breastfeeding to improve let-down.
- Lactation consultants suggest the use of gentle breast massage techniques to increase milk supply.[77]
- Galactagogues are medications or herbs that aid in initiating and maintaining adequate milk production, and are particularly useful for women who are unable to produce adequate breast milk. They are also used when a woman wishes to breastfeed in cases of adoption or surrogate motherhood.[78] Pharmaceutical and botanical galactagogues are discussed in the following.

Medical Treatment

In addition to the general strategies described in the preceding, medical intervention includes the use of dopamine antagonists as galactagogues to augment lactation. Most exert their pharmacologic effects through interactions with dopamine receptors, resulting in increased prolactin levels and thereby augmenting milk supply. Metoclopramide (Reglan) is the preferred pharmaceutical agent because of its documented record of efficacy and safety in women and infants. Domperidone crosses the blood–brain barrier and enters the breast milk to a lesser extent than metoclopramide, decreasing the risk of toxicity to both mother and infant, possibly making it an attractive alternative. Traditional antipsychotics sulpiride and chlorpromazine have been evaluated, but adverse events limit their use. Human growth hormone, thyrotrophin-releasing hormone (TRH), and oxytocin have also been studied. There are insufficient studies on the safety and efficacy of growth hormone in the infant, TRH is not commonly used for this purpose, and although it was highly effective at increasing milk production in limited studies, oxytocin is no longer available on the market.[78]

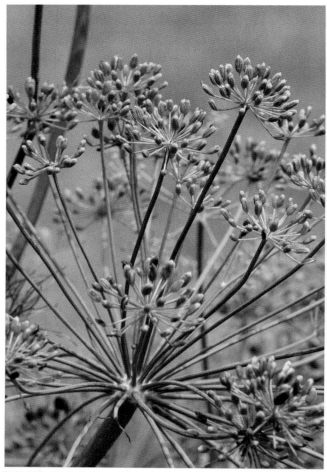

FIGURE 22-2 Fennel *(Foeniculum vulgare)*. (Photo by Martin Wall.)

BOX 22-3   Recipe from *The Ladies' Dispensatory*

To increase milk abundantly:
Leaves of sea-purslane eaten with meat
Seed of agnus-castus drunk
French barley boiled with fennel seed, eaten often
Decoction of mallows drunk
Juice of sow-thistle drunk
Lettuce eaten often
Anise drunk
Dry dill seed drunk, or the decoction of the tops
Fennel eaten (Fig. 22-2)

From Balaban C, Erlen J, Siderits R: *Ladies' Dispensatory*, New York, 2002, Routledge.

Herbal Treatment

The use of galactagogues to enhance milk production and relaxing herbs (i.e., nervines, anxiolytics) to promote let-down is as old as the proverbial hills, with traditional herbals and "recipe" books nearly ubiquitously containing recipes for these purposes (Box 22-3). The use of aromatic spices such as aniseed, caraway, cinnamon, dill, fennel, and fenugreek

TABLE 22-3 Herbs Commonly Used to Increase Milk Supply

Therapeutic Goal	Therapeutic Activity	Botanical Name	Common Name
Increase breast milk production	Galactagogue	*Althea officinalis*	Marshmallow root
		Anethum graveolens	Dill
		Avena sativa	Oats
		Carum carvi	Caraway
		Cnicus benedictus	Blessed thistle
		Foeniculum vulgare	Fennel seed
		Galega officinalis	Goat's rue
		Hordeum vulgare	Barley
		Humulus lupulus	Hops
		Pimpinella anisum	Anise seed
		Trigonella foenum-graecum	Fenugreek
		Vitex agnus-castus	Chaste berry
Promote relaxation to disinhibit let-down	Nervine Anxiolytic	*Humulus lupulus*	Hops
		Lavandula officinalis	Lavender
		Leonurus cardiaca	Motherwort
		Matricaria recutita	Chamomile
		Verbena officinalis	Blue vervain

remains popular today.[56] Other commonly used galactagogues include chaste berry, barley, goat's rue, blessed thistle, oats, hops, nettle leaf, slippery elm bark, and marshmallow root, many of which are discussed in the following. Nervines and anxiolytics are important adjuncts to improving breast milk production and delivery to the baby. Specific herbs for this purpose are listed in Table 22-3.

Discussion of Botanicals
Anise Seed, Fennel Seed, Caraway, and Dill
In the Netherlands, anise seed cookies are a traditional gift to bring to new mothers to ensure a plentiful milk supply.[77] Aromatic herbs including anise seed, fennel seed, dill, and caraway are traditionally used to improve milk supply.[56,77] They can be included in foods or taken as teas, and are common ingredients in tea products marketed as "mother's milk" blends. These herbs are approved by the German Commission E for another of their traditional uses—treatment of indigestion, abdominal bloating, mild cramping, and flatulence.[3] ESCOP also supports similar uses for fennel, anise, and caraway (dill is not discussed in the monographs.)[52] No trials have been conducted on the use of these herbs to promote lactation; however, they are generally considered a safe addition to the diet.[56] Little information is available on the culinary or medicinal use of fennel seed; however, one animal study observed an estrogenic effect (i.e., vaginal cornification and estrus) in female rats fed an oral preparation of an acetone extract of fennel seed (dose not available in abstract) for 10 days. Moderate doses increased the weight of the mammary glands and higher doses increased the weight of the oviduct, endometrium, myometrium, cervix, and vagina.[79] Transanethole from anise seed also has demonstrated estrogen activity in animal models.[52] Theoretically it may be prudent to avoid the use of these herbs in breastfeeding women with a history or risk of estrogen-dependent breast cancer. Note: It is the whole herbs that are used as galactagogues; essential oils

are not safe for internal use. Star anise is not the same herb as anise seed, cannot be substituted, and has been associated with toxicity.

MOTHER'S MILK SUPPORT TEA

Combine the following herbs:

1 oz dried chamomile flowers	(*Matricaria recutita*)
1 oz dried catnip	(*Nepeta cataria*)
¼ oz fennel seeds	(*Foeniculum vulgare*)
⅛ oz dried lavender blossoms	(*Lavandula officinalis*)

Place 1 tablespoon of the dried herbs in a cup or teapot and cover with 1 cup of boiling water. Cover the cup or pot and steep the herbs for 10 minutes. Strain and lightly sweeten if desired.

Blessed Thistle

Blessed thistle is an aromatic bitter used to stimulate digestive secretions and improve appetite.[3,57] It is a popular ingredient in galactogogue formulae, although not widely reported for its efficacy compared with fenugreek and the other aromatic seeds discussed in the preceding. The AHPA considers it safe when used appropriately; its use is contraindicated in pregnancy.[10] Although there are cautions about possible allergic reactions in patients who are sensitive to plants in the *Asteraceae* family, no allergic reactions have been reported.[3] No research has been conducted on the use of blessed thistle for promoting lactation.

Chaste Berry

The use of chaste berry to promote breast milk production dates back to ancient Greece, recommended by both Dioscorides and Pliny.[56] Its efficacy as a galactogogue, however, is somewhat controversial against modern evidence that demonstrates that the efficacy of this herb for the treatment of other gynecologic complaints, including mastodynia and amenorrhea, is believed to be in part related to its prolactin-inhibiting effects, which would seem to be directly contradictory to the promotion of breast milk.[80-84] No modern studies of the efficacy of chaste berry on lactation have been conducted. A 1954 trial compared the use of chaste berry with vitamin B_1 and no treatment; however, because of the significant methodological flaws of the study, no conclusions can be made. Animal studies using subcutaneous injection of *Vitex agnes-castus* extract demonstrates decreased milk production. Low Dog and Micozzi stated that lactogenic activity may be dose-dependent; however, the only study demonstrating lactogenic effect is that of 20 healthy males in whom prolactin secretion was increased at a dose of 120 mg and decreased at 480 mg.[56] Madaus, the manufacturer of the most widely studied *V. agnes-castus* product, Agnolyt, states that chaste berry is contraindicated for use during lactation, and lactation has been used as an exclusion criterion in other human clinical trials studying chaste berry.[56,85]

Fenugreek

Fenugreek is a traditionally used herbal galactagogue that continues to be discussed in contemporary medical and herbal literature and widely used by midwives, herbalists, lactation consultants, and the general public.[56,57,77,78] The seeds contain 40% mucilage along with coumarin compounds, diosgenin, and alkaloids such as trigonelline, gentianin, and carpaine, and make a pleasant-tasting tea—the seeds themselves being generally regarded as safe (GRAS) and used as a food flavoring. Fenugreek is thought to act via stimulation of sweat production, enhancing milk secretion. (The breast is a modified sweat gland.) Anecdotal reports of its successful use as a galactogogue date back to 1945. In one remarkable anecdotal report, 1200 women reported increased milk production within 24 to 72 hours. Adverse effects are extremely rare and include diarrhea; a maplelike aroma in urine, breast milk, or sweat (fenugreek has a maple syrup–like flavor and scent); and aggravation of asthmatic symptoms.[86] One report states that this side effect could lead to a mistaken diagnosis of maple syrup urine disease, a rare metabolic disease, in the infant, so the infant's pediatrician should be informed of the mother's consumption of the herb.[87] There is a single oral report of a premature infant having a side effect of GI bleeding. However, this is purely speculative because premature infants may have GI bleeding secondary to infection. One clinical trial was identified. A 2011 study tested an herbal tea containing fenugreek for breast milk production and infants' early postnatal weight gain. Sixty-six women were randomized into three groups: herbal tea treatment group ($n = 22$) and two control groups ($n = 22$ each). The primary outcomes measured were birth weight, loss of birth weight, time of regain of birth weight, and breast milk amount. The results suggest that maximum weight loss was lower in group 1 infants compared with control groups, and regainment of birth weight was earlier (both $p < .05$). Mean breast milk volume was also high in the maternal tea group compared with controls ($p < .05$)[Dose and tea ingredients not available].[88]

Caution is often advised when using fenugreek in diabetic or hypoglycemic patients because the herb has been shown to lower blood glucose; however, this does not appear to be a significant effect, with blood sugar changes only minimal, even in non–insulin-dependent diabetic patients.[87] Fenugreek is often used in conjunction with metoclopramide or domperidone.[86] The AHPA gives this herb a high safety rating, and does not contraindicate its use during lactation. However, it cautions about keeping doses within 5 grams of seeds per day, although substantially larger doses (30 to 40 g/day) have been used safely with diabetic patients.[10,56] The German Commission E supports the use of fenugreek for loss of appetite.[3] It is typically taken in capsule or tea forms. Fenugreek tea should not be taken during pregnancy in medicinal amounts.[87]

Goat's Rue

Goat's rue has a long history of use as a galactogogue. It was reported to the French Academy in 1873 after it was observed that this herb increased milk production in cows, a fact that was later cited in *The Dispensatory of the United States of America*, 1918.[89] It has been used traditionally as an antidiabetogenic herb; however, evidence of efficacy is lacking. Scant evidence for its efficacy as a galactogogue is found in contemporary botanical literature, and some toxicity has been demonstrated in livestock fed the herb. Nonetheless, goat's rue is sometimes used by midwives and herbalists, and its use is commonly recommended on Internet sites. Case reports of maternal ingestion of a galactogogue tea containing goat's rue, licorice, fennel, and anise seed were associated with drowsiness, hypotonia, lethargy, emesis, and poor sucking in two newborns with no evidence of infection or other illness present. Symptoms resolved after maternal discontinuation of the tea and a 2-day hiatus from breastfeeding.[34] Given even the potential for toxicity, and safer alternatives, it may be prudent to reserve this herb for short-term use only, and only for cases when other herbs have not been effective.

Oats, Barley, and Marshmallow Root

Mucilaginous herbs have long been used for their nutritive properties and to increase breast milk supply. Oats and barley are both foods traditionally given to new mothers as porridge, as well as barley in stew. They are safe for daily consumption in food quantities. Marshmallow root is considered a safe herb when used as recommended.[35] It is typically included in galactogogue infusions. There are no known contraindications to the use of marshmallow root; however, the absorption of other medications taken simultaneously might be inhibited by marshmallow root.[52]

NUTRITIONAL CONSIDERATIONS

A full discourse on the nutritional needs of the mother during breastfeeding is beyond the scope of this book. However, it cannot be overstated that optimal nutrition, adequate fluid intake, unrestricted nursing patterns, minimization of stress, and avoidance of cigarette smoke are all first-line approaches to ensuring optimal breast milk production in otherwise healthy mothers.

23

Menopausal Health

PERIMENOPAUSE AND MENOPAUSE: AN OVERVIEW

In other cultures women do not report severe symptoms of menopause and menopause is not managed medically. Relying solely on a medical perspective (or disease model) of menopause does not account for the impact of culture and other social influences and may ignore the variety of patient perspectives on the menopausal transition.[1]

Women's opinions and experience of menopause are changing. Until recent decades, menopause was a hushed topic for the 40 million American women going through "the change." Times have changed and women today are openly looking for strategies to maintain their health and minimize discomforts. Women are also concerned about preventing the problems that commonly arise during and after menopause; for example, cardiovascular disease and osteoporosis, which may occur partly as a result of the decline in estrogen that is the hormonal hallmark of menopause. Although perimenopause—the commonly symptomatic phase leading to the permanent cessation of the menses—may be associated with varying degrees of discomfort from mild to severe, it is important to remember that this can be the beginning of a welcomed new phase of life for women. Social factors are sometimes more predictive than biological factors of whether women will develop symptoms. A number of studies have found that women who report increased freedom, social status, and mobility after menopause are less likely to report negative symptoms.[2-6] In the United States, fear of aging and higher socioeconomic status are more frequently associated with negative menopausal symptoms than are body mass index or history of bilateral oophorectomy. A definition of menopause must take into account the effect of "social/cultural factors to encompass the range of experiences that women experience at the menopause transition. This biocultural definition permits exploration of the worldwide differences in menopause within the framework of the human life cycle and appropriately accounts for the influence of medico-cultural definitions of the menopausal transition."[1]

WHAT IS MENOPAUSE?

Although the menopause refers to the permanent cessation of menstruation after 1 year of complete absence of the menses, the term *menopause* is typically used to refer to what are actually three distinct phases: perimenopause, menopause, and postmenopause (Fig. 23-1).

Perimenopause refers to the period of 2 to 8 years before the cessation of menstruation, during which regular cycles of ovulation and menses become irregular before terminating, a natural result of declining hormone levels, until 1 year after the cessation of menstruation. An elevated follicle-stimulating hormone (FSH) level of 60 to 100 mIU/L on two tests done at least 1 month apart is considered indicative of menopause, although not definitive. Other hormonal indicators of the perimenopause are a luteinizing hormone (LH) level greater than 50 mIU/L and an estradiol level less than 50 pg/mL. The complete termination of menstrual bleeding for 12 months in the absence of another cause of amenorrhea heralds menopause and indicates that reproductive capabilities have ceased.

Postmenopause is the time after complete cessation of menses; technically, this is the menopause. Despite ethnic, racial, and cultural variations, the median age around the world of 51 years for menopause indicates there are some common biological elements, although individuals range from ages 40 to 58 years old. However, there is a great deal of cultural disparity related to symptoms that arise during this period. For example, according to the World Health Organization (WHO), menopausal vasomotor symptoms are not as problematic for women worldwide as they are for women in the United States and other Westernized nations. Along with diet and exercise patterns, cultural attitude differences toward menopause may play some role in these epidemiologic differences.[7]

The editor wishes to thank *Botanical Medicine for Women's Health*, ed 1 contributors Susun S. Weed, Paulaqaa Gardiner, Bhaswati Bhattacharya, Clara A. Lennox, Roberta Lee, Wendy Grube, Robin DiPasquale, Margi Flint, and David Winston for their original contributions to this chapter.

Stages/Nomenclature of Normal Reproductive Aging in Women
Recommendations for Stages of Reproductive Aging Workshop (STRAW), Park City, Utah, USA, July 2001

Stages:	5	4	3	2	1	0	1	2
Terminology:	Reproductive			Menopausal transition			Postmenopause	
	Early	Peak	Late	Early	Late*		Early*	Late
				Perimenopause				
Duration of stage:	Variable			Variable		ⓐ 1 yr	ⓑ 4 yrs	Until demise
Menstrual cycles:	Variable to regular	Regular		Variable cycle length (7 days different from normal)	2 skipped cycles and an interval of amenorrhea (60 days)	Aman 12ms	None	
Endocrine:	Normal FSH		↑ FSH	↑ FSH		↑ FSH		

Medscape®

* Stages most likely to be characterized by vasomotor symptoms   ↑ elevated
FSH, Follicle-stimulating hormone.

FIGURE 23-1 The Stages of Reproductive Aging Workshop (STRAW) staging system. (From Soules MR et al: *Fertil Steril* 76:874, 2001.)

Rather than view menopause as the end of a woman's life, it is important to remember that life expectancies in the developed countries around 80 give women an estimated equal number of years in the menopausal chapter of their lives as in the 25–35 years of fertility they experience. This positive emphasis on a woman's post-fertile years is celebrated by progressive women's health advocates. Terms such as the perimenopausal decline, past the prime of life, crone, and post-fertile do not address the new chapters of a woman's life that begin when her child-conceiving capacities have altered. The impact of patient-directed advertising and marketing that impedes the redefining of mid-life for women is disheartening. The implicit reference to women primarily as childbearers, mothers, and caretakers for upbringing focuses away from the other roles women dream of in their lives: purposes, spiritual journeys, and ambitions on nonreproductive levels that women also embody.

Bhaswati Bhattacharya

The "diagnosis" of menopause is based on clinical history and physical examination. The cessation of menses for 12 months is usually accompanied by symptoms of estrogen loss. During perimenopause, the menstrual cycle can become erratic, as can the quantity and quality of the menstrual flow. In eliciting a good history, the client might note vasomotor symptoms, including hot flashes and night sweats. Hot flashes usually last 1 to 2 years but may persist for as long as 5 years. The severity of hot flashes increases with fatigue and stress. The most severe hot flashes usually occur at night and may adversely affect sleep. Other problems seen in perimenopausal and menopausal women are depression, decreased libido, irritability, nervousness, and insomnia, which may be related to poor sleep patterns associated with night sweats. Women may report difficulties with memory and concentration, or feeling fatigued or moody.

On physical examination, there are numerous changes in the female body accompanying the perimenopause. Women present with dry skin, smaller breast tissue, and smaller ovaries. With advancing age, the walls of the vagina become thinner, dryer, and less elastic. These changes can make sexual intercourse uncomfortable, leading to dyspareunia, or she may experience pain or urgency with urination. During menopause the bone density decreases, leading to increased risk of osteoporosis. Women are also at increased risk for heart disease, with decreases in high-density lipoprotein (HDL) cholesterol, glucose tolerance, and an increase in blood pressure.

There are changes in women's social fabric as well. In losing their ability to reproduce, some women see it is a time of sexual freedom, whereas for others a time of mourning and reflection. There is a transition in the woman's role as a mother, partner, or daughter.

In terms of preventative care, in addition to her pap smears, mammogram, and blood work (lipid profile), a dual-energy x-ray absorptiometry (DEXA) scan can screen for osteoporosis. Some physicians find an FSH and LH level helpful for the diagnosis of menopause.

SYMPTOMS OF PERI/MENOPAUSE FOR WHICH WOMEN COMMONLY SEEK HERBAL CARE

Hot flashes, insomnia, memory problems, fatigue, heart palpitations, depression, anxiety, vaginal dryness, heavy vaginal bleeding, and incontinence are some of the most common problems for which women seek botanical therapies during the perimenopause and after. Women encounter new concerns about their heart and bones after menopause. Heart disease and osteoporosis raise the question of whether to use hormone replacement therapy (HRT) for protection. The sections in this chapter present the reader with current botanical thinking, allowing practitioners to help their patients sort through the myriad of options available.

HERBAL STRATEGIES: AN OVERVIEW

Following is an introduction to the most common menopausal complaints and concerns, and the herbs most commonly used by menopausal women. The herbs are presented comprehensively throughout the other parts in this chapter of the textbook.

A number of botanicals are used in the symptomatic relief or treatment of perimenopausal and postmenopausal complaints and problems—some of these, for example, soy, red clover, and black cohosh, have become almost household names. Though the use of many herbs and supplements is supported by solid scientific, clinical, and historical evidence, caution is advised when considering and purchasing herbs and supplements marketed for menopause-related complaints. Menopause is a cash cow for the pharmaceutical and supplement industries, which recognize the product sales potential in the vast number of women desiring relief from menopausal symptoms.

Botanical treatments must also be placed in the context of a holistic approach that recognizes and addresses social, emotional, psychological, and other factors that can affect women, and must be proactive in helping women to prevent the development of symptoms during this time in their lives, especially heart disease and osteoporosis.

Hot Flashes and Night Sweats

Approximately 80% of US women experience hot flashes; 15% have severe symptoms. This may lead to embarrassment, physical discomfort, and night waking, which can aggravate insomnia and related problems such as depression. Botanical therapies commonly used include motherwort (*Leonurus cardiaca*), sage (*Salvia officinalis*), black cohosh (*Actaea racemosa*), and red clover (*Trifolium pratense*) (Table 23-1).

Memory Problems

Memory difficulties may be a function of hormonal changes, and are worsened by lack of sleep and emotional stress. They can be extremely disconcerting, prompting many women to fear that they have Alzheimer's disease or another serious disorder. Botanical therapies commonly used include ginkgo (*Ginkgo biloba*), bacopa (*Bacopa monnieri*), peony (*Paeonia lactiflora*), ginseng (*Panax ginseng*), and rosemary (*Rosmarinus officinalis*). Aromatherapy is also a popular option for stimulating cognition and memory.

Insomnia

Insomnia is a common and sometimes debilitating problem for perimenopausal women, worsened by night waking caused by hot flashes and night sweats. Lack of sleep aggravates stress, memory loss, depression, and many physical discomforts. Botanical therapies commonly used to treat insomnia include skullcap (*Scutellaria lateriflora*), motherwort (*Leonurus cardiaca*), passionflower (*Passiflora incarnata*), lavender (*Lavandula angustifolia*), California poppy (*Eschscholzia californica*), kava kava (*Piper methysticum*), and valerian (*Valeriana officinalis*).

Heart Palpitations

Heart palpitations are common among otherwise healthy perimenopausal women, although cardiac and thyroid problems should be ruled out. Botanical therapies commonly used include motherwort (*Leonurus cardiaca*), hawthorn (*Crataegus laevigata*), lemon balm (*Melissa officinalis*), and black cohosh (*Actaea racemosa*).

Depression and Anxiety

The question about menopause as an etiology for depression in women has been hotly debated for years. The association between the two has been described since antiquity, and a

TABLE 23-1   Herbs for Relief of Hot Flashes, Night Sweats, and Accompanying Symptoms

Therapeutic Goal	Therapeutic Activity	Botanical Name	Common Name
Relieve hot flashes and night sweats	Serotinergic activity	*Angelica sinensis* *Actaea racemosa* *Glycine max* *Humulus lupulus* *Salvia officinalis* *Trifolium pratense*	Dong quai Black cohosh Soy Hops Sage Red clover
Relieve hot flashes and night sweats Improve sleep	Phytoestrogen SERM Nervine Sedative	See Chapter 23	
Improve mood/relieve fatigue, irritability	Adaptogen Antidepressant Nervine	See: • Chapter 5 • Chapter 23 • Chapter 23	

causal relationship had been assumed. The preponderance of current medical evidence demonstrates that depressive disorders that meet *Diagnostic and Statistical Manual of Mental Disorders*, ed 4 *(DSM-IV)* criteria are not more frequent during menopause.[8] In fact, the prevalence of depressed mood is actually greater among young adults than midlife women.[8,9]

A theory of subthreshold depression describes depressive symptoms that are less severe or fewer than required for classification of depression[8]; the similarity between climacteric symptoms and depressive symptoms also may account for the apparent relationship between menopause and depression, leading to a postulated menopausally related mood syndrome that involves less-severe depressed mood, anxiety, insomnia, irritability, fatigue, forgetfulness, decreased self-esteem, and decreased libido, possibly related to vasomotor symptoms.[10,11] Other factors strongly associated with depression in menopause include impaired health, vasomotor symptoms (e.g., hot flashes, sweats, insomnia), physical inactivity, a past history of depression and stressful life circumstances (e.g., problems with family, money, or work), or premenstrual dysphoric disorder.[8-17]

Hormonal changes, worries about aging, personal concerns, loss of sleep, inadequate nutrition, memory problems, and other physical complaints can fuel feelings of frustration and depression, and new concerns about health can lead to anxiety. Botanical therapies commonly used include adaptogens (see Chapter 5, the section Stress, Adaptation, the Hypothalamic-Pituitary-Adrenal Axis, and Women's Health), ashwagandha *(Withania somnifera)*, eleuthero *(Eleutherococcus senticosus)*, ginkgo *(Ginkgo biloba)*, ginseng *(Panax ginseng)*, dong quai *(Angelica sinensis)*, motherwort *(Leonurus cardiaca)*, St. John's wort *(Hypericum perforatum)*, and blue vervain *(Verbena officinalis)*.

Vaginal Dryness

Vaginal dryness, caused by reduced endogenous estrogen levels, is uncomfortable, increases susceptibility to infection, and has a negative effect on sexual experience with both physical and psychoemotional ramifications. Botanical therapies include topical emollient therapies to moisten and lubricate the vagina, as well as internal botanical protocol to increase estrogen, such as red clover *(Trifolium pratense)*, chaste berry *(Vitex agnus castus)*, licorice *(Glycyrrhiza glabra)*, calendula *(Calendula officinalis)*, American ginseng *(Panax quinquefolius)*, wild yam *(Dioscorea villosa)*, and black cohosh *(Actaea racemosa)*.

Heavy Bleeding

Many women experience at least one episode of heavy vaginal bleeding, or "flooding," during perimenopause in the absence of pathology. Nonetheless, incidences of abnormal vaginal bleeding in a perimenopausal or menopausal woman should be investigated to rule out gynecologic cancer. Botanicals commonly used to manage dysfunctional uterine bleeding include yarrow *(Achillea millefolium)*, lady's mantle *(Alchemilla vulgaris)*, tienchi ginseng *(Panax notoginseng)*, and shepherd's purse *(Capsella bursa pastoris)*, among others.

SUMMARY

Menopause is a time of tremendous physical, emotional, and social change for women. It can be a major life milestone for some—a time of psychoemotional reckoning, evaluation, introspection, and integration, as well as a time of starting a new phase in life. For some women, this is a smooth transition; for others, it is a rocky time, accompanied by varying degrees of symptoms, some physical, others emotional. It is also a time of increased vulnerability to developing heart disease and osteoporosis, both of which can lead to major future debility and hardship. Therefore this is a time that practitioners working with women must be aware of and address the many nuances of change women face and the enormous opportunity for preventative care. Botanicals are but one option for helping to support or restore health and balance as women face the beginning of the rest of their lives.

REFRAMING MENOPAUSE: THE WISE WOMAN PERSPECTIVE

Wise Woman model:

The joy of menopause is the world's best-kept secret. Like venturing through the gateway to enter an ancient temple, in order to claim that joy a woman must be willing to pass beyond the monsters who guard its gate...as thousands of women from all cultures throughout history have whispered to each other, it is the most exciting passage a woman ever makes.[18]

Medical model:

[Menopause] is not a natural condition; it is an endocrine disorder and should be treated medically with the same seriousness we treat other endocrine disorders, such as diabetes or thyroid disease.[19]

Theresa L. Crenshaw

The medical definition of menopause is the end of menstruation. However, this definition fails to recognize women's experience: that menopause, like puberty, is not a moment, not an end, but a metamorphosis that may take 5 to 10 years.[1] Many practitioners—from both the scientific and alternative communities—define menopause as a state of loss, or an abnormal state. Menopause is described in disease terms as an endocrine disorder, estrogen deficiency, or simply hormonal imbalance. "This insistence on viewing menopause as a disease … defines older women as aberrant."[20] In contrast, the *Wise Woman tradition* (i.e., woman-centered herbal medicine based on principles of nourishing the whole woman) defines menopause as a natural event occurring over several years, and during which the hormonal and nervous systems undergo cumulative and profound changes. In this woman-centered view, the menopausal years are an opportunity for conscious change and increased personal power, not a time of failure.

... the conventional view of menopause as a scary transition heralding 'the beginning of the end' couldn't be farther from the truth.[21]

THE MEDICALIZATION OF MENOPAUSE

During the 1960s, with the popularization of hormone replacement, menopause became a treatable medical problem—and big business. Hormones became "the cure," enabling women to remain "forever female." The norm of care for middle- and upper-class white menopausal women in the United States from the mid 1960s to the present has been some form of hormonal supplementation: a combination of estrogen and progesterone for women who still have their uterus, estrogen for those without. It is now recognized that HRT increases the risk of endometrial and breast cancer.[22-26]

Given the volumes of press devoted to HRT, one might assume that most US women use hormonal therapies at menopause; however, this is not the truth. One survey found that 52% of women wanted to avoid the use of hormones and 58% preferred alternative therapies for menopausal symptoms.[27] Even before the recent cancellation of one large double-blind study of HRT, only half of all women over 50 had ever filled a prescription for estrogen or hormone replacement, and only one third of those ever refilled the prescription. It is estimated that as many as 85% of the 37 million postmenopausal women in the United States do not want to use HRT.[28] With growing concerns over the safety of HRT, many women—and even some physicians—are turning to alternatives. An understanding of the appropriate use of herbal medicines to nourish women during this transitional time and address common complaints associated with menopause can ease this transition and promote health for women entering their "wisdom years."

REFRAMING MENOPAUSE: WOMEN'S MYSTERY STORIES

Menopause is not simply an artifact of technology that has allowed us to expand our life expectancy and outlive our usefulness. Kristen Hawkes of the University of Utah studies hunter-gatherer cultures. Her "grandmother hypothesis," based on observing the vigor and effectiveness of postmenopausal women in these cultures, demonstrates that postmenopausal women were critical to the health of their grandchildren, their community members, and the culture as a whole, and suggests that the presence of menopausal women in a society provides a survival advantage.[29] The most industrious members of the Hadza culture (i.e., the last remaining hunter-gatherer culture) are women in their fifties, sixties, and seventies: "The older woman knows the land, and its water, the seasons, the movements of the game, and the time to harvest each plant, she is not a sentiment, she is a requirement."[29] "Among many non-Western groups, the older woman enjoys increased status in the family and greater freedom in society at large. Menopause and the cessation of childbearing become positive events in a woman's life."[30] Reframing menopause from a "problem" to a "gift" is a direct help to most women. Women in cultures in which menopause is regarded as a gift have fewer problems with the physical and emotional changes that accompany it.[31] A vigorous life keeps women vital. Vigorous exercise and a whole foods diet can help us live longer; reframing menopause can help us enjoy each passing year, gray hair, wrinkles, and all.

Women's mysteries are the great events of a woman's life—menarche, pregnancy, lactation, menopause—and the stories and ceremonies associated with these life-changing times. Women's mystery stories reveal important and surprising truths from a woman-centered perspective that has been lacking in "modern" medicine. The stories, ceremonial themes, and herbal remedies that are shared here from these mystery teachings evoke and rely on the millions of careful observations and experiments made by wise women over hundreds of generations. The mystery stories of menopause are gifts to modern women from their foremothers, the ancient healers: women who were deeply intuitive and in tune with women's needs, emotional and spiritual as well as physical.

Using the mystery stories of menopause, we can ease a woman's menopausal distress by reframing her experience. Reframing is done in a variety of effective ways, including one-on-one counseling, peer group sessions, teaching, performance arts, storytelling, and through the written word. Reframing menopause allows women to think outside the box of victim-centered cultural beliefs. Because both orthodox and alternative practitioners in the United States believe that menopausal symptoms indicate a lack or an imbalance, they frequently prescribe hormones for healthy, but symptomatic, menopausal women. This makes it easy for women to remain in the role of victim: She is a victim of menopause, a victim of a body that is undependable and unable to age without medical intervention.

We have come to believe, patient and practitioner alike, that normal aging is a failure of our glands and that hormones—not just estrogen, but progesterone, testosterone, dehydroepiandrosterone (DHEA), and melatonin—are fountains of youth that will provide for us when our bodies fail. Reframing our view leads not only to a different attitude about normal menopausal symptoms, but to radically different treatments, in which herbs are not used as natural hormones, but as sources of the rich variety of helpful phytochemicals available from nature. Reframing menopause gives women a greater sense of self-worth. We reframe "loss of fertility" into "acquisition of postmenopausal zest." This gives women something to look forward to; a reward for passing through the gates of menopause. One manifestation of this reframing is the "Crone's Crowning Ceremony." This honoring ceremony, which celebrates a woman's passage through the menopausal years, has become increasingly popular in the United States, especially among "the culturally creative" and women engaged in natural lifestyles.[2,32]

We reframe mood swings and depression into "menopausal women need more time alone," validating a core need experienced by many menopausal women. Taking quality alone time during menopause appears to be a critical factor for mental and physical health. Time out can give the menopausal woman an opportunity to try out new ways of dressing, being, and serving her community. It provides the freedom to experiment, and the privacy to feel safe doing it. Quiet time alone in nature, or sitting in a comfortable chair listening to soothing music, allows the hidden thoughts and feelings that have accumulated since menarche to arise. Menopause encourages us to sort through those "holdings" and discard those that are no longer needed.

Women also find ways to reframe the "aggravating hot flash" into a "movement of energy." Women have described themselves riding hot flashes like a surfer on a wave, skiing them like a snowboarder on a fresh snowy slope, luxuriating in them like a hot bath, and enjoying them like an especially intense orgasm. Women who reframe their hot flashes often report that doing so gives them an increased sense of empowerment.

MENOPAUSE SUPPORT GROUPS

Menopause support groups help women form alliances and are a natural extension of the groups women tend to form throughout different stages of their lives, for example, alliances of young mothers at the playground sharing the joys and challenges of child rearing, or breast cancer support groups. Menopause support groups give women a safe place to tell their stories without interference or judgment. Support groups help women share remedies, ways of coping, and prevent isolation as women experience shifting roles in their personal lives, which may include having an "empty nest," divorce, or changes in work or social life. Talking about and listening to others helps us to remember that we are not the only ones going through changes, that we are part of the web of women.

A WHOLE FOODS DIET FOR MENOPAUSE AND BEYOND

The healthiest diet for most women before, during, and after menopause is a whole foods diet including whole grains and beans, nuts, seeds, a variety of organic fruits and vegetables, organic lean meats, cold-water fish, good-quality oils, and organic dairy products. A whole foods diet is heart-healthy and less likely to promote diabetes, cardiovascular, and nutritional deficiencies that become more common as we age.

Adequate, high-quality fat intake is essential; human steroid hormones are synthesized from cholesterol. Interestingly, studies have shown an inverse correlation between milk consumption and breast cancer. After tracking 4697 Finnish women ages 15 to 90 for 25 years, researchers discovered that those "women who habitually drank the most milk had only half the breast cancer risk of those who drank the least."[33] A recent study done in the United States came to the same conclusion: Women who drank milk as children and continued to drink at least three glasses a day as adults had half the rate of breast cancer as those who drank little or no milk.[34] Is it possible that cholesterol-rich foods eaten as part of a healthy

whole foods diet are health promoting, and that hydrogenated and partially hydrogenated vegetable fats are the real culprits in heart disease?[35] A study of 61,000 Swedish women between the ages of 40 and 76 found that consumption of the monounsaturated fats, even from meat, milk, cheese, and butter, lowered the risk of breast cancer. For each 10 grams of monounsaturated fat (from dairy products and meat), the risk of breast cancer fell by 55%. For each 5 grams of polyunsaturated fat (from vegetable oil), the risk rose by 70%.[36] Studies on the relationship between dairy and cancer, however, are often conflicting, with other studies demonstrating a direct correlation between dairy consumption and ovarian cancer.

The healthiest women in the world may be the women of Greece. They have some of the lowest rates of heart disease and breast cancer in the world.[37] Their diets contain lavish amounts of olive oil, goat cheese, nuts, fresh vegetables, and meat. There is an inverse correlation between the amount of olive oil a Greek woman eats and her risk of breast cancer.[38]

HERBAL MEDICINES FOR THE MENOPAUSAL YEARS

Goals for helping women experience a healthy menopausal transition may include:
- Relief from or help with bothersome symptoms; for example, hot flashes, insomnia
- Maintenance and repair of bones; prevention of fractures
- Prevention of cardiovascular disease
- Prevention of breast cancer
- Prevention and treatment of incontinence, pelvic laxity, vaginal dryness, and sexual debility

The core approach to a healthy menopause achieves these goals through the use of nourishing herbal infusions; reframing counterproductive menopausal beliefs via counseling and/or group support; a whole foods diet that includes good-quality oils, calcium sources (e.g., organic yogurt), and healthy sources of phytoestrogens (not concentrated soy isolate supplements); and incorporating consistent, adequate exercise. Personal empowerment, time for reflection, and pursuing one's dreams are also important for ease during this transition.

Nourishing Herbal Infusions

Nourishing herbal infusions provide nutritional, phytochemical support for menopausal and postmenopausal women with low cost and little effort. There is generally a high acceptance and follow-through rate among women of many ethnicities, cultures, education levels, and economic abilities.[3] When amply extracted into boiling water, herbs such stinging nettle, oat straw, and red clover release generous amounts of vitamins, minerals, proteins, phytoestrogens, and other important constituents.[39-41] If the menopausal and postmenopausal diet is not mineral-rich, the entire woman suffers; not just her bones, but her heart, blood vessels, and immune and nervous systems. Minerals may be difficult to get, even in an adequate diet.[40] Mineral values in commercial foodstuffs have decreased dramatically since the early part of the twentieth century.[40] Regular use of nourishing herbal infusions can help to close this gap.[40,42-44]

Cooked greens are also a rich source of minerals, as are edible seaweeds. Herbal vinegars are another great source of minerals and a way to encourage women to consume herbs daily, along with a healthful salad. Minerals are poorly absorbed from encapsulated herbs, and the amount taken is very small. Mineral-rich herbs are more like foods than medicines or drugs, and need to be consumed in dietary quantities—1 to 4 cups of infusion, not tea, or 1 to 3 tablespoons of infused vinegar daily. One cup of nourishing herbal infusion, prepared by steeping 35 g of dried herb in a liter of boiling water overnight, provides 100 to 400 mg of calcium. A tablespoon of medicinal herbal vinegar, prepared by macerating fresh herbs in vinegar for 6 weeks, may provide up to 50 to 100 mg of calcium.[45]

Supporting the Adrenals

Adrenal stress is often overlooked as a factor possibly contributing to a number of menopausal complaints including increased stress and irritability, panic attacks, emotional lability, fatigue, night waking, and possibly even night sweats.[46,47] Stinging nettle (*Urtica dioica*) is an excellent herbal ally. Fresh nettle leaves are eaten in soups, or as a cooked green or fresh or dried herb; 2 to 4 cups is a daily nourishing infusion. There is no scientific evidence exploring the effects of nettle on the adrenals; however, many herbalists corroborate the observation that nettle improves many symptoms associated with chronic stress and has rapid, reliable effects. Adaptogenic herbs are also important for providing adrenal support. See Chapter 5 for a comprehensive discussion of adaptogens.

Supporting the Liver, Nourishing the Blood: A Vital Component of Menopausal Health

Traditional Chinese Medicine (TCM) sees menopausal symptoms such as night sweats, hot flashes, memory loss, sleep disturbances, emotional swings, and sometimes even heart disease, as a result of liver qi stagnation, excess liver fire, and blood and yin deficiency.[48] Many herbs are used in TCM to treat these "imbalances." Among the most commonly used by Western herbalists as analogs for the Chinese herbs for moving liver qi and cooling heat are dandelion (*Taraxacum officinale*), yellow dock root (*Rumex crispus*), burdock root (*Arctium lappa*), motherwort (*Leonurus cardiaca*), and bupleurum (*Bupleurum falcatum*). Dong quai (*Angelica sinensis*) is perhaps the most popularly used herb for nourishing the blood. For use of traditional Chinese herbs, women can be referred to acupuncturists and TCM herbalists.

Phytoestrogens and Menopause

Phytoestrogens are hormones made by plants for their own biological needs. They weakly activate estrogen receptors in mammals and are found in ordinary foodstuffs such as whole grains, many legumes (not just soy), root vegetables including carrots and yams, seeds (e.g., flax), and nuts, as well as in herbs.[49,50] A diet rich in phytoestrogens confers benefits such as reduction of breast cancer risk, with little effect on premenopausal women's cycles.[51-54] Phytoestrogens may also help prevent osteoporosis, high blood pressure, heart disease, and senility.[55,56] Phytoestrogens are ubiquitous in plants; only a totally plant-free diet would prevent exposure to them. Thus phytoestrogenic foods are generally considered safe for long-term, daily use. Phytoestrogenic herbs and supplements, however, may not be safe for daily or long-term use for women at risk of developing estrogen-dependent cancers.[57]

A FEW WORDS ON EXERCISE

Although exercise alone is not sufficient to prevent heart attacks, osteoporosis, or fractures, it is vitally and tremendously important in their prevention and for the promotion of healthy hearts, healthy bones, and longevity.[58] Exercise not only strengthens bone, it also increases muscular flexibility and improves balance. A broken bone can cause a fall, but poor balance leads to more falls and more broken bones. Plus, of course, exercise improves the functioning of the heart, counters depression, and may even help prevent breast cancer. The amount of exercise needed varies, but 30 minutes daily is a goal most women can easily achieve and maintain. Any kind of exercise helps, but best results are found with a mix of strength building (such as weight training), simple walking—brisk if possible, and flexibility improvement with tai chi and yoga. Best of all, we are never too old and never too unfit to begin benefiting from some form of exercise.

SUMMARY

Menopause is a natural transition for most women. Reframing the menopause into a life and age affirming opportunity and transformation can improve women's experiences of this time. Emotional and nutritional supports—including nourishing herbal infusions and a whole foods–based, phytoestrogen-rich diet plus exercise—are often sufficient to alleviate mild to moderate acute symptoms and provide a basis for long-term health of bones, heart, and breasts, and the whole, wise woman.

HORMONE REPLACEMENT THERAPY: RISKS, BENEFITS, ALTERNATIVES

HRT has been a standard treatment for menopausally related symptoms for decades, with equivocal findings as to effectiveness, tolerability, and safety. The history of HRT is quite instructive because it illustrates many of the pitfalls of orthodox drug use. Initially, HRT was ERT (i.e., estrogen replacement therapy), and menopause was regarded as a deficiency state to be corrected by the use of the hormone. In the 1960s and 1970s, many women were advised by their physicians to take estrogen.

By 1975, medical reports were documenting an increased risk of endometrial cancer (5 to 15 times more likely).[59] At this point, for women with a uterus, a synthetic progestin (usually Provera) was added for 10 days of the month ("sequential" pattern), followed by a week of no "hormone replacement" during which withdrawal bleeding would occur. The risk of endometrial cancer was reduced, but other problems surfaced quickly. Women did not feel as well on HRT as they had on ERT.[60] Many women did not want to have bleeding every month indefinitely; the "premenstrual syndrome (PMS)" side effects during the 10 days on the progestin and the return of menopausal symptoms on the week of no hormones made them miserable. The regimen was changed again to smaller doses of progestin to be taken every day, along with estrogen. Bleeding patterns changed from predictable to unpredictable, requiring endometrial biopsies and other even more invasive tests. Many women opted out of HRT, despite hypothetical benefits postulated by the medical establishment, mostly subsequently disproved. Data from 1992 showed that despite evidence supporting the benefits of HRT, only 15% of postmenopausal women currently used HRT.[5] Of those who began HRT, fewer than 50% continued beyond 1 year.

The leading reasons for women's "refusal or discontinuation of HRT are fear of malignancy, side effects such as vaginal bleeding, weight gain, depressed mood, and breast tenderness, and social reasons such as regarding menopause as a natural transition, not as a disease that requires treatment."[61] The controversy surrounding HRT use continues, with women concerned about its safety and eager for alternatives for the symptoms.

Estrogen has a modulating effect on serotonin, dopamine, and possibly norepinephrine,[11] likely explaining its antidepressant effects. Unfortunately, progestin, which also has a theoretical basis for antidepressant effect in that it increases monoamine oxidase levels, has been shown in several studies to worsen depression.[10,11] Pearlstein reminds us, "The negative mood effects of progesterone are well-known in premenopausal women using oral contraceptives. Depressed mood has been reported in as many as 30% of OCP users and may occur less frequently with lower-dose OCPs."[60] She also points out, "Most controlled studies have reported that progesterone sequentially added to estrogen has a negative effect on mood."[60] There are studies showing that estrogen alone does improve mood and control vasomotor symptoms, especially during perimenopause and if the depressed mood is mild.[11,60,62-64]

Much of the data derive from studies involving Anglo-American women who had chosen to use estrogen, who were younger, more likely to be married, less likely to live alone, and better educated; they were more physically active, thinner, had better cognitive function and functional status, and were more likely to have a primary care doctor; other studies were done on women who chose to seek help from menopause or psychiatric clinics, who had longstanding severe symptoms.[16,65] What do these studies tell us about the rest of us? There are a very small number of studies showing improvement in depressed mood with progestin or testosterone, but many are equivocal or describe worsening of mood symptoms.[11,60,64] Please note that the progesterone in most of these studies was almost always Provera, which is actually synthetic medroxyprogesterone, not human bioidentical progesterone, which is being studied now.

Many studies have found no evidence of effectiveness of HRT (i.e., estrogen plus progestin) on alleviating depressed mood.[16,66-69] A very interesting study showed no difference in psychological or psychiatric symptoms (including depression, insomnia, forgetfulness, irritability, lethargy, and sexual difficulties) in women who received estrogen or placebo implants.[67] Cognitive function was unrelated to menopause or HRT; sexual activity and satisfaction were almost identical in estrogen- and placebo-treated groups.[62] Two studies of positive mood and life satisfaction during the menopausal transition showed that life satisfaction was predicted by earlier attitudes; positively associated with feelings for partner and exercise; negatively associated with stress and smoking; and unaffected by menopause status, hormone levels, or HRT; "the most important predictor of positive mood at the phase of late perimenopause or postmenopause was positive mood in the premenopause."[70,71]

In addition to the lack of solid proof of efficacy, the risks of HRT that were well documented before 2002 included stroke, venous thromboembolism, worsening of hypertriglyceridemia, cholelithiasis, deterioration of liver function in women with liver disease, and increased pain in benign breast disease[72]; abnormal bleeding, weight gain, fluid retention, blood pressure elevation, glucose intolerance, and headache.[73] Caution was advised in women with sickle cell anemia, obesity, and tumors.[74]

The most serious risk, however, is the increased risk of breast cancer, which becomes significant even after only 1 year of use[75]; by 10 years the relative risk of developing breast cancer is 30% higher in women taking estrogen[72]; "adding a progestin may further increase risk substantially above this"[72,76]; and "there was a 43% increase in deaths from breast cancer in patients who took HRT for longer than 10 years."[73] In 2002, results of two randomized trials of HRT (i.e., the Women's Health Initiative [WHI] and the Heart and Estrogen/Progestin Replacement Study [HERS] trials) showed that it was not cardioprotective, and may increase risk of cardiovascular disease.[72,77,78] Premarin (i.e., conjugated equine estrogens [CEEs]) may be more risky than estradiol because it causes levels of equilin estrogens that are many times higher than the levels of estrone and estradiol that occur,[79] but there is still no evidence that estradiol is effective. The summary of current evidence about the overall clinical relevance of currently prescribed HRT in treatment of depression is that it is unproven[80] to be effective, and proven to be hazardous.

HRT remains a cornerstone of allopathic treatment of menopausal symptoms. Since HRT was introduced 70 years ago, a steady flow of studies has produced evidence of both harmful and beneficial effects. Recent studies show HRT to be associated with an increased risk of breast cancer, myocardial infarction, cerebrovascular disease, and thromboembolic disease. Based on these new data, HRT prescribing practices are rapidly changing; health care professionals are no longer recommending it as a "preventative medicine."

Today, the main reasons for prescribing HRT are relief of menopausal symptoms and prevention or management of osteoporosis. Strong evidence from both observational studies and randomized controlled trials (RCTs) show estrogen to be highly effective for controlling hot flashes and genitourinary symptoms.[81] Urogenital atrophy and vasomotor instability are improved with HRT.

CONVENTIONAL TREATMENT APPROACHES

Until relatively recently, the allopathic gold standard of treatment for menopause has been HRT. Approximately 38% of postmenopausal women in the United States in 1995 used HRT—estrogen with or without progestin—to treat symptoms of menopause and prevent chronic conditions such as cardiovascular disease and osteoporosis.[82] In 2000, 46 million prescriptions were written for Premarin (CEEs), making it the second most frequently prescribed drug in the United States.[83] HRT was indicated for the classic symptoms of hot flashes and night sweats, which related to declining estrogen levels and are reported by 85% of US menopausal women.[84,85] HRT can effectively treat menopausal symptoms such as vasomotor instability (e.g., hot flashes), mood swings, concentration difficulties, dyspareunia, and vaginal irritation caused by dryness.[86]

For women with an intact uterus, HRT includes both an estrogenic agent and a progestin. Progestins are generally indicated to offset the increased risk of endometrial cancer with the use of unopposed estrogen. For women using both an estrogenic agent and a progestin, there is a choice between cyclic and continuous dosing regimens. With the cyclic dosing regimens (i.e., intermittent high-dose progestin and estrogenic withdrawal), women can anticipate resuming a predictable (but artificial) menstrual cycle. With the continuous regimens (i.e., continual estrogen and low-dose progestin, without withdrawal), women can anticipate amenorrhea with occasional erratic spotting. Progestins are usually not recommended for women who have had a hysterectomy.[87]

The preventive effects of HRT on long-term health outcomes are now challenged by new data from clinical studies. In terms of beneficial effects, randomized clinical trials have proved that HRT is effective for vasomotor and urogenital symptoms.[88] A meta-analysis of estrogen treatment (oral or intravaginal) for urinary incontinence revealed a significant improvement in subjective symptoms, but no improvement in objective measures such as urodynamic testing.[89] It is unclear if HRT helps directly with depression and other nervous system disorders. A "domino" effect may occur; for example, relieving hot flashes may improve sleep, which may improve mood.[90]

Other allopathic treatments for hot flashes include a combination of ergotamine, belladonna alkaloids, and phenobarbital, which has been used for many years to relieve climacteric symptoms. Alpha-adrenergic agents (e.g., clonidine), are used for the relief of vasomotor symptoms. Physicians also prescribe selective serotonin reuptake inhibitors (SSRIs) to treat depression and mood disturbances related to menopause. Off-label use of megestrol acetate may help control hot flashes.

Osteoporosis

Another area where HRT was found to be helpful was for the treatment of osteoporosis. Osteoporosis is estimated to affect 200 million women worldwide.[91] The consequence is that more than 250,000 hip fractures occur annually, with a health care cost of approximately $14 billion per year. Hip fracture carries a 10% to 20% risk of death within a year and a 25% chance of institutionalization.[92] After age 35 men and women start to lose approximately 1% of bone mass each year. However, bone loss is accelerated during the first 3 to 4 years after menopause. Estrogen therapy inhibits age-related bone loss after menopause by acting on osteoclasts (i.e., bone-resorbing cells) and osteoblasts (i.e., bone-building cells) to decrease bone resorption. Estrogen also helps calcium to be absorbed in the gut. The daily dosage required to prevent bone loss is 0.625 mg of conjugated estrogen, but even 0.3 mg may suffice if taken with adequate calcium supplements.[86] Estrogen must be taken for at least 7 years to provide significant benefit and the risk of osteoporosis reverts back to baseline once the estrogen is discontinued.[81] Bone loss resumes within a year after stopping HRT, however, and bone turnover rises to the level of that in untreated women within 3 to 6 months.[93] RCTs have shown that HRT reduces bone loss at clinically relevant sites such as the spine and neck of the femur.[94] The WHI study was the first randomized controlled trial to show a reduction in hip fracture with HRT.[95] No herbal product studied has been proven effective in the prevention or treatment of osteoporosis.[96]

Nonhormonal therapies such as bisphosphates (e.g., Fosamax) and selective estrogen receptor modulators (SERMS) are as effective as HRT for preventing fractures. Bisphosphates inhibit osteoclast activity in the bone. RCTs have demonstrated Fosamax efficacy increasing bone mineral density (BMD) and reducing fractures.[97] Etidronate (Didronel) is another bisphosphate. It is Food and Drug Administration (FDA)–labeled for the treatment of Paget's disease, but has had an off-label use as a treatment for osteoporosis in patients who cannot tolerate Fosamax. Intranasal calcitonin is a polypeptide hormone that also inhibits osteoclastic activity; an intranasal form is now available for treatment of established osteoporosis. A SERM, raloxifene (Evista), has been FDA labeled for prophylactic treatment of osteoporosis. For women whose main interest is prevention of osteoporosis, this agent offers an alternative to traditional HRT. Other SERMs pending FDA labeling include droloxifene and idoxifene.[86]

Colorectal Cancer

Observational studies have consistently suggested that HRT reduces the risk of colorectal cancer. The WHI study, however, was the first randomized controlled trial to confirm this, reporting six fewer colorectal cancers each year per every 10,000 women taking HRT compared with the placebo group.[95]

Cardiac Disease

Recent studies have cast doubt on the cardioprotective effects of HRT, the most frequently cited reason for starting women on HRT—further undermining conventional recommendations. Today, the results of the WHI have radically changed the way doctors are prescribing HRT. The WHI, the largest randomized trial of HRT, showed that long-term use of HRT poses more risks than benefits for healthy postmenopausal women. The WHI studied the use of estrogen plus progestin for prevention of coronary heart disease in 16,608 postmenopausal women age 50 to 79 years. After 5 years of follow-up, this arm of the study was stopped because of the adverse effects of the intervention. The researchers found that HRT increases the risk of several events: coronary heart disease events, invasive breast cancer, stroke, venous thromboembolic events, and pulmonary embolism.[95]

HERS examined the effects of HRT in postmenopausal women with coronary artery disease. HERS was a large randomized controlled trial of 2763 women with an average follow-up time of 4.1 and 6.8 years. It showed no statistically significant difference between the HRT (estrogen plus medroxyprogesterone) group compared with the placebo group in either of the primary outcomes (nonfatal myocardial infarction or coronary heart disease death) or in the secondary outcomes (coronary revascularization, unstable angina, congestive heart failure, resuscitated cardiac arrest, stroke or transient ischemic attack, and peripheral arterial disease). However, further analysis showed a significant time trend, with more coronary heart disease events in the hormone group than in the placebo group during the first year of treatment and fewer in years 3 to 5. The recommendation after the HERS study was that postmenopausal HRT should not be used for reducing risk of coronary heart disease.[98] Thus the WHI and HERS trials have shown that continuous treatment with 0.625 mg of CEEs plus 2.5 mg of medroxyprogesterone increases the risk of heart disease events by 29% (37 versus 30 per 10,000 person years) and stroke by 41% (29 versus 21 per 10,000 person years).[95,98]

Thromboembolic Disease

Studies generally show an increased risk of deep venous thrombosis and pulmonary embolus in women taking HRT.[99,100] History of or risk factors for these conditions are contraindications to the use of HRT.

Endometrial Cancer

More than 30 observational studies have shown that unopposed estrogen therapy increases the risk of endometrial cancer. Progestin use in women with a uterus mitigates the risk of cancer associated with estrogen.[81]

Breast Cancer

A large meta-analysis of data from 51 observational studies reported that the risk of breast cancer increased by 2.3% for every year of use of HRT.[22] This increased risk does not become significant unless HRT is taken for longer than 5 years. The risk of breast cancer falls after stopping HRT and returns to baseline within 5 years.

Because the WHI study stopped early, it could not examine the risk of death from breast cancer. However, it did confirm the excess risk of breast cancer with HRT. There was a 15% increase in invasive breast cancer in women taking estrogen plus progestogen for less than 5 years and a 53% increase in those taking it for longer than 5 years. The study concluded that for every 10,000 women taking estrogen and progestogen, there would be eight more cases of invasive breast cancer a year.[22,95]

Mood and Cognitive Changes

Studies have also indicated that many cases of depression relate more to life stresses or "midlife crises" than to the hormonal changes of menopause.[87] Menopause is not only a physical change but also a social transition. These transitions include an alteration in family roles, grown children leaving home; a changing social support network; a changing relationship with one's partner; deaths of parents or other close relatives; and changes in finances as one looks to retirement. Dysphorias, irritability, anger, memory loss, and losses of clarity of thought are among the most frequent symptoms reported by menopausal women, although the research data on the role of estrogen loss to depression and cognitive changes are mixed.[87] It is often the presence of mood- or memory-related symptoms that motivates a woman to request HRT. Physicians are now prescribing SSRIs to help women with these symptoms.

SIDE EFFECTS OF HORMONE REPLACEMENT THERAPY

There are many reasons for noncompliance with HRT, but the most commonly cited include thrombotic complications, side effects on mood, and changes in the breasts.[87] Only about one in three women stay on HRT after a year as a result of the side effects. Adverse effects attributed to HRT include breast tenderness, breakthrough bleeding, and thromboembolic disorders. In addition, there are relative and absolute contraindications to the use of HRT (Box 23-1).

BOX 23-1 Relative and Absolute Hormone Replacement Therapy Contraindications

Relative Contraindications
- Gallbladder conditions
- Uterine fibroids
- Poorly controlled high blood pressure
- Endometriosis
- Chronic liver dysfunction
- History of thrombotic disease
- Acute intermediate porphyria

Absolute Contraindications
- Breast cancer
- Estrogen-sensitive cancers
- Endometrial cancers
- Undiagnosed vaginal bleeding
- Active liver disease
- Active thrombotic disease

WOMEN'S OPINIONS OF HORMONE REPLACEMENT THERAPY

Women's experiences of menopausal symptoms vary widely and have been found to relate to factors such as social class, ethnicity, and culture. The most common reason motivating women to take HRT is the relief of menopausal symptoms. Before the WHI, women who were trying HRT were having serious concerns about its use, and discontinuation was a major issue.[101,102] In 1995, a survey of women aged 50 to 80 found that 50% of women who had never used HRT believed that hormones were unnecessary, and 18% believed that menopause was a natural event not requiring medication. Safety concerns were expressed by nearly 30% of women who never used HRT, including fear of cancer (15.3%) and fear of side effects (12.9%).[103] Only a third to a half of women who leave their physician's office with a prescription for HRT are still taking it 1 year later. Women express concerns about the prospect of having menses indefinitely, the potential side effects of HRT, and the increased risk of cancer.[104,105] Forty percent of women discontinue HRT within 8 months of initial therapy or never fill the prescription.[106] Women who are currently using HRT are more likely to have had a hysterectomy than women who have never used HRT. In one survey of women who had undergone a hysterectomy, 50% of women were using HRT, 37% of women had used it in the past, and 24% of women never used HRT.[103]

NATURAL HORMONES

The most frequently prescribed estrogen in the traditional HRT regimen is CEE. As public awareness of the source of CEE has grown, more women find this choice objectionable, whether out of concern for animal rights or out of an aversion to ingesting hormones that come from horse urine.[107] There has been a demand for natural sources of estrogen.

The three most common forms of estrogen produced by the body are estradiol (E2), estrone (E1), and estriol (E3). Estradiol, produced by the ovaries, is the most potent. Estrone becomes the most plentiful estrogen after menopause. Estriol is the weakest and is the estrogen that becomes more plentiful during pregnancy.[108] Estradiol can be produced from plants, and there is a growing market for such products. These estrogens are referred to as "natural" or "bioidentical" hormones, and are formulated by compounding pharmacies. There is little in the medical literature about these hormones. Additionally, among the lay public, there has been a growing demand for individually compounded hormone regimens. This demand is in response to the work of Wright and Morgenthaler and others who argue that HRT should mimic the ratios of E1, E2, and E3 naturally found in the body, or roughly 3%, 7%, and 90%, respectively.[108,109] This combination is known by the name of triestrogen or Tri-Est, which may consist of 1 mg estriol (E3), 0.125 mg estrone (E1), and 0.125 mg estradiol (E2) taken twice daily. This is equivalent to 0.625 mg CEE. There is also a product on the market called Bi-Est or biestrogen, which is estriol and estradiol. Bioidentical estrogens are compounded into sublingual troches, transdermal creams, and gels. Although only recently gaining popularity in the United States, these products have been used extensively in Europe, where they are very popular. Although these estrogens are compounded in doses equivalent to prescription estrogens, and appear to have equivalent effects in regards to stimulation of the endometrium, there are, thus far, no studies that look at their safety or efficacy, particularly in regard to preventing or treating osteoporosis.[108] Although these are "natural" products, the safety of this estrogen and progesterone is being questioned after the publication of results from the WHI.

If many of the first-line measures are ineffective, such as clonidine, megestrol acetate, and antidepressants, low doses of bioidentical hormones may be initiated and titrated upward as needed for symptom control. Topical estrogen can be applied to the vagina for vaginal dryness or thinning, or painful intercourse.

PROGESTERONE

Progesterone plays a very important role in the shedding of the endometrium to avoid endometrial hyperplasia in postmenopausal women after they are exposed to estrogen in HRT. Therefore it is now standard care to prescribe some form of progesterone with HRT in women with an intact uterus. It is also believed that progesterone has additional benefits and risks. Synthetic progestins such as medroxyprogesterone and norethindrone have been shown to decrease vasomotor symptoms.[110,111] Reported androgenic effects of synthetic progestins include fluid retention, glucose metabolism, reduction of HDL cholesterol levels, headaches, and mood disturbance.[112] Furthermore, it was recently reported that women who were given HRT using a synthetic progestin had an increased rate of breast cancer compared with women who took estrogen alone.[25]

Natural progesterone taken by mouth is inactivated in the gastrointestinal (GI) tract. However, micronizing progesterone is a process designed to increase the half-life of progesterone and reduce its destruction in the GI tract. Micronization decreases particle size and enhances the dissolution of progesterone.[112] Unlike synthetic progestins, micronized progesterone has not been shown to affect mood or lipid profile (or adversely affect pregnancy outcome).[112,113] The most commonly reported side effects are fatigue and sedation. Extensive use in Europe has shown that the micronized form can be taken once daily and is as effective as the synthetic progestins in controlling endometrial growth, but displays significantly fewer metabolic side effects.[108,114]

A number of compounding pharmacies make natural progesterone products as alternatives to medroxyprogesterone acetate. Certain plants, including wild yam and soybeans, produce sterols called saponins that have chemical structures similar to progesterone. These sterols can be used as precursors for progesterone in the pharmacy. Most preparations that contain bioidentical progesterone contain United States Pharmacopeia (USP)–grade progesterone, formulated from these plant sterols, and sold in bulk.[108] The hormone is not available from any natural source without extraction and synthesis. The body is not able to convert plants such as wild yam into progesterone on its own. Contrary to popular understanding, wild yam creams provide no active hormones because the sterols in plants cannot be converted into active steroidal compounds.[115] Only wild yam creams to which bioidentical progesterone has been added will exert a progestogenic effect. Bioidentical progesterone is sold as a topical cream, a vaginal gel, and rectal or vaginal suppositories. The transdermal cream is formulated to contain 400 mg progesterone per ounce and is easily absorbed into the skin. The usual doses are ¼ and ½ teaspoon once or twice a day. Recent research has cast doubt on whether the transdermal creams, even in prescription strengths, provide serum levels sufficient to protect the endometrium.[116]

In a double-blind placebo-controlled trial, 102 healthy women within 5 years of menopause applied 20 mg transdermal progesterone cream or placebo daily for 1 year. Each woman received daily multivitamins and 1200 mg of calcium and was seen every 4 months for review of symptoms. Improvement or resolution of vasomotor symptoms, as determined by review of weekly symptom diaries, was noted in 83% of treatment subjects and 19% placebo subjects. However, the number of women who showed gain in BMD exceeding 1.2% did not differ.[117]

BOTANICAL ALTERNATIVES TO HORMONE REPLACEMENT THERAPY

In the past several years, more than 100 over-the-counter (OTC) products targeted for menopausal women have reached the market, and women spend an estimated $600 million per year on these products. For nearly 70% of women, the transition into menopause is smooth[118]; however, many women seek advice for management of symptoms such as hot flashes or vaginal dryness. Women also seek information on the prevention of associated long-term health problems such as osteoporosis and coronary artery disease. It is essential that the practitioner address the whole woman. An individual assessment of her health risk factors and preferences for supportive care are chosen based on the symptoms she experiences and her risk of heart disease, breast cancer, and osteoporosis. This section addresses the clinical findings for

botanicals commonly used as substitutes for HRT, or as treatments for menopausal concerns (Table 23-2). Specific menopausal concerns are also addressed in individual chapters.

Red Clover

Red clover was not traditionally used on a long-term basis for hot flashes, but today it is commonly used as an "estrogen substitute" for menopausal symptoms and the prevention of osteoporosis. Red clover contains phytoestrogenic isoflavones such as formononetin, biochanin A, daidzein, and genistein. Red clover has estrogenic properties on endometrial and breast cancer cells in vitro.[119,120] It is unknown whether long-term use has an estrogenic effect on the breast or endometrium. One small double-blind, randomized controlled pilot study looked at the effect of a 3-month course of a 33 mg red clover isoflavone supplement on endometrial cells taken between days 8 and 11 of the menstrual cycle. In this study of 30 late-reproductive age and perimenopausal women, there was no difference in endometrial index or thickness compared with the placebo groups.[121] Red clover extract is marketed as Promensil in Europe; it contains 40 mg isoflavones per tablet, which is approximately equivalent to the isoflavone content of a cup of soy milk or 5 cups of chickpeas. Promensil showed significant estrogenic activity, equivalent to 10 to 8 mol/L estradiol.[122] A 30-week small double-blind, randomized crossover trial of 43 perimenopausal and menopausal women with three hot flashes daily found no significant difference between Promensil (40 mg) or placebo to manage hot flashes.[123] A randomized, double-blind placebo-controlled prospective trial of 37 postmenopausal women with symptoms of estrogen deficiency was performed over a 12-week period. The women were randomized to three treatment groups: placebo, 40 mg, or 160 mg (isoflavone extract containing red clover isoflavones). There was no significant difference in the incidence of flashes among the three groups. There was no significant difference between the groups in Greene Menopause Symptom Scores, vaginal pH, levels of FSH, sex hormone–binding globulin (SHBG), or total cholesterol, liver function, or blood parameters. A statistically significant increase in HDL cholesterol of 18.1% ($p = .038$) occurred in the 40-mg group.[124] Isoflavones have been found to increase arterial compliance in postmenopausal women,[125] thus presumably reducing heart disease risk. In another double-blind, randomized study, 60 postmenopausal

TABLE 23-2	Botanicals Commonly Used for Treating Menopausal Symptoms		
Botanical Name	**Common Name**	**Dose**	**Symptom/Purpose**
Actaea racemosa	Black cohosh	40-200 mg dried root daily	For vasomotor complaints such as hot flashes, vaginal dryness
Angelica sinensis	Dong quai	200 mg standardized extract daily	For vasomotor complaints such as hot flashes, vaginal dryness
Melissa officinalis	Lemon balm	1-3 cups of tea daily	To improve mood and insomnia, relieve anxiety
Panax ginseng	Ginseng	100-300 mg standardized extract daily	To improve energy and mood
Trifolium pratense	Red clover	40 mg daily	For vasomotor complaints such as hot flashes, vaginal dryness
Valeriana officinalis	Valerian	200 mg extract at bedtime	For sleep disturbances

women received either a commercially available red clover isoflavone supplement (80 mg/day) or placebo for 90 days. In this trial, red clover isoflavone supplementation significantly decreased the rate of menopausal symptoms and had a positive effect on vaginal cytology.[126] A recent meta-analysis and systematic review showed mixed benefits in reducing hot flashes compared with placebo.[127,128]

Although clinical research is lacking, the phytoestrogenic effects of red clover may, in theory, produce undesirable or unpredictable effects in the face of hormone-dependent tumors. Therefore caution is advised in patients with estrogen receptor–positive neoplasia,[129] and patients taking hormonal or antihormonal medications such as tamoxifen.[129,130] Use with caution in patients susceptible to bleeding problems or those taking anticoagulants.[129]

Dong Quai

For the past 3 years, sales of Rejuvex, the most popular health remedy containing dong quai, have been extensive among hundreds of thousands of users in the United States.[131] In the Chinese materia medica, dong quai is indicated for disorders of the women's reproductive system, including menopausal symptoms, dysmenorrhea and irregular periods, and menstrual cramps, and is used to "strengthen the blood." The symptoms of "deficient blood" listed in Chinese texts are similar to those that Western medicine associates with menopause: menstrual flow abnormalities, nervousness, dizziness, insomnia, and forgetfulness.[87] Dong quai, traditionally prescribed as a tonic for women, is most commonly used as part of a mixture. It is sold in the United States for use alone or as part of newly formulated, nontraditional herbal combinations.

Its chemical constituents include furocoumarins, beta-sitosterol, flavonoids, and others. However, its presumed mechanism of action remains unknown. In a double-blind, randomized controlled study, 71 postmenopausal women ages 40 to 65 were instructed to take three capsules three times daily, equivalent to taking 4.5 g of dong quai root daily (standardized to 0.5 mg/kg ferulic acid). There was no difference in Kupperman Index scores, number of hot flashes, or endometrial thickness and vaginal maturation. A recent systematic review found dong quai to be ineffective in ameliorating menopausal symptoms at the dosages and preparations in the clinical trials reviewed.[127]

It would be valuable to study TCM formulae prescribed in accordance with TCM diagnostic methods. Dong quai does not contain the typically reported phytoestrogens, and the data on stimulation of estrogen receptor–positive breast cancer cells or binding to estrogen receptors are conflicting.[61,119,120] Dong quai contains coumarins and can cause bleeding when administered concurrently with warfarin; the furocoumarins contained in dong quai can cause photosensitization.

Black Cohosh

Black cohosh (Fig. 23-2) is widely used in Europe and has become increasingly popular in the United States as a treatment for menopausal symptoms (e.g., hot flashes, vaginal dryness). Since 1956, more than 1.5 million women in Germany have used black cohosh extract, and in 1994 menopausal women in Germany, Scandinavia, and Austria used over 6.5 million monthly dosages of black cohosh extract.[132] It is an indigenous North American plant long used by Native American populations. Black cohosh contains several triterpenes and isoflavonoids. Other constituents are ascorbic acid, beta-carotene, butyric acid, calcium, chromium, selenium, thiamine, zinc, and salicylic acid. The German Commission E recommends it for premenstrual discomfort and dysmenorrhea as well as climacteric neurovegetative complaints.[133]

Studies of black cohosh's physiologic effects have had mixed results. Originally, it was believed that black cohosh had estrogenic effects, but now there is evidence to dispute this claim.[61,119,134,135] Data that suggest a nonestrogenic or estrogen-antagonistic effect of the herb on human breast cancer cells may lead to the conclusion that treatment may be a safe natural remedy for menopausal symptoms in breast cancer, but the data are mixed.[136,138] There are no long-term safety studies using black cohosh in women who have had breast cancer.[139]

In numerous case studies, standardized black cohosh monodrug preparations have been used to treat menopausal symptoms, menstrual disorders (e.g., amenorrhea, oligomenorrhea, dysmenorrhea, polymenorrhea, PMS), and complaints during

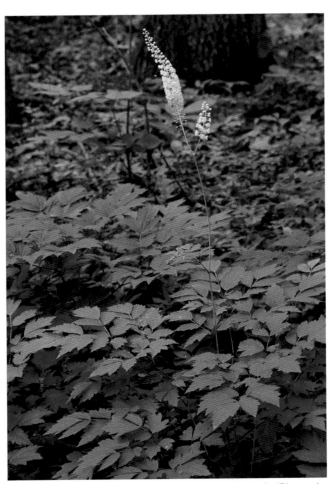

FIGURE 23-2 Black cohosh *(Actaea racemosa)*. (Photo by Martin Wall.)

pregnancy. The literature describes the efficacy of black cohosh in approximately 1500 patients with menopausal disorders, citing distinct and clear improvements in the clinical picture and good to very good therapeutic responses.[134,140] By 1960, 1256 case reports in 111 published studies by gynecologists, general practitioners, internists, and neurologists had evaluated the use of black cohosh for the treatment of menopausal symptoms with positive effects and few side effects.[140] Most of the clinical trials assessing the use of black cohosh for menopausal complaints have been carried out using Remifemin (Schwabe North America, Green Bay, WI). Remifemin (Schwabe North America, Green Bay, WI) is standardized with respect to triterpene glycoside content, with each 20-mg tablet containing 1 mg of 27 deoxyactein; it is also available in a standardized liquid extract. Remifemin is the most clinically studied black cohosh product and has been the subject of more than 20 trials over the last 40 years. For an assessment tool, many studies have used the Kupperman Menopausal Index, which is a weighted sum of 10 individual symptoms: hot flashes, outbreaks of sweating, sleep disorders, nervousness, irritability, dizziness, difficulty in concentration, joint pains, headaches, and palpitations.[141] The clinical trials are generally of poor methodically quality, small, and lack a control group. The results are mixed but most studies show benefit.[142-151] Recent systematic reviews demonstrate that the majority of studies indicated that extract of black cohosh (Actaea racemosa) improved menopause-related symptoms.[127,152,153]

Black cohosh is not usually used on a long-term basis, and no clinical trials have lasted for more than 6 to 12 months. However, the safety profile is reassuring and black cohosh is well tolerated.[154,155] Tolerability of Remifemin appears to be good, with mild GI symptoms being the only significant adverse effect. Although black cohosh may be useful for menopausal symptoms, long-term use cannot be presumed to be safe until appropriate safety studies are conducted. Research by the German manufacturer has shown that black cohosh supplements have no effect on FSH, LH, estrone, estradiol, progesterone, SHBG, the vaginal maturation index, or endometrial thickness.[156] To date, four case reports of possible hepatotoxicity have been published, although previous safety reviews suggest that black cohosh is well tolerated and adverse events are rare when it is used appropriately.[127,153,157] Additionally, there is one case report of a woman with severe asthenia and very high blood levels of creatine phosphokinase and lactate dehydrogenase after using black cohosh.[158]

Evening Primrose Oil

Evening primrose, borage, and black currant produce seeds that contain gamma-linolenic acid (GLA). A 6-month randomized double-blind placebo-controlled trial was conducted with 56 menopausal women who reported having hot flashes three or more times a day. Participants were randomized to receive evening primrose oil 2000 mg with 40 mg vitamin E or placebo twice daily. Twenty-one women discontinued the study because of a poor clinical response to the treatment, 10 taking evening primrose oil and 11 taking placebo. This study showed that evening primrose oil had no benefit over placebo

in the alleviation of vasomotor symptoms.[159] A recent systematic review found no benefit.[127]

Panax Ginseng

Ginseng is reputed to be an aphrodisiac and to have estrogenic actions that improve menopausal symptoms. The Ginsana Corporation in Switzerland, the largest manufacturer of ginseng products worldwide, conducted a 16-week placebo-controlled trial in almost 400 postmenopausal women.[160] Although vasomotor complaints were not reduced, improvements were noted on scales used to rate depression and general health and well-being. Assessments of estrogenic effects, including the maturation index and measurement of plasma FSH and estradiol over the 16-week period, showed that there was no difference between the effects of ginseng and those of placebo.[161] A randomized, multicenter, double-blind, parallel study on symptomatic postmenopausal women assessed the effects of 16 weeks of treatment of standardized ginseng extract or placebo on quality of life and on physiologic parameters. To assess the efficacy of ginseng on postmenopausal symptoms, physiologic parameters (i.e., FSH and estradiol levels, endometrial thickness, maturity index, vaginal pH) were recorded at the same time points. Of the 384 randomized patients (mean age 53.5 ± 4.0 years), the questionnaires were completed by 193 women treated with ginseng and 191 treated with placebo. No differences were found between treatment subjects and placebo control in vasomotor symptoms, but significant improvements were reported on the quality measures for depression and well-being in favor of ginseng compared with placebo. Physiologic parameters such as FSH and estradiol levels, endometrial thickness, maturity indexes, and vaginal pH were not affected by the treatment.[162] In a double-blind placebo-controlled study, 57 postmenopausal women were randomly assigned to 12 weeks of treatment with Gincosan (320 mg/day, containing 120 mg ginkgo biloba and 200 mg Panax ginseng) or placebo. The researchers found no significant effects of Gincosan treatment on ratings of mood, bodily symptoms of somatic anxiety, menopausal symptoms, sleepiness or on any of the cognitive measures of attention, memory, or frontal lobe function. Additionally, a recent systematic review found no benefit to using ginseng for menopause symptoms.[127] Ginseng's adverse reactions include nervousness, GI upset or diarrhea, insomnia, dizziness, headache, euphoria, blood pressure effects, and vaginal bleeding.[163] Case reports link ingestion of ginseng with postmenopausal bleeding.[164,165] One case of postmenopausal bleeding occurred after topical use of a ginseng-containing face cream.[166]

Soy

Lower estrogen levels and longer menstrual cycles have been reported with soy-rich diets. Menopausal symptoms are reported to be less problematic in cultures (particularly Asian cultures) in which the diet is predominantly plant based and contains a lot of soy. Soy protein appears to be effective in reducing hot flashes, bone loss, and total and low-density lipoprotein (LDL) cholesterol level.[167] The consumption

TABLE 23-3 Lifestyle Modification

Treatment	How it Helps
Diet	
High fiber	Decreases heart disease, decreases constipation, helps maintain weight
Low fat	Improves cholesterol, helps maintain weight
Rich in antioxidants	May decrease hot flashes and other menopausal symptoms
Increase soy	May decrease hot flashes, part of a heart-healthy diet
Exercise	
Cardiovascular	Decreases CAD risk, improves mood, aids sleep, helps maintain weight
Weight-bearing and strengthening	Improves bone health, may decrease hot flashes, helps maintain weight
Other Lifestyle Factors	
Smoking cessation	Decreases heart disease, decreases smoking-related cancers, decreases osteoporosis risk, may decrease hot flashes
Decrease alcohol consumption	May decrease hot flashes, decreases osteoporosis risk
Maintain regular sexual activity	May decrease vaginal dryness (i.e., use it or lose it), may improve depressive symptoms

CAD, Coronary artery disease.

of soy may reduce the frequency, severity, and incidence of hot flashes, but clinical studies and systematic reviews have showed mixed results.[168-174] The majority of phytoestrogens found in human diets are divided into two classes: isoflavones and lignins. Isoflavones are found predominantly in soy foods and other legumes such as chickpeas, pinto beans, and lima beans. Lignins are found in whole grains, seeds (particularly flax), and some fruits and vegetables. Soy supplement products are not recommended; whole food sources are optimal.

ADDITIONAL THERAPIES

For women with mild to moderate menopausal complaints, simple lifestyle modifications (Table 23-3) may be enough to cope with the discomforts of this change without medications of any kind. Diet, exercise, and comfort measures can reduce hot flashes and other discomforts mildly to significantly.

Key dietary recommendations include the following:

- Diet: low fat and high fiber, increased variety of fruits and veggies (five servings a day)
- Whole grain foods
- Monounsaturated fats such as olive oil and canola oil
- Essential fatty acid and multivitamin supplements

Some have suggested that regular aerobic exercise lessens the frequency and severity of hot flashes.[175] Studies show that women who regularly exercise are less likely than their counterparts to experience severe hot flashes. In one observational study of 1323 women in Sweden, 15% of sedentary women experienced "severe" hot flashes, compared with only 5% of the subjects who exercised.[176]

There are many simple lifestyle changes women can make to help with hot flashes. The practice of wearing light, "breathable" cotton clothing helps, as does layering clothing. Other suggestions include keeping the ambient temperature of a room low; and avoiding hot and spicy foods, caffeine, and alcohol. Women also can benefit from stress reduction. In one study, women were taught "paced breathing," a biofeedback technique that lowered their rate of hot flashes.[177] Good diet and exercise also decrease bone loss. Other benefits can be derived from stopping smoking, decreasing soda and alcohol consumption, and improving dietary calcium intake.

Several studies have shown a benefit of calcium on improving bone density in both adults and children. There is no definitive evidence, however, that it lowers fracture risk. Calcium remains an important adjunct to the prevention and treatment of osteoporosis. Women should be encouraged to get their calcium through dietary intake of calcium-rich or fortified foods, but most women have trouble getting enough through diet. The aim for postmenopausal women should be a daily intake of 1000 to 1500 mg. Vitamin D supplementation should be a part of any osteoporosis prevention program. Studies have shown a decrease in fracture rates in older people treated with vitamin D, compared with those on placebo.[178,179] Present evidence suggests a daily dose of 400 to 800 IU may be required. Research has shown that people whose diets are rich in both magnesium and potassium have denser bones.[180]

CASE HISTORY

Clare, a 50-year-old woman, presented with complaints of irritability, mood swings, hot flashes, and insomnia. She had had irregular periods for the past year, and now they had stopped for several months. "Doc, I think that I am going crazy. Could I be going through menopause?" She did not want to use hormone replacement therapy (HRT) because her mother had a history of breast cancer.

Her medical history included a family history of breast cancer, hypertension, and diabetes. Clare had mild hypertension and type 2 diabetes. She had no history of anxiety or depression. She had recently lost her job, and described being under extreme stress at home caused by financial hardship. Her husband was employed. Her son had broken his leg in a skiing accident.

She was currently taking Glucophage (500 mg bid), Atenolol (10 mg daily), a daily multivitamin, and calcium (1500 mg daily).

The following herbal protocol was recommended for anxiety and insomnia:

- Remifemin (standardized black cohosh) 40 mg twice daily
- Oat straw, chamomile, and lemon balm tea for sleep, as needed
- Sage aromatherapy mist to be sprayed near her bed or in her immediate vicinity for symptomatic relief of hot flashes

A follow-up in 3 months found Clare with symptoms much improved, and still taking the Remifemin.

Common and Botanical Medicine Names
Quick Reference Dose Chart

HERB		DOSAGE RANGE	
Common Name	Botanical Name	Dried Herb (or Infused/Decocted) G/Dose/× Per Day	Tincture mL/Dose/× Per Day
American ginseng	*Panax quinquefolius*	3-6 g/day	3-12 mL/day
Anise seed	*Pimpinella anisum*	1-5 g/2-3×/day	1-3 mL/2-3×/day
Ashwagandha	*Withania somnifera*	3-6 g powder/day	4-10 mL/day
Astragalus	*Astragalus membranaceus*	9-30 g/day	5-10 mL/day
Bacopa	*Bacopa monnieri*	N/A	4-7 mL/day
Barberry	*Berberis vulgaris*	1-2/3×/day	1-2 mL/3×/day
Bayberry	*Myrica cerifera*	1-2/3×/day	1-2 mL/3×/day
Beth root	*Trillium erectum*	0.5-2 g/day	1-4 mL/day
Birch	*Betula* spp.	2-3 g/day	1-2 mL/day
Black cohosh	*Actaea racemosa*	0.04-0.2 g, up to 1-3 g/day	Tincture: 0.4 mL liquid extract up to 20 drops/day
Black haw	*Viburnum prunifolium*	N/A	3-10 mL/day
Bladderwrack	*Fucus vesiculosus*	5-10/3×/day	Liquid extract: 4-8/3×/day
Blood root	*Sanguinaria canadensis*	Topical use only	
Blue cohosh	*Caulophyllum thalictroides*	0.3-1 g/3×/day	0.5-2.5 mL/3×/day
Blue flag	*Iris versicolor*	0.6-2 g/2×/day	1-2 mL/3×/day
Blue vervain	*Verbena officinalis*	2-4 g/1-3×/day	2-4 mL/1-3×/day
Bugle weed	*Lycopus* spp.	N/A	1-3/1-2×/day
Bupleurum	*Bupleurum falcatum*	1.5-12 g/day	3-7 mL/day
Burdock root	*Arctium lappa*	3-18 g/day	3-5 mL/2-3×/day
Butterbur	*Petasites hybridus*	Recommended in PA–free standardized form	
Calendula	*Calendula officinalis*	1-4 g/3g/day	0.3-1.2 mL/day
California poppy	*Eschscholzia californica*	N/A	2-4 mL/2-3×/day
Celandine (greater)	*Chelidonium majus*	1-2 g/3×/day	1-2 mL/3×/day
Centaury	*Centaurium erythraea*	2-4 g/3×/day	2-4 mL/3×/day
Chamomile	*Matricaria recutita*	2-8 g/3×/day	1-4 mL/3×/day
Chaste berry	*Vitex agnus-castus*	30-40 mg/day up to 500-1000 mg daily	0.2 mL/2-3×/day up to 3-5 mL/day
Chinese skullcap	*Scutellaria baicalensis*	N/A	4-7 mL/1-2×/day
Cinnamon	*Cinnamomum* spp.	0.5-1 g/3×/day	Liquid extract: 0.5-1.5 mL/day; tincture: 2-4 mL/day
Cleavers	*Galium aparine*	N/A	4-10 mL/day
Coleus	*Coleus forskohlii*	N/A	1.5-4 mL/day
Cordyceps	*Cordyceps sinensis*	3-15 g/day	N/A
Corn silk	*Zea mays*	4-8 g/in infusion 3×/day	5-15 mL/3×/day
Corydalis	*Corydalis ambigua*	5-10 g/day	5-20 mL/day
Cotton root	*Gossypium herbaceum*	N/A	2-4 mL/2×/day
Couch grass	*Elymus repens*	4-8 g/day in decoction	5-15 mL/3×/day
Cramp bark	*Viburnum opulus*	N/A	3-10 mL/day
Cranberry	*Vaccinium macrocarpon*		300 mL cranberry juice daily for up to 6 months
Cranesbill geranium	*Geranium maculatum*	N/A	2-5 mL/day
Damiana	*Turnera diffusa*	2-4 g/3×/day	2-4 mL/day

HERB		DOSAGE RANGE	
Common Name	**Botanical Name**	**Dried Herb (or Infused/Decocted) G/Dose/× Per Day**	**Tincture mL/Dose/× Per Day**
Dandelion leaf	*Taraxacum officinale*	4-10 g/3×/day	Liquid extract: 4-10 mL/3×/day; tincture: 2-5 mL/3×/day; Fresh juice: 5-10 mL/2×/day
Dandelion root	*Taraxacum officinale*	2-8 g/3×/day	Liquid extract: 2-8 mL/day; tincture: 5-10 mL/day
Dong quai	*Angelica sinensis*	3-9 g/day	5-15 mL/day
Echinacea	*Echinacea* spp.	1-3 g/3×/day	Liquid extract 0.5-1 mL/3×/day; tincture: 2-5 mL/3×/day
Eleuthero	*Eleutherococcus senticosus*	0.6-3 g daily for up to 3 months	2-16 mL/day up to 1 month
Evening primrose	*Oenothera biennis*	Taken as a dietary supplement oil, 1500 mg/day	
False unicorn	*Chamaelirium luteum*	1-2 g/3×/day	Liquid extract: 1-2 mL/3×/day; tincture: 2-5 mL/3×/day
Fennel	*Foeniculum vulgare*	2.5 g/2×/day in tea	2-4 mL/2×/day
Fenugreek	*Trigonella foenum-graecum*	1-6 g/3×/day	2-4 mL/3×/day
Feverfew	*Tanacetum parthenium*	Freeze-dried: 0.05 g/1× after meals; dried: 5-200 g/day	Liquid extract: 6.25 mg/3×/day; tincture: 1-40 drops every 2-3 hours
Figwort	*Scrophularia nodosa*	2-8 g/day	Liquid extract: 2-8 mL/day; tincture: 2-4 mL/day
Flax	*Linum usitatissimum*	10-50 g seeds/day	N/A
Fringe tree	*Chionanthus virginicus*	N/A	2-5 mL/day
Garlic	*Allium sativum*	2-4 g/3×/day	2-4 mL/3×/day
Gentian	*Gentiana lutea*	0.6-2 g/3×/day	1-4 mL/3×/day
Ginger	*Zingiber officinale*	0.25-1 g/3×/day	1.5-3 mL/3×/day
Ginkgo	*Ginkgo biloba*	120-240 mg extract	120-240 mg extract/day in 2-3 divided doses
Ginseng	*Panax ginseng*	1-9 g/day in 2-3 divided doses	1-6 mL/day
Goldenrod	*Solidago canadensis*	3-5 g/2-3×/day	2-3 mL/2-3×/day
Goldenseal	*Hydrastis canadensis*	0.5-1 g/3×/day	Liquid extract: 0.3-1 mL/2-3×/day; tincture: 2-4 mL/2-3×/day
Green tea	*Camellia chinensis*	1-4 cups/day	
Gromwell	*Lithospermum officinale*	N/A	2-4 mL/day
Guggul	*Commiphora mukul*	500-1000 mg guggulipid standardized to 2.5% guggulsterones 2-3×/day or an equivalent dose of prepared guggulsterone 25 mg 3×/day	
Gymnema	*Gymnema sylvestre*	200 mg 2-3×/day	2 mL/2-3×/day
Hawthorn	*Crataegus monogyna*	0.3-1 g/3×/day	Liquid extract: 0.5-1 mL/3×/day; tincture: 1-2 mL/3×/day
Hollyhock	*Alcea rosea*	N/A	1-3 mL/2×/day
Hops	*Humulus lupulus*	0.5-2 g/2-4×/day	Liquid extract: 0.5-3 mL/3×/day; tincture: 1-2 mL/3×/day
Horse chestnut	*Aesculus hippocastanum*	1-2 g/3×/day	Liquid extract: 2-6 mL
Horsetail	*Equisetum arvense*	1.5 g of herb taken as infusion, 2-3×/day	Liquid extract: 1-3 mL 1-4×/day
Jamaican dogwood	*Piscidia piscipula*	1-2 g/3×/day	2-8 mL/day

Continued

HERB		DOSAGE RANGE	
Common Name	Botanical Name	Dried Herb (or Infused/Decocted) G/Dose/× Per Day	Tincture mL/Dose/× Per Day
Kava kava	*Piper methysticum*	1.5 g-3 g to 60-120 mg kava lactones/day	Liquid extract 3-6 mL/day; standardized preparations:100 mg-200 mg kava lactones/day; 60 mg kava lactones 2-4×/day
Ladies' mantle	*Alchemilla vulgaris*	2-4 g/3×/day	2-4 mL/3×/day
Lavender	*Lavandula officinalis*	1-3 g/2-3×/day	2-4 mL×/day
Lemon balm	*Melissa officinalis*	1.5-4.5 g/2-3×/day	2-4 mL/2-3×/day
Licorice	*Glycyrrhiza glabra*	1-4 g/2×/day	0.6-2 mL/2-3×/day
Lobelia	*Lobelia inflata*	0.2-0.6 g/3×/day	Liquid extract: 0.2-0.6 mL/3×/day; tincture: 0.6-2 mL/3×/day
Marijuana	*Cannabis sativa*	*Dose not specified*	
Marshmallow root	*Althea officinalis*	2-5 g/3×/day	2-5 mL/3×/day
Meadowsweet	*Filipendula ulmaria*	4-6 g/3×/day	Liquid extract: 1.5-6 mL/3×/day; tincture: 3-4 mL/3×/day
Milk thistle	*Silybum marianus*	12-15 g/day	2-4 mL/2-3×/day
Milky oats	*Avena sativa*	N/A	3-5 mL/2-3×/day
Motherwort	*Leonurus cardiaca*	2-4 g/3×/day	Liquid extract: 2-4 mL/3×/day; tincture: 2-6 mL/3×/day
Mugwort	*Artemisia vulgaris*	1-3 g/2×/day	1-2 mL/2×/day
Mullein leaf	*Verbascum thapsus*	3-6 g/day	2-4 mL/2-3×/day
Myrrh	*Commiphora molmol*	N/A	1-2.5 mL/day
Nettle leaf	*Urtica dioica*	2-4 g/3×/day	Liquid extract: 3-4 mL/3×/day; tincture: 2-6 mL/3×/day; fresh juice: 1-15 mL/3×/day
Ocotillo	*Fouquieria splendens*	N/A	2-4 mL/2×/day
Oregano	*Origanum vulgaris*	Essential oil for topical use only	
Oregon grape	*Mahonia aquifolium*	1.5-3 g/2-3 mL/day	2.5-5 g/2-3×/day
Osha	*Lomatium dissectum*	1-3 g/2×/day	1-3 mL/2×/day
Partridge berry	*Mitchella repens*	N/A	2-4 mL/2×/day
Passionflower	*Passiflora incarnata*	4-8 g/day	1-4 mL/3×/day
Peony	*Paeonia lactiflora*	3-6 g/day	3-5 mL/1-2×/day
Peppermint	*Mentha piperita*	3-5 g/1-3×/day as tea	0.5-2 mL/1-2×/day
Picrorrhiza	*Picrorhiza kurroa*	N/A	2-4 mL/2-3×/day
Poke root	*Phytolacca americana*	For topical use only	
Pulsatilla	*Anemone pulsatilla*	NA	Tincture: 3-5 drops every 15 minutes until symptoms abate
Quaking aspen	*Populus tremuloides*	N/A	1-3 mL/2×/day
Red clover	*Trifolium pratense*	3-5 g/3×/day	1-2 mL/3×/day
Red raspberry	*Rubus idaeus*	4-8 g/3×/day	4-8 mL/3×/day
Red root	*Ceanothus americanus*	N/A	2-4 mL/1-2×/day
Rehmannia	*Rehmannia glutinosa*	2-6 g/day	4-12 mL/day
Reishi	*Ganoderma lucidum*	6-12g/day	10 mL/3×/day
Rhaponticum	*Rhaponticum carthamoides*	N/A	
Rhodiola	*Rhodiola rosea*	50-500 mg/day × 2 weeks	
Rosemary	*Rosmarinus officinalis*	2-4 g/3×/day	Liquid extract: 2-4 mL/3×/day
Sage	*Salvia officinalis*	1-4 g/3×/day	Tincture: 1-4 mL/3×/day
Saw palmetto	*Serenoa repens*	320 mg lipophilic compounds (160 mg/2×/day)	
Schisandra	*Schisandra chinensis*	1.5-15 g/day	3-7 mL/1-2×/day
Shatavari	*Asparagus racemosa*	N/A	4-7 mL/1-2×/day
Shepherd's purse	*Capsella bursa-pastoris*	2-5 g/3×/day	2-4 mL/3×/day
Skullcap	*Scutellaria lateriflora*	1-2 g/3×/day	Tincture: 1-2 mL/3×/day

HERB		DOSAGE RANGE	
Common Name	**Botanical Name**	**Dried Herb (or Infused/Decocted) G/Dose/x Per Day**	**Tincture mL/Dose/x Per Day**
Slippery elm	*Ulmus rubra*	2-5 g/1-3×/day	Not typically taken in these forms
St. John's wort	*Hypericum perforatum*	2-4 g/3×/day	2-4 mL/3×/day
Tea tree	*Melaleuca alternifolia*	N/A	Used topically as an essential oil
Thuja*	*Thuja occidentalis*	N/A	1.5-2.5 mL/day
Thyme	*Thymus vulgaris*	1-4 g/3×/day	2-3 mL/1-3×/day
Tienchi ginseng	*Panax notoginseng*	2-9 g/day	4-18 mL/day
Tribulus	*Tribulus terrestris*	N/A	3-5 mL/2×/day
Tumeric	*Curcuma longa*	750 mg - 3 g/day in divided doses	N/A
Usnea	*Usnea barbata*	N/A	2-4 mL/2-3×/day
Uva ursi	*Arctostaphylos uva ursi*	3-12 g daily in divided doses	2-4 mL/2-4×/day
Valerian	*Valeriana officinalis*	1-3 g/3×/day	3-5 mL/3×/day
Wild yam	*Dioscorea villosa*	2-4 g/day in divided doses	2-4 mL/day in 3-5 divided doses
Willow	*Salix* spp.	1-3 g/3×/day up to 60-120 mg salicin/day	1-3 mL/3×/day
Witch hazel	*Hamamelis virginiana*	2 g/3×/day	2-4 mL/3×/day
Yarrow	*Achillea millefolium*	2-5 g/3×/day	2-4 mL/3×/day
Yellow dock	*Rumex crispus*	3-5 g/3×/day	2-4 mL/3×/day
Yellow sweet clover	*Melilotus officinalis*	2-4 g/day in tea form to no greater than 3-30 mg coumarin daily	
Yerba mansa	*Anemopsis californica*	N/A	3-5 mL
Ziziphus	*Ziziphus spinosa*	5-10 g/day	5-10 mL/day[1]

N/A, Not applicable; *PA,* pyrrolizidine alkaloid.

References
1. Barnes J, Anderson L, Phillipson J: *Herbal medicines,* ed 3, London, 2007, Pharmaceutical Press.
2. Barrett M: *The handbook of clinically tested herbal remedies,* Binghamton, 2004, Haworth Press.
3. Basch E, Ulbricht C: *Natural standard herb and supplement reference: evidence-based clinical reviews,* St. Louis, 2005, Mosby.
4. Blumenthal M: *The ABC clinical guide to herbs,* Austin, 2003, American Botanical Council.
5. Blumenthal M, Busse W, Goldberg A, et al, editors: *The complete German Commission E monographs,* Austin, 1998, American Botanical Council: Integrative Medicine Communications.
6. Bone K: *A clinical guide to blending liquid herbs: herbal formulations for the individual patient,* St. Louis, 2003, Churchill Livingstone.
7. Bone K: *Clinical applications of Ayurvedic and Chinese herbs,* Queensland, 2000, Phytotherapy Press.
8. European Scientific Cooperative on Phytotherapy: *ESCOP monographs: the scientific foundation for herbal medicinal products,* Stuttgart, 2003, Thieme.
9. McKenna D, et al: *Botanical medicines: the desk reference for major herbal supplements,* New York, 2002, Haworth Press.
10. Upton R: *American herbal pharmacopoeia and therapeutic compendium series,* Santa Cruz, 2000-2007, American Herbal Pharmacopoeia.
11. Wichtl M: *Herbal drugs and phytopharmaceuticals: a handbook for practice on a scientific basis,* ed 4, Stuttgart, 2004, Medpharm.
12. Bone K, Mills S: *Principles and practice of phytotherapy,* ed 2, Edinburgh, 2013, Churchill Livingstone.

II APPENDIX

Chemical Constituents of Medicinal Plants

An understanding of herbal constituents can help practitioners develop greater discernment in preparing and using botanical medicines. Phytochemistry focuses on the physical aspect of a plant's healing powers—the molecules and compounds behind observable qualities, actions, and clinical effects. These structures are readily identifiable on a sensory level, permitting organoleptic analysis of many herbs, imparting, for example, scent resulting from the small, volatile compounds in essential oils; bitter taste from certain lactones or alkaloids; colorful hues of light reflected by the antioxidant flavonoid pigments; and the slippery texture of the heteropolysaccharides known as mucilages. When approaching the study of phytochemistry in a holistic way, we transcend the world of dry abstraction and experience the tangible realm of what plants really do: We integrate sensory experience, beauty, and practical application with knowledge of the unseen architecture of life.

Naming an herbal constituent gives only a bare hint of its character, classification, relationships, and properties. No molecule exists naturally in isolation, and so must always be considered within the broader context of its biosynthetic origin, its companion molecules, and the plant matrix from which it arises. At the same time, the science of chemistry enables us to make fine distinctions on a very small scale. A sense of balance between details and context is important for incorporating phytochemical information into our knowledge base as practitioners. We must consider not only the structure of an individual compound, but also how this compound behaves in relationship to other molecules in the plant, the extract, the herbal formula, and the individual consuming the product.

Molecules are, profoundly and literally, patterns of energy in relationship. These patterns of energy interact with other patterns of energy—biological molecules—in the human body to effect changes in health. When reading the following material, try to keep this in mind. The molecular world is far more mystical, fluid, and dynamic than college chemistry classes might have suggested.

SYNERGY AND VARIABILITY

A living plant contains myriad compounds that work synergistically to protect the plant from harm and carry out all the processes of its metabolism. Interestingly, many of these molecules have similar functions in plants and humans. For instance, the berberine in *Mahonia aquifolium* (Oregon grape; Fig. A-1) is an example of an antimicrobial compound that protects against fungal and bacterial infection in both plants and humans. Another example is the class of molecules known as flavonoids, which occur in all green plants. In the

chloroplasts, flavonoids act as primary antioxidants to protect the delicate light-harvesting compounds from ultraviolet and free radical damage. In the human body, these same compounds act as antioxidants, anticarcinogens, and antiinflammatories by virtue of their radical-quenching activities.

From a practitioner's perspective, an herb is chosen for therapeutic effects based on its particular "personality." Physically, this characteristic is encoded within the unique blend of constituents inside the plant. Rather than investing in the concept of active ingredients, we can more usefully entertain the idea of synergistic activity complexes: sets of constituents that may potentiate, stabilize, or attenuate each other to produce a characteristic set of herbal actions. As we discuss phytochemicals on an individual basis, we must always remember that the reductionist perspective provides

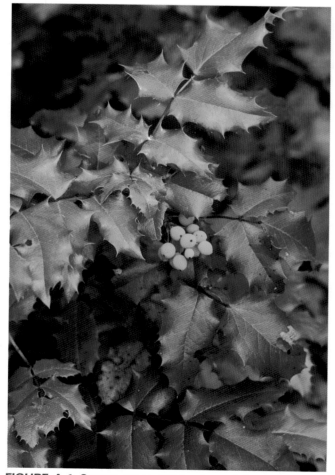

FIGURE A-1 Oregon grape (*Mahonia aquiolium*). (Photo by Martin Wall.)

only a small and relatively static snapshot of a dynamic and complex process. The scientific information concerning the properties of isolated phytochemicals must always be interpreted within a larger context.

Phytochemical variability is an important concern for the herbal practitioner. We must keep in mind that the chemical profile of a living plant is a system that constantly adapts to conditions in the environment. For example, seasonal variability is demonstrated in *Taraxacum officinalis* (dandelion) by levels of the therapeutic oligosaccharide inulin (a soluble fiber) known to range from 2% to 40% in spring and fall roots, respectively. In this same herb, the levels of sesquiterpene lactones (i.e., digestive bitters) vary tremendously among the seasons, accounting for the sweetness of early spring leaves as opposed to their pronounced bitterness later in the summer. Along with seasonal variation, the herbalist must consider phytochemical variations owing to time of day; rainfall; soil composition; growing location; companion plants, fungi, and insects; developmental stage of the herb; and, traditionalists might argue, phases of the moon, vitality of the plant, and energetic or spiritual relationships between the plant and the people who harvest and use its medicine. In addition, many species have chemotypes, or significantly differing chemical races, which may be difficult to distinguish visually. Therefore proper growing conditions and harvesting time and techniques largely determine the efficacy of individual herb products, and any assessment of product quality must consider these variables.

It is interesting and important to consider that traditional rituals and prescriptions for botanical harvest and preparation have often taken such factors into account based on intuitive knowledge or empirical observations. Today, these abilities are supplemented by data from precise analytic evaluation. The three perspectives of tradition, organoleptics, and science can be combined to develop a holistic understanding of constituents and their significance in herbal medicine.

CONSTITUENT CLASSIFICATION

Constituents may be classified according to structural similarities, biosynthetic relationships, or therapeutic actions. For example, hamamelitannin, a compound from witch hazel (*Hamamelis virginiana*) could be classified as a hydrolyzable tannin (i.e., structural), a polyphenol (i.e., biosynthetic), or an astringent (i.e., action). In this scheme, the compounds are classified mainly from a biosynthetic perspective, which overarches and includes structural considerations; therapeutic actions often, but not always, fall in line with this approach. This classification helps us to understand the place of an individual compound within the entire panoply of medicinal metabolites.

A Word About Glycosides

There is often confusion about the meaning of the term *glycoside*. There is not a distinct phytochemical category for glycosides; rather, any type or class of molecule may occur in the form of a glycoside. Simply put, a glycoside is any molecule with one or more sugar groups attached. The molecule without its additional sugar group(s) is called an *aglycone*. For example, the purple anthocyanin compound called cyanidin can occur as a free aglycone, or in the form of numerous glycosides with various different sugar groups attached. Well-known groups of compounds such as the cyanogenic glycosides and the cardiac glycosides are best classified according to the structure of their aglycons: The former are amino acid derivatives, whereas the latter are steroidal compounds.

Herbal Constituent Categories

The main categories of herbal constituents are:
- Carbohydrates and derivatives
- Lipids
- Amino acids and derivatives
- Phenolic compounds
- Terpenes
- Steroidal compounds
- Alkaloids

Although there is considerable variation within each of these categories, the compounds are related by biosynthetic origin and basic structural organization. Within each major category are a number of distinct subcategories (because of space limitations, only the most prominent are listed here). Although they are related chemically, we cannot necessarily assume that all of the compounds within a subcategory have similar physiologic actions. For example, the beneficial anticancer lignans in flax (*Linum usitatissimum*) have a completely different character than the powerful cytotoxic lignan podophyllotoxin from mayapple (*Podophyllum peltatum*) or the suspected adaptogenic lignans in schisandra (*Schisandra chinensis*).

1. Carbohydrates and derivatives
   a. Monosaccharides: simple sugars, for example, glucose (i.e., first product of photosynthesis; human blood sugar) and fructose (i.e., fruit sugar)
   b. Disaccharides: composed of two simple sugars bonded together, for example, sucrose in *Saccharum* (sugar cane)
   c. Oligosaccharides: short chains of simple sugars, for example, inulin in dandelion (*Taraxacum officinale*) (Fig. A-2) and chicory (*Cichorium intybus*)
   d. Polysaccharides: long chains of simple sugars, for example, mucilage in marshmallow (*Althea officinalis*), immunomodulating polysaccharides in echinacea (*Echinacea* spp.) (Fig. A-3) or medicinal mushrooms; starch and cellulose
   e. Organic acids: derived from monosaccharides, for example, oxalic acid in sheep sorrel (*Rumex* spp.); formic acid in nettle (*Urtica dioica*) stingers
2. Lipids (sometimes called polyketides)
   a. Fatty acids: simple lipids, for example, alpha-linolenic acid (ALA), gamma linolenic acid (GLA), docosahexaenoic acid (DHA), eicosapentaenoic acid (EPA)
   b. Triglycerides (i.e., triacylglycerols, neutral fats): main component of dietary oils such as olive oil

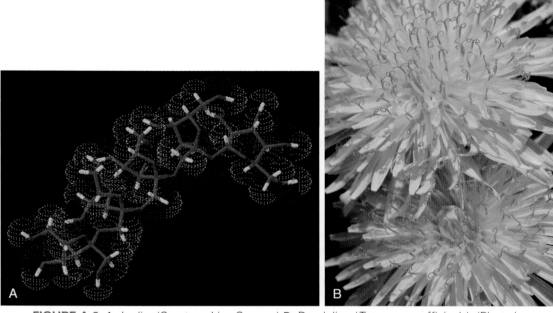

FIGURE A-2 **A,** Inulin. (Courtesy Lisa Ganora.) **B,** Dandelion (*Taraxacum officinale*). (Photo by Martin Wall.)

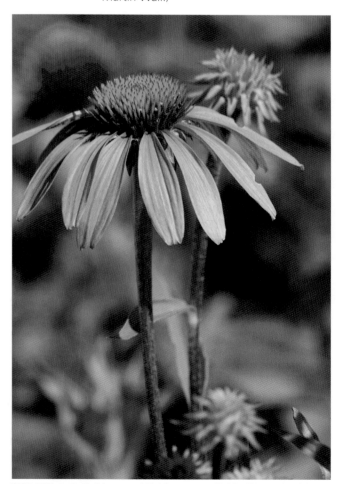

FIGURE A-3 Echinacea (*Echinacea pollida*). (Photo by Martin Wall.)

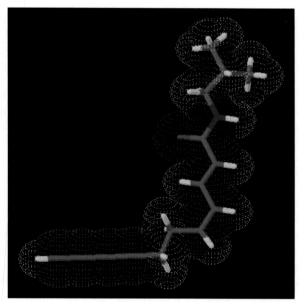

FIGURE A-4 Isobutylamide molecule. (Courtesy Lisa Ganora.)

c. Phospholipids: main component of cell membranes in plants and animals; for example, phosphatidylcholine (PC), phosphatidylserine (PS)

d. Alkylamides: nitrogenous lipids with actions on the immune system, for example, isobutylamides in echinacea *(Echinacea angustifolia; E. purpurea)* (Fig. A-4)

e. Polyacetylenes: antimicrobial or toxic molecules with carbon-carbon triple bonds, for example, arctinal in burdock *(Arctium lappa)* seed

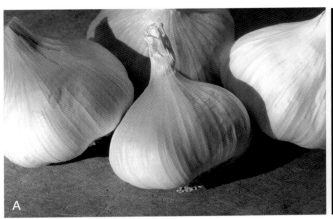
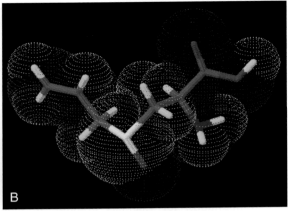

FIGURE A-5 A, Garlic (*Allium sativum*). (Photo by Martin Wall.) B, Alliin molecule. (Courtesy Lisa Ganora.)

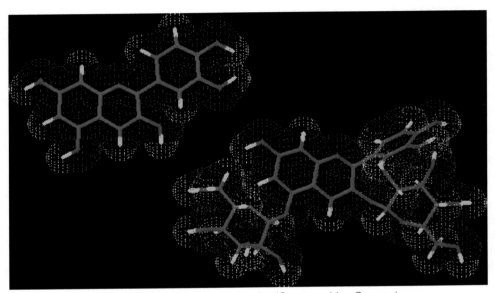

FIGURE A-6 Cyanidin molecule. (Courtesy Lisa Ganora.)

3. Amino acids and derivatives
   a. Amino acids: building blocks of proteins; precursors of many types of molecules; for example, phenylalanine, cysteine, lysine
   b. Sulfated amino acid derivatives: sulfur compounds in garlic and onions (*Allium* spp.) (Fig. A-5), for example, allicin; glucosinolates and derivatives in cabbages, broccoli, mustard (*Brassica* spp.) species, for example, sulforaphane
   c. Cyanogenic glycosides: cyanide-generating compounds, for example, prunasin in wild cherry (*Prunus serotina*) (Fig. A-6)
   d. Amines
      i. Aromatic amines: neuroactive compounds, for example, ephedrine in ephedra (*Ephedra sinensis*); histamine in nettle stingers
      ii. Methylxanthines: central nervous system stimulants, for example, caffeine in coffee (*Coffea theobroma*); theophylline in tea (*Camellia sinensis*)

4. Phenolic compounds (sometimes called polyphenols)
   a. Phenolic acids and phenylpropanoids: variety of actions, for example, antioxidant chlorogenic acid in, for example, blueberry, cranberry (*Vaccinium* spp.); carminative anethole in fennel (*Foeniculum vulgare*) seeds
   b. Phenylpropanoid derivatives: for example, vasoactive capsaicin in cayenne (*Capsicum annum*); antiinflammatory curcumin in tumeric (*Curcuma longa*)
   c. Coumarins: venotonics such as aesculin in horse chestnut (*Aesculus hippocastanum*); melilotoside in sweet clover (*Melilotus* spp.). Note: coumarins per se are not blood thinners; dicoumarol, formed from them by fungal action in moldy dried plant material, is a potent anticoagulant and the molecular basis for the drug Coumadin.
   d. Lignans: anticarcinogenic phytoestrogens, for example, secoisolariciresinol in flax (*Linum usitatissimum*); antioxidants, for example, nordihydroguaiaretic acid (NDGA) in chaparral (*Larrea* spp.); wide variety of activities; some are toxic

e. Stilbenoids: antioxidant, antiinflammatory, antimutagenic compounds, for example, resveratrol in grape skins and seed

f. Xanthones: yellow pigments, for example, the antidepressant synergist norathyriol in St. John's wort *(Hypericum perforatum)*; the hepatoprotective gentisin from gentian *(Gentiana lutea)*

g. Styrylpyrones: for example, the antispasmodic kavalactones in kava kava *(Piper methysticum)*

h. Flavonoids: thousands of compounds, generally antioxidant, antiinflammatory, cardioprotective, or hepatoprotective, and anticarcinogenic/carcinostatic; some are antispasmodic and antiallergenic as well

   i. Anthocyanins: for example, cyanidin in blue/purple/red fruits and berries such as elder berries *(Sambucus* spp.)

   ii. Chalcones and aurones: for example, the licochalcones from licorice *(Glycyrrhiza glabra)* root

   iii. Flavonols: for example, catechin from green tea

   iv. Flavanones: for example, hesperidin from *Citrus* species; flavanones are sometimes called citrus bioflavonoids or vitamin P

   v. Flavonols: for example, quercetin from onion *(Allium cepa)*

   vi. Flavones: for example, apigenin from parsley *(Petroselinum* spp.)

   vii. Hydrolyzable tannins: for example, ellagitannins in strawberry *(Fragaria* spp.); gallotannins in oak bark *(Quercus* spp.)

   viii. Condensed tannins (including proanthocyanidins): for example, OPCs (oligomeric proanthocyanidin complexes) in grape skins and seeds; the flavins in black tea

i. Isoflavonoids: phytoestrogenic compounds, for example, genistein in soybean *(Glycine* spp.), biochanin A in red clover *(Trifolium pratense)*

j. Benzofurans: rare; for example, the antibacterial usnic acid from usnea *(Usnea barbata)*

k. Chromones: also rare; for example, the cardiotonic and bronchodilatory khellin from khella *(Ammi visnaga)*

l. Quinones

   i. Benzoquinones: for example, the cardioprotective coenzyme Q10

   ii. Naphthoquinones: for example, antifungal juglone from black walnut *(Juglans nigra)*

   iii. Anthraquinones: for example, aperient emodin in yellow dock *(Rumex crispus),* cascarosides in cascara sagrada *(Frangulas purshiana)*

m. Phloroglucinol derivatives: rare; for example, the antidepressant synergist hyperforin in St. John's wort; the psychoactive tetrahydrocannabinol (THC) in *Cannabis* spp.

5. Terpenes (sometimes called isoprenoids)

a. Monoterpenes: small volatile molecules in the essential oils of many plants; for example, the anticarcinogenic limonene in *Citrus* peel; the antiemetic menthol in peppermint *(Mentha x piperita)*

   i. Iridoids (monoterpene lactones): for example, the mosquito-repellant nepetalactone from catnip *(Nepeta cataria)*

   ii. Secoiridoids: bitter compounds, for example, gentiopicrin from yellow gentian *(Gentiana luteum)*

b. Sesquiterpenes: heavier volatile compounds in many essential oils; for example, the antiinflammatory alpha-bisoprolol in chamomile *(Matricaria recutita)*

   i. Sesquiterpene lactones: digestive bitters such as lactucin from chicory; antiinflammatory parthenolide from feverfew *(Tanacetum parthenium)*

c. Diterpenes: resinous compounds, for example, the antitussive, antimicrobial grindelic acid in gumweed *(Grindelia* spp.)

d. Triterpenes (including triterpene saponins): for example, triterpene glycosides in black cohosh *(Actaea racemosa);* saponins such as the antiinflammatory, hepatoprotective, immunomodulant glycyrrhizin in licorice

e. Tetraterpenes (carotenoids): oil-soluble antioxidant and anticarcinogenic compounds

f. Lycopene, from tomatoes

   i. Carotenes: alpha-, beta-, delta-, and gamma-carotenes in orange/yellow vegetables and flowers and in green leaves

   ii. Xanthophylls (oxygenated carotenoids): including lutein and capsanthin (from red peppers, sweet or hot)

6. Steroidal compounds

a. Phytosterols: cell-membrane plant steroids analogous to cholesterol; for example, beta-sitosterol in saw palmetto *(Serenoa repens)* (Fig. A-7)

b. Steroidal saponins: for example, the adaptogenic ginsenosides from *Panax* species; the venotonic ruscogenin in butcher's broom *(Ruscus aculeatus)*

c. Cardiac glycosides (cardenolides): potent cardioactive compounds including convallatoxin from lily of the valley *(Convallaria majalis)* and digitoxin from foxglove *(Digitalis purpurea)*

7. Alkaloids (there are many subcategories; these are the most commonly encountered in herbalism)

a. Betalain alkaloids: potent antioxidants/anticarcinogens including red/purple betalains from beets, pokeweed *(Phytolacca americana)* berries, and yellow betaxanthins from yellow beets and prickly pear cactus *(Opuntia ficus-indica)*

b. Indole alkaloids: a large and varied class that includes potent compounds such as yohimbine from yohimbe *(Pausinystalia yohimbe)*; the ergoline alkaloids from morning glory *(Ipomoea* spp.) and ergot fungus *(Claviceps* spp.) fungi; quinine from *Cinchona* species; and reserpine from Indian snakeroot *(Rauwolfia serpentina)*

c. Isoquinoline alkaloids: a large class that includes the familiar protoberberines, for example, berberine and hydrastine from goldenseal *(Hydrastis canadensis);* also includes sanguinarine from bloodroot *(Sanguinaria canadensis)* and eschscholzidine from California poppy *(Eschscholzia californica)* (Fig. A-8); the morphinan

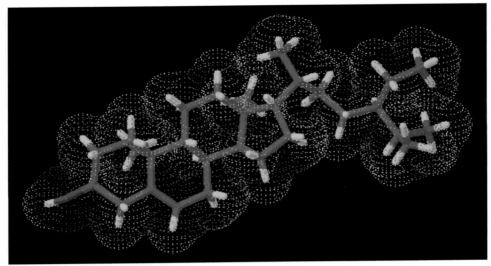

FIGURE A-7 Beta-sitosterol molecule. (Courtesy Lisa Ganora.)

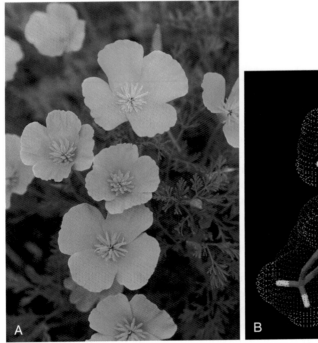
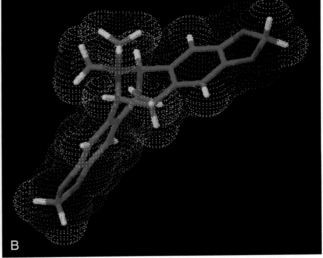

FIGURE A-8 A, California poppy (*Eschscholzia californica*). (Photo by Martin Wall.) B, Californi-dine molecule. (Courtesy Lisa Ganora.)

alkaloids from opium poppy (*Papaver somniferum*) are isoquinoline derivatives

d. Piperidine alkaloids: varied compounds including the bronchodilatory, antispasmodic lobeline from lobelia (*Lobelia inflata*); the highly toxic coniine from poison hemlock (*Conium* spp.); and the pungent, absorption-enhancing piperine from black pepper (*Piper nigrum*)

e. Pyrrolizidine alkaloids: toxicity varies considerably; the most toxic (for example, macrocyclic esters: senkirkine, retrorsine) are found in *Senecio, Heliotropium,* and *Crotalaria* spp.; others (for example, symphytine,

intermedin) occur in comfrey (*Symphytum officinale*), borage (*Borago officinalis*), and other *Boraginaceae* spp.; nontoxic pyrrolizidine alkaloids (PAs) (for example, tussilagine) occur in *Echinacea* spp.

f. Steroidal alkaloids: structurally related to steroidal saponins, these include the narcotic or toxic *Solanaceous* (nightshade family) alkaloids such as solanine, solasodine, and tomatine

g. Tropane alkaloids: potent neuroactive or psychoactive compounds such as hyoscyamine and scopolamine in deadly nightshade (*Atropa belladonna*), sacred jimsonweed (*Datura inoxia*), and henbane (*Hyoscyamus niger*)

TABLE A-1   Solubility

Liquid	Soluble Constituents
Water	Most carbohydrates (monosaccharides, oligosaccharides, polysaccharides); mucilages and gums in cold water; starch in hot water
	Organic acids (especially in basic solutions)
	Many polyphenols (especially glycosides) and flavonoids (generally more soluble in alkaline solutions); tannins (hydrolyzable and condensed) in hot water
	B complex vitamins and vitamin C
	Some alkaloids, including betalains and berberine (alkaloids in general are more soluble in acidic solutions)
	Aromatic amines (i.e., ephedrine), more so in acidic solutions
	Amino acids and proteins (including enzymes)
	Saponins (often foam when shaken in water)
	Salts of fatty acids in a basic solution (soaps)
	Monoterpenes and sesquiterpenes are soluble in steam (e.g., steam-distilled essential oils)
Ethanol or ethanol/water	Many alkaloids (generally around 50% ethanol/water ratio)
	Some polyphenols (especially aglycons) including stilbenoids, lignins
	Terpenes (including monopenes, sesquipenes, dipenes, and triterpenes), generally above 50% ethanol/water ratio
	Resins (need high ethanol to water ratio, approximately 90%)
Oil	Lipids, including fatty acids
	Terpenes (including carotenoids and xanthophylls)
	Some polyphenols (especially aglycons), including some phenylpropanoids and derivatives
	Steroidal compounds (including phytosterols)
	Vitamins D, E (tocopherols, tocotrienols), A, K

SOLUBILITY

The question often arises concerning whether the herbalist should use a water extraction (e.g., infusion, decoction, tea, soup) versus an alcohol extraction (e.g., tincture, extract, fluid extract) or some other type of material. There is a definite difference between these preparations; one brings a different range and concentration of constituents out of a plant than does another. Much of this difference is based on the solubility of the constituents within the herb. The solubilities of isolated constituents can be found in tables, but those values are subject to change within the matrices of different plants. In fact, they can vary considerably. Solubility is influenced by many factors, including pH, heat, concentration, and the presence of salts, tannins, and various other constituents. It can be difficult to predict; practical experience, organoleptic evaluation, and analytical analysis must be used to determine which extraction methods are most efficacious for which compounds (see **Botanical Preparation Forms**).

Sometimes when different extracts are combined (or an extract is mixed with water), a precipitate forms; this cloudy or granular matter contains constituents that have suddenly become insoluble owing to changes in the overall properties of the solution. For example, polysaccharides often precipitate out of solution as the ethanol content is increased. Conversely, a high-alcohol resinous extract produces a milky precipitate in water as the resins fall out of solution. Another example is when alkaloids precipitate out of an acidic water solution as it becomes more basic.

The list given in Table A-1 is oversimplified; there are numerous exceptions. It should be kept in mind that most compounds have at least some degree of solubility in water, alcohol, and oil menstrua. It is often more helpful to think of solubility on a continuum, rather than in absolute terms such as soluble or insoluble. For example, we may think of certain compounds as being only alcohol soluble or only oil soluble; but a small concentration of these molecules can dissolve in water as well.

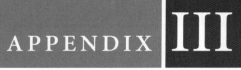

Summary Table of Herbs for Women's Health

Common Name	Botanical Name	Part Used	Dried Herb (In Capsules, Tea, Infusion, Decoction)	Tincture	Actions	Women's Health Indications Described in This Book	Safety Concerns
Albizia	Albizia lebbeck	Leaves and stem bark	3-6g/day	4-8 mL/day	Antiallergic Antimicrobial Hypocholesterolemic Mild mood enhancement	Depression, grief Eczema Fertility problems Inflammation Irritability Memory deficits Pruritus	• LS/LD • ØP
Alfalfa	Medicago sativa	Above-aerial parts	5-10 g/3×/day	5-10 mL/3×/day	Nutritive Phytoestrogen	Iron-deficiency anemia Osteoporosis prevention Vaginal dryness and atrophy	• KSw/C • In large amounts, alfalfa seeds may exacerbate SLE in patients with SLE • Case report of pancytopenia with use of the seeds; not an expected adverse effect with the leafy parts
Aloe vera	Aloe spp.	Gel from leaf	Topical use		Antiinflammatory Antiviral Vulnerary	HSV 1 and 2 (topical) PUPPP Sore, cracked nipples in lactating mothers Vulvovaginitis	• KSw/C • Case report of delayed wound healing following complicated gynecologic surgery • Case report of photodermatitis with use after dermabrasion treatment
American ginseng	Panax quinquefolius	Root	3-6 g/day	3-12 mL/day	Adaptogen	Debility Fatigue HPA dysregulation HSV Memory deficits Mild depression PCOS Stress Stress-related illness	• KSw/C • H-D! • Diabetics may need to adjust insulin doses because of the reported hypoglycemic effect of the herb • Adverse events associated with American ginseng use include headache, weakness, apathy, aversion to cold, distended abdomen, vomiting, and delayed menstruation • One study showed it significantly induced the growth of an ER-positive breast cancer cell line (MCF-7) in vitro; however, there was no evidence of estrogenic activity in the α- or β-estrogen receptors and no increase in uterine weight was observed
Anise	Pimpinella anisum	Seed	1-5 g/2-3×/day	1-3 mL/2-3×/day	Carminative Flavoring Lactagogue Spasmolytic	Flatulence, intestinal cramping Increase milk supply	• May potentiate warfarin action • KSw/C • LSP/L-culinary use • Contact dermatitis with large exposure to seeds and oil • Do not substitute with star anise, which has known toxicity

Common name	Scientific name	Part	Dose	Actions	Indications	Safety notes
Ashwagandha	*Withania somnifera*	Root	3-6 g powder/day 4-10 mL/day	Adaptogen Analgesic Antiinflammatory Hematopoietic Sedative (mild)	Acute and chronic pain Anxiety Depression Fatigue, lassitude Frequent colds Headache HPA dysregulation HSV Insomnia Hypothyroidism Iron-deficiency anemia Mental/emotional exhaustion Musculoskeletal pain PCOS PMS Postpartum depression PUPPP Stress Stress-related illness	• LS • H-D! • ∅P • Possible respiratory depression in excessive doses • Possible additive effects with sedative herbs and medications
Astragalus	*Astragalus membranaceus*	Root	9-30 g/day 5-10 mL/day	Adaptogen Cardiotonic Hypotensive Immunomodulator Qi tonic	Convalescence (e.g., postpartum, postsurgical) Endometriosis Fatigue HSV Susceptibility to infection	• KSw/C • H-D! • Traditionally, use is not recommended during acute infection and acute inflammatory conditions • Caution in diabetics because of possible hypoglycemic effects • Caution with patients on anticoagulant therapy because of possible increase in bleeding risk
Bacopa	*Bacopa monnieri*	Aerial parts	4-7 mL/day	Adaptogen Nootropic	Depression Memory Uterine fibroids	• LS/LD
Barberry	*Berberis vulgaris*	Bark	1-2 g /3x/day 1-2 mL/3x/day	Antimicrobial Hepatic		• LSw/C/LD • ∅P/L • Not recommended for use in individuals with liver disease, elevated liver enzymes, jaundice, or biliary disease
Barley	*Hordeum vulgare*	Seed (grain)	1.5-3 g/day	Demulcent Lipid-lowering effects Nutritive	Increase milk supply Hypercholesterolemia	• KSw/C • Contraindicated in patients with celiac disease
Bayberry	*Myrica cerifera*	Bark	1-2 g/3x/day 1-2 mL/3x/day	Astringent	DUB Leukorrhea Menorrhagia Postnatal perineal care Uterine fibroids	• LS/LD • ∅P

Continued

Common Name	Botanical Name	Part Used	Dried Herb (In Capsules, Tea, Infusion, Decoction)	Tincture	Actions	Women's Health Indications Described in This Book	Safety Concerns
Bethroot	*Trillium erectum*	Root	0.5-2 g/day	1-4 mL/day	Astringent Uterine tonic	DUB Leukorrhea Menorrhagia Uterine fibroids	• LS/LD • ⊘ P
Bilberry	*Vaccinium myrtillus*	Fruit	50-115 mg fresh fruit daily 80-480 mg standardized to 25% anthocyanoside daily of extract in three divided doses		Urinary complaints Vasoprotective	Treatment of UTI (see cranberry) Varicosities (treat/prevent)	• KSw/C • H-D! • Possible decreased platelet aggregation and increased bleeding time in preclinical studies, so caution is advised with anticoagulant therapies • Caution advised for diabetic patients because of possible hypoglycemic effects • Bilberry anthocyanin extract given to pregnant women at doses of 80 or 160 mg 2 to 3 times/day for 3 months for the treatment of lower-limb venous stasis and acute-phase hemorrhoids led to no adverse effects
Birch	*Betula* spp.	Bark	2-3 g/day	1-2 mL/day	Antiinflammatory Diuretic	Interstitial cystitis	• LS/LD
Black cohosh	*Actaea racemosa* syn. *Cimicifuga racemosa*	Root and rhizome	0.3-2 g twice daily	Tincture: 3-7.5 mL Liquid extract (1:1): 0.9-6 mL daily	Antihypertensive Possible antiproliferative effects Possible serotonergic or dopaminergic action Spasmolytic SERM activity has been proposed, but this is not currently considered a likely mechanism of action	Amenorrhea Anxiety Breast cancer Chronic pelvic pain DUB Dysfunctional labor/labor augmentation Dysmenorrhea Endometriosis Hypertension Osteoporosis prevention Musculoskeletal pain or spasms Painful labor PMS Uterine fibroids Vaginal dryness and atrophy Vasomotor and vegetative complaints of perimenopause and menopause	• LSw/C • RHT • ⊘ P/L • Generally well tolerated as directed for up to 6 months • Possible hepatotoxicity associated with herb; warnings now accompany products sold in Europe and Canada; FDA has not required warning labels as of publication • Headache, dizziness, nausea in excessive doses • Theoretical risk of stimulation in ER-sensitive cancers; therefore should be used under supervision of a qualified care provider

Common name	Latin name	Part used	Dose (dried herb)	Dose (tincture)	Actions	Indications	Cautions
Black haw	*Viburnum prunifolium*	Bark	N/A	3-10 mL/day	Hypotensive Spasmolytic	Abdominal pain associated with endometriosis and chronic pelvic pain After-birth pains Chronic pelvic pain Dysmenorrhea Endometriosis Hypertension Incoordinate uterine contractions Irritable uterus Painful labor Premature labor (threatened) Threatened miscarriage Uterine fibroids	• KS/LD • Long history of traditional use for threatened miscarriage, uterine irritability, and painful labor suggests possible safety during pregnancy • Acute toxicity studies in animals at high doses led to respiratory paralysis and death by cardiac arrest at doses of 5 to 7 g of extract administered subcutaneously
Black horehound	*Ballota nigra*	Herb	Infusion: 2-4 g/3×/day	1-2 mL/3×/day	Antiemetic Sedative	NVP	• LS/LD • No known major side effects and no reported herb–drug interactions
Bladderwrack	*Fucus vesiculosus*	Herb	5-10 g/3×/day	4-8 mL/3×/day	Demulcent Thyroid stimulant Weight reducing	Hypothyroidism because of iodine deficiency	• LSw/C • ⊘ P/L • Excess intake may lead to hyperthyroidism • May contain concentrated heavy metals found in the ocean • High sodium content may make use inadvisable for patients with heart or renal failure • Not for medicinal use during pregnancy and lactation (modest food use acceptable) because iodides can cross the placenta and enter into breast milk
Blessed thistle	*Cnicus benedictus*	Herb	1.5-3 g/3×/day	7.5-10 mL/3×/day	Appetite stimulant Emmenagogue Lactagogue	Anorexia Increase milk supply	• LSw/C/LD • H-D! • ⊘ P • Gastric irritation and vomiting at high doses • Possible reduction in the efficacy of antacids, H₂-receptor antagonists, PPIs, and sucralfate if taken with blessed thistle • Possible decrease in platelet aggregation and increase in bleeding time • Tannins in the herb theoretically increase risk of gastric and esophageal cancer, hepatotoxicity, and nephrotoxicity if taken chronically

Continued

Common Name	Botanical Name	Part Used	Dried Herb (In Capsules, Tea, Infusion, Decoction)	Tincture	Actions	Women's Health Indications Described in This Book	Safety Concerns
Blood root	*Sanguinaria canadensis*	Root	Topical use only		Antimicrobial Antitumorigenic	Cervical dysplasia	• ⊘P/L • No toxic effects documented from topical use; however, all use during pregnancy is contraindicated because of possible absorption and toxicity to the fetus • Topically, the herb has been shown to be nonirritant and nonallergenic
Blue cohosh	*Caulophyllum thalictroides*	Root	0.3-1 g/3×/day	0.5-2.5 mL/3×/day	Emmenagogue Oxytocic Uterine and ovarian tonic	Amenorrhea Benign breast disorder Chronic pelvic pain DUB Dysfunctional labor/ labor augmentation Dysmenorrhea Endometriosis Hypomenorrhea Oligomenorrhea Ovarian cysts Postdates pregnancy Uterine fibroids	• ⊘P • RHT • Overdose can cause symptoms similar to nicotine poisoning • Maternal use during pregnancy has been associated with case reports of neonatal MI, cerebral ischemia, increased meconium, and fetal tachycardia. Should be used only by skilled midwives and obstetric care providers
Blue flag	*Iris versicolor*	Rhizome	0.6-2g/2×/day	1-2 mL/3×/day	Antiinflammatory Dermatologic	Interstitial cystitis	• ⊘P/L • RHT • The safety of internal consumption is in question because isolated components have been reported to be toxic in humans and livestock • Use of fresh plant has been reported to cause nausea and vomiting • Volatile oils in the plant have been reported to cause irritation of the throat and eyes, as well as headache
Blue vervain	*Verbena* spp.	Herb	2-4 g/1-3×/day	2-4 mL/1-3×/day	Nervine Possible lactagogue Spasmolytic Uterine stimulant	Benign breast disorder Depression Endometriosis Headache Improve let-down reflex/ increase milk supply Irritability Mental/emotional exhaustion PMS-like symptoms	• LS/LD • ⊘P • Small amounts of verbalin stimulated the uterus in a frog model; the herb is contraindicated in pregnancy because of possible abortifacient/oxytocic activity

Common name	Botanical name	Part	Dosage (dried)	Dosage (tincture)	Actions	Indications	Safety/Notes
Bugleweed	*Lycopus virginiana*	Herb	3-9 g/day	3-9 mL/2×/day	Sedative (mild) / TSH antagonist	Anxiety / Hyperthyroidism / Night sweats / Palpitations / Possibly Graves' disease	• ⊘ P/L • Possible thyroid suppression • Do not give concurrently with thyroid medications
Bupleurum	*Bupleurum falcatum*	Root	3-12 g/day	4-8 mL/day	Antiinflammatory / Constrained liver qi / Hepatoprotective / Immunomodulator / Sedative (mild)	Dysmenorrhea / Irritability and emotional lability / Premenstrual and menstrual headache / PMS	• ⊘ P • Flatulence, nausea, vomiting • Sedation • Cases of hepatotoxicity have occurred after consumption of TCM formulae containing bupleurum; however, the formulae also contained other herbs and no causality has been established with this herb
Burdock	*Arctium lappa*	Root	3-18 g/day	3-5 mL/2-3×/day	Alterative / Antimicrobial / Aperient	Acne / Eczema / PUPPS	• KSw/C/LD • ⊘ P—first trimester • Caution advised in diabetic patients because of possible hypoglycemic effects of the herb • Three case reports of allergic dermatitis associated with topical use • Limited clinical evidence in HIV patients suggested possible additive effects with estrogens • In vivo uterine stimulant activity has been reported; this has not been observed clinically; however, medicinal use of burdock should be avoided during the first trimester
Butterbur	*Petasites hybridus*	Aerial parts / Rhizome / Root	Recommended in PA-free standardized form. PA intake is not to exceed 1 µg daily, and not to exceed intake for longer than 4-6 weeks/year		Antiinflammatory / Spasmolytic	Migraine headache	• LS/LD • ⊘ P/L • RHT • PAs found in this herb are known to be hepatotoxic, carcinogenic, and mutagenic • PA-free products used for short duration (up to 4 months) and in the recommended dosage are likely safe; however, there are limited safety data on this herb. As product quality may vary, it is possible that toxic amounts of PAs may be present in poorly processed products

Continued

Common Name	Botanical Name	Part Used	Dried Herb (In Capsules, Tea, Infusion, Decoction)	Tincture	Actions	Women's Health Indications Described in This Book	Safety Concerns
Calendula	*Calendula officinalis*	Flower	1-2 g/3/day	0.3-1.2 mL/day	Antiinflammatory Antimicrobial Lymphatic Vulnerary	Acne, inflammatory skin conditions Benign breast disorder Cervical dysplasia Endometriosis Hemorrhoids HSV (topical) Nipple thrush and cracked nipples Lymphadenopathy Postpartum perineal care UTI Vaginal dryness and atrophy (topical) Vulvovaginitis	• Internal use: LSw/C/LD • Topical use: KSw/C • ⊘ P—internal use • Allergic sensitivity has been reported, including cross-sensitivity in patients with latex allergy • Because calendula was traditionally used to affect the menstrual cycle, and in vitro uterotonic activity has been reported, internal consumption during pregnancy is not recommended • May have spermatocide activity
California poppy	*Eschscholzia californica*	Herb	N/A	2-4 mL/2-3×/day	Analgesic Anxiolytic Sedative (mild)	Anxiety Chronic pelvic pain DUB Dysmenorrhea Endometriosis Insomnia Menorrhagia Migraine/headache Musculoskeletal tension PMS	• LS/LD • ⊘ P
Canada fleabane, erigeron	*Erigeron canadense*	Aerial parts	N/A	1-2 mL 2-4×/day	Antihemorrhagic Astringent	Uterine fibroids	• LS/LD • ⊘ P
Caraway	*Carum carvi*	Seed	2-5 g/2×/day	2-3 mL/2×/day	Lactagogue	Increase milk supply	• LS/LD • ⊘ P • Do not use caraway oil internally
Castor	*Ricinus castor*	Oil extracted from seed	This herb is toxic for internal use. The pharmaceutical grade oil is used internally up to 4 oz spread over two doses as a laxative and uterine stimulant to induce labor		Stimulating laxative	Labor induction	• ⊘ P/L • Castor is a highly toxic plant and should not be taken internally other than in commercially prepared oil extract products • Castor is contraindicated in pregnancy other than to stimulate labor • Causes diarrhea

Common name	Latin name	Part	Dose	Actions	Indications	Cautions/Notes
Cat's claw	*Uncaria tomentosa*	Bark	2-30 g/day in decoction	Antiinflammatory Antimicrobial Immunostimulant	HSV	• H-D! • LD • ⊘P/L—internal use • Contraindicated with concurrent administration of immunosuppressive medications, passive vaccines, immunoglobulin therapy, cryoprecipitates, and fresh plasma products • It should not be taken by patients who have recently received or are awaiting organ or bone marrow transplantation • Should not be taken by women trying to conceive—it is traditionally used as a contraceptive agent
Catnip	*Nepeta cataria*	Leaf	5 g/3×/day 2-4 mL/3×/day	Nervine Sedative (mild) Spasmolytic	After-birth pains Dysmenorrhea Insomnia Nervousness	• KS/LD
Celandine	*Chelidonium majus*	Aerial part Root	1-2 g/2×/day 1-2 mL/3×/day	Alterative Antiinflammatory Hepatic/biliary action Immunomodulatory Laxative Spasmolytic	Endometriosis Hemorrhoids Uterine fibroids	• LD • ⊘P/L • RHT • Internal consumption of celandine has been associated with a total of 47 case reports of adverse events to the WHO Uppsala Monitoring Center up to the July 2005, including several case reports of hepatotoxicity including symptoms such as hepatitis, jaundice, and elevated liver enzymes. In 2003, the Australian government's Therapeutic Goods Administration recommended that *C. majus* preparations intended for oral intake be labeled with a warning to seek the advice of a health care professional before using if there is a history of liver disease and to discontinue use if symptoms of liver disease occur • Nausea, abdominal pain, diarrhea, discolored stool, and vomiting may result from use
Centaury	*Centaurium erythraea*	Herb	2-4 g/3×/day 2-4 mL/3×/day	Hepatic	PMS	• LD

Continued

Common Name	Botanical Name	Part Used	Dried Herb (In Capsules, Tea, Infusion, Decoction)	Tincture	Actions	Women's Health Indications Described in This Book	Safety Concerns
Chamomile	Matricaria recutita	Flowers	2-8 g/3×/day	1-4 mL/3×/day	Antiinflammatory, Carminative, Nervine, Sedative (mild), Spasmolytic	Abdominal pain associated with endometriosis and chronic pelvic pain, Acne (topical), Amenorrhea, Anxiety, Chronic pelvic pain, Dysmenorrhea, Endometriosis, GI spasm; Headache, Insomnia, PMS-related digestive symptoms, Restlessness, Topical for skin inflammation	• KS/LD • Skin rash occasionally with topical application • While chamomile is commonly cited as a contraindicated herb during pregnancy, this is based on a study conducted in 1979 that found teratogenic effects using a concentrated extract of α-bisoprolol at high doses. No teratogenic effects were seen at lower doses and the dose of the oil constituent required to cause teratogenicity is far greater than it would ever be possible for someone drinking the tea to ever approximate
Chaste berry	Vitex agnus-castus	Fruit	0-40 mg/day up to 30-40 mg/day	0.2 mL/2-3×/day up to 3-5 mL/day	Dopaminergic agonist (↓FSH), Galactogogue, Indirect progestogenic activity, Prolactin inhibitor	Benign breast disorder, Corpus luteal insufficiency, Endometriosis, Fertility problems, Habitual miscarriage, Hyperprolactinemia, Increase milk supply, Mastalgia, Menstrual irregularities, PCOS, Relieve PMS symptoms, Sometimes used for treatment of symptoms of perimenopause, Teenage acne, Uterine fibroids	• H-D! • KSwC/LD • ∅P • Adverse effects include nausea, headache, acne, and GI symptoms • According to a German postmarket surveillance study of 1634 women taking the herb, a total of 23 women became pregnant while using chaste tree; 19 of the 23 reported having been previously unsuccessful in trying to conceive • Theoretical inhibition of breast milk, though traditionally used to increase breast milk supply • May exacerbate depression in some women with progesterone deficiency or PMS-D • Possible interference with dopaminergic drugs
Chinese skullcap	Scutellaria baicalensis	Aerial parts	6-15 g in decoction	4-7 mL/1-2×/day	Antiinflammatory, Antimicrobial	Acne, HSV, PUPPP	• LS/LD

Common name	Botanical name	Part used	Dose	Liquid dose	Actions	Indications	Safety/Cautions
Cinnamon	*Cinnamomum zeylanicum*	Bark	1-4 g taken up to 4× daily	Liquid extract: 0.5-1.5 mL/day; Tincture: 2-4 mL/day	Astringent; Carminative; Flavoring	DUB; Menorrhagia; Uterine fibroids	• KS/LD • H-D! • Caustic with prolonged exposure to skin and mucosa • Because of possible hypoglycemic action, caution is advised in diabetics • No known contraindications to cinnamon during pregnancy as long as taken in amounts not greater than food amounts
Cleavers	*Galium aparine*	Herb	N/A	4-10 mL/day	Alterative	Acne; Benign breast disorder	• KS/LD
Coleus	*Coleus forskohlii*	Root	N/A	1.5-4 mL/day	Antihypertensive; Antiplatelet; Cardiotonic; Spasmolytic	CHF; Hypertension; Hypothyroidism; Ischemic heart disease	• LSw/C/LD • ⊘P/L • Not for use without medical supervision • Not to be used by patients with bleeding/clotting disorders • Do not combine with BP, cardiac, peptic ulcer, or antiplatelet medications
Comfrey	*Symphytum officinale*	Root and leaf	External use only		Demulcent; Vulnerary	Postpartum perineal care; Nipple thrush and cracked nipples; Vaginal dryness and atrophy (topical); Vulvovaginitis	• LSw/C • ⊘P/L—internal or extended topical • Comfrey products are safe for topical application. While there is some transdermal absorption of PAs, which can be hepatotoxic when taken internally, the amount absorbed when used on unbroken skin is likely to be insignificant, and even on broken skin, minimal. Nonetheless, regular use on broken skin is not recommended. The German Commission E recommends not exceeding 1000 µg/day of PAs transdermally, and not using topical applications of comfrey products for longer than 4 to 6 weeks total per year
Coptis	*Coptis chinensis*	Rhizome	2-4 g/3×/day	2-4 mL/3×/day	Antimicrobial	GBS; Vulvovaginitis	• LSw/C/LD • ⊘P/L • See Barberry • As with other berberine-containing herbs (e.g., barberry, goldenseal), internal use is generally not recommended during pregnancy; however, topical use in suppositories appears to be safe
Cordyceps	*Cordyceps sinensis*	Fruit body or mycelium	3-15 g/day	2-6 mL daily	Adaptogen; Immunomodulator	Endometriosis	• LS/LD

Continued

Common Name	Botanical Name	Part Used	Dried Herb (In Capsules, Tea, Infusion, Decoction)	Tincture	Actions	Women's Health Indications Described in This Book	Safety Concerns
Corn silk	*Zea mays*	Stigma, style	4-8 g/in infusion 3×/day	5-15 mL/3×/ day	Demulcent Diuretic Mucilage	Interstitial cystitis	• KS/LD • An isolated crystalline component from corn silk has been shown to have hypotensive and uterine-stimulating activity in rabbits, likely because of cholinergic effects. Although the herb is not typically contraindicated during pregnancy, it is prudent to be cautious given this observation.
Corydalis	*Corydalis ambigua*	Rhizome	5-10 g/day	5-20 mL/day	Analgesic Antispasmodic	Chronic pelvic pain Dysmenorrhea Endometriosis HA HSV 1 and 2—pain	• H-D! • ∅ P • Possible additive effects with antiarrhythmic medications • Oral administration of 1 to 50 mg/kg of gindarin to rats from the first to the second day of gestation led to significant embryotoxicity
Cotton root	*Gossypium herbaceum*	Root	N/A	2-4 mL/2×/ day	Abortifacient Emmenagogue	Amenorrhea Dysfunctional labor/labor augmentation Endometriosis Uterine fibroids	• ∅ P/LD • Because of the known abortifacient activity of this herb, it is contraindicated during pregnancy
Couch grass	*Elymus repens*	Rhizome	4-8 g/day in decoction	5-15 mL/3×/ day	Antimicrobial Demulcent Mucilage	Interstitial cystitis UTI	• LS/LD
Cramp bark/ black haw	*Viburnum opulus/ V. prunifolium*	Root	N/A	3-10 mL/day	Antihypertensive Spasmolytic	Abdominal pain associated with endometriosis and chronic pelvic pain After-birth pains Chronic pelvic pain Dysmenorrhea Endometriosis Hypertension Incoordinate uterine contractions Irritable uterus Painful labor Premature labor (threatened) Restless legs Threatened miscarriage Uterine fibroids	• KS/LD • Long history of traditional use for threatened miscarriage, uterine irritability, and painful labor suggests possible safety during pregnancy

Common name	Botanical name	Part	Dose (dried)	Dose (liquid)	Actions	Indications	Safety/Notes
Cranberry	Vaccinium macrocarpon	Fruit		Up to 400 mL cranberry juice daily for up to 6 months, or equivalent capsules	Urinary antiseptic	Reduction of odor associated with urinary incontinence; UTI	• H-D! • KSw/C • In clinical trials, there is a high dropout rate of cranberry juice users because of taste • Contrary to some claims, it is unlikely that regular consumption of cranberry juice will lead to the development of uric acid or oxalate stones; however, individuals who tend to form such stones may wish to avoid regular consumption and/or consumption of large amounts of cranberry juice • There are several reports of interaction with warfarin • There are no known contraindications to the use of cranberry juice during pregnancy and lactation
Cranesbill geranium	Geranium maculatum	Leaf	N/A	2-5 mL/day	Astringent	Menorrhagia; Uterine fibroids	• LS/LD • Because of high tannin content, use cautiously in inflammatory and ulcerative GI conditions
Damiana	Turnera diffusa	Leaf	2-4 g/3×/day	2-4 mL/day	Aphrodisiac; Nervine	Anxiety; Depression; Low libido; Vaginal dryness and atrophy	• LD • Ø P/L • Mild stimulating effects may possibly lead to insomnia • Because of possible cyanogenetic constituents, use during pregnancy and lactation is not recommended
Dandelion	Taraxacum officinale	Leaf	4-10 g/3×/day	Liquid extract: 4-10 mL/3×/day; Tincture: 2-5 mL/3×/day; Fresh juice: 5-10 mL/2×/day	Bitter tonic; Choleretic; Diuretic	Acne; Constipation; Mastalgia; PMS symptoms; UTI	• KS/LD • Contraindicated in bile duct and intestinal obstructions • Diuresis is not appropriate during pregnancy; use of dandelion leaf as a food is acceptable • Dandelion leaf should be treated as a prescription diuretic in terms of precautions with other medications; dandelion is K+ rich
Dandelion	Taraxacum officinale	Root	2-8 g/3×/day	Liquid extract: 2-8 mL/day; Tincture: 5-10 mL/day	Alterative; Aperient; Bitter tonic	Acne; Benign breast disorders; Constipation; Endometriosis; NVP/Related anorexia; PUPPS; Uterine fibroids	• KS/LD • Contraindicated for patients with gallbladder obstruction and obstructive ileus • No known contraindications during pregnancy when used in amounts comparable to food use

Continued

Common Name	Botanical Name	Part Used	Dried Herb (In Capsules, Tea, Infusion, Decoction)	Tincture	Actions	Women's Health Indications Described in This Book	Safety Concerns
Dong quai	*Angelica sinensis*	Root	3–9 g/day	5–15 mL/day	Antiinflammatory Antithrombotic Reproductive tonic TCM: yin and blood deficiency, blood moving	Amenorrhea Benign breast disorder Chronic pelvic pain Constipation Dysmenorrhea Endometriosis Fertility problems Hypomenorrhea Irregular menstruation Menstrual migraines Oligomenorrhea/ Uterine fibroids Vasomotor complaints of perimenopause and menopause Weakness, fatigue, lassitude	• KSw/C • Ø P/L • Increased bleeding • Not to be taken with blood-thinning medications • In TCM, dong quai is always combined with other herbs • GI symptoms, including nausea, laxative effects, vomiting, and bloating may occur • Photosensitivity with severe reactions may occur because of furocoumarin, psoralen, and bergapten contents • Dong quai may have hypotensive action; a limited body of research suggests possible interference with antiarrhythmic medications, β-blockers, and calcium channel blockers • Avoid during pregnancy unless under the care of a qualified TCM practitioner • Two case reports of rash in breastfeeding infants of mothers who took dong quai, including reappearance with discontinuation and retrial
Echinacea	*Echinacea* spp.	Herb root	1–3 g/3×/day	Liquid extract: 0.5–3 mL/3×/day Tincture: 2–5 mL/3×/day	Alterative Antiinflammatory Antimicrobial Immunomodulating Lymphatic	Acne Cervical dysplasia Endometriosis GBS HSV 1 and 2 Interstitial cystitis Lymphadenopathy Mastitis Recurrent UTI Upper respiratory infection Vulvovaginitis	• KS • Transitory tingling of the tongue is a normal effect of this herb • Possible allergy when flowering tops are given to allergic patients; use of root product only usually prevents allergy • Should not be taken by transplant patients or patients taking immunomodulatory medications • There is no clear evidence from either basic science or human reports that echinacea causes significant hepatotoxicity • Oral intake of echinacea is considered safe during pregnancy based on preliminary studies

Common name	Botanical name	Part used	Dosage	Actions	Uses/Indications	Safety/Notes
Eleuthero	*Eleutherococcus senticosus*	Root	1-4 g daily for up to 3 months; 2-16 mL/day up to 1 month	Adaptogen Immunomodulator	Convalescence Depression Exhaustion Fatigue, lassitude HSV Illness exacerbated by stress Improve mental stamina Improve physical stamina Physical or nervous stress	• KS • Insomnia has been rarely observed in clinical studies • Some sources recommend a limitation on the duration of use from 1 to 3 months; however, this is based on the need to reevaluate for possible health conditions rather than risks associated with the herb • Contrary to some reports, there does not appear to be a significant need for concern over the development of hypertension from the use of eleuthero • Eleuthero has been known to be adulterated with *Periploca sepium*, a plant that contains cardioactive glycosides and was associated with a case of fetal androgenization ("hairy baby syndrome") in a woman who unknowingly consumed an adulterated product during pregnancy
Evening primrose	*Oenothera biennis*	Oil from seeds	Dietary supplement oil: 1500 mg/day	Antiinflammatory Rich in EFAs, especially GLA	Benign breast disorder Chronic pelvic pain Dysfunctional labor/labor augmentation Endometriosis Improves quality of breast milk Migraines PMS symptoms	• KSw/C/LD • Contraindicated in patients with seizure disorders; use of the oil may trigger undiagnosed temporal lobe epilepsy, particularly in schizophrenic patients, or those taking epileptogenic medications • Possible GI upset • No teratogenicity has been demonstrated during pregnancy; however, data are limited. Because linoleic and gamalenic acids are components of breast milk, it seems safe for breastfeeding mothers to consume EPO; however, data are limited and concerns have been raised whether maternal consumption would cause excess consumption in the breastfeeding infant
False unicorn root	*Chamaelirium luteum*	Root	1-2 g/3×/day; Liquid extract: 1-2 mL/3×/day; Tincture: 2-5 mL/3×/day	Ovarian tonic Uterine tonic	Amenorrhea Fertility problems Irregular menstruation Ovarian pain PCOS Threatened miscarriage Uterine atony	• LD • Although this herb has traditionally been used to improve fertility, there are no safety data on intake during pregnancy. The herb possesses uterotonic activity. Therefore the herb should be discontinued when pregnancy has been achieved and care taken in women with a prior history of first-trimester miscarriage • This plant is considered endangered and therefore should only be used from cultivated sources

Continued

Common Name	Botanical Name	Part Used	Dried Herb (In Capsules, Tea, Infusion, Decoction)	Tincture	Actions	Women's Health Indications Described in This Book	Safety Concerns
Fennel	*Foeniculum vulgare*	Seeds	2.5 g/2×/day in tea	2-4 mL/2×/day	Carminative Estrogenic Lactagogue Spasmolytic	DUB Increase milk supply PMS-related digestive symptoms	• LSw/C/LD • EO not for internal use • Not for medicinal use during pregnancy because of possible estrogenic effects • Caution is recommended in women with a history or risk of ER-positive cancer
Fenugreek	*Trigonella foenum-graecum*	Seed	1-6 g/3×/day	2-4 mL/3×/day	Aphrodisiac Flavoring Lactagogue Lipid-lowering effects	Hypercholesterolemia Increase milk supply Low libido in menopausal years	• Sw/C • ⊘P • Caution in diabetics because of hypoglycemic effects • Caution in patients taking hypokalemic agents, cardiac glycoside medications, or with cardiac disease because of risk of hypokalemia from consumption • Theoretical risk of increased bleeding; caution advised in patients taking anticoagulants • Possible estrogenic activity requires caution when combined with estrogenic medications and oral contraceptives • Possible reduction in serum thyroid hormone concentrations; therefore caution is required for patients with hypothyroidism • Not for medicinal use during pregnancy because of possible hypoglycemic and hypothyroid effects • Possible potentiation of MAOIs in patients taking these medications • If a nursing mother consumes a large amount, the baby's urine may have a maple syrup–like odor that could be confused with maple syrup urine disease • Possible interference with iron absorption with long-term use
Feverfew	*Tanacetum parthenium*	Leaf	Freeze-dried: 0.05 g/1× after meals Dried: 50-200 mg/day	Liquid extract: 0.7-2 mL/day Tincture: 3-5 mL/day	Antiinflammatory Emmenagogue	Amenorrhea Dysmenorrhea Headaches: PMS, tension, and migraine	• LSw/C • ⊘P/L • Contact dermatitis (including oral ulcers/sore mouth) from fresh leaves • Reported side effects include GI complaints, tingling sensation on the tongue, headache, diarrhea, nausea, abdominal pain, flatulence, dizziness, and skin rash • No adverse effects seen in rats and pigs receiving 100 to 150 times the human dose daily • Because of reported abortifacient activity, feverfew is contraindicated during pregnancy. It has been reported to induce uterine contractions in full-term pregnant women

Common name	Latin name	Part used	Dose		Actions	Indications	Cautions
Figwort	*Scrophularia nodosa*	Aerial parts	2-8g/day	Liquid extract: 2-8 mL/day Tincture: 2-4 mL/day	Antiinflammatory Dermatologic	Acne	• LD
Flax seed	*Linum usitatissimum*	Seed	10-50 g seeds/day	N/A	Laxative Lipid-lowering effects: 1-3 Tbsp/day 1000 mg/tid Nutritional supplement: EFA source (omega-3) Phytoestrogen	Benign breast disorder Constipation Hot flashes Hypercholesterolemia Uterine fibroids Vaginal dryness and atrophy	• LSw/C • ∅P • Avoid in patients with bleeding disorders and those on anticoagulant/antiplatelet therapies • May interfere with absorption of medications; take 2 hours apart from other medications • Use cautiously in patients with irritable bowel disorders, chronic diarrhea, or diverticulitis • Caution advised in patients with diabetes because of case series showing elevated glucose levels in patients taking omega-3 fatty acids, which are found in flax seeds • Drink plenty of water when taking soaked or ground flax seed to prevent constipation and bowel obstruction • Has uncertain effects on triglyceride levels (may raise or lower); avoid in patients with hypertriglyceridemia • Immature flax seeds are neurotoxic and should not be taken. Symptoms of toxicity include ataxia, tachycardia, and weakness • Possible interactions with NSAIDs, mood stabilizers, oral hypoglycemic agents (including insulin), antihyperlipidemic agents, oral contraceptives, HRT, and antihypertensive drugs • Animal studies show possible harmful effects when taken during pregnancy and lactation, including increased levels of LH and testosterone, increased epididymal weight, and decreased prostate weight in males; altered mammary structure, delayed or early onset puberty depending on dose, and reduced or lengthened number of estrous cycles in females exposed to flax seeds in utero
Fringe tree	*Chionanthus virginicus*	Root bark	N/A	2-5 mL/day	Cholagogue/choleretic Laxative	Benign breast disorder Endometriosis	• LD

Continued

Common Name	Botanical Name	Part Used	Dried Herb (In Capsules, Tea, Infusion, Decoction)	Tincture	Actions	Women's Health Indications Described in This Book	Safety Concerns
Garlic	*Allium sativum*	Bulb	2-4 g/3×/day	Liquid extract: 0.5-2 mL/ 3×/day	Antiatherosclerotic Antihypertensive Antimicrobial (if fresh) Lipid-lowering effects	Atherosclerosis CAD GBS Hypercholesterolemia Hypertension Postpartum perineal care Trichomoniasis Vulvovaginitis	• KSw/C • Direct or prolonged exposure to skin can lead to irritation and ulceration • GI upset when taken raw internally; also garlic odor from ingesting fresh garlic • Possible interactions with anticoagulant and antiplatelet medications • Possible increased bleeding time; therefore discontinuation 2 weeks prior to surgery is recommended • In vitro increase in uterine activity; therefore caution when taking medicinally in pregnancy; no expected adverse effects when taken as a food in pregnancy • Altered odor of breast milk in breastfeeding mothers consuming garlic has led to alterations in infant feeding in a blinded, placebo-controlled study. Amniotic fluid odor is also influenced by maternal garlic consumption • There are no known adverse clinical or experimental effects of garlic on pregnancy or lactation
Gentian	*Gentiana lutea*	Rhizome	0.6-2 g/3×/day	1-4 mL/3×/ day	Hepatic	PMS	• KS/LD • ⊘P/L • Contraindicated in pregnancy and lactation because of mutagenic effects seen on Ames test
Ginger	*Zingiber officinale*	Rhizome	0.25-1 g/3×/day	1.5-3 mL/3×/ day	Antiemetic Antiinflammatory Antinauseant Antiplatelet Carminative Flavoring Spasmolytic	Amenorrhea Digestive complaints associated with endometriosis and chronic pelvic pain Dysmenorrhea Nausea with HIV, chemotherapy NVP Pelvic pain and congestion Reduce nausea associated with herbs and medications Uterine fibroids	• KSw/C • May increase absorption of other medications • Contraindicated in patients with gallstones • Caution in patients with peptic ulcer disease or GERD • Contraindicated in patients with bleeding disorders, on medications for bleeding disorders, and before and after surgery • During pregnancy dose should not exceed 1 g/day because of possible abortifacient activity; doses up to this amount considered safe for the treatment of NVP

Ginkgo	*Ginkgo biloba*	Leaf	Extract: 120-240 mg/day Extract: 120-240 mg/day in 2-3 divided doses	Antioxidant Anti-PAF Circulatory stimulant Cognition enhancing	Dysmenorrhea Headache Memory loss and cognitive decline Pelvic congestion	• LSw/C • ⊘ P/L • Possible GI upset, headache, dizziness • Case reports of spontaneous bleeding have led to a high level of caution pre- and post-surgery and in patients on antiplatelet/anticoagulant therapies
Ginseng	*Panax ginseng*	Root	1-9 g/day in 2-3 divided doses 1-6 mL/day	Adaptogen TCM: Tonify qi, spleen, stomach, heart	Convalescence Endometriosis Fatigue, poor stamina PCOS Physical, mental fatigue Poor concentration Susceptibility to colds, infection Vaginal dryness and atrophy	• KSw/C • ⊘ P/L • Generally well tolerated in most clinical trials • Caution advised in diabetic patients because of possible hypoglycemic effects • May cause or exacerbate hypertension, insomnia, anxiety, palpitations, and tachycardia in some individuals. Patients with any of these as pre-existing conditions should avoid ginseng use unless under the supervision of a qualified TCM practitioner • Limited case reports of epistaxis, increased vaginal bleeding, and a single report of reduced effectiveness of warfarin. Based on these reports, caution has been advised for patients on antiplatelet/anticoagulant medications and pre- and post-surgically • Although no adverse effects, mutagenicity, or teratogenicity have been reported, and the herb is traditionally used during pregnancy and for postpartum convalescence, it is generally recommended that ginseng only be used under the supervision of a qualified health professional during pregnancy

Continued

Common Name	Botanical Name	Part Used	Dried Herb (In Capsules, Tea, Infusion, Decoction)	Tincture	Actions	Women's Health Indications Described in This Book	Safety Concerns
Globe artichoke	*Cynara scolymus*	Fruit	250-750 mg of cymarin daily or 4-9 g leaves daily	3-8 mL daily	Lipid-lowering effects	Hypercholesterolemia	• LS/LD • Considered well tolerated, with no known contraindications or major adverse effects • Individuals may experience nonspecific GI complaints when taking globe artichoke • Likely safe when taken for short periods • Because of lack of toxicity data, excessive use should be avoided in pregnancy and lactation
Goat's rue	*Galega officinalis*	Herb	3-6 g/day of dried herb in infusion	4-8 mL/day	Lactagogue	Increase milk supply	• ⊘ P/LD • Goat's rue has caused poisoning and death in sheep; however, there is no evidence of human poisoning by goat's rue reported in the literature. Oral administration of goat's rue to pregnant ewes at various stages of gestation produced no noticeable damage in the offspring • Caution is advised in diabetic patients because goat's rue may enhance the hypoglycemic effects of hypoglycemic drugs; however, there are no documented cases of this effect • Goat's rue taken with mineral salts increased milk production in lactating women in a controlled trial from 1968; however, no safety or toxicity studies have been done on use during lactation
Goldenrod	*Solidago virgaurea*	Herb	3-5 g/2-3×/day	2-3 mL/2-3×/day	Antiinflammatory Diuretic	Interstitial cystitis UTI	• LS/LD • Possible sensitivity in patients allergic to plants in the *Compositae* family, and specifically to goldenrod; contact dermatitis

| Goldenseal | *Hydrastis canadensis* | Root/rhizome | 0.5-1 g/3×/day | Liquid extract: 0.3-1 mL/ 2-3×/day Tincture: 2-4 mL/2-3×/ day | Antiinflammatory Antihemorrhagic Antimicrobial Astringent | Cervical dysplasia GBS Menorrhagia Nipple thrush Pelvic congestion Vaginal discharge Vaginal infection Vulvovaginitis | • H-DI
 • LSw/C/LD
 • There is limited research on goldenseal herb; however, much is known about isolated constituents from the herb, most notably, berberine and hydrastine
 • Although one cannot extrapolate the effects of isolated constituents to the whole plant, cautions are suggested when using this herb regularly or in high doses
 • Consumption of isolated berberine alkaloids in goldenseal is toxic
 • High doses of hydrastine have caused elevated blood pressure after intravenous administration in animal studies; lower doses of berberine and hydrastine have hypotensive effects. Caution is suggested in use with hypertensive patients, and those on antihypertensive medications
 • No reported clinical herb–drug interactions
 • In vitro berberine has been reported to decrease the anticoagulant effects of heparin in dog and human blood, and although no sedative activity has been reported, increased barbiturate sleeping time has been reported
 • Berberine is reported to increase coronary blood flow, and at high doses is reported to inhibit cardiac muscle activity
 • Caution is advised in patients with cardiac arrhythmias
 • Antihistamine and antimuscarine activity has been reported
 • The use of goldenseal during pregnancy is controversial. Typically contraindicated, this is based on limited reports of increased activity of the in vitro increase of uterine stimulant activity on guinea pig and rat uterine tissue from the isolated fraction canadine. However, the total alkaloid fraction of goldenseal has demonstrated anticonvulsant activity in vitro. The issue of contraindication in pregnancy appears to have less to do with the effects of the herb as a uterine tonic and more to do with the potential toxicity of long-term intake of the alkaloids. At this time, goldenseal is not recommended for regular or high-dose intake during pregnancy; however, based on current literature, it is premature to entirely contraindicate its use during pregnancy and lactation
 • This herb is considered ecologically endangered; therefore only products made from cultivated herb should be used |

Continued

Common Name	Botanical Name	Part Used	Dried Herb (In Capsules, Tea, Infusion, Decoction)	Tincture	Actions	Women's Health Indications Described in This Book	Safety Concerns
Gotu kola	*Centella asiatica*	Herb	1–10 g/3×/day	20–40 mL/day	Connective tissue repair Nervine tonic	Anxiety, stress Chronic venous insufficiency and varicosities Fatigue Improve memory, cognitive function PUPPP/prevent striae	• H-DI • LS/LD • Well tolerated when taken for up to 6 to 12 months for chronic insufficiency and wound healing • Numerous case reports of allergic reactions and contact dermatitis • Limited reports of adverse effects of gastric irritation and nausea have been reported • Conflicting reports state both possible lipid-lowering and lipid-elevating effects with this herb • Animal studies suggest possible sedating effects • Caution in diabetics based on animal evidence of possible ability to raise blood glucose • Safety unknown during pregnancy and lactation
Green tea	*Camellia sinensis*	Leaf	2–4 cups/day		Antidyslipidemic Antioxidant Antiviral	Endometriosis HSV Improve mood, memory, concentration Nipple thrush and cracked nipples Osteoporosis prevention Reduce LDL, raise HDL Uterine fibroids Varicosities, hemorrhoids	• KSw/C • Diuresis • More than 500 mg/day of caffeine is associated with insomnia, palpitations, anxiety, agitation, delirium, psychosis, and detrusor muscle instability. Withdrawal commonly accompanies cessation of chronic use • Preliminary research suggests a possible reduction in estrogen associated with regular green tea consumption • Regular consumption of high tannin beverages may interfere with iron absorption • Numerous interactions with caffeine and medications are known; the effects of green tea as a source of herb–drug interactions has not been well studied • Regular caffeine consumption is best avoided in pregnancy, especially in the first trimester, because caffeine crosses the placenta. Consumption of more than 400 mg/day of caffeine during pregnancy has been associated with increased rates of SIDS; more than 1100 mg/day has been associated with congenital birth defects • Caffeine is readily transferred into breast milk and may lead to sleep disturbances in infants. Infants of breastfeeding mothers consuming more than 500 mg caffeine/day have been reported to have tremors and cardiac dysrhythmias • Green tea extracts and other concentrated green tea products are not recommended and are not considered safe during pregnancy and lactation

Common Name	Latin Name	Part	Dose	Actions	Indications	Safety & Interaction Codes / Notes
Gromwell	*Lithospermum officinale*	Herb	N/A; 2-4 mL/day		Hyperthyroidism	LD
Guggul	*Commiphora mukul*	Resin	500-1000 g guggulipid standardized to 2.5% gugulsterones or/2-3 day or an equivalent dose of prepared gugulsterone 25 mg/3×/day	Antidyslipidemic, Antioxidant, Antiplatelet aggregation	Acne, Atherosclerosis prevention, Reduce LDL, raise HDL	H-DI!, LSw/C, ⊘P/L • Considered safe when used in recommended doses for up to 6 months • Reversible inhibition of platelet aggregation; possible interference with anticoagulant and antiplatelet medications; discontinue 1 week prior to surgery • Mild thyroid stimulation; not recommended in patients with thyroid disorders • Possible hypersensitivity reactions • May increase bioavailability of propranolol (β-blocker) and decrease the bioavailability of diltiazem (calcium channel blocker) • Adverse effects include GI upset and headache • Not recommended during pregnancy because of possible abortive effects; not recommended during lactation
Gymnema	*Gymnema sylvestris*	Leaf	2-3 g/2-3×/day; 3-5 mL/2-3×/day	Antidiabetic, Hypocholesterolemic, Hypoglycemic	PCOS	LS/LD, ⊘P/L • No known adverse effects or herb–drug interactions have been associated with this herb other than the possible glucose-lowering effects and possible potentiation of hypoglycemic agents and antihyperlipidemic effects and possible potentiation of lipid-lowering drugs
Hawthorn	*Crataegus oxyacantha*	Fruit	0.3-1 g/3×/day; Liquid extract: 0.5-2 mL/3×/day; Tincture: 1-6 mL/3×/day	Antihypertensive, Cardiotonic, Peripheral vasodilator	Cardiac insufficiency, Heart palpitations with anxiety, Hypertension, Tachycardia	KSw/C • Hawthorn is exceptionally well tolerated and safe as recommended • Theoretical concerns exist regarding potentiation of the actions of other cardiovascular medications; however, this has not been demonstrated clinically, including in a trial comparing digoxin alone compared with digoxin plus hawthorn. Potentiation of inotropic effects without toxicity was observed in guinea pig hearts. Use of the herb concurrently with cardiac glycosides has been suggested as a means to lower cardiac glycoside dose and toxicity • Theoretical potentiation of effect on medications with coronary dilatory effects was seen in animal studies • Rare reported side effects include nausea, headache, dizziness, and palpitations • Unspecified hawthorn extracts have demonstrated reduction in uterine tissue tone and motility in vitro. The clinical significance of this is unknown in pregnancy

Continued

Common Name	Botanical Name	Part Used	Dried Herb (In Capsules, Tea, Infusion, Decoction)	Tincture	Actions	Women's Health Indications Described in This Book	Safety Concerns
Hollyhock	Alcea rosea		N/A	1-3 mL/2×/day	Demulcent, mucilage	Interstitial cystitis	• LS/LD
Hops	Humulus lupulus	Strobile	0.5-2 g/2-4×/day	Liquid extract: 0.5-3 mL/3×/day. Tincture: 1-2 mL/3×/day	Anxiolytic, Estrogenic, Sedative (mild), Spasmolytic	Amenorrhea, Anxiety, Chronic pelvic pain, Dysmenorrhea, Headache, Insomnia, Lactation—improve let down reflex, Increase milk supply	• H-D! • KSw/C • ⊘P • May exacerbate depression in some patients. Do not use concurrently with antidepressant medications or in patients with moderate to severe depression • High doses may be significantly sedating • Direct estrogenic effects of phytoestrogens have been observed in vitro. Caution is advised in patients with ER–positive cancer and those using hormonal contraception or HRT • Hops may increase serum glucose levels; therefore caution is advised in diabetic patients • Not for use during pregnancy
Horse chestnut	Aesculus hippocastanum	Seed	1-2 g/day	Extracts equivalent to 50-150 mg triterpenes (aescin) in divided doses	Antiinflammatory, Venotonic	Chronic pelvic pain, Chronic venous insufficiency, varicosities, hemorrhoids, Pelvic congestion syndrome, Vaginal dryness and atrophy	• LS • Possible GI irritation • No documented herb–drug interactions • Improperly prepared products may contain aescin, which has theoretical additive effects with anticoagulant and antiplatelet drugs • Limited data suggest no adverse reactions or toxicity during pregnancy and possible safety for the treatment of venous insufficiency and varicosities
Horsetail	Equisetum arvense	Herb	50-75 mg aescin twice daily from standardized product; equivalent to 300 mg standardized product/day	Extracts equivalent to 50-150 mg triterpenes/day	Antiinflammatory, Diuretic, Urinary astringent	Interstitial cystitis, Osteoporosis prevention, UTI	• H-D! • LSw/C • ⊘P/L • Horsetail is generally very well tolerated with few reports of adverse effects • Theoretical herb–drug interactions include: —Thiamine depletion because of thiaminase in the herb —Adverse effects with cardiac glycosides, diuretics, steroids, and laxatives because of potassium-depleting effects of horsetail • The nicotine content in horsetail is theoretically suggested to cause side effects associated with nicotine use and has theoretically suggested ability to have additive effects with other CNS stimulants • Not for internal use during pregnancy

Common name	Botanical name	Part used	Dosage	Actions	Indications	Cautions
Jamaican dogwood	*Piscidia piscipula*	Root bark	1-2 g/3×/day; 2-8 mL/day	Analgesic, Sedative, Spasmolytic	Chronic pelvic pain, Dysmenorrhea, Endometriosis, Headache/migraine, Insomnia	• LD • LSw/C • Rotenone, a constituent in Jamaican dogwood, is a known toxin. Symptoms of overdose may include numbness, tremors, salivation, and sweating. In vivo oral doses of up to 1.5 mg/kg have not been shown to be toxic in animal studies • Caution is advised in patients with hypotension, cardiac insufficiency, and bradycardia • Jamaican dogwood has been reported to have a potent depressant effect on the uterus in vivo and in vitro, possibly equivalent to papaverine • Use is generally not recommended in pregnancy because of limited safety data; however, cautious use under the supervision of a qualified practitioner may be acceptable for a limited number of conditions. Use is not recommended during the first trimester of pregnancy
Kava kava	*Piper methysticum*	Root	1.5-3 g/day, equivalent to 60-120 mg kavalactones/day; Liquid extract: 3-6 mL/day; Standardized preparations: 100-200 kavalactones/day; 60 mg kavalactones 2-4×/day	Analgesic, Anxiolytic, Sedative, Spasmolytic	Anxiety; tension, Chronic pelvic pain, Endometriosis, Headache, Hot flashes, Insomnia, Interstitial cystitis, Musculoskeletal tension, PMS symptoms, UTI	• H-D! • LSw/C • ⊘P/L • Associated with risk of hepatotoxicity; contraindicated in patients with history of liver disease. Periodic evaluation of liver enzymes may be prudent with chronic use • Should not be taken in conjunction with CNS-affecting drugs because of possible potentiation; possible interaction with benzodiazepines • Possible extrapyramidal effects with kava use • Kava dermopathy may occur with abuse; it is reversible on discontinuation
Ladies' mantle	*Alchemilla vulgaris*	Herb	2-4 g/3×/day; 2-4 mL/3×/day	Astringent, Uterotonic	Chronic pelvic pain, Endometriosis, Menorrhagia, Uterine fibroids	• LS/LD
Lavender	*Lavandula officinalis*, *L. angustifolia*	Flower	1-3 g/2-3×/day; 2-4 mL/1-2×/day	Antidepressant (mild), Antimicrobial, Antiseptic, Anxiolytic, Carminative, Sedative (mild), Spasmolytic	Acne (topical), Anxiety, Cervical dysplasia, Headache, Insomnia, Irritability, Mild depression, PMS, Postpartum perineal care (topical), Restlessness, Vaginal dryness and atrophy (topical), Vulvovaginitis (topical)	• H-D! • LSw/C • Theoretical additive effects with CNS depressants, antidepressant drugs, and antiseizure medications • Possible lipid-lowering effects may be additive with lipid-lowering medications • EO for topical use only • Because of the ability of volatile oils to cross the placenta and the CNS effects of lavender, use of not more than an occasional cup of beverage tea with lavender is recommended during the first trimester

Continued

Common Name	Botanical Name	Part Used	Dried Herb (In Capsules, Tea, Infusion, Decoction)	Tincture	Actions	Women's Health Indications Described in This Book	Safety Concerns
Lemon balm	Melissa officinalis	Leaf	1.5-4.5 g/2-3×/day	2-4 mL/2-3×/day	Antiviral Anxiolytic Nervine Spasmolytic	Anxiety Depression (mild) Headache Hot flashes HSV Hyperthyroidism Insomnia	• KS • Possible TSH/thyroxin antagonist effects
Licorice	Glycyrrhiza glabra	Root	1-4 g/2×/day	0.6-2 mL/2-3×/day	Adaptogen Antiinflammatory Antitussive Antiviral	Cardiac insufficiency Constipation HSV Interstitial cystitis PCOS (with peony) PUPPS UTI Vulvovaginitis (topical)	• H-D! • Ø P/L • Serious side effects include hypertension, symptoms of hyperaldosteronism, electrolyte imbalances (and associated sequelae), and hormonal dysregulation including elevated prolactin and estrogen levels in women, which may affect fertility or menstrual regularity • Hypokalemia with chronic use/overdose; also blocked aldosterone/renin response, lethargy, hypertension, headache, sodium retention, and in rare cases pulmonary hypertension and CHF (not caused by the DGL form) • Caution should be exercised with patients on digoxin because of potential decreases in potassium associated with licorice intake • May reduce the effects of diuretics such as hydrochlorothiazide and spironolactone, affecting blood pressure and CHF control, and may cause hypokalemia when combined with furosemide, insulin, or Kayexalate • May theoretically interfere with hormonal contraceptives and HRT • Contraindicated in patients with hypertension or mineralocorticoid disorders • Increased risk of premature labor when used regularly during pregnancy. Generally not recommended for use during pregnancy; exceptions may be considered for short-term use under supervision of a qualified practitioner for specific conditions

Common Name	Botanical Name	Part Used	Dose (dried)	Dose (liquid)	Actions	Indications	Safety/Interactions
Lily of the valley	*Convallaria majalis*	Flower	N/A	0.5-1 mL/2×/day	Cardiotonic	Cardiac insufficiency	• H-DI! • ∅ P/L • Side effects associated with cardiac glycosides including vomiting, diarrhea, nausea, visual disturbances, hypotension, serious arrhythmias, and sinoatrial block • Risk of interactions/potentiation with other cardiac glycoside drugs
Linden (Lime blossom)	*Tilia* spp.	Flower	2-4 g/2×/day	1-2 mL/2×/day	Diuretic Sedative (mild) Spasmolytic	Anxiety Headache Hypertension Insomnia See which other uses in text	• LS/LD • There are limited data on the safety and efficacy of linden, an herb with a long history of use in European herbal medicine. Prior allegations that the herb should be avoided in patients with a cardiac disorder do not appear to have any scientific basis
Lobelia	*Lobelia inflata*	Herb	0.2-0.6 g/3×/day	Liquid extract: 0.2-0.6 mL/3×/day Tincture: 0.6-2 mL/3×/day	Analgesic Sedative Spasmolytic	Acute anxiety Cervical dilatation Dysmenorrhea (severe) Endometrial pain Insomnia Interstitial cystitis	• ∅ P/L • Lobelia acts on nicotinic receptors and may cause respiratory stimulation in low doses and respiratory depression in high doses • Tachycardia may occur at higher doses; if it does, discontinue and resume only at a lower dose with close monitoring, if at all • Other side effects include nausea, vomiting, dizziness, hypotension, diaphoresis, and palpitations • Some midwives use this herb to relax the cervix during a difficult labor with failure to progress; there are no data on the efficacy or safety of this practice. The herb should not be used in pregnancy prior to labor and should only be used in labor, if at all, under the supervision of a qualified practitioner
Marijuana	*Cannabis* spp.	Flower Resin	Dose not specified		Anodyne Appetite stimulant Sedative Spasmolytic	Chemotherapy: nausea Chronic pelvic pain Dysmenorrhea Endometrial pain HIV: pain, appetite Insomnia Interstitial cystitis NVP	• LS • Sedation • Decreased reflexes • Risks associated with smoking • Risks of dependency • Because of illegality, use is not recommended
Marshmallow	*Althaea officinalis*	Root	2-5 g/3×/day	2-5 mL/3×/day	Antiinflammatory Demulcent	Increase milk supply Interstitial cystitis UTI Vulvovaginitis	• KS/LD • There are no reported side effects or herb-drug interactions. The high mucilage content has been purported to possibly reduce the absorption of other medications

Continued

Common Name	Botanical Name	Part Used	Dried Herb (In Capsules, Tea, Infusion, Decoction)	Tincture	Actions	Women's Health Indications Described in This Book	Safety Concerns
Meadow-sweet	Filipendula ulmaria	Herb	4-6 g/3×/day	Liquid extract: 1.5-6 mL/3×/day Tincture: 3-4 mL/3×/day	Antacid Antiinflammatory Urinary antiseptic	See how used in book	• H-D! • ⊘ P/L • Avoid in patients with salicylate sensitivity, G6PD deficiency, and bleeding disorders • Toxicity and fetal malformations have been seen in animal studies; therefore use of this herb is contraindicated during pregnancy and lactation
Milk thistle	Silybum marianum	Seed	4-9 g/day	2-4 mL/2-3×/day	Antioxidant Hepatoprotective	See how used in book PUPPP	• H-D! • KSw/C • Well tolerated with no expected side effects with the exception of reports of hypersensitivity reactions • Rarely, headache, pruritus, or GI upset have been reported • Hypoglycemic effects have been reported; thus caution is advised in diabetic patients • Possible herb–drug interactions include interference with medications metabolized by CYP via inhibition of the enzyme, theoretical decreased clearance of glucuronidated agents, increased clearance of estrogens, and increased efficacy of chemotherapeutic drugs, including platinums and anthracyclines • Two separate clinical trials of milk thistle in pregnant women yielded positive results with no evidence of harmful effects on the pregnancy or offspring. In one study, 400 mg of silymarin was used to treat mothers for 60 days for intrahepatic cholestasis. The women experienced improvements in symptoms and blood work. In another study, a 15-day trial of milk thistle was shown to attenuate pruritus associated with intrahepatic cholestasis
Milky oats	Avena sativa	Milk Seed	N/A	3-5 mL/2-3×/day	Nervine	Increase milk supply Insomnia Nervous exhaustion PUPPP Stress, tension, irritability	• KS/LD

Common name	Botanical name	Part	Dose	Actions	Dose (extract)	Indications	Safety / Notes
Motherwort	*Leonurus cardiaca*	Herb	2-4 g/3×/day	Bitter Cardiotonic Hypotensive Nervine Spasmolytic Uterine tonic	Liquid extract: 2-4 mL/3×/day Tincture: 2-6 mL/3×/day	Amenorrhea Anxiety, stress, irritability Benign breast disorder Dysfunctional labor/labor augmentation Dysmenorrhea Endometriosis Hypertension Improve let-down reflex/increase milk supply Irregular menstruation Menstrual headache Palpitations (e.g., because of stress, hyperthyroidism) PMS Uterine fibroids	• LS/LD • ∅P • No adverse effects or herb–drug interactions are expected. There is a general lack of clinical and safety data on this herb, although there is a significant record of historical use • No warnings or cautions have been reported in association with the purported cardioactivity of the herb, which was found to have inhibitory effects on myocardial function • Motherwort is traditionally not recommended for use during pregnancy because of purported uterotonic effects. Leonurine, a constituent, is reported to have uterotonic effects; stachydrine, another constituent, is reported to have oxytocic effects
Mugwort	*Artemisia vulgaris*	Aerial parts	1-3 g/2×/day	Emmenagogue	1-2 mL/2×/day	Amenorrhea	• LD • ∅P
Mullein	*Verbascum thapsus*	Leaf	3-6 g/day	Demulcent Mucilage	2-4 mL/2-3×/day	Interstitial cystitis	• LS/LD
Myrrh	*Commiphora molmol*	Resin	N/A	Antiinflammatory Antimicrobial Antitumorigenic Vulnerary	1.5-4.5 mL/day	Cervical dysplasia GBS HSV ulcers (topical) Hypothyroidism Postpartum perineal care Vulvovaginitis (topical)	• LS/LD • ∅P • Prolonged topical use may cause contact dermatitis—limit topical use to 7 days consecutively
Nettle	*Urtica dioica*	Leaf	2-4 g/3×/day	Antiallergic Diuretic Nutritive Vascular tonic	Liquid extract: 3-4 mL/3×/day Tincture: 2-6 mL/3×/day Fresh juice: 1-15 mL/3×/day	Acne Anemia DUB Fatigue Iron-deficiency anemia Menstrual irregularities Osteoporosis prevention Pelvic congestion Sugar, caffeine cravings Varicosities	• KS/LD • Nettle has a long historic use as a food and tonic. It is considered well tolerated but is almost entirely lacking in clinical data • Uterotonic activity has been reported in vivo in pregnant and nonpregnant murine models, with betaine and serotonin considered the active ingredients. The clinical relevance of this is unknown. Although this has been a purported basis for contraindication of use during pregnancy, nettle has been consumed in large quantities by pregnant women as a uterine tonic with no reported increase in uterine activity, miscarriage, or malformations in the offspring

Continued

Common Name	Botanical Name	Part Used	Dried Herb (In Capsules, Tea, Infusion, Decoction)	Tincture	Actions	Women's Health Indications Described in This Book	Safety Concerns
Oregano	*Origanum vulgare*	Leaf	Used topically as a diluted EO	N/A	Antimicrobial Antiviral	Cervical dysplasia GBS	• KSw/C • ØP • Oregano is considered safe when used in amounts comparable with use in foods • The EO is for topical use only. Prolonged topical use may lead to contact dermatitis • Not for internal medicinal use during pregnancy and lactation because the volatile oils can cross the placenta and enter into breast milk
Oregon grape root	*Berberis aquifolium* syn. *Mahonia aquifolium*	Root	1.5-3 g/2-3 mL/day	2.5-5 g/2-3×/day	Antiinflammatory Antimicrobial Bitter	Acne (topical/internal) Benign breast disorder GBS Nipple thrush PUPPS (topical) UTI Vulvovaginitis (topical)	• LSw/C • See Goldenseal for cautions associated with berberine, which is found in Oregon grape root
Osha	*Lomatium dissectum*	Root	1-3 g/2×/day	1-3 mL/2×/day	Antiviral	Cervical dysplasia	• LD • ØP
Partridge berry	*Mitchella repens*		N/A	2-4 mL/2×/day	Uterine astringent/tonic	Chronic pelvic pain Dysmenorrhea Uterine fibroids	• LS/LD
Passionflower	*Passiflora incarnata*	Herb	4-8 g/day	1-4 mL/3×/day	Analgesic Antispasmodic Anxiolytic Sedative (mild)	Anxiety, stress, tension Dysmenorrhea Endometrial pain Headache Insomnia Nervous irritability PMS	• KSw/C/LD • No known contraindications or herb–drug interactions reported in the literature; excessive doses may theoretically cause sedation • At the highest concentrations of extract, passionflower increased spontaneous uterine contractions on isolated rat uteri, and caused a statistically significant reduction in tissue response to acetylcholine when compared with control
Pau d'Arco	*Tabebuia impetiginosa*	Bark	1-2 g/2×/day	Liquid extract (1:2) 3-7 mL/day	Antimicrobial	Vaginal infections (topical) Vulvovaginitis (topical)	• LSw/C • ØP/L • Safe when used for topical use, including for acute use as a suppository during pregnancy
Peony	*Paeonia lactiflora*	Root	3-6 g/day	3-5 mL/1-2×/day	Spasmolytic	Amenorrhea Dysmenorrhea Endometriosis Fertility problems Interstitial cystitis Iron-deficiency anemia PCOS Threatened miscarriage Uterine fibroids	• LSw/C • Possible anticoagulant activity; caution should be used with patients with bleeding problems or on anticoagulant/antiplatelet medications

Common name	Botanical name	Part	Dose	Dose	Actions	Indications	Notes
Peppermint	*Mentha piperita*	Leaf	2-3 g/1-3× day as tea	2-5.5 mL/1-2× day	Antiemetic	Digestive complaints associated with PMS NVP	• KS • Contraindicated in patients with esophageal reflux disease • Caution recommended for patients with salicylate allergy • Caution recommended for patients with gallstones • EO not for internal use • For use as a beverage tea only during the first trimester of pregnancy; the volatile oils can cross the placenta
Picrorhiza	*Picrorhiza kurroa*	Root	N/A	2-4 mL/2-3× day	Antiinflammatory Antioxidant Hepatoprotective Immunomodulatory	Benign breast disorder	• LSw/C/LD • ⊘P • Side effects include GI symptoms and skin rash
Pipsissewa	*Chimaphila umbellata*	Aerial parts	N/A	2-3 mL/2-3× day	Astringent tonic	Interstitial cystitis	• LS/LD
Poke root	*Phytolacca americana*	Root	For topical use only	N/A	Alterative Antiinflammatory Cytotoxic Lymphatic	Benign breast disorder	• ⊘P/L • Known toxicity associated with internal use of all parts of the plant with both internal and topical use. Peripheral blood changes have been observed with ingestion, including eosinophilia • Toxicity symptoms include nausea, vomiting, cramping, weakness, diarrhea, hematemesis, hypotension, and tachycardia • Limited topical use under qualified supervision only • Not for internal or topical use at any time during pregnancy or lactation
Psyllium	*Plantago ovata*	Seed	20-35 g/day	N/A	Bulk laxative	Constipation	• LSw/C • Serious allergic reactions have been reported after ingestion • Bowel obstruction has been reported after ingestion, particularly in individuals who have had prior bowel surgery or when psyllium has been taken with inadequate quantities of water • GI side effects include bloating, gas, and diarrhea, as well as constipation (as a result of obstruction) • Caution is suggested in diabetic patients because of the hypoglycemic effects of psyllium • Pregnancy and lactation warnings include those described above for this herb. No other known contraindications exist during pregnancy for any of the trimesters; however, pregnancy safety studies are lacking

Continued

Common Name	Botanical Name	Part Used	Dried Herb (In Capsules, Tea, Infusion, Decoction)	Tincture	Actions	Women's Health Indications Described in This Book	Safety Concerns
Pulsatilla (Pasque flower)	*Anemone pulsatilla*	Herb	0.12–0.3 g/3×/day	Liquid extract: 0.12–0.3 mL/3×/day Tincture: 0.3–1 mL/3×/day	Analgesic	Chronic pelvic pain Dysmenorrhea Endometriosis Interstitial cystitis Migraines	• LSw/C/LD • ⊘ P/L • Only preparations made from *dried* plant material should be used—fresh plant is toxic • Increased uterine activity has been documented
Quaking aspen	*Populus tremelloids*	Bark	1–4 g/2–3×/day as a decoction	1–3 mL/2×/day	Antiinflammatory Antiseptic Astringent	Interstitial cystitis	• LD • The high salicylates and tannin levels in this herb suggest that use during pregnancy is not appropriate; however, there are no studies of pregnancy/lactation safety with this herb, and a dearth of research on this herb generally
Red clover	*Trifolium pratense*	Flower Herb	3–5 g/3×/day	1–2 mL/3×/day	Alterative Phytoestrogen (isoflavones) Spasmolytic	Acne Benign breast disorder Osteoporosis prevention Uterine fibroids Vaginal dryness and atrophy Vasomotor complaints of perimenopause and menopause	• KSw/C • Some consider caution advisable for patients with a risk/history of ER–positive cancer • Standardized isoflavone products should not be used during pregnancy and lactation because of the potential for estrogenic activity • Possible cautionary use when taking hormonal contraceptives or HRT. Red clover may enhance estrogenic effects via ER binding
Red raspberry	*Rubus idaeus*	Leaf	4–8 g/3×/day	4–8 mL/3×/day	Astringent Nutritive Partus preparator Uterine tonic	Chronic pelvic pain DUB Dysfunctional labor/labor augmentation Dysmenorrhea Pregnancy uterine tonic Uterine fibroids	• KS • Safety of use during pregnancy has been demonstrated • There are no known contraindications or expected side effects or herb–drug interactions; however, any herb with a high tannin content can theoretically interfere with nutrient absorption, particularly iron, when taken in high doses or for extended periods • Some women report nausea when taking raspberry leaf tea during the first trimester of pregnancy, likely because of the astringency of the herb
Red root, New Jersey tea	*Ceanothus americanus*	Root	N/A	2–4 mL/1–2×/day	Antiviral Astringent Lymphatic	Cervical dysplasia Fibrocystic breasts	• LSw/C • ⊘ P/L • Not to be used for patients with coagulation disorders or those taking anticoagulant/antiplatelet medications

Common Name	Botanical Name	Part	Dose	Actions	Uses	Safety/Cautions
Rehmannia	Rehmannia glutinosa	Root	2-20 g/day; Liquid extract (1:2): 4-12 mL/day	Antihemorrhagic, Antiinflammatory	DUB, Endometriosis	• LSw/C • Digestive complaints have been reported • Caution is advised in patients with immune dysfunction, autoimmune disorders, and those taking immunosuppressive medications • Safety in pregnancy is not established • There is no expected contraindication in lactation
Reishi	Ganoderma lucidum	Fruiting body and mycelium	6-12 g/day; 10 mL/3×/day	Adaptogen, Cardiotonic, Immunomodulator	Cervical dysplasia, Frequent colds, susceptibility to infection, GBS, HSV 1 and 2, Hypertension, Palpitations, Prevent atherosclerosis, Stress	• LSw/C • Side effects are uncommon; rashes are one of the most common side effects • Caution is advised in patients with immune dysfunction, autoimmune disorders, and those taking immunosuppressive medications • Safety in pregnancy is not established • There is no expected contraindication in lactation
Rhaponticum	Rhaponticum carthamoides	Root	150/kg daily; In process of locating dose	Adaptogen	Benign breast disorder, Cervical dysplasia, Chronic pelvic pain, Endometriosis, PCOS, PMS, Uterine fibroids	• LS/LD
Rhodiola	Rhodiola rosea	Root	50-500 mg/day × 2 weeks; Liquid extract (1:2): 10-20 mL/day	Adaptogen, Antidepressant, Cardiotonic/cardioprotective	Benign breast disorder, Cardiovascular protection, Cervical dysplasia, Chronic pelvic pain, Depression, Endometriosis, PCOS, PMS, Uterine fibroids	• LS/LD • Limited data show this to be a well-tolerated herb with no expected side effects or herb–drug interactions • Safety in pregnancy is not established • There is no expected contraindication in lactation
Rosemary	Rosmarinus officinalis	Leaf	2-4 g/3×/day; Liquid extract: 2-4 mL/3×/day	Antiinflammatory, Antioxidant, Antimicrobial, Circulatory stimulant, Neuroprotective, Spasmolytic	Depression, Endometriosis, Headache, Memory difficulties with menopause, Postpartum perineal care (bath), Vaginal infection (topical)	• KSw/C • ØP • Overall, this herb is reported to have low toxicity • Because of reputed abortifacient effects and ability to affect the menstrual cycle, this herb is not recommended for internal use during pregnancy beyond the normal amount found in food use • EO is for topical use only; extended topical use may lead to irritation

Continued

Common Name	Botanical Name	Part Used	Dried Herb (In Capsules, Tea, Infusion, Decoction)	Tincture	Actions	Women's Health Indications Described in This Book	Safety Concerns
Sage	Salvia officinalis	Leaf	1-4 g/3×/day	Tincture (1:1): 1-4 mL/3×/day	Anhidrotic Antimicrobial Antiseptic Carminative/spasmolytic Emmenagogue Estrogenic	Hot flashes/night sweats Inhibits breast milk secretion Postpartum perineal care (topical) Vulvovaginitis (topical)	• LSw/C • ⊘P/L • Sage products should not be used internally during pregnancy beyond minimal amounts found as seasoning in foods. The herb is strongly abortifacient and emmenagogic • Sage oil is toxic and is not meant for internal consumption
Salvia	Salvia miltiorrhiza	Root	2-6 g/day dried root	1-4 mL/3×/day	Antihypertensive Antithrombotic	CAD Hypertension	• ⊘P/L • Contraindicated for patients with bleeding disorders or on anticoagulant/antiplatelet medications • May increase risk of bleeding and should be discontinued 1 week prior to surgical procedures • LD • No side effects or drug interactions have been reported; overall, there are limited data on this herb
Sarsaparilla	Smilax ornata	Root	1-4 g 3×/day as decoction	N/A	Antiinflammatory Hepatoprotective	Benign breast disorder	• H-DI
Saw pal-metto	Serenoa repens, S. serrulata	Fruit	1.5-3 g/day	320 mg of lipophilic compounds (160 mg 2x/day)	Antiandrogenic Estrogenic	Acne (adult) Fertility problems PCOS	• ⊘P/L • Not for use with adolescents because of possible hormonal effects; treatment of acne may be an exception under qualified supervision • May cause GI upset • Possible interference with hormonal contraception and HRT
Schisandra	Schisandra chinensis	Fruit	1.5-15 g/day	3-7 g/1-2×/day	Adaptogen Antioxidant Hepatoprotective Nervine Oxytocic	Benign breast disorder Depression (mild) DUB Fatigue Frequent colds, susceptibility to infection Improve memory Improve stamina Insomnia Labor augmentation PCOS PMS Stress-related illness Uterine fibroids	• Not for use in pregnancy because of potential for stimulating uterine contractions • Caution recommended with barbiturates, which may be potentiated; may antagonize the effects of stimulants

Common name	Latin name	Part	Dose (solid)	Dose (liquid)	Actions	Indications	Safety/Contraindications
Senna	*Senna alexandrina*	Leaf	3-12 pods in 150 g warm water for 6-12 hours	0.5-2 mL/day	Laxative	Constipation	• LSw/C • Contraindicated in patients with intestinal obstruction, stenosis, atony inflammatory bowel diseases, appendicitis, and undiagnosed GI disorders • Contraindicated in patients with electrolyte disturbances and dehydration • Excessive use can lead to dependency • Long-term use can lead to hypokalemia with resultant cardiac and neuromuscular dysfunction, particularly when combined with cardiac glycosides, diuretics, or steroids • Although there have been no documented adverse effects from the use of senna during pregnancy or lactation, use during pregnancy and lactation is generally not recommended because of potentially genotoxic anthracoids (emodin and physcione) contained in the herb
Shatavari	*Asparagus racemosa*	Root	N/A	Liquid extract (1:2): 4-7 mL/1-2×/day	Adaptogen Aphrodisiac/tonic Lactagogue	Decreased libido Depression Fatigue, lassitude Fertility problems Insufficient breast milk Oligomenorrhea Susceptibility to infection	• ∅ P • Because of the high saponin content, this herb is not recommended for patients with cholestasis, fat malabsorption, and upper GI irritation, or inflammation. Gastric irritation and reflux are possible side effects • In a murine model using oral administration of the herb, Kupffer cell enlargement, liver congestion, bile plugs, mild cellular degeneration, fibrosis, and leukocytic infiltration were observed • Although this herb is used traditionally to promote fertility, it is also used as an abortifacient; therefore use in pregnancy is not recommended and if used as a fertility agent, use should be discontinued upon conception. There is no known increase in harmful effects on the fetus from limited use in women
Shepherd's purse	*Capsella bursa-pastoris*	Herb	2-5 g/3×/day	2-4 mL/3×/day	Antihemorrhagic	DUB Menorrhea, metrorrhagia Uterine fibroids	• LSw/C/LD • ∅ P • There is a general lack of safety and toxicity data available for this herb. Low toxicity was shown in a single murine study in vitro of intraperitoneally and subcutaneously injected extract, at doses of 1.5 g/kg and 31.5 g/kg, respectively. Toxicity signs included sedation, pupil dilatation, hind limb paralysis, dyspnea, and death because of respiratory paralysis • Generally contraindicated in pregnancy because of reported oxytocin activity, possibly a result of tyramine contained in the plant

Continued

Common Name	Botanical Name	Part Used	Dried Herb (In Capsules, Tea, Infusion, Decoction)	Tincture	Actions	Women's Health Indications Described in This Book	Safety Concerns
Skullcap	*Scutellaria lateriflora*	Herb	1-2 g/3×/day	Tincture: 1-2 mL/3×/day	Nervine Sedative (mild)	Anxiety, stress, tension Headache Insomnia PMS-related symptoms	• LSw/C/LD • There is a general lack of safety and toxicity data for skullcap, with no reported contraindications or herb–drug interactions • Adulterations of skullcap with the toxic herb *Teucrium* have occurred; thus caution is advised and a reliable product source should be obtained. This is of particular importance in pregnancy. Ingestion of *Teucrium* has led to reports of hepatitis • Overdose of skullcap tincture may lead to the following symptoms: giddiness, stupor, confusion, and seizures. This is most likely a result of adulteration with *Teucrium*
Slippery elm	*Ulmus rubra*	Inner bark	2-5 g/1-3×/day	5 mL/3×/day	Demulcent	Acid reflux Interstitial cystitis Vaginal infections (topical in suppository mix)	• KS/LD • There are no known contraindications or toxicity issues associated with slippery elm use • Any contraindications to use of slippery elm during pregnancy are a vestige of the use of slippery elm sticks to dilate the cervix mechanically to induce abortion. Oral intake of slippery elm is not known to be abortifacient and is considered safe during pregnancy • Slippery elm was traditionally used as a supplement for newborns, and also to increase the supply and quality of breast milk. There are no expected contraindications to use during lactation
Soy	*Glycine max*	Fruit	Used as a food from sources such as tofu, soy milk, and tempeh		Phytoestrogen	Hot flashes Osteoporosis prevention Uterine fibroids Vaginal dryness and atrophy	• KSw/C • Gas, indigestion • Possible goitrogenic effects (>30 g/day) • Fermented products contraindicated with MAOIs • Concentrated soy products are not recommended for use during pregnancy and lactation because of possible estrogenic effects

Common name	Botanical name	Part used	Dosage		Actions	Indications	Cautions
St. John's wort	*Hypericum perforatum*	Flower Herb	2-5 g/3×/day	2-5 mL/3×/day	Antidepressant Antiviral Nervine Vulnerary	Cervical dysplasia Chronic pelvic pain Depression Endometriosis HSV (internal and topical) Insomnia Neuromuscular pain Nipple thrush and cracked nipples PMS Postpartum perineal care Psychological complaints associated with perimenopause Vaginal dryness and atrophy (topical) Vulvovaginitis	• H-DI • LSw/C • Not for treatment of severe depression • Potential herb–drug interactions with anticoagulants (e.g., warfarin), immunosuppressives (e.g., cyclosporine), oral contraceptives, indinavir and other HIV medications, digoxin, and other drugs metabolized by the CYP oxidase system, and SSRIs • Theoretical effects on serum hormone levels because of actions on CYP metabolism • Photosensitivity has been reported in patients taking high doses of hypericin; caution should be observed for patients using high-dose St. John's wort or taking the herb for a prolonged duration • Safety during pregnancy has not been established • The detrimental effect of untreated depression on the mother and fetus are increasingly well accepted. There is no known contraindication to use during lactation. Prenatal and postpartum depression should be treated by a qualified health professional • Safety during pregnancy and lactation is discussed in detail in Plant Profiles: St. John's Wort
Sweet sumach	*Rhus aromatica*	Leaf	3-5 g/1-3×/day in infusion	2-4 mL/1-3×/day	Astringent tonic	Interstitial cystitis	• LD
Tea tree	*Melaleuca alternifolia*	Leaf	Used topically as an EO	N/A	Antimicrobial	Acne Cervical dysplasia GBS Nipple thrush and cracked nipples Vaginal infection Vulvovaginitis	• KSw/C • Not for internal use • Prolonged topical use may cause irritation
Thuja	*Thuja occidentalis*	Leaf	N/A	1.5-2.5 mL/day	Antimicrobial	Cervical dysplasia HPV infection HSV (topical)	• Ø P/L • Known neurotoxicity • Not for internal use • Avoid even topical use during pregnancy and lactation

Continued

Common Name	Botanical Name	Part Used	Dried Herb (In Capsules, Tea, Infusion, Decoction)	Tincture	Actions	Women's Health Indications Described in This Book	Safety Concerns
Thyme	*Thymus vulgaris*	Leaf	1-2 g/1-2×/day	1-2 mL/1-3×/ day	Antimicrobial	Cervical dysplasia GBS HPV infection HSV infection Vulvovaginitis	• LSw/C • ⊘ P/L • Not for internal use during pregnancy (topical and suppository use is acceptable), other than amounts typically consumed in foods • Not to exceed 10 g dried leaf containing 0.03% thymol/day • Thyme oil is highly toxic and not intended for internal use (dilute use in suppositories is acceptable)
Tribulus	*Tribulus terrestris*	Aerial parts	3-10 g/day	3-5 mL/2×/ day	Aphrodisiac Estrogenic Tonic	Fertility problems Menstrual irregularities PCOS	• LS/LD • ⊘ P/L • Tribulus is used as a fertility agent in both men and women. Because it has demonstrated an increase in fetal damage in animal studies, discontinuation immediately upon conception is recommended. No increase in frequency of malformation or other harmful fetal effects have been seen in women using it to increase fertility; however, studies are very limited and animal evidence of harm is significant • In vivo mouse studies have suggested a very low toxicity from this herb. Staggers (a neuromuscular disease), cholestasis, and photosensitivity have all been observed in sheep that have consumed tribulus • The high saponin content may cause gastric irritation and reflux as side effects

		Part	Dose	Actions	Uses	Notes
Turmeric	Curcuma longa	Rhizome	1.5-3 g/day in divided doses; Liquid extract (1:1) 5-15 mL/day	Antidepressant, Antiinflammatory, Antioxidant, Hepatoprotective, Hypolipidemic, Neuroprotective	Depression, Endometriosis	• H-D! • KSw/C • ∅P • Overall, turmeric has a very good safety profile, even in high doses • High doses and prolonged use may be associated with gastric irritation and are not recommended for individuals with peptic ulcer disease or gastric hyperacidity • Turmeric should not be taken by individuals with bile duct obstruction, gallstones, or those taking immunosuppressant medications • In vitro studies demonstrate inhibition of platelet aggregation and thus the herb may potentiate the effects of anticoagulant/antiplatelet medications. Caution is also advised with discontinuation of the herb 1 week prior to surgical procedures • Curcumin potently inhibits CYP in rats. There are no human data • Curcumin (200 mg/kg) protected against doxorubicin myocardial toxicity in rats • Because of lipid-lowering effects, turmeric may potentiate the effects of lipid-lowering medications • It is traditionally considered emmenagogic; therefore, it is not recommended for internal use in pregnancy in doses higher than those typically found in food
Usnea	Usnea barbata	Herb (lichen)	N/A; 2-4 mL/2-3x/day	Antimicrobial	Cervical dysplasia, GBS, Trichomoniasis, Vaginal infection	• LS/LD • Safety in pregnancy is not established; therefore, use topically (including in vaginal suppositories) only
Uva ursi	Arctostaphylos uva ursi	Leaf	3-12 g daily in divided doses; 2-4 mL/2-4x/day	Astringent, Antiinflammatory, Urinary antiseptic	Postnatal perineal care, UTI, Vulvovaginitis	• LSw/C • Many references state that uva ursi is not to be used in pregnancy; however, there is no evidence direct evidence to support this claim. See Plant Profiles: Uva Ursi • Not for use more than 7 days consecutively • Some authorities claim that the herb is most effective when urinary pH is alkaline; therefore it is often given with two 00-sized capsules of baking soda

Continued

Common Name	Botanical Name	Part Used	Dried Herb (In Capsules, Tea, Infusion, Decoction)	Tincture	Actions	Women's Health Indications Described in This Book	Safety Concerns
Valerian	*Valeriana officinalis*	Root	1-3 g/2-3x/day	3-5 mL/3x/day	Anxiolytic Carminative Sedative Spasmolytic	Anxiety Gastric distress related to endometriosis or PMS Headache Insomnia	• H-DI! • LSw/C • ⊘P • Valerian effects possibly enhanced by alcohol consumption—avoid excessive alcohol consumption concurrently with this herb • Intake of valerian preparations is not recommended within 2 hours before driving or operating machinery because of possibly impaired response time • Herbalists have reported a paradoxic effect of stimulation rather than relaxation in a small percentage of patients using valerian • In vitro experiments suggest that valerian may inhibit CYP activity • Caution is recommended when using in combination with CNS-depressing medications • Even overdose with large quantities of the herb have not led to fatality; however, side effects have included tremor, GI upset, chest tightness, and when injected, cardiac disturbance, blurred vision, and excitability, among other less significant symptoms • The safety of valerian during pregnancy and lactation has not been established. In a limited number of cases of valerian intoxication during pregnancy, no teratogenic effects have been observed. Degradation products of valepotriates have demonstrated cytotoxicity and mutagenicity in vitro, but have not caused birth defects in a limited number of animal studies. They are poorly absorbed
White oak	*Quercus alba*	Bark	Topical use only	N/A	Astringent	Postnatal perineal care Varicosities and hemorrhoids (topical)	• Topical use only for use during pregnancy for the treatment of varicosities, hemorrhoids, and postnatal perineal care

Common name	Latin name	Part	Dose	Actions	Uses	Cautions/Notes
Wild yam	*Dioscorea villosa*	Root	2-4 g/day in divided doses 2-10 mL/3×/day in 3-5 divided doses	Antiinflammatory Possible estrogenic effects Spasmolytic	Chronic pelvic pain Dysmenorrhea Endometriosis Fertility problems Interstitial cystitis NVP Threatened miscarriage UTI Vaginal dryness and atrophy	• H-DI • LSw/C • Possible GI complaints with long-term use of high doses • Although hormonal effects are not supported by scientific research, internal use is not recommended in individuals with a history of sex hormone–dependent cancers • Possible/theoretical interactions with steroids, hormonal contraception, HRT, and lipid-lowering agents (potentiation) • Caution is advised in avoiding products that may have been adulterated with progesterone
Willow	*Salix* spp.	Bark	1-3 g/3×/day equivalent up to 60-120 mg salicin/day 1-3 mL/3×/day	Analgesic Antiinflammatory	Headache	• H-DI • LSw/C • ⊘P/L • Minor adverse effects include GI upset, dizziness, sweating, and rash. Adverse effects associated with salicylates may be associated with this herb • Precautions similar to those with other salicylate-containing medications are advised, including avoiding if there is salicylate sensitivity, asthma, peptic ulcer disease, gout, bleeding disorders, and kidney or liver disease • Drug interactions associated with salicylates are theoretically possible with the use of willow bark • Safety during pregnancy is not known, and in fact, the safety of aspirin in pregnancy is somewhat uncertain. Salicylates excreted in breast milk have been observed to cause skin rash in the breastfeeding infant
Witch hazel	*Hamamelis virginiana*	Bark	2 g/3×/day 2-4 mL/3×/day	Astringent Antiinflammatory	Acne DUB Hemorrhoids (topical) Menorrhagia Postnatal perineal care PUPPP Uterine fibroids Varicosities (topical)	• LSw/C • ⊘P • Data on the internal use of witch hazel are limited. • No side effects or contraindications are reported for this herb other than possible GI irritation in some individuals • Excessive ingestion is not recommended because of the high tannin content of the herb • No problems are expected with the topical use of witch hazel during pregnancy and lactation. Internal use is not recommended

Continued

Common Name	Botanical Name	Part Used	Dried Herb (In Capsules, Tea, Infusion, Decoction)	Tincture	Actions	Women's Health Indications Described in This Book	Safety Concerns
Yarrow	*Achillea millefolium*	Flower Herb	2-5 g/3×/day	2-4 mL/3×/day	Antihemorrhagic Antimicrobial Astringent Spasmolytic urinary antiseptic Vulnerary	Benign breast disorder Chronic pelvic pain DUB Dysmenorrhea Endometriosis Hemorrhoids Menorrhagia Pelvic congestion Postnatal perineal care Uterine fibroids UTI Vulvovaginitis	• LSw/C/LD • ∅ P • Limited safety and clinical data available; considered to have low toxicity with toxic principles in too low a concentration to be clinically significant in humans • Contraindicated in those with known allergy to plants in the *Compositae* family • Not for internal use during pregnancy because of thujone content and purported abortifacient activity
Yellow dock	*Rumex crispus*	Root	3-5 g/3×/day	2-4 mL/3×/day	Alterative Aperient	Acne Constipation Iron-deficiency anemia	• LSw/C/LD • Limited data available for this herb; excessive and prolonged use of laxatives may lead to abdominal cramping, diarrhea, and hypokalemia • Avoid if there is intestinal obstruction, as with all laxatives • Although no safety data exist for use during pregnancy and lactation, caution is advised during pregnancy because of anthraquinone contents; anthraquinones can be passed into the breast milk
Yellow sweet clover	*Melilotus officinalis*	Aerial parts	2-4 g/day in tea form to no greater than 3-30 mg coumarin daily	2-4 mL/day	Antiinflammatory	Benign breast disorder Interstitial cystitis	• LD
Yerba mansa	*Anemopsis californica*	Root	N/A	3-5 mL/day	Antiinflammatory Antimicrobial Astringent tonic	Interstitial cystitis Vulvovaginitis	• LS/LD

Yohimbe	*Pausinystalia yohimbe*	Bark	16-20 g yohimbine hydrochloride (standardized) per day	Aphrodisiac CNS stimulant	Low libido	• H-D! • ⊘ P/L • Multiple adverse effects are associated with use. Side effects include nausea, vomiting, tachycardia, hypertension, hypotension, dizziness, and irritability. Toxicity is associated with lupuslike syndrome • Avoid in patients with renal disease, hypertension, CAD, PTSD, panic disorder, ulcers (active), bipolar disorder, and hepatic insufficiency • Multiple possible herb–drug interactions include drugs metabolized by CYP, alcohol, androgenic and antiandrogenic drugs, benzodiazepines, antihypertensive medications, MAOIs, opioid antagonists, and sympathomimetics, as well as other theoretic contraindications • Not for long-term use • Should only be used by trained practitioners
Ziziphus	*Ziziphus spinosa*	Seed	5-10 g/day 5-10 mL/day	Antihidrotic Anxiolytic Hypotensive Sedative (mild)	Anxiety Insomnia Irritability Nervous exhaustion Night sweats Palpitations	• LS/LD • In vivo mouse models showed low toxicity. Limited human clinical and safety data • Commonly used in TCM, including in formulae used during pregnancy • No reported contraindications or herb–drug interactions

BP, Blood pressure; *CAD*, coronary artery disease; *CHF*, congestive heart failure; *CNS*, central nervous system; *CYP*, cytochrome P450; *DGL*, deglycyrrhizinated licorice; *DUB*, dysfunctional uterine bleeding; *EFAs*, essential fatty acids; *EO*, essential oil; *EPO*, evening primrose oil; *ER*, estrogen receptor; *FDA*, Food and Drug Administration; *FSH*, follicle-stimulating hormone; *G6PD*, glucose-6-phosphate deficiency; *GBS*, group B streptococcus; *GERD*, gastroesophageal reflux disease; *GI*, gastrointestinal; *GLA*, gamma-linolenic acid; *H₂*, histamine-2; *H-DI*, herb–drug interaction; *HDL*, high-density lipoprotein; *HIV*, human immunodeficiency virus; *HPA*, hypothalamic-pituitary-adrenal; *HRT*, hormone replacement therapy; *HSV*, herpes simplex virus; *K⁺*, potassium; *KS*, known safe; *KS/LD*, known safe/limited data; *KSw/C*, known safe with cautions; *KSwC/LD*, known safe with cautions/limited data; *LDL*, low-density lipoprotein; *LH*, luteinizing hormone; *LS*, likely safe; *LS/LD*, likely safe/limited data; *LSP/L*-culinary use, likely safe during pregnancy and lactation-culinary use; *LSw/C*, likely safe with cautions; *LSw/C/LD*, likely safe with cautions/limited data; *MAOI*, monoamine oxidase inhibitor; *MI*, myocardial infarction; *N/A*, not applicable; *NSAID*, nonsteroidal antiinflammatory drug; *NVP*, nausea and vomiting of pregnancy; *P*, pregnancy; *P/L*, pregnancy/lactation; *P/LD*, pregnancy/limited data; *PA*, pyrrolizidine alkaloid; *PAF*, platelet-activating factor; *PCOS*, polycystic ovarian syndrome; *PMS*, premenstrual syndrome; *PMS-D*, premenstrual syndrome-depression; *PPI*, proton pump inhibitor; *PTSD*, posttraumatic stress disorder; *PUPPP*, pruritic urticarial papules and plaques of pregnancy; *RHT*, reported human toxicity; *SERM*, selective estrogen receptor modulator; *SIDS*, sudden infant death syndrome; *SLE*, systemic lupus erythematosus; *SSRI*, selective serotonin reuptake inhibitor; *TCM*, Traditional Chinese Medicine; *TSH*, thyroid-stimulating hormone; *UTI*, urinary tract infection; *WHO*, World Health Organization.

Bibliography

CHAPTER 1

1. Sakala C. Content of care by independent midwives: assistance with pain in labor and birth. *Soc Sci Med*. 1988;26(11):1141–1158.
2. Clarke TC, Black LI, Stussman BJ, et al. *Trends in the use of complementary health approaches among adults: united States, 2002-2012. National health statistics reports; no 79*. Hyattsville, MD: National Center for Health Statistics; 2015.
3. Gahche J, Bailey R, Burt V, et al. *Dietary supplement use among U.S. adults has increased since NHANES III (1988–1994). NCHS data brief, no 61*. Hyattsville, MD: National Center for Health Statistics; 2011.
4. Jonas W. Advising patients on the use of complementary and alternative medicine. *Appl Psychophysiol Biofeedback*. 2001;26(3):205–213.
5. Kohatsu W. *Complementary and Alternative Medicine Secrets*. Philadelphia: Hanley & Belfus; 2002.
6. NCCAM: National Center for Complementary and Alternative Medicine: What Is Complementary and Alternative Medicine (CAM)? National Institutes of Health National Center for Complementary and Alternative Medicine.
7. Jonas W, Linde K. Evaluating research in complementary and alternative medicine. In: Weintraub M, eds. *Alternative and Complementary Treatment in Neurologic Illness*. New York: Churchill Livingstone; 2001.
8. Barrett B. Complementary and alternative medicine: what's it all about? *Wisc Med J*. 2001;100(7):20–26.
9. Eisenberg D, Ettner S. Trends in alternative medicine use in the United States, 1990-1997: results of a follow-up national survey. *JAMA*. 1998;280(18):1569–1575.
10. Peregoy JA, Clarke TC, Jones LI, et al. *Regional variation in use of complementary health approaches by U.S. adults. NCHS data brief, no 146*. Hyattsville, MD: National Center for Health Statistics; 2014.
11. Chambliss L. Alternative and complementary medicine: an overview. *Clin Obstet Gynecol*. 2001;44(4):640–652.
12. WHO. *World Health Organization: Traditional Medicine Fact Sheet*. Geneva: World Health Organization; May 2003. 134.
13. Snyderman R, Weil A. Integrative medicine: bringing medicine back to its roots. *Arch Int Med*. 2002;162:395.
14. Chez R, Jonas W, Crawford C. A survey of medical students' opinions about complementary and alternative therapies. *Am J Obstet Gynecol*. 2001;185(5):754–757.
15. Ernst E. Research into complementary/alternative medicine: an attempt to dispel the myths. *Int J Clin Pract*. 2001;55(6):376–379.
16. DSEA. Barometer survey: exploring consumer attitudes about dietary supplements, an executive summary, press release, Dietary Supplement Education Alliance; August 6, 2001.
17. Hughes E: Overview of complementary, alternative, and integrative medicine, Clin Obstet Gynecol 44(4):774–779.
18. Epstein K. New studies show alternative therapies don't stand alone. *Nat Foods Merch*. 1999.
19. Bauer B. Herbal therapy: what a clinician needs to know to counsel patients effectively. *Mayo Clin Proc*. 2000;75(8):835–841.
20. US Congress. Dietary Supplement Health and Education Act. *US Statutes*. 1994;108:4325–4335.
21. Astin JA. Why patients use alternative medicine: results of a national study. *JAMA*. 1998;279:1548–1553.
22. Brokaw J, Tunnicliff G, Raess B. The teaching of complementary and alternative medicine in U.S. medical schools: a survey of course directors. *Acad Med*. 2002;77(9):876–881.
23. Hughes EF. Integrating complementary and alternative medicine into clinical practice. *Clin Obstet Gynecol*. 2001;44(4):902–906.
24. Skiba-King E. Vitamins, herbs, and supplements: tools of empowerment. *J Psychosocial Nursing Mental Health Serv*. 2001;39(4):34–41.
25. Gawande A. *Complications: A Surgeon's Notes on an Imperfect Science*. New York: Picador; 2002.
26. Chez R, Jonas W. The challenge of complementary and alternative medicine. *Am J Obstet Gynecol*. 1997;177(5):1156–1161.
27. Furnham A. *Can Alternative Medicine Be Integrated into Mainstream Care?* London: NCCAM and the Royal College of Physicians; 2001:23–24. January.
28. Sloan E. Women's health market, potential and direction. *Nat Foods Merch*. 2001:42–44.
29. Belenky M. *Women's Ways of Knowing*. San Francisco: HarperCollins; 1986.
30. Roberts H. *Women's Health Matters*. London: Routledge; 1992.
31. Konrad TR, Link CL, Shackelton RJ, et al. It's about time. *Medical Care*. 2010;48(2):95–100.
32. Achterberg J. *Woman as Healer*. Boston: Shambala; 1990.
33. Jonas W. Alternative medicine and the conventional practitioner. *JAMA*. 1998;279(9):708–710.
34. AARP, NCCAM. *Complementary and Alternative Medicine: What people aged 50 and older discuss with their health care providers*. Consumer Survey Report; April 13, 2010.
35. Smolinske S. Dietary supplement-drug interactions. *J Amer Med Women's Assoc*. 1999;54(4):191–195.
36. Ness J. Dietary supplements: important component of alternative medicine curricula. *J Gen Int Med*. 1999;69(1).
37. Lee Y, Georgiou C, Raab C. The knowledge, attitudes and practices of dieticians licensed in Orgeon regarding functional foods, nutrient supplements, and herbs as complementary medicine. *J Am Diet Assoc*. 2000;100(5):543–548.
38. Neal R. Report by David M. Eisenberg, M.D. on educational issues pertaining to complementary and alternative medicine in the United States. *JACM*. 2001;7(suppl 1):S41–S43.

39. Wetzel MS, Kaptchuk TJ, Haramati A, Eisenberg DM. Complementary and alternative medical therapies: implications for medical education. *Anna los Internal Medicine.* 2003;138(3):191–196.

40. Kligler B, Lee R. Integrative medicine. In: Kligler B, Lee R, eds. *Integrative Medicine.* New York: McGraw-Hill; 2004:609–621.

41. Rakel D. *Integrative Medicine.* Philadelphia: Saunders; 2003.

CHAPTER 2

1. Bennett J. *Lilies of the Hearth.* Ontario: Camden House; 1991.

2. Achterberg J. *Woman as Healer: A Panoramic Survey of the Healing Activities of Women from Prehistoric Times to the Present.* Boston: Shambhala; 1990.

3. Brooke E. *Women Healers, Portraits of Herbalists, Physicians, and Midwives.* Rochester, VT: Healing Arts Press; 1995.

4. Ehrenreich B, English D. *Witches, Midwives, and Nurses.* New York: The Feminist Press/SUNY College; 1973.

5. O'Dowd M. *The History of Medications for Women: Materia Medica Woman.* New York: Parthenon Publishing Group; 2001.

6. Harley D. Historians as demonologists: the myth of the midwife-witch. *J Soc Social History Med.* 1990;3(1):1–26.

7. Purkiss D. *The Witch in History: Early Modern and Twentieth-Century Representations.* London: Routledge; 1996.

8. Merchant C. *The Death of Nature: Women, Ecology, and the Scientific Revolution.* San Francisco: Harper San Francisco; 1980.

9. Green M. *The Trotula: An English Translation of the Medieval Compendium of Women's Medicine.* Philadelphia: University of Pennsylvania Press; 2002.

10. Withering W. *An Account of Foxglove and Some of Its Medical Uses.* Birmingham: England: M. Swinney; 1785.

11. Weisman C. *Women's Health Care: Activist Traditions and Institutional Change.* Baltimore: Johns Hopkins University Press; 1998.

12. Reed M. *Margaret Sanger: Her Life in Her Words.* Fort Lee, NJ: Barricade Books; 2003.

13. Balaban C, Erlen J, Siderits R. *The Ladies' Dispensatory.* New York: Routledge; 2003.

14. Berman A. The Heroic Approach in 19(th) Century Therapeutics. *Bull Am Soc Hosp Pharm.* 1954;11:321–327.

15. Shryock RH. *Medicine and Society in America: 1660–1860.* New York: New York University Press; 1960.

CHAPTER 3

1. Brokaw J, Tunnicliff G, Raess B. The teaching of complementary and alternative medicine in U.S. medical schools: a survey of course directors. *Acad Med.* 2002;77(9):876–881.

2. Astin J. Complementary and alternative medicine and the need for evidence-based criticism. *Acad Med.* 2002;77(9):864–868.

3. Kroll D. Concerns and needs for research in herbal supplement pharmacotherapy and safety. *J Herb Pharmacother.* 2001;1(2):3–23.

4. Barrett B. Complementary and alternative medicine: what's it all about? *Wisc Med J.* 2001;100(7):20–26.

5. Jonas W. Advising patients on the use of complementary and alternative medicine. *Appl Psychophysiol Biofeed.* 2001;26(3):205–213.

6. Mills S, Bone K. *Principles and Practice of Phytotherapy: Modern Herbal Medicine.* London: Churchill Livingstone; 2000.

7. Sackett D, Rosenberg W, Gray J, et al. Evidence-base medicine: what it is and what it isn't. *BMJ.* 1996;312:71–72.

8. Mills S. Extract database: an appropriate application of evidence-based medicine? http://www.phytotherapy.info/papers/tradevidence.htm; 2003.

9. Singh B, et al. Research in complementary and alternative medicine. In: Kohatsu W, ed. *Complementary and Alternative Medicine Secrets.* Philadelphia: Hanley & Belfus; 2002:6–15.

10. McDermott JH, Motyka TM. *Assessing the Quality of Botanical Preparations.* Medscape Pharmacology; 2000.

11. World Health Organization. *Regulatory Situation of Herbal Medicine: A Worldwide Review.* Geneva, Switzerland: WHO/TRM; 1998.

12. LowDog TiB. Determining Efficacy of Herbal Preparations. In: Barrett M, ed. *Handbook of Clinically Tested Herbal Remedies.* New York: Haworth; 2004.

13. Juni P, Witschi A, Bloch R, et al. The hazards of scoring the quality fo clinical trials for meta-analysis. *JAMA.* 1999;282(12):1054–1060.

14. Hart A. Randomized controlled trials: the control group dilemma revisited. *Comp Ther Med.* 2001;9:40–44.

15. Blackweilder R. Allopathic medicine. In: Kohatsu W, ed. *Complementary and Alternative Medicine Secrets.* Philadelphia: Hanley & Belfus; 2002:84–91.

16. Chambliss L. Alternative and complementary medicine: an overview. *Clin Obstet Gynecol.* 2001;44(4):640–652.

17. Rotblatt M, Ziment I. *Evidence-Based Herbal Medicine.* Philadelphia: Hanley & Belfus; 2000.

18. Mansi I, Frei C, Chen-Pin W, et al. Statins and new-onset diabetes mellitus and diabetic complications: a retrospective cohort study of US healthy adults. *J Gen Intern Med.* April 2015. http://dx.doi.org/10.1007/s11606-015-3335-1. Accessed on line.

19. Shin J-Y, Park M-J, Lee SH. Risk of intracranial haemorrhage in antidepressant users with concurrent use of non-steroidal anti-inflammatory drugs: nationwide propensity score matched study. *BMJ.* 2015;351:h3517. Published 14 July 2015.

20. Lo W, Friedman J. Teratogenicity of recently introduced medications in human pregnancy. *Obstet Gynecol.* 2002;100(3):465–473.

21. Kohatsu W. *Complementary and Alternative Medicine Secrets.* Philadelphia: Hanley & Belfus; 2002.

22. Imrie R, Ramey DW. The evidence for evidence-based medicine. *Comp Ther Med.* 2000;8:123–126.

23. Jonas W, Linde K. Evaluating research in complementary and alternative medicine. In: Weintraub M, ed. *Alternative and Complementary Treatment in Neurologic Illness.* New York: Churchill Livingstone; 2001.

24. Houghton P. Traditional plant knowledge helps guide drug development. *Chem Ind.* 1999;4:15–19.

25. Mills S. Extract database: are herbs actually effective? http://www.phytotherapy.info/papers/tradevidence.htm.

26. Bone K. Writing about herbs: prioritizing and interpreting information. *J Amer Herb Guild.* 2000;1(1).

27. Weiss RF, Fintelmann V. *Herbal Medicine.* 2nd ed. New York: Thieme; 2000.

28. Cabrera C. *Selection Criteria: unpublished document;* 2004.

29. Hoffmann D. *Medical Herbalism: The Science and Practice of Herbal Medicine.* Rochester, VT: Healing Arts Press; 2003.

30. Upton R. *Angelica sinensis.* Santa Cruz: American Herbal Pharmacopoeia; 2003.

31. Romm A, Upton R. Angelica sinensis: survey of the American Herbalists Guild. *JAHG.* 2005;5(2).

32. Kraft K, Hobbs C. *Pocket Guide to Herbal Medicine.* Stuttgart: Thieme; 2004.

33. Bone K. *A Clinical Guide to Blending Liquid Herbs: Herbal Formulations for the Individual Patient.* St. Louis: Churchill Livingstone; 2003.

34. Romm A. Vitex agnus castus: survey of the American Herbalists Guild. *JAHG.* 2005;5(2).

35. Balansard G. *Plant Med Phytother.* 1983;17:123. [in French].

36. Bilia AR, Bergonzi MC, Gallori S, et al. Stability of the constituents of Calendula, milk-thistle and passionflower tinctures by LC-DAD and LC-MS. *J Pharm Biomed Anal.* 2002;30:613–624.

37. Hobbs C. St. John's wort. Hypericum perforatum L. *HerbalGram.* 1989;18/19:24–33.

38. Bone KM. Echinacea: what makes it work? *Alt Med Rev.* 1997;2(2):87–93.

39. Yousif AN, Durance TD, Scaman CH, et al. Headspace volatiles and physical characteristics of vacuum-microwave, air, and freeze-dried oregano (Lippia berlandieri Schauer). *J Food Sci.* 2000;65(6):926–930.

40. Diaz-Maroto MC, Perez-Coello MS, Gonzalez-Vinas MA, et al. Influence of drying on the flavor quality of spearmint (Mentha spicata L.). *J Agric Food Chem.* 2003;51:1265–1269.

41. Di Cesare LF, Forni E, Viscardi D, et al. Changes in the chemical composition of basil caused by different drying procedures. *J Agric Food Chem.* 2003;51(12):3575–3581.

42. Chan JCC, Cheung PCK, Ang PO. Comparative studies on the effect of three drying methods on the nutritional composition of seaweed Sargassum hemiphyllum (Turn.). *C. Ag, J Agric Food Chem.* 1997;45(8):3056–3059.

43. Mittman P. Randomized double-blind study of freeze-dried urtica dioica in the treatment of allergic rhinitis. *Planta Med.* 1990;56(1):44–47.

44. Baetgen D. Effects in treatment of whooping cough with Echinacin. *Therapiewoche.* 1984;34:5115–5119. [in German].

45. Kleijnen J, Knipschild P. Mistletoe treatment for cancer. Review of controlled trials in humans. *Phytomedicine.* 1994;1:255–260.

46. Suzuki H, Ohta Y, Takino T. Effects of glycyrrhizin on biochemical tests in patients with chronic hepatitis. *Double blind trial, Asian Med J.* 1983;26:423–438.

47. Arase Y, Ikeda K, Murashima N. The long term efficacy of glycyrrhizin in chronic hepatitis C patients. *Cancer.* 1997;79:1494–1500.

48. Mori K, Sakai H, Suzuki S. Effects of glycyrrhizin (SNMC: Stronger Neo-Minophagen C) in hemophilia patients with HIV-1 infection. *Tohoku J Exp Med.* 1990;162:183–193.

49. Hruby K, Fuhrmann M, Csomós G, et al. Pharmacotherapy of Amanita phalloides poisoning with silybin. *Wien klin Wschr.* 1983;95:3–9.

50. Chang HM, But PP. *Pharmacology and applications of Chinese Materia Medica.* Singapore: World Scientific; 1986.

51. Bergner P: personal communication.

FURTHER READING

Bruneton J. *Pharmacognosy Phytochemistry Medicinal Plants.* 2nd ed. Paris: Lavoisier Publishing; 1999.

Dewick PM. *Medicinal Natural Products: A Biosynthetic Approach.* 2nd ed. Chichester: John Wiley & Sons, Ltd; 2002.

Harborne J, Baxter H, Moss G. *Phytochemical Dictionary: A Handbook of Bioactive Compounds from Plants.* 2nd ed. London: Taylor & Francis Ltd; 1999.

Heinrich M, ed. *Fundamentals of Pharmacognosy and Phytotherapy.* St. Louis: Churchill Livingstone; 2004.

van Wyk BE, Wink M. *Medicinal Plants of the World.* Portland DR: Timber Press; 2004.

The Phytochemistry of Herbs. http://www.herbalchem.net.

CHAPTER 4

1. Snyderman R, Weil A. Integrative medicine: bringing medicine back to its roots. *Arch Int Med.* 2002;162:395.

2. Hughes E: Overview of complementary, alternative, and integrative medicine, Clin Obstet Gynecol 44(4):774–779.

3. Kohatsu W. *Complementary and Alternative Medicine Secrets.* Philadelphia: Hanley and Belfus; 2002.

4. Chambliss L. Alternative and complementary medicine: an overview. *Clin Obstet Gynecol.* 2001;44(4):640–652.

5. Ernst E. Research into complementary/alternative medicine: an attempt to dispel the myths. *Int J Clin Pract.* 2001;55(6):376–379.

6. Chez R, Jonas W, Crawford C. A survey of medical students' opinions about complementary and alternative therapies. *Am J Obstet Gynecol.* 2001;185(5):754–757.

7. Smolinske S. Dietary supplement-drug interactions. *J Amer Med Women's Assoc.* 1999;54(4):191–195.

8. Ness J. Dietary supplements: important component of alternative medicine curricula. *J Gen Int Med.* 1999;69(1).

9. AARP

10. WHO. *Requirements for adverse reaction reporting.* Geneva: World Health Organization; 1975.

11. Kessler D. Introducing MedWatch, using FDA form 3500, a new approach to reporting medication and device adverse effects and product problems. *JAMA.* 1993;269: 2765–2768.

12. Pharmacists ASoH S. ASHP guidelines on adverse drug reaction monitoring and reporting. *Am J Health-Syst Pharm.* 1995;52(52):417–419.

13. Fucik H, Backlund A, Farah M. Building a computerized herbal substance register for implementation and use in the World Health Organisation International Drug Monitoring Programme. *Drug Inf J.* 2002;36:839–854.

14. Ernst E. Safety of Herbal Medicines. *Amer J Med.* 1998;104:170–178.

15. Barnes J, Mills SY, Abbot NC, Willoughby M, Ernst E. Different standards for reporting ADRs to herbal remedies and conventional OTC medicines: face-to-face interviews with 515 users of herbal remedies. *British Journal of Clinical Pharmacology.* 1998;45(5):496–500. http://dx.doi.org/10.1046/j.1365-2125.

16. Hazell L, Shakir S. Under-Reporting of Adverse Drug Reactions. *Drug Safety:* 385–396. Retrieved January 10, 2016, http://www.ncbi.nlm.nih.gov/pubmed/16689555

17. Palmer M, Haller C, McKinney P. Adverse events associated with dietary supplements: an observational study. *Lancet.* 2003;361:101–106.

18. DIETARY SUPPLEMENTS FDA May Have Opportunities to Expand Its Use of Reported Health Problems to Oversee Products. Retrieved January 11, 2016. http://www.gao.gov/assets/660/653113.pdf; 2013, March 1.

19. Shaw D, Leon C, Kolev S and Murray V: Traditional remedies and food supplements; a five year toxicologic study (1991–1995), *Drug Safety*. 1997;17:342–356.

20. Mills S, Bone K. *The Essential Guide to Herbal Safety*. St. Louis: Elsevier Churchill Livingstone; 2005.

21. Upton R, Petrone C. *American Herbal Pharmacopoeia and Therapeutic Compendium: Valerian root (Valeriana officinalis)*. Santa Cruz, CA: American Herbal Pharmacopoeia; 1999.

22. Stoller R. Liver damage and kava extracts. *Schweizerische Ärztezeitung*. 2000;81(24):1335–1336.

23. Pokhrel P, Ergil K. Aristolochic acid: a toxicologic review. *Clin Acupunct Orient Med*. 2000;1:161–166.

24. Herbal Dietary Supplements. Examples of Deceptive or Questionable Marketing Practices and Potentially Dangerous Advice. *GAO*. 2010, May 26:10–662T.

25. Romm A. *Scientific Approaches to Quality Assessment of Botanical Products: Determination of Botanical Medicine Quality by Herbal Practitioners and Small Manufacturers*. Oxford, MS: National Center for Natural Products Research (NCNPR), School of Pharmacy, The University of Mississippi; September 7-9, 2004.

26. Saper R, Kales S, Paquin J, et al. Heavy metal content of ayurvedic herbal medicine products. *JAMA*. 2004;292(23):2868–2873.

27. Ernst E. Review of adulteration of Chinese herbal medicines with synthetic drug. *J Int Med*. 2002;252:107–113.

28. WebIndia123.com. Testing of heavy metals in herbal medicine a must. Accessed October 24, 2005.

29. Ko R, Au A. *Compendium of Asian Patent Medicines*. Sacramento: California Department of Health Services; 1997-1998.

30. Eisenberg D, Davis R, Ettner S. Trends in alternative, medicine use in the United States, 1990-97. *JAMA*. 1998;280:1569–1575.

31. Hensrud D, Engle B, Scheitel S. Underreporting the use of dietary supplements and nonprescription medications among patients undergoing periodic health examination. *Mayo Clin Proc*. 1999;74(5):443–447.

32. Hardy M. Herb-drug interactions: an evidence-based table. *Alt Med Alert*. 2000:64–69. June.

33. Izzo A, Ernst E. Interactions between herbal medicines and prescribed drugs. *Drugs*. 2001;51(15):2163–2175.

34. Upton R, Cott J, Flannery M. *Ginkgo Leaf & Ginkgo Leaf Dry Extract Monograph*. Scotts Valley, CA: American Herbal Pharmacopoeia; 2003.

35. Upton R, Lawson L, Graff A. *Garlic monograph (draft)*. Scotts Valley, CA: American Herbal Pharmacopoeia; 2003.

36. Page R, Lawrence J. Potentiation of warfarin by dong quai. *Pharmacotherapy*. 1999;19(7):870–876.

37. Heck A, DeWitt B, Lukes A. Potential interactions between alternative therapies and warfarin. *Am J Health-Syst Pharm*. 2000;57:1221–1227.

38. Gundling K, Ernst E. Herbal medicines: influences on blood coagulation. *Perfusion*. 2001;14:336–342.

39. Budzinski J, Foster B, Vandenhoek S, Arnason J. An in vitro evaluation of human cytochrome P450 3A4 inhibition by selected commercial herbal extracts and tinctures. *Phytomedicine*. 2000;7(4):273–282.

40. Hall 2003

41. Barone G, Gurley B, Ketel B, Abul-Ezz S. Herbal supplements: a potential for drug interactions in transplant recipients. *Transplantation*. 2001;71:239–241.

42. Upton R, Barrett M, Wadlington C. *Astragalus Root*. Santa Cruz, CA: American Herbal Pharmacopoeia; 1999.

43. Upton R, Mattioda J, Mutch J. *Reishi Mushroom*. Santa Cruz, CA: American Herbal Pharmacopoeia; 2000.

44. Upton R, Barrett M, Mattioda J. *Schisandra Berry Root*. Santa Cruz, CA: American Herbal Pharmacopoeia; 1999.

45. Weiger W, Smith M, Boon H. Advising patients who seek complementary and alternative medical therapies for cancer. *Ann Int Med Comp Alt Med Ser*. 2003;137(11):891–911.

46. Boullata J, Nace A. Safety issues with herbal medicines. *Pharmacotherapy*. 2000;20(3):257–269.

47. GAO/PEMB. *FDA Drug Review: Postapproval Risks*; April 1990. 1976-85.

48. Doucet J, Chassagne P, Trivalle C. Drug-drug interactions related to hospital admissions in older adults: a prospective study of 1000 patients. *J Am Ger Soc*. 1996;44:944–948.

49. Lazarou J, Pomeranz B, Corey P. Incidence of adverse drug reactions in hospitalized patients: a meta-analysis of prospective studies. *JAMA*. 1998;279(15):1200–1205.

50. Starfield B. *Is United States health really the best in the world?* 2000;320:1362.

51. Zhan C, et al. Ambulatory Care Visits for Treating Adverse Drug Effects in the United States, 1995–2001. *Jt Comm J Qual Patient Saf*. July 2005;31(7):372–378 (7).

52. Jones CM, Mack KA, Paulozzi LJ. Pharmaceutical Overdose Deaths, United States, 2010. *JAMA*. 2013;309(7):657–659. http://dx.doi.org/10.1001/jama.2013.272.

53. Pennachio D. Drug-herb interactions: how vigilant should you be? *Patient Care*. 2000;19:41–68.

54. Kelly K. Complementary and alternative medical therapies for children with cancer. *Eur J Cancer*. September 2004;40(14):2041–2046. Kelly 2004 p.39.

55. Nobili Stefania. Natural compounds for cancer treatment and prevention. *Pharmacological Research*. June 2009;59(6):365–378.

56. McColloch M, et al. Astragalus-Based Chinese Herbs and Platinum-Based Chemotherapy for Advanced Non–Small-Cell Lung Cancer: Meta-Analysis of Randomized Trials. *JCO*. January 20, 2006;24(3):419–430.

57. Boon 2004

58. Olaku O, White JD. Herbal therapy use by cancer patients: a literature review on case reports. *Eur J Cancer*. 2011;47(4):508–514.

59. Yarnell E, Meserole L. Toxic Botanicals: is the Poison in the Plant or Its Regulation? Alt Comp Ther

60. Letzel H, Haan J, et al. *Nootropics: Efficacy and tolerability of products from three active substance classes*. 1996;8:77–94.

61. Wettstein A. Cholinesterase inhibitors and Ginkgo extracts—are they comparable in the treatment of dementia? *Phytomedicine*. 2000;6(6):393–401.

62. Linde K, Ramirez G, Mulrow C, Pauls A, Weidenhammeer W, Melchart D. St John's wort for depression-an overview and meta-analysis of randomised clinical trials. *BMJ*. 1996;313:253–258.

63. Schulze J, Raasch W, Siegers C. Toxicity of kava pyrones, drug safety and precautions—a case study. *Phytomedicine*. 2003;10(suppl 4):68–73.

64. Adams K, Cohen M, Eisenberg D, et al. Ethical considerations of complementary and alternative medical therapies in conventional medical settings. *Ann Int Med*. 2002;137(8):660–664.

65. Sugarman J. Physicians' ethical obligations regarding alternative medicine. *JAMA*. 2000;280(18):1623–1625.

66. Jonas W. Advising patients on the use of complementary and alternative medicine. *Appl Psychophysiol Biofeed*. 2001;26(3):205–213.

67. Nutrition, 1995

68. Association #7902

69. Awang DV. Maternal use of ginseng and neonatal androgenization. *JAMA*. 1991;266(3):363.

70. www.crnusa.org/NYAG/quotes.html)

CHAPTER 5

1. Strieder T, Prummel M, Tijssen J, Endert E, Wiersinga W. Risk factors for and prevalence of thyroid disorders in a cross-sectional study among healthy female relatives of patients with autoimmune thyroid disease. *Clin Endocrinol*. 2003;59:396–401.

2. Helfand M. Screening for subclinical thyroid dysfunction in nonpregnant adults: a summary of the evidence for the U.S. Preventive Services Task Force. *Ann Int Med*. 2004;140(2):128–141.

3. Redmond G. Thyroid dysfunction and women's reproductive health. *Thyroid*. 2004;14(suppl1):S5–S15.

4. Poppe K, Glinoer D. Thyroid autoimmunity and hypothyroidism before and during pregnancy. *Hum Reprod Update*. 2003;9(2):149–161.

5. Poppe K, Velkeniers B. Thyroid and infertility (abstract). *Verhandelingen—Koninklijke Academie voor Geneeskunde van Belgie*. 2002;6:389–399, 400-402.

6. Mitchell M, Klein R. The sequelae of untreated maternal hypothyroidism. *Eur J Endocrinol*. 2004;151(suppl 3):45–48.

7. Speroff L, Glass R, Kase G. *Clinical Gynecologic Endocrinology and Infertility*. Baltimore: Lippincott Williams & Wilkins; 1999.

8. Roberts C, Ladenson P. Hypothyroidism. *Lancet*. 2004;363:793–803.

9. Vanderpump M, Turnbridge M. Epidemiology and prevention of clinical and subclinical hypothyroidism. *Thyroid*. 2002;12(10):839–847.

10. Hollowell J, Staehling N, Flanders W, et al. Serum TSH, T(4), and thyroid antibodies in the United States population (1988 to 1994): National Health and Nutrition Examination Survey (NHANES III). *J Clin Endocrinol Metab*. 2002;87(2). 489–489.

11. Nicholson W, Robinson K, Smallridge R, Ladenson P, Powe N. Prevalence of Postpartum Thyroid Dysfunction: a Quantitative Review. *Thyroid*. 2006;16:573–582.

12. Nygaard B. Hypothyroidism (primary). *Clinical Evidence*. 2014;02:605.

13. Low Dog T. Integrative approach to endocrinology. In: Kligler B, Lee R, eds. *Integrative Medicine: Principles for Practice*. New York: McGraw-Hill; 2004:433–455.

14. Buchberger W, Holler W, Winsauer K. Effects of sodium bromide on the biosynthesis of thyroid hormones and brominated/iodinated thyronines. *J Trace Elem Electrolytes Health Dis*. 1990;4(1):25–30.

15. Peckham S, Lowery D, Spencer S. Are fluoride levels in drinking water associated with hypothyroidism prevalence in England? A large observational study of GP practice data and fluoride levels in drinking water. *J Epidemiol Community Health*. http://dx.doi.org/10.1136/jech-2014-204971

16. Badenhoop K, Dieterich W, Segni M, et al. HLA DQ2 and/or DQ8 is associated with celiac disease-specific autoantibodies to tissue transglutaminase in families with thyroid autoimmunity. *Am J Gastroenterol*. 2001;96(5):1648–1649.

17. Counsell C, Taha A, Ruddell W. Coeliac disease and autoimmune thyroid disease. *Gut*. 1994;35(6):844–846.

18. Stagnaro-Green A. Postpartum thyroiditis. *Best Pract Res Clin Endocrinol Metab*. 2004;18(2):303–316.

19. Turken O, NarIn Y, DemIrbas S, et al. Breast cancer in association with thyroid disorders. *Breast Cancer Res*. 2003;5(5):110–113.

20. Cengiz O, Bozkurt B, Unal B, et al. The relationship between prognostic factors of breast cancer and thyroid disorders in Turkish women. *J Surg Oncol*. 2004;87(1):19–25.

21. Flynn R, Macdonald T, Morris A, Jung R, Leese G. The Thyroid Epidemiology, Audit, and Research Study: thyroid dysfunction in the general population. *J Clin Endocrinol Metab*. 2004;89(8):3879–3884.

22. Jatwa R, Kar A. Amelioration of metformin-induced hypothyroidism by Withania somnifera and Bauhinia purpurea extracts in Type 2 diabetic mice. *Phytother Res*. 2009, Aug;23(8):1140–1145.

23. Panda S, Kar A. Changes in thyroid hormone concentrations after administration of ashwagandha root extract to adult male mice. *J Pharm Pharmacol*. 1998;50(9):1065–1068.

24. Mills S, Bone K. *The Essential Guide to Herbal Safety*. St. Louis: Churchill Livingstone; 2005.

25. Basch E, Ulbricht C. *Natural Standard Herb and Supplement Handbook*. St. Louis: Mosby; 2000.

26. Bone K. *A Clinical Guide to Blending Liquid Herbs: Herbal Formulations for the Individual Patient*. St. Louis: Churchill Livingstone; 2003.

27. Ding X, Staudinger J. Induction of drug metabolism by forskolin: the role of the pregnane X receptor and the protein kinase a signal transduction pathway. *JPET*. 2005;312:849–856.

28. Bone K. *Clinical Applications of Ayurvedic and Chinese Herbs*. Queensland, Australia: Phytotherapy Press; 2000.

29. Singh AK, Prasad GC. Effect of some chemical agents on thyroid gland in vitro. *J Exp Zool*. 1998;1(2):131–141.

30. Sathyapalan T, Manuchehri AM, Thatcher NJ, et al. The effect of soy phytoestrogen supplementation on thyroid status and cardiovascular risk markers in patients with subclinical hypothyroidism: a randomized, double-blind, crossover study. *J Clin Endocrinol Metab*. 2011, May;96(5):1442–1449.

31. Rakel D. *Integrative Medicine*. Philadelphia: Saunders; 2003.

32. Greenspan F, Gardner D. *Basic and Clinical Endocrinology*. 6th ed. New York: McGraw-Hill; 2001.

33. Biondi B, Palmieri E, Klain M, Schlumberger M, Filetti S, Lombardi G. Subclinical hyperthyroidism: clinical features and treatment options. *Eur J Endocrinol*. 2005;152(1):1–9.

34. Wallach J. *Interpretation of Diagnostic Tests*. New York: Little, Brown; 1996.

35. Briancon-Scheid F, Stierle A. Inhibition of human platelet cyclic AMP phosphodiesterase and of platelet aggregation by a hemisynthetic flavanoid, amentoflavone hexacetate. *Biochem Pharmacol*. 1986;35(2):257–262.

36. Blumenthal M. *The ABC Clinical Guide to Herbs*. Austin: American Botanical Council; 2003.

37. Weiss RF, Fintelmann V. *Herbal Medicine*. 2th ed. Stuttgart: Thieme; 2000.

38. BHMA. *British Herbal Pharmacopoeia*. Keighley, UK: British Herbal Medicine Association; 1983.

39. Priest A, Priest L. *Herbal Medication*. London: Fowler and Co; 1982.

40. Hoffmann D. *Medical Herbalism: The Science and Practice of Herbal Medicine*. Rochester, VT: Healing Arts Press; 2003.

41. Beer AM, Wiebelitz KR, Schmidt-Gayk H. Lycopus europaeus (Gypsywort): effects on the thyroidal parameters and symptoms associated with thyroid function. *Phytomedicine*. 2008, Jan;15(1-2):16–22.

42. Eiling R, Wieland V, Niestroj M. [Improvement of symptoms in mild hyperthyroidism with an extract of Lycopus europaeus (Thyreogutt® mono)]. *Wien Med Wochenschr*. 2013, Feb;163(3-4):95–101.

43. Kelly G. Peripheral metabolism of the thyroid hormones: a review. *Alt Med Rev*. 2005;5(4):307–333.

44. Auf'mkolk M, Ingbar J, Kubota K. Extracts and auto-oxidized constituents of certain plants inhibit the receptor-binding and the biological activity of Graves' immunoglobulins. *Endocrinology*. 1985;116:1687–1693.

45. Blumenthal M, Busse W, Goldberg A, et al. *The Complete German Commission E Monographs: Therapeutic Guide to Herbal Medicine*. Boston: American Botanical Council; 1998.

46. Felter H, Lloyd J. *King's American Dispensatory, Cincinnati, reprinted by Eclectic Medical Publications*; 1983:1898.

47. Winterhoff H, Sourgens H, Kemper F. Antihormonal effects of plant extract: pharmacodynamic effects of Lithospermum officinale on the thyroid gland of rats; comparison with the effects of iodide. *Hormone Metab Res*. 1983;15:503–507.

48. Kohrle J, Spanka M, Irmscher K, Hesch R. Flavonoid effects on transport, metabolism and action of thyroid hormones. *Prog Clin Biol Res*. 1988;280:323–340.

49. Mills S, Bone K. *Principles and Practice of Phytotherapy*. London: Churchill Livingstone; 2000.

50. Oliviero O, Girelli D, Azzini M. Low selenium status in older adults influences thyroid hormones. *Clin Sci*. 1995;89:637–642.

51. Gartner R, Gasnier B, Johannes W. Selenium supplementation in patients with autoimmune thyroiditis decreases thyroid peroxidase antibodies concentrations. *J Clin Endocrinol Metab*. 2002;87(4):1687–1691.

52. Sapolsky R. *Why Zebras Don't Get Ulcers*. New York: Henry Holt; 2004.

53. McEwen B. Protection and damage from acute and chronic stress: allostasis and allostatic overload and relevance to the pathophysiology of psychiatric disorders [biobehavioral stress response: protective and damaging effects: Part I. Novel paradigms for considering stress- hormone response]. *Ann NY Acad Sci*. 2004;1032:1–7.

54. Strike P, Steptoe A. Psychosocial factors in the development of coronary artery disease. *Progr Cardiovasc Dis*. 2004;46(4):337–347.

55. Beishuizen A, Thijs L. The immunoneuroendocrine axis in critical illness: beneficial adaptation or neuroendocrine exhaustion? *Curr Opin Crit Care*. 2004;10:461–467.

56. Chrousos G, Torpy D, Gold P. Interactions between the hypothalamic-pituitary-adrenal axis and the female reproductive system: clinical implications. *Ann Int Med*. 1998;129(3):229–240.

57. Panossian A. Adaptogens: a historical overview and perspective. *Nat Pharm*. 2003;7(4):19–20.

58. Chrousos G. Stressors, stress, and neuroendocrine integration of the adaptive response: the 1997 Hans Selye Memorial Lecture. *Ann NY Acad Sci*. 1998;851:311–335.

59. Jacobs G. The physiology of mind-body interactions: the stress response and the relaxation response. *J Alt Comp Med*. 2001;7(suppl 1):S83–S92.

60. Szabo S. Hans Selye and the development of the stress Concepta: special reference to gastroduodenal ulcerogenesis [stress of life: from molecules to mana: Hans Selye and his legacy today]. *Ann NY Acad Sci*. 1998;851:19–27.

61. Engelmann M, Landgrafb R, Wotjakb C. The hypothalamic-neurohypophysial system regulates the hypothalamic-pituitary-adrenal axis under stress: an old concept revisited. *Frontiers Neuroendocrinol*. 2004;25:132–149.

62. Panossian A, Wikman G, Wagner H. Plant adaptogens. III. Earlier and more recent aspects and concepts on their mode of action. *Phytomedicine*. 1999;6(4):287–300.

63. Van Voorhees E, Scarpa A. The effects of child maltreatment on the hypothalamic-pituitary-adrenal axis. *Trauma Violence Abuse Rev J*. 2004;5(4):333–352.

64. Mackinnon L, Hooper S, Jones S, Gordon R. Bachmann A: Hormonal, immunological, and hematological responses to intensified training in elite swimmers. *Med Sci Sports Exerc*. 1997;29(12):1637–1645.

65. Singh B, Chandan B, Gupta D. Adaptogenic activity of a novel withanolidefree aqueous fraction from the roots of withania somnifera dun (Part II). *Phytother Res*. 2003;17:531–536.

66. Coven M. *Parasympathomimetics and adaptogens: Tonic therapy for chronic stress*. Albuquerque: Paper presented at American Herbalists Guild Building Knowledge, Building Community; 2003.

67. Low Dog T. *The endocrine system*. Albuquerque: Found Herbal Med; 2000.

68. Spoerke D, Rouse J. *Ashwagandha*; 2005.

69. Devi P, Sharada A, Solomon F. Antitumor and radiosensitizing effects of Withania somnifera (Ashwagandha) on a transplantable mouse tumor, Sarcoma 180. *Ind J Exp Biol*. 1993;31(7):607–611.

70. Upton R. *Ashwagandha root: withania somnifera*. Santa Cruz, CA: American Herbal Pharmacopoeia; 2000.

71. Tohda C, Kuboyama T, Komatsu K. Dendrite extension by methanol extract of Ashwagandha (roots Withania somnifera) in SK-N-SH cells. *Neuroreport*. 2000;11(9):1981–1985.

72. Dhuley J. Effect of ashwagandha on lipid peroxidation in stress-induced animals. *J Ethnopharmacol*. 1998;60(2):173–178.

73. Dhuley J. Nootropic-like effect of ashwagandha (Withania somnifera L.) mice. *Phytother Res*. 2001;15(6):524–528.

74. Dhuley JN. Therapeutic efficacy of Ashwagandha against experimental aspergillosis mice. *Immunopharmacol Immunotoxicol*. 1998;20(1):191–198.

75. Bhattacharya S, Bhattacharya A, Sairam K, Ghosal S. Anxiolytic-antidepressant activity of Withania somnifera glycowithanolides: an experiment study. *Phytomedicine*. 2000;7(6):463–469.

76. Bhattacharya A, Muruganandam A, Kumar V, Bhattacharya S. Effect of poly herbal formulation, EuMil, on neurochemical perturbations induced by chronic stress. *Indian J Exp Biol*. 2002;40(10):1161–1163.

77. Davis L, Kuttan G. Immunomodulatory activity of Withania somnifera. *J Ethnopharmacol*. 1999;71:193–200.

78. Gautam M, Diwanayb S, Gairolac S, et al. Preliminary report. Immune response modulation to DPT vaccine by aqueous extract of Withania somnifera in experimental system. *Immunopharmacology*. 2004;4:841–849.

79. Upton R. *American Herbal Pharmacopoeia and Therapeutic Monographs: Ashwagandha Root.* Santa Cruz, CA: American Herbal Pharmacopoeia; 2000.

80. Nagashayana N, Sankarankutty P, Nampoothiri M, Mohan P, Mohanakumar K. Association of L-DOPA with recovery following Ayurveda medication in Parkinson's disease. *J Neurol Sci.* 2000;176(2):124–127.

81. McGuffin M, Hobbs C, Upton R, Goldberg A. Boca Raton: CRC Press; 1997.

82. Wichtl M. *Herbal drugs and phytopharmaceuticals: A handbook for practice on a scientific basis.* 4th ed. Stuttgart: Medpharm; 2004.

83. Fulder S. Ginseng and the hypothalamic pituitary control of stress. *Am Journ Chinese Med.* 1981;9(2):112–118.

84. Chang H. *Botanical pharmacology and applications of Chinese materia medica.* Singapore: Chinese University of Hong Kong; 1987.

85. Davydov M, Krikorian AD. Eleutherococcus senticosus (rupr & maxim) maxim. (Araliaceae) as an adaptogen: a closer look. *J Ethnopharmacol.* 2000;72(3):345–393.

86. Kimura T, Saunders PA, Kim HS, Rheu HM, Oh KW, Ho IK. Interactions of ginsenosides with ligand-bindings of GABA(A) and GABA(B) receptors. *Gen Pharmacol.* 1994;25(1):193–199.

87. Szolomicki J, Samochowiec L, Wojcicki J, Drozdzik M, Szolomicki S. The influence of active components of Eleutherococcus senticosus on cellular defence and physical fitness in man. *Phytother Res.* 2000;14(1):30–35.

88. Gaffney BT, Hugel HM, Rich PA. Panax ginseng and Eleutherococcus senticosus may exaggerate an already existing biphasic response to stress via inhibition of enzymes which limit the binding of stress hormones to their receptors. *Med Hypotheses.* 2001;56(5):567–572.

89. Hartz AJ, Bentler S, Noyes R, et al. Randomized controlled trial of Siberian ginseng for chronic fatigue. *Psychol Med.* 2004;34(1):51–61.

90. Schulz V, Hansel R, Blumenthal M, Tyler V. *Rational Phytotherapy: A Reference Guide for Physicians and Pharmacists.* 5th ed. Berlin: Springer-Verlag; 2004.

91. Spelman K. *Adaptogens.* Baltimore; 2005.

92. Yance D. Adaptogens. In: Romm A, ed. Ashland, OR; 2005.

93. McKenna D, Jones K, Hughes K, Humphrey S. *Botanical medicines: the desk reference for major herbal supplements.* New York: Haworth Press; 2002.

94. Avakian E. Effect of Panax ginseng extract on energy metabolism during exercise in rats. *Planta Med.* 1984;50(12):151–154.

95. Yun A. A case control study of ginseng intake and cancer. *Int J Epidemiol.* 1990;19(4):871–876.

96. Yun T. Anticarcinogenic effect of long-term oral administration of red ginseng on newborn mice exposed to various chemical carcinogens. *Cancer Det Prev.* 1983;6:515–525.

97. Scaglione F, Cogo R, Cocuzza C, Arcidiacono M, Beretta A. Immunomodulatory effects of Panax ginseng: C.A. Meyer (G115) on alveolar macrophages from patients suffering with chronic bronchitis. *Int J Immunother.* 1994;10(1):21–24.

98. Kenarova B. Immunomodulating activity of ginsenoside Rg1 from Panax ginseng. *Jpn J Pharmacol.* 1990;54(4):447–454.

99. Jie Y, Cammisuli S, Baggiolini M. Immunomodulatory effects of Panax ginseng C.A. Meyer in the mouse. *Agents Actions.* 1984;15(3-4):386–391.

100. Scaglione F. Immunomodulatory effects of two extracts of Panax ginseng. *Drugs Exp Clin Res.* 1990;16(10):537–542.

101. Salvati G, Genovesi G, Marcellini L. *Paniminerva Med.* 1996;38(4):249–254.

102. Cheng-chai L, Ching-ch'u T. *Chin Med J.* 1973;11:156.

103. Attele AS, Wu JA, Yuan C-S. Ginseng pharmacology: multiple constituents and multiple actions. *Biochem Pharmacol.* 1999;58(11):1685–1693.

104. Sievenpiper JL, Arnason JT, Leiter LA, Vuksan V. Variable effects of American ginseng: a batch of American ginseng (Panax quinquefolius L.) with a depressed ginsenoside profile does not affect postprandial glycemia. *Eur J Clin Nutr.* 2003;57(2):243–248.

105. Bhattacharya S, Mitra S. Anxiolytic activity of Panax ginseng roots: an experimental study. *J Ethnopharmacol.* 1991;34:87–92.

106. Basch E, Ulbricht C. *Natural Standard Herb and Supplement Handbook.* St. Louis: Mosby; 2000.

107. Takeda A, Katoh N, Yonezawa M. Restoration of radiation injury by ginseng. III. Radioprotective effect of thermostable fraction of ginseng extract on mice, rats and guinea pigs. *J Radiat Res (Tokyo).* 1982;23(2):150–167.

108. Chen J, Chen T. *Ren sheni (radix ginseng), Chinese Medical Herbology and Pharmacology.* City of Industry, CA: Art of Medicine Press; 2004:836–840.

109. Kim HJ, Woo DS, Lee G, Kim JJ. The relaxation effects of ginseng saponin in rabbit corporal smooth muscle: is it a nitric oxide donor? *Br J Urol.* 1998;82(5):744–748.

110. ESCOP: *Radix Ginseng. ESCOP Monographs: The Scientific Foundation for Herbal Medicinal Products.* 2nd ed. Exeter, UK: European Scientific Cooperative on Phytotherapy & Thieme; 2003:211–225.

111. WHO. Geneva: World Health Organization; 1999:168–182.

112. Janetzky K, Morreale AP. Probable interaction between warfarin and ginseng. *Am J Health Syst Pharm.* 1997;54(6):692–693.

113. Krausse R, Bielenberg J, Blaschek W, Ullmann U. In vitro anti-Helicobacter pylori activity of Extractum liquiritiae, glycyrrhizin and its metabolites. *J Antimicrob Chemother.* 2004;54(1):243–246.

114. Cohen J. Licking latency with licorice. *J Clin Invest.* 2005;115(3):591–593.

115. Somjen D, Katzburg S, Vaya J, et al. Estrogenic activity of glabridin and glabrene from licorice roots on human osteoblasts and prepubertal rat skeletal tissues. *J Steroid Biochem Mol Biol.* 2004;91(4-5):241–246.

116. Nakagawa K, Kishida H, Arai N, Nishiyama T, Mae T. Licorice flavonoids suppress abdominal fat accumulation and increase in blood glucose level in obese diabetic KK-A(y) mice. *Biol Pharm Bull.* 2004;27(11):1775–1778.

117. Parle M, Dhingra D, Kulkarni S. Memory-strengthening activity of Glycyrrhiza glabra in exteroceptive and interoceptive behavioral models. *J Med Food.* 2004;7(4):462–466.

118. Association BHM: *British Herbal Compendium.* Bournemouth, UK: BHMA; 1992.

119. Saratikov A, Tuzov S. Influence of Leuzea carthamoides on the physical work ability and some functional indicators of the organism. *Ser Biomed Sci.* 1963;12(3):126–132.

120. Yance D. Rhaponticum carthamoides (syn. Leuzea carthamoides): monograph and review of the literature. *J Amer Herb Guild.* 2005;5(2).

121. Krasnov E, Saratikov A, Yakunina G. Active substances of Leuzea carthamoides. *Ser Biol.* 1977;5(1):93–95.

122. Krasnov E, Saratikov A, Yakunin G. Incosterone and ecdysterone from Rhaponticum carthamoides. *Chem Nat Comp.* 1976;4:550.

123. Azizov A, Seifulla R. The effect of antioxidants Elton and Leveton on the physical work capacity of athletes. *Eksp Klin Farmakol.* 1998;61(1):61–62.

124. Kokoska L, Polesny Z, Rada V, Nepovim A, Vanek T. Screening of some Siberian medicinal plants for antimicrobial activity. *J Ethnopharmacol.* 2002;82(1):51–53.

125. Kolmakova L, Kutolina N. Clinical observation for action Leuzea, Eleuterococcus and golden root extracts in diabetes patients. In: Tomsk, ed. *Stimulants of the Central Nervous System.* 1966:131–132.

126. Galambosi B, Varga Z, Jokela K. Introduction of Leuzea carthamoides DC as an adaptive medical plant in the Nordic climate. *Drogenreport J.* 1997;10(1):6–9.

127. Gerasyuta M, Koval T. *The experience of prolonged use of Leuzea carthamoides extract for the purposes of preservation and increase of mental and physical work capacity in New Data on Eleutherococcus and Other Adaptogens, Proceedings of the 1st International Symposium on Eleutherococcus.* Hamburg: Paper presented at 1st International Symposium on Eleutherococcus; 1981.

128. Yakunina G, Krasnov E. Leuzea carthamoides as a prospective resource of new remedies. Herbal remedies in traditional and folk medicine. *Ulan Ude.* 1996:155–156.

129. Syrov V, Kurmukov A. On the anabolic activity of phytoecdisone-ecdisterone extracted from Rhaponticum carthamoides. *Pharmacol Toxicol.* 1976;39(6):690–693.

130. Lupandin A. *Adaptation and rehabilitation in sports.* Khabarovsk: USSRInstitute of Physical Culture; 1991.

131. Gadzhieva R, Portugalov S, Paniushkin V, Kondrat'eva I. A comparative study of the anabolic action of ecdysten, leveton and Prime Plus, preparations of plant origin. *Eksp Klin Farmakol.* 1995;58(5):46–48.

132. Logvinov S, Pugachenko N. Ischemia-induced changes in synaptoarchitectonics of brain cortex and their correction with ascovertin and Leuzea extract. *Bull Exp Biol Med.* 2001;132(4):1017–1020.

133. Jankulow J, Issaew I, Bojadjiewa M, Petkow W, Owtscharow R. Preparations with stimulating effect from the roots of Rhaponticum carthamoides (WILLD) ILJIN cultivated in Bulgaria. *Pharmazie.* 1964;19:345–347.

134. Bespalov V, Aleksandrov V, Iaremenko K. The inhibiting effect of phytoadaptogenic preparations from bioginseng, Eleuterococcus senticosus and Rhaponticum carthamoides on the development of nervous system tumors in rats induced by N nitrosomethylurea. *Vopr Onkol.* 1992;38(9):1073–1080.

135. Maimeskulova L, Maslov L. Anti-arrhythmic effect of phytoadaptogens. *Eksp Klin Farmakol.* 2000;63(4):29–31.

136. Kholodova I, Tugai V, Zimina V. Effect of vitamin D3 & 20-hydroxyecdysone on the content of ATP, creatine phosphate, carnosine and Ca2+ in skeletal muscles. *Ukr Biokhim Zh.* 1997;69(3):3–9.

137. Chobot V, Buchta V, Jahodarova H, et al. Antifungal activity of a thiophene polyene from Leuzea carthamoides. *Fitoterapia.* 2003;74(3):288–290.

138. Vavilova P, Kondratyev A. New plants for feeding in animal husbandry. *Ros Selkhoz Izdat.* 1975:123–126.

139. Mirzaev I, Syrov V, Khrushev S, et al. Effect of ecdistene on parameters of the sexual function under experimental and clinical conditions. *Eksp Klin Farmakol.* 2000;63(4):35–37.

140. Azizov A. Effects of eleutherococcus, elton, leuzea, and leveton on the blood coagulation system during training in athletes. *Eksp Klin Farmakol.* 1997;60(5):58–60.

141. Lamer-Zarawska E, Gasiorowwski K, Brocos B: Immunomodulatory activity of polysaccharide-rich fraction from Rhaponticum carthamoides leaves, Fitoterapia 4:371–372.

142. De Bock K, Eijinde B, Ramaekers M, Hespel P. Acute Rhodiola rosea intake can improve endurance exercise performance. *Int J Sport Nutr Exerc Metabol.* 2004;14:292–301.

143. Review AM. Rhodioloa rosea monograph. *Alt Med Rev.* 2002;7(5):421–423.

144. Brown R, Gerberg P, Ramazanov Z. Rhodiola rosea: a phytomedicinal overview. *HerbalGram.* 2002;56:40–52.

145. Kelly GS. Rhodiola rosea: a possible plant adaptogen. *Alt Med Rev.* 2001;6(3):302–393.

146. Shevtsov V, Zholus B, Shervarly V, et al. A randomized trial of two different doses of a SHR-5 Rhodiola rosea extract versus placebo and control of capacity for mental work. *Phytomedicine.* 2003;10(2-3):95–105.

147. Abidov M, Crendal F, Grachev S, et al. Effect of extracts from Rhodiola rosea and Rhodiola crenulata (Crassulaceae) roots on ATP content in mitochondria of skeletal muscles. *Bull Exp Biol Med.* 2003;136(6):585–587.

148. Bucci L. Selected herbals and human exercise performance. *Am J Clin Nutr.* 2000;72(suppl):624S–636S.

149. Abidov M, Grachev S, Seifulla R, Ziegenfuss T. Extract of Rhodiola rosea radix reduces the level of C-reactive protein. *Bull Exp Biol Med.* 2004;138(1):63–64.

150. Provalova N, Skurikhin E, Pershina O, et al. Mechanisms underling the effects of adaptogens on erythropoiesis during paradoxical sleep deprivation. *Bull Exp Biol Med.* 2002;133(5):428–432.

151. Maimeskulova L, Maslov L. [Anti-arrhythmic effect of phytoadaptogens] [Russian]. *Eksp Klin Farmakol.* 2000;63(4):29–31.

152. Razina T, Zueva E, Amosova E, Krylov AS. [Medicinal plant preparations used as adjuvant therapeutics in experimental oncology] [Russian]. *Eksp Klin Farmakol.* 2000;63(5):59–61.

153. Upton R. Schisandra berry: schisandra chinensis, American Herbal Pharmacopoeia and Therapeutic Compendium, Santacruz; 1999.

154. Bensky D, Gamble A. *Chinese Herbal Medicine Materia Medica.* Seattle: Eastman Press; 1993.

155. Song WZ, Tong GY. Occurrence and assay of some important lignins in Schisandra chinensis and its allied species. *Acta Pharm Sin.* 1983;18(2):138–143.

156. Bone K. *Clinical applications of Ayurvedic and Chinese herbs.* Queensland, Australia: Phytotherapy Press; 2000.

157. Zhu M, Lin KF, Yeung RY, Li RC. Evaluation of the protective effects of Schisandra chinensis on phase I drug metabolism using a CCl4 intoxication model. *Journ of Ethropharmacology.* 1999;67:61–68.

158. Bone K. Schisandra chinensis-Schisandra. *MediHerb Prof Rev.* 2000;74:1–4.

159. Dex AM. *Schizandra chinensis.* Micromedex; 2005.

160. Birkenhager-Gillesse E, Derksen J, Lagaay A. DHEAS in the oldest old, aged 85 and over. *Ann NY Acad Sci.* 1994;179:543–551.

161. Pepping J. DHEA: dehydroepiandrosterone [alternative therapies]. *Am J Health-System Pharm.* 2000;57(22):2048. 2050, 2053–2054, 2056.

162. Mortola J, Yen S. The effects of oral dehydroepiandrosterone on endocrine-metabolic parameters in postmenopausal women. *Clin Endocrinol Metab.* 1990;71:696–704.

163. Wei A, Pritts E. Therapy for polycystic ovarian syndrome. *Curr Opin Pharmacol.* 2003;3:678–682.

164. Richardson M. Current perspectives in polycystic ovary syndrome. *Am Fam Physician.* 2003;68(4):697–704.

165. Speroff L, Glass R, Kase G. *Clinical Gynecologic Endocrinology and Infertility.* Baltimore: Lippincott Williams & Wilkins; 1999.

166. Solomon C. The epidemiology of polycystic ovary syndrome: prevalence and associated disease risks. *Endocrinol Metab Clin North Am.* 1999;28(2):247–263.

167. Fraser I, Kovacs G. Current recommendations for the diagnostic evaluation and follow-up of patients presenting with symptomatic polycystic ovary syndrome. *Best Pract Res Clin Obstet Gynaecol.* 2004;18(5):813–823.

168. Guzick D. Polycystic ovary syndrome: symptomatology, pathophysiology, and epidemiology. *Am J Obstet Gynecol.* 1998;196(6 Pt 2):S89–S93.

169. Talbott E, Clerici A, Berga S, et al. Adverse lipid and coronary heart disease risk profiles in young women with polycystic ovary syndrome: results of a case-control study. *J Clin Epidemiol.* 1998;51(5):415–422.

170. Holte J, Gennarelli G, Wide L, et al. High prevalence of polycystic ovaries and associated clinical, endocrine, and metabolic features in women with previous gestational diabetes. *J Clin Endocr Metab.* 1998;83(4):1143–1150.

171. deVries M, Dekker G, Schoemaker J. Higher risk of preeclampsia in the polycystic ovary syndrome: a case control study. *Eur J Obstet Gynecol Reprod Biol.* 1998;76(1):91–95.

172. Holte J. Polycystic ovary syndrome and insulin resistance: thirty genes struggling with over-feeding and sedentary lifestyle? *J Endocrinol Invest.* 1998;21(9):601–689.

173. Cresswell J, Barker D, Osmond C, et al. Fetal growth, length of gestation, and polycystic ovaries in adult life. *Lancet.* 1997;350(9085):1131–1135.

174. Goudas V, Dumesic D. Polycystic ovary syndrome. *Endocrinol Metab Clin North Am.* 1997;26(4):893–912.

175. Hopkinson Z, Satar N, Fleming R, et al. Polycystic ovarian syndrome: the metabolic syndrome comes to gynecology. *BMJ.* 1998;317:329–332.

176. Ehrmann D, Barnes R, Rosenfield R, et al. Prevalence of impaired glucose tolerance and diabetes in women with polycystic ovary syndrome. *Diabetes Care.* 1999;22(1):141–146.

177. Ostrzens A. *Gynecology: Integrating Conventional, Complementary, and Natural Alternative Therapy.* Philadelphia: Lippincott Williams & Wilkins; 2002.

178. D'Hooghe T, Hill J. *Infertility. Novak's Gynecology.* Philadelphia: Lippincott Williams & Wilkins; 2002.

179. Parades A, Galvez A, Leyton V, et al. Stress promotes development of ovarian cysts in rats: the possible role of sympathetic activation. *Endocrine.* 1998;8(3):309–315.

180. Weiner C, Primeau M, Ehrmann D. Androgens and mood dysfunction in women: comparison of women with polycystic ovarian syndrome to healthy controls. *Psychosomat Med.* 2004;66:356–362.

181. Stenchever M. *Comprehensive Gynecology.* 4th ed. St. Louis: Mosby; 2001.

182. Fleming R, Hopkinson Z, Michael Wallace M, et al. Ovarian function and metabolic factors in women with oligomenorrhea treated with metformin in a randomized double-blind placebo controlled trial. *J Clin Endocrinol Metab.* 2003;87(2):557–569.

183. Lord J, Flight I, Norman R. Insulin-sensitizing drugs (metformin, troglitazone, rosiglitazone pioglitazone, D-chiro-inositol) for polycystic ovarian syndrome. *Cochrane Database Syst Rev.* 2003;3(CD003053).

184. McCarthy E, Walker S, McLachlan K, et al. Merformin in obstetric and gynecologic practice: a review, Obstetrical and Gynecologic Survey CME Review Article; 2004.

185. Crosignani P, Colombo M, Vegetti W. Overweight and obese anovulatory patients with polycystic ovaries: parallel improvements in anthropometric indices, ovarphysiology and fertility rate by diet. *Hum Reprod.* 1928-1932;18(9).

186. Jakubowicz D, Nestler J. 17-Alpha-hydroxyprogesterone responses to leuprolide and serum androgens in obese women with and without polycystic ovary syndrome offer dietary weight loss. *J Clin Endocr Metab.* 1997;82(2):556–560.

187. Pasquali R, Casimirri F, Vicennati V. Weight control and its benefits on fertility in women with obesity and polycystic ovary syndrome. *Hum Reprod.* 1997;12(suppl 1):82–87.

188. Kahn JA, Gordon C. Polycystic ovary syndrome. *Adolesc Med.* 1999;10(2):231–236.

189. Van Dam E, Roelfsema F, Veldhuis J, et al. Increase in daily LH secretion in response to short-term caloric restriction in obese women. *Am J Physiol Endocrinol Metab.* 2001;282:865–872.

190. Low Dog T. *The endocrine system.* Albuquerque: Foundations in Herbal Medicine; 2000. Foundations in Herbal Medicine.

191. Bone K. *Clinical Applications of Ayurvedic and Chinese Herbs.* Queensland, Australia: Phytotherapy Press; 2000.

192. McKenna D, Jones K, Hughes K, et al. *Botanical Medicines: The Desk Reference for Major Herbal Supplements.* New York: Haworth Press; 2002.

193. Wuttke W, Jarry H, Christoffel V, et al. Chaste tree (Vitex agnus castus)—Pharmacology and clinical indications. *Phytomedicine.* 2003;10:348–357.

194. Mills S, Bone K. *Principles and Practice of Phytotherapy.* London: Churchill Livingstone; 2000.

195. Ye Q, Zhang QY, Zheng CJ, Wang Y, Qin LP. Casticin, a flavonoid isolated from Vitex rotundifolia, inhibits prolactin release in vivo and in vitro. *Acta Pharmacol Sin.* 2010, Dec;31(12):1564–1568.

196. Bone K. *A Clinical Guide to Blending Liquid Herbs: Herbal Formulations for the Individual Patient.* St. Louis: Churchill Livingstone; 2003.

197. Yaginuma T, Izumi R, Yasui H, et al. Effects of traditional herbal medicines on serum testosterone levels and it's induction of regular ovulation in hyperandrogenic and oligomenorrheic women (author's transl). *Nippon Sanka Fujinka Gakkai Zasshi.* 1998;34(7):939–944.

198. Takahashi K, Kitao M. Effects of TJ-68 (shakuyaku-kanzo-to) on polycystic ovarian disease. *Int J Fertil Menopausal Stud.* 1994;39(2):69–76.

199. Yang H, Ko W, Kim J, et al. Paeoniflorin: an antihyperlipidemic agent from Paeonia lactiflora. *Fitoterapia.* 2004;75(1):45–49.

200. Hsu F, Lai C, Cheng J. Antihyperglycemic effects of paeoniflorin and 8-debenzoylpaeoniflorin, glucosides from the root of Paeonia lactiflora. *Planta Medica.* 1997;63(4):323–325.

201. Sakai A, Kondo Z, Kamei K, et al. Induction of ovulation by Sairei-to for polycystic ovary syndrome patients. *Endocr J.* 1999;46(1):217–220.

202. Bone K. Tribulus terrestis. *Professional Review.* 2001;76.

203. Adimoelja A. Phytochemicals and the breakthrough of traditional herbs in the management of sexual dysfunction. *Int J Androl.* 2000;2:23.

204. Kamel HH. Role of phyto-oestrogens in ovulation induction in women with polycystic ovarian syndrome. *Eur J Obstet Gynecol Reprod Biol.* 2013 May;168(1):60–63.

205. Wang JG, Anderson RA, Graham GM, et al. The effect of cinnamon extract on insulin resistance parameters in polycystic ovary syndrome: a pilot study. *Fertil Steril*. 2007, Jul;88(1):240–243.

206. A scientific review: the role of chromium in insulin resistance. *Diabetes Educator*. 2004;(suppl):2–14.

207. Low Dog T. The Endocrine System: Diabetes. *Foundations in Herbal Medicine*. 2000. Foundations in Herbal Medicine.

208. Oner G, Muderris I. Clinical, endocrine and metabolic effects of metformin vs N-acteyl-cytseine in women with polycystic ovary syndrome. *Eur J Obstet Gynecol Reprod Biol*. 2011;159:127–131.

209. Davis A, Christiansen M, Horowitz J, et al. Effect of pinitol treatment on insulin action in subjects with insulin resistance. *Diabetes Care*. 2000;23:1000–1005.

210. Galletta M, Grasso S, Vaiarelli A, Roseff SJ. Bye-bye chiro-inositol – myo-inositol: true progress in the treatment of polycystic ovary syndrome and ovulation induction. *Eur Rev Med Pharmacol Sci*. 2011 Oct;15(10):1212–1214.

211. Lydic M, McNurlan M, Bembo S, Mitchell L, Komaroff E, Gelato M. Chromium picolinate improves insulin sensitivity in obese subjects with polycystic ovary syndrome. *Fertil Steril*. 2006;86:243–246.

212. Mavropoulos JC, Yancy WS, Hepburn J, Westman EC. The effects of a low-carbohydrate, ketogenic diet on the polycystic ovary syndrome: a pilot study. *Nutr Metab (Lond)*. 2005;2:35.

213. Nestler J, Jakubowicz D, Reamer P, Gunn R, Allan G. Ovulatory and metabolic effects of d-chiro-inositol in the polycystic ovary syndrome. *N Engl J Med*. 1999;340:1314–1320.

214. Nordio M, Proietti E. The combined therapy with myo-inositol and D-chiro-inositol reduces the risk of metabolic disease in PCOS overweight patients compared to myo-inositol supplementation alone. *Eur Rev Med Pharmacol Sci*. 2012;16(5):575–581.

215. Ramarao P, Bhargava HN. Antagonism of the acute pharmacological actions of morphine by panax ginseng extract. *Gen Pharmacol*. 1990;21(6):877–880.

216. Mehta A, Binkley P, Gandhi S, Tick M. Pharmacological effects of Withania somnifera root extract on GABAA receptors complex. *Ind J Med Res*. 1991;94:312–315.

217. Russo A, Izzo A, Cardile V, Borrelli F, Vanella A. Indian medicinal plants as antiradicals and DNA cleavage protectors. *Phytomedicine*. 2001;8(2):125–132.

218. Chakraborti S, Barun DeK, Bandyopadhyay T. Variations in the antitumor constituents of Winthania somnifera. *Experientia*. 1974;30(8):852–853.

219. Devi P, Aharada A, Solomon F, Kamath M. In vivo growth inhibitory effect of Withania somnifera on a transplantable mouse tumor, Sarcoma 180. *Indian J Exp Biol*. 1992;30(3):169–172.

220. Shukla S, Jain S, Sharma K, Bhatnagar M. Stress induced neuron degeneration and protective effects of Semecarpus anacardium Linn. and Withania somnifera Dunn. hippocampus of albino rats: an ultrastructural study. *Indian J Exp Biol*. 2000;38(10):1007–1013.

CHAPTER 6

1. Ringdahl E, Pereira S, Delzell J. Treatment of primary insomnia. *J Am Board Fam Pract*. 2004;17:212–219.

2. Becker P. Insomnia: prevalence, impact, pathogenesis, differential diagnosis, and evaluation. *Psychiatr Clin North Am*. 2006;29:855–870.

3. Mellman T. Sleep and anxiety disorders. *Psychiatr Clin North Am*. 2006;29:1047–1058.

4. Soares CN, Murray BJ. Sleep disorders in women: clinical evidence and treatment strategies. *Psychiatr Clin North Am*. 2006;29(4):1095–1113. abstract xi.

5. Sahota P, Jainb S, Dhandb R. Sleep disorders in pregnancy. *Curr Opin Pulm Med*. 2003;9:477–483.

6. Yang C, Spielman A, Glovinsky P. Nonpharmacologic strategies in the management of insomnia. *Psychiatr Clin North Am*. 2006;29:895–919.

7. Brevoort P. The booming U.S. botanical market: a new overview. *Herbal Gram*. 1998;44:33–48.

8. Wheatley D. Medicinal plants for insomnia: a review of their pharmacology, efficacy and tolerability. *J Psychopharmacol*. 2005;19(4):414–421.

9. Low Dog T. *Women's Health in Complementary and Integrative Medicine: A Clinical Guide*. St. Louis: Elsevier; 2004.

10. Hoffmann D. *Medical Herbalism: The Science and Practice of Herbal Medicine*. Rochester, VT: Healing Arts Press; 2003.

11. Bone K. *A Clinical Guide to Blending Liquid Herbs: Herbal Formulations for the Individual Patient*. St. Louis: Churchill Livingstone; 2003.

12. Rolland A, Fleurentin J, Lanhers MC, et al. Behavioural effects of the American traditional plant *Eschscholzia californica*: sedative and anxiolytic properties. *Planta Medica*. 1991;57(3):212–216.

13. Rolland A, Fleurentin J, Lanhers MC, et al. Neurophysiological effects of an extract of Eschscholzia californica Cham. (Papaveraceae). *Phytother Res*. 2001;15(5):377–381.

14. ESCOP. *ESCOP Monographs: The Scientific Foundation for Herbal Medicinal Products*. Stuttgart: Thieme; 2003.

15. Blumenthal M. *The complete German Commission E monographs; therapeutic guide to herbal medicines*. Austin: American Botanical Council; 1998.

16. Schiller H, Forster A, Vonhoff C, Hegger M, Biller A, Winterhoff H. Sedating effects of *Humulus lupulus* L. extracts. *Phytomedicine*. 2006;13:535–541.

17. Basch E, Ulbricht C. *Natural Standard Herb and Supplement Reference: Evidence-Based Clinical Reviews*. St. Louis: Elsevier/Mosby; 2005.

18. Masago R, Matsuda T, Kikuchi Y, et al. Effects of inhalation of essential oils on EEG activity and sensory evaluation. *J Physiol Anthropol Appl Hum Sci*. 2000;19(1):35–42.

19. Avallone R, Zanoli P, Corsi L. Benzodiazepine compounds and GABA in flower heads of matricaria chamomilla. *Phytother Res*. 1996;10:177–179.

20. Zick SM, Wright BD, Sen A, Arnedt JT. Preliminary examination of the efficacy and safety of a standardized chamomile extract for chronic primary insomnia: a randomized placebo-controlled pilot study. *BMC Complement Altern Med*. 2011:1178.

21. Blumenthal M. *The ABC Clinical Guide to Herbs*. New York: Thieme Press; 2002.

22. Wheatley D. Kava and valerian in the treatment of stress-induced insomnia. *Phytother Res*. 2001;15(6):549–555.

23. Davies LP, Drew CA, Duffield P, Johnston GA, Jamieson DD. Kava pyrones and resin: studies on GABAA, GABAB and benzodiazepine binding sites in rodent brain. *Pharmacol Toxicol*. 1992;71(2):120–126.

24. Jussofie A, Schmiz A, Hiemke C. Kavapyrone enriched extract from Piper methysticum as modulator of the GABA binding site in different regions of rat brain. *Psychopharmacology*. 1994;116(4):469–474.

25. Boonen G, Haberlein H. Influence of genuine kavapyrone enantiomers on the GABA-A binding site. *Planta Medica*. 1998;64(6):504–506.

26. Singh YN, Singh NN. Therapeutic potential of kava in the treatment of anxiety disorders. *CNS Drugs*. 2006;16(11):731–743.

27. Gleitz J, Friese J, Beile A, Ameri A, Peters T. Anticonvulsive action (of ±kavain) estimated from its properties on stimulated synaptosomes and Na+ channel receptor sites. *Eur J Pharmacol*. 1996;315(1):89–97.

28. Schirrmacher K, Busselberg D, Langosch JM, Walden J, Winter U, Bingmann D. Effects (of ±kavain) on voltage-activated inward currents of dorsal root ganglion cells from neonatal rats. *Eur Neuropsychopharmacol*. 1999;9(1-2):171–176.

29. Grunze H, Langosch J, Schirrmacher K, Bingmann D, Von Wegerer J, Walden J. Kava pyrones exert effects on neuronal transmission and transmembraneous cation currents similar to established mood stabilizers— a review. *Progr Neuro-Psychopharmacol Biol Psychiatr*. 2001;25(8):1555–1570.

30. Müller SF, Klement S. A combination of valerian and lemon balm is effective in the treatment of restlessness and dyssomnia in children. *Phytomedicine*. 2006, Jun;13(6):383–387.

31. Kennedy D, Little W, Scholey A. Effects of Melissa officinalis (lemon balm) on mood changes during acute psychological stress. *Pharmacol Biochem Behav*. 2003;72:953–964.

32. Wichtl M. *Herbal Drugs and Phytopharmaceuticals: A Handbook for Practice on a Scientific Basis*. 4th ed. Stuttgart: Medpharm; 2004.

33. Linck VM, da Silva AL, Figueiró M, Piato AL, Herrmann AP, Dupont Birck F, et al. Inhaled linalool-induced sedation in mice. *Phytomedicine*. 2009, Apr;16(4):303–307.

34. Lytle J, Mwatha C, Davis KK. Effect of lavender aromatherapy on vital signs and perceived quality of sleep in the intermediate care unit: a pilot study. *Am J Crit Care*. 2014;23(1):24–29. United States.

35. Lee IS, Lee GJ. Effects of lavender aromatherapy on insomnia and depression in women college students. *Taehan Kanho Hakhoe Chi*. 2006, Feb;36(1):136–143.

36. Ma H, Jo YJ, Ma Y, Hong JT, Kwon BM, Oh KW. Obovatol isolated from Magnolia obovata enhances pentobarbital-induced sleeping time: possible involvement of GABAA receptors/chloride channel activation. *Phytomedicine*. 2009, Apr;16(4):308–313.

37. Koetter U, Barrett M, Lacher S, Abdelrahman A, Dolnick D. Interactions of Magnolia and Ziziphus extracts with selected central nervous system receptors. *J Ethnopharmacol*. 2009, Jul 30;124(3):421–425.

38. Mucci M, Carraro C, Mancino P, et al. Soy isoflavones, lactobacilli, Magnolia bark extract, vitamin D3 and calcium. Controlled clinical study in menopause. *Minerva Ginecol*. 2006, Aug;58(4):323–334.

39. Dhawan K, Dhawan S, Sharma A. Passiflora: a review update. *J Ethnopharmacol*. 2004;94(1):1–23.

40. Soulimani R, Younos C, Jarmouni S, Bousta D, Misslin R, Mortier F. Behavioural effects of *Passiflora incarnata L.* and its indole alkaloid and flavonoid derivatives and maltol in the mouse. *J Ethnopharmacol*. 1997;57(1):11–20.

41. Ngan A, Conduit R. A double-blind, placebo-controlled investigation of the effects of *Passiflora incarnata* (passionflower) herbal tea on subjective sleep quality. *Phytother Res*. 2011, Aug;25(8):1153–1159.

42. Grodstein F. Postmenopausal hormone therapy and mortality. *NEJM*. 1997;336:1769–1775.

43. Fisher A, Purcell P, Le Couteur D. Toxicity of Passiflora incarnata. *Clin Toxicol*. 2000;38(1):63–66.

44. Miyasaka L, Atallah A, Soares B. Passiflora for anxiety disorder. *Cochrane Database Syst Rev*. 2007;3.

45. Awad R, Arnason JT, Trudeau V, et al. Phytochemical and biological analysis of skullcap (*Scutellaria lateriflora L.*): a medicinal plant with anxiolytic properties. *Phytomedicine*. 2003;10(8):640–649.

46. AltMedDex: RPS Herbal Medicines: A guide for Health-Care Professionals: Skullcap, Montvale, NJ, Thomson Micromedex.

47. Upton R. Valerian Root: valeriana officinalis. *Analytical, Quality Control and Therapeutic Monograph*. Santa Cruz, CA: American Herbal Pharmacopoeia; 1999.

48. Werner C, ASSESSMENT REPORT ON VALERIANA OFFICINALIS L. RADIX [Internet]. European Medicines Agency. Available from: http://www.ema.europa.eu/docs/en_GB/document_library/Herbal_-_HMPC_assessment_report/2009/12/WC500017929.pdf; 2007, Nov 29.

49. World Health Organization. Valeriana radix. *WHO Monographs on Selected Medicinal Plants*. vol. 1. Geneva: World Health Organization; 1999.

50. Stevinson C, Ernst E. Valerian for insomnia: a systematic review of randomized clinical trials. *Sleep Med*. 2000;1:91–99.

51. Fugh-Berman A, Cott J. Dietary supplements and natural products as psychotherapeutic agents. *Psychosom Med*. 1999;61:712–728.

52. Barton DL, Atherton PJ, Bauer BA, Moore DF, Mattar BI, Lavasseur BI, et al. The use of Valeriana officinalis (Valerian) in improving sleep in patients who are undergoing treatment for cancer: a phase III randomized, placebo-controlled, double-blind study (NCCTG Trial, N01C5). *J Support Oncol*. 2011;9(1):24–31.

53. Taavoni S, Ekbatani N, Kashaniyan M, Haghani H. Effect of valerian on sleep quality in postmenopausal women: a randomized placebo-controlled clinical trial. *Menopause*. 2011, Sep;18(9):951–955.

54. Cuellar NG, Ratcliffe SJ. Does valerian improve sleepiness and symptom severity in people with restless legs syndrome? *Altern Ther Health Med*. 2009;15(2):22–28.

55. Taavoni S, Nazem Ekbatani N, Haghani H. Valerian/lemon balm use for sleep disorders during menopause. *Complement Ther Clin Pract*. 2013;19(4):193–196. England.

56. Maroo N, Hazra A, Das T. Efficacy and safety of a polyherbal sedative-hypnotic formulation NSF-3 in primary insomnia in comparison to zolpidem: a randomized controlled trial. *Indian J Pharmacol*. 2013;45(1):34–39.

57. Koetter U, Schrader E, Käufeler R, Brattström A. A randomized, double blind, placebo-controlled, prospective clinical study to demonstrate clinical efficacy of a fixed valerian hops extract combination (Ze 91019) in patients suffering from non-organic sleep disorder. *Phytother Res*. 2007, Sep;21(9):847–851.

58. Salter S, Brownie S. Treating primary insomnia - the efficacy of valerian and hops. *Aust Fam Physician*. 2010, Jun;39(6):433–437.

59. Mucclough M. *Hope or hype? Philadelphia Enquirer*; May 13, 1996.

60. Taibi DM, Vitiello MV, Barsness S, Elmer GW, Anderson GD, Landis CA. A randomized clinical trial of valerian fails to improve self-reported, polysomnographic, and actigraphic sleep in older women with insomnia. *Sleep Med.* 2009, Mar;10(3):319–328.

61. Hadley S, Petry JJ. Valerian. *Am Fam Physician.* 2003;67(8):1155–1158.

62. Anderson GD, Elmer GW, Taibi DM, Vitiello MV, Kantor E, Kalhorn TF, et al. Pharmacokinetics of valerenic acid after single and multiple doses of valerian in older women. *Phytother Res.* 2010, Oct;24(10):1442–1446.

63. Jiang JG, Huang XJ, Chen J, Lin QS. Comparison of the sedative and hypnotic effects of flavonoids, saponins, and polysaccharides extracted from Semen Ziziphus jujube. *Nat Prod Res.* 2007, Apr;21(4):310–320.

64. Cao JX, Zhang QY, Cui SY, Cui XY, Zhang J, Zhang YH, et al. Hypnotic effect of jujubosides from Semen Ziziphi Spinosae. *J Ethnopharmacol.* 2010, Jul 6;130(1):163–166.

65. Wang LE, Cui XY, Cui SY, Cao JX, Zhang J, Zhang YH, et al. Potentiating effect of spinosin, a C-glycoside flavonoid of Semen Ziziphi spinosae, on pentobarbital-induced sleep may be related to postsynaptic 5-HT(1A) receptors. *Phytomedicine.* 2010, May;17(6):404–409.

66. Rondanelli M, Opizzi A, Monteferrario F, Antoniello N, Manni R, Klersy C. The effect of melatonin, magnesium, and zinc on primary insomnia in long-term care facility residents in Italy: a double-blind, placebo-controlled clinical trial. *J Am Geriatr Soc.* 2011, Jan;59(1):82–90. tsynaptic 5-HT(1A) receptors. *Phytomedicine.* 2010, May;17(6):404-9.

67. Geddes J, Butler R. Depressive disorders. *Clin Evid.* 2001;6:727.

68. Banger M. Affective syndrome during perimenopause. *Maturitas.* 2002;41(suppl 1):S13.

69. Lett, 2005.

70. Goroll A, May L, Mulley A. *Primary Care Medicine: Office Evaluation and Management of the Adult Patient.* 4th ed. Philadelphia: Lippincott; 2000.

71. American Psychiatric Association. *Diagnostic and Statistical Manual of Mental Disorders, Text Revision.* 4th ed. Washington, DC: American Psychiatric Association; 2000.

72. Center C, Davis M, Detre T, et al. Confronting Depression and Suicide in Physicians: a Consensus Statement. *JAMA.* 2003;289(23):3161–3166.

73. Santen R. Treatment of menopausal symptoms in women not taking estrogen. UpToDateOnline10.3. 2002 Aug:8.

74. MISSING

75. Vollmer S. Depression: meeting the clinical challenge. *Fam Prac Recert.* 2002;24(9):31.

76. *Drug Facts and Comparisons.* 55th ed. St. Louis: Facts and Comparisons; 2001.

77. Strohecker J, Strohecker NS. *Natural Healing for Depression, Solutions from the World's Great Health Traditions and Practitioners.* New York: Penguin Putnam; 1999.

78. Packard CC. The sustainable herbalist: the sustainable life. *J Northeast Herbal Assoc Summer/Fall.* 2002:3.

79. Nhat Hanh T. *Being Peace.* Berkeley: Parallax Press; 1987.

80. Greenspan M. *Healing through the dark emotions: the wisdom of grief, fear, and despair.* Boston: Shambhala; 2003.

81. Weil Andrew, *Natural Health, Natural Medicine.* Boston: Houghton Mifflin; 1998.

82. Irvine KN, Warber SL. Greening healthcare: practicing as if the natural environment really mattered. *Altern Ther Health Med.* 2002;8(5):76–83.

83. Tierra M. Mimosa (*Albizzia julibrissin*). http://www.planetherbs.com/mimosa.htm.

84. Rosenberg Z: op. cit., p. 76.

85. Kang TH, Jeong SJ, Kim NY, et al. Sedative activity of two flavonol glycosides isolated from the flowers of *Albizzia julibrissin Durazz. J Ethnopharm.* 2000;71(1-2):321–323.

86. Kasture VS, Chopde CT, Deshmukh VK. Anticonvulsive activity of *Albizzia lebbeck, Hibiscus rosa sinensis*, and *Butea monosperma* in experimental animals. *J Ethnopharmacol.* 2000;71(1-2):65–75.

87. Jung MJ, Chung HY, Kang SS, et al. Antioxidant activity from the stem bark of *Albizzia julibrissin. Arch Pharm Res Korea.* 2003;26(6):458–462.

88. Chintawar SD, Somani RS, Kasture VS, et al. Nootropic activity of *Albizzia lebbeck* in mice. *J Ethnopharmacol.* 2002;81(3):299–305.

89. Une HD, Sarveiya VP, Pal SC, et al. Nootropic and anxiolytic activity of saponins of *Albizzia lebbeck* leaves. *Pharmacol Biochem Behav.* 2001;69(3-4):439–444.

90. Tierra M. *Ashwagandha: Wonder Herb of India*; 1996. p6. http://www.planetherbs.com/articles/ashwagandha.htm.

91. McIntyre A. Ashwagandha: Winter Cherry, *Withania somnifera*, Positive Health Complementary Medicine Magazine. http://www.positivehealth.com/permit/Articles/Regular/mcintyre77.htm. Positive Health Publications Ltd, 2002, pp 1–2.

92. Takasugi N, et al. Effect of *Eleutherococcus senticosus* and its components on rectal temperature, body and grip tones, motor coordination, and exploratory and spontaneous movements in acute stressed mice. *Shoyakugaku Zasshi.* 1985;39(3):232–237.

93. Mishra LC, Singh BB, Dagenais S. Scientific basis for the therapeutic use of *Withania somnifera* (Ashwagandha): a review. *Altern Med Rev.* 2000;5(4):334–346.

94. Vaidya A. The status and scope of Indian medicinal plants acting on the central nervous system. *Ind J Pharmacol.* 1997;29:S340–S343.

95. Bhattacharya SK, Bhattacharya A, Sairam K, et al. Anxiolytic-antidepressant activity of *Withania somnifera glycowithanolides*: an experimental study. *Phytomedicine.* 2000;7(6):463–469.

96. Gupta YK, Sharma SS, Rai K, et al. Reversal of paclitaxel-induced neutropenia by *Withania somnifera* in mice. *Indian J Physiol Pharmacol.* 2001;45(2):253–257.

97. Dhuley JN. Nootropic-like effect of ashwagandha (*Withania somnifera L.*) in mice. *Phytother Res.* 2001;15(6):524–528.

98. Rege NN, Thatte UM, Dahanukar SA. Adaptogenic properties of six rasayana herbs used in Ayurvedic medicine. *Phytother Res.* 1991;13(4):275–291.

99. Bhattacharya SK, Muruganandam AV. Adaptogenic activity of *Withania somnifera*: an experimental study using a rat model of chronic stress. *Pharmacol Biochem Behav.* 2003;75(3):547–555.

100. Bhattacharya SK, Muruganandam AV, Kumar V, Bhattacharya SK: op. cit., pp 1161–1163.

101. Muruganandam AV, Kumar V, Bhattacharya SK: op. cit., pp 1151–1160.

102. Bhattacharya SK, Bhattacharya A, Chakrabarti A. Adaptogenic activity of Siotone, a polyherbal formulation of Ayurvedic rasayanas. *Ind J Exp Biol.* 2000;38(2):119–128.

103. Buhrman S. op. cit., pp 5–7.

104. Gerson S. *Bacopa monniera*, National Institute of Ayurvedic Medicine: Medicinal Plants. http://www.niam.com/corp-web/bacopa.htm.

105. Mishra SK. Ayurveda and yoga for depression and promoting mental health. In: Strohecker J, Strohecker NS, eds. *Natural Healing for Depression, Solutions from the World's Great Health Traditions and Practitioners.* New York: Penguin Putnam; 1999.

106. Roodenrys S, Booth D, Bulzomi S, et al. Chronic effects of Brahmi (*Bacopa monniera*) on human memory. *Neuropsychopharmacology.* 2002;27(2):279–281.

107. Singh HK, Dhawan BN. Neuropsychopharmacological effects of the Ayurvedic nootropic *Bacopa monniera* (brahmi). *Indian J Pharmacol.* 1997;29:S359–S365.

108. Stough C, Lloyd J, Clarke J, et al. The chronic effects of an extract of *Bacopa monniera* (Brahmi) on cognitive function in healthy human subjects. *Psychopharmacol (Berl).* 2001;156(4):481–484.

109. Bhattacharya SK, Bhattacharya A, Kumar A, et al. Antioxidant activity of Bacopa monniera in rat frontal cortex, striatum, and hippocampus. *Phytother Res.* 2000;14(3):174–179.

110. Devi A. op. cit., pp 69–70.

111. Sairam K, Dorababu M, Goel RK, et al. Antidepressant activity of standardized extract of *Bacopa monniera* in experimental models of depression in rats. *Phytomedicine.* 2002;9(3):207–211.

112. Dhawan BN: Centrally acting agents from Indian plants. In: Koslow SH, Murthy RS, Coelho GV, eds. Decade of the Brain: India/USA Research in Mental Health and Neurosciences. Rockville, MD: National Institute of Mental Health; 1995.

113. Kidd PM. A review of nutrients and botanicals in the integrative management of cognitive dysfunction. *Alt Med Rev.* 1999;4(3):144–161.

114. Sumathy T, Govindasamy S, Balakrishna K, et al. Protective role of *Bacopa monniera* on morphine-induced brain mitochondrial enzyme activity in rats. *Fitoterapia.* 2002;73(5):381–385.

115. Vohora D, Pal SN, Pillai KK. Protection from phenytoin-induced cognitive deficit by *Bacopa monniera*, a reputed Indian nootropic plant. *J Ethnopharmacol.* 2000;71(3):383–390.

116. Chowdhuri DK, Parmar D, Kakkar P, et al. Antistress effects of bacosides of *Bacopa monniera*: modulation of Hsp70 expression, superoxide dismutase and cytochrome P450 activity in rat brain. *Phytother Res.* 2002;16(7):639–645.

117. Rai D, Bhatia G, Palit G, et al. Adaptogenic effect of *Bacopa monniera* (Brahmi). *Pharmacol Biochem Behav.* 2003;75(4):823–830.

118. Ellingwood F. American Materia Medica. *Therapeutics and Pharmacognosy.* 1919.

119. Dentali S. In: Mischoulon D, Rosenbaum JF, eds. *Natural Medications for Psychiatric Disorders: Considering the Alternatives.* Philadelphia: Lippincott Williams & Wilkins; 2002.

120. Wuttke W, Seidlova-Wuttke D, Gorkow C. The Cimicifuga preparation BNO 1055 vs. conjugated estrogens in a double-blind placebocontrolled study: effects on menopause symptoms and bone markers. *Maturitas.* 2003;44(suppl 1):S67–S77.

121. Oktem M, Eroglu D, Karahan HB, Taskintuna N, Kuscu E, Zeyneloglu HB. Black cohosh and fluoxetine in the treatment of postmenopausal symptoms: a prospective, randomized trial. *Adv Ther.* 2007;24(2):448–461.

122. Huang YX, Song L, Zhang X, Lun WW, Pan C, Huang YS. Clinical study of combined treatment of remifemin and paroxetine for perimenopausal depression. *Zhonghua Yi Xue Za Zhi.* 2013, Feb 26;93(8):600–602.

123. McKenna DJ, Jones K, Humphrey S, et al. Black cohosh: efficacy, safety, and use in clinical and preclinical applications. *Altern Ther Health Med.* 2001;7(3):93–100.

124. Kligler B. Black cohosh. *Am Fam Physician.* 2003;68(1):114–116.

125. Jarry H, Metten M, Spengler B, et al. In vitro effects of the *Cimicifuga racemosa* extract BNO 1055. *Maturitas.* 2003;44(suppl 1):S31–S38.

126. Amato P, Christophe S, Mellon PL. Estrogenic activity of herbs commonly used as remedies for menopausal symptoms. *Menopause.* 2002;9(2):145–150.

127. Mahady GB. Is black cohosh estrogenic? *Nutr Rev.* 2003;61(5 Pt 1):183–186.

128. Einer-Jensen N, Zhao J, Andersen KP, et al. *Cimicifuga* and *Melbrosia* lack oestrogenic effects in mice and rats. *Maturitas.* 1996;25(2):149–153.

129. Beck V, Unterrieder E, Krenn L, et al. Comparison of hormonal activity (estrogen, androgen and progestin) of standardized plant extracts for large scale use in hormone replacement therapy. *J Steroid Biochem Mol Biol.* 2003;84(2-3):259–268.

130. Freudenstein J, Dasenbrock C, Nisslein T. Lack of promotion of estrogen- dependent mammary gland tumors in vivo by an isopropanolic *Cimicifuga racemosa* extract. *Cancer Res.* 2002;62(12):3448–3452.

131. Dixon-Shanies D, Shaikh N. Growth inhibition of human breast cancer cells by herbs and phytoestrogens. *Oncol Rep.* 1999;6(6):1383–1387.

132. Bodinet C, Freudenstein J. Influence of *Cimicifuga racemosa* on the proliferation of estrogen receptor-positive human breast cancer cells. *Breast Cancer Res Treat.* 2002;76(1):1–10.

133. Dog TL, Powell KL, Weisman SM. Critical evaluation of the safety of *Cimicifuga racemosa* in menopause symptom relief. *Menopause.* 2003;10(4):299–313.

134. Huntley A, Ernst E. A systematic review of the safety of black cohosh. *Menopause.* 2003;10(1):58–64.

135. Hoffmann D. *An Herbal Guide to Stress Relief.* Rochester: Healing Arts Press; 1991.

136. Wang Y, Han T, Zhu Y, et al. Antidepressant properties of bioactive fractions from the extract of Crocus sativus L. *J Nat Med.* 2010, Jan;64(1):24–30.

137. Moshiri E, Basti AA, Noorbala AA, Jamshidi AH, Hesameddin Abbasi S, Akhondzadeh S. Crocus sativus L. (petal) in the treatment of mild-to-moderate depression: a double-blind, randomized and placebo-controlled trial. *Phytomedicine.* 2006, Nov;13(9-10):607–611.

138. Akhondzadeh Basti A, Moshiri E, Noorbala AA, Jamshidi AH, Abbasi SH, Akhondzadeh S. Comparison of petal of Crocus sativus L. and fluoxetine in the treatment of depressed outpatients: a pilot double-blind randomized trial. *Prog Neuropsychopharmacol Biol Psychiatry.* 2007, Mar 30;31(2):439–442.

139. Tierra L. PMS, Depression and Menopause, 6th International Herb Symposium; 2002:174–176.

140. Huang KC. *The Pharmacology of Chinese Herbs.* Boca Raton: CRC Press; 1993.

141. Bloomfield H. op. cit., pp 107–108.

142. Leung AY, Foster S. *Encyclopedia of Common Natural Ingredients Used in Food, Drugs, and Cosmetics.* 2nd ed. New York: John Wiley & Sons; 1996.

143. Asano K, et al. Effect of *Eleutherococcus senticosus* extract on human physical working capacity. *Planta Med.* 1986;3:175–177.

144. Wagner H, Hikino H, Farnsworth NR. *Economic and Medicinal Plant Research*. London: Academic Press; 1985.

145. Bohn B, Nebe C, Birr C. Flow-cytometric studies with E. Senticoccus extract as an immunomodulatory Agent. *Arzneimforsch*. 1987;37(10):1193–1196.

146. Bradley PR. British Herbal Compendium. vol. 1. Bournemouth, UK: British Herbal Medicine Association; 1992.

147. Fang J, et al. Immunologically active polysaccharides of E. senticosus. *Phytochemistry*. 1985;24:2619–2622.

148. Yonezawa M, et al. Radiation protection by Shigoka extract on split dose irradiation in mice. *J Radiation Res*. 1989;30(3):247–254.

149. Winther K, et al. Russian root (Siberian ginseng) improves cognitive functions in middle-aged people, whereas Ginkgo biloba seems effective only in the elderly. *J Neurol Sci (XVI World Congress of Neurology, Buenos Aires)*. 1997;150:S90.

150. Gladstar R. Rosemary Gladstar's Family Herbal. op. cit.

151. Kleijnen J, Knipschild P. Ginkgo biloba for cerebral insufficiency. *Br J Clin Pharmacol*. 1992;34(4):352–358.

152. Kleijnen J, Knipschild P. Ginkgo biloba. *Lancet*. 1992;340(8828):1136–1139.

153. Ernst E, Pittler MH. Ginkgo biloba and dementia: a systematic review of double-blind, placebo-controlled trials. *Clin Drug Invest*. 1999;17(4):301–308.

154. Hopfenmuller W. Proof of the therapeutic effectiveness of a Ginkgo biloba special extract: meta-analysis of 11 clinical trials in aged patients with cerebral insufficiency [in German]. *Arzneimforsch*. 1994;44(9):1005–1013.

155. Oken BS, Storzbach DM, Kaye JA. The efficacy of Ginkgo biloba on cognitive function in Alzheimer disease. *Arch Neurol*. 1998;55(11):1409–1415.

156. Hofferberth B. The efficacy of Egb 761 in patients with senile dementia of the Alzheimer type: a double-blind placebo-controlled study on different levels of investigation. *Hum Psychopharmacol*. 1994;9:215–222.

157. Kanowski S, Hermann WM, Stephan K, et al. Proof of the efficacy of the Ginkgo biloba special extract Egb 761 in outpatients suffering from mild to moderate dementia of the Alzheimer's type or multiinfarct dementia. *Phytomedicine*. 1997;4(1):3–13.

158. Le Bars PL, Katz MM, Berman N, et al. A placebo-controlled, doubleblind, randomized trial of an extract of Ginkgo biloba for dementia. *JAMA*. 1997;278(16):1327–1332.

159. Russo E. op. cit., p 144.

160. Itil TM, Martorano D. Natural substances in psychiatry: ginkgo biloba in dementia. *Psychopharm Bull*. 1995;31(1):147–158.

161. Itil TM, Eralp E, Ahmed I, et al. The pharmacological effects of Ginkgo biloba, a plant extract, on the brain of dementia patients in comparison with tacrine. *Psychopharmacol Bull*. 1998;34(3):391–397.

162. Letzel H, Haan J, Feil WB. Nootropics: efficacy and tolerability of products from three active substance classes. *J Drug Dev Clin Pract*. 1996;8:77–94.

163. Mix JA, Crews WD. A double-blind, placebo-controlled, randomized trial of Ginkgo biloba extract Egb 761 in a sample of cognitivelyintact older adults: neuropsychological findings. *Hum Psychopharmacol*. 2002;17(6):267–277.

164. Kennedy DO, Scholey AB, Wesnes KA. The dose-dependent cognitive effects of acute administration of Ginkgo biloba to healthy young volunteers. *Psychopharmacology (Berl)*. 2000;151(4):416–423.

165. Kennedy DO, Scholey AB, Wesnes KA. Differential dose-dependent changes in cognitive performance following acute administration of a Ginkgo biloba/Panax ginseng combination to healthy young volunteers. *Nutr Neurosci*. 2001;4(5):399–412.

166. Scholey AB, Kennedy DO. Acute, dose-dependent cognitive effects of Ginkgo biloba, Panax ginseng, and their combination in healthy young volunteers: differential interactions with cognitive demand. *Hum Psychopharmacol*. 2002;17(1):35–44.

167. Das A, Shanker G, Nath C, et al. A comparative study in rodents of standardized extracts of *Bacopa monniera* and Ginkgo biloba anticholinesterase and cognitive enhancing activities. *Pharmacol Biochem Behav*. 2002;73(4):893–900.

168. Vorberg G. Ginkgo biloba extract (GBE): a long-term study of chronic cerebral insufficiency in geriatric patients. *Clin Trials J*. 1986;22:149–157.

169. Lesser IM, Mena I, et al. Reduction in cerebral blood flow in older depressed patients. *Arch Psychiatr*. 1994;51:677–686.

170. Schubert H, Halama P. Depressive episode primarily unresponsive to therapy in elderly patients: efficacy of ginkgo biloba extract (Egb 761) in combination with antidepressants. *Geriatr Forsch*. 1993;3:45–53.

171. Huguet F, et al. Decreased cerebral 5-HT receptors during aging: reversal by Ginkgo biloba extract (EGb 761). *J Pharm Pharmacol*. 1994;46:316–318.

172. Kass-Annese B. Alternative therapies for menopause. *Clin Obstet Gynecol*. 2000;43(1):174.

173. Kennedy DO, Scholey AB, Wesnes KA. Modulation of cognition and mood following administration of single doses of Ginkgo biloba, ginseng, and a ginkgo/ginseng combination to healthy young adults. *Physiol Behav*. 2002;75(5):739–751.

174. Hemmeter U, Annen B, Bischof R, et al. Polysomnographic effects of adjuvant Ginkgo biloba therapy in patients with major depression medicated with imipramine. *Pharmacopsychiatry*. 2001;34(2):50–59.

175. Zhang XY, Zhou DF, Su JM, Zhang PY. The effect of extract of Ginkgo biloba added to haloperidol on superoxide dismutase in inpatients with chronic schizophrenia. *J Clin Psychopharmacol 2001 Feb*. 2001;21(1):85–88.

176. Cohen A. Treatment of antidepressant-induced sexual dysfunction: a new scientific study shows benefits of Ginkgo biloba. *Healthwatch*. 1996;5.

177. Cohen A. Ginkgo biloba for drug-induced sexual dysfunction (abstract 35). In: *Syllabus and Proceedings Summary*. San Diego: American Psychiatric Association Annual Meeting; 1997, 5.

178. Ellison JM, DeLuca P. Fluoxetine-induced genital anesthesia relieved by Ginkgo biloba extract. *J Clin Psychiatry*. 1998;59(4):199–200.

179. Davidson J, Connor K. *Herbs for the Mind: What Science Tells Us about Nature's Remedies for Depression, Stress, Memory Loss, and Insomnia*. New York: Guilford Press; 2000.

180. Birks J, Grimley EV, Van Dongen M. Ginkgo biloba for cognitive impairment and dementia. *Cochrane Database Syst Rev*. 2002;4:CD003120.

181. Israel D, Youngkin E. Herbal therapies for perimenopausal and menopausal complaints. *Pharmacotherapy*. 1997;17(5):977.

182. Engelsen J, Nielsen JD, Hansen KF. Effect of Coenzyme Q10 and Ginkgo biloba on warfarin dosage in patients on long-term warfarin treatment; a randomized, double-blind placebo-controlled crossover trial. *Ugeskr Laeger*. 2003;165(18):1868–1871.

183. Kalus JS, Piotrowski AA, Fortier CR, et al. Hemodynamic and electrocardiographic effects of short-term Ginkgo biloba. *Ann Pharmacother.* 2003;37(3):345–349.

184. Northrup C. *The Wisdom of Menopause.* New York: Bantam; 2001.

185. Schoenbeck L, Gibson C, Barss MB. *Menopause: bridging the Gap Between Natural and Conventional Medicine.* New York: Kensington Publishing; 2002.

186. Gerson S. Centella asiatica, National Institute of Ayurvedic Medicine: Medicinal Plants. http://www.niam.com/corp-web/centella.htm.

187. Apparao MVR, Srinivasan K, Rao K: The effect of Mandukapami on the general mental ability on mentally retarded children, *J Res Ind Med.*

188. Kuppurajen K, Srinivasan K, Janak K. A double-blind study of the effect of Mandukapami on the general mental ability of normal children. *J Res Ind Med Yog Homeopath.* 1978;13: 37–41.

189. Singh RH, Singh L. Studies on antianxiety effect of an indigenous drug: Brahmi—part 1 (Clinical Studies). *J Res Ayu Siddha.* 1980;1:138–148.

190. Veerendra Kumar MH. Gupta YK: Effect of different extracts of Centella asiatica on cognition and markers of oxidative stress in rats. *J Ethnopharmacol.* 2002;79(2):253–260.

191. Goodman-Gilman A, Rall T, Nies A, Palmer T. *The Pharmacological Basis of Therapeutics.* 8th ed. New York: Pergamon Press; 1990.

192. Cesarone MR, Laurora G, DeSanctis MT, et al. The microcirculatory activity of Centella asiatica in venous insufficiency: a double-blind study. *Minerva Cardioangiol.* 1994;42(6): 299–304.

193. Bradwejn J, Zhou Y, Koszycki D, Shlik J. A double-blind placebocontrolled study on the effects of Gotu Kola (Centella asiatica) on acoustic startle response in healthy subjects. *J Clin Psychopharmacol.* 2000;20(6):680–684.

194. Keville K. *The Illustrated Herb Encyclopedia.* New York: BDD Promotional Book Co; 1991.

195. Chatterjee M, Verma P, Maurya R, Palit G. Evaluation of ethanol leaf extract of Ocimum sanctum in experimental models of anxiety and depression. *Pharm Biol.* 2011, May;49(5): 477–483.

196. Blumenthal M, Goldberg A, Brinckmann J. Herbal Medicine: Expanded Commission E Monographs, American Botanical Council. *Integrative Medicine Communications.* 2000.

197. Mojay G. op. cit., p 91.

198. Felter HW. The Eclectic Materia Medica. *Pharmacol Therapeut.* 1922.

199. Lorig TS, Schwartz GE. EEG activity during fine fragrance administration. *Psychophysiol.* 1987;24:599.

200. Lorig TS, Herman KB, Schwartz GE, Cain WS. EEG activity during administration of low-concentration odors. *Bull Psychonomic Soc.* 1990;28:405–408.

201. Diego M, Jones NA, Field T, et al. Aromatherapy reduces anxiety and enhances EEG patterns associated with positive mood and alertness. *Int J Neurosci.* 1998;96:217–224.

202. Buchbauer B, Jirovetz L, Jager W, et al. Aromatherapy: evidence for sedative effects of the essential oils of lavender after inhalation. *Naturforschung.* 1991;46:1067–1072.

203. Van Toller S. Emotion and the Brain. In: Van Toller S, Dodd GH, eds. *Perfumery: the psychology and biology of fragrance.* London: Chapman and Hall; 1988.

204. Kikuchi A, Tanida M, Uenoyama S, Yamaguchi H. Effect of odors on cardiac response patterns in a reaction time test. *Chem Senses.* 1991;16(2):183.

205. Buckle J. op. cit., p 44.

206. Styles JL. op. cit., pp 16–20.

207. Woolfson A, Hewitt D. Intensive aromacare. *Int J Aroma.* 1992;4(2):12–14.

208. Brownfield A. Aromatherapy in arthritis: a study. *Nurs Stand.* 1998;13(5):34–35.

209. Dunn C, Sleep J, Collett D. Sensing an improvement: an experimental study to evaluate the use of aromatherapy, massage, and periods of rest in an ICU. *J Adv Nurs.* 1995;21:34–40.

210. Moss M, Cook J, Wesnes K, Duckett P. Aromas of rosemary and lavender essential oils differentially affect cognition and mood in healthy adults. *Int J Neurosci.* 2003;113(1):15–38.

211. Holmes P. Lavender Oil: A Study in Contradictions. *Int J Aromather.* 1992;4(2):20–22.

212. Lawless J. *Lavender Oil: the New Guide to Nature's Most Versatile Remedy.* London: Thorsons; 1994.

213. Martin T. op. cit., pp 38–40.

214. Hutchens A. *Indian Herbology of North America.* Boston: Shambhala; 1991.

215. Newall C, Anderson LA, Phillipson JD. *Herbal Medicines: A Guide for Health Care Professionals.* London: The Pharmaceutical Press; 1996.

216. Kuo-Hsiung L, et al. The cytotoxic principles of *Prunella vulgaris, Psychotria serpens,* and *Hyptis capitata*: ursolic acid and related derivatives. *Planta Med.* 1988;54:308.

217. Xia XX. Leonurus. *J Trad Chin Med.* 1983;3:185.

218. Milkowska-Layck K, Filipek B, Strzelecka H. Pharmacological effects of lavandulifolioside from *Leonurus cardiaca.* *J Ethnopharmacol.* 2002;80(1):85–90.

219. Stansbury J. Botanical Medicines Acting on the Female Reproductive System, p 35.

220. Zou QZ, Bi RG, Li JM, et al. Effect of motherwort on blood hyperviscosity. *Am J Chin Med.* 1989;17(1-2):65–70.

221. Crawford AM. The Herbal Menopause Book: Herbs, Nutrition, & other Natural Therapies. Freedom: The Crossing Press; 1996.

222. Hudson T. *Gynecology and Naturopathic Medicine: a Treatment Manual.* 3rd ed. Aloha, HI: TK Publications; 1994.

223. Mao QQ, Ip SP, Tsai SH, Che CT. Antidepressant-like effect of peony glycosides in mice. *J Ethnopharmacol.* 2008a, Sep 26;119(2):272–275.

224. Mao Q, Huang Z, Ip S, Che C. Antidepressant-like effect of ethanol extract from Paeonia lactiflora in mice. *Phytother Res.* 2008b, Nov;22(11):1496–1499.

225. Mao QQ, Ip SP, Xian YF, Hu Z, Che CT. Anti-depressant-like effect of peony: a mini-review. *Pharm Biol.* 2012a, Jan;50(1):72–77.

226. Mao QQ, Ip SP, Ko KM, Tsai SH, Xian YF, Che CT. Effects of peony glycosides on mice exposed to chronic unpredictable stress: further evidence for antidepressant-like activity. *J Ethnopharmacol.* 2009, Jul 15;124(2):316–320.

227. Mao QQ, Huang Z, Ip SP, Xian YF, Che CT. Peony glycosides reverse the effects of corticosterone on behavior and brain BDNF expression in rats. *Behav Brain Res.* 2012b, Feb 1; 227(1):305–309.

228. Mannucci C, Navarra M, Calzavara E, Caputi AP, Calapai G. Serotonin involvement in Rhodiola rosea attenuation of nicotine withdrawal signs in rats. *Phytomedicine.* 2012, Sep 15;19(12):1117–1124.

229. Mattioli L, Perfumi M. Evaluation of Rhodiola rosea L. extract on affective and physical signs of nicotine withdrawal in mice. *J Psychopharmacol*. 2011, Mar;25(3):402–410.

230. Chen QG, Zeng YS, Qu ZQ, Tang JY, Qin YJ, Chung P, et al. The effects of Rhodiola rosea extract on 5-HT level, cell proliferation and quantity of neurons at cerebral hippocampus of depressive rats. *Phytomedicine*. 2009, Sep;16(9):830–838.

231. Darbinyan V, Aslanyan G, Amroyan E, Gabrielyan E, Malmström C, Panossian A. Clinical trial of Rhodiola rosea L. extract SHR-5 in the treatment of mild to moderate depression. *Nord J Psychiatry*. 2007;61(5):343–348.

232. Field T. op. cit., pp 116–120.

233. Machado DG, Cunha MP, Neis VB, Balen GO, Colla A, Bettio LE, et al. Antidepressant-like effects of fractions, essential oil, carnosol and betulinic acid isolated from Rosmarinus officinalis L. *Food Chem*. 2013, Jan 15;136(2):999–1005.

234. Machado DG, Cunha MP, Neis VB, Balen GO, Colla AR, Grando J, et al. Rosmarinus officinalis L. hydroalcoholic extract, similar to fluoxetine, reverses depressive-like behavior without altering learning deficit in olfactory bulbectomized mice. *J Ethnopharmacol*. 2012, Aug 30;143(1):158–169.

235. McIntyre A. *The Complete Woman's Herbal: A Manual of Healing Herbs and Nutrition for Personal Well-being and Family Care*. New York: Henry Holt; 1995.

236. Snow JM: *Hypericum perforatum L*. (Hyperiaceae), Prot J Botan Med 2(1):16–21.

237. Muller WE. Current St. John's wort research from mode of action to clinical efficacy. *Pharmacol Res*. 2003;47(2):101–109.

238. Chen F, Rezvani AH, Lawrence AJ. Autoradiographic quantification of neurochemical markers of serotonin, dopamine, and opioid systems in rat brain mesolimbic regions following chronic St. John's wort treatment. *Naunyn Schmiedebergs Arch Pharmacol*. 2003;367(2):126–133.

239. Greeson JM, Sanford B, Monti DA. St. John's wort (*Hypericum perforatum*): a review of the current pharmacological, toxicological, and clinical literature. *Psychopharmacology (Berl)*. 2001;153(4):402–414.

240. Butterweck V. Mechanism of action of St. John's wort in depression: what is known? *CNS Drugs*. 2003;17(8):539–562.

241. Murck H. Atypical depression and related illnesses—neurobiological principles for their treatment with Hypericum extract. *Wien Med Wochenschr*. 2002;152(15-16):398–403.

242. Noldner M, Schotz K. Rutin is essential for the antidepressant activity of *Hypericum perforatum* extracts in the forced swimming test. *Planta Med*. 2002;68(7):577–580.

243. Wurglics M, Schubert-Zsilavecz M. Hypericum perforatum: a 'modern' herbal antidepressant: pharmacokinetics of active ingredients. *Clin Pharmacokinet*. 2006;45(5):449–468.

244. Leuner K, Kazanski V, Müller M, Essin K, Henke B, Gollasch M, et al. Hyperforin–a key constituent of St. John's wort specifically activates TRPC6 channels. *FASEB J*. 2007, Dec;21(14):4101–4111.

245. Reichling J, Hostanska K, Saller R. St. John's wort (*Hypericum perforatum L.*)—multicompound preparations vs. single substances. *Forsch Komplementarmed Klass Naturheilkd*. 2003;10(suppl 1):28–32.

246. Linde K, Ramirez G, Mulrow C, et al. St. John's wort for depression - an overview and meta-analysis of randomised clinical trials. *BMJ*. 1996;313:253–258.

247. Kim HL, Streltzer J, Goebert D. St. John's wort for depression: a metaanalysis of well-defined clinical trials. *J Nerv Ment Dis*. 1999;187:532–538.

248. Williams JW, Mulrow CD, Chiquette E, et al. A systematic review of newer pharmacotherapies for depression in adults: evidence report summary. *Ann Intern Med*. 2000;132:743–756.

249. Linde K, Mulrow CD. St. John's wort for depression. *Cochrane Database Syst Rev*. 2000;(2):CD000448.

250. Whiskey E, Werneke U, Taylor D. A systemic review and meta-analysis of *Hypericum perforatum* in depression: a comprehensive clinical review. *Int Clin Psychopharmacol*. 2000;16(5):239–252.

251. Laakmann G, Jahn G, Schule C. *Hypericum perforatum* extract in treatment of mild to moderate depression: clinical and pharmacological aspects. *Nervenarzt*. 2002;73(7):600–612.

252. Hammerness P, Basch E, Ulbricht C, et al. St. John's wort: a systematic review of adverse effects and drug interactions for the consultation psychiatrist. *Psychosomatics*. 2003;44(4):271–282.

253. Cirigliano MD. Clinical Use of St. John's wort, UpToDate Online 10.3. www.uptodate.com; 2003.

254. Linde K, Berner MM, Kriston L. St John's wort for major depression. *Cochrane Database Syst Rev*. 2008;(4):CD000448.

255. Kalb R, Trautmann-Sponsel RD, Kieser M. Efficacy and tolerability of hypericum extract WS 5572 versus placebo in mildly to moderately depressed patients: a randomized double-blind multicenter clinical trial. *Pharmacopsychiatry*. 2001;34(3):96–103.

256. Rychlik R, Siedentop H, von den Driesch V, Kasper S. St. John's wort extract WS 5572 in minor to moderately severe depression: effectiveness and tolerance of 600 and 1200 mg active ingredient daily. *Fortschr Med Orig*. 2001;119(3-4):119–128.

257. Lecrubier Y, Clerc G, Didi R, Kieser M. Efficacy of St. John's wort extract WS 5570 in major depression: a double-blind placebo-controlled trial. *Am J Psychiatry*. 2002;159(8):1361–1366.

258. Brenner R, Azbel V, Madhusoodanan S, et al. Comparison of an extract of hypericum (LI 160) and sertraline in the treatment of depression: a double-blind, randomized pilot study. *Clin Ther*. 2000;22:411–419.

259. Schrader E, et al. Equivalence of St. John's wort extract (Ze 117) and fluoxetine: a randomized, controlled study in mild-moderate depression. *Int Clin Psychopharmacol*. 2000;15:61–68.

260. Mannel M, Kuhn U, Schmidt U, Ploch M, Murck H. St. John's wort extract LI160 for the treatment of depression with atypical features - a double-blind, randomized, and placebo-controlled trial. *J Psychiatr Res*. 2010, Sep;44(12):760–767.

261. Sarris J, Fava M, Schweitzer I, Mischoulon D. St John's wort (Hypericum perforatum) versus sertraline and placebo in major depressive disorder: continuation data from a 26-week RCT. *Pharmacopsychiatry*. 2012, Nov;45(7):275–278.

262. Rapaport MH, Nierenberg AA, Howland R, Dording C, Schettler PJ, Mischoulon D. The treatment of minor depression with St. John's Wort or citalopram: failure to show benefit over placebo. *J Psychiatr Res*. 2011, Jul;45(7):931–941.

263. Mischoulon D. *St. John's wort: a review of the evidence*. In: *Integrating Complementary Therapies into Clinical Practice: Cases and Evidence*. Boston: Harvard Medical School; 2003.

264. Behnke K, Jensen GS, Graubaum HJ, Gruenwald J. Hypericum perforatum vs. Fluoxetine in the treatment of mild to moderate depression. *Adv Ther*. 2002;19(1):43–52.

265. Kasper S, Anghelescu IG, Szegedi A, Dienel A, Kieser M. Superior efficacy of St John's wort extract WS 5570 compared to placebo in patients with major depression: a randomized, double-blind, placebo-controlled, multi-center trial [IS-RCTN77277298]. *BMC Med.* 2006:414.

266. Randløv C, Mehlsen J, Thomsen CF, Hedman C, von Fircks H, Winther K. The efficacy of St. John's Wort in patients with minor depressive symptoms or dysthymia—a double-blind placebo-controlled study. *Phytomedicine.* 2006, Mar;13(4):215–221.

267. Gastpar M, Singer A, Zeller K. Comparative efficacy and safety of a once-daily dosage of hypericum extract STW3-VI and citalopram in patients with moderate depression: a double-blind, randomised, multicentre, placebo-controlled study. *Pharmacopsychiatry.* 2006, Mar;39(2):66–75.

268. Anghelescu IG, Kohnen R, Szegedi A, Klement S, Kieser M. Comparison of Hypericum extract WS 5570 and paroxetine in ongoing treatment after recovery from an episode of moderate to severe depression: results from a randomized multicenter study. *Pharmacopsychiatry.* 2006, Nov;39(6):213–219.

269. Kasper S, Anghelescu IG, Szegedi A, Dienel A, Kieser M. Placebo controlled continuation treatment with Hypericum extract WS 5570 after recovery from a mild or moderate depressive episode. *Wien Med Wochenschr.* 2007;157(13-14):362–366.

270. Moreno RA, Teng CT, Almeida KM, Tavares Junior H. Hypericum perforatum versus fluoxetine in the treatment of mild to moderate depression: a randomized double-blind trial in a Brazilian sample. *Rev Bras Psiquiatr.* 2006, Mar;28(1):29–32.

271. Melzer J, Brignoli R, Keck ME, Saller R. A hypericum extract in the treatment of depressive symptoms in outpatients: an open study. *Forsch Komplementmed.* 2010;17(1):7–14. Switzerland.

272. Brattström A. Long-term effects of St. John's wort (Hypericum perforatum) treatment: a 1-year safety study in mild to moderate depression. *Phytomedicine.* 2009, Apr;16(4):277–283.

273. Khan A, Khan S, Brown WA. Are placebo controls necessary to test new antidepressants and anxiolytics? *Int J Neuropsychopharmacol.* 2002;5(3):193–197.

274. Grube B, Walper A, Wheatley D. St. John's wort extract: efficacy for menopausal symptoms of psychological origin. *Adv Ther.* 1999;16:177–186.

275. Schultz H, Jobert M. Effects of hypericum extract on the sleep EEG in older volunteers. *J Geriatr Psychiatry Neurol.* 1994;7(suppl 1):S39–S43.

276. Rezvani AH, Overstreet DH, Yang Y, Clark E. Attenuation of alcohol intake by extract of *Hypericum perforatum* (St. John's wort) in two different strains of alcohol-preferring rats. *Alcohol Alcohol.* 1999;34(5):699–705.

277. Perfumi M, Ciccocioppo R, Angeletti S, et al. Effects of *Hypericum perforatum* extract on alcohol intake in Marchigian Sardinian alcohol-preferring rats. *Alcohol.* 1999;34(5):690–698.

278. Panocka I, Perfumi M, Angeletti S, et al. Effects of *Hypericum perforatum* extract on ethanol intake, and on behavioral despair: a search for the neurochemical systems involved. *Pharmacol Biochem Behav.* 2000;66(1):105–111.

279. Beijamini V, Andreatini R. Effects of *Hypericum perforatum* and paroxetine on rat performance in the elevated T-maze. *Pharmacol Res.* 2003;48(2):199–207.

280. Stevinson C, Ernst E. A pilot study of *Hypericum perforatum* for the treatment of premenstrual syndrome. *BJOG.* 2000;107(7):870–876.

281. Kumar V, Singh PN, Bhattacharya SK. Anti-stress activity of Indian *Hypericum perforatum* L. *Indian J Exp Biol.* 2001;39(4):344–349.

282. Khalifa AE. *Hypericum perforatum* as a nootropic drug: enhancement of retrieval memory of a passive avoidance conditioning paradigm in mice. *J Ethnopharmacol.* 2001;76(1):49–57.

283. Widy-Tyszkiewicz E, Piechal A, Joniec I, Blecharz-Klin K. Long term administration of *Hypericum perforatum* improves spatial learning and memory in the water maze. *Biol Pharm Bull.* 2002;25(10):1289–1294.

284. Singh A, Naidu PS, Gupta S, Kulkarni SK. Effect of natural and synthetic antioxidants in a mouse model of chronic fatigue syndrome. *J Med Food.* 2002;5(4):211–220.

285. Taylor LH, Kobak KA. An open-label trial of St. John's wort (Hypericum perforatum) in obsessive-compulsive disorder. *J Clin Psychiatry.* 2000;61(8):575–578.

286. Barnes J, Anderson LA, Phillipson JD. St. John's wort (*Hypericum perforatum* L.): a review of its chemistry, pharmacology and clinical properties. *J Pharm Pharmacol.* 2001;53(5): 83–600.

287. Raso GM, Pacilio M, Di Carlo G, et al. In-vivo and in-vitro antiinflammatory effect of Echinacea purpurea and Hypericum perforatum. *J Pharm Pharmacol.* 2002;54(10):1379–1383.

288. Hostanska K, Reichling J, Bommer S, et al. Aqueous ethanolic extract of St. John's wort (*Hypericum perforatum* L.) induces growth inhibition and apoptosis in human malignant cells in vitro. *Pharmazie.* 2002;57(5):323–331.

289. Schempp CM, Muller KA, Winghofer B, et al. St. John's wort (*Hypericum perforatum* L.): a plant with relevance for dermatology. *Hautarzt.* 2002;53(5):316–321.

290. Fiebich BL, Knörle R, Appel K, Kammler T, Weiss G. Pharmacological studies in an herbal drug combination of St. John's Wort (Hypericum perforatum) and passion flower (Passiflora incarnata): in vitro and in vivo evidence of synergy between Hypericum and Passiflora in antidepressant pharmacological models. *Fitoterapia.* 2011, Apr;82(3):474–480.

291. Sarris J, Kavanagh DJ, Deed G, St Bone KM. John's wort and Kava in treating major depressive disorder with comorbid anxiety: a randomised double-blind placebo-controlled pilot trial. *Hum Psychopharmacol.* 2009, Jan;24(1):41–48.

292. De Smet PA, Nolen WA. St. John's wort as an antidepressant. *BMJ.* 1996;313(7052):241–242.

293. Schultz V. Incidence and clinical relevance of interactions and side effects of hypericum preparations. *Schweiz Rundsch Med Prax.* 2000;89(50):2131–2140.

294. Kasper S. *Hypericum perforatum*: a review of clinical studies. *Pharmacopsychiatry.* 2001;34(suppl 1):S51–S55.

295. Nierenberg AA, Mischoulon D, DeCecco L, In: Mischoulon D, Rosenbaum JF eds. op. cit., p 5.

296. Lawrence Review of Natural Products. *St. John's Wort.* St. Louis: Facts and Comparisons; 1997.

297. Vorbach EU, Arnoldt KH, Wolpert E. St. John's wort: a potential therapy for elderly depressed patients? *Drugs Aging.* 2000;16(3):189–197.

298. Hippius H. St. John's wort (*Hypericum perforatum*)—an herbal antidepressant. *Current Med Res Opinion.* 1998;14(8):181.

299. Brockmoller J, Reum T, Bauer S, et al. Hypericin and pseudohypericin: pharmacokinetics and effects on photosensitivity in humans. *Pharmacopsychiat (suppl).* 1997;30:94–101.

300. Schempp CM, Winghofer B, Muller K, et al. op. cit., pp 141–146.

301. Ernst E, Rand JI, Stevinson C. Adverse effects profile of the herbal antidepressant St. John's wort (*Hypericum perforatum* L.). *Eur J Clin Pharmacol*. 1998;54:589–594.

302. Bilia AR, Gallori S, Vincieri FF. St. John's wort and depression: efficacy, safety, and tolerability—an update. *Life Sci*. 2002;70(26):3077–3096.

303. Johne A, Brockmoller J, Bauer S, et al. Pharmacokinetic interaction of digoxin with an herbal extract of St. John's wort (Hypericum perforatum). *Clin Pharmacol Ther*. 1999;66:338–345.

304. Piscitelli SC, Burstein AH, Chaitt D, et al. Indinavir concentrations and St. John's wort. *Lancet*. 2000;355(9203):547–548.

305. Ruschitzka F, Meier PJ, Turina M, et al. Acute heart transplant rejection caused by St. John's wort. *Lancet*. 2000;355(9203):548–549.

306. Moore LB, Goodwin B, Jones SA, et al. St. John's wort induces hepatic metabolism through activation of the pregnane X receptor. *Proc Natl Acad Sci USA*. 2000;97(13):7500–7502.

307. Mathijssen R, Verweij J, de Bruijn P, et al. Effects of St. John's wort on irinotecan metabolism. *J Natl Cancer Inst*. 2002;94:1247–1249.

308. Andelic S. Bigeminy—the result of interaction between digoxin and St. John's wort. *Vojnosanit Pregl*. 2003;60(3):361–364.

309. Sugimoto K, Ohmori M, Tsuruoka S, et al. Different effects of St. John's wort on the pharmacokinetics of simvastatin and pravastatin. *Clin Pharmacol Ther*. 2001;70(6):518–524.

310. Lantz M, Buchalter E, Giambanco V. St. John's wort and antidepressant drug interactions in the elderly. *J Geriatr Psychiatry Neurol*. 1999;12:7–10.

311. Klier CM, Schafer MR, Schmid-Siegel B, et al. St. John's wort (Hypericum perforatum)—is it safe during breastfeeding? *Pharmacopsychiatry*. 2002;35(1):29–30.

312. Hammerly M. *Depression: The New Integrative Approach; How to Combine the Best of Traditional and Alternative Therapies*. Avon, UK: Adams Media; 2001.

313. McIntyre A. Flower Power: op. cit., p 67.

314. Taylor AM, Castonguay A, Taylor AJ, et al. Microglia disrupt mesolimbic reward circuitry in chronic pain. *J Neurosci*. 2015;35(22):8442–8450. United States.

315. Kulkarni SK, Akula KK, Deshpande J. Evaluation of antidepressant-like activity of novel water-soluble curcumin formulations and St. John's wort in behavioral paradigms of despair. *Pharmacology*. 2012;89(1-2):83–90.

316. Kumar A, Singh A. Possible nitric oxide modulation in protective effect of (Curcuma longa, Zingiberaceae) against sleep deprivation-induced behavioral alterations and oxidative damage in mice. *Phytomedicine*. 2008, Aug;15(8):577–586.

317. Xia X, Cheng G, Pan Y, Xia ZH, Kong LD. Behavioral, neurochemical and neuroendocrine effects of the ethanolic extract from Curcuma longa L. in the mouse forced swimming test. *J Ethnopharmacol*. 2007, Mar 21;110(2):356–363.

318. Xia X, Pan Y, Zhang WY, Cheng G, Kong LD. Ethanolic extracts from Curcuma longa attenuates behavioral, immune, and neuroendocrine alterations in a rat chronic mild stress model. *Biol Pharm Bull*. 2006, May;29(5):938–944.

319. Xu Y, Ku B, Tie L, et al. Curcumin reverses the effects of chronic stress on behavior, the HPA axis, BDNF expression and phosphorylation of CREB. *Brain Res*. 2006, Nov 29;1122(1):56–64.

320. Werbach M, In: Strohecker J, Strohecker NS, eds. op. cit., pp 92–111.

321. Murray M. op.cit., pp 106–107.

322. Pearlstein TB. Hormones and depression: what are the facts about premenstrual syndrome, menopause, and hormone replacement therapy? *Am J Obstet Gynecol*. 1995;173(2):650.

323. Brown MA, Robinson J. *When Your Body Gets the Blues: The Clinically Proven Program for Women Who Feel Tired and Stressed and Eat Too Much*. New York: Berkley; 2002.

324. Muskin P. Complementary and Alternative Medicine and Psychiatry (Review of Psychiatry Series, vol. 19, no. 1; Oldham JM, Riba MB, series eds.) Washington, DC: American Psychiatric Press; 2000:125–126.

325. Hobbs C, Haas E. *Vitamins for Dummies*. Foster City: IDG Books Worldwide; 1999.

326. Pochwat B, Szewczyk B, Sowa-Kucma M, Siwek A, Doboszewska U, Piekoszewski W, et al. Antidepressant-like activity of magnesium in the chronic mild stress model in rats: alterations in the NMDA receptor subunits. *Int J Neuropsychopharmacol*. 2014, Mar;17(3):393–405.

327. Zarate C, Duman RS, Liu G, Sartori S, Quiroz J, Murck H. New paradigms for treatment-resistant depression. *Ann N Y Acad Sci*. 2013, Jul:129221–129231.

328. Derom ML, Sayón-Orea C, Martínez-Ortega JM, Martínez-González MA. Magnesium and depression: a systematic review. *Nutr Neurosci*. 2013, Sep;16(5):191–206.

329. Barragán-Rodríguez L, Rodríguez-Morán M, Guerrero-Romero F. Efficacy and safety of oral magnesium supplementation in the treatment of depression in the elderly with type 2 diabetes: a randomized, equivalent trial. *Magnes Res*. 2008, Dec;21(4):218–223.

330. Mischoulon D, Rosenbaum JF. *Natural Medications for Psychiatric Disorders: Considering the Alternatives*. Philadelphia: Lippincott Williams & Wilkins; 2002.

331. Haag, 2003.

332. Otto, 2003.

333. Ohara, 2005.

334. Maes, 1996.

335. Mischoulon, 2000.

336. Brown MA, Goldstein-Shirley J, Robinson J, et al. The Effects of a multi-modal intervention trial of light, exercise, and vitamins on women's mood. *Women and Health*. 2001;34(3):94.

337. Moore KA, Blumenthal JA. Exercise Training as an alternative treatment for depression among older adults. *Altern Ther Health Med*. 1998;4(1):48–56.

338. Blumenthal JA, Babyak MA, Moore KA, et al. Effects of exercise training in older patients with major depression. *Arch Intern Med*. 1999;159(19):349–356.

339. Hammar M, Berg G, Lindgren R. Does Physical exercise influence the frequency of postmenopausal hot flushes? *Acta Obstet Gynecol Scand*. 1990;69:409–412.

340. Slaven L, Lee C. Mood and symptom reporting among middleaged women: the relationship between menopausal status, hormone replacement therapy, and exercise participation. *Health Psychol*. 1997;16(3):203–208.

341. Martinsen E. Physical fitness, anxiety and depression. *Br J Hosp Med*. 1990;43:199.

342. Kabat-Zinn J. *Mindfulness Meditation*. New York: Nightingale- Conant Corp. [audiotape]; 1995.

343. Benson H, Stuart E. *The Wellness Book: The Comprehensive Guide to Maintaining Health and Treating Stress-Related Illness*. New York: Birch Lane Press; 1992.

344. Irvin J, Domar A, Clark C, et al. The effects of relaxation response training on menopausal symptoms. *J Psychosom Obstet Gynaecol*. 1996;17(4):202–207.

345. Goleman D, Gurin J. *Mind-Body Medicine: How to Use Your Mind for Better Health*. New York: Consumer Reports Books; 1993.

346. Pizzorno J. In: Strohecker J, Strohecker NS eds. op. cit., pp 58–59.

347. Rost K, Nutting P, Smith J, et al. Managing depression as a chronic disease: a randomized trial of ongoing treatment in primary care. *BMJ*. 2002;325:934–937.

348. Keller M. Past, present, and future directions for defining optimal treatment outcome in depression: remission and beyond. *JAMA*. 2003;289(23):3152–3160.

349. Raffensperger C. op. cit., pp 111–115.

350. Kaplan H, Sadock B. Anxiety Disorders. In: *Kaplan and Sadock's Synopsis of Psychiatry*. 8th ed. Baltimore: Williams & Wilkins; 1998.

351. Jetty P, Charney D, Goddard A. Generalized anxiety disorder. *Psychiatric Clin North Am*. 2001;24(1).

352. Ferrarese C, Appollonio I, Frigio M, et al. Decreased density of benzodiazepine receptors in lymphocytes of anxious patients: reversal after chronic diazepam treatment. *Acta Psychiatr Scand*. 1990;82:169–173.

353. Mathew RJ, Ho BT, Francis DJ, et al. Catecholamines and anxiety. *Acta Psychiatr Scand*. 1982;65:142–147.

354. King D, Hunter M. Psychologic and spiritual aspects of menopause. *Clin Fam Practice*. 2002;4(1).

355. Cawood EHH, Bancroft J. Steroid hormones, the menopause, sexuality and well-being of women. *Psychol Med*. 1996;26:925–936.

356. Dossey MF, Dossy MA. The climacteric woman. *Patient Counsel Health Educ*. 1980;2:14.

357. Uphold CR, Susman EJ. Self reported climacteric symptoms as a function of the relationships between marital adjustment and childrearing stage. *Nurs Res*. 1981;30:84.

358. Costello EJ. Married with children. Predictors of mental and physical health in middle-aged women. *Psychiatry*. 1991;54:292.

359. Menopause Guidebook: Helping Women Make Informed Healthcare Decisions Through Menopause and Beyond. The North American Menopause Society. http://www.menopause.org/edumaterials/guidebook/perimenopausalchanges.pdf. Accessed 5/26/03.

360. Brawman-Mintzer O. Generalized anxiety disorder: Pharmacologic Treatment of generalized anxiety disorder. *Psychiatr Clin North Am*. 2001;24(1).

361. Gladstar R. *Herbs for Reducing Stress & Anxiety*. Pownal, VT: Storey Books; 1999.

362. Foster S. Black cohosh, Cimicifuga racemosa, a literature review. *Herbalgram*. 1999;35–49.

363. Stoll W. Phytotheraopeutickum beeinflusst atrophisches Vaginal epith. Doppelblindversuch Cimicifuga vs. oestrogenpraeparat [Phytopharmaceutic vaginal epithelium. Double-blind study on Cimicifuga vs an estrogen preparation]. *Therapeutickon*. 1987;1:23.

364. Borrelli F, Ernst E. *Cimicifuga racemosa*: a systematic review of its clinical and pharmacological effects. *Eur J Clin Pharmacol*. 2002;58(4):235.

365. http://www.naturalstandard.com. Black cohosh. Accessed 8/20/03.

366. Liu J, Burdette JE, Xu H, et al. Evaluation of estrogenic activity of plant extracts for the potential treatment of menopausal symptoms. *J Agric Food Chem*. 2001;49(5):2472–2479.

367. Fugh- Berman A. Black Cohosh. In: *The Five Minute Herb & Dietary Supplement Consult*. Philadelphia: Lippincott Williams & Wilkins; 2003.

368. Kruse SO, Loohning A, Pauli GF, et al. Fukiic and piscidic acid esters from the rhizome of Cimucifuga racemosa and the in vitro estrogenic activity of fukinolic acid. *Planta Med*. 1999;65:763.

369. Liske E, Hanggi W. Henneicke-von Zepelin H: Physiological investigation of a unique extract of black cohosh (*Cimicifugae racemosae rhizoma*): a 6-month clinical study demonstrates no systemic estrogenic effect. *J Women's Health Gend Based Med*. 2002;11(2):163–174.

370. McGuffin M, Hobbs C, Upton R, et al. *American Herbal Products Association's Botanical Safety Handbook*. Boca Raton: CRC Press; 1997.

371. Brinker F. *Herb Contraindications and Drug Interactions*. 3rd ed. Sandy, OR: Eclectic Medical Publications; 2001.

372. Amsterdam JD, Shults J, Soeller I, Mao JJ, Rockwell K, Newberg AB. Chamomile (Matricaria recutita) may provide antidepressant activity in anxious, depressed humans: an exploratory study. *Altern Ther Health Med*. 2012;18(5):44–49.

373. Balick M, Lee R. Traditional use of sakau (kava): lessons for integrative medicine. *Alt Ther Health Med*. 2002;8(4).

374. Pittler M, Ernest E. Efficacy of kava extract for treating anxiety: systematic review and meta-analysis. *J Clin Psychopharmacol*. 2000;20:84.

375. Warnecke G. Psychosomatic dysfunctions in the female climacteric: Clinical effectiveness and tolerance of kava Extract WS 1490. *Forschr Med*. 1991;109(4):119.

376. De Leo V, La Marca A, Lanzetta D, et al. Assessment of the association of Kava-kava extract and hormone replacement therapy in the treatment of postmenopausal anxiety. *Minerva Ginecol*. 2000;52:263. [In Italian].

377. Leo De, La Marca A, Morgante G, et al. Evaluation of combining kava extract with hormone replacement therapy in the treatment of postmenopausal anxiety. *Maturitas*. 2001;39(2):185.

378. Sarris J, Kavanagh DJ, Byrne G, Bone KM, Adams J, Deed G. The Kava Anxiety Depression Spectrum Study (KADSS): a randomized, placebo-controlled crossover trial using an aqueous extract of Piper methysticum. *Psychopharmacology (Berl)*. 2009, Aug;205(3):399–407.

379. Justofie A, Schmiz A. Hiemke: Kava pyrone enriched extract from Piper methysticum as a modulator of the GABA binding site in different regions of rat brain. *Psychopharmacology*. 1994;116:469.

380. Walden J, Von wegerer J, Winter U, et al. Effects of kawain and dihydromethysticin on field potential changes in the hippocampus. *Prog Neuropsychol Psychiatry*. 1997;21(4):697.

381. Seitz U, Schule A, Gleitz J. [3H]-monoamine uptake inhibition properties of kava pyrones. *Planta Med*. 1997;63(6):548.

382. Baum SS, Hill R, Rommelspacher H. Effect of Kava extract and individual kavapyrones on neurotransmitter levels in the nucleus accumbens of rats. *P Neuropsychopharmacol Biol Psychiatry*. 1998;22(7):1105.

383. Holm E, Staedt U, Heep J, et al. The action profile of D, L-Kavain. Cerebral sites and sleep-wakefulness-rhythm in animals. *Arneimittelforschung*. 1991;41(7):673.

384. www.naturalstandard.com/monographs/herbalsupplements/kava.asp. accessed 3/20/03.

385. Ruze P. Kava induced dermopathy: a niacin deficiency? *Lancet*. 1990;335(8703):1442.

386. American Botanical Council (ABC). *Kava product warning label issued by leading herbal association [press release]*. Austin: TX; 2001.

387. Waller DP. *Report on kava and liver damage*. Silver Spring, MD: American Herbal Products Assn; 2002.

388. Buckle J. Aromatherapy. *Nurs Times*. 1993;89(20):32–35.

389. http://www.naturalstandard.com. accessed 7/18/03. Last updated January 2002.

390. Elisabetsky E, Marschner J, Souza DO. Effects of linalool on glutamatergic system in the rat cerebral cortex. *Neurochem Res*. 1995;0(4):461.

391. Linck VM, da Silva AL, Figueiró M, Caramão EB, Moreno PR, Elisabetsky E. Effects of inhaled Linalool in anxiety, social interaction and aggressive behavior in mice. *Phytomedicine*. 2010, Jul;17(8-9):679–683.

392. Jager W, Buchbauer G, Jirovetz L, et al. Percutaneous absorption of lavender oil from massage oil. *J Soc Cosm Chem*. 1992;43:49.

393. Radmaker M. Allergic contact dermatitis from lavender fragrance in Dfflam gel. *Contact Dermatitis*. 1994;31(1):58.

394. Ripple GH, Gould MN, Steward JA, et al. Phase I clinical trail of perillyl alcohol administered daily. *Clin Cancer Res*. 1998;4(5):1159.

395. Guillemain J, Rousseau A, Delaveu P. Neurodepressive effects of the essential oil of *Lavandula angustifolia Mill*. *Ann Pharm Fr*. 1989;47(6):337.

396. Ripple GH, Gould MN, Arzoomanian RZ, et al. Phase I clinical and pharmacokinetic study of perillyl alcohol administration. *Clin Cancer Res*. 2000;6(2):390.

397. Ibarra A, Feuillere N, Roller M, Lesburgere E, Beracochea D. Effects of chronic administration of Melissa officinalis L. extract on anxiety-like reactivity and on circadian and exploratory activities in mice. *Phytomedicine*. 2010, May;17(6): 397–403.

398. Kennedy DO, Little W, Haskell CF, Scholey AB. Anxiolytic effects of a combination of Melissa officinalis and Valeriana officinalis during laboratory induced stress. *Phytother Res*. 2006, Feb;20(2):96–102.

399. www.naturalstandard.com, passionflower. Accessed 8/20/03.

400. Akhondzadeh S, Naghavi HR, Vazirian M, et al. Passionflower in the treatment of generalized anxiety: a pilot double-blind randomized controlled trial with oxazepam. *J Clin Pharm Ther*. 2001;26(5):363.

401. Bourin M, Bougerol T, Guitton B, et al. A combination of plant extracts in the treatment of outpatients with adjustment disorder with anxious mood: controlled study versus placebo. *Fund Clin Pharmacol*. 1997;11(2):27–32.

402. Trompetter I, Krick B, Weiss G. Herbal triplet in treatment of nervous agitation in children. *Wien Med Wochenschr*. 2013, Feb;163(3-4):52–57.

403. Miyasaka LS, Atallah ÁN, Soares B. Passiflora for anxiety disorder. *Cochrane Database Syst Rev*. 2007; Issue 1. Art. No.: CD004518. http://dx.doi.org/10.1002/14651858.CD004518.pub2.

404. Brock C, Whitehouse J, Tewfik I, Towell T. American Skullcap (Scutellaria lateriflora): a randomised, double-blind placebo-controlled crossover study of its effects on mood in healthy volunteers. *Phytother Res*. 2014;28(5):692–698. England.

405. www.naturalstandard.com, valerian. Accessed 8/20/03.

406. Sousa MPd, Pacheco P, Rodao V. Double-blind comparative study of the efficacy and safety of Valdispert vs. clozepam. *KaliChemi Med Res Info (Report)*. 1992.

407. Andreatinini R, Sartori VA, Seabra ML, et al. Effect of valpotriates (valerian extract) in generalized anxiety disorder: a randomized placebo- controlled pilot study. *Phytotherapy*. 2002;16(7):650.

408. Tang JY, Zeng YS, Chen QG, Qin YJ, Chen SJ, Zhong ZQ. Effects of Valerian on the level of 5-hydroxytryptamine, cell proliferation and neurons in cerebral hippocampus of rats with depression induced by chronic mild stress. *Zhong Xi Yi Jie He Xue Bao*. 2008, Mar;6(3):283–288.

409. Ortiz JG, Nieves-Natal J, Chavez P. Effects of Valeriana officinalis extracts on [3H]flunitrazepam binding, synaptosomal [3H] GABA uptake and hippocampal [3H] GABA release. *Neurochem Res*. 1999;24(11):1373.

410. Del Valle-Mojica LM, Ortíz JG. Anxiolytic properties of Valeriana officinalis in the zebrafish: a possible role for metabotropic glutamate receptors. *Planta Med*. 2012, Nov;78(16):1719–1724.

411. Shultz V, Hansel R, Tyler VE. *Valerian in Rational Phytotherapy: A Physicians' Guide to Herbal Medicine*. 4th ed. Berlin: Springer; 2001.

412. Facklemann K. Medicine for menopause, researchers study herbal remedies for hot flashes. *Sci News*. 1998;153:392–393.

413. Tharakan B, Manyam B. Botanical therapies in sexual dysfunction. *Phytother Res*. 2005;19:457–463.

414. Muniyappa R, Norton M, Dunn ME, Banerji MA. Diabetes and female sexual dysfunction: moving beyond "benign neglect". *Curr Diabetes Repts*. 2005;5:3230–3236.

415. Rosen RC, Barsky JL. Normal sexual response in women. *Obstet Gynecol Clin North Am*. 2006;33:4515–4526.

416. Basson R, Berman J, Burnett A, et al. Report of the international consensus development conference on female sexual dysfunction: definitions and classifications. *J Urol*. 2000;163:3888–3893.

417. Carey C. Disorders of sexual desire and arousal. *Obstet Gynecol Clin North Am*. 2006;33:549–564.

418. Laumann E, Paik A, Rosen R. Sexual dysfunction in the United States: prevalence and predictors. *JAMA*. 1999;281: 6537–6544.

419. Moynihan R. The marketing of a disease: female sexual dysfunction. *BMJ*. 2005;330(7484):192–194.

420. Berman JR, Berman LA, Werbin TJ, Goldstein I. Female sexual dysfunction: anatomy, physiology, evaluation and treatment options. *Curr Opin Urol*. 1999;9:6563–6568.

421. Bernardo A. Sexuality in patients with coronary disease and heart failure. *Herz*. 2001;26:5353–5359.

422. Modelska K, Cummings S. Female sexual dysfunction in postmenopausal women: systematic review of placebo-controlled trials [see comment]. *Am J Obstet Gynecol*. 2003;188:1286–1293.

423. Altman A. Etiology and diagnosis of sexual dysfunction in women, UpToDate. 2007.

424. Cope D. The sexual history and approach to the patient with sexual dysfunction, UpToDate. 2007.

425. Anantharaman P, Schmidt RJ. Sexual function in chronic kidney disease. *Adv Chro Kidney Dis* 14:2119-2125. 2007.

426. Ottem DP, Carr LK, Perks AE, Lee P, Teichman JMH. Interstitial cystitis and female sexual dysfunction. *Urology*. 2007;69:4608–4610.

427. Shabsigh R, Anastasiades A, Cooper KL, Rutman MP. Female sexual dysfunction, voiding symptoms and depression: common findings in partners of men with erectile dysfunction. *World J Urol*. 2006;24:6653–6656.

428. Verit FF, Verit A, Yeni E. The prevalence of sexual dysfunction and associated risk factors in women with chronic pelvic pain: a crosssectional study. *Arch Gynecol Obstet.* 2006;274:5297–5302.

429. Amato P. Categories of female sexual dysfunction. *Obstet Gynecol Clin North Am.* 2006;33:4527–4534.

430. Gregersen N, Hilmand CB, Jensen PT, Giraldi AGE. Sexual dysfunction in the menopause. Incidence, pharmacological treatment and side effects. *Ugeskrift for Laeger.* 2006;168:6559–6563.

431. Heiman JR. Psychologic treatments for female sexual dysfunction: are they effective and do we need them? *Arch Sex Behav.* 2002;31:5445–5450.

432. Rowland D, Tai W. A review of plant-derived and herbal approaches to the treatment of sexual dysfunctions. *J Sex Marital Ther.* 2003;29:3185–3205.

433. O'Dowd M. *The History of Medications for Women: Materia Medica Woman.* New York: Parthenon Publishing Group; 2001.

434. Aung H. Alternative therapies for male and female sexual dysfunction. *Am J Chin Med.* 2004;32:2161–2173.

435. Jayne C. *An Evidence-Based Review of Herbal Therapies for the Treatment of Female Sexual Dysfunction*; 2006.

436. Ito TY, Trant AS, Polan ML. A double-blind placebo-controlled study of ArginMax, a nutritional supplement for enhancement of female sexual function. *J Sex Marital Ther.* 2001;27(5):541–549.

437. Ito TY, Polan ML, Whipple B, Trant AS. The enhancement of female sexual function with ArginMax, a nutritional supplement, among women differing in menopausal status. *J Sex Marital Ther.* 2006;32(5):369–378.

438. Bottari A, Belcaro G, Ledda A, Luzzi R, Cesarone MR, Dugall M. Lady Prelox® improves sexual function in generally healthy women of reproductive age. *Minerva Ginecol.* 2013, Aug;65(4):435–444.

439. Zava DT, Dollbaum CM, Blen M. Estrogen and progestin bioactivity of foods, herbs, and spices. *Proc Soc Exp Biol Med.* 1998;217(3):369–378.

440. Szewczyk K, Zidorn C. Ethnobotany, phytochemistry, and bioactivity of the genus Turnera (Passifloraceae) with a focus on damiana-Turnera diffusa. *J Ethnopharmacol.* 2014, Mar 28;152(3):424–443.

441. Smith E. Maca root: modern rediscovery of an ancient Andean fertility food. *J Am Herbalists Guild.* 2003;4:215–221.

442. Dording CM, Fisher L, Papakostas G, et al. A double-blind, randomized, pilot dose-finding study of maca root (L. meyenii) for the management of SSRI-induced sexual dysfunction. *CNS Neurosci Ther.* 2008;14(3):182–191.

443. Shin BC, Lee MS, Yang EJ, Lim HS, Ernst E. Maca (L. meyenii) for improving sexual function: a systematic review. *BMC Complement Altern Med.* 2010:1044.

444. Cohen A, Bartlik B. Ginkgo biloba for antidepressant-induced sexual dysfunction. *J Sex Marital Ther.* 1998;24:139–143.

445. Waynberg J, Brewster S. Effects of herbal *** on libido and sexual activity in premenopausal and postmenopausal women. *Adv Ther.* 2000;17:255–262.

446. Meston CM, Rellini AH, Telch MJ. Short- and long-term effects of Ginkgo biloba extract on sexual dysfunction in women. *Arch Sex Behav.* 2008, Aug;37(4):530–547.

447. Maciocia G. *Obstetrics and Gynecology in Chinese Medicine.* London: Churchill Livingstone; 1998.

CHAPTER 7

1. Society NAM. Management of osteoporosis in postmenopausal women: 2006 position statement of the North American Menopause Society. *Menopause.* 2006;13(3):340–367.

2. Lobo R, Kelsey J, Marcus R. *Menopause: Biology and Pathobiology.* San Diego: Academic Press; 2000.

3. Mizra F, Prestwood K. Bone health and aging: implications for menopause. *Endocrinol Metab Clin North Am.* 2004;33:741–759.

4. Mosekilde L, Vestergaard P, Langdahl B. Fracture prevention in postmenopausal women. *BMJ Clin Evid.* 2007;8:1109.

5. Brown J, Josse R. Scientific Advisory Council of the Osteoporosis Society of Canada: clinical practice guidelines for the diagnosis and management of osteoporosis in Canada. *CMAJ.* 2002;167(90100).

6. Nieves J. Osteoporosis: the role of micronutrients. *Am J Clin Nutr.* 2005;81(suppl):1232S–1239S.

7. Fernando G, Martha R, Evangelina R. Consumption of soft drinks with phosphoric acid as a risk factor for the development of hypocalcemia in postmenopausal women. *J Clin Epidemiol.* 1999;52(10):1007.

8. Wyshak G. Teenaged girls, carbonated beverage consumption, and bone fractures. *Arch Pediatr Adolesc Med.* 2000;154(6):610.

9. Kanis J. Assessment of fracture risk and its application to screening for postmenopausal osteoporosis: synopsis of a WHO report: WHO Study Group. *Osteoporos Int.* 1994;4:368–381.

10. Tang BMP, Eslick GD, Nowson C, Smith C, Bensoussan A. Use of calcium or calcium in combination with vitamin D supplementation to prevent fractures and bone loss in people aged 50 years and older: a meta-analysis [see comment]. *Lancet.* 2007;370(9588):657–666.

11. Warensjö, Eva, Liisa Byberg, Håkan Melhus, et al. Dietary Calcium Intake and Risk of Fracture and Osteoporosis: Prospective Longitudinal Cohort Study. *BMJ.* 2011;342:d1473.

12. Lai CY, Yang JY, Rayalam S, Della-Fera MA, Ambati S, Lewis RD, et al. Preventing bone loss and weight gain with combinations of vitamin D and phytochemicals. *J Med Food.* 2011, Nov;14(11):1352–1362.

13. Shuback D. Update in osteoporosis and metabolic bone disorders. *J Clin Endocrinol Metab.* 2007;92(3):747–753.

14. Riggs B, Hodgson S, O'Fallon W. Effects of fluoride treatment on the fracture rate in postmenopausal women with osteoporosis. *NEJM.* 1990;322:802.

15. Eftekhari MH, Rostami ZH, Emami MJ, Tabatabaee HR. Effects of "vitex agnus castus" extract and magnesium supplementation, alone and in combination, on osteogenic and angiogenic factors and fracture healing in women with long bone fracture. *J Res Med Sci. Iran.* 2014;19(1):1–7.

16. Hannan M, Tucker K, Dawson-Hughes B, Cupples L, Felson D, Kiel D. Effect of dietary protein on bone loss in elderly men and women: the Framingham osteoporosis study. *J Bone Miner Res.* 2000;15:2504–2512.

17. Setchell K, Lydeking-Olsen E. Dietary phytoestrogens and their effect on bone: evidence from in vitro and in vivo, human observational, and dietary intervention studies. *Am J Clin Nutr.* 2003;78(suppl):593S–609S.

18. Notoya K, Yoshida K, Taketomi S. Inhibitory effect of ipriflavone on osteoclast-mediated bone resorption and new osteoclast formation in long-term cultures of mouse infractionated bone cells. *Calcif Tissue Int.* 1993;16(suppl):S349.

19. Benvenuti S, Tanini A, Fediani U. Effects of ipriflavone and its metabolites on a clonal osteoblastic cell line. *J Bone Miner Res.* 1991;6:987.

20. Adami S, Bufalino L, Cervetti R. Ipriflavone prevents radial bone loss in postmenopausal women with low bone mass over 2 years. *Osteoporos Int.* 1997;7:119.

21. Valente M, Bufalino L, Castiglione G. Effects of 1-year treatment with ipriflavone on bone in postmenopausal women with low bone mass. *Calcif Tissue Int.* 1994;54:377.

22. Agnusdei D, Crepaldi G, Isaia G. A double-blind placebo-controlled trial of ipriflavone for prevention of postmenopausal spinal bone loss. *Calcif Tissue Int.* 1997;61(S):19.

23. Alexandersen P, Toussaint A, Christiansen C, Devogelaer J. Ipriflavone in the treatment of postmenopausal osteoporosis: a randomized controlled trial. *JAMA.* 2001;285(11):482.

24. Low Dog T. *Women's Health in Complementary and Integrative Medicine: A Clinical Guide.* St. Louis: Elsevier; 2004.

25. Bonaiuti D, Shea B, Iovine R, Negrini S. Exercise for preventing and treating osteoporosis in postmenopausal women (Cochrane review). *The Cochrane Library.* 2003.

26. Kelley G. Aerobic exercise and bone density at the hip in postmenopausal women: a meta-analysis. *Prev Med.* 1998;27:789.

27. Black D, Cummings S, Karpf D. Randomized trial of effect of Alendronate on risk of fracture in women with existing vertebral fractures. *Lancet.* 1996;348:1535.

28. Graham D, Malaty H. Alendronate gastric ulcers. *Alim Pharmacol Therapeut.* 1999;13(4):515.

29. Rico H, Revilla M, Hernandez E. Total and regional bone mineral content and fracture rate in postmenopausal osteoporosis treated with salmon calcitonin: a prospective study. *Calcif Tiss Int.* 1995;56(3):181.

30. Investigators, 2002.

31. Riggs B, Hartmann L. Selective estrogen-receptor modulators—mechanisms of action and application to clinical practice. *NEJM.* 2003;348:618.

32. Clifton-Bligh P, Baber R, Fulcher G, Nery M, Moreton T. The effect of isoflavones extracted from red clover (rimostil) on lipid and bone metabolism. *Menopause.* 2001;8(4):259.

33. Labos G, Trakakis E, Pliatsika P, Augoulea A, Vaggopoulos V, Basios G, et al. Efficacy and safety of DT56a compared to hormone therapy in Greek post-menopausal women. *J Endocrinol Invest.* 2013;36(7):521–526.

34. Shedd-Wise KM, Alekel DL, Hofmann H, et al. The soy isoflavones for reducing bone loss study: 3-yr effects on pQCT bone mineral density and strength measures in postmenopausal women. *J Clin Densitom.* 2011;14(1):47–57.

35. Levis S, Strickman-Stein N, Ganjei-Azar P, Xu P, Doerge DR, Krischer J. Soy isoflavones in the prevention of menopausal bone loss and menopausal symptoms: a randomized, double-blind trial. *Arch Intern Med.* 2011, Aug 8;171(15):1363–1369.

36. Wuttke W, Seidlova-Wuttke D, Gorkow C. The Cimicifuga preparation BNO 1055 vs. conjugated estrogens in a double-blind placebo-controlled study: effects on menopause symptoms and bone markers. *Maturitas.* 2003;44(suppl 1):S67–S77.

37. Nisslein T, Freudenstein J. Effects of an isopropanolic extract of *Cimicifuga racemosa* on urinary crosslinks and other parameters of bone quality in ovariectomized rats. *J Bone Min Metab.* 2003;21(6):370.

38. Seidlova-Wuttke D, Jarry H, Becker T, Christoffel V, Wuttke W. Pharmacology of *Cimicifuga racemosa* extract BNO 1055 in rats: bone, fat, uterus. *Maturitas.* 2003;44(suppl 1):S39.

39. Seidlova-Wuttke D, Stecher G, Kammann M, Haunschild J, Eder N, Stahnke V, et al. Osteoprotective effects of Cimicifuga racemosa and its triterpene-saponins are responsible for reduction of bone marrow fat. *Phytomedicine.* 2012, Jul 15;19(10):855–860.

40. Kolios L, Daub F, Sehmisch S, Frosch KH, Tezval M, Stuermer KM, et al. Absence of positive effect of black cohosh (Cimicifuga racemosa) on fracture healing in osteopenic rodent model. *Phytother Res.* 2010a, Dec;24(12):1796–1806.

41. Kolios L, Schumann J, Sehmisch S, Rack T, Tezval M, Seidlova-Wuttke D, et al. Effects of black cohosh (Cimicifuga racemosa) and estrogen on metaphyseal fracture healing in the early stage of osteoporosis in ovariectomized rats. *Planta Med.* 2010b, Jun;76(9):850–857.

42. Li JX, Liu J, He CC, et al. Triterpenoids from Cimicifugae rhizoma, a novel class of inhibitors on bone resorption and ovariectomy-induced bone loss. *Maturitas.* 2007, Sep 20;58(1):59–69.

43. Wuttke W, Jarry H, Heiden I, et al. Selective estrogen receptor modulator (SERM) activity of the *Cimicifuga racemosa* extract BNO 1055: pharmacology and mechanisms of action. *Phytomedicine.* 2000;7(suppl 2).

44. Avsar U, Karakus E, Halici Z, Bayir Y, Bilen H, Aydin A, et al. Prevention of bone loss by Panax ginseng in a rat model of inflammation-induced bone loss. *Cell Mol Biol (Noisy-le-grand).* 2013;59 SupplOL1835-41.

45. Gong YS, Chen J, Zhang QZ, Zhang JT. Effect of 17beta-oestradiol and ginsenoside on osteoporosis in ovariectomised rats. *J Asian Nat Prod Res.* 2006;8(7):649–656.

46. Li XD, Wang JS, Chang B, Chen B, Guo C, Hou GQ, et al. Panax notoginseng saponins promotes proliferation and osteogenic differentiation of rat bone marrow stromal cells. *J Ethnopharmacol.* 2011, Mar 24;134(2):268–274.

47. Gautam J, Kushwaha P, Swarnkar G, Khedgikar V, Nagar GK, Singh D, et al. EGb 761 promotes osteoblastogenesis, lowers bone marrow adipogenesis and atherosclerotic plaque formation. *Phytomedicine.* 2012, Sep 15;19(12):1134–1142.

48. Lucinda LM, Aarestrup BJ, Peters VM, Reis JE, Oliveira RS, Guerra Mde O. The effect of the Ginkgo biloba extract in the expression of Bax, Bcl-2 and bone mineral content of Wistar rats with glucocorticoid-induced osteoporosis. *Phytother Res.* 2013, Apr;27(4):515–520.

49. Lucinda LM, de Oliveira TT, Salvador PA, Peters VM, Reis JE, Guerra Mde O. Radiographic evidence of mandibular osteoporosis improvement in Wistar rats treated with Ginkgo biloba. *Phytother Res.* 2010b, Feb;24(2):264–267.

50. Lucinda LM, Vieira BJ, Oliveira TT, et al. Evidences of osteoporosis improvement in Wistar rats treated with Ginkgo biloba extract: a histomorphometric study of mandible and femur. *Fitoterapia.* 2010a, Dec;81(8):982–987.

51. Oh SM, Kim HR, Chung KH. Effects of ginkgo biloba on in vitro osteoblast cells and ovariectomized rat osteoclast cells. *Arch Pharm Res.* 2008, Feb;31(2):216–224.

52. Shen CL, Chyu MC, Pence BC, Yeh JK, Zhang Y, Felton CK, et al. Green tea polyphenols supplementation and Tai Chi exercise for postmenopausal osteopenic women: safety and quality of life report. *BMC Complement Altern Med.* 2010:1076.

53. Shen CL, Chyu MC, Yeh JK, Zhang Y, Pence BC, Felton CK, et al. Effect of green tea and Tai Chi on bone health in postmenopausal osteopenic women: a 6-month randomized placebo-controlled trial. *Osteoporos Int.* 2012, May;23(5):1541–1552.

CHAPTER 8

1. Association of Women's Health OANN. *Postmenopausal Health Risks and the Importance Of Prevention (Monograph I)*; 1999. Chicago.

2. National Heart LaBI: International position paper on women's health and menopause: a comprehensive approach, National Institutes of Health.

3. Misra DEThe women's health data book. *a profile of women's health in the United States*. 3rd ed. Washington: DC: Jacobs Institute of Women's Health & the Henry J. Kaiser Family Foundation; 2001.

4. Fitzgerald M, Winland-Brown J. Cardiovascular problems. In: Dunphy L, ed. *Primary Care*. Philadelphia: FA Davis; 2001.

5. North American Menopause Society. Treatment of menopause-associated vasomotor symptoms: position statement of The North American Menopause Society. *Menopause*. 2004;11(1):31–33.

6. Trial TwGftP. Effects of estrogen or estrogen/progestin regimens on heart disease risk factors in postmenopausal women. *JAMA*. 1995;273:199–208.

7. Wynne A, Woo T, Millard M. *Pharmacotherapeutics for nurse practitioner prescribers*. Philadelphia: FA Davis; 2002.

8. Mansi I, Frei CR, Wang CP, Mortensen EM. Statins and new-onset diabetes mellitus and diabetic complications: a retrospective cohort study of US healthy adults. *J Gen Int Med*. http://dx.doi.org/10.1007/s11606-015-3335.

9. Low Dog T. *Women's Health in Complementary and Integrative Medicine: A Clinical Guide*. St. Louis: Elsevier; 2004.

10. Upton R. *American Herbal Pharmacopoeia and Therapeutic Compendium: Black Cohosh*. Santa Cruz: American Herbal Pharmacopoeia; 2002.

11. Mills S, Bone K. *Principles and Practice of Phytotherapy*. London: Churchill Livingstone; 2000.

12. Bone KA. *Clinical Guide to Blending Liquid Herbs: Herbal Formulations for the Individual Patient*. St. Louis: Churchill Livingstone; 2003.

13. Upton R. *American Herbal Pharmacopoeia and Therapeutic Monographs: Cramp Bark*. Santa Cruz: American Herbal Pharmacopoeia; 2000.

14. Upton R. *American Herbal Pharmacopoeia and Therapeutic Compendium: Dang gui Root Angelica sinensis (Oliv.) Diels*. Santa Cruz: AHP; 2003.

15. Thompson Coon J, Ernst ME. Herbs for serum cholesterol reduction: a systematic review. *J Fam Pract*. 2003;52(6):468–478.

16. Blumenthal M. *The complete German Commission E monographs; therapeutic guide to herbal medicines*. Austin: American Botanical Council; 1998.

17. Lawson L. Garlic: a review of its medicinal effects and indicated active compounds. In: Lawson L, Bauer R, eds. *Phytomedicines of Europe: Chemistry and Biological Activity*. Washington, DC: American Chemical Society; 1998:176–209.

18. Rahman K, Lowe GM. Garlic and cardiovascular disease: a critical review. *J Nutr*. 2006;136(3 suppl):736S–740S.

19. Liu L, Yeh Y-Y. S-alk(en)yl cysteines of garlic inhibit cholesterol synthesis by deactivating HMG-CoA reductase in cultured rat hepatocytes. *J Nutr*. 2002;132(6):1129–1134.

20. Yeh YY, Yeh SM. Garlic reduces plasma lipids by inhibiting hepatic cholesterol and triacylglycerol synthesis. *Lipids*. 1994;29(3):189–193.

21. Yeh YY, Liu L. Cholesterol-lowering effect of garlic extracts and organosulfur compounds: human and animal studies. *J Nutr*. 2001;131(3s):989S–993S.

22. Gebhardt R. Multiple inhibitory effects of garlic extracts on cholesterol biosynthesis in hepatocytes. *Lipids*. 1993;28(7):613–619.

23. Gebhardt R. Inhibition of cholesterol biosynthesis by a water-soluble garlic extract in primary cultures of rat hepatocytes. *Arzneimittel-Forschung*. 1991;41(8):800–804.

24. Matsuura H. Saponins in garlic as modifiers of the risk of cardiovascular disease. *J Nutr*. 2001;131(3s):1000S–1005S.

25. Rahman K, Billington D. Dietary supplementation with aged garlic extract inhibits ADP-induced platelet aggregation in humans. *J Nutr*. 2000;130(11):2662–2665.

26. Li L, Sun T, Tian J, Yang K, Yi K, Zhang P. Garlic in clinical practice: an evidence-based overview. *Crit Rev Food Sci Nutr*. 2013;53(7):670–681. England.

27. Stabler SN, Tejani AM, Huynh F, Fowkes C. Garlic for the prevention of cardiovascular morbidity and mortality in hypertensive patients. *Cochrane Database Syst Rev*. 2012;8:CD007653. England.

28. Blumenthal M. *The ABC Clinical Guide to Herbs*. New York: Thieme Press; 2002.

29. Piscitelli S, Burstein A, Welden N. The effect of garlic supplements on the pharmacokinetics of saquinivir. *Clin Infect Dis*. 2002;34(2).

30. ESCOP. *ESCOP Monographs: The Scientific Foundation for Herbal Medicinal Products*. Stuttgart: Thieme; 2003.

31. Kim SY, Seo SK, Choi YM, et al. Effects of red ginseng supplementation on menopausal symptoms and cardiovascular risk factors in postmenopausal women: a double-blind randomized controlled trial. *Menopause*. 2012;19(4):461–466. United States.

32. Mucalo I, Jovanovski E, Rahelić D, Božikov V, Romić Z, Vuksan V. Effect of American ginseng (Panax quinquefolius L.) on arterial stiffness in subjects with type-2 diabetes and concomitant hypertension. *J Ethnopharmacol*. 2013;150(1):148–153. Ireland.

33. Lupattelli G, Marchesi S, Lombardini R, et al. Artichoke juice improves endothelial function in hyperlipemia. *Life Sci*. 2004;76(7):775–782.

34. Thompson Coon JS, Ernst E. Herbs for serum cholesterol reduction: a systematic view. *J Fam Pract*. 2003;52(6):468–478.

35. Ulbricht C, Basch E, Szapary P, et al. Guggul for hyperlipidemia: a review by the Natural Standard Research Collaboration. *Compl Ther Med*. 2005;13(4):279–290.

36. Urizar NL, Moore DD. Gugulipid: a natural cholesterol-lowering agent. *Annu Rev Nutr*. 2003;23:303–313.

37. Abell S, El Tahir K, Hammerly M, Murray M. *Guggul*. Montvale, NJ: Thomson Micromedex; 2004.

38. Upton R. *Hawthorn leaf with flower Crataegus spp*; 1999. Santa Cruz.

39. Hoffmann D. *Medical Herbalism: The Science and Practice of Herbal Medicine*. Rochester, VT: Healing Arts Press; 2003.

40. Mozaffari-Khosravi H, Jalali-Khanabadi BA, Afkhami-Ardekani M, Fatehi F, Noori-Shadkam M. The effects of sour tea (Hibiscus sabdariffa) on hypertension in patients with type II diabetes. *J Hum Hypertens*. 2009;23(1):48–54. England.

41. Evans W. *Trease and Evans' Pharmacognosy*. 14th ed. London: Saunders; 1998.

43. Weiss RF, Fintelmann V. *Herbal Medicine*. 2nd ed. Stuttgart: Thieme; 2000.

44. Bruneton J. *Pharmacognosy: Phytochemistry of Medicinal Plants*. London: Technique and Documentation; 1999.

45. Chedraui P, San Miguel G, Hidalgo L, Morocho N, Ross S. Effect of Trifolium pratense-derived isoflavones on the lipid profile of postmenopausal women with increased body mass index. *Gynecol Endocrinol*. 2008;24(11):620–624. England.

46. Bensky D, Gamble A. *Chinese Herbal Medicine Materia Medica*. Seattle: Eastman Press; 1993.

47. Cheng TO. Danshen: what every cardiologist should know about this Chinese herbal drug. *Int J Cardiol*. 2006;110(3):411–412.

48. Zhou L, Zuo Z, Chow MSS. Danshen: an overview of its chemistry, pharmacology, pharmacokinetics, and clinical use. *J Clin Pharmacol*. 2005;45(12):1345–1359.

49. Oh SH, Cho K-H, Yang B-S, Roh YK. Natural compounds from Danshen suppress the activity of hepatic stellate cells. *Arch Pharmacol Res*. 2006;29(9):762–767.

50. Lam FFY, Yeung JHK, Cheung JHY, Or PMY. Pharmacological evidence for calcium channel inhibition by danshen (*Salvia miltiorrhiza*) on rat isolated femoral artery. *J Cardiovasc Pharmacol*. 2006;47(1):139–145.

51. Lam FY, Ng SCW, Cheung JHY, Yeung JHK. Mechanisms of the vasorelaxant effect of Danshen (*Salvia miltiorrhiza*) in rat knee joints. *J Ethnopharmacol*. 2006;104(3):336–344.

52. Wang W, Hu G-Y, Wang Y-P. Selective modulation of L-type calcium current by magnesium lithospermate B in guinea-pig ventricular myocytes. *Life Sci*. 2006;78(26):2989–2997.

53. Yue KKM, Lee K-W, Chan KKC, Leung KSY, Leung AWN, Cheng CHK. Danshen prevents the occurrence of oxidative stress in the eye and aorta of diabetic rats without affecting the hyperglycemic state. *J Ethnopharmacol*. 2006;106(1):136–141.

54. Zhang M, Li X, Qin G, Liu Y, Zhao X. Effects of Danshen injection on the reserve of tissue plasminogen activator and nitric oxide in endothelium and vasodilatation in diabetic patients. *Zhong Yao Cai*. 2005;28(6):529–532.

55. Hu Z, Yang X, Ho PCL, et al. Herb-drug interactions: a literature review. *Drugs*. 2005;65(9):1239–1282.

56. Chan TY. Interaction between warfarin and danshen (*Salvia miltiorrhiza*). *Ann Pharmacother*. 2001;35(4):501–504.

57. Bailey RL, Fakhouri TH, Park Y, et al. Multivitamin-mineral use is associated with reduced risk of cardiovascular disease mortality among women in the United States. *J Nutr*. 2015;145(3):572–578. United States.

58. Chiuve SE, Fung TT, Rexrode KM, et al. Adherence to a low-risk, healthy lifestyle and risk of sudden cardiac death among women. *JAMA*. 2011;306(1):62–69. United States.

59. Rakel D. *Integrative medicine*. Philadelphia: Saunders; 2003.

60. Ding E, Hutfless S, Ding X, Girota S. Chocolate and the prevention of cardiovascular disease. *Nutr Metab*. 2006;2(2):1–12.

61. Kim JH, Yoon JW, Kim KW, et al. Increased dietary calcium intake is not associated with coronary artery calcification. *Int J Cardiol*. 2012;157(3):429–431. Elsevier.

62. Bolland MJ, Barber PA, Doughty RN, et al. Vascular events in healthy older women receiving calcium supplementation: randomised controlled trial. *BMJ*. 2008;336(7638):262–266. England.

63. Yokoyama M, Origasa H, Matsuzaki M, et al. Effects of eicosapentaenoic acid on major coronary events in hypercholesterolaemic patients (JELIS): a randomised open-label, blinded endpoint analysis. *The Lancet*. 2007;369(9567):1090–1098. Elsevier.

64. Lavie CJ, Dinicolantonio JJ, Milani RV, O'Keefe JH. Vitamin D and cardiovascular health. *Circulation*. 2013;128(22):2404–2406. United States.

65. Gangwisch JE, Rexrode K, Forman JP, Mukamal K, Malaspina D, Feskanich D. Daytime sleepiness and risk of coronary heart disease and stroke: results from the Nurses' Health Study II. *Sleep Med*. 2014;15(7):782–788. Netherlands.

CHAPTER 9

1. Speroff L, Glass R, Kase G. *Clinical Gynecologic Endocrinology and Infertility*. Baltimore: Lippincott Williams & Wilkins; 1999.

2. Shuttle P, Redgrove P. *The Wise Wound: The Myths, Realities, and Meanings of Menstruation*. New York: Grove Press; 1986.

3. Green M. *The Trotula: An English Translation of the Medieval Compendium of Women's Medicine*. Philadelphia: University of Pennsylvania Press; 2002.

4. Secundus Plinius C. *Historia Naturalis*. Carbondale, IL: Southern Illinois University Press; 1962.

5. Achterberg J. *Woman as Healer*. Boston: Shambhala; 1990.

6. Bennett J. *Lilies of the Hearth: The Historical Relationship Between Women and Plants. Willowdale*. Ontario: Camden House; 1991.

7. Baker S. Menstruation and Related Problems and Concerns. In: Youngkin E, Davis M, eds. *Women's Health: A Primary Care Clinical Guide*. Stamford, CT: Appleton & Lange; 1998:140–160.

8. Trickey R. *Women, Hormones, and the Menstrual Cycle*. St. Leonards, Australia: Allen and Unwin; 1998.

9. Marianne E, McPherson B, Korfine L. Menstruation across time: menarche, menstrual attitudes, experiences, and behaviors. *Women's Health Issues*. 2004;14:193–200.

10. Kridli A-O. Health Beliefs and Practices Among Arab Women. *MSN*. 2002;27(3):278–303.

11. Harlow S. Menstruation and Menstrual Disorders. In: Goldman M, Hatch M, eds. *Women and Health*. San Diego: Academic Press; 2000.

12. Solomon C, Hu F, Dunaif A, et al. Long or highly irregular menstrual cycles as a marker for risk of type 2 diabetes mellitus. *JAMA*. 2001;286(19):2421–2426.

13. Goldman M, Hatch C. *Women and Health*. San Diego: Academic Press; 2000.

14. Youngkin E, Davis M. *Women's Health: A Primary Care Clinical Guide*. Stamford: Appleton & Lange; 1998.

15. Harmon K. Evaluating and treating exercise-related menstrual irregularities. *Phys Sports Med*. 2002;30:35–39.

16. Kaunitz A. Menstruation: choosing whether and when. *Contraception*. 2000;62:277–284.

17. McLean J, Barr S. Research report: cognitive dietary restraint is associated with eating behaviors, lifestyle practices, personality characteristics and menstrual irregularity in college women. *Appetite*. 2003;40:185–192.

18. Lebenstedt M, Platte P, Pirke K. Reduced resting metabolic rate in athletes with menstrual disorders. *Med Sci Sports Exerc*. 1999;31(9):1250–1256.

19. Manore M. Dietary recommendations and athletic menstrual dysfunction. *Sports Med*. 2002;32(14):87–90.

20. Eliakim A, Beyth Y. Exercise training, menstrual irregularities and bone development in children and adolescents. *J Pediatr Adolesc Gynecol*. 2003;16(4):201–206.

21. Koebnick C, Strassner C, Hoffmann I, et al. Consequences of a long-term raw food diet on body weight and menstruation: results of a questionnaire survey. *Ann Nutr Metab.* 1999;43(2):69–79.

22. Barr SI. Vegetarianism and menstrual cycle disturbances: is there an association? *Am J Clin Nutr.* 1999;70(suppl): 549S–554S.

23. Balbi C, Musone R. Influence of menstrual factors and dietary habits on menstrual pain in adolescence age. *Eur J Obstet Gynecol Reprod Biol.* 2000;91(2):143–148.

24. Douchi T, Kuwahata R, Yamamoto S, et al. Relationship of upper body obesity to menstrual disorders. *Acta Obstet Gynecol Scand.* 2002;81(2):147.

25. Fujiwara T. Skipping breakfast is associated with dysmenorrhea in young women in Japan. *Int J Food Sci Nutr.* 2003;54(6):505–509.

26. Beals K, Manore M. Behavioral, psychological, and physical characteristics of female athletes with subclinical eating disorders. *Int J Sport Nutr Exerc Metab.* 2000;10(2):128–143.

27. Beals K. Eating behaviors, nutritional status, and menstrual function in elite female adolescent volleyball players. *J Am Diet Assoc.* 2002;102(9):1293–1296.

28. Newton T, Philhower C. Socioemotional correlates of self-reported menstrual cycle irregularity in premenopausal women. *Psychosomat Med.* 2003;65:1065–1069.

29. Loucks AL, Thuma JT. Luteinizing hormone pulsatility is disrupted at a threshold of energy availability in regularly menstruating women. *J Clin Endocrinol Metab.* 2003;88(1):297–311.

30. Klebanoff N. *Menstrual synchronization.* Denton, Texas: Texas Woman's University; 1994.

31. Harlow S, Campbell B. Ethnic differences in the duration and amount of menstrual bleeding during the postmenarchal period. *Am J Epidemiol.* 1996;144(110):980–988.

32. Low Dog T. *Women's Health in Complementary and Integrative Medicine: A Clinical Guide.* St. Louis: Elsevier; 2004.

33. Tampons, Asbestos D, Toxic Shock Syndrome. http://www.fda.gov/cdrh/consumer/tamponsabs.html. accessed May 10, 2007.

34. Smith C, Noble V, Bensch R, et al. Bacterial flora of the vagina during the menstrual cycle: findings in users of tampons, napkins, and sea sponges. *Ann Intern Med.* 1982;96(6 Pt 2):948–951.

35. Friedman E. Menstrual and lunar cycles. *Am J Obstet Gynecol.* 1981;140(3):350.

36. Hillard P. Menstruation in young girls: a clinical perspective. *Obstet Gynecol.* 2002;4(99):655–662.

37. Ostrzens A. *Gynecology: Integrating Conventional, Complementary, and Natural Alternative Therapy.* Philadelphia: Lippincott Williams & Wilkins; 2002.

38. Goldman M, Hatch C. *Women and Health.* San Diego: Academic Press; 2000.

39. Kuczynski A. *Teenage magazines mostly reject breast enlargements ads.* The New York Times; August 13, 2001. C1.

40. Gardiner P, Conboy L, Kemper K. Herbs and adolescent girls: avoiding the hazards of self-treatment. *Contemp Pediatr.* March 1 2000.

41. Braun C, Halcon L, Bearinger L. Adolescent use of alternative and complementary therapies. *J Holistic Nurs.* 2000;18(2): 176–191.

42. Wilson K, Klein J. Adolescents' use of complementary and alternative medicine. *Ambul Pediatr.* 2002;2(2):104–110.

43. McKenna D, Jones K, Hughes K, et al. *Botanical Medicines: The Desk Reference for Major Herbal Supplements.* New York: Haworth Press; 2002.

44. Blumenthal M. *The Complete German Commission E Monographs: Therapeutic Guide to Herbal Medicine.* Boston: American Botanical Council; 1998.

45. Rosblatt M, Ziment I. *Evidence-Based Herbal Medicine.* Philadelphia: Hanley and Belfus; 2002.

46. Bone K. *Clinical Applications of Ayurvedic and Chinese Herbs.* Queensland, Australia: Phytotherapy Press; 2000.

47. Low Dog T. Premenstrual Syndrome. *An Integrative Approach to Women's Health.* Albuquerque: Integrative Medicine Education Associates; 2000.

48. McGuffin M, Hobbs C, Upton R, et al. Boca Raton: CRC Press; 1997.

49. Upton R. *American Herbal Pharmacopoeia and Therapeutic Compendium: Cramp Bark.* Santa Cruz: American Herbal Pharmacopoeia; 2000.

50. Low Dog T. *Dysmenorrhea. An Integrative Approach to Women's Health.* Albuquerque: Integrative Medicine Education Associates; 2000.

51. Upton R. *American Herbal Pharmacopoeia and Therapeutic Compendium: Black Cohosh.* Santa Cruz: American Herbal Pharmacopoeia; 2002.

52. Mills S, Bone K. *Principles and Practice of Phytotherapy.* London: Churchill Livingstone; 2000.

53. Lithgow D, Politzer W. Vitamin A in the treatment of menorrhagia. *South African Medical Journal.* 1997;51(7):191–193.

54. Hanna S, Sharma J, Klotz J. Acne vulgaris: more than skin deep. *Dermatol Online J.* 2003;9(3).

55. Lee D, Van Dyke G, Kim J. Update on pathogenesis and treatment of acne. *Current Opin Pediatr.* 2003;15(4):405–410.

56. Berson D, Chalker D, Harper J, et al. Current concepts in the treatment of acne. *Cutis.* 2003;72(suppl 1):5–13.

57. Baldwin H. The interaction between acne vulgaris and the psyche. *Cutis.* 2002;70(2):133–139.

58. Rudy S. Overview of the evaluation and management of acne vulgaris. *Pediatr Nurs.* 2003;29(4):287–293.

59. Krowchuk D, Stancin T, Keskinen R, et al. The psychosocial effects of acne on adolescents. *Pediatr Dermatol.* 1991;8(4):332–338.

60. Atkan S, Ozmen E, Sanli B. Anxiety, depression, and nature of acne vulgaris in adolescents. *Int J Dermatol.* 2000;39(5):274–279. May.

61. Tan J, Vasey K, Fung K. Attitudes of female patients regarding oral contraceptives. *J Cutan Med Surg.* 2001;5(6):471–474.

62. Bergfeld W. A lifetime of healthy skin: implications for women. *Int J Fertil Women's Med.* 1999;44(2):93–95.

63. Gouden V, Stables G, Cunliffe W. Prevalence of facial acne in adults. *J Am Acad Dermatol.* 1999;41(4):577–580.

64. Thiboutot DF. New treatments and therapeutic strategies for acne. *Arch Fam Med.* 2000;9:179–187.

65. Ostrzens A. *Gynecology: Integrating Conventional, Complementary, and Natural Alternative Therapy.* Philadelphia: Lippincott Williams & Wilkins; 2002.

66. Rakel D. *Integrative Medicine.* Philadelphia: Saunders; 2003.

67. Hull S. Acne vulgaris and acne rosacea. In: Rakel D, ed. *Integrative Medicine.* Philadelphia: Saunders; 2003.

68. Poli F, Dreno B, Verschoore M. An epidemiological study of acne in female adults: results from France. *J Euro Dermatol Venereol.* 2001;15(6):541–545.

69. Chiu A, Chon S, Kimball A. The response of skin disease to stress: changes in the severity of acne affected by examination stress. *Arch Dermatol.* 2003;139(7):897–900.

70. Redmond G. Androgens and women's health. *Int J Fertil Women's Med.* 1998;43(2):81–97.

71. Derman R. Androgen excess in women. *Int J Fertil Menopausal Stud.* 1996;41(2):172–176.

72. Krowchuk D, Lucky A. Managing adolescent acne. *Adolesc Med.* 2001;12(2):ii355–ii374.

73. Leyden J. A review of the use of combination therapies for the treatment of acne. *J Am Acad Dermatol.* 2003;49(suppl 3):S200–S210.

74. Larsen T, Jemec G. Acne: comparing hormonal approaches to antibiotics. *Expert Opin Pharmacother.* 2003;4(7):1097–1103.

75. Fouladi RF. Aqueous extract of dried fruit of Berberis vulgaris L. in acne vulgaris, a clinical trial. *J Diet Suppl.* 2012, Dec;9(4):253–261.

76. Felter H, Lloyd J. *King's American Dispensatory.* Cincinnati: 1898, reprinted by Eclectic Medical Publications; 1983.

77. Wichtl M. *Herbal Drugs and Phytopharmaceuticals: A Handbook for Practice on a Scientific Basis.* 4th ed. Stuttgart: Medpharm; 2004.

78. Hoffmann D. *Medical Herbalism: The Science and Practice of Herbal Medicine.* Rochester, VT: Healing Arts Press; 2003.

79. Burgess N. Calendula officinalis. *Modern Phytotherapist.* 1995;1(3):11–13.

80. Bone K. *A Clinical Guide to Blending Liquid Herbs: Herbal Formulations for the Individual Patient.* St. Louis: Churchill Livingstone; 2003.

81. Gardiner P. Calendula (Calendula officinalis). http://www.children'shospital.org/holistic/. accessed Nov, 2003.

82. Morgan M. Chamomile from a clinical perspective. *Modern Phytother.* 1996;3(1):19–21.

83. Low Dog T. The Integumentary System. *Foundations in Herbal Medicine.* Albuquerque: Foundations in Herbal Medicine; 2001.

84. Romm A. J. T. Vitex agnus castus: Survey of the American Herbalists Guild. *JAHG.* 2001;12(2):27–31.

85. Upton R. *American Herbal Pharmacopoeia and Therapeutic Monographs: Ashwagandha Root.* Santa Cruz: American Herbal Pharmacopoeia; 2000.

86. Giss G. *Rothenburg W Z Haut Geschlechtsler.* 1968;43(1 5):645–647.

87. Gardiner P. Dandelion (Taraxacum officinalis). http://www.children'shospital.org/holistic/. accessed Nov, 2003.

88. Sharma M, Schoop R, Suter A, Hudson JB. The potential use of Echinacea in acne: control of Propionibacterium acnes growth and inflammation. *Phytother Res.* 2011, Apr;25(4):517–521.

89. Thappa D, Dogra J. Nodulocystic acne: oral gugulipid versus tetracycline. *J Dermatol.* 1994;21(10):729–731.

90. Basch E, Ulbricht C. *Natural Standard Herb and Supplement Handbook.* St. Louis: Mosby; 2005.

91. Bone K. Licorice: the universal herb Part 1. *MediHerb Professional Review.* April 1989;10.

92. European Scientific Cooperative on Phytotherapy E. *Monographs on the Medicinal Uses of Plant Drugs: Hamameils folium.* New York: Thieme; 2003.

93. Brown D, Dattner A. Phytotherapeutic approaches to common dermatologic conditions. *Archives of Dermatology.* 1998;134(11):1401–1404.

94. Bone K. Oregon grape and acne. *MediHerb Professional Monitor.* 1996;19:4.

95. AltMedDex: AltMedDex(TM) Protocols: ACNE.

96. Dattner A. From medical herbalism to phytotherapy in dermatology: back to the future. *Dermatol Ther.* 2003;16(2):106–113.

97. Kraft K, Hobbs C. *Pocket Guide to Herbal Medicine.* Stuttgart: Thieme; 2004.

98. Mitchell W. *Plant Medicine in Practice: Using the Teachings of John Bastyr.* St. Louis: Churchill Livingstone; 2004.

99. Bassett I, Pannowitz D, Barnetson R. A comparative study of tea-tree oil versus benzoyl peroxide in the treatment of acne. *Med J Austr.* 1990;153:455–458.

100. Enshaieh S, Jooya A, Siadat AH, Iraji F. The efficacy of 5% topical tea tree oil gel in mild to moderate acne vulgaris: a randomized, double-blind placebo-controlled study. *Indian J Dermatol Venereol Leprol.* 2007;73(1):22–25.

101. Kohani R. Acne. In: Kohatsu W, ed. *Complementary and Alternative Medicine Secrets.* Philadelphia: Hanley and Belfus; 2002.

102. Yarnell E, Abascal K, Hooper C. *Clinical Botanical Medicine.* Larchmont, NY: Mary Ann Liebert Publishers; 2003.

103. Evans W. *Trease and Evans' Pharmacognosy.* 14th ed. London: WB Saunders; 1998.

104. He Z, Wang D, Shi L, et al. Treating amenorrhea in vital energy-deficient patients. *J Trad Chin Med.* 1986;6(3):187–190.

105. Yamada K, Kanba S, Yagi G, et al. Herbal Medicine (Shakuyaku-kanzo-to) in the Treatment of Risperidone-Induced Amenorrhea. *J Clin Psychopharmacol.* 1999;19:380–381.

106. Ciganda C, Laborde A. Herbal infusions used for induced abortion. *J Toxicol Clin Toxicol.* 2003;41(3):235–239.

107. Brinker F. Blue cohosh. *JAHG.* 2001;2(2):4–8.

108. Felter H. The Eclectic Materia Medica. *Pharmacology and Therapeutics.* Cincinatti: Electic Medical Publications; 1922.

109. McFarlin B, Gibson M, O'Rear J, et al. A national survey of herbal preparation use by nurse-midwives for labor stimulation. Review of the literature and recommendations for practice. *J Nurse Midwif.* 1999;44:205–216.

110. Betz J, Andrzejewski D, Troy A, et al. Gas chromatographic determination of toxic quinolizidine alkaloids in blue cohosh Caulophyllum thalictroides (L.) Michx. *Phytochem Anal.* 1998;9:232–236.

111. Kennylly E, Flynn T, Mazzola E, et al. Detecting potential teratogenic alkaloids from blue cohosh rhizomes using and in vitro rat embryo culture. *J Nat Prod.* 1999;62(10):1385–1389.

112. Romm A, Treasure J. AHG Professional Member Botanical Therapeutics Survey: vitex agnus castus. *JAHG.* 2001;2(2):27–31.

113. AltMedDex. *AltMedDex(TM) Protocols: Amenorrhea*; 2004.

114. Petersen FJ. *Materia Medica and Clinical Therapeutics.* Los Olivos, CA: F. J. Petersen; 1905.

115. (BHMA) BHMA. *British Herbal Pharmacopoeia.* Keighley, UK: British Herbal Medicine Association; 1983.

116. AltMedDex. *AltMedDex(TM) Protocols: Gossypol*; 2003.

117. Nath D, Sethi N, Srivastava S, et al. Teratogenic evaluation of an indigenous antifertility medicinal plant Gossypium herbaceum in rat. *Fitoterapia.* 1997;68(2):137–139.

118. Upton R. *American Herbal Pharmacopoeia and Therapeutic Compendium: Dang gui Root Angelica sinensis (Oliv.) Diels.* Santa Cruz: AHP; 2003.

119. (ESCOP) ESCoP. *ESCOP Monographs: The Scientific Foundation for Herbal Medicinal Products.* Stuttgart: Thieme; 2003.

120. Blumenthal M. *The ABC Clinical Guide to Herbs.* Austin: American Botanical Council; 2003.

121. Weiss RF, Fintelmann V. *Herbal Medicine.* 2nd ed. Stuttgart: Thieme; 2000.

122. Ellingwood F. Cincinnati: Eclectic Medical Publications; 1919.

123. O'Dowd M. *The History of Medications for Women: Materia Medica Woman.* New York: Parthenon Publishing Group; 2001.

124. Bruneton J. *Pharmacognosy: Phytochemistry of Medicinal Plants.* London: Technique and Documentation; 1999.

125. Gladstar R. *Herbal Healing for Women.* New York: Simon and Schuster; 1993.

126. Upton R. *American Herbal Pharmacopoeia and Therapeutic Compendium: Schisandra berry.* Santa Cruz: American Herbal Pharmacopoeia; 1999.

127. Bensky D, Gamble A. *Chinese Herbal Medicine Materia Medica.* Seattle: Eastman Press; 1993.

128. Yuan HN, Wang CY, Sze CW, Tong Y, Tan QR, Feng XJ, et al. A randomized, crossover comparison of herbal medicine and bromocriptine against risperidone-induced hyperprolactinemia in patients with schizophrenia. *J Clin Psychopharmacol.* 2008, Jun;28(3):264–370.

129. Brinker F. A comparative review of eclectic female regulators. *J Naturopath Med.* 1997;7(1):21–26.

130. Ostad SN, Soodi M, Shariffzadeh M, et al. The effect of fennel essential oil on uterine contraction as a model for dysmenorrhea, pharmacology and toxicology study. *J Ethnopharmacol.* 2001;76:299–304.

131. AltMedDex. AltMedDex(TM) Protocols: Dysmenorrhea, 2004.

132. Aksoy AN, Gözükara I, Kabil Kucur S. Evaluation of the efficacy of Fructus agni casti in women with severe primary dysmenorrhea: a prospective comparative Doppler study. *J Obstet Gynaecol Res.* 2014;40(3):779–784. Australia.

133. Upton R. *American Herbal Pharmacopoeia and Therapeutic Monographs: Black Haw.* Santa Cruz, Ca: American Herbal Pharmacopoeia; 2000.

134. Beretz A, Briançon-Scheid F, Stierlé A, Corre G, Anton R, Cazenave J. Inhibition of human platelet cyclic AMP phosphodiesterase and of platelet aggregation by a hemisynthetic flavonoid, amentoflavone hexaacetate. *Biochem Pharmacol.* 1986;35(2):257–262.

135. Du J, Bai B, Kuang X, Yu Y, Wang C, Ke Y, et al. Ligustilide inhibits spontaneous and agonists- or K+ depolarization-induced contraction of rat uterus. *J Ethnopharmacol.* 2006, Nov 3;108(1):54–58.

136. Tanaka S, Kano Y, Tabata M, et al. Effects of "toki" (Angelica acutiloba) extracts on writhing and capillary permeability in mice (analgesic and anti-inflammatory effects). *Yakugaku Zassh.* 1971;91:1098–1104.

137. Harada M, Suzuki M, Ozake Y. Effect of Japanese Angelica root and Peony root in uterine contraction in the rabbit in situ. *J Pharm Dyn.* 1984;7:304–311.

138. Yoshiro K. The physiologic actions of Tang Kuei and Cnidium. *Bull Oriental Healing Arts Inst.* 1985;10:269–278.

139. Zhu D. Dong Quai. *Am J Chinese Med Am J Chinese Med.* 1987;15(3-4):117–125.

140. Namavar J, Tartifizadeh A, Khabnadideh S. Comparison of fennel and mefenamic acid for the treatment of primary dysmenorrhea. *Int J Gynecol Obstet.* 2003;80:153–157.

141. Ghodsi Z, Asltoghiri M. The effect of fennel on pain quality, symptoms, and menstrual duration in primary dysmenorrhea. *J Pediatr Adolesc Gynecol.* 2014;27(5):283–286. United States.

142. Choi E, Hwang J. Antiinflammatory, analgesic and antioxidant activities of the fruit of Foeniculum vulgare. *Fitoterapia.* 2004;75(6):557–565.

143. Locock R. Fennel. *Can Pharm J.* 1994;126(10):503–504.

144. Younesy S, Amiraliakbari S, Esmaeili S, Alavimajd H, Nouraei S. Effects of fenugreek seed on the severity and systemic symptoms of dysmenorrhea. *J Reprod Infertil.* 2014;15(1):41–48. Iran.

145. Jenabi E. The effect of ginger for relieving of primary dysmenorrhoea. *J Pak Med Assoc.* 2013, Jan;63(1):8–10.

146. Halder A. Effect of progressive muscle relaxation versus intake of ginger powder on dysmenorrhoea amongst the nursing students in Pune. *Nurs J India.* 2012;103(4):152–156.

147. Rahnama P, Montazeri A, Huseini HF, Kianbakht S, Naseri M. Effect of Zingiber officinale R. rhizomes (ginger) on pain relief in primary dysmenorrhea: a placebo randomized trial. *BMC Complement Altern Med.* 2012:1292.

148. Ozgoli G, Goli M, Moattar F. Comparison of effects of ginger, mefenamic acid, and ibuprofen on pain in women with primary dysmenorrhea. *J Altern Complement Med.* 2009, Feb;15(2):129–132.

149. Imai A, Horibe S, Fuseya S, et al. Possible evidence that the herbal medicine shakuyaku-kanzo-to decreases prostaglandin levels through suppressing arachidonate turnover in endometrium. *J Med.* 1995;26(3-4):163–174.

150. Hsieh L, Suen H, Lee S. The effect of I-mu-ts'ao on a partially purified prostaglandin E 9-ketoreductase from swine kidney. *Proc Natl Sci Counc Repub China.* 1985;9(3):197–201.

151. Lee C, Jiang L, Shang H, et al. Prehispanolone, a novel platelet activating factor receptor antagonist from Leonurus heterophyllus. *Br J Pharmacol.* 1991;103(3):1719–1724.

152. Isaev L, Bojadzieva M. Obtaining Galenic and neogalenic preparations and experiments on the isolation of active substances from Leonurus cardiaca. *Nauchni Tr Visshiya Med Inst Sofiya.* 1960;37(5):145–152.

153. Shi M, Chang L, He G. Stimulating action of Carthamus tinctorius L., Angelica sinensis (Oliv.) Diels and Leonurus sibiricus L. on the uterus. *Zhongguo Zhong Yao Za Zhi.* 1995;20(3):173–175.

154. Bird GW, Wingham J. Anti-Cad lectin from the seeds of Leonurus cardiaca. *Clin Lab Haematol.* 1979;1(1):57–59.

155. Senatore F. Sterols from Leonurus cardiaca L., growing in different geographical areas. *Herba Pol.* 1991;37:3–7.

156. Gulubov A. Structure of alkaloids from Leonurus cardiaca. *Khim Biol.* 1970;8:129–132.

157. Weinges K. Natural products from medicinal plants, XVIII, Isolation and structure elucidation of a new c15-irodoid glucoside from Leonurus cardiaca. *Justus Liebigs Ann Chem.* 1973;4:566–572.

158. Kong Y, Yeung H, Cheung Y, et al. Isolation of the uterotonic principle from Leonurus artemisia, the Chinese motherwort. *Am J Chin Med.* 1976;4(4):373–382.

159. Cheng K, Yip C, Yeung H, et al. Leonurine, and improved synthesis. *Experientia.* 1979;35(5):571–572.

160. Kartnig T. Flavinoid-O-Glycosides form the herbs of Leonurus cardiaca. *J Nat Prod.* 1985;48:494–507.

161. Sakamoto S, Kudo H, Kawasaki T, et al. Effects of a Chinese herbal medicine, keishi-bukuryo-gan, on the gonadal system of rats. *J Ethnopharmacol.* 1988;23(2):51–158.

162. Mirabi P, Dolatian M, Mojab F, Majd HA. Effects of valerian on the severity and systemic manifestations of dysmenorrhea. *Int J Gynaecol Obstet.* 2011, Dec;115(3):285–288.

163. Hoerhammer L. Flavone concentration of medicinal plants with regard to their spasmolytic action. *Chem Abstr.* 1988;61(19):578–588.

164. Petcu P, Andoronescu E, Gheorheci V, et al. Treatment of juvenile meno-metrorrhagia with Alchemilla vulgaris fluid extract. *Clucul Med.* 1979;52(3):266–267.

165. Hosseinlou A, Alinejad V, Alinejad M, Aghakhani N. The effects of fish oil capsules and vitamin B1 tablets on duration and severity of dysmenorrhea in students of high school in Urmia-Iran. *Glob J Health Sci.* 2014;6(7 Spec No):124–129. Canada.

166. Moghadamnia AA, Mirhosseini N, Abadi MH, Omranirad A, Omidvar S. Effect of Clupeonella grimmi (anchovy/kilka) fish oil on dysmenorrhoea. *East Mediterr Health J.* 2010, Apr;16(4):408–413.

167. Lasco A, Catalano A, Benvenga S. Improvement of primary dysmenorrhea caused by a single oral dose of vitamin D: results of a randomized, double-blind, placebo-controlled study. *Archives of internal medicine.* 2012;172(4):366–367.

168. Han SH, Hur MH, Buckle J, Choi J, Lee MS. Effect of aromatherapy on symptoms of dysmenorrhea in college students: a randomized placebo-controlled clinical trial. *J Altern Complement Med.* 2006;12(6):535–541.

169. Raisi Dehkordi Z, Hosseini Baharanchi FS, Bekhradi R. Effect of lavender inhalation on the symptoms of primary dysmenorrhea and the amount of menstrual bleeding: a randomized clinical trial. *Complement Ther Med.* 2014;22(2):212–219. Scotland.

170. Rapkin A. A review of treatment of premenstrual syndrome & premenstrual dysphoric disorder. *Psychoneuroendocrinology.* 2003;28:39–53.

171. ACOG Practice Bulletin 15, Premenstrual Syndrome, *Obst & Gyn.* 2000;95(15):1–9.

172. Stevinson C, Ernst E. Complementary/alternative therapies for premenstrual syndrome: a systematic review of randomized controlled trials. *AJOG.* 2001;185(1):227–235.

173. Girman A, Lee R, Kligler B. An integrative medicine approach to premenstrual syndrome. *Am J Obstet Gynecol.* 2003;188(5):56–65.

174. Steiner M. Premenstrual syndrome and premenstrual dysphoric disorder: guidelines for management. *J Psychiatry Neurosci.* 2000;25(5):459–468.

175. Steiner M. Premenstrual dysphoric disorder. An update. *Gen Hosp Psychiatry.* 1996;18(4):244–250.

176. Association AP. *Diagnostic and Statistical Manual of Mental Disorders.* 4th ed. Arlington: American Psychiatric Association; 1994.

177. Chrousos G, Torpy D, Gold P. Interactions between the hypothalamic-pituitary-adrenal axis and the female reproductive system: clinical implications. *Ann Intern Med.* 1998;129:229–240.

178. Reid R, Yen S. Premenstrual syndrome. *Am J Obstet Gynecol.* 1981;139:85–104.

179. Lurie S, Borenstein R. The premenstrual syndrome. *Obst Gyn Surv.* 1990;45(4):220–228.

180. Shaugn O'Brien P, Symonds E. Prolactin levels in the premenstrual syndrome. *Br J Obstet Gyn.* 1982;89:306–308.

181. Shaw S, Wyatt K, Thompson J, et al. Vitex agnus castus for premenstrual syndrome. *The Cochrane Database of Systematic Reviews.* 2005;1.

182. D'Amico J, Greendale G, Lu J. Induction of hypthalamic opioid activity with transdermal estradiol administration in postmenopausal women. *Fertil Steril.* 1991;55:754–758.

183. Morissette M, Lévesque D, Di Piaolo T. Effect of chronic estradiol treatment on brain dopamine receptor reappearance after irreversible blockade: an autoradiographic study. *Mol Pharmacol.* 1992;42:480–488.

184. Bethea C, Lu N, Gundlah C. Diverse actions of ovarian steroids in the serotonin neural system. *Front Neuroendocrinol.* 2002;23(1):41–100.

185. Arpels J. The female brain hypoestrogenic continuum from the premenstrual syndrome to menopause: a hypothesis and review of supporting data. *J Reprod Med.* 1996;41:633–639.

186. Boyd R, Amsterdam J. Mood disorders in women from adolescence to late life: an overview. *Obstetrics Andgynecology.* 2004;47(3):515–526.

187. Halbreich U, Bergeron R, Yonkers K, et al. Efficacy of intermittent, luteal phase sertraline treatment of premenstrual dysphoric disorder. *Obstetrics & Gynecology.* 2002;100(6):1219–1230.

188. Kessel B. Premenstrual syndrome. Advances in diagnosis and treatment. *Obstet Gynecol Clin North Am.* 2000;27(3):625–639.

189. Hammerback S, Damer J, Backstrom T. Relationship between symptom severity and hormone changes in women with premenstrual syndrome. *J Clin Endocr Metab.* 1989;125-30:125–130.

190. Dalton K. The aetiology of premenstrual syndrome is with the progesterone receptors. *Med Hypotheses.* 1990;31:323–327.

191. Roca C, Schmidt P, Altemus M, et al. Differential menstrual cycle regulation of hypothalamic-pituitary-adrenal axis in women with premenstrual syndrome and controls. *J Clin Endocrinol Metab.* 2003;88(7):3057–3063.

192. Freeman E, Frye C, Rickels K, et al. Allopregnenalone levels and symptom improvement in severe premenstrual syndrome. *J Clin Psychopharmacol.* 2002;22(5):516–520.

193. Symonds C, Gallagher P, Thompson J, et al. Effects of the menstrual cycle on mood, neurocognitive, and neuroendocrine function in health premenopausal women. *Psychol Med.* 2004;34(1):93–102.

194. Halbreich U. Premenstrual syndromes: closing the 20th century chapters. *Curr Opin Obstet Gynecol.* 1999;11(3):265–270.

195. Gottheil M, Steinberg R, Granger L. An exploration of the clinician's diagnostic approaches to PMS symptomatology. *Can J Behav Sci.* 1999;31(4):254–262.

196. Steiner M, Born L. Diagnosis and treatment of premenstrual dysphoric disorder: an update. *Int Clin Psychopharmacol Supp.* 2000;1(3):15–17.

197. Nogueira Pires M, Calil H. Clinical utility of the premenstrual assessment form as an instrument auxiliary to the diagnosis of premenstrual dysphoric disorder. *Psychiatry Res.* 2000;94(3):211–219.

198. Backstrom T, Hansson-Malmstrom Y, Lindhe B. Oral contraceptives in premenstrual syndrome: a randomised comparison of triphasic and monophasic preparations. *Contraception.* 1992;46(3):253–268.

199. Watts J, Butt W, Edwards R. A clinical trial using danazol for the treatment of premenstrual tension. *Br J Obstet Gynaecol.* 1987;94:30–34.

200. Halbreich U, Rojansky N, Palter S. Elimination of ovulation and menstrual cyclicity (with danazol) improves dysphoric premenstrual syndromes. *Fertil Steril.* 1991;56:1066–1099.

201. Mortolla J, Girton L, Fischer U. Successful treatment of severe premenstrual syndrome by combined use of gonadotrophin releasing hormone agonist and estrogen/progestin. *J Clin Endocrinol Metab*. 1991;72(2). 252A–252F.

202. West C, Hillier H. Ovarian suppression with the gonadotropin-releasing hormone agonist goserelin (Zoladex): in management of the premenstrual tension syndrome. *Hum Reprod*. 1994;9:1058–1063.

203. Mira M, McNeil D, Fraser I. Mefenamic acid in the treatment of premenstrual syndrome. *Obstet Gynecol*. 1986;68(3):395–398.

204. Thomas J, ed. *Australian Prescription Products Guide*. Hawthorn, Australia: Australian Pharmaceutical Publishing Company Ltd; 1995.

205. Carr R, Ensom M. Fluoxetine in the treatment of premenstrual dysphoric disorder. *Ann Pharmacother*. 2002;36(4):713–717.

206. Freeman E, Jabara S, Sondheimer S. Citalopram in PMS patients with prior SSRI treatment failure: a preliminary study. *J Women's Health Gend Based Med*. 2002;11(5):459–464.

207. Freeman E, Rickels K, Yonkers K. Venlafaxine in the treatment of premenstrual dysphoric disorder. *Obstet Gynecol*. 2001;98(5 Pt 1):737–744.

208. Redei E, Freeman E. Preliminary evidence for plasma adrenocorticotropin levels as biological correlates of premenstrual symptoms. *Acta Endocrinol (Copenh)*. 1993;128(6):536–542.

209. Daiber W. Climacteric complaints: success without using hormones! *Arztl Prax*. 1985;35(65):1946–1947.

210. Vorberg G. Treatment of menopausal complaints. *Z Allgeinmed*. 1984;60(13):626–629.

211. Stoll W. Phytopharmacon influences atrophic vaginal epithelium. Double-blind study—Cimicifuga vs estrogenic substances. *Therapeutikon*. 1987;1:23–31.

212. Lehmann-Willenbrock E, Riedel H. Clinical and endocrinologic examinations concerning therapy of climacteric symptoms following hysterectomy with remaining ovaries. *Zent Bl Gynakol*. 1988;110(611-618).

213. McKenna DJ, Jones K, Humphrey S. Black cohosh: efficacy, safety, and use in clinical and preclinical applications. *Altern Ther Health Med*. 2001;7(3):93–100.

214. Lieberman S. A review of the effectiveness of Cimicifuga racemosa (black cohosh): for the symptoms of menopause. *J Women's Health*. 1998;7(5):525–529.

215. Liske E, Hanggi W, Henneicke-von Zepelin H. Physiologic investigation of a unique extract of black cohosh (Cimicifugae racemosae rhizoma): a 6-month clinical study demonstrates no systemic estrogenic effect. *J Women's Health Gend Based Med*. 2002;11(2):163–174.

216. van Die MD, Burger HG, Teede HJ, Bone KM. Vitex agnus-castus extracts for female reproductive disorders: a systematic review of clinical trials. *Planta Med*. 2013;79(7):562–575.

217. Schellenberg R, Zimmermann C, Drewe J, Hoexter G, Zahner C. Dose-dependent efficacy of the Vitex agnus castus extract Ze 440 in patients suffering from premenstrual syndrome. *Phytomedicine*. 2012, Nov 15;19(14):1325–1331.

218. Zamani M, Neghab N, Torabian S. Therapeutic effect of Vitex agnus castus in patients with premenstrual syndrome. *Acta Med Iran*. 2012;50(2):101–106.

219. Ma L, Lin S, Chen R, Wang X. Treatment of moderate to severe premenstrual syndrome with Vitex agnus castus (BNO 1095) in Chinese women. *Gynecol Endocrinol*. 2010, Aug;26(8):612–616.

220. van Die MD, Bone KM, Burger HG, Reece JE, Teede HJ. Effects of a combination of Hypericum perforatum and Vitex agnus-castus on PMS-like symptoms in late-perimenopausal women: findings from a subpopulation analysis. *J Altern Complement Med*. 2009, Sep;15(9):1045–1048.

221. He Z, Chen R, Zhou Y, Geng L, Zhang Z, Chen S, et al. Treatment for premenstrual syndrome with Vitex agnus castus: a prospective, randomized, multi-center placebo controlled study in China. *Maturitas*. 2009, May 20;63(1):99–103.

222. Daniele C, Thompson Coon J, Pittler M, Ernst E. Vitex agnus castus. *Drug Safety*. 2005;28(4):319–332.

223. Turner S, Mills S. A double-blind clinical trial on a herbal remedy for premenstrual syndrome: a case study. *Compl Ther Med*. 1993;1:73–77.

224. Lauritzen C, Reuter H, Repges R. Treatment of premenstrual tension syndrome with Vitex agnus-castus Controlled, double-blind study versus pyridoxine. *Phytomedicine*. 1997;4(3):183–189.

225. Halaska M, Raus K, Beles P. Treatment of cyclical mastodynia using an extract of Vitex agnus-castus: results of a double-blind comparison with a placebo. *Ceska Gynekol*. 1998;63(5):388–392.

226. Berger D, Schaffner W, Schrader E. Efficacy of Vitex agnus-castus L. extract Ze 440 in patients with pre-menstrual syndrome (PMS). *Arch Gynecol Obstet*. 2000;264(3):150–153.

227. Schellenberg R. Treatment for the premenstrual syndrome with agnus castus fruit extract: prospective, randomised, placebo controlled study. *BMJ*. 2001;322(7279):134–137.

228. India Go. New Delhi: Government of India, Ministry of Health and Family Welfare; 1989.

229. Sharifi F, Simbar M, Mojab F, Majd HA. Comparison of the effects of Matricaria chamomila (Chamomile) extract and mefenamic acid on the intensity of premenstrual syndrome. *Complement Ther Clin Pract*. 2014;20(1):81–88. England.

230. Pittler M, Ernst E. Efficacy of kava for treating anxiety: systematic review and metaanalysis. *J Clin Psychopharmacol*. 2000;20:84–90.

231. Vernet-Maury E, Alaoui-Isma'ili O, Dittmar A. Basic emotions induced by odorants: a new approach based on autonomic pattern results. *J Auton Nerv Syst*. 1999;75(2-3):83–86.

232. Stevinson C, Ernst E. A pilot study of Hypericum perforatum for the treatment of premenstrual syndrome. *Br J Obstet Gynecol*. 2000;107:870–876.

233. Shelton R, Keller M, Gelenberg A. Effectiveness of Hypericum in major depression: a randomized controlled trial. *JAMA*. 2001;285(15):1978–1986.

234. Lecrubier Y, Clerc G, Didi R. Efficacy of St. John's wort extract WS 5570 in major depression: a double-blind, placebo-controlled trial. *Am J Psychiatry*. 2002;159(8):1361–1366.

235. Kalb R, Trautmann-Sponsel R, Kieser M. Efficacy and tolerability of Hypericum extract WS 5572 versus placebo in mildly to moderately depressed patients. a randomized double-blind multicenter clinical trial. *Pharmacopsychiatry*. 2001;34(3):96–103.

236. Rychlik R, Siedentop H, von den Driesch V. St. John's wort extract WS 5572 in minor to moderately severe depression. Effectiveness and tolerance of 600 and 1200 mg active ingredient daily. *Fortschr Med Orig*. 2001;119(3-4):119–128.

237. Canning S, Waterman M, Orsi N, Ayres J, Simpson N, Dye L. The efficacy of Hypericum perforatum (St John's wort) for the treatment of premenstrual syndrome: a randomized, double-blind, placebo-controlled trial. *CNS Drugs*. 2010, Mar;24(3):207–225.

238. van Gurp G, Meterissian G, Haiek L. St. John's Wort or sertraline? Randomized controlled trial in primary care. *Can Fam Physician.* 2002;48:905–912.

239. Group HDTS. Effect of Hypericum (St. John's wort) in major depressive disorder: a randomized controlled trial. *JAMA.* 2002;287(14):1807–1814.

240. Behnke K, Jensen G, Graubaum H. Hypericum versus fluoxetine in the treatment of mild to moderate depression. *Adv Ther.* 2002;19(1):43–52.

241. Schrader E. Equivalence of Hypericum extract (Ze 117) and fluoxetine: a randomized, controlled study in mild-moderate depression. *Int Clin Psychopharmacol.* 2000;15(2):61–68.

242. Timoshanko A, Stough C, Vitetta L. A preliminary investigation on the acute pharmacodynamic effects of Hypericum on cognitive and psychomotor performance. *Behav Pharmacol.* 2001;12(8):35–64.

243. Thys-Jacobs S, Starkey P, Bernstein D, et al. Calcium carbonate and the premenstrual syndrome: effects on premenstrual and menstrual symptoms. *AJOG.* 1998;179(2):444–452.

244. Thys-Jacobs S. Micronutrients and the premenstrual syndrome: the case for calcium. *J Am Coll Nutr.* 2000;19:220–227.

245. Facchinetti F, Borella P, Sances G. Oral magnesium successfully relieves premenstrual mood changes. *Obstet Gynecol.* 1991;78:177–181.

246. Chocano-Bedoya PO, Manson JE, Hankinson SE, Willett WC, Johnson SR, Chasan-Taber L, et al. Dietary B vitamin intake and incident premenstrual syndrome. *Am J Clin Nutr.* 2011, May;93(5):1080–1086.

247. Wilson S. Calcium therapy for treating PMS. *J Fam Pract.* 1998;47(6):410–411.

248. Williams M, Harris R, Dean B. Controlled trial of pyridoxine in the premenstrual syndrome. *J Int Med Res.* 1985;13:174–179.

249. Brush M, Bennet T, Hansen K. Pyridoxine in the treatment of premenstrual syndrome: a retrospective survey of 630 patients. *Br J Clin Prac.* 1998;42(11):448–452.

250. Fuchs N, Hakim M, Abraham G. The effect of a nutritional supplement, Optivite for women, on pre-menstrual tension syndromes: 1. Effect on blood chemistry and serum steroid levels during the mid luteal phase. *J Appl Nutr.* 1985;37:1–11.

251. Fugh-Berman A, Kronenberg F. Review complementary and alternative medicine (CAM) in reproductive-age women: a review of randomized controlled trials. *Reprod Toxicol.* 2003;17:137–152.

252. Parry G, Bredesen D. Sensory neuropathy with low-dose pyridoxine. *Neurology.* 1985;35:1466–1468.

253. Moller S. Serotonin, carbohydrates, and atypical depression. *Pharmacol Toxicol.* 1992;71(71 suppl 1):61–71.

254. Steinberg S, Annable L, Young SN, et al. A placebo-controlled clinical trial of tryptophan in premenstrual dysphoria. *Biol Psychiatry.* 1999;45:313–320.

255. Sayegh R, Schiff I, Wurtman J. The effect of a carbohydrate-rich beverage on mood, appetite, and cognitive function in women with premenstrual syndrome. *Obstet Gynecol.* 1995;86(4 Pt 1):520–528.

256. Tanskanen A, Hibbeln J, Tuomilehto J. Fish consumption and depressive symptoms in the general population in Finland. *Psychiatr Serv.* 2001;52(4):529–531.

257. Mischoulon D, Fava A. Docosahexanoic acid and omega-3 fatty acids in depression. *Psychiatr Clin North Am.* 2000;23(4):785–794.

258. Goldin B, Gorbach S. The relationship between diet and rat fecal bacterial enzymes implicated in colon cancer. *J Natl Cancer Inst.* 1976;57:371–375.

259. Goldin B, Adlercreutz H, Gorbach S. The relationship between estrogen levels and diets of Caucasian American and Oriental immigrant women. *Am J Clin Nutr.* 1986;44(6):945–953.

260. Longcope C, Gorbach S, Goldin B. Effect of low fat diet on oestrogen metabolism. *J Clin Endocrinol Metab.* 1987;64(6):1246–1249.

261. Goldin B, Woods M, Spiegelman D. The effect of dietary fat and fiber on serum estrogen concentrations in premenopausal women under controlled dietary conditions. *Cancer.* 1994;74(suppl 3):1125–1131.

262. Rose D, Goldman M, Connolly J. High-fiber diet reduces serum estrogen concentrations in premenopausal women. *Am J Clin Nutr.* 1991;54(3):520–525.

263. Woods M, Gorbach S, Longcope C. Low-fat, high-fiber diet and serum estrone sulfate in premenopausal women. *Am J Clin Nutr.* 1989;49(6):1179–1183.

264. Goldin B, Gorbach S. The effect of milk and lactobacillus feeding on human intestinal bacterial enzyme activity. *Am J Clin Nutr.* 1984;39:756–761.

265. Gorbach S. Estrogens, breast cancer and intestinal flora. *Rev Inf Dis.* 1984;6(S 1):S85–S90.

266. Steege J, Blumenthal J. The effects of aerobic exercise on premenstrual symptoms in middle-aged women: a preliminary study. *J Psychosom Res.* 1993;37:127–133.

267. Aganoff J, Boyle G. Aerobic exercise, mood states and menstrual cycle symptoms. *J Psychosom Res.* 1994;38:183–192.

268. Choi P, Salmon P. Symptom changes across the menstrual cycle in competitive sportswomen, exercisers and sedentary women. *Br J Clin Psychol.* 1995;34(Pt3):447–460.

269. Prior J, Vigna Y. Conditioning exercise and premenstrual symptoms. *Reprod Med.* 1987;32:423–428.

270. Goodale I, Domar A, Benson H. Alleviation of premenstrual syndrome symptoms with the relaxation response. *Obstet Gynecol.* 1990;75:649–655.

271. Groer M, Ohnesorge C. Menstrual cycle lengthening and reduction in premenstrual distress through guided imagery. *J Holist Nurs.* 1993;11:286–294.

272. Oleson T, Flocco W. Randomized controlled study of premenstrual symptoms treated with ear, hand, and foot reflexology. *Obstet Gynecol.* 1993;82:906–911.

273. Hernandez-Reif M, Martinez A, Field T. Premenstrual symptoms are relieved by massage therapy. *J Psychosom Obstet Gynecol.* 2000;21(1):9–15.

274. Blake F, Salkovskis P, Gath D. Cognitive therapy for premenstrual syndrome: a controlled trial. *J Psychosom Res.* 1998;45:307–318.

275. Hamelsky S, Stewart W, Lipton R. Epidemiology of Headache in Women: emphasis on Migraine. In: Goldman M, Hatch M, eds. *Women and Health.* San Diego: Academic Press; 2000:1084–1097.

276. Parker-Falzoi J, Ferrary E. Common Medical Problems: musculoskeletal Injuries through Uninary Tract Disorders. In: Youngkin E, Davis M, eds. *Women's Health: A Primary Care Clinical Guide.* Stamford, CT: Appleton & Lange; 1998:785–865.

277. Lipton R, Stewart W, Diamond S, et al. Prevalence and burden of migraine in the United States: data from the American Migraine Study II. *Headache.* 2001;41:646–657.

278. Boyle C. Management of menstrual migraine [Women's Health Initiatives: Management of Migraine & Epilepsy Throughout the Reproductive Cycle: Articles]. *Neurology*. 1999;54(4, suppl 1):S14–S18.

279. Silberstein S, Merriam G. Sex hormones and headache 1999 (menstrual migraine). *Neurology*. 1999;53(4, suppl 1): S3–S13.

280. Silberstein S, Merriam G. Physiology of the menstrual cycle. *Cephalgia*. 2000:148–154.

281. Kelman L. Use of topiramate for headache prophylaxis in clinical practice. *Headache*. 2004;44:2–7.

282. MacGregor E. "Menstrual" migraine: toward a definition. *Cephalgia*. 1996;16:11–21.

283. Rapkin A, Morgan M, Goldman L, et al. Progesterone metabolite allopregnenolone in women with premenstrual syndrome. *Obstet Gynecol*. 1997;90(5):709–715.

284. Silberstein S. Hormone-related headache. *Med Clin North Am*. 2001;85(4):1017–1035.

285. Spierings E, Sorbi M, Haimowitz B, et al. Changes in daily hassles, mood, and sleep in the 2 days before a migraine headache. *Clin J Pain*. 1996;12(1):38–42.

286. Ben-Yehuda A, Bentov Y, Bar G. Headaches in women undergoing in vitro fertilization and embryo-transfer treatment. *Headache*. 2005;45:215–219.

287. Silberstein S, Freitag F. Preventive treatment of migraine. *Neurology*. 2003;60(suppl 2):S38–S44.

288. Mann D, Coeytaux R. Migraine and Tension-Type Headache. In: Rakel D, ed. *Integrative Medicine*. Philadelphia: Saunders; 2003:65–75.

289. Ambrosini A, Di Lorenzo C, Coppola G, Pierelli F. Use of Vitex agnus-castus in migrainous women with premenstrual syndrome: an open-label clinical observation. *Acta Neurol Belg*. 2013;113(1):25–29. Italy.

290. Grossman W, Schimidramsl H. An extract of Petasites hybridus is effective in the prophylaxis of migraine. *Alt Med Rev*. 2001;6(3):303–310.

291. Thomet O, Simon HU. Petasins in the treatment of allergic diseases: results of preclinical and clinical studies. *Int Arch Allergy Immunol*. 2002;129(2):108–112.

292. Danesch U. Petasites hybridus (butterbur root) extract in the treatment of asthma—an open trial. *Alt Med Rev*. 2004;9(1):54–62.

293. Lipton R, Göbel H, Einhäupl K, et al. Petasites hybridus root (butterbur) is an effective preventive treatment for migraine. *Neurology*. 2004;63:2240–2244.

294. Rapoport A, Bigal M. Preventive migraine therapy: what is new. *Neurol Sci*. 2004;25:S177–S185.

295. Diener H, Rahlfs V, Danesch U. The first placebo-controlled trial of a special butterbur root extract for the prevention of migraine: reanalysis of efficacy criteria. *Eur Neurol*. 2004;51(2):89–97.

296. Holland S, Silberstein SD, Freitag F, Dodick DW, Argoff C, Ashman E. Quality Standards Subcommittee of the American Academy of Neurology and the American Headache Society. Evidence-based guideline update: NSAIDs and other complementary treatments for episodic migraine prevention in adults: report of the Quality Standards Subcommittee of the American Academy of Neurology and the American Headache Society. *Neurology*. 2012;78(17):1346–1353. United States.

297. Agosti R, Duke RK, Chrubasik JE, Chrubasik S. Effectiveness of Petasites hybridus preparations in the prophylaxis of migraine: a systematic review. *Phytomedicine*. 2006;13(9-10): 743–746. Germany.

298. Oelkers-Ax R, Leins A, Parzer P, et al. Butterbur root extract and music therapy in the prevention of childhood migraine: an explorative study. *Eur J Pain*. 2008;12(3):301–313. http://dx.doi.org/10.1016/j.ejpain.2007.06.003.

299. Schulz V, Hansel R, Blumenthal M, et al. *Rational Phytotherapy: A Reference Guide for Physicians and Pharmacists*. 5th ed. Berlin: Springer-Verlag; 2004.

300. Murphy J, Heptinstall S, Mitchell J. Randomized, double-blind placebo controlled trial of fever few in migraine prevention. *Lancet*. 1988;2:189–192.

301. Johnson E, Kadam N, Hylands D, et al. Efficacy of fever few as prophylactic treatment of migraine. *BMJ*. 1985;291:569–573.

302. Palevitch D, Earon G, Caraao R. Fever few (tanacetum parthenium) as a prophylactic treatment for migraine in a double-blind placebo controlled study. *Phyto Ther Res*. 1997;11:508–511.

303. Ferro EC, Biagini AP, da Silva ÍE Silva ML, Silva JR. The combined effect of acupuncture and Tanacetum parthenium on quality of life in women with headache: randomised study. *Acupunct Med*. 2012;30(4):252–257. England.

304. Cady RK, Goldstein J, Nett R, Mitchell R, Beach ME, Browning R. A double-blind placebo-controlled pilot study of sublingual feverfew and ginger (LipiGesic™ M) in the treatment of migraine. *Headache*. 2011;51(7):1078–1086. United States.

305. Shrivastava R, Pechadre JC, John GW. Tanacetum parthenium and Salix alba (Mig-RL) combination in migraine prophylaxis: a prospective, open-label study. *Clin Drug Investig*. 2006;26(5):287–296. New Zealand.

306. Ernst E, Pittler M. The efficacy and safety of feverfew (Tanacetum parthenium L.): an update of a systematic review. *Public Health Nutr*. 2000;3(4A):509–514.

307. Saranitzky E, White CM, Baker EL, Baker WL, Coleman CI. Feverfew for migraine prophylaxis: a systematic review. *J Diet Suppl. England*. 2009;6(2):91–103.

308. Pittler M, Vogler B, Ernst E. Feverfew for preventing migraine. *The Cochrane Library*. 2002;4.

309. Review AM. Monograph: Zingiber officinale. *Alt Med Rev*. 2003;8(3):331–335.

310. Langner E, Greifenberg S, Gruenwald J. Ginger: history and Use. *Adv Nat Ther*. 1998;15(1):35–44.

311. Ernst E, Pittler M. Systematic Review og Ginger for Nausea and Vomiting. *Br J Anaesthes*. 2000;84(3):367–371.

312. Afzal M, Al-Hadidi D, Menon M, et al. Ginger: an ethnomedical, chemical, and pharmacological review. *Drug Metabol Drug Interact*. 2001;18(3-4):159–174.

313. Bone K. Ginger: the Herbal Aspirin? *Part 2, MediHerb Professional Review*. 1996;53:1–3.

314. Maghbooli M, Golipour F, Moghimi Esfandabadi A, Yousefi M. Comparison between the efficacy of ginger and sumatriptan in the ablative treatment of the common migraine. *Phytother Res*. 2014;28(3):412–415. England.

315. Bone K. Corydalis ambigua—Corydalis. *MediHerb Professional Review*. 2002;78:1–3.

316. Henkes H, Franz M, Kendall O, et al. Evaluation of the anxiolytic properties of tetrahydropalmatine, a Corydalis yanhusuo compound, in the male Sprague-Dawley rat. *AANA J*. 2011 Aug;79(suppl 4):S75–S80.

317. Singh Y, Singh N. Therapeutic potential of kava in the treatment of anxiety disorders. *CNS Drugs*. 2002;16(11):731–743.

318. Gobel H, Heinze A, Dworschak M, et al. Analgesic efficacy and tolerability of locally applied oleum menthae piperitae preparation LI 170 in patients with migraine or tension-type headache [Abstract]. *Zeitschrift fur Allgemeinmedizin*. 2001;77(6):287–295.

319. Gobel H, Schmidt G. Effect of peppermint and eucalyptus oil preparations on headache parameters [Abstract]. *Z Phytother*. 1995;16(1):23–26, 29-33.

320. Mills S, Bone K. *The Essential Guide to Herbal Safety*. St. Louis: Churchill Livingstone; 2005.

321. Moerman D. *Native American Ethnobotany*. 3rd ed. Portland, OR: Timber Press; 2000.

322. Upton R. *Willow Bark (Salix spp.), American Herbal Pharmacopoeia and Therapeutic Compendium*; December 1999.

323. Ribnicky D, Poulev A, Raskin I. Wintergreen (Gaultheria procumbens): a rich source of salicylates, Journal of Nutraceuticals. *Funct Med Foods*. 2003;4(1):39–52.

324. Chrubasik S, Eisenberg E, Balan E, et al. Treatment of low back pain exacerbations with willow bark extrac: a randomized double-blind study. *Amer J Med*. 2000;109:9–14.

325. Burke B, Olson R, Cusack B. Randomised controlled trial of phytoestrogen in the prophylactic treatment of menstrual migraine. *Biomed Pharmacother*. 2002;56(6):283–288.

326. Basch E, Foppa I, Liebowitz R, et al. Lavender (Lavandula angustifolia). *J Herb Pharmacopther*. 2004;4(2):73–77.

327. Cavanagh H. Biological activities of lavender essential oil. *Phytother Res*. 2002;16:301–308.

328. Schattner P, Randerson D. Tiger balm as a treatment for tension headache: a clinical trial in general practice. *Aust Fam Physician*. 1996;25(2):216–222.

329. Köseoglu E, Talaslioglu A, Gönül AS, Kula M. The effects of magnesium prophylaxis in migraine without aura. *Magnes Res*. 2008;21(2):101–108. England.

330. Mauskop A, Altura B, Altura B. Serum ionized magnesium levels and serum ionized calcium/ionized magnesium ratios in women with menstrual migraine. *Headache: J Head Face Pain*. 2004;42(4):242.

331. Facchinetti F, Sances G, Borella P, et al. Magnesium prophylaxis of menstrual migraine: effects on intracellular magnesium. *Headache*. 1992;31(5):298–301.

332. Rozen T, Oshinsky M, Gebeline C, et al. Open label trial of coenzyme Q10 as a migraine preventive. *Cephalalgia*. 2002;22(2):137–141.

333. Maizels M, Blumenfeld A, Burchette R. A combination of riboflavin, magnesium, and feverfew for migraine prophylaxis: a randomized trial, Headache. *J Head Face Pain*. 2004;9:885.

334. Bianchi A, Salomone S, Caraci F, et al. Role of magnesium, coenzyme Q10, riboflavin, and vitamin B12 in migraine prophylaxis [Review]. *Vitamins & Hormones*. 2004;69:297–312.

335. Thys-Jacobs S. Vitamin D and calcium in menstrual migraine. *Headache*. 1994;34(9):544–546.

336. Strid J, Jepson R, Moore V, et al. Evening primrose oil or other essential fatty acids for the treatment of pre-menstrual syndrome (PMS) [Protocol]. *Cochrane Database Syst Rev*. 2005;1.

337. Vernon H, McDermaid C, Hajino C. Systematic review of randomized clinical trials of complementary/alternative therapies in the treatment of tension-type and cervicogenic headache. *Complement Ther Med*. 1999;7:142–155.

CHAPTER 10

1. Kletzky O. Amenorrhea and Abnormal Uterine Bleeding. In: Hacker N, Moore J, eds. *Essentials of Obstetrics and Gynecology*. 2nd ed. Philadelphia: WB Saunders; 1992.

2. Baker S. Menstruation and Related Problems and Concerns. In: Youngkin E, Davis M, eds. *Women's health: A Primary Care Clinical Guide*. Stamford, CT: Appleton & Lange; 1998:140–160.

3. Bosker GE. Menstrual Abnormalities. In: Bosker G, ed. *The Textbook of Primary and Acute Care Medicine: Principles, Protocols, Pathways*. Atlanta: Thomson American Health Consultants; 2002.

4. Stenchever M, Droegemueller W, Herbst A, et al. Abnormal uterine bleeding. In: Stenchever M, Droegemueller W, Herbst A, eds. *Comprehensive Gynecology*. 4th ed. St. Louis: Mosby; 2001:157–158, 1079-1097.

5. Speroff L, Glass R, Kase G. *Clinical Gynecologic Endocrinology and Infertility*. Baltimore: Lippincott Williams & Wilkins; 1999.

6. Kelly R, Lumsden M, Abel M, et al. The relationship between menstrual blood loss and prostaglandin production in the human: evidence for increased availability of arachidonic acid in women suffering from menorrhagia. *Prostaglandins Leukotrienes Med*. 1984;16(1):69–78.

7. Nurse-Midwives ACo. Clinical Bulletin No 6. *J Midwif Women's Health*. 2002;47(3):207–213.

8. Harlow S. Menstruation and Menstrual Disorders. In: Goldman M, Hatch M, eds. *Women and Health*. San Diego: Academic Press; 2000.

9. Riggs S. Abnormal vaginal bleeding secondary to iron deficiency in a thirteen year old. *J Adolesc Health Care*. 1990;10(6):567–569.

10. Achterberg J. *Woman as Healer*. Boston: Shambhala; 1990.

11. Irvine G, Cameron I. Medical management of dysfunctional uterine bleeding. *Baillieres Best Pract Res Clin Obstet Gynaecol*. 2000;13(2):189–202.

12. Cameron I. Dysfunctional uterine bleeding. *Baillieres Clin Obstet Gynaecol*. 1990;3(2):315–327.

13. Hallberg L. Menstrual blood loss: a population study. *Acta Scand Obstet Gynecol*. 1966;45:321–351.

14. Magos A. Management of menorrhagia. *BMJ*. 1990;300:1537–1538.

15. Jennings J. Abnormal uterine bleeding. *Med Clin North Am*. 1995;79:1357–1376.

16. Bayer S, Cherney A. Clinical manifestations and treatment of dysfunctional uterine bleeding. *JAMA*. 1993;269:1823–1828.

17. Ferenczy A. Pathophysiology of endometrial bleeding. *Maturitas*. 2003;45(1):1–14.

18. Jaffe R. Importance of angiogenesis in reproductive physiology. *Semin Perinatol*. 2000;24(1):79–81.

19. Trickey R. *Women, Hormones, and the Menstrual Cycle*. St. Leonards, Australia: Allen and Unwin; 1998.

20. Xiao E, Xia-Zhang L, Ferin M. Inadequate luteal function is the initial clinical cyclic defect in a 12-day stress model that includes apsychogenic component in the Rhesus monkey. *J Clin Endocrinol Metab*. 2002;87(5):2232–2237.

21. Meseguer A, Puche C, Cabero A. Sex steroid biosynthesis in white adipose tissue. *Horm Metab Res*. 2003;34(11):731–736.

22. Serdar S. Effects of hypertension and obesity on endometrial thickness. *Eur J Obstet Gynecol Reprod Biol*. 2003;109:72–75.

23. Mills S, Bone K. *Principles and Practice of Phytotherapy*. London: Churchill Livingstone; 2000.

24. Bumbulien A. Casual analysis of menstrual disorders in adolescent girls. *Ginekol Pol*. 2003;74(4):267–273.

25. Ding J. High serum cortisol levels in exercise-associated amenorrhea. *Ann Int Med*. 1988;108(4):530–534.

26. Strickler R. Dysfunctional uterine bleeding in ovulatory women. *Postgrad Med*. 1985;77(1):235–247.

27. Doufas A, Mastorakos G. The hypothalamic-pituitary-thyroid axis and the female reproductive system. *Ann NY Acad Sci*. 2000;900:65–76.

28. Slap G. Menstrual disorders in adolescence. *Best Pract Res Clin Obstet Gynaecol.* 2003;17(1):75–92.
29. O K, Schrager S. Abnormal uterine bleeding. *Am Fam Physician.* 1999;60:1371–1382.
30. Schneider H, Goeser R, Cirkel U. Lisuride and Other Dopamine Agonists. *Prolactin and the inadequate corpus luteum*NY: Raven Press; 1983.
31. Loucks A. Effects of exercise training on the menstrual cycle: existence and mechanisms. *Med Sci Sports Exerc.* 1990;22(3):275–280.
32. Sowers M. Menopause: its Epidemiology. In: Goldman M, Hatch M, eds. *Women and Health.* San Diego: Academic Press; 2000.
33. Albers J, Hull S, Wesley R. Abnormal uterine bleeding. *Am Fam Physician.* 2004;69(8):1915–1926.
34. Dickersin K, Munro M, Langenberg P, et al. Design paper Surgical Treatments Outcomes Project for Dysfunctional Uterine Bleeding (STOP-DUB): design and methods. *Control Clin Trials.* 2003;24:591–609.
35. Marlies Y, Bongers A, Ben W, et al. Current treatment of dysfunctional uterine bleeding. *Maturitas.* 2004;47:159–174.
36. Iglesias E, Coupey S. Menstrual cycle abnormalities: diagnosis and management. *Adolesc Med.* 1999;10(2):255–273.
37. Agarwal N, Kriplani A. Brief communication: medical management of dysfunctional uterine bleeding. *Int J Gynecol Obstet.* 2001;199(2):199–201. 75.
38. Upton R. *American Herbal Pharmacopoeia and Therapeutic Compendium: dang gui Root Angelica sinensis (Oliv.) Diels.* Santa Cruz: AHP; 2003.
39. Bone K. *A Clinical Guide to Blending Liquid Herbs: herbal Formulations for the Individual Patient.* St. Louis: Churchill Livingstone; 2003.
40. (ESCOP) ESCoP. *ESCOP Monographs: the Scientific Foundation for Herbal Medicinal Products.* Stuttgart: Thieme; 2003.
41. Romm A, Treasure J. AHG professional member botanical therapeutics survey: vitex agnus castus. *JAHG.* 2001;2(2):27–31.
42. Milewicz A. Vitex agnus castus extract in the treatment of luteal phase defects owing to hyperprolactinemia: results of a randomized placebo-controlled double-blind study. *Arzneim-Forsch Drug Res.* 1993;43(7):752–756.
43. Kayser H, Istanbulluglu S. Eine behandlung von menstruationsstorungen ohne hormone. *Hippokrates.* 1954;25:717–718.
44. AltMedDex. *Menorrhagia*; 2004.
45. Blumenthal M. *The Complete German Commission E Monographs: therapeutic Guide to Herbal Medicine.* Boston: American Botanical Council; 1998.
46. Bone K. *Clinical Applications of Ayurvedic and Chinese Herbs.* Queensland, Australia: Phytotherapy Press; 2000.
47. Ellingwood F. American Materia Medica. *Therapeutics and Pharmacognosy.* vol. 2. Cincinnati: Eclectic Medical Publications; 1919.
48. Association BHM. *British Herbal Pharmacopoeia (BHP).* vol. 1. Bournemouth, UK: British Herbal Medicine Association; 1990.
49. Wichtl M. *Herbal Drugs and Phytopharmaceuticals: a Handbook for Practice on a Scientific Basis.* 4th ed. Stuttgart: Medpharm; 2004.
50. Steinberg A, Segal H, Parris H. Role of oxalic acid and certain related dicarboxylic acids in the control of hemorrhage. *Annals Oto Rhino Laryngo.* 1940;49:1008–1021.
51. McGuffin M, Hobbs C, Upton R, et al. *Botanical Safety Handbook.* vol. 231. Boca Raton: CRC Press; 1997.
52. Aksoy A, Hale W, Dixon J. Capsella bursa-pastoris (L.) Medic. as a biomonitor of heavy metals. *Sci Total Environ.* 1999;226(2-3):177–186.
53. White C, Fan C, Song J, et al. An evaluation of the hemostatic effects of hydrophilic, alcohol and lipophilic extracts of noto-ginseng. *Pharmacotherapy.* 2001;21(7):773–777.
54. LeMone P. Vitamins and Minerals. *J Obstet Gynecol Neonatal Nurs.* 1999;28(5):520–533.

CHAPTER 11

1. Moore J. Benign Diseases of the Uterus. In: Hacker N, Moore J, eds. *Essentials of Obstetrics and Gynecology.* 2nd ed. Philadelphia: Saunders; 1992:347–355.
2. Ryan G, Syrop C, Van Voorhis B. Role, epidemiology, and natural history of benign uterine mass lesions. *Clin Obstet Gynecol.* 2005;48(2):312–324.
3. Speroff L, Glass R, Kase G. *Clinical Gynecologic Endocrinology and Infertility.* Baltimore: Lippincott Williams & Wilkins; 1999.
4. Girman A, Lee R, Kligler B. An integrative medicine approach to premenstrual syndrome. *Am J Obstet Gynecol.* 2003;188(5):56–65.
5. Chez R. Etiology and treatment of uterine fibroids. *Alt Ther.* 2002;8(2):32–33.
6. De Leo V, Morgante G. Uterine fibromas and the hormonal pattern. *Minerva Gynecol.* 1996;48(12):533–538.
7. Vollenhoven B, Pearce P, Herington A, Healy D. Steroid receptor binding and messenger RNA expression in fibroids from untreated and gonadotrophin-releasing hormone agonist pretreated women. *Clin Endocrinol.* 1994;40(4):537–544.
8. Trickey R. *Women, Hormones, and the Menstrual Cycle.* St. Leonards, Australia: Allen and Unwin; 1998.
9. Vollenhoven B, Herington A, Healy D. Messenger ribonucleic acid expression of the insulin-like growth factors and their binding proteins in uterine fibres and myometrium. *J Clin Endocrinol Metab.* 1993;76(5):1106–1110.
10. Day B, Dunson D. Why is parity protective for uterine fibroids? *Epidemiology.* 2003;14(2):247–250.
11. LeRoy N. Uterine fibroids: an integrative approach. *Orient Med J.* 2003;11(2):2–18.
12. Riquelme J. Uterine fibroids (Leiomyomata). In: Rakel D, ed. *Integrative Medicine.* Philadelphia: Saunders; 2003:389–392.
13. Bradley L. New endometrial ablation techniques for treatment of menorrhagia. *Surg Technol Int.* 2004;12:161–170.
14. Olive D, Lindheim S, Pritts E. Non-surgical management of leiomyoma: impact on fertility [Fertility]. *Curr Opin Obstet Gynecol.* 2004;16(3):239–243.
15. Mehl-Madrona L. Complementary medicine treatment of uterine fibroids: a pilot study. *Alt Ther.* 2002;8(2):44–46.
16. Cramer D, Willett W, Bell D. Galactose consumption and metabolism in relation to the risk of ovarian cancer. *Lancet.* 1989;2(66-71).
17. Larsson S, Bergkyst L, Wolk A. Milk and lactose intakes and ovarian risk in the Swedish mammography cohort. *Am J Clin Nutr.* 2004;80(5):1353–1357.
18. McIntyre A. *The Complete Woman's Herbal.* New York: Henry Holt; 1995.
19. McQuade-Crawford A. *Herbal Remedies for Women.* Rocklin, CA: Prima Publishing; 1997.

20. Maciocia G. *Obstetrics and Gynecology in Chinese Medicine.* London: Churchill Livingstone; 1998.

21. Bone K. Chinese herbal formula shrinks fibroids. *MediHerb Professional Monitor.* 1996;18:2–3.

22. Mills S, Bone K. *Principles and Practice of Phytotherapy.* London: Churchill Livingstone; 2000.

23. Wuttke W, Jarry H, Christoffel V, Spengler B, Seidlova-Wuttke D. Chaste tree (Vitex agnus-castus)—Pharmacology and clinical indications. *Phytomedicine.* 2003;10:348–357.

24. Xi S, Liske E, Wang S, et al. Effect of Isopropanolic Cimicifuga racemosa Extract on Uterine Fibroids in Comparison with Tibolone among Patients of a Recent Randomized, Double Blind, Parallel-Controlled Study in Chinese Women with Menopausal Symptoms. *Evid Based Complement Alternat Med.* 2014;2014:717686. United States.

25. Cassidy A. Potential tissue selectivity of dietary phytoestrogens and estrogens. *Curr Opin Lipidol.* 1999;10:47–52.

26. Low Dog T. *Women's Health in Complementary and Integrative Medicine: a Clinical Guide.* St. Louis, MO: Elsevier; 2004.

27. Zava D, Dollbaum C, Blen M. Estrogen and progestin bioactivity of foods, herbs, and spices. *Proc Soc Exp Biol Med.* 1998;217:369–378.

28. Liu J, Burdette J, Xu H, et al. Evaluation of estrogenic activity of plant extracts for the potential treatment of menopausal symptoms. *J Agric Food Chem.* 2001;49(5):2472–2479.

29. Schulz V, Hansel R, Blumenthal M, Tyler V. *Rational Phytotherapy: a Reference Guide for Physicians and Pharmacists.* 5th ed. Berlin: Springer-Verlag; 2004.

30. Wichtl M. *Herbal Drugs and Phytopharmaceuticals: A Handbook for Practice on a Scientific Basis.* 4th ed. Stuttgart: Medpharm; 2004.

31. Ellingwood F. Cincinnati: Eclectic Medical Publications; 1919.

32. Petersen FJ. *Materia Medica and Clinical Therapeutics.* Los Olivos, CA: F. J. Petersen; 1905.

33. Remington J, Wood H. *The Dispensatory of the United States of America*; 1918.

34. Roshdy E, Rajaratnam V, Maitra S, Sabry M, Allah AS, Al-Hendy A. Treatment of symptomatic uterine fibroids with green tea extract: a pilot randomized controlled clinical study. *Int J Womens Health.* 2013;5:477–486. New Zealand.

35. Zhang D, Al-Hendy M, Richard-Davis G, Montgomery-Rice V, Rajaratnam V, Al-Hendy A. Antiproliferative and proapoptotic effects of epigallocatechin gallate on human leiomyoma cells. *Fertil Steril.* 2010;94(5):1887–1893. United States.

36. Bensky D, Gamble A. *Chinese Herbal Medicine Materia Medica.* Seattle: Eastman Press; 1993.

37. Bone K. *Influence of Herbs on Detoxification by the Liver. Medicines from the Earth.* Brevard, NC: Gaia Herbal Research Institute; 2003.

38. Tilgner S. *Herbal Medicine from the Heart of the Earth.* Creswell, OR: Wise Acres Press; 1999.

39. Zylstra S. Office Management of Benign Breast Disease. *Clin Obstet Gynecol.* 1999;42(2):234–248.

40. Horner NK, Lampe JW. Potential mechanisms of diet therapy for fibrocystic breast conditions show inadequate evidence of effectiveness. *J Am Diet Assoc.* 2000;100(11):1368–1380.

41. Marchant D. Benign breast disease. *Obstet Gynecol Clin.* 2002;29:1–20.

42. Gateley C, Miers M, Mansel R, Hughes L. Drug treatments for mastalgia: 17 years experience in the Cardiff mastalgia clinic. *J R Soc Med.* 1992;85:12–15.

43. Goodwin, Pamela J. et al. Elevated high-density lipoprotein cholesterol and dietary fat intake in women with cyclic mastopathy, American Journal of Obstetrics & Gynecology, Volume 179, Issue 2, 430 – 437.

44. van Die MD, Burger HG, Teede HJ, Bone KM. Vitex agnus-castus extracts for female reproductive disorders: a systematic review of clinical trials. Planta Med. *Germany.* 2013;79(7):562–575.

45. Halaska M, Beles P, Gorkow CCS. Treatment of cyclic mastalgia with a solution containing a Chaste berryangus castus extract: results of a placebo-controlled double-blind study. *Breast.* 1999;8:175–181.

46. Barrett M. *The Handbook of Clinically Tested Herbal Remedies.* 12th ed. Binghamton, NY: Haworth Press; 2004.

47. Wuttke W, Splitt G, Gorkow C, Sieder C. Treatment of a cyclic mastalgia with a medicinal product containing agnus castus: results of a randomized, placebo-controlled, double-blind study. *Geburtshilfe und Frauenheilkunde.* 1997;57(1):569–574.

48. Halaska M, Raus K, Beles P. Treatment of cyclical mastodynia using an extract of Chaste berryagnus-castus: results of a double-blind comparison with a placebo. *Ceska Gynekol.* 1998;63(5):388–392.

49. Kubista E, Muller GJS. Treatment of mastopathies with cyclic mastodynia. Clinical results and hormonal profiles. *Rev Francaise Gyn Obstet.* 1987;82:221–227.

50. Hirata J, Swiersz L, Zell B. Does dong quai have estrogenic effects in postmenopausal women? A double-blind, placebo-controlled trial. *Fertil Steril.* 1997;68:981–986.

51. Amato P, Christophe S, Mellon P. Estrogenic activity of herbs commonly used as remedies for menopausal symptoms. *Menopause.* 2002;9:145–150.

52. Kang H, Ansbacher R, Hammoud M. Use of alternative and complementary medicine in menopause. *Int J Gyn Obstet.* 2002;79:195–207.

53. Kronenberg F, Fugh-Berman A. Complementary and alternative medicine for menopausal symptoms: a review of randomized, controlled trials. *Ann Intern Med.* 2002;137:805–813.

54. Ozaki Y. Antitiinflammatory effect of tetramethylpyrazine and ferulic acid. *Chem Pharm Bull.* 1992;40:954–956.

55. Thompson L. Flaxseeds, lignins, and cancer. In: Cunnane S, Thompson L, eds. *Flaxseed in Human Nutrition.* Chicago: AOCS Publishing; 1995.

56. Tou J, Thompson L. Exposure to flaxseed or its lignin component during different developmental stages influences rat mammary gland structures. *Carcinogenesis.* 1999;20:1831–1835.

57. Wang C, Kurzer M. Phytoestrogen concentration determines effects on DNA synthesis in human breast cancer cells. *Nutr Cancer.* 1997;28:236–247.

58. Wanasundara P, Shahidi F. *Process-Induced Chemical Changes in Food.* New York: Plenum Press; 1998.

59. Sidani M, Campbell J. Gynecology: select topics, Prim Care. *Clin Office Pract.* 2002;20(20):297–321.

60. Warber S, Zick S. Peripheral vascular disease. In: Rakel D, ed. *Integrative Medicine.* Philadelphia, WB: Saunders; 2003.

61. Pashby N. A clinical trial of evening primrose oil in mastalgia. *Br J Surg.* 1981;68:801–824.

62. Pye J, Mansel R, Hughes L. Clinical experience of drug treatments for mastalgia. *Lancet.* 1985;2:373–377.

63. Pruthi S, Wahner-Roedler DL, Torkelson CJ, et al. Vitamin E and evening primrose oil for management of cyclical mastalgia: a randomized pilot study. *Altern Med Rev.* 2010;15(1):59–67. United States.

64. Jellin J, Gregory P, Batz F, Hitchens K. *Pharmacist's Letter/Presciber's Letter Natural Medicines Comprehensive Database.* 4th ed. Stockton: Therapeutic Research Faculty; 2002.

65. Bullough B, Hindi-Alexander M, Fetouh S. Methylxanthines and fibrocystic breast disease: a study of correlations. *Nurse Pract.* 1990;15:36–44.

66. Boyle C, Berkowitz G, LiVolsi V. Caffeine consumption and fibrocystic breast disease: a case-control epidemiologic study. *J Natl Cancer Inst.* 1984;72:1015–1019.

67. Levinson W, Dunn P. Nonassociation of caffeine and fibrocystic breast disease. *Arch Intern Med.* 1986;146:1773–1775.

68. Heyden S, Muhlbaier L. Prospective study of "fibrocystic breast disease" and caffeine consumption. *Surgery.* 1984;96:479–484.

69. Parazzini F, LaVecchia C, Riundi R. Methylxanthine, alcohol-free diet and fibrocystic breast disease: a factorial clinical trial. *Surgery.* 1986;99:576–580.

70. Lubin F, Ron E, Wax Y. A case-control study of caffeine and methylxanthines in benign breast disease. *JAMA.* 1985;253:2388–2392.

71. Ernster V, Mason L, Goodson W. Effects of caffeine-free diet on benign breast disease: a randomized trial. *Surgery.* 1982;91:263–267.

72. Minton J, Abou-Issa HNR. Clinical and biochemical studies on methylxanthine-related fibrocystic breast disease. *Surgery.* 1981;90:299–304.

73. Hudson T. Natural approaches to treating fibrocystic breasts. *Altern Complement Ther.* 2000;6:145–148.

74. Ghent WR, Eskin BA, Low DA, et al. Iodine replacement in fibrocystic disease of the breast. *Can J Surg.* 1993;36:453–460.

75. Crofford L, Clauw D. Fibromyalgia: where are we a decade after the American College of Rheumatology classification criteria were developed? *Arthritis Rheum.* 2002;46:1136–1138.

76. Rawson J. Prevalence of endometriosis in asymptomatic women. *J Reprod Med.* 1991;36(7):513–515.

77. Mahmood T, Templeton A. Prevalence and genesis of endometriosis. *Hum Reprod.* 1991;6(4):544–549.

78. Wheeler J. Epidemiology of endometriosis-associated infertility. *J Reprod Med.* 1989;34(1):41–46.

79. Vercellini P, Ragni G, Trespidi L. Does contraception modify the risk of endometriosis? *Hum Reprod.* 1993;8:547–551.

80. Ramcharan S, Pellegrin F, Ray R. Bethesda: National Institutes of Health: center for Population Research Monograph; 1981.

81. Parazzini F, Ferraroni M, Bocciolone L. Contraceptive methods and risk of pelvic endometriosis. *Contraception.* 1994;49:47–55.

82. Vercellini P, Ragni G, Trespidi L. Does contraception modify the risk of endometriosis? *Hum Reprod.* 1993;8:547–551.

83. Konickx P, Oosterlynck D, D'Hooghe T, Meuleman C. Deeply infiltrating endometriosis is a disease whereas mild endometriosis could be considered a non-disease. *Ann NY Acad Sci.* 1994;734:333–341.

84. Jones D. *Textbook of Functional Medicine.* Gig Harbor, WA: Institute of Functional Medicine; 2005.

85. Ishikawa M, Nakata T, Yaginuma Y, Nishiwaki K, Goishi K, Saitoh S. Expression of superoxide dismutase (SOD) in adenomyosis. *Am J Obstet Gynecol.* 1993;169(3):730–734.

86. Rier S, Martin D, Bowman R, Becker J. Immunoresponsiveness in endometriosis: implications of estrogen toxicants. *Environ Health Persp.* 1995;103(7):151–156.

87. Berkkanoglu M, Arici A. Immunology and endometriosis. *Am J Reprod Immunol.* 2003;50(1):58–59.

88. Mathur S-P. Autoimmunity in endometriosis: relevance to infertility. *Am J Reprod Immunol.* 2000;44(2):89–95.

89. Ho HW, Wu MY, Yang YS. Peritoneal cellular immunity and endometriosis. *Am J Reprod Immunol.* 1997;38(6):400–412.

90. Schaffner W, Schrader E, Meier B, Brattström A. Efficacy of Vitex agnus castus L. extract Ze. 440 in patients with pre-menstrual syndrome (PMS). *Arch Gynecol Obstet.* 2000;264(3):150–153.

91. D'Hooghe T, Bambra C, Raeymaekers B, Jonge De, Hill J, Konickx P. The effects of immunosuppression on the development and progression of endometriosis in baboons (Papio anubis). *Fertil Steril.* 1995;64(1):172–178.

92. Nichols T, Lamb K, Arkins J. The association of atopic diseases with endometriosis. *Ann Allerg.* 1987;59:360–363.

93. Mol B, Bayram N, Lijmer J, et al. The performance of CA-125 measurement in the detection of endometriosis: a meta-analysis. *Fertil Steril.* 1998;70(6):1101–1108.

94. Youngkin E, Davis M. *Women's Health: A Primary Care Clinical Guide.* Stamford, CT: Appleton and Lange; 1998.

95. Ylanen K, Laatikainen T, Lahteenmaki P, Moo-Young A. Subdermal progestin implant (Nestorone) in the treatment of endometriosis: clinical response to various doses. *Acta Obstet Gynecol Scand.* 2003;82(2):167–172.

96. Hornstein M. Retreatment with nafarelin for recurrent endometriosis symptoms: efficacy, safety, and bone mineral density. *Fertil Steril.* 1997;67(6):1013–1018.

97. Adamson G, Nelson H. Surgical treatment of endometriosis. *Obstet Gynecol Clin North Am.* 1997;24(2):375–409.

98. Droegemueller W. *Comprehensive Gynecology.* St. Louis: Mosby; 2001:531–564.

99. Upton R. *American Herbal Pharmacopoeia and Therapeutic Compendium: Dong quai Root Angelica sinensis (Oliv.) Diels.* Santa Cruz, CA: AHP; 2003.

100. Arndt D, Bobermien K, Heyer H, Hinken B, Schwesinger G, Köhler G. Die kombinierte Endometriosetherapie–Langzeitergebnisse in Abhängigkeit vom Aktivitätszustand der Endometriose. Geburtshilfe und Frauenheilkunde. 67(S 1):PO_E_03_09.

101. Blumenthal M. *The Complete German Commission E Monographs: Therapeutic Guide to Herbal Medicine.* Boston: American Botanical Council; 1998.

102. Speroni E, Govoni P, Guizzardi S, et al. Anti-inflammatory and cicatrizing activity of Echinacea pallida Nutt root extract. *J Ethnopharmacol.* 2002;79(2):265–272.

103. ESCOP. *ESCOP Monographs: The Scientific Foundation for Herbal Medicinal Products.* Stuttgart: Thieme; 2003.

104. Hobbs C. Feverfew, Tanacetum parthenium: a review. *HerbalGram.* 1989;20:26–35.

105. Felter H, Lloyd J. *King's American Dispensatory.* Cincinnati: Reprinted by Eclectic Medical Publications., (1898); 1983.

106. Blumenthal M. *The ABC Clinical Guide to Herbs.* Austin: American Botanical Council; 2003.

107. Elias G, Rao M. Inhibition of albumin denaturation and antiinflammatory activity of dehydroaingerone and its analogs. *Ind J Exp Biol.* 1988;26(7):540–542.

108. Srivastava K, Mustafa T. Ginger (Zingiber officinale) in rheumatism and musculoskeletal disorders. *Med Hypoth.* 1992;39(4):342–348.

109. Gajera H, Patel S, Golakiya B. Antioxidant properties of some therapeutically active medicinal plants—an overview. *J Med Aromat Plant Sci.* 2005;27(1):91–100.

110. Arora R, Gupta D, Chawla R, et al. Radioprotection by plant products: present status and future prospects. *Phytother Res.* 2005;19(1):21–22.

111. Yoshida M. Antiproliferative constituents from Umbelliferae plants VII. Active triterpenes and rosmarinic acid from Centella asiatica. *Biol Pharm Bull.* 2005;28(1):173–175.

112. Somchit M, Sulaiman M, Zuraini A, et al. Antinociceptive and anti inflammatory effects of Centella asiatica. *Ind J Pharmacol.* 2004;36(6):377–380.

113. Incandela L, Cesarone MR, Cacchio M, et al. Total triterpenic fraction of Centella asiatica in chronic venous insufficiency and in high-perfusion microangiopathy. *Angiology.* 2001;52(suppl):S9–S13.

114. Bone K. *A Clinical Guide to Blending Liquid Herbs: Herbal Formulations for the Individual Patient.* St. Louis: Churchill Livingstone; 2003.

115. Koo M, Cho C. Pharmacological effects of green tea on the gastrointestinal system. *Eur J Pharmacol.* 2004;500(1): 177–185.

116. Sur P, Chaudhuri T, Vedasiromoni J, et al. Antiinflammatory and antioxidant property of saponins of tea [Camellia sinensis (L) O. Kuntze] root extract. *Phytother Res.* 2001;15(2): 174–176.

117. Herold A, Cremer L, Calugaru A, et al. Hydroalcoholic plant extracts with anti-inflammatory activity. *Roum Arch Microbiol Immunol.* 2003;1(62):117–129.

118. Tall J, Seeram N, Zhao C, et al. Tart cherry anthocyanins suppress inflammation-induced pain behavior in rat. *Behav Brain Res.* 2004;153(1):181–188.

119. Seeram N, Momin R, Nair M, Bourquin L, Nair M. Cyclooxygenase inhibitory and antioxidant cyanidin glycosides in cherries and berries. *Phytomedicine.* 2001;8(5):362–369.

120. Klein K, Janfaza M, Wong J, Chang J. Estrogen bioactivity in fo-ti and other herbs used for their estrogen-like effects as determined by a recombinant cell bioassay. *J Clin Endocrinol Metab.* 2003;88(9):4077–4079.

121. Chen J, Gao H, Li Q, et al. Efficacy and safety of remifemin on peri-menopausal symptoms induced by post-operative GnRH-a therapy for endometriosis: a randomized study versus tibolone. *Med Sci Monit.* 2014;20:1950–1957. United States.

122. Haensel R, Kallmann S. Verbascoside: a main constituent of Verbena officinalis. (German). *Archiv der Pharmazie (Weinheim).* 1986;319:227–230.

123. Upton R. *American Herbal Pharmacopoeia and Therapeutic Monographs: Chaste Tree Fruit (Vitex agnus Castus).* Santa Cruz, CA: American Herbal Pharmacopoeia; 2001.

124. Dharmananda S. Therapeutic approaches to endometriosis: traditional Chinese specific condition review. *Prot J Botanic Med.* 1996;1(4):36–44.

125. Kohama T, Herai K, Inoue M. Effect of French maritime pine bark extract on endometriosis as compared with leuprorelin acetate. *J Reprod Med.* 2007;52(8):703–708. United States.

126. Donovan J, DeVane -C, Lewis J, et al. Effects of St. John's Wort (Hypericum perforatum L.) extract on plasma androgen concentrations in healthy men and women: a pilot study. *Phytother Res.* 2005;19(10):901–906.

127. Simmen U, Burkard W, Berger K, et al. Extracts and constituents of Hypericum perforatum inhibit the binding of various ligands to recombinant receptors expressed with the Semliki forest virus system. *J Recept Signal Transduct Res.* 1999;19(1-4):59–74.

128. Grimm H, Mayer K, Mayser P, et al. Regulatory potential of n-3 fatty acids in immunological and inflammatory processes. *Br J Nutr.* 2002;87(suppl. 1):S59–S67.

129. Schwertner A, Conceição Dos Santos CC, Costa GD, et al. Efficacy of melatonin in the treatment of endometriosis: a phase II, randomized, double-blind, placebo-controlled trial. *Pain.* 2013;154(6):874–881. Netherlands.

130. Porpora MG, Brunelli R, Costa G, et al. A promise in the treatment of endometriosis: an observational cohort study on ovarian endometrioma reduction by N-acetylcysteine. *Evid Based Complement Alternat Med.* 2013;2013:240702. United States.

131. Fowler G, Milburn A, Reiter R, Robinson J. How to help women with chronic pelvic pain. *Patient Care.* 1994:22–39.

132. Forrest D. Common gynecologic pelvic disorders. In: Youngkin E, Davis M, eds. *Women's Health: A Primary Care Clinical Guide.* Stamford, CT: Appleton and Lange; 1998:313–362.

133. Rapkin A. Chronic pelvic pain. In: Hacker N, Moore J, eds. *Essentials of Obstetrics and Gynecology.* Philadelphia: Saunders; 1992.

134. Reed B, Haefner H, Punch M, et al. Psychosocial and sexual functioning in women with vulvodynia and chronic pelvic pain: a comparative evaluation. *J Reprod Med.* 2000;45(8):624–632.

135. Thomson J. Chronic inflammation of the peritoneum and vagina—review of its significance, immunologic pathogenesis, investigation and rationale for treatment. *J Reprod Med.* 2005;50(7):507–512.

136. Mathias S, Kuppermann M, Liebermann R, Lipschutz R, Steege J. Chronic pelvic pain: prevalence, health-related quality of life, and economic correlates. *Obstet Gynecol.* 1996;87(3):321–327.

137. Berkley K. A life of pelvic pain. *Physiol Behav.* 2005;86(3):272–280.

138. Smith C. Chronic pelvic pain: why empathy and listening are keys to diagnosis. *Consultant.* 1997:161–170.

139. Ostrzens A. *Gynecology: integrating Conventional, Complementary, and Natural Alternative Therapy.* Philadelphia: Lippincott Williams & Wilkins; 2002.

140. Gutta S. Perioperative preparation: chronic pelvic pain in women. *Gen Surg Laparosc News.* 1995;16(10):45–51.

141. Loffredo V. Clinical aspects and complementary tests in pelvic congestive states [French]. *Revue Francaise de Gynecologie et d Obstetrique.* 1991;86(2 Pt. 2):191–194.

142. Almeida R, Navarro D, Barbosa-Filho J. Plants with central analgesic activity. *Phytomedicine.* 2001;8(4):310–322.

143. Dillard J. Integrative approach to pain. In: Rakel D, ed. *Integrative Medicine.* Philadelphia: Saunders; 2003.

144. Moerman D. *Native American Ethnobotany.* 3rd ed. Portland, OR: Timber Press; 2000.

145. Felter H, Lloyd J. *King's American Dispensatory.* Cincinnati: reprinted by Eclectic Medical Publications., (1898); 1983.

146. Huang Ke. *The Pharmacology of Chinese Herbs.* 2nd ed. Boca Raton, FL: CRC Press; 1999.

147. Yeung H. *Handbook of Chinese Herbs.* Rosemead, CA: Institute of Chinese Medicine; 1996.

148. Della-Loggia R, Zilli C, Del-Negro R, Redaelli C, Tubaro A, Cody V. Isoflavones as spasmolytic principles of Piscidea Erythrina. Paper presented at: progress in Clinical and Biological Research, Vol. 280. *Plant Flavonoids in Biology and Medicine II: Biochemical, Cellular, and Medicinal Properties, Meeting,* Strasbourg, France, August 31-September 3, 1987.

149. McKenna D, Jones K, Hughes K, Humphrey S. *Botanical Medicines: The Desk Reference for Major Herbal Supplements*. New York: Haworth Press; 2002.

150. Yoshiro K. The physiological actions of Tang Kuei and Cnidium. *Bull Oriental Healing Arts Inst*. 1985;10:269–278.

151. Harada M, Suzuki M, Ozake Y. Effect of Japanese Angelica root and Peony root on uterine contraction in the rabbit in situ. *J Pharm Dyn*. 1984;7:304–311.

152. Zhu D. Dong quai. *Am J Chinese Med*. 1987;15(3-4):17–125.

153. Russo E. Cannabis treatments in obstetrics and gynecology: a historical review. In: Russo E, Dreher M, Mathre M, eds. *Women and Cannabis: Medicine, Science, and Sociology*. Binghamton, NY: Haworth Herbal Press; 2002:5–20035.

154. Ma Y, Yang D, Tian Z, Qu S, Ding Y, Wei Y. Effect of motherwort herb on the myoelectric activity of uterus in rats. *Zhongguo-Zhongyao-Zazhi*. 2000;25(6):364–366.

155. Reed B, Haefner H, Punch M, Chen C, Kwan C. Endothelium-independent vasorelaxation by Leonurine, a plant alkaloid purified from Chinese motherwort. *Life Sci*. 2001;68(8):953–960.

156. Reed B, Haefner H, Punch M, Zou Q. Effect of motherwort on blood hyperviscosity. *Am J Chin Med*. 1989;17(1):65–70.

157. Khishova O, Shcherbinin I, Kravchenko Y-V, Petrov P, Dunets L. Soporific activity of a preparation based on valerian (Valeriana L.), motherwort (Leonurus L.), and haw (Crataegus L.). *Farmatsiya [Russian]*. 2004;3:38–39.

158. Upton R. *American Herbal Pharmacopoeia and Therapeutic Monographs: Cramp Bark*. Santa Cruz, CA: American Herbal Pharmacopoeia; 2000.

159. Upton R. *American Herbal Pharmacopoeia and Therapeutic Monographs: Black Haw*. Santa Cruz, CA: American Herbal Pharmacopoeia; 2000.

160. Mills S, Bone K. *The Essential Guide to Herbal Safety*. St. Louis: Churchill Livingstone; 2005.

161. Kennelly E, Flynn T, Mazzola E, et al. Detecting potential teratogenic alkaloids from blue cohosh rhizomes using and in vitro rat embryo culture. *J Nat Prod*. 1999;62(10):1385–1389.

162. BHMA. *British Herbal Pharmacopoeia*. Keighley, UK: British Herbal Medicine Association; 1983.

163. Basch E, Ulbricht C. *Natural Standard Herb and Supplement Reference: Evidence-Based Clinical Reviews*. St. Louis: Mosby; 2005.

164. Ripoll E, Mahowald D. Hatha Yoga therapy management of urologic disorders. *World J Urol*. 2002;20(5):306–309.

165. Baker P. Musculoskeletal origins of chronic pelvic pain. *Obstet Gynecol Clin North Am*. 1993;20(4):719–742.

166. Glazer H, Rodke G, Swencionis C, Hertz R, Young A. Treatment of vulvar vestibulitis syndrome with electromyographic biofeedback of pelvic floor musculature. *J Reprod Med*. 2000;40(4):1.

167. Yount J, Solomons C, Willems J, St. Amand R. Effective nonsurgical treatments for vulvar pain. *Women's Health Dig*. 1997;3(2):98–103.

168. de-Oliveira-Bernardes N and Bahamondes L. Intravaginal electrical stimulation for the treatment of chronic pelvic pain. *J Reprod Med*. 2005;50(4):267–272.

169. Hudson T. *Women's Encyclopedia of Natural Medicine*. Los Angeles: McGraw-Hill; 1999.

170. Hrushesky W, Sothern R, Rietveld W, Du-Quiton JB, Mathilde E. Cancer-epidemiology-biomarkers-and-prevention. *Season, sun, sex, and cervical cancer*. 2005;14(8):1940–1947.

171. Cook W. *The Physio-Medical Dispensatory: A Treatise of Therapeutics, Materia Medica and Pharmacy*. Sandy, OR: Eclectic Medical Publications; 1985.

172. Ahmad N, Gupta S, Husain MM, Heiskanen KM, Mukhtar H. Differential antiproliferative and apoptotic response of sanguinarine for cancer cells versus normal cells. *Clin Cancer Res*. 2000;6(4):1524–1528.

173. Adhami VM, Aziz MH, Mukhtar H, Ahmad N. Activation of prodeath Bcl-2 family proteins and mitochondrial apoptosis pathway by sanguinarine in immortalized human HaCaT keratinocytes. *Clin Cancer Res*. 2003;9(8):3176–3182.

174. Begne M, Yslas N, Reyes E, Quiroz V, Santana J, Jimenez G. Clinical effect of a Mexican Sanguinaria extract (Polygonum aviculare L.) on gingivitis. *J Ethnopharmacol*. 2001;74(1):45–51.

175. Eversole L, Eversole G, Kopcik J. Sanguinaria-associated oral leukoplakia: comparison with other benign and dysplastic leukoplakic lesions. *Oral Surg Oral Med Oral Pathol Oral Radiol Endod*. 2000;89(4):455–464.

176. Allen C, Loudon J, Mascarenhas A. Sanguinaria-related leukoplakia: epidemiologic and clinicopathologic features of a recently described entity. *Gen Dentist*. 2001;49:608–614.

177. Munro I, Delzell E, Nestmann E, Lynch B. Viadent usage and oral leukoplakia: a spurious association. *Regul Toxicol Pharmacol*. 1999;30(3):182–196.

178. Kopczyk R, Abrams H, Brown A, Matheny J, Kaplan A. Clinical and microbiologica effects of a sanguinaria containing mouthrinse and dentifrice with and without fluoride during. 6 months of use. *J Periodontolog*. 1991;62(10):617–622.

179. Hannah J, Johnson J, Kuftinec M. Long-term clinical evaluation of toothpaste and oral rinse containing sanguinaria extract in controlling plaque, gingival inflammation and sulcular bleeding during orthodontic treatment. *Am J Orthodont Dentofac Orthop*. 1989;96(3):199–207.

180. Becci P, Schwartz H, Barnes H, Southard G. Short-term toxicity studies of sanguinarine and of two alkaloid extracts of Sanguinaria canadensis. *J Toxicol Environ Health*. 1987;20(1):199–208.

181. Keller K, Meyer D. Reproductive and developmental toxicological evaluation of sanguinaria extract. *J Clin Dent*. 1989;1(3):59–66.

182. Sepkovic DW, Stein J, Carlisle AD, Ksieski HB, Auborn K, Bradlow HL. Diindolylmethane inhibits cervical dysplasia, alters estrogen metabolism, and enhances immune response in the K14-HPV16 transgenic mouse model. *Cancer Epidemiol Biomarkers Prev*. 2009;18(11):2957–2964. United States.

183. Chen DZ, Qi M, Auborn KJ, Carter TH. Indole-3-carbinol and diindolylmethane induce apoptosis of human cervical cancer cells and in murine HPV16-transgenic preneoplastic cervical epithelium. *J Nutr*. 2001;131(12):3294–3302. United States.

184. Del Priore G, Gudipudi DK, Montemarano N, Restivo AM, Malanowska-Stega J, Arslan AA. Oral diindolylmethane (DIM): pilot evaluation of a nonsurgical treatment for cervical dysplasia. *Gynecol Oncol*. 2010;116(3):464–467. United States.

185. Hale L, Greer P, Trinh T, James C. Proteinase activity and stability of natural bromelain preparations. *Int Immunopharmacol*. 2005;5(4):783–793.

186. Gaspani L, Limiroli E, Ferrario P, Bianchi M. In vivo and in vitro effects of bromelain on PGE2 and SP concentrations in the inflammatory exudate in rats. *Pharmacology*. 2002;65(2):83–86.

187. Kumakura S, Yamashita M, Tsurufuji S. Effect of bromelain on kaolin-induced inflammation in rats. *Eur J Pharmacol*. 1988;10(150):295–301.

188. Katori M, Hori Y, Uchida Y, Tanaka K, Harada Y. Different modes of interaction of bradykinin with prostaglandins in pain and acute inflammation. *Adv Exp Med Biol. B*. 1986:393–398. 198 Pt.

189. Vellini M, Desideri D, Milanese A, et al. Possible involvement of eicosanoids in the pharmacological action of bromelain. *Arzneimittel-Forschung*. 1986;36(1):110–112.

190. Kleef R, Delohery TM, Bovbjerg DH. Selective modulation of cell adhesion molecules on lymphocytes by bromelain protease, 5. *Pathobiology*. 1996;64(6):339–346.

191. Batkin S, Taussig SJ, Szekerezes J. Antimetastatic effect of bromelain with or without its proteolytic and anticoagulant activity. *J Cancer Res Clin Oncol*. 1988;114(5):507–508.

192. Desser L, Zavadova E, Herbacek I. Oral enzymes as additive cancer therapy. *Int J Immunother*. 2001;17(2):153–161.

193. Eckert K, Grabowska E, Stange R, Schneider U, Eschmann K, Maurer HR. Effects of oral bromelain administration on the impaired immunocytotoxicity of mononuclear cells from mammary tumor patients. *Oncol Repts*. 1999;6(6):1191–1199.

194. Sanders H. Therapy of chlamydia infections with tetracyclines. *Int J Exp Clin Chemother*. 1990;3(2):101–106.

195. Bogdanova NS, Nikolaeva IS, Shcherbakova LI, Tolstova TI, Moskalenko N, Pershin GN. Study of antiviral properties of Calendula officinalis. *Farmakologiia i Toksikologiia*. 1970;33(3):349–355.

196. Schmidgall J, Schnetz E, Hensel A. Evidence for bioadhesive effects of polysaccharides and polysaccharide-containing herbs in an ex vivo bioadhesion assay on buccal membranes. *Planta Medica*. 2000;66(1):48–53.

197. Hore SK, Koley KM, Maiti SK. Modulatory role of Calendula officinalis on thermal stimulus-induced nociception and carrageenin-induced inflammation in rats. *Ind Vet J*. 1997;74(10):844–846.

198. Jorge Neto J, Fracasso JF, Neves MDCLC, Santos LED, Banuth VL. Treatment of varicose ulcer and skin lesions with Calendula officinalis L. or Stryphnodendron barbadetiman (Vellozo) Martius. *Revista de Ciencias Farmaceuticas*. 1996;17:181–186.

199. Hamburger M, Adler S, Baumann D, Forg A, Weinreich B. Preparative purification of the major anti-inflammatory triterpenoid esters from Marigold (Calendula officinalis). *Fitoterapia*. 2003;74(4):328–338.

200. Akihisa T, Yasukawa K, Oinuma H, et al. Triterpene alcohols from the flowers of compositae and their anti-inflammatory effects. *Phytochemistry*. 1996;43(6):1255–1260.

201. Shipochliev T, Dimitrov A, Aleksandrova E. [Anti-inflammatory action of a group of plant extracts]. *Veterinarno-Meditsinski Nauki*. 1981;18(6):87–94.

202. Pommier P, Gomez F, Sunyach MP, D'Hombres A, Carrie C, Montbarbon X. Phase III randomized trial of Calendula officinalis compared with trolamine for the prevention of acute dermatitis during irradiation for breast cancer. *J Clin Oncol*. 2004;22(8):1447–1453.

203. Tang XD, Zhou X, Zhang QZ, Le AD, Zhou KY. [Effects of green tea extract on expression of human papillomavirus type 16 oncoproteins-induced hypoxia-inducible factor-1alpha and vascular endothelial growth factor in human cervical carcinoma cells]. *Zhonghua Yi Xue Za Zhi*. 2008;88(40):2872–2877. China.

204. Stockfleth E, Beti H, Orasan R, et al. Topical Polyphenon E in the treatment of external genital and perianal warts: a randomized controlled trial. *Br J Dermatol*. 2008;158(6):1329–1338. England.

205. Tatti S, Swinehart JM, Thielert C, Tawfik H, Mescheder A, Beutner KR. Sinecatechins, a defined green tea extract, in the treatment of external anogenital warts: a randomized controlled trial. *Obstet Gynecol*. 2008;111(6):1371–1379. United States.

206. Scazzocchio F, Cometa MF, Tomassini L, Palmery M. Antibacterial activity of Hydrastis canadensis extract and its major isolated alkaloids. *Planta Medica*. 2001;67(6):561–564.

207. Hwang BY, Roberts SK, Chadwick LR, Wu CD, Kinghorn AD. Antimicrobial constituents from goldenseal (the Rhizomes of Hydrastis canadensis) against selected oral pathogens. *Planta Med*. 2003;69(7):623–627.

208. Anonymous. Berberine. *Alt Med Rev*. 2000;5(2):175–177.

209. Villinski JR, Dumas ER, Chai H-B, Pezzuto JM, Angerhofer CK, Gafner S. Antibacterial activity and alkaloid content of Berberis thunbergii, Berberis vulgaris and Hydrastis canadensis. *Pharm Biol*. 2003;41(8):551–557.

210. Rehman J, Dillow JM, Carter SM, Chou J, Le B, Maisel AS. Increased production of antigen-specific immunoglobulins G and M following in vivo treatment with the medicinal plants Echinacea angustifolia and Hydrastis canadensis. *Immunol Letts*. 1999;68(2):391–395.

211. Okimasu E, Moromizato Y, Watanabe S. Inhibition of phospholipase A2 and platelet aggregation by glycyrrhizin, an anti-inflammatory drug. *Acta Med Okayama*. 1983;37:355–391.

212. Cohen JI. Licking latency with licorice [comment]. *J Clin Invest*. 2005;115(3):591–593.

213. Lin J-C. Mechanism of action of glycyrrhizic acid in inhibition of Epstein-Barr virus replication in vitro. *Antiviral Res*. 2003;59(1):41–47.

214. Jeong HG, Kim JY. Induction of inducible nitric oxide synthase expression by 18beta-glycyrrhetinic acid in macrophages. *FEBS Letts*. 2002;513(2):208–212.

215. Yoshida T, Kobayashi M, Li X-D, Pollard RB, Suzuki F. Inhibitory effect of glycyrrhizin on the replication of M-tropic HIV in cultures of peripheral blood monocytes stimulated with neutrophils. *FASEB J*. 2005;19(5, suppl S, Part. 2):A1433.

216. Begami N. Prophaylactic effects of long-term oral administration of glycyrrhizin on aids development of asymptomatic patients. *Int Conf AIDS*. 1993;9(1):34 (abstract no. PO-A225-0596).

217. Hattori T. Preliminary evidence for inhibitory effect of glyrhhizin on HIV replication in patients with AIDS. *Antiviral Res*. 1989;11:255.

218. Begami N. Clinical Evaluation of Glycyrrhiza on HIV-Infected Asymptomatic Patients Hemophiliac Patients in Japan. *Paper presented at Fifth International Conference on AIDS*. June, 1989.

219. Mori K. Effects of glycyrrhizin (SNMC: Stonger Neo-Minophagen C) in hemophilia patients with HIV-1 infection. *Tohoku J Esp Med*. 1996;162:183–193.

220. Susuki H. Effects of glycyrrhizin on biochemical tests in patients with chronic hepatitis double blind trial. *Asian Med J*. 1984;26:423–438.

221. Partridge M, Posswillo D. Topical Carbonosolone sodium in management of herpes simplex infections. *Br J Oral Maxillofac Surg*. 1984;22:138–145.

222. Shibata S. A drug over the millennia: pharmacognosy, chemistry, and pharmacology of licorice. *Yakugaku Zasshi J Pharmaceut Soc Jpn.* 2000;120(10):849–862.

223. Fujisawa Y, Sakamoto M, Matsushita M, Fujita T, Nishioka K. Glycyrrhizin inhibits the lytic pathway of complement: possible mechanism of its anti-inflammatory effect on liver cells in viral hepatitis. *Microbiol Immunol.* 2000;44(9):799–804.

224. Brinker F. *Eclectic Dispensatory of Botanical Therapeutics: botanical Medicine Research Summaries: Lomatium dissectum.* Sandy OR: Eclectic Medical Publications; 1995:83–84.

225. McCutcheon A, Roberts T, Gibbons E, et al. Antiviral screening of British Columbian medicinal plants. *J Ethnopharmacol.* 1995;49(2):101–110.

226. Lee T, Kashiwada Y, Huang L. Suksdorfin: an anti-HIV principle from Lomatium suksdorfii, its structure-activity correlation with related coumarins, and synergistic effects with anti-AIDS nucleosides. *Bioorg Med Chem.* 1994;2(10):1051–1056.

227. Huang L, Kashiwada Y, Cosentino L. 3(,4(-DI-(camphanoyl-+ is-kelectome and related compounds: a new class of potential-HIV agents. *Bioorg Med Chem Lett.* 1994;4(4):593–598.

228. Moore M. *Medicinal plants of the Pacific west.* Santa Fe, NM: Red Crane Books; 1995.

229. Rountree R, Abascal K. *Lomatium, Micromedex;* 2001.

230. Schelz ZS, Molnar J, Hohmann J. Antimicrobial activity of volatile oils. *Int J Antimicrob Agents.* 2004:S205.

231. Nascimento GGF, Locatelli J, Freitas PC, Silva GL. Antibacterial activity of plant extracts and phytochemicals on antibiotic-resistant bacteria. *Brazilian J Microbiol.* 2000;31(4):247–256.

232. Lai PK, Roy J. Antimicrobial and chemopreventive properties of herbs and spices. *Curr Med Chem.* 2004;11(11):1451–1460.

233. Siddiqui YM, Ettayebi M, Haddad AM, Al-Ahdal MN. Effect of essential oils on the enveloped viruses: antiviral activity of oregano and clove oils on herpes simplex virus type 1 and Newcastle disease virus. *Med Sci Res.* 1996;24(3):185–186.

234. Upton R. *American Herbal Pharmacopoeia and Therapeutic Compendium: reishi Mushroom (Ganoderma lucidum).* Santa Cruz: American Herbal Pharmacopoeia; 2000.

235. Mistrangelo M, Cornaglia S, Pizzio M, et al. Immunostimulation to reduce recurrence after surgery for anal condyloma acuminata: a prospective randomized controlled trial. *Colorectal Dis.* 2010;12(8):799–803. England.

236. Lin ZB. Cellular and molecular mechanisms of immuno-modulation by Ganoderma lucidum. *J Pharmacol Sci.* 2005;99(2):144–153.

237. Gao Y, Tang W, Dai X, et al. Effects of water-soluble Ganoderma lucidum polysaccharides on the immune functions of patients with advanced lung cancer. *J Med Food.* 2005;8(2):159–168.

238. Lai LK, Abidin NZ, Abdullah N, Sabaratnam V. Anti-Human Papillomavirus (HPV) 16 E6 Activity of Ling Zhi or Reishi Medicinal Mushroom, Ganoderma lucidum (W. Curt.: Fr.) P. Karst. (Aphyllophoromycetideae) Extracts. International Journal of Medicinal Mushrooms. *Begel House Inc.* 2010;(3):12.

239. Hernandez-Marquez E, Lagunas-Martinez A, Bermudez-Morales VH, et al. Inhibitory Activity of Lingzhi or Reishi Medicinal Mushroom, Ganoderma lucidum (Higher Basidiomycetes) on Transformed Cells by Human Papillomavirus. *Int J Med Mushrooms.* 2014;16(2):179–187. United States.

240. Cao QZ, Lin ZB. Ganoderma lucidum polysaccharides peptide inhibits the growth of vascular endothelial cell and the induction of VEGF in human lung cancer cell. *Life Sci.* 2006;78(13):1457–1463.

241. Stanley G, Harvey K, Slivova V, Jiang J, Sliva D. Ganoderma lucidum suppresses angiogenesis through the inhibition of secretion of VEGF and TGF-beta1 from prostate cancer cells. *Biochem Biophys Res Commun.* 2005;330(1):46–52.

242. Lai SW, Lin JH, Lai SS, Wu YL. Influence of Ganoderma lucidum on blood biochemistry and immunocompetence in horses. *Amer J Chin Med.* 2004;32(6):931–940.

243. Hu H, Ahn NS, Yang X, Lee YS, Kang KS. Ganoderma lucidum extract induces cell cycle arrest and apoptosis in MCF-7 human breast cancer cell. *Int J Cancer.* 2002;102(3):250–253.

244. Mau JL, Lin HC, Chen CC. Antioxidant properties of several medicinal mushrooms. *J Agric Food Chem.* 2002;50(21):6072–6077.

245. McGuffin M, Hobbs C, Upton R, Goldberg A. Boca Raton: CRC Press; 1997.

246. Basu P, Dutta S, Begum R, et al. Clearance of cervical human papillomavirus infection by topical application of curcumin and curcumin containing polyherbal cream: a phase II randomized controlled study. *Asian Pac J Cancer Prev.* 2013;14(10):5753–5759. Thailand.

CHAPTER 12

1. Egan ME, Lipsky MS. Diagnosis of vaginitis. *Am Fam Physician.* 2000;62(5):1095–1104.

2. Say PJ, Jacyntho C. Difficult-to-manage vaginitis. *Clin Obstet Gynecol.* 2005;48(4):753–768.

3. Wilson C. Recurrent vulvovaginitis candidiasis; an overview of traditional and alternative therapies [see comment]. *Adv Nurse Pract.* 2005;13(5):24–29. quiz 30.

4. Kent H. Epidemiology of vaginitis. *Am J Obstet Gynecol.* 1991;165(4 pt 2):1168–1176.

5. Ressel G. CDC releases 2002 guidelines for treating STDs: part I. Diseases characterized by vaginal discharge and PID. *Am Fam Physician.* 2002;66(9).

6. Nyirjesy P. Chronic vulvovaginal candidiasis. *Am Fam Physician.* 2001;63(4):697–702.

7. Owen MK, Clenney TL. Management of vaginitis. *Am Fam Physician.* 2004;70(11):2125–2132.

8. Anderson MR, Klink K, Cohrssen A. Evaluation of vaginal complaints [see comment]. *JAMA.* 2004;291(11):1368–1379.

9. Schaaf V, Perez-Stable E, Borchardt K. The limited value of symptoms and signs in the diagnosis of vaginal infections. *Arch Intern Med.* 2001;150:1929–1933.

10. Ferris D. Management of bacterial vaginosis during pregnancy. *Amer Acad Fam Phys.* 1998;57(6).

11. Cram L, Zapata M, Toy E, Baker B. Genitourinary infections and their association with preterm labor. *Am Fam Physician.* 2002;65(2):241–248.

12. McDonald H, Brocklehurst P, Parsons J, Vigneswaran R. Antibiotics for treating bacterial vaginosis during pregnancy. *Cochrane Database.* 2006;1(CD000262).

13. Gynecologists ACoOa. Assessment of risk factors for preterm birth. *ACOG Pract Bull.* 2001.

14. Okun N, Gronau KA, Hannah ME. Antibiotics for bacterial vaginosis or Trichomonas vaginalis in pregnancy: a systematic review. *Obstet Gynecol.* 2005;105(4):857–868.

15. Ringdahl E. Treatment of recurrent vulvovaginal candidiasis. *Am Acad Fam Phys*. 2000;61:11.

16. Nyirjesy P, Weitz MV, Grody MH, Lorber B. Over-the-counter and alternative medicines in the treatment of chronic vaginal symptoms. *Obstet Gynecol*. 1997;90(1):50–53.

17. Harris JC, Cottrell SL, Plummer S, Lloyd D. Antimicrobial properties of Allium sativum (garlic). *Appl Microbiol Biotechnol*. 2001;57(3):282–286.

18. Watson CJ, Grando D, Fairley CK, et al. The effects of oral garlic on vaginal candida colony counts: a randomised placebo controlled double-blind trial. *BJOG*. 2014;121(4):498–506. England.

19. Sandhu D, Warraich M, Singh S. Sensitivity of yeasts isolated from cases of vaginitis to aqueous extracts of garlic. *Mykosen*. 1980;23:691–698.

20. Van Kessel K, Assefi N, Marrazzo J, Eckert L. Common complementary and alternative therapies for yeast vaginitis and bacterial vaginosis: a systematic review. *Obstet Gynecol Surv*. 2003;58(5):351–358.

21. McKenna D, Jones K, Hughes K, Humphrey S. *Botanical Medicines: The Desk Reference for Major Herbal Supplements*. New York: Haworth Press; 2002.

22. Anonymous. Berberine. *Alt Med Rev*. 2000;5(2):175–177.

23. Scazzocchio F, Cometa MF, Tomassini L, Palmery M. Antibacterial activity of Hydrastis canadensis extract and its major isolated alkaloids. *Planta Med*. 2001;67(6):561–564.

24. Villinski JR, Dumas ER, Chai H-B, Pezzuto JM, Angerhofer CK, Gafner S. Antibacterial activity and alkaloid content of Berberis thunbergii, Berberis vulgaris and Hydrastis canadensis. *Pharmaceut Biol*. 2003;41(8):551–557.

25. Rehman J, Dillow JM, Carter SM, et al. Increased production of antigen-specific immunoglobulins G and M following in vivo treatment with the medicinal plants Echinacea angustifolia and Hydrastis canadensis. *Immunol Letts*. 1999;68(2-3):391–395.

26. Low Dog T. *Women's Health in Complementary and Integrative Medicine: A Clinical Guide*. St. Louis: Elsevier; 2004.

27. Kalemba D, Kunicka A. Antibacterial and antifungal properties of essential oils [review]. *Curr Med Chem*. 2003;10(10):813–829.

28. D'Auria FD, Laino L, Strippoli V, et al. In vitro activity of tea tree oil against Candida albicans mycelial conversion and other pathogenic fungi. *J Chemother*. 2001;13(4):377–383.

29. Faleiro M, Miguel M, Ladeiro F, et al. Antimicrobial activity of essential oils isolated from Portuguese endemic species of Thymus. *Lett Appl Microbiol*. 2003;36(1):35–40.

30. Carson CF, Hammer KA, Riley TV. Melaleuca alternifolia (Tea Tree) oil: a review of antimicrobial and other medicinal properties. *Clin Microbiol Rev*. 2006;19(1):60–62.

31. Carson CF, Riley TV. Antimicrobial activity of the major components of the essential oil of Melaleuca alternifolia. *J Appl Bacteriol*. 1995;78(3):264–269.

32. Hammer KA, Carson CF, Riley TV. In vitro susceptibilities of lactobacilli and organisms associated with bacterial vaginosis to Melaleuca alternifolia (tea tree) oil. *Antimicrob Agents Chemother*. 1999;43(1):96.

33. Hammer KA, Carson CF, Riley TV. Melaleuca alternifolia (tea tree) oil inhibits germ tube formation by Candida albicans. *Med Mycol*. 2000;38(5):355–362.

34. Cox SD, Mann CM, Markham JL, et al. The mode of antimicrobial action of the essential oil of Melaleuca alternifolia (tea tree oil). *J Appl Microbiol*. 2000;88(1):170–175.

35. Blackwell AL. Tea tree oil and anaerobic (bacterial) vaginosis. *Lancet*. 1991;337(8736):300.

36. Hammer KA, Carson CF, Riley TV. In vitro activity of Melaleuca alternifolia (tea tree) oil against dermatophytes and other filamentous fungi. *J Antimicrob Chemother*. 2002;50(2):195–199.

37. Mondello F, De Bernardis F, Girolamo A, Cassone A, Salvatore G. In vivo activity of terpinen-4-ol, the main bioactive component of Melaleuca alternifolia Cheel (tea tree) oil against azole-susceptible and -resistant human pathogenic Candida species. *BMC Infect Dis*. 2006;6:158. England.

38. Hammer KA, Carson CF, Riley TV. Antifungal activity of the components of Melaleuca alternifolia (tea tree) oil. *J Appl Microbiol*. 2003;95(4):853–860.

39. Hammer KA, Carson CF, Riley TV. In vitro activities of ketoconazole, econazole, miconazole, and Melaleuca alternifolia (tea tree) oil against Malassezia species. *Antimicrob Agents Chemother*. 2000;44(2):467–469.

40. Cox SD, Gustafson JE, Mann CM, et al. Tea tree oil causes K+ leakage and inhibits respiration in Escherichia coli. *Letts Appl Microbiol*. 1998;26(5):355–358.

41. Hada T, Inoue Y, Shiraishi A, Hamashima H. Leakage of K+ ions from Staphylococcus aureus in response to tea tree oil. *J Microbiol Meth*. 2003;53(3):309–312.

42. Carson CF, Mee BJ, Riley TV. Mechanism of action of Melaleuca alternifolia (tea tree) oil on Staphylococcus aureus determined by time-kill, lysis, leakage, and salt tolerance assays and electron microscopy. *Antimicrob Agents Chemother*. 2002;46(6):1914–1920.

43. Nelson RR. Selection of resistance to the essential oil of Melaleuca alternifolia in Staphylococcus aureus. *J Antimicrob Chemother*. 2000;45(4):549–550.

44. Gustafson JE, Liew YC, Chew S, et al. Effects of tea tree oil on Escherichia coli. *Letts Appl Microbiol*. 1998;26(3):194–198.

45. Madamombe IT, Afolayan AJ. Evaluation of antimicrobial activity of extracts from South African Usnea barbata. *Pharmaceut Biol*. 2003;41(3):199–202.

46. Tosun F, Kizilay CA, Sener B, Vural M: The evaluation of plants from Turkey for in vitro antimycobacterial activity, *Pharmaceut Biol*. 43(1):58–63.

47. Bone K. *A Clinical Guide to Blending Liquid Herbs: Herbal Formulations for the Individual Patient*. St. Louis: Churchill Livingstone; 2003.

48. (ESCOP) ESCoP. *ESCOP Monographs: The Scientific Foundation for Herbal Medicinal Products*. Stuttgart: Thieme; 2003.

49. Wichtl M. *Herbal Drugs and Phytopharmaceuticals: A Handbook for Practice on a Scientific Basis*. 4th ed. Stuttgart: Medpharm; 2004.

50. Blumenthal M, Busse W, Goldberg A, et al., eds. *The Complete German Commission E Monographs*. Austin: American Botanical Council: Integrative Medicine Communications; 1998.

51. Reid G. Probiotics for urogenital health. *Nutr Clin Care*. 2002;5(1):3–8.

52. Hilton E, Isenberg H, Alperstein P. Ingestion of yogurt containing Lactobacillus acidophilus as prophylaxis for candidal vaginitis. *Arch Fam Med*. 1992;116:353–357.

53. Youngkin E, Davis M. *Women's Health: A Primary Care Clinical Guide*. Stamford: Appleton and Lange; 1998.

54. Jovanovic R, Congema E, Nguyen HT. Antifungal agents vs. boric acid for treating chronic mycotic vulvovaginitis. *J Reprod Med*. 1991;36(8):593–597.

55. Van Slyke K, Michel V, Rein M. Treatment of vulvovaginal candidiasis with boric acid powder. *Am J Obstet Gynecol.* 1981;141:145–148.

56. Sobel JD, Chaim W. Treatment of Torulopsis glabrata vaginitis: retrospective review of boric acid therapy. *Clin Infect Dis.* 1997;24(4):649–652.

57. Swate T, Weed J. Boric acid treatment of vulvovaginal candidiasis. *Obstet Gynecol.* 1974;43:893–895.

58. Workowski K, Levine W. Sexually transmitted diseases treatment guidelines. *Morbid Mortal Wkly Rept.* 2002; 51(RR-6).

59. Beutner K, Conant M, Friedman-Kien A. Patient applied podofilox for treatment of genital warts. *Lancet.* 1989;1(Apr 15):831–834.

60. Lassus A. Comparison of podophyllotoxin and podophyllin in treatment of genital warts. *Lancet.* 1987;2(Aug 29):512–513.

61. Welander C, Homesley H, Smiles K, Peets E. Intralesional interferon alfa-2b for the treatment of genital warts. *Am J Obstet Gynecol.* 1990;162:348–354.

62. Chang H. Singapore: World Scientific; 1987.

63. Zhi-wei Q, Shu-juan M, Xiao-chen C. Viral etiology of chronic cervicitis and its therapeutic response to a recombinant interferon. *Chin Med J.* 1990;103(8):647.

64. Luettig B, Steinmuller C, Gifford G, Wagner H, Lohmann-Mathes M. Macrophage activity by the polysaccharide arabinogalactan isolated from plant cell cultures of Echinacea purpurea. *J Natl Cancer Inst.* 1989;81(9):669–676.

65. Vonau B, Chard S, Mandalia S, Wilkinson D, Barton S. Does the extract of the plant Echinacea purpurea influence the clinical course of recurrent genital herpes? *Int J STD AIDS.* 2001;12:154–158.

66. Binns S, Hudson J, Merali S, Arnason J. Antiviral activity of characterized extracts from Echinacea spp. (Heliantheae: Asteraceae) against Herpes simplex virus (HSV-1). *Planta Med.* 2002;68:780–783.

67. Stockfleth E, Beti H, Orasan R, et al. Topical Polyphenon E in the treatment of external genital and perianal warts: a randomized controlled trial. *Br J Dermatol.* 2008;158(6):1329–1338. England.

68. Tatti S, Swinehart JM, Thielert C, Tawfik H, Mescheder A, Beutner KR. Sinecatechins, a defined green tea extract, in the treatment of external anogenital warts: a randomized controlled trial. *Obstet Gynecol.* 2008;111(6):1371–1379. United States.

69. Litvinenko V, Popova T, Simonjan A, Zoz I, Sokolov V. "Gerbstoffe" und Oxyzimtsaureabkommlinge in Labiaten. *Planta Medica.* 1975;27:372–380.

70. Chalbicz J, Galasinski W. The components of Melissa officinalis that influence protein biosynthesis in vitro. *J Pharm Pharmacol.* 1986;38(11):791–794.

71. Koytchev R, Alken R, Dundarov S. Lemon balm cream reduces outbreak of oral herpes in clinical study. *Phytomedicine.* 1999;6(4):225–230.

72. Cerny A, Schmid K. Tolerability and efficacy of valerian/lemon balm in health volunteers (a double-blind, placebo-controlled, multicentre study). *Fitoterapia.* 1999;70:221–228.

73. Siddiqui YM, Ettayebi M, Haddad AM, Al-Ahdal MN. Effect of essential oils on the enveloped viruses: antiviral activity of oregano and clove oils on herpes simplex virus type 1 and Newcastle disease virus. *Med Sci Res.* 1996;24(3):185–186.

74. Lai PK, Roy J. Antimicrobial and chemopreventive properties of herbs and spices. *Curr Med Chem.* 2004;11(11):1451–1460.

75. Mills S, Bone K. *The Essential Guide to Herbal Safety.* St. Louis: Elsevier Churchill Livingstone; 2005.

76. McGuffin M, Hobbs C, Upton R, Goldberg A. Boca Raton: CRC Press; 1997.

77. Fleming D. Herpes simplex virus type 2 in the United States. *NEJM.* 1997;337(16):1105–1111.

78. Committee on Infectious Diseases. *Red Book: Report of the committee on infectious diseases.* Elk Grove: Am Acad of Ped; 2000.

79. Miller KE, Ruiz DE, Graves JC. Update on the prevention and treatment of sexually transmitted diseases. *Am Fam Physician.* 2003;67(9):1915–1922.

80. Roe VA. Living with genital herpes: how effective is antiviral therapy? *J Perinat Neonat Nurs.* 2004;18(3):206–215.

81. Priddy K. Immunologic adaptations during pregnancy. *J Obstet Gynecol Neonatal Nurs.* 1997;26(4):288–394.

82. Holmes KK, Levine R, Weaver M. Effectiveness of condoms in preventing sexually transmitted infections. *Bull WHO.* 2004;82(6):454–461.

83. Alvarez-Lafuente R, Fernandez-Gutierrez B, de Miguel S, et al. Potential relationship between herpes viruses and rheumatoid arthritis: analysis with quantitative real time polymerase chain reaction. *Ann Rheum Dis.* 2005;64(9):1357–1359.

84. Steben M. Genital herpes simplex virus infection. *Clin Obstet Gynecol.* 2005;48(4):838–844.

85. Cone R, Hobson A, Brown Z. Frequent detection of genital herpes simplex virus DNA by polymerase chain reaction among pregnant women. *JAMA.* 1994;272:792–796.

86. Jacobs R. Neonatal herpes simplex virus infections. *Semin Perinatol.* 1998;22:64–71.

87. Kimberlin D, Lin C, Jacobs R. Safety and efficacy of high-dose intravenous acyclovir in the management of neonatal herpes simplex virus infections. *Pediatrics.* 2001;108:230–238.

88. Brown A, Selke S, Zeh J, et al. The acquisition of herpes simplex virus during pregnancy. *NEJM.* 1997;337(8):509–515.

89. Braig S, Luton D, Sibony O, et al. Acyclovir prophylaxis in late pregnancy prevents recurrent genital herpes and viral shedding. *Eur J Obstet Gynecol Reprod Biol.* 2001;96(1):55–58.

90. Kesson A. Management of neonatal herpes simplex virus infection. *Paediatr Drugs.* 2001;3(2):81–90.

91. Scott L, Hollier L, McIntire D, Sanchez P, Jackson G, Wendel GJ. Acyclovir suppression to prevent clinical recurrences at delivery after first episode genital herpes in pregnancy: an open-label trial. *Infect Dis Obstet Gynecol.* 2001;9(2):75–80.

92. Saller R, Buechi S, Meyrat R, Schmidhauser C. Combined herbal preparation for topical treatment of Herpes labialis. *Forsch Komplementarmed Klass Naturheilkd.* 2001;8(6):373–382.

93. Carson CF, Ashton L, Dry L, Smith DW, Riley TV. Melaleuca alternifolia (tea tree) oil gel (6%) for the treatment of recurrent herpes labialis. *J Antimicrob Chemother.* 2001;48(3):450–451.

94. Pollara G, Katz DR, Chain BM. The host response to herpes simplex virus infection. *Curr Opin Infect Dis.* 2004;17(3):199–203.

95. Felter H, Lloyd J. *King's American Dispensatory.* Cincinnati: reprinted by Eclectic Medical Publications; 1983. 1898.

96. Syed T, Cheema K, Ashfaq A, Holt A. Aloe vera extract 0.5% in a hydrophilic cream versus Aloe vera gel for the management of genital herpes in males: a placebo controlled, double-blind, comparison study [letter]. *J Eur Acad Dermatol Venereol.* 1996:294–295.

97. Syed T, Afzal M, Ashfaq A, Ahmad S. Management of genital herpes in men with 0.5% Aloe vera extract in a hydrophilic cream: a placebo controlled double-blind study. *J Dermatol Treat.* 1997;8:99–102.

98. Ghaemi A, Soleimanjahi H, Gill P, Arefian E, Soudi S, Hassan Z. Echinacea purpurea polysaccharide reduces the latency rate in herpes simplex virus type-1 infections. *Intervirology.* 2009;52(1):29–34. Switzerland.

99. Gallo M, Sarkar M, Au W, et al. Pregnancy outcome following exposure to echinacea: a prospective controlled study. *Arch Int Med.* 2000;160:3141–3143.

100. Allahverdiyev A, Duran N, Ozguven M, Koltas S. Antiviral activity of the volatile oils of Melissa officinalis L. against Herpes simplex virus type-2. *Phytomedicine.* 2004;11 (7-8):657–661.

101. Koytchev R, Alken RG, Dundarov S. Balm mint extract (Lo-701) for topical treatment of recurring herpes labialis. *Phytomedicine.* 1999;6(4):225–230.

102. Astani A, Reichling J, Schnitzler P. Melissa officinalis extract inhibits attachment of herpes simplex virus in vitro. *Chemotherapy.* 2012;58(1):70–77. Switzerland.

103. Nolkemper S, Reichling J, Stintzing FC, Carle R, Schnitzler P. Antiviral effect of aqueous extracts from species of the Lamiaceae family against Herpes simplex virus type 1 and type 2 in vitro. *Planta Med.* 2006;72(15):1378–1382. Germany.

104. Astani A, Navid MH, Schnitzler P. Attachment and penetration of acyclovir-resistant herpes simplex virus are inhibited by Melissa officinalis extract. *Phytother Res.* 2014;28(10):1547–1552. England.

105. Utsunomiya TKM, Herndon DN. Glycyrrhizin (20 beta-carboxy-11-oxo-30-norolean-12-en-3 beta-yl-2-O-beta-D-glucopyranuronosyl-alpha-D-glucopyranosiduronic acid) improves the resistance of thermally injured mice to opportunistic infection of herpes simplex virus type 1. *Immunol Lett.* 1995;44(1):59–66.

106. Hirabayashi K, Iwata S, Matsumoto H. Antiviral activities of glycyrrhizin and its modified compounds against human immunodeficiency virus type 1 (HIV-1) and herpes simplex virus type 1 (HSV-1) in vitro. *Chem Pharm Bull (Tokyo).* 1991;39(1):112–115.

107. Pompei R, Flore O, Marccialis MA, Pani A, Loddo B. Glycyrrhizic acid inhibits virus growth and inactivates virus particles. *Nature.* 1979;281(5733):689–690.

108. Wang Z, Nixon D. Licorice and cancer (review). *Nutr Cancer.* 2001;39(1):1–11.

109. Shibata S. A drug over the millennia: pharmacognosy, chemistry, and pharmacology of licorice. *Yakugaku Zasshi—J Pharmaceut Soc Jpn.* 2000;120(10):849–862.

110. Sekizawa T, Yanagi K, Itoyama Y. Glycyrrhizin increases survival of mice with herpes simplex encephalitis. *Acta Virol.* 2001;45(1):51–54.

111. Cohen J. Licking latency with licorice. *J Clin Invest.* 2005;115(3):591–593.

112. Li Z, Liu J, Zhao Y. Possible mechanism underlying the antiherpetic activity of a proteoglycan isolated from the mycelia of Ganoderma lucidum in vitro. *J Biochem Mol Biol.* 2005;38(1):34–40.

113. Eo SK, Kim YS, Lee CK, Han SS. Possible mode of antiviral activity of acidic protein bound polysaccharide isolated from Ganoderma lucidum on herpes simplex viruses. *J Ethnopharmacol.* 2000;72(3):475–481.

114. Kim YS, Eo SK, Oh KW, Lee C, Han SS. Antiherpetic activities of acidic protein bound polysaccharide isolated from Ganoderma lucidum alone and in combinations with interferons. *J Ethnopharmacol.* 2000;72(3):451–458.

115. Eo SK, Kim YS, Lee CK, Han SS. Antiherpetic activities of various protein bound polysaccharides isolated from Ganoderma lucidum. *J Ethnopharmacol.* 1999;68(1-3):175–181.

116. Oh KW, Lee CK, Kim YS, Eo SK, Han SS. Antiherpetic activities of acidic protein bound polysaccharide isolated from Ganoderma lucidum alone and in combinations with acyclovir and vidarabine. *J Ethnopharmacol.* 2000;72(1-2):221–227.

117. Hijikata Y, Yasuhara A, Sahashi Y. Effect of an herbal formula containing Ganoderma lucidum on reduction of herpes zoster pain: a pilot clinical trial. *Am J Chin Med.* 2005;33(4):517–523.

118. Andersen DO, Weber ND, Wood SG, Hughes BG, Murray BK, North JA. In vitro virucidal activity of selected anthraquinones and anthraquinone derivatives. *Antiviral Res.* 1991;16(2):185–196.

119. Sydiskis RJ, Owen DG, Lohr JL, Rosler KH, Blomster RN. Inactivation of enveloped viruses by anthraquinones extracted from plants. *Antimicrob Agents Chemother.* 1991;35(12):2463–2466.

120. Mannel M, Koytchev R, Dundarov S. Oral hypericum extract LI 160 is an effective treatment of recurrent herpes genitalis and herpes labialis. *Phytomedicine.* 2000;7(suppl 2):17.

121. Schnitzler P, Schon K, Reichling J. Antiviral activity of Australian tea tree oil and eucalyptus oil against herpes simplex virus in cell culture. *Pharmazie.* 2001;56(4):343–347.

122. Singha PK, Roy S, Dey S. Antimicrobial activity of Andrographis paniculata. *Fitoterapia.* 2003;74(7-8):692–694.

123. Ji LL, Wang Z, Dong F, Zhang WB, Wang ZT. Andrograpanin, a compound isolated from anti-inflammatory traditional Chinese medicine Andrographis paniculata, enhances chemokine SDF-1alpha-induced leukocytes chemotaxis. *J Cell Biochem.* 2005;95(5):970–978.

124. Burgos RA, Seguel K, Perez M, et al. Andrographolide inhibits IFN-gamma and IL-2 cytokine production and protects against cell apoptosis. *Planta Medica.* 2005;71(5):429–434.

125. Rakel D. *Integrative Medicine.* Philadelphia: Saunders; 2003.

126. Wiart C, Kumar K, Yusof MY, Hamimah H, Fauzi ZM, Sulaiman M. Antiviral properties of ent-labdene diterpenes of Andrographis paniculata nees, inhibitors of herpes simplex virus type 1. *Phytother Res.* 2005;19(12):1069–1070.

127. Glatthaar-Saalmuller B, Sacher F, Esperester A. Antiviral activity of an extract derived from roots of Eleutherococcus senticosus. *Antiviral Res.* 2001;50(3):223–228.

128. Ellingwood F. Cincinnati: Eclectic Medical Publications; 1919.

129. Hoffmann D. *Medical Herbalism: The Science and Practice of Herbal Medicine.* Rochester, VT: Healing Arts Press; 2003.

130. Schulz V, Hansel R, Blumenthal M, Tyler V. *Rational Phytotherapy: A Reference Guide for Physicians and Pharmacists.* 5th ed. Berlin: Springer-Verlag; 2004.

131. Wolfson P, Hoffmann DL. An investigation into the efficacy of Scutellaria lateriflora in healthy volunteers. *Alt Ther Health Med.* 2003;9(2):74–78.

132. Awad R, Arnason JT, Trudeau V, et al. Phytochemical and biological analysis of skullcap (Scutellaria lateriflora L.): a medicinal plant with anxiolytic properties. *Phytomedicine.* 2003;10(8):640–649.

133. Corina P, Dimitris S, Emanuil T, Nora R. [Treatment with acyclovir combined with a new Romanian product from plants]. *Oftalmologia*. 1999;46(1):55–57.

134. Greenway FL, Frome BM, Engels TM, McLellan A. Temporary relief of postherpetic neuralgia pain with topical geranium oil. *Am J Med*. 2003;115(7):586–587.

135. McCune M. Treatment of recurrent herpes simplex infection with L-lysine monohydrochloride. *Cutis*. 1984;34(4):366–373.

136. Choi B, Lee ES, Sohn S. Vitamin D3 ameliorates herpes simplex virus-induced Behçet's disease-like inflammation in a mouse model through down-regulation of Toll-like receptors. *Clin Exp Rheumatol*. 2011;29(4 suppl 67):S13–S19. Italy.

137. De Luca C, Kharaeva Z, Raskovic D, Pastore P, Luci A, Korkina L. Coenzyme Q(10), vitamin E, selenium, and methionine in the treatment of chronic recurrent viral mucocutaneous infections. *Nutrition*. 2012;28(5):509–514. United States.

138. Mikhail IS, DiClemente R, Person S, et al. Association of complementary and alternative medicines with HIV clinical disease among a cohort of women living with HIV/AIDS. *JAIDS*. 2004;37(3):1415–1422.

139. Foote-Ardah CE. The meaning of complementary and alternative medicine practices among people with HIV in the United States: strategies for managing everyday life. *Soc Health Illness*. 2003;25(5):481–500.

140. Thorne S, Paterson B, Russell C, Schultz A. Complementary/alternative medicine in chronic illness as informed self-care decision making. *Int J Nurs Stud*. 2002;39(7):671–683.

141. Mills E, Singh R, Kawasaki M, et al. Emerging issues associated with HIV patients seeking advice from health food stores. *Can J Pub Health Rev Canadienne de Sante Publique*. 2003;94(5):363–366.

142. Leonard B, Huff H, Merryweather B, Lim A, Mills E. Knowledge of safety and herb-drug interations among HIV+ individuals: a focus group study. *Can J Pub Health Rev Canadienne de Sante Publique*. 2004;11(2):227–231.

143. Fairfield KM, Eisenberg DM, Davis RB, Libman H, Phillips RS. Patterns of use, expenditures, and perceived efficacy of complementary and alternative therapies in HIV-infected patients. [see comment]. *Arch Int Med*. 1998;158(20): 2257–2264.

144. Hsiao AF, Wong MD, Kanouse DE, et al. Complementary and alternative medicine use and substitution for conventional therapy by HIV-infected patients. *JAIDS*. 2003;33(2):157–165.

145. Furler MD, Einarson TR, Walmsley S, Millson M, Bendayan R. Use of complementary and alternative medicine by HIV-infected outpatients in Ontario, Canada. *AIDS Pat Care Stds*. 2003;17(4):155–168.

146. de Visser R, Grierson J. Use of alternative therapies by people living with HIV/AIDS in Australia. *AIDS Care*. 2002;14(5):599–606.

147. Kirksey KM, Goodroad BK, Kemppainen JK, et al. Complementary therapy use in persons with HIV/AIDS. *J Hol Nurs*. 2002;20(3):264–278.

148. Jernewall N, Zea MC, Reisen CA, Poppen PJ. Complementary and alternative medicine and adherence to care among HIV-positive Latino gay and bisexual men. *AIDS Care*. 2005;17(5):601–609.

149. Tsao JC, Dobalian A, Myers CD, Zeltzer LK. Pain and use of complementary and alternative medicine in a national sample of persons living with HIV. *J Pain Sympt Mgmt*. 2005;30(5):418–432.

150. Meneilly G, Carr R, Brown L. *Alternative therapy use in HIV-positive women [abstract MOB-301]*. Vancouver, BC: Paper presented at: 11th International Conference on AIDS; 1996.

152. Pawluch D, Cain R, Gillett J. Lay constructions of HIV and complementary therapy use. *Soc Sci Med*. 2000;51:251–264.

151. Foote-Ardah CE. Sociocultural barriers to the use of complementary and alternative medicine for HIV. *Qual Health Res*. 2004;14(5):593–611.

153. Mills E, Wu P, Ernst E. Complementary therapies for the treatment of HIV: in search of the evidence. *Int J STD AIDS*. 2005;16(6):395–403.

154. Liu J, Manheimer E, Yang M. Herbal medicine for treating HIV infection and AIDS. *Cochrane Database*. 2005;3 (Art. No.: CD003937.pub2. http://dx.doi.org/10.1002/14651858).

155. Burack J, Cohen M, Hahn J, Abrams D. Pilot randomized controlled trial of Chinese herbal treatment for HIV-associated symptoms. *J AIDS Hum Retrovirol*. 1996;12(4):386–393.

156. Weber R, Christen L, Loy M, Schaller S, Christen S, Joyce C. Randomized, placebo-controlled trial of Chinese herb therapy for HIV-infected individuals. *JAIDS*. 1999;22(1):56–64.

157. Durant J, Chantre P, Gonzalez G, Vandermander J, Halfon P, Rousse B. Efficacy and safety of Buxus semperirens L. preparations (SPV 30) in HIV-infected asymptomatic patients: a multicentre, randomized, double-blind, placebo-controlled trial. *Phytomedicine*. 1998;5(1):1–10.

158. Holodniy M, Koch J, Mistal M, Schmidt J, Khandwala A, Pennington J. A double blind, randomized, placebo-controlled phase II study to assess the safety and efficacy of orally administered SP-303 for the symptomatic treatment of diarrhea in patients with AIDS. *Am J Gastroenterol*. 1999;94(11):3267–3273.

CHAPTER 13

1. Goldman M, Hatch C. *Women and Health*. San Diego: Academic Press; 2000.

2. Youngkin E, Davis M. *Women's Health: A Primary Care Clinical Guide*. Stamford: Appleton and Lange; 1998.

3. Kasper D, Braunwald E, Fauci A, et al. *Harrison's Principles of Internal Medicine*. 16th ed. New York: McGraw-Hill; 2005.

4. Reid G, Bruce AW. Urogenital infections in women: can probiotics help? *Postgrad Med J*. 2003;79(934):428–432.

5. Howes D, Henry S. Urinary tract infection, female. *eMedicine*. 2005.

6. Reid G, Burton J, Devillard E. The rationale for probiotics in female urogenital healthcare. *Medgenmed [computer file]: Medscape Gen Med*. 2004;6(1):49.

7. McKenna D, Jones K, Hughes K, Humphrey S. *Botanical Medicines: The Desk Reference for Major Herbal Supplements*. New York: Haworth Press; 2002.

8. Upton R. Cranberry fruit: vaccinium macrocarpon. American Herbal Pharmacopoeia and Therapeutic Compendium. *American Herbal Pharmacopoeia and Therapeutic Compendium*. 2002.

9. Ofek I, Zafriri D, Adar R, Lis H, Sharon N. Inhibition of Escherichia coli Adherences to Eukaryotic Cells by Fruit Juices. *Abstracts of the Annual Meeting of the American Society for Microbiology*. 1989;38.

10. Raz R, Chazan B, Dan M. Cranberry juice and urinary tract infection. *Clin Infect Dis*. 2004;38(10):1413–1419.

11. Ahuja SK, Kaak B, Roberts JA. Loss of fimbrial adhesion with the addition of vaccinium macrocarpon to the growth media of P-fimbriated *E. coli*. *J Urol*. 1996;155(suppl 5):674A.

12. Kontiokari T. The effect of dietary factors on the risk of developing urinary tract infection: reply. *Pediatr Nephrol*. 2004;19(11):1304.

13. Habash MB, Van der Mei HC, Busscher HJ, Reid G. The effect of water, ascorbic acid, and cranberry derived supplementation on human urine and uropathogen adhesion to silicone rubber. *Can J Microbiol*. 1999;45(8):691–694.

14. Jepson R, Mihaljevic L, Craig J. Cranberries for preventing urinary tract infections. *Cochrane Database*. 2004;(2). Art. No.: CD001321. http://dx.doi.org/001310.100214651858. CD100214001321.pub100214651853.

15. Takahashi S, Hamasuna R, Yasuda M, et al. A randomized clinical trial to evaluate the preventive effect of cranberry juice (UR65) for patients with recurrent urinary tract infection. *J Infect Chemother*. 2013;19(1):112–117. Japan.

16. Lee Y, Najm W, Owens J, et al. Anti-microbial activitiy of urine after ingestion of cranberry: a pilot study. *Epublication prior to print publication: eCAM*. 2010;7(2):227–232. http://dx.doi.org/10.1093/ecam/nem183.

17. Efros M, Bromberg W, Cossu L, Nakeleski E, Katz AE. Novel concentrated cranberry liquid blend, UTI-STAT with Proantinox, might help prevent recurrent urinary tract infections in women. *Urology*. 2010;76(4):841–845. United States.

18. Cadková I, Doudová L, Nováčková M, Huvar I, Chmel R. [Effect of cranberry extract capsules taken during the perioperative period upon the post-surgical urinary infection in gynecology]. *Ceska Gynekol*. 2009;74(6):454–458. Czech Republic.

19. McMurdo ME, Argo I, Phillips G, Daly F, Davey P. Cranberry or trimethoprim for the prevention of recurrent urinary tract infections? A randomized controlled trial in older women. *J Antimicrob Chemother*. 2009;63(2):389–395. England.

20. Mazokopakis EE, Karefilakis CM, Starakis IK. Efficacy of cranberry capsules in prevention of urinary tract infections in postmenopausal women. *J Altern Complement Med*. 2009;15(11): 1155–1155. Mary Ann Liebert, Inc. 140 Huguenot Street, 3rd Floor New Rochelle, NY 10801 USA.

21. Wing DA, Rumney PJ, Preslicka CW, Chung JH. Daily cranberry juice for the prevention of asymptomatic bacteriuria in pregnancy: a randomized, controlled pilot study. *J Urol*. 2008;180(4):1367–1372. United States.

22. Low Dog T. *Women's Health in Complementary and Integrative Medicine: A Clinical Guide*. St. Louis: Elsevier; 2004.

23. Lynch D. Cranberry for prevention of urinary tract infections [see comment]. *Am Fam Physician*. 2004;70(11):2175–2177.

24. Upton R. *Uva ursi leaf: Arctostaphylos uva ursi*. Santa Cruz: Am Herb Pharm; 2006.

25. Blumenthal M, Busse W, Goldberg A, et al. *The Complete German Commission E Monographs: Therapeutic Guide to Herbal Medicine*. Boston: American Botanical Council; 1998.

26. (ESCOP) ESCoP. *ESCOP Monographs: The Scientific Foundation for Herbal Medicinal Products*. Stuttgart: Thieme; 2003.

27. Jahodar L, Jilek P, Paktova M, Dvorakova V. [Antimicrobial effect of arbutin and an extract of the leaves of Arctostaphylos Uva ursi in vitro]. *Ceskoslovenska Farmacie*. 1985;34(5):174–178.

28. Matsuda H, Tanaka T, Kubo M. [Pharmacological studies on leaf of Arctostaphylos Uva ursi (L.) Spreng. III. Combined effect of arbutin and indomethacin on immuno-inflammation]. *Yakugaku Zasshi J Pharmaceut Soc Jpn*. 1991;111(4-5):253–258.

29. Matsuda H, Nakata H, Tanaka T, Kubo M. [Pharmacological study on Arctostaphylos Uva ursi (L.) Spreng. II. Combined effects of arbutin and prednisolone or dexamethazone on immuno-inflammation]. *Yakugaku Zasshi J Pharmaceut Soc Jpn*. 1990;110(1):68–76.

30. Larsson B, Jonasson A, Fianu S. Prophylactic effect of uva-e in women with recurrent cystitis: a preliminary report. *Curr Therapeut Res*. 1993;53:441–443.

31. Weiss RF, Fintelmann V. *Herbal Medicine*. 2nd ed. Stuttgart: Thieme; 2000.

32. Yarnell E. Botanical medicines for the urinary tract. *World J Urol*. 2002;20(5):285–293.

33. McGuffin M, Hobbs C, Upton R, Goldberg A. Boca Raton: CRC Press; 1997.

34. Mills S, Bone K. *The Essential Guide to Herbal Safety*. St. Louis: Churchill Livingstone; 2005.

35. Brinker F. *Herb Contraindications and Drug Interactions*. 3rd ed. Sandy: OR, Eclectic Medical Publications; 2001.

36. Bove M. *Personal communication*; 2006. ***.

37. Stojanovi G, Radulovi N, Hashimoto T, Pali R. In vitro antimicrobial activity of extracts of four Achillea species: the composition of Achillea clavennae L. (Asteraceae) extract. *J Ethnopharmacol*. 2005;101:185–190.

38. Candan F, Unlu M, Tepe B, Daferera D, Polissiou M, Sokmen H. Antioxidant and antimicrobial activity of the essential oil and methanol extracts of Achillea millefolium subsp. millefolium Afan. (Asteraceae). *J Ethnopharmacol*. 2003;87:215–220.

39. Wichtl M. *Herbal Drugs and Phytopharmaceuticals: A Handbook for Practice on a Scientific Basis*. 4th ed. Stuttgart: Medpharm; 2004.

40. Nascimento G, Locatelli J, Freitas P, Silva G. Antibacterial activity of plant extracts and phytochemicals on antibiotic resistant bacteria. *J Microbiol*. 2000;31:247–256.

41. Holetz FB, Pessini GL, Sanches NR, Cortez DA. Screening of some plants used in the Brazilian folk medicine for the treatment of infectious diseases. *Mem Inst Oswaldo Cruz*. 2002;9(7):1027–1031.

42. Bone K. *A Clinical Guide to Blending Liquid Herbs: Herbal Formulations for the Individual Patient*. St. Louis: Churchill Livingstone; 2003.

43. Melzig MF. [Goldenrod—a classical exponent in the urological phytotherapy]. *Wiener Medizinische Wochenschrift*. 2004;154(21-22):523–527.

44. Reid G. Potential preventive strategies and therapies in urinary tract infection. *World J Urol*. 1999;17(6):359–363.

45. Reid G. Probiotics for urogenital health. *Nutr Clin Care*. 2002;5(1):3–8.

46. Kontiokari T, Laitinen J, Jarvi L, Pokka T, Sundqvist K, Uhari M. Dietary factors protecting women from urinary tract infection. *Am J Clin Nutr*. 2003;77(3):600–604.

47. Mombelli B, Gismondo MR. The use of probiotics in medical practice. *Int J Antimicrob Agents*. 2000;16(4):531–536.

48. Stapleton AE, Au-Yeung M, Hooton TM, et al. Randomized, placebo-controlled phase 2 trial of a Lactobacillus crispatus probiotic given intravaginally for prevention of recurrent urinary tract infection. *Clin Infect Dis*. 2011;52(10):1212–1217. United States.

49. Czaja CA, Stapleton AE, Yarova-Yarovaya Y, Stamm WE. Phase I trial of a Lactobacillus crispatus vaginal suppository for prevention of recurrent urinary tract infection in women. *Infect Dis Obstet Gynecol*. 2007;2007:35387. Egypt.

50. Carlsson S, Wiklund NP, Engstrand L, Weitzberg E, Lundberg JO. Effects of pH, nitrite, and ascorbic acid on nonenzymatic nitric oxide generation and bacterial growth in urine. *Nitric Oxide*. 2001;5(6):580–586.

51. Hanno PM. Interstitial cystitis and related disorders. In: Walsh PC, ed. *Campbell's Urology*. 8th ed. Philadelphia: Elsevier; 2002.

52. Parsons CL, Albo M. Intravesical potassium sensitivity in patients with prostatitis. *J Urol*. 2002;168:1054–1057.

53. Parsons CL, Hurst RE. Decreased urinary uronic acid levels in individuals with interstitial cystitis. *J Urol*. 1990;143:690–693.

54. Smith SD, Wheeler MA, Foster HE, Weiss RM. Urinary nitric oxide synthase activity and cyclic GMP levels are decreased with interstitial cystitis and increased with urinary infections. *J Urol*. 1996;155:1432–1435.

55. Theoharides T. Hydroxyzine in the treatment of interstitial cystitis. *Urol Clin North Am*. 1994;21:113.

56. Parsons CL. Effective treatments for interstitial cystitis. *Hospital Med*. 1996:24–31. Feb.

57. Mills S, Bone K. *Principles and Practice of Phytotherapy: Modern Herbal Medicine*. Edinburgh: Churchill Livingstone; 2000.

58. Moore M. *Herbs for the urinary tract*. New Canaan, CT: Keats Publishing; 1998.

59. Hudson T. Treating interstitial cystitis: a natural medicine approach. *Altern Complemen Ther*. 2001;7(2):88–90.

60. Brinker F. *Herb contraindications and drug interactions*. 2nd ed. Sandy, OR: Eclectic Medical Publications; 1998.

61. Katske F, Shoskes DA, Sender M, et al. Treatment of interstitial cystitis with a quercetin supplement. *Techniq Urol*. 2001;7(1):44–46.

62. Mori S, Ojima Y, Hirose T, et al. The clinical effect of proteolytic enzyme containing bromelain and trypsin on urinary tract infection evaluated by double blind method. *Acta Obstet Gynaecol Jpn*. 1972;19(3):47–53.

63. Borchers AT, Keen CL, Stern JS, Gershwin ME. Inflammation and Native American medicine: the role of botanicals. *Am J Clin Nutr*. 2000;72:339–347.

64. Felter HW, Lloyd JU. *King's American Dispensatory*. 18th ed. Vol. 2. Portland, OR: Eclectic Medical Publications; 1983; 1898.

65. Krivoy N, Pavlotzky E, Chrubasik S, et al. Effect of salicis cortex extract on human platelet aggregation. *Planta Med*. 2001;67:209–212.

66. Kroes BH, Beukelman CJ, van den Berg AJJ, et al. Inhibition of human complement by beta-glycyrrhetinic acid. *Immunology*. 1997;90:115–120.

67. Haraguchi H, Yoshida N, Ishikawa H, et al. Protection of mitochondrial functions against oxidative stresses by isoflavones from *Glycyrrhiza glabra*. *J Pharm Pharmacol*. 2000;52:219–223.

68. Davis EA, Morris DJ. Medicinal uses of licorice through the millennia: the good and plenty of it. *Mol Cell Endocrinol*. 1991;78:1–6.

69. Tang W, Eisenbrand G. *Chinese drugs of plant origin*. Berlin: Springer-Verlag; 1992.

70. Pittler MH, Ernst E. Efficacy of kava extract for treating anxiety: systematic review and meta-analysis. *J Clin Psychopharmacol*. 2000;20:84–89.

71. Hanno P. Interstitial cystitis and related diseases. In: Walsh PC, Retik AB, Vaughan Jr Ed, Wein AJ, eds. *Campbell's urology*. 7th ed. Philadelphia: Saunders; 1998:631–661.

72 Gessner B, Cnota P, Steinbach T. Extract of the kava-kava rhizome in comparison with diazepam and placebo. *Z Phytother*. 1994;15:30–37. [in German].

73. Hoffmann D. *The complete illustrated herbal*. New York: Barnes & Noble Books; 1996.

74. Lemus I, García R, Erazo S, et al. Diuretic activity of an Equisetum bogotense tea (platero herb): Evaluation in healthy volunteers. *J Ethnopharmacol*. 1996;54:55–558.

75. Shrivastava SC, Sisodia CS. Analgesic studies on Vitex negundo and Valeriana wallichii. *Indian Vet J*. 1970;47(2):170–175.

76. Albrecht M, Berger W, et al. Psychopharmaceuticals and safety in traffic. *Z Allegmeinmed*. 1995;71:1215–1221. [in German].

77. Turner NJ. Counter-irritant and other medicinal uses of plants in Ranunculaceae by native peoples in British Columbia and neighbouring areas. *J Ethnopharmacol*. 1984;11(2):181–201.

78. Buxbaum D, Sanders-Bush E, Efron DH. Analgesic activity of tetrahydrocannabinol in the rat and mouse. *Fed Proc*. 1969;28:735.

79. Joy JE, Watson SJ, Benson Jr JA, eds. *Marijuana and medicine, assessing the science base*. Washington, DC: Institution of Medicine, National Academy Press; 1999.

80. Formukong EA, Evans AT, Evans FJ. Analgesic and anti-inflammatory activity of constituents of *Cannabis sativa L*. *Inflammation*. 1988;41:705–709.

81. McPartland JM, Pruitt PL. Side effects of pharmaceuticals no elicited by comparable herbal medicines: the case of tetrahydrocannabinol and marijuana. *Altern Ther*. 1999;5:57–62.

82. Evans AT, Formukong EA, Evans FJ. Actions of Cannabis constituents on enzymes of prostaglandin synthesis: antiinflammatory potential. *Biochem Pharmacol*. 1987;36:2035–2037.

83. Smith SD, Wheeler MA, Foster HE, Weiss RM. Improvement in interstitial cystitis symptom scores during treatment with oral L-arginine. *J Urol*. 1997;158:703–708.

84. Ehren I, Lundberg JON, Adolfsson J, Wiklund P. Effects of L-arginine treatment on symptoms and bladder nitric oxide levels in patients with interstitial cystitis. *Urology*. 1998;52:1026–1029.

85. Korting GE, Smith SD, Wheeler MA, et al. A randomized double-blind trial of oral L-arginine for treatment of interstitial cystitis. *J Urol*. 1999;161:558–565.

86. Whitmore KE. Self-care regimens for patients with interstitial cystitis. *Urol Clin North Am*. 1994;21:121–130.

87. Weiss JM. Pelvic floor myofascial trigger points: manual therapy for interstitial cystitis and the urgency-frequency syndrome. *J Urol*. 2001;166:2226–2231.

88. Doggweiler-Wiygul R, Wiygul JP. Interstitial cystitis, pelvic pain, and the relationship to myofascial pain and dysfunction: a report on four patients. *World J Urol*. 2002;20:310–314.

89. Chang PL. Urodynamic studies in acupuncture for women with frequency, urgency and dysuria. *J Urol*. 1988;140:563–566.

90. Fall M, Lindstrom S. Transcutaneous electrical nerve stimulation in classic and nonulcer interstitial cystitis. *Urol Clin North Am*. 1994;21:131–139.

91. Geirsson G, Wang YH, Lindstrom S, et al. Traditional acupuncture and electrical stimulation of the posterior tibial nerve: a trial in chronic interstitial cystitis. *Scand J Urol Nephrol*. 1993;27:67–70.

CHAPTER 14

1. Balneaves LG, Truant TLO, Kelly M, et al. Bridging the gap: decision-making processes of women with breast cancer using complementary and alternative medicine (CAM). *Support Care Cancer*. 2007;15(8):973–983.

2. Fauci A, Braunwald E, Kasper D, et al. *Harrison's Principles of Internal Medicine*. 17th ed. New York: McGraw-Hill; 2008.

3. Knutson D, Steiner E. Screening for breast cancer: current recommendations and future directions. *Am Fam Physician*. 2007;75(11):1660–1666.

4. Pruthi S, Brandt KR, Degnem AC, et al. A multidisciplinary approach to the management of breast cancer, part 1: prevention and diagnosis. *Mayo Clin Proc*. 2007;82(8):999–1012.

5. Holmes M, Willett W. Does diet affect breast cancer risk? *Breast Cancer Res*. 2004;6:170–178.

6. Steiner E, Klubert D, Hayes M, et al. Clinical inquiries. Does a low-fat diet help prevent breast cancer? *J Fam Pract*. 2007;56(7):583–584.

7. Carmichael AR. Obesity as a risk factor for development and poor prognosis of breast cancer. *BJOG*. 2006;113(10):1160–1166.

8. Brody JG, Rudel RA, Michels KB, et al. Environmental pollutants, diet, physical activity, body size, and breast cancer: where do we stand in research to identify opportunities for prevention? *Cancer*. 2007;109(suppl 12):2627–2634.

9. Brody JG, Moysich KB, Humblet O, et al. Environmental pollutants and breast cancer: epidemiologic studies. *Cancer*. 2007;109(suppl 12):2667–2711.

10. Newman LA, Vogel VG. Breast cancer risk assessment and risk reduction. *Surg Clin North Am*. 2007;87(2):307–316.

11. Chen WY, Rosner B, Colditz GA. Moving forward with breast cancer prevention. *Cancer*. 2007;109(12):2387–2391.

12. Malin J, Schuster M, Kahn K, et al. Quality of breast cancer care: what do we know? *J Clin Oncol*. 2002;20(21):4381–4393.

13. Humphrey L, Helfand M, Chan B, et al. Breast cancer screening: a summary of the evidence for the U.S. Preventive Services Task Force. *Ann Intern Med*. 2002;137:347–360.

14. Nystrom L, Andersson I, Bjurstam N, et al. Long-term effects of mammography screening: updated overview of the Swedish randomised trials. *Lancet*. 2002;359:909–919.

15. Olsen O, Gotzsche P. Cochrane review on screening for breast cancer with mammography [Letter]. *Lancet*. 2001;358:1340–1342.

16. Bjurstam N, Bjorneld L, Duffy S, et al. The Gothenburg breast screening trial: first results on mortality, incidence, and mode of detection for women ages 39-49 years at randomization. *Cancer*. 1997;80:2091–2099.

17. Frisell J, Lidbrink E, Hellstrom L, et al. Followup after 11 years-update of mortality results in the Stockholm mammographic screening trial. *Breast Cancer Res Treat*. 1997;45:263–270.

18. Andersson I, Janzon L. Reduced breast cancer mortality in women under age 50: updated results from the Malmo Mammographic Screening Program. *J Natl Cancer Inst Monogr*. 1997;22:63–67.

19. Alexander F, Anderson T, Brown H, et al. 14 years of follow-up from the Edinburgh randomised trial of breast-cancer screening. *Lancet*. 1999;353:1903–1908.

20. Miller A, Baines C, To T, et al. Canadian National Breast Screening Study: 2. Breast cancer detection and death rates among women aged 50 to 59 years. *CMAJ*. 1992;147:1477–1488.

21. Miller A, Baines C, To T, et al. Canadian National Breast Screening Study: 1. Breast cancer detection and death rates among women aged 40 to 49 years. *CMAJ*. 1992;147:1459–1476.

22. Pruthi S, Boughey JC, Brandt KR, et al. A multidisciplinary approach to the management of breast cancer, part 2: therapeutic considerations. *Mayo Clin Proc*. 2007;82(9):1131–1140.

23. Tilyou S. BEIR V report. Experts urge cautious interpretation of higher risk estimates. *J Nucl Med*. 1990;31:13A–19A.

24. Feig S. Radiation risk from mammography: is it clinically significant? *Am J Roentgenol*. 1984;143:469–475.

25. Feig S. Hypothetical breast cancer risk from mammography. *Recent Results Cancer Res*. 1984;90:1–10.

26. Brewer NT, Salz T, Lillie SE. Systematic review: the long-term effects of false-positive mammograms [see comment]. *Ann Int Med*. 2007;146(7):502–510.

27. Teh W, Wilson A. The role of ultrasound in cancer screening. A consensus statement by the European Group for Breast Cancer Screening. *Eur J Cancer*. 1998;34:449–450.

28. Kolb T, Lichy J, Newhouse J. Comparison of the performance of screening mammography, physical examination, and breast United States and evaluation of factors that influence them: an analysis of 27,825 patient evaluations. *Radiology*. 2002;225:165–175.

29. Society AC.

30. de Lemos M, John L, Nakashima L, et al. Advising cancer patients on natural health products-a structured approach. *Ann Pharmacother*. 2004;38:1406–1411.

31. Richardson M. Research of complementary/alternative medicine therapies in oncology: promising but challenging. *J Clin Oncol*. 1999;17(11):38–43.

32. Von Gruenigen V, White L, Kirven M, et al. A comparison of complementary and alternative medicine use by gynecology and oncology patients. *Int J Gynecol Cancer*. 2001;11:205–209.

33. Cassileth B. Complementary and alternative cancer medicine. *J Clin Oncol*. 1999;17(11):44–52.

34. DiGianni LM, Garber JE, Winer EP. Complementary and alternative medicine use among women with breast cancer. *J Clin Oncol*. 2002;20(suppl 18):34S–38S.

35. Richardson M, Sanders T, Palmer L, et al. Complementary/alternative medicine use in a comprehensive cancer center and the implications for oncology. *J Clin Oncol*. 2000;18(13):2505–2514.

36. Growing interest in complementary and alternative cancer therapies. *CA Cancer J Clin*. 2004;54:286–288.

37. Jacobson JS, Workman SB, Kronenberg F. Research on complementary/alternative medicine for patients with breast cancer: a review of the biomedical literature. *J Clin Oncol*. 2000;18(3):668–683.

38. Ernst E. CAM for cancer? *Support Care Cancer*. 2005;13:669–670.

39. Chatwin J, Tovey P. Complementary and alternative medicine (CAM), cancer and group-based action: a critical review of the literature. *Eur J Cancer*. 2004;13:210–218.

40. Markham M. Safety issues in using complementary and alternative medicine. *J Clin Oncol*. 2002;20(18):39–41.

41. Cabrera C. *Treatment of Breast Cancer with Herbal Medicine and Nutrition*. Ashland; 2003.

42. Cassileth B, Vickers A. High prevalence of complementary and alternative medicine use among cancer patients: implications for research and clinical care. *J Clin Oncol*. 2005;23(12):2590–2592.

43. Ladas E, Jacobson J, Kennedy D, et al. Antioxidants and cancer therapy: a systematic review. *J Clin Oncol.* 2004;22(3):517–524.

44. Boon HS, Olatunde F, Zick SM. Trends in complementary/alternative medicine use by breast cancer survivors: comparing survey data from 1998 and 2005. *BMC Women's Health.* 2007;7:4.

45. Khan N, Mukhtar H. Tea polyphenols for health promotion. *Life Sci.* 2007;81(7):519–533.

46. Zhang M, Holman CDAJ, Huang J-P, et al. Green tea and the prevention of breast cancer: a case-control study in Southeast China. *Carcinogenesis.* 2007;28(5):1074–1078.

47. Sun C-L, Yuan J-M, Koh W-P, et al. Green tea, black tea and breast cancer risk: a meta-analysis of epidemiological studies. *Carcinogenesis.* 2006;27(7):1310–1315.

48. Thangapazham RL, Singh AK, Sharma A, et al. Green tea polyphenols and its constituent epigallocatechin gallate inhibits proliferation of human breast cancer cells in vitro and in vivo. *Cancer Letters.* 2007;245(1-2):232–241.

49. Carlson JR, Bauer BA, Vincent A, et al. Reading the tea leaves: anticarcinogenic properties (of-epigallocatechin)-3-gallate. *Mayo Clinic Proc.* 2007;82(6):725–732.

50. Wu AH, Arakawa K, Stanczyk FZ, et al. Tea and circulating estrogen levels in postmenopausal Chinese women in Singapore. *Carcinogenesis.* 2005;26(5):976–980.

51. Fujiki H, Suganuma M, Okabe S, et al. Mechanistic findings of green tea as cancer preventive for humans. *Proc Soc Exp Biol Med.* 1999;220(4):225–228.

52. Low Dog T. *Women's Health in Complementary and Integrative Medicine: A Clinical Guide.* St. Louis: Elsevier; 2004.

53. Gikas PD, Mokbel K. Phytoestrogens and the risk of breast cancer: a review of the literature. *Int J Fertil Womens Med.* 2005;50(6):250–258.

54. Duffy C, Perez K, Partridge A. Implications of phytoestrogen intake for breast cancer. *CA.* 2007;57(5):260–277.

55. Ha TC, Lyons-Wall PM, Moore DE, et al. Phytoestrogens and indicators of breast cancer prognosis. *Nutr Cancer.* 2006;56(1):3–10.

56. Atkinson C, Warren R, Bingham SA, et al. Mammographic patterns as a predictive biomarker of breast cancer risk: effect of tamoxifen. *Cancer Epidemiol Biomarkers Prev.* 1999;8(10):863–866.

57. Nagel G, Mack U, von Fournier D, et al. Dietary phytoestrogen intake and mammographic density-results of a pilot study. *Eur J Med Res.* 2005;10(9):389–394.

58. Atkinson C, Bingham SA. Mammographic breast density as a biomarker of effects of isoflavones on the female breast. *Breast Cancer Res.* 2002;4(1):1–4.

59. Jakes RW, Duffy SW, Ng FC, et al. Mammographic parenchymal patterns and self-reported soy intake in Singapore Chinese women. *Cancer Epidemiol Biomarkers Prev.* 2002;11(7):608–613.

60. Tempfer CB, Bentz E-K, Leodolter S, et al. Phytoestrogens in clinical practice: a review of the literature. *Fertil Steril.* 2007;87(6):1243–1249.

61. Wagner JD, Anthony MS, Cline JM. Soy phytoestrogens: research on benefits and risks. *Clin Obstet Gynecol.* 2001;44(4):843–852.

62. Setchell K, Brown N, Desai P. Bioavailability of pure isoflavones in healthy humans and analysis of commercial soy isoflavone supplements. *J Nutr.* 2001;131(suppl):1362S–1375S.

63. Tew BY, Xu X, Wang HJ, et al. A diet high in wheat fiber decreases the bioavailability of soybean isoflavones in a single meal fed to women. *J Nutr.* 1996;126(4):871–877.

64. Tham DM, Gardner CD, Haskell WL. Clinical review 97: potential health benefits of dietary phytoestrogens: a review of the clinical, epidemiological, and mechanistic evidence. *J Clin Endocrinol Metab.* 1998;83(7):2223–2235.

65. COT (Committee on Toxicity of Chemicals in Food, Consumer Products and the Environment). UK Ministry of Health; 2002.

66. Touillaud MS, Thiebaut ACM, Fournier A, et al. Dietary lignin intake and postmenopausal breast cancer risk by estrogen and progesterone receptor status. *J Natl Cancer Inst.* 2007;99(6):475–486.

67. Thanos J, Cotterchio M, Boucher BA, et al. Adolescent dietary phytoestrogen intake and breast cancer risk (Canada). *Cancer Causes Contr.* 2006;17(10):1253–1261.

68. Deng G, Cassileth B. Integrative oncology: complementary therapies for pain, anxiety, and mood disturbance. *CA Cancer J Clin.* 2005;55(2):109–116.

69. Jacobson JS, Troxel AB, Evans J, et al. Randomized trial of black cohosh for the treatment of hot flashes among women with a history of breast cancer. *J Clin Oncol.* 2001;19(10):2739–2745.

70. Standish LJ, Greene K, Greenlee H, et al. Complementary and alternative medical treatment of breast cancer: a survey of licensed North American naturopathic physicians. *Alt Ther Health Med.* 2002;8(5):68–70, 72-765.

71. Russell N. *Herbal/Plant Therapies.* Hoxsey: University of Texas MD Anderson Cancer Center; 2007.

72. Zick SM, Sen A, Feng Y, et al. Trial of Essiac to ascertain its effect in women with breast cancer (TEA-BC). *J Altern Complement Med.* 2006;12(10):971–980.

73. Kulp KS, Montgomery JL, Nelson DO, et al. Essiac and Flor-Essence herbal tonics stimulate the in vitro growth of human breast cancer cells. *Breast Cancer Res Treat.* 2006;98(3):249–259.

CHAPTER 15

1. Fugh-Berman A, Lione A, Scialli AR. Do no harm: avoidance of herbal medicines during pregnancy [comment]. *Obstet Gynecol.* 2005;106(2):409–410. author reply 410–411.

2. Hepner DL, Harnett M, Segal S, et al. Herbal medicine use in parturients. *Anesthes Analges.* 2002;94(3):690–693.

3. Ernst E. Herbal medicinal products during pregnancy: are they safe? *BJOG.* 2002;109:227–235.

4. Gibson P. Herbal and alternative medicine use during pregnancy: a cross-sectional survey. *Obstetrics and Gynecology.* 2001;97(suppl 4):44.

5. Pinn G, Pallett L. Herbal medicine in pregnancy. *Comp Ther Nursing Midwif.* 2002;8:77–80.

6. Glover DD, Amonkar M, Rybeck BF, et al. Prescription, over-the-counter, and herbal medicine use in a rural, obstetric population. *Am J Obstet Gynecol.* 2003;188(4):1039–1045.

7. Ranzini A. Use of complementary medicines and therapies among obstetric patients. *Obstet Gynecol.* 2001;97(suppl 4):46.

8. Mabina M, Ptiso S, Moodley J. The effect of traditional herbal medicines on pregnancy outcome. *SAMJ.* 1997;87(8).

9. Allaire AD, Moos M-K, Wells SR. Complementary and alternative medicine in pregnancy: a survey of North Carolina certified nurse-midwives. *Obstet Gynecol.* 2000;95(1):19–23.

10. Beal M. Women's use of complementary and alterna-tive therapies in reproductive health care. *J Nurs Midwif.* 1998;43(3):224–234.
11. Lee L. Introducing conventional medicine into conventional health care settings. *J Nurs Midwif.* 1999;44(3):253–266.
12. Raisler J. Complementary and alternative healing in midwifery care. *J Nurs Midwif.* 1999;44(3):189–191.
13. Tiran D. Midwives turn to alternative therapies. *R Coll Midwives J.* 1998;1(1).
14. Lo W, Friedman J. Teratogenicity of recently intro-duced medications in human pregnancy. *Obstet Gynecol.* 2002;1000(3):465–473.
15. Stapleton H. The use of herbal medicine in pregnancy and labour. Part II: events after birth, including those affecting the health of babies. *Comp Ther Nurs Midwif.* 1995;1:165–167.
16. Tiran D. Complementary strategies in antenatal care. *Comp Ther Nurs Midwif.* 2001;7:19–24.
17. Kennedy H, Lowe N. Science and midwifery: paradigms and paradoxes. *J Midwif Women's Health.* 2001;46(2):91–97.
18. Tiran D. Complementary therapies education in midwifery. *Comp Ther Nurs Midwif.* 1995;1:41–43.
19. Bunce K. The use of herbs in midwifery. *J Nurs Midwif.* 1987;32(4):255–259.
20. Ehudin E, Paluzzi P, Ivory L, et al. The use of herbs in nurse-midwifery practice. *J Nurs Midwif.* 1987;32:460–462.
21. McFarlin B, Gibson M, O'Rear J, et al. A national survey of herbal preparation use by nurse-midwives for labor stim-ulation: review of the literature and recommendations for practice. *J Nurse Midwifery.* 1999;44(3):205–216.
22. Kane Low L. Letters to the editor. *J Nurs Midwif.* 1999;44(6):602.
23. Ernst E, Schmidt K. Health risks over the internet: advice offered by "medical herbalists" to a pregnant woman. *Wien Med Wschr.* 2002;152:190–192.
24. Chez RA, Jonas WB. Complementary and alternative medi-cine. Part I: Clinical studies in obstetrics. *Obstet Gynecol Surv.* 1997;52(11):704–708.
25. Hardy M. Herbs of special interest to women. *J Amer Pharma-ceut Assoc.* 2000;40(2):234–239.
26. Mills S, Bone K. *The Essential Guide to Herbal Safety.* St. Lou-is: Churchill Livingstone; 2005.
27. Mazzotta P, Magee L. Pharmacological and non-pharmaco-logical management of nausea and vomiting of pregnancy (NVP); a systematic critical review of the literature on safety and effectiveness of treatment; 1998. http://www.nvp-volumes.org/p1_11.htm.
28. Hansten P. Managing drug interactions with herbal products. *ASHP Midyear Clinical Meeting.* 2000;35:102.
29. Simpson M, Parsons M, Greenwood J, et al. Raspberry leaf in pregnancy: its safety and efficacy in labor. *J Midwif Women's Health.* 2001;46:51–59.
30. Gallo M, Sarkar M, Au W, et al. Pregnancy outcome following exposure to echinacea: a prospective controlled study. *Arch Int Med.* 2000;160:3141–3143.
31. Bryer E. A literature review of the effectiveness of ginger in alleviating mild-to-moderate nausea and vomiting of preg-nancy. *J Midwifery Women's Health.* 2005;50:1–3.
32. Awang D. Maternal use of ginseng and neonatal androgeniza-tion. *JAMA.* 1991;266:363.
33. Bone K. Safe use of herbs in pregnancy. *Mod Phytother.* 1999:12–18.
34. Chan E. Displacement of bilirubin from albumin by berber-ine. *Biol Neonate.* 1993;63:201–208.
35. Wright I. Neonatal effects of maternal blue cohosh consump-tion. *J Pediatr.* 1999;134(3):384.
36. Jones T, Lawson B. Profound neonatal congestive heart failure caused by maternal consumption of blue cohosh herbal medi-cation. *J Pediatr.* 2003;132:3.
37. McKenna D, Jones K, Hughes K, et al. *Botanical Medicines: The Desk Reference for Major Herbal Supplements.* New York: Haworth Press; 2002.
38. Low Dog T. *Women's Health in Complementary and Integra-tive Medicine: A Clinical Guide.* St. Louis: Elsevier; 2004.
39. McGuffin M, Hobbs C, Upton R, et al. Boca Raton: CRC Press; 1997.
40. Strandberg T, Andersson S, Jarvenpaa A, et al. Preterm birth and licorice consumption during pregnancy. *Am J Epidemiol.* 2002;156(9):803–805.

CHAPTER 16

1. Cedars M. *Practical Pathways Series in Obstetrics and Gynecol-ogy.* Columbus: McGraw-Hill; 2005.
2. De Cherney A, Nathan L. Infertility. *Current Obstetrics and Gynecologic Diagnosis and Treatment.* 9th ed. New York: McGraw-Hill; 2003.
3. D'Hooghe T, Hill J. Infertility. Philadelphia: Lippincott Wil-liams & Wilkins; 2002.
4. Promotion CfDCaPNCfCDPaH. *2002 Assisted Reproductive Technology Success Rate: National Summary and Fertility Clinic Report.* U.S. Department of Health and Human Services Centers for Disease Control and Prevention; December 2004.
5. Youngkin E, Davis M. *Women's Health: A Primary Care Clini-cal Guide.* Stamford: Appleton and Lange; 1998.
6. Evers J, Land J. Chlamydia infections and subfertility, best practice result. *Clin Obstet Gynecol.* 2002;6:16.
7. Barbieri R. Management of infertility caused by ovulatory dysfunction. *Am Coll Obstet Gynecol Pract Bull.* 2002;2:34.
8. Bone K. *A Clinical Guide to Blending Liquid Herbs: Herbal Formulations for the Individual Patient.* St. Louis: Churchill Livingstone; 2003.
9. McKenna D, Jones K, Hughes K, et al. *Botanical Medicines: The Desk Reference for Major Herbal Supplements.* New York: Haworth Press; 2002.
10. Blumenthal M. *The ABC Clinical Guide to Herbs.* Austin: American Botanical Council; 2003.
11. Milewicz A. Vitex agnus castus extract in the treatment of luteal phase defects due to hyperprolactinemia: results of a randomized placebo-controlled double-blind study. *Arzneim-Forsch Drug Res.* 1993;43(7):752–756.
12. Westphal 2006.
13. Frawley D, Lad V. *The Yoga of Herbs.* Twin Lakes, WI: Lotus Press; 1988.
14. Mills S, Bone K. *The Essential Guide to Herbal Safety.* St. Lou-is: Churchill Livingstone; 2005.
15. Adaikan P, Gauthaman K, Prasad R. Proerectile pharmaco-logical effects of Tribulus terrestris extract on the rabbit cor-pus cavernosum. *Ann Acad Med Singapore.* 2000;29(1):22–26.
16. Zafar R, Lalwani M. Tribulus terrestris Linn—a review of the current knowledge. *Ind Drugs.* 1989;27(3):148–153.
17. Bourke C, Stevens G, Carrigan M. Locomotor effects in sheep of alkaloids identified in Australian Tribulus terrestris. *Aust Vet J.* 1992;69(7):163–165.

18. Takahashi K, Kitao M. Effects of TJ-68 (shakuyaku-kanzo-to) on polycystic ovarian disease. *Int J Fertil Menopausal Stud.* 1994;39(2):69–76.

19. Bone K. Echinacea. What makes it work? *Mod Phytother.* 1997;3(2):19.

20. Bone K. *Clinical Applications of Ayurvedic and Chinese Herbs.* Queensland, Australia: Phytotherapy Press; 2000.

21. Ward N. Preconceptual care and pregnancy outcome; 2006.

22. Stanton C, Gray R. Effects of caffeine consumption on delayed conception. *Am J Epidemiol.* 1995;142(12):1322–1329.

23. Bolumer F, Olsen J, Rebagliato M, et al. Caffeine intake and delayed conception: a European multicenter study on infertility and subfecundity. *Am J Epidemiol.* 1997;145(4):324–334.

24. Curtis K, Savitz D, Arbuckle T. Effects of smoking, caffeine consumption, and alcohol intake on fecundability. *Am J Epidemiol.* 1997;146(1):12–41.

25. Ruder EH, Hartman TJ, Reindollar RH, Goldman MB. Female dietary antioxidant intake and time to pregnancy among couples treated for unexplained infertility. *Fertil Steril.* 2014;101(3):759–766. United States.

26. Hammiche F, Vujkovic M, Wijburg W, et al. Increased preconception omega-3 polyunsaturated fatty acid intake improves embryo morphology. *Fertil Steril.* 2011;95(5):1820–1823. United States.

27. Paffoni A, Ferrari S, Viganò P, et al. Vitamin D deficiency and infertility: insights from in vitro fertilization cycles. *J Clin Endocrinol Metab.* 2014;99(11):E2372–E2376. United States.

28. Aleyasin A, Hosseini MA, Mahdavi A, et al. Predictive value of the level of vitamin D in follicular fluid on the outcome of assisted reproductive technology. *Eur J Obstet Gynecol Reprod Biol.* 2011;159(1):132–137. Ireland.

29. Garbedian K, Boggild M, Moody J, Liu KE. Effect of vitamin D status on clinical pregnancy rates following in vitro fertilization. Canadian Medical Association Open Access Journal. *Canadian Medical Association.* 2013;1(2):E77–E82.

30. Ozkan S, Jindal S, Greenseid K, et al. Replete vitamin D stores predict reproductive success following in vitro fertilization. *Fertil Steril.* 2010;94(4):1314–1319. United States.

31. Anagnostis P, Karras S, Goulis DG. Vitamin D in human reproduction: a narrative review. *Int J Clin Pract.* 2013;67(3):225–235. England.

32. Grzechocinska B, Dabrowski FA, Cyganek A, Wielgos M. The role of vitamin D in impaired fertility treatment. *Neuro Endocrinol Lett.* 2013;34(8):756–762. Sweden.

33. Pludowski P, Holick MF, Pilz S, et al. Vitamin D effects on musculoskeletal health, immunity, autoimmunity, cardiovascular disease, cancer, fertility, pregnancy, dementia and mortality-a review of recent evidence. *Autoimmun Rev.* 2013;12(10):976–989. Netherlands.

34. Lynch CD, Sundaram R, Maisog JM, Sweeney AM, Buck Louis GM. Preconception stress increases the risk of infertility: results from a couple-based prospective cohort study–the LIFE study. *Hum Reprod.* 2014;29(5):1067–1075. England.

35. Domar A, Seibel M, Benson H. The mind/body program for infertility: a new behavioral treatment approach for women with infertility. *Fertil Steril.* 1990;53(2):246–249.

36. Sheiner E, Sheiner E, Hammel R. Effects of occupational exposure on male fertility: literature review. *Ind Health.* 2003;41(2):55–62.

37. Premalatha G, Ravindram J. Reproductive problems in the workforce. *Med J Malaysia.* 2000;55(1):146–151.

38. Choy C, Lam C, Cheung L. Infertility, blood mercury concentration and dietary seafood consumption: a case control. *BJOG.* 2002;109(10):1121–1125.

39. Smith E, Hammonds-Ehlers M, Clark M. Occupational exposure and risk of female infertility. *J Occup Med.* 1997;39(2):138–147.

40. Kovacic P, Jacintho J. Reproductive toxins: pervasive theme of oxidative stress and electron transfer. *Curr Med Chem.* 2001;8(7):863–892.

41. Burgess N. Clinical notes on Silybum marianum. *Mod Phytother.* 1996;2(2).

42. Zhang H, Wang G. Preliminary report of the treatment of luteal phase defect by replenishing kidney. An analysis of 53 cases. *Zhongguo Zhong Xi Yi Jie He Za Zhi.* 1992;12(8):473–474.

43. Lian F. TCM Treatment of luteal phase defect—an analysis of 60 cases. *J Trad Chin Med.* 1991;11(2):115–120.

CHAPTER 17

1. Northrup C. *Women's Bodies, Women's Wisdom.* New York: Bantam Books; 1994.

2. Enkin M. *A Guide to Effective Care in Pregnancy and Childbirth.* Oxford: Oxford University Press; 1995.

3. Goer H. *Obstetric Myths Versus Research Realities.* Westport, CT: Bergin and Garvey; 1995.

4. Suarez S. Midwifery is not the practice of medicine. *Yale J Law Feminism Spring.* 1993;5(2).

5. Woodcock H. A matched cohort study of planned home and hospital births in Western Australia: 1981-1987. *Midwifery.* 1994;10(3):125–135.

6. Wagner M. Is homebirth dangerous? *Birth Gazette.* 1989; 5(4).

7. Cunningham J. Experiences of Australian mothers who gave birth either at home, at a birth center, or in hospital labor wards. *Soc Sci Med.* 1993;36(4):475–483.

8. Durand M. The safety of home birth: the farm study. *J Amer Public Health Assoc.* 1992;82:450–452.

9. Janssen P. Licensed midwife-attended, out-of-hospital births in Washington State: are they safe? *Birth.* 1994;21(3):141–148.

10. Ernst E. Herbal medicinal products during pregnancy: are they safe? *BJOG.* 2002;109:227–235.

11. Weed S. *Wise woman herbal for the childbearing years.* Woodstock, NY: Ash Tree Publishing; 1986.

12. Simpson M, Parsons M, Greenwood J, Wade K. Raspberry leaf in pregnancy: its safety and efficacy in labor. *J Midwif Women's Health.* 2001;46:51–59.

13. Parsons M, Simpson M, Ponton T. Raspberry leaf and its effect on labor: safety and efficacy. *Aust Coll Midwives J.* 1999;12(20-25).

14. Gallo M, Sarkar M, Au W, et al. Pregnancy outcome following exposure to echinacea: a prospective controlled study. *Arch Int Med.* 2000;160:3141–3143.

15. Fischer-Rasmussen W, Kjaer S, Dahl C, Asping U. Ginger treatment of hyperemesis gravidarum. *Eur J Obstet Gyn Reprod Biol.* 1990;38(1):19–24.

16. Vutyavanich T, Kraisarin T, Ruangsri R. Ginger for nausea and vomiting in pregnancy: randomized, double-masked, placebo-controlled trial. *Obstet Gynecol.* 2001;97(4):577–582.

17. Low Dog T. *Women's health in complementary and integrative medicine: a clinical guide.* St. Louis: Elsevier; 2004.

18. Wang X, Chen C, Wang L, Chen D, Guang W, French J. Conception, early pregnancy loss, and time to clinical pregnancy: a population-based prospective study. *Fertil Steril.* 2003;79(3):577–584.

19. Wilcox A, Weinberg C, O'Connor J, et al. Incidence of early loss of pregnancy. *NEJM.* 1988;319(4):189–194.

20. Hacker N, Moore J. *Essentials of obstetrics and gynecology.* 2nd ed. Philadelphia: WB Saunders; 1992.

21. Upton R. *American Herbal Pharmacopoeia and Therapeutic Monographs: Cramp Bark.* Santa Cruz: American Herbal Pharmacopoeia; 2000.

22. Upton R. *American Herbal Pharmacopoeia and Therapeutic Monographs: Black Haw.* Santa Cruz: American Herbal Pharmacopoeia; 2000.

23. Wichtl M. *Herbal Drugs and Phytopharmaceuticals: A Handbook for Practice on a Scientific Basis.* 4th ed. Stuttgart: Medpharm; 2004.

24. Treasure J. American Herbalists Guild clinical survey on the use of Vitex agnus castus. *J Am Herbalists Guild.* 2001;2(2).

25. Upton R. *American Herbal Pharmacopoeia and Therapeutic Monographs: Chaste Tree Fruit (Vitex agnus castus).* Santa Cruz: American Herbal Pharmacopoeia; 2001.

26. Wuttke W, Jarry H, Christoffel V, Spengler B, Seidlova-Wuttke D. Chaste tree (Vitex agnus castus)—pharmacology and clinical indications. *Phytomedicine.* 2003;10:348–357.

27. Sliutz G, Speiser P, Schultz AM, Spona J, Zeillinger R. Agnus castus extracts inhibit prolactin secretion of rat pituitary cells. *Horm Metab Res.* 1993;25(5):253–255.

28. Schellenberg R. Treatment for the premenstrual syndrome with agnus castus fruit extract: prospective, randomised, placebo controlled study. *BMJ.* 2001;322(7279):134–137.

29. Milewicz A, Gejdel E, Sworen H, et al. Vitex agnus castus extract in the treatment of luteal phase defects due to latent hyperprolactinaemia: results of a randomized placebo-controlled double blind study. *Arzneimittel Forschung.* 1993;43(7):752–756.

30. Loch EG, Selle H, Boblitz N. Treatment of premenstrual syndrome with a phytopharmaceutical formulation containing Vitex agnus castus. *J Women's Health Gender-Based Med.* 2000;9(3):315–320.

31. Fairweather D. Nausea and vomiting in pregnancy. *Am J Obstet Gynecol.* 1968;102:135.

32. Tierson FD, Olsen CL, Hook EB. Nausea and vomiting of pregnancy and association with pregnancy outcome. *Am J Obstet Gynecol.* 1986;155(5):1017–1022. [erratum appears in Am J Obstet Gynecol 160(2):518-519, 1989].

33. Association of professor of Gynecology and Obstetrics. Nausea ans vomiting of pregnancy. *Assoc Prof Gyn Obstet.* 2001. Washington DC.

34. Deuchar N. Nausea and vomiting in pregnancy: a review of the problem with particular regard to psychological and social aspects. *Br J Obstet Gynaecol.* 1995;102:6.

35. O'Brien B, Evans M, White-McDonald E. Isolation from "being alive": coping with severe nausea and vomiting of pregnancy. *Nurs Res.* 2002;51(5):302–308.

36. Flaxman S, Sherman P. Morning sickness: a mechanism for protecting mother and embryo. *Q Rev Biol.* 2000;75(2):113–148.

37. Sherman PW, Flaxman SM. Nausea and vomiting of pregnancy in an evolutionary perspective. *Am J Obstet Gynecol.* 2002;186(suppl 5):S190–S197.

38. Goodwin T. Hyperemesis gravidarum. *Clin Obstet Gynecol.* 1998;41(3):597–605.

39. Bailit J. Hyperemesis gravidarum: epidemiologic findings from a large cohort. *Am J Obstet Gynecol.* 2005;193(3 Pt 1):811–814.

40. Kallen B. Hyperemesis during pregnancy and delivery outcome: a registry study. *Eur J Obstet Gynecol Reprod Biol.* 1987;26:292.

41. Hallak M, Tsalamandris K, Dombrowski M. Hyperemesis gravidarum: effects on fetal outcome. *J Reprod Med.* 1996;41:871.

42. Tsang I, Katz V, Wells S. Maternal and fetal outcomes in hyperemesis gravidarum. *Int J Gynaecol Obstet.* 1996;55:231.

43. Boneva R, Moore C, Botto L, Wong L, Erickson J. Nausea during pregnancy and congenital heart defects: a population-based case-control study. *Am J Epidemiol.* 1999;149(8):717–725.

44. Paauw J, Bierling S, Cook C, Davis A. Hyperemesis gravidarum and fetal outcome. *J Parenter Enteral Nutr.* 2005;29:93.

45. Depue R, Bernstein L, Ross R, Judd H, Henderson B. Hyperemesis gravidarum in relation to estradiol levels, pregnancy outcome, and other maternal factors: a seroepidemiologic study. *Am J Obstet Gynecol.* 1987;156(5):1137–1141.

46. Dodds L, Fell D, Joseph K, Allen V, Butler B. Outcomes of pregnancies complicated by hyperemesis gravidarum. *Obstet Gynecol.* 2006;107(2 Pt 1):285–292.

47. Fell D, Dodds L, Joseph K, Allen V, Butler B. Risk factors for hyperemesis gravidarum requiring hospital admission during pregnancy. *Obstet Gynecol.* 2006;107(2 Pt 1):277–284.

48. Broussard C, Richter J. Nausea and vomiting of pregnancy. *Gastroenterol Clin North Am.* 1998;27(1):123–151.

49. Koch KL. Gastrointestinal factors in nausea and vomiting of pregnancy. *Am J Obstet Gynecol.* 2002;186(suppl 5):S198–S203.

50. Buckwalter JG, Simpson SW. Psychological factors in the etiology and treatment of severe nausea and vomiting in pregnancy. *Am J Obst Gynecol.* 2002;186(suppl 5):S210–S214.

51. Lagiou P, Tamimi R, Mucci LA, Trichopoulos D, Adami H-O, Hsieh C-C. Nausea and vomiting in pregnancy in relation to prolactin, estrogens, and progesterone: a prospective study. *Obstet Gynecol.* 2003;101(4):639–644.

52. Goodwin T, Montoro M, Mestman J, Pekary A, Hershman J. The role of chorionic gonadotropin in transient hyperthyroidism of hyperemesis gravidarum. *J Clin Endocrinol Metab.* 1992;75(5):1333–1337.

53. Goodwin TM. Nausea and vomiting of pregnancy: an obstetric syndrome. *Am J Obstet Gynecol.* 2002;186(suppl 5):S184–S189.

54. Frigo P, Lang C, Reisenberger K, Kolbl H, Hirschl A. Hyperemesis gravidarum associated with *Helicobacter pylori* seropositivity. *Obstet Gynecol.* 1998;91(4):115–117.

55. Jacoby E, Porter K. *Helicobacter pylori* infection and persistent hyperemesis gravidarum. *Am J Perinatol.* 1999;16(2):85–88.

56. Jewell D, Young G. Interventions for nausea and vomiting in early pregnancy. *Cochrane Database Syst Rev.* 2003. CD000145.

57. Seto A, Einarson T, Koren G. Pregnancy outcome following first trimester exposure to antihistamines: meta-analysis. *Am J Perinatol.* 1997;14:119.

58. Magee LA, Mazzotta P, Koren G. Evidence-based view of safety and effectiveness of pharmacologic therapy for nausea and vomiting of pregnancy (NVP). *Am J Obstet Gynecol.* 2002;186(suppl 5):S256–S261.

59. Koren G, Levichek Z. The teratogenicity of drugs for nausea and vomiting of pregnancy: perceived versus true risk. *Am J Obstet Gynecol.* 2002;186(suppl 5):S248–S252.

60. Safari H, Alsulyman O, Gherman R. Experience with oral methylprednisolone in the treatment of refractory hyperemesis gravidarum. *Am J Obstet Gynecol.* 1998;178:1054.

61. Taylor R. Successful management of hyperemesis gravidarum using steroid therapy. *QJM.* 1996;89:103.

62. Nelson-Piercy C, Fayers P, de Swiet M. Randomised, double-blind, placebo-controlled trial of corticosteroids for the treatment of hyperemesis gravidarum. *BJOG.* 2001;108(1):9–15.

63. Moran P, Taylor R. Management of hyperemesis gravidarum: the importance of weight loss as a criterion for steroid therapy. *QJM.* 2002;95(3):153–158.

64. Yost N, McIntire D, Wians FJ. A randomized, placebo-controlled trial of corticosteroids for hyperemesis due to pregnancy. *Obstet Gynecol.* 2003;102:1250.

65. Shepard T, Brent R, Friedman J. Update on new developments in the study of human teratogens. *Teratology.* 2002;65:153.

66. Park-Wyllie L, Mazzotta P, Pastuszak A. Birth defects after maternal exposure to corticosteroids: prospective cohort study and meta-analysis of epidemiological studies. *Teratology.* 2000;62:385.

67. ACOG. Nausea and vomiting of pregnancy. *Obstet Gynecol.* 2004;103:803.

68. Mazzotta P, Magee LA. A risk-benefit assessment of pharmacological and nonpharmacological treatments for nausea and vomiting of pregnancy. *Drugs.* 2000;59(4):781–800.

69. Heinrichs L. Linking olfaction with nausea and vomiting of pregnancy, recurrent abortion, hyperemesis gravidarum, and migraine headache. *Am J Obstet Gynecol.* 2002;186(suppl 5):S215–S219.

70. Erick M. Hyperolfaction and hyperemesis gravidarum: what is the relationship? *Nutr Rev.* 1995;53(10):289–295.

71. Muller A, Verhoeff A, Mantel M. Thyroid autoimmunity and abortion: a prospective study in women undergoing in vitro fertilisation. *Fertil Steril.* 1999;71(1):30–34.

72. Niebyl J, Goodwin T. Overview of nausea and vomiting of pregnancy with an emphasis on vitamins and ginger. *Am J Obstet Gynecol.* 2002;186(suppl 5):S253–S255.

73. Koren G, Maltepe C. Pre-emptive therapy for severe nausea and vomiting of pregnancy and hyperemesis gravidarum. *J Obstet Gynaecol.* 2004;24(5):530–533.

74. Roscoe J, Matteson S. Acupressure and acustimulation bands for control of nausea: a brief review. *Am J Obstet Gynecol.* 2002;186(suppl 5):S244–S247.

75. Mazzotta P, Magee L. Pharmacological and non-pharmacological management of nausea and vomiting of pregnancy (NVP): a systematic critical review of the literature on safety and effectiveness of treatment. http://www.nvp-volumes.org/p1_11.htm; 1998.

76. Carlsson C. Manual acupuncture reduces hyperemesis gravidarum: a placebo-controlled, randomized, single-blind cross-over study. *Pain Symp Manage.* 2000;20(4):273–279.

77. Norheim A, Pedersen E, Fonnebo V, Berge L. Acupressure treatment of morning Sickness in pregnancy: a randomised, double blind, placebo-controlled study. *Scand J Prim Health Care.* 2001;19(1):43–47.

78. Stern R, Jokerst M, Muth E, Hollis C. Artsomsaaga ATHM: acupressure relieves the symptoms of motion sickness and abnormal gastric activity. *Alt Ther Health Med.* 2001;7(4):91–94.

79. Davis M. Nausea and vomiting of pregnancy: an evidence-based review. *J Perinat Neonat Nursing.* 2004;18(4):312–328.

80. Jakobovits AA, Szekeres L. Interactions of stress and reproduction—a personal view. *Zentralblatt fur Gynakologie.* 2002;124(4):189–193.

81. Slotnick R. Safe, successful nausea suppression in early pregnancy with P-6 acustimulation. *J Reprod Med.* 2001;46(9):811–814.

82. Ho C, Hseu S, Tsai S, Lee T. Effect of P-6 acupressure on prevention of nausea and vomiting after epidural morphine for post-Cesarean section pain relief. *Acta Anaesthesiol Scand (Denmark).* 1996;40(3):372–375.

83. Yavari Kia P, Safajou F, Shahnazi M, Nazemiyeh H. The effect of lemon inhalation aromatherapy on nausea and vomiting of pregnancy: a double-blinded, randomized, controlled clinical trial. *Iran Red Crescent Med J.* 2014;16(3):e14360. United Arab Emirates.

84. Simon E, Schwartz J. Medical hypnosis for hyperemesis gravidarum. *Birth.* 1999;26(4):248–254.

85. Zechnich R, Hammer T. Brief psychotherapy for hyperemesis gravidarum. *Am Fam Physician.* 1982;26(5):179–181.

86. Borrelli F, Capasso R, Aviello G, Pittler MH, Izzo AA. Effectiveness and safety of ginger in the treatment of pregnancy-induced nausea and vomiting. *Obstet Gynecol.* 2005;105(4):849–856.

87. Aikins Murphy P. Alternative therapies for nausea and vomiting of pregnancy. *Obstet Gynecol.* 1998;91(1):149–155.

88. Strong T. Alternative therapies of morning sickness. *Clin Obstet Gynecol.* 2001;44(4):653–660.

89. Wilkinson JM. What do we know about herbal morning sickness treatments? *A literature survey, Midwifery.* 2000;1(693):224–228.

90. Schulz V, Hansel R, Blumenthal M, Tyler V. *Rational Phytotherapy: A Reference Guide for Physicians and Pharmacists.* 5th ed. Berlin: Springer-Verlag; 2004.

91. Vutyavanich T, Kraisarin T, Ruangsri R. Ginger for nausea and vomiting in pregnancy: randomized, double-masked, placebo-controlled trial. *Obstet Gynecol.* 2001;97(4):577–582.

92. Keating A, Chez R. Ginger syrup as an antiemetic in early pregnancy. *Altern Ther Health Med.* 2002;8:89–91.

93. Sripramote M, Lekhyananda N. A randomized comparison of ginger and vitamin B6 in the treatment of nausea and vomiting of pregnancy. *J Med Assoc Thai.* 2003;86:846–853.

94. Willetts K, Ekangaki A, Eden J. Effect of a ginger extract on pregnancy-induced nausea: a randomised controlled trial. *Aust NZ J Obstet Gynaecol.* 2003;43:139–144.

95. Smith C, Crowther C, Willson K, Hotham N, McMillian V. A randomized controlled trial of ginger to treat nausea and vomiting in pregnancy. *Obstet Gynecol.* 2004;103:639–645.

96. Hoffmann D. *Medical Herbalism: The Science and Practice of Herbal Medicine.* Rochester, VT: Healing Arts Press; 2003.

97. Ozgoli G, Goli M, Simbar M. Effects of ginger capsules on pregnancy, nausea, and vomiting. *J Altern Complement Med.* 2009;15(3):243–246. United States.

98. Ensiyeh J, Sakineh MA. Comparing ginger and vitamin B6 for the treatment of nausea and vomiting in pregnancy: a randomised controlled trial. *Midwifery.* 2009;25(6):649–653. Scotland.

99. Chittumma P, Kaewkiattikun K, Wiriyasiriwach B. Comparison of the effectiveness of ginger and vitamin B6 for treatment of nausea and vomiting in early pregnancy: a randomized double-blind controlled trial. *J Med Assoc Thai.* 2007;90(1):15–20. Thailand.

100. Tate S. Peppermint oil: a treatment for postoperative nausea. *J Adv Nurs.* 1997;26(3):543–549.

101. Kurzthaler I, Hummer M, Miller C, et al. Effect of cannabis use on cognitive functions and driving ability. *J Clin Psychiat.* 1999;60(6):395–399.

102. Romm A. *The Natural Pregnancy Book.* San Francisco: Celestial Arts; 2003.

103. McGuffin M, Hobbs C, Upton R, Goldberg A. *Botanical safety handbook.* Boca Raton: CRC Press; 1997.

104. Blumenthal M. *The Complete German Commission E Monographs: Therapeutic Guide to Herbal Medicine.* Boston: American Botanical Council; 1998.

105. Felter H, Lloyd J. *King's American Dispensatory.* Cincinnati: reprinted by Eclectic Medical Publications., 1898; 1983.

106. Cook W. *The Physio-Medical Dispensatory: A Treatise of Therapeutics, Materia Medica and Pharmacy.* Sandy, OR: Eclectic Medical Publications; 1985.

107. Westfall RE. Use of anti-emetic herbs in pregnancy: women's choices, and the question of safety and efficacy. *Comp Ther Nurs Midwifery.* 2004;10(1):30–36.

108. Mills E, Duguoa J, Perri D, Koren G. *Herbal Medicines in Pregnancy and Lactation: An Evidence-Based Approach.* Boca Raton: Taylor and Francis; 2006.

109. Fischer-Rasmussen W, Kjaer S, Dahl C, Asping U. Ginger treatment of hyperemesis gravidarum. *Eur J Obstet Gyn Reprod Biol.* 1990;38(1):19–24.

110. Russo E, Dreher M, Mathre M. *Women and Cannabis: Medicine, Science, and Sociology.* Binghamton, NY: Haworth Herbal Press; 2002.

111. Russo E. Cannabis treatments in obstetrics and gynecology: a historical review. In: Russo E, Dreher M, Mathre M, eds. *Women and Cannabis: Medicine, Science, and Sociology.* Binghamton, NY: Haworth Herbal Press; 2002:5–35.

112. Di Marzo V, Petrocellis LD. Plant, synthetic, and endogenous cannabinoids in medicine. *Annu Rev Med.* 2006;57:553–574.

113. Wright T. Correspondence. *Cincinnati Lancet Observe.* 1862;5(4):246–247.

114. Darmani NA, Crim JL. Delta-9-tetrahydrocannabinol differentially suppresses emesis versus enhanced locomotor activity produced by chemically diverse dopamine D2/D3 receptor agonists in the least shrew *(Cryptitis parva). Pharmacol Biochem Behav.* 2005;80(1):35–44.

115. Di Carlo G, Izzo AA. Cannabinoids for gastrointestinal diseases: potential therapeutic applications. *Exp Opin Invest Drugs.* 2003;12(1):39–49.

116. Izzo AA, Coutts AA. Cannabinoids and the digestive tract. *Handb Exp Pharmacol.* 2005;(168):573–598.

117. Walsh D, Nelson KA, Mahmoud FA. Established and potential therapeutic applications of cannabinoids in oncology [see comment]. *Support Care Cancer.* 2003;11(3):137–143.

118. Woolridge E, Barton S, Samuel J, Osorio J, Dougherty A, Holdcroft A. Cannabis use in HIV for pain and other medical symptoms. *J Pain Sympt Mgmt.* 2005;29(4):358–367.

119. Goodman M. Risk factors and antiemetic management of chemotherapy-induced nausea and vomiting. *Oncol Nurs Forum.* 1997;24(suppl 7):20–32.

120. de Jong BC, Prentiss D, McFarland W, et al. Marijuana use and its association with adherence to antiretroviral therapy among HIV-infected persons with moderate to severe nausea. *JAIDS.* 2005;38(1):43–46.

121. Tramer MR, Carroll D, Campbell FA, et al. Cannabinoids for control of chemotherapy induced nausea and vomiting: quantitative systematic review [see comment]. *BMJ.* 2001;323(7303):16–21.

122. Haney M, Rabkin J, Gunderson E, Foltin RW. Dronabinol and marijuana in HIV+ marijuana smokers: acute effects on caloric intake and mood. *Psychopharmacology.* 2005;181(1):170–178.

123. Kalant H. Medicinal use of cannabis: history and current status. *Pain Res Mgmt.* 2001;6(2):90–91.

124. Martin BR, Wiley JL. Mechanism of action of cannabinoids: how it may lead to treatment of cachexia, emesis, and pain. *J Support Oncol.* 2004;2(4):305–314. discussion 314–306.

125. Page SA, Verhoef MJ. Medicinal marijuana use: experiences of people with multiple sclerosis. *Can Fam Physician.* 2006;52:64–65.

126. Duran M, Laporte JR, Capella D. [News about therapeutic use of Cannabis and endocannabinoid system]. *Medicina Clinica.* 2004;122(10):390–398.

127. Andrews PL, Sanger GJ. Abdominal vagal afferent neurones: an important target for the treatment of gastrointestinal dysfunction. *Curr Opin Pharmacol.* 2002;2(6):650–656.

128. Gorter RW. Cancer cachexia and cannabinoids. *Forsch Komplementarmed.* 1999;6(suppl 3):21–22.

129. Karila L, Cazas O, Danel T, Reynaud M. [Short- and long-term consequences of prenatal exposure to cannabis]. *J Gynecol Obstet Biol Reprod.* 2006;35(1):62–70.

130. Park B, McPartland JM, Glass M. Cannabis, cannabinoids and reproduction. *Prostaglandins Leukot Essent Fatty Acids.* 2004;70(2):189–197.

131. Westfall RE, Janssen PA, Lucas P, Capler R. Survey of medicinal cannabis use among childbearing women: patterns of its use in pregnancy and retroactive self-assessment of its efficacy against 'morning sickness'. *Comp Ther Clin Pract.* 2006;12(1):27–33.

132. Connell C, Fried P. An investigation of prenatal cannabis exposure and minor physical anomalies in a low risk population. *Neurobehav Toxicol Teratol.* 1984;6:345–350.

133. English D, Hulse G, Milne E, Holman C, Bower C. Maternal cannabis use and birth weight: a meta-analysis. *Addiction.* 1987;92:1553–1560.

CHAPTER 18

1. Berkow R, ed. *The Merck Manual of Diagnosis and Therapy.* 16th ed. Rahway, NJ: Merck Research Laboratories; 1992.

2. Blackburn S. *Maternal, Fetal, & Neonatal Physiology—A Clinical Perspective.* 2nd ed. St. Louis: Saunders; 2003.

3. Richter JE. Review article: the management of heartburn in pregnancy. *Alim Pharmacol Therapeut.* 2005;22(9):749–757.

4. Marrero J, Goggin P, de Caestecker J. Determinants of pregnancy heartburn. *Br J Obstet Gynaecol.* 1992;99:731–734.

5. Lind JF, Smith AM, Mciver DK, Coopland AT, Crispin JS. Heartburn In Pregnancy—A Manometric Study. *Obstet Gynecol Surv.* 1968;23(9):845–847. http://dx.doi.org/10.1097/00006254-196809000-00005.

6. Leite L, Johnston B, Garrett J. Nonspecific esophageal motility disorder is primarily ineffective esophageal motility: is it associated with abnormal recumbent acid exposure? *Dig Dis Sci.* 1997;42:1859–1865.

7. Koenig CJ, Marquardt DN. Clinical inquiries. What medications are safe and effective for heartburn during pregnancy? *J Fam Pract*. 2001;50(4):304–305.

8. Gaedderrt A. How do you treat heartburn and GERD? *Townsend Lett Doctor Patient*. 2001;155.

9. Rayburn W, Liles E, Christensen H, Robinson M. Antacids vs. antacids plus non-prescription ranitidine for heartburn during pregnancy. *Int J Gynaecol Obstet*. 1999;66:35–37.

10. Murphy D, Castell D. Chocolate and heartburn: evidence of increased esophageal acid exposure after chocolate ingestion. *Am J Gastroenterol*. 1988;83:633–636.

11. Feldman M, Barnett C. Relationships between the acidity and osmolality of popular beverages and reported postprandial heartburn. *Gastroenterology*. 1995;108:125–131.

12. Sigmund C, McNally E. The action of a carminative on the lower esophageal sphincter. *Gastroenterology*. 1969;56:56–58.

13. Kaltenbach T, Crockett S, Gerson L. Are lifestyle measures effective in patients with gastroesophageal reflux disease? An evidence-based approach. *Arch Intern Med*. 2006;166:965–971.

14. Austin GL, Thiny MT, Westman EC, Yancy WS, Shaheen NJ. A very low-carbohydrate diet improves gastroesophageal reflux and its symptoms. *Dig Dis Sci*. 2006;51(8):1307–1312. United States.

15. Basch E, Ulbricht C. *Natural Standard Herb and Supplement Reference: Evidence-Based Clinical Reviews*. St. Louis: Elsevier/Mosby; 2005.

16. Baker W. Iron deficiency in pregnancy, obstetrics, and gynecology. *Hematol Oncol Clin North Am*. 2000;14(5):1061–1077.

17. Centers for Disease Control and Prevention. Recommendations to prevent and control iron deficiency in the United States. *MMWR*. 1998;47(RR-3):1–36.

18. Perry G, Yip R, Zyrkowski C. Nutritional risk factors among low-income pregnant US women: the Centers for Disease Control and Prevention (CDC) Pregnancy Nutrition Surveillance System. *1979 through 1993 Semin Perinatol*. 1995;19(3):211–221.

19. Young S, Ali S. Linking traditional treatment of maternal anemia to iron supplement use: an ethnographic case study from Pemba Island, Zanzibar. *Maternal and Child Nutrition*. 2005;1:51–58.

20. Allen LH. Multiple micronutrients in pregnancy and lactation: an overview. *Am J Clin Nutr*. 2005;81(5):1206S–1212S.

21. Mills E, Duguoa J, Perri D, Koren G. *Herbal medicines in pregnancy and lactation: An Evidence-Based Approach*. Boca Raton: FL: Taylor and Francis; 2006.

22. Farnsworth N, Bingel A, Cordell G, Crane F, Fong H. Potential value of plants as sources of new antifertility agents. *Int J Pharm Sci*. 1975;64:535–598.

23. Romm A. The natural pregnancy book, berkeley: Celestial Arts; 2003.

24. Weed S. *Wise woman herbal for the childbearing years*. woodstock, NY: Ash Tree Publishing; 1986.

25. Remington J, Wood H. *The dispensatory of the United States of America*. Philaelphia: Lippincott; 1918.

26. Arias E, MacDorman M, Strobino D, Guyer B. Annual summary of vital statistics—2002. *Pediatrics*. 2003;112:1215.

27. Weismiller D. Preterm labor. *Am Fam Physician*. 1999;59(3):593–604.

28. Newton E. Preterm labor, eMedicine.

29. Dimes Mo. Preterm labor. *Pregnancy and Newborn Health Education Center*; 2007.

30. Siega-Riz A, Herrmann T, Savitz D, Thorp J. Frequency of eating during pregnancy and its effect on preterm delivery. *Am J Epidemiol*. 2001;153(7):647–652.

31. Olsen S, Secher N. Low consumption of seafood in early pregnancy as a risk factor for preterm delivery: prospective cohort study. *BMJ*. 2002;324(7335):447–450.

32. Siega-Riz A, Promislow J, Savitz D. Vitamin C intake and the risk of preterm birth. *Am J Obstet Gynecol*. 2001;185(6):S138.

33. Sosa CFA, Belizan J, Bergel E. Bed rest in singleton pregnancies for preventing preterm birth. *Cochrane Database Syst Rev YR*. 2004;1(CD003581).

34. Mittendorf R, Dammann O, Lee KS. Brain lesions in newborns exposed to high-dose magnesium sulfate during preterm labor. *J Perinatol*. 2006;26(1):57–63.

CHAPTER 19

1. Jewell D, Young G. Interventions for treating constipation in pregnancy (Cochrane Review). *The Cochrane Library*. 2002;(4).

2. Kahn D, Koos B. Maternal Physiology during Pregnancy. In: DeCherney A, Nathan L, eds. *Curr Diagn Treat Obstet Gynecol*. 10th ed. New York: McGraw-Hill; 2007.

3. Derbyshire E, Davies J, Costarelli V, et al. Diet, physical inactivity and the prevalence of constipation throughout and after pregnancy. *Maternal Child Nutr*. 2006;2(3):127.

4. Prather CM. Pregnancy-related constipation. *Curr Gastroenterol Rpts*. 2004;6(5):402–404.

5. Schulz V, Hansel R, Blumenthal M, et al. *Rational Phytotherapy: A Reference Guide for Physicians and Pharmacists*. 5th ed. Berlin, Germany: Springer-Verlag; 2004.

6. Thukral C, Wolf JL. Therapy insight: drugs for gastrointestinal disorders in pregnant women. *Nat Clin Pract Gastroenterol Hepatol*. 2006;3(5):256–266.

7. Wald A. Constipation, diarrhea and symptomatic hemorrhoids during pregnancy. *Gastroenterol Clin North Am*. 2003;32:309–322.

8. Greenhalf J, Leonard H. Laxatives in the treatment of constipation in pregnant and breast-feeding mothers. *Practitioner*. 1973;210:259–263.

9. Low Dog T. *Women's Health in Complementary and Integrative Medicine: A Clinical Guide*. St. Louis: Elsevier; 2004.

10. Attaluri A, Donahoe R, Valestin J, Brown K, Rao SS. Randomised clinical trial: dried plums (prunes) vs. psyllium for constipation. *Aliment Pharmacol Ther*. 2011;33(7):822–828. England.

11. Weiss RF, Fintelmann V. *Herbal Medicine*. 2nd ed. Stuttgart: Thieme; 2000.

12. Bub S, Brinckmann J, Cicconetti G, Valentine B. Efficacy of an herbal dietary supplement (Smooth Move) in the management of constipation in nursing home residents: a randomized, double-blind, placebo-controlled study. *J Am Med Dir Assoc*. 2006;7(9):556–561. United States.

13. (ESCOP) ESCoP. *ESCOP Monographs: The Scientific Foundation for Herbal Medicinal Products*. Stuttgart: Thieme; 2003.

14. Brusick D, Mengs U. Assessment of the genotoxic risk from laxative senna products. *Environ Mol Mutagen*. 1997;29:1–9.

15. Heidermann A, Miltenburger H, Mengs U. The genotoxicity status of senna. *Pharmacology*. 1993;47(suppl 1):178–186.

16. Mills E, Duguoa J, Perri D, et al. *Herbal Medicines in Pregnancy and Lactation: An Evidence-Based Approach*. Boca Raton: Taylor and Francis; 2006.

17. Acs N, Bánhidy F, Puhó EH, Czeizel AE. No association between severe constipation with related drug treatment in pregnant women and congenital abnormalities in their offspring: A population-based case-control study. *Congenit Anom (Kyoto)*. 2010;50(1):15–20. Japan.

18. Gattuso J, Kamm M. Adverse effects of drugs used in the management of constipation and diarrhoea. *Drug Saf*. 1994;10:47–65.

19. McGuffin M, Hobbs C, Upton R, et al. Boca Raton: CRC Press; 1997.

20. Mills S, Bone K. *The Essential Guide to Herbal Safety*. St. Louis: Churchill Livingstone; 2005.

21. Wichtl M. *Herbal Drugs and Phytopharmaceuticals: A Handbook for Practice on a Scientific Basis*. 4th ed. Stuttgart: Medpharm; 2004.

22. Hawrelak JA, Myers SP. Effects of two natural medicine formulations on irritable bowel syndrome symptoms: a pilot study. *J Altern Complement Med*. 2010;16(10):1065–1071. United States.

23. Strandberg T, Andersson S, Jarvenpaa A, et al. Preterm birth and licorice consumption during pregnancy. *Am J Epidemiol*. 2002;15(699):803–805.

24. Strandberg T, Jarvenpaa A, Vanhanen H, et al. Birth outcome in relation to licorice consumption during pregnancy. *Am J Epidemiol*. 2001;153:1085–1099.

25. Frishman WH, Schlocker SJ, Awad K, et al. Pathophysiology and medical management of systemic hypertension in pregnancy. *Cardiol Rev*. 2005;13(6):274–284.

26. Report of the National High Blood Pressure Education Program Working Group on High Blood Pressure in Pregnancy. *Am J Obstetr Gynecol*. 2000;183:175–183.

27. Gynecologists ACoOa. Technical Bulletin No 219. Hypertension in pregnancy. *Int J Gynecol and Obstet*. 1996;53:175–183.

28. Lopez-Jaramillo P, Garcia R, Lopez M. Preventing pregnancy-induced hypertension: are there regional differences for this global problem? *J Hypertens*. 2005;23:1121–1129.

29. Knuist M, Bonsel G, Zonder van H, et al. Low sodium diet and pregnancy-induced hypertension: a multicentre randomized controlled trial. *Br J Obstet Gynecol*. 1998;105:430–434.

30. Sibai B. Treatment of hypertension in pregnant women. *NEJM*. 1996;335:257–265.

31. Dekker G, Sibai B. Low-dose aspirin in the prevention of preeclampsia and fetal growth retardation: rationale, mechanisms, and clinical trials. *Am J Obstet Gynecol*. 1993;168:214–227.

32. Louden K, Pipkin F, Hepinstall S. Neonatal platelet reactivity and serum thromboxane B2 production in whole blood: the effect of maternal low-dose aspirin. *Br J Obstet Gynaecol*. 1994;101(203-208).

33. Duley L, Henderson-Smart D, Knight M. Antiplatelet drugs for prevention of preeclampsia and its consequences: systematic review. *BMJ*. 2001;322:323–333.

34. Klockenbusch W, Rath W. Prevention of preeclampsia by low-dose acetylsalicylic acid—a critical appraisal [German]. *Geburtshilfe Neonatal*. 2002;206:125–130.

35. Hermida R, Ayala D, Iglesias M. Administration time-dependent influence of aspirin on blood pressure of pregnant women. *Hypertension*. 2003;41(3 pt 2):651–656.

36. Levine R, Hauth J, Curet L. Trial of calcium to prevent preeclampsia. *NEJM*. 1997;337:69–76.

37. Atallah A, Hofmeyr G, Duley L. Calcium supplementation during pregnancy for preventing hypertensive disorders and related problems. *Cochrane Database Syst Rev*. 2002;1. CD001059.

38. Sibai B, Abdella T, Anderson G. Pregnancy outcomes in 211 patients with mild chronic hypertension. *Obstet Gynecol*. 1983;61:571–576.

39. Varma T. Serum uric acid levels as an index of fetal prognosis in pregnancies complicated by preexisting hypertension and preeclampsia of pregnancy. *Intl J Gynecol Obstet*. 1987;25:35–40.

40. Sibai B, Mabie W, Shamsa F, et al. A comparison of no medication vs. methyldopa or labetalol in chronic hypertension during pregnancy. *Am J Obstet Gynecol*. 1998;162:960–965.

41. Monton S, Anandakumar C, Arulkumaran S, et al. Effects of Methyldopa and utero-placental and fetal hemodynamics in pregnancy-induced hypertension. *Am J Obstet Gynecol*. 1993;168:152–156.

42. Magloire L, Funai E. Gestational hypertension. http://www.uptodateonline.com; August 16, 2006 accessed December 27, 2006.

43. Upton R. *American Herbal Pharmacopoeia and Therapeutic Monographs: Cramp Bark*. Santa Cruz, Ca: American Herbal Pharmacopoeia; 2000.

44. Upton R. *American Herbal Pharmacopoeia and Therapeutic Monographs: Black Haw*. Santa Cruz, Ca: American Herbal Pharmacopoeia; 2000.

45. Blumenthal M. *The Complete German Commission E Monographs: Therapeutic Guide to Herbal Medicine*. Boston: American Botanical Council; 1998.

46. McKenna D, Jones K, Hughes K, et al. *Botanical Medicines: The Desk Reference for Major Herbal Supplements*. New York: Haworth Press; 2002.

47. McGuffin M, Hobbs C, Upton R, et al. Boca Raton: CRC Press; 1997.

48. Ziaei S, Hantoshzadeh S, Rezasoltani P, et al. The effect of garlic tablets on plasma lipids and platelet aggregation in nulliparous pregnants at high risk of preeclampsia. *Eur J Obstet Gynec Reprod Biol*. 2001;99:201–206.

49. Mennella J, Johnson A, Beauchamp G. Garlic ingestion by pregnant women alters the odor of amniotic fluid. *Chem Senses*. 1995;20:207–209.

50. Meher S, Duley L. Garlic for preventing preeclampsia and its complications. *Cochrane Database Syst Rev*. 2006;3. CD006065.

51. Low Dog T. *Women's Health in Complementary and Integrative Medicine: A Clinical Guide*. St. Louis: Elsevier; 2004.

52. Bae W-C, Kim Y-S, Lee J-W. Bioactive substances from *Ganoderma lucidum*. *Korean J Microbiol Biotechnol*. 2005;33(2):75–83.

53. Lee KH, Jeong H, Kim YI, et al. Production of antihypertensive constituents from *Ganoderma-Lucidum* Iy005 by fermentation using industrial wastes. *Korean J Mycol*. 1991;19(1):79–84.

54. Rhee HM, Lee SY. Cardiovascular effects of mycelium extract of Ganoderma-Lucidum inhibition of sympathetic efferent nerve activity. *Eur J Pharmacol*. 1990;183(3):1010–1011.

55. Futrakul N, Boonyen M, Patumraj S, et al. Treatment of glomerular endothelial dysfunction in steroid-resistant nephrosis with *Ganoderma lucidum*, vitamins C, E and vasodilators. *Clin Hemorheol Microcirc*. 2003;29(3-4):205–210.

56. Chen AF, Luo J-D, Lin Z-B. Ganoderma lucidum polysaccharides improve endothelial function via reducing NADPH oxidase-derived superoxide in mineralocorticoid hypertension. *FASEB J.* 2004;18(4-5):816.

57. Kanmatsuse K, Kajiwara N, Hayashi K, et al. Studies on *Ganoderma-Lucidum* I. Efficacy against hypertension and side effects. *Yakugaku Zasshi.* 1985;105(10):942–947.

58. Chu TT, Benzie IF, Lam CW, Fok BS, Lee KK, Tomlinson B. Study of potential cardioprotective effects of Ganoderma lucidum (Lingzhi): results of a controlled human intervention trial. *Br J Nutr.* 2012;107(7):1017–1027. England.

59. Upton R. *American Herbal Pharmacopoeia and Therapeutic Compendium: Reishi Mushroom (Ganoderma lucidum).* Santa Cruz: American Herbal Pharmacopoeia; 2000.

60. Parrish MR, Martin JN, Lamarca BB, et al. Randomized, placebo controlled, double blind trial evaluating early pregnancy phytonutrient supplementation in the prevention of preeclampsia. *J Perinatol.* 2013;33(8):593–599. United States.

61. O'Brien PM, Pipkin FB. The effect of essential fatty acid and specific vitamin supplements on vascular sensitivity in the mid-trimester of human pregnancy. *Clin Exp Hyperten B, Hypertens Pregnancy.* 1983;2(2):247–254.

62. Johri AK, Paoletti LC, et al. "Group B Streptococcus: global incidence and vaccine development." *Nat Rev Microbiol.* 2006;4(12):932–942.

63. Schrag S, Zell E, Lynfield R. A population-based comparison of strategies to prevent early-onset group B streptococcal disease in neonates. *NEJM.* 2002;347(233-239).

64. Tudela CM, Stewart RD, et al. "Intrapartum evidence of early-onset group B streptococcus." *Obstet Gynecol.* 2012;119(3):626–629.

65. Crombleholme W. Obstetrics. In: Tierney L, McPhee S, Papadakis M, eds. *Current Medical Diagnosis and Treatment.* New York: McGraw-Hill; 2007.

66. Feigin RD, Cherry JD, et al. *Textbook of Pediatric Infectious Diseases.* Saunders; 2009.

67. CDC. "Prevention of perinatal group b streptococcal disease." *MMWR.* 2010;59:1–32.

68. Libster R, Edwards KM, et al. "Long-term outcomes of group B streptococcal meningitis." *Pediatrics.* 2012;130(1):e8–e15.

69. Ohlsson A, Shah VS. "Intrapartum antibiotics for known maternal Group B streptococcal colonization." *Cochrane Database Syst Rev.* 2013;1:CD007467.

70. ACOG Committee Opinion. Prevention of early-onset group B streptococcal disease in newborns. *Int J Gyn.* 1996;54(2):197–205.

71. American Academy of Pediatrics. Committee on Fetus and Newborn: revised guidelines for prevention of early-onset group B streptococcal (GBS) infection. *Pediatrics.* 1997;99:489–496.

72. Schuchat A. Epidemiology of Group B Streptococcal Disease in the United States: shifting Paradigms. *Clin Microbiol Rev.* 1998;11(3):497–513.

73. Facchinetti F, Piccinini F, Mordini S. Chlorhexidine vaginal flushings vs. systemic ampicillin in the prevention of vertical transmission of neonatal group B streptococcus, at term. *J Matern Fetal Neonatal Med.* 2002;11(2):84–88.

74. Zarate G, Nader-Macias ME. "Influence of probiotic vaginal lactobacilli on in vitro adhesion of urogenital pathogens to vaginal epithelial cells." *Lett appl Microbiol.* 2006;43(2):174–178.

75. Ronnqvist PD, Forsgren-Brusk UB, et al. "Lactobacilli in the female genital tract in relation to other genital microbes and vaginal pH." *Acta Obstet Gynecol Scand.* 2006;85(6):726–735.

76. Wolff K, Johnson R, Surmond D. *Fitzpatrick's Color Atlas and Synopsis of Clinical Dermatology.* 5th ed. New York: McGraw-Hill; 2005.

77. Kroumpouzos G, Cohen L. Specific dermatoses of pregnancy: an evidence-based systematic review. *Am J Obstet Gynecol.* 2003;188:1083.

78. Matz H, Orion E, Wolf R. Pruritic urticarial papules and plaques of pregnancy: polymorphic eruption of pregnancy (PUPPP). *Clin Dermatol.* 2006;24(2):105–108.

79. Beckett M, Goldberg N. Pruritic urticarial plaques and papules of pregnancy and skin distention. *Arch Dermatol.* 1991;127:125–126.

80. Cohen L, Capeless E, Krusinski P, et al. Pruritic urticarial papules and plaques of pregnancy and its relationship to maternal-fetal weight gain and twin pregnancy. *Arch Dermatol.* 1989;125:378–381.

81. Blumenthal M. *The Complete German Commission E Monographs: Therapeutic Guide to Herbal Medicine.* Boston: American Botanical Council; 1998.

82. Bensky D, Gamble A. *Chinese Herbal Medicine Materia Medica.* Seattle: Eastman Press; 1993.

83. Lim H, Son K, Chang H, et al. Inhibition of chronic skin inflammation by topical anti-inflammatory flavonoid preparation, Ato Formula. *Arch Pharm Res.* 2006;29(6):503–507.

84. Mills S, Bone K. *The Essential Guide to Herbal Safety.* St. Louis: Churchill Livingstone; 2005.

85. Young G, Jewell D. Creams for preventing stretch marks in pregnancy. *Cochrane Database Syst Rev.* 2006;1. http://dx.doi.org/10.1002/14651858.CD000066. Art. No.: CD000066.

86. Morisset R, Cote N, Panisset J. Evaluation of the healing activity of Hydrocotyle tincture in the treatment of wounds. *Phytother Res.* 1987;1:117–121.

87. Eun H, Lee A. Cont Dermat due to Madecassol. *Cont Dermat.* 1985;13:310–313.

88. Danese P, Carnevali C, Bertazzoni M. Allergic Cont Dermat due to Centella asiatica extract. *Cont Dermat.* 1994;31:201.

89. Cramer D, Rouse J, Rountree R. Oats, Montvale, NJ: Micromedex Healthcare Series; 2002. Thomson.

90. Schulz V, Hansel R, Tyler VE. *Rational Phytotherapy: A Physicians' Guide to Herbal Medicine.* 3rd ed. Berlin: Springer; 1997.

91. Schempp C, Windeck T, Hezel S, et al. Topical treatment of atopic dermatitis with St. John's wort cream: a randomized, placebo-controlled, double-blind half-side comparison. *Phytomedicine.* 2003;10(suppl 4):31–37.

92. Schempp C, Winghofer B, Lutke R. Topical application of St. John's wort (Hypericum perforatum) and of its metabolite hyperforin inhibits the allostimulatory capacity of epidermal cells. *Br J Dermatol.* 2000;142:979–984.

93. ESCOP. *ESCOP Monographs: The Scientific Foundation for Herbal Medicinal Products.* Stuttgart: Thieme; 2003.

94. Basch E, Ulbricht C. *Natural Standard Herb and Supplement Reference: Evidence-Based Clinical Reviews.* St. Louis: Mosby; 2005.

95. Mills E, Duguoa J, Perri D, et al. *Herbal Medicines in Pregnancy and Lactation: An Evidence-Based Approach.* Boca Raton: Taylor and Francis; 2006.

96. Low Dog T. *The Integumentary System, in Foundations in Herbal Medicine*. Albuquerque, NM: Foundations in Herbal Medicine; 2001.

97. Gardiner P. Dandelion (*Taraxacum officinalis*). http://www.children'shospital.org/holistic/ Accessed Nov 2003.

98. McKenna D, Jones K, Hughes K, et al. *Botanical Medicines: The Desk Reference for Major Herbal Supplements*. New York: Haworth Press; 2002.

99. Strandberg T, Andersson S, Jarvenpaa A, et al. Preterm birth and licorice consumption during pregnancy. *Am J Epidemiol*. 2002;156(9):803–805.

100. Strandberg T, Jarvenpaa A, Vanhanen H, et al. Birth outcome in relation to licorice consumption during pregnancy. *Am J Epidemiol*. 2001;153:1085–1099.

101. Elling SV, Powell FC. Physiological changes in the skin during pregnancy. *Clin Dermatol*. 1997;15(1):35–43.

102. Stansby G. Women, pregnancy, and varicose veins. *Lancet*. 2000;355(9210):117–118.

103. Fan C-M. Epidemiology and pathophysiology of varicose veins. *Techn Vasc Intervent Radiol*. 2003;6(3):108–110.

104. Young GL, Jewell D. Interventions for varicosities and leg oedema in pregnancy. *Cochrane Database Syst Rev*. 2000: 2D001066.

105. Basch E, Ulbricht C. *Natural Standard Herb and Supplement Reference: Evidence-Based Clinical Reviews*. St. Louis: Elsevier/Mosby; 2005.

106. Morisset R, Cote N, Panisset J. Evaluation of the healing activity of Hydrocotyle tincture in the treatment of wounds. *Phytother Res*. 1987;1:117–121.

107. Eun H, Lee A. Cont Dermat due to Madecassol. *Cont Dermat*. 1985;13:435–436.

108. Danese P, Carnevali C, Bertazzoni M. Allergic Cont Dermat due to Centella asiatica extract. *Cont Dermat*. 1994;31:201.

109. Schulz V, Hansel R, Blumenthal M, et al. *Rational Phytotherapy: A Reference Guide for Physicians and Pharmacists*. 5th ed. Berlin, Germany: Springer-Verlag; 2004.

110. McKenna D, Jones K, Hughes K, et al. *Botanical Medicines: The Desk Reference for Major Herbal Supplements*. New York: Haworth Press; 2002.

111. Pittler MH, Ernst E. Horse chestnut seed extract for chronic venous insufficiency. *Cochrane Database Syst Rev*. 2012;11:CD003230. England.

112. Mills S, Bone K. *The Essential Guide to Herbal Safety*. St. Louis: Churchill Livingstone; 2005.

113. Steiner M. Untersuchungen zur odervermindernden und odemportektiven wirking vonrokastaniensamenextrakt. *Phlebol Prokto*. 1990;19:230–242.

114. Westfall E. Herbal medicine in pregnancy and childbirth. *Adv Ther*. 2001;18(1):47–55.

115. Belcaro G, Gizzi G, Pellegrini L, et al. Pycnogenol® in postpartum symptomatic hemorrhoids. *Minerva Ginecol*. 2014;66(1):77–84. Italy.

116. Cesarone MR, Belcaro G, Rohdewald P, et al. Improvement of signs and symptoms of chronic venous insufficiency and microangiopathy with Pycnogenol: a prospective, controlled study. *Phytomedicine*. 2010;17(11):835–839. Germany.

117. Abt L, Lutz B, Rouse J. *Rutin*. Montvale, NJ: Micromedex; 2002.

118. Pien GW, Schwab RJ. Sleep disorders during pregnancy. *Sleep*. 2004;27(7):1405–1417.

119. Soares CN, Murray BJ. Sleep disorders in women: clinical evidence and treatment strategies. *Psychiatr Clin North Am*. 2006;29(4):1095–1113. abstract xi.

120. Sahota P, Jainb S, Dhandb R. Sleep disorders in pregnancy. *Curr Opin Pulm Med*. 2003;9:477–483.

121. Miller EH. Women and insomnia. *Clinical Cornerstone*. 2004;6(suppl 1B):S8–S18.

122. Speroff L, Glass R, Kase G. *Clinical Gynecologic Endocrinology and Infertility*. Baltimore: Lippincott Williams & Wilkins; 1999.

123. Manconi M, Govoni V, De Vito A, et al. Restless legs syndrome and pregnancy. *Neurology*. 2004;63(6):1065–1069.

124. Tarsy D, Sheon R. Restless legs syndrome; 2007.

125. Wheatley D. Medicinal plants for insomnia: a review of their pharmacology, efficacy and tolerability. *J Psychopharmacol*. 2005;19(4):414–421.

126. Zick SM, Wright BD, Sen A, Arnedt JT. Preliminary examination of the efficacy and safety of a standardized chamomile extract for chronic primary insomnia: a randomized placebo-controlled pilot study. *BMC Complement Altern Med*. 2011:1178.

127. (ESCOP) ESCoP. *ESCOP Monographs: The Scientific Foundation for Herbal Medicinal Products*. Stuttgart: Thieme; 2003.

128. Low Dog T. *Women's Health in Complementary and Integrative Medicine: A Clinical Guide*. St. Louis: Elsevier; 2004.

129. Upton R. *American Herbal Pharmacopoeia and Therapeutic Monographs: Cramp Bark*. Santa Cruz: American Herbal Pharmacopoeia; 2000.

130. Felter H. *The Eclectic Materia Medica, Pharmacology and Therapeutics*. Portland, Oregon: Eclectic Medical Publications., [1922]; 1985.

131. Felter H, Lloyd J. *King's American Dispensatory*. Cincinnati: 1898, reprinted by Eclectic Medical Publications; 1983.

132. Buchbauer G, Jirovetz L, Jaeger W, et al. Aromatherapy Evidence For Sedative Effects Of The Essential Oil Of Lavender After Inhalation: zeitschrift fuer Naturforschung Section C. *J Biosci*. 1991;46(11-12):1067–1072.

133. Guillmain J, Rousseau A, Delaveau P. Effets neurodepresseurs de l'huile essentielle de lavandula augustifolia Mill. *Ann Pharmaceutiques*. 1989;47:337–343.

134. Hardy M, Kirk-Smith M, Stretch D. Replacement of drug treatment for insomnia by ambient odour. *Lancet*. 1995;346:493–496.

135. Diego M, Jones N, Field T, et al. Aromatherapy positively affects mood, EEG patterns of alertness and math computations. *Int J Neurosci*. 1998;96:217–224.

136. Lytle J, Mwatha C, Davis KK. Effect of lavender aromatherapy on vital signs and perceived quality of sleep in the intermediate care unit: a pilot study. *Am J Crit Care*. 2014;23(1):24–29. United States.

137. Lee IS, Lee GJ. [Effects of lavender aromatherapy on insomnia and depression in women college students]. *Taehan Kanho Hakhoe Chi*. 2006, Feb;36(1):136–143.

138. Henley D, Lipson N, Korach K, et al. Pubertal gynecomastia linked to lavender and tea tree oils. *NEJM*. 2007;356:479–485.

139. Blumenthal M, Busse W, Goldberg A, et al., eds. *The Complete German Commission E Monographs*. Austin, American Botanical Council: Integrative Medicine Communications; 1998.

140. Kennedy D, Little W, Scholey A. Effects of Melissa officinalis (lemon balm) on mood changes during acute psychological stress. *Pharmacol Biochem Behav*. 2003;72:953–964.

141. Hofmeyr GJ, Hannah ME. Planned caesarean section for term breech delivery [update of Cochrane Database Syst Rev, 1D000166; PMID: 11279680]. *Cochrane Database Syst Rev*. 2003;(3):D000166.

142. Practice ACoO. Mode of term singleton breech delivery. *ACOG Committee Opinion.* 2006;340:1–3.

143. Amon E, Sibai BM, Anderson GD. How perinatologists manage the problem of the presenting breech. *Am J Perinatol.* 1988;5(3):247–250.

144. Goffinet F, Carayol M, Foidart J, et al. Is planned vaginal delivery for breech presentation at term still an option? Results of an observational prospective survey in France and Belgium. *Am J Obstet Gynecol.* 2006;194:1002–1011.

145. Glezerman M. Five years to the term breech trial: The rise and fall of a randomized controlled trial. *Am J Obstet Gynecol.* 2006;194:20–25.

146. Alarab M, Regan C, O'Connell M. Singleton vaginal breech delivery at term: still a safe option. *Obstet Gynecol.* 2004;103(3):407–412.

147. Vangsgaard K, Gronlund A. [Breech presentation, vaginal delivery or cesarean section?] [see comment]. *Ugeskrift for Laeger.* 1996;158(47):6752–6755.

148. Gifford DS, Keeler E, Kahn KL. Reductions in cost and cesarean rate by routine use of external cephalic version: a decision analysis [see comment]. *Obstet Gynecol.* 1995;85(6):930–936.

149. Ben-Arie A, Kogan S, Schachter M, et al. The impact of external cephalic version on the rate of vaginal and cesarean breech deliveries: a 3-year cumulative experience. *Eur J Obstet Gynecol Reprod Biol.* 1995;63(2):125–129.

150. Megory E, Ohel G, Fisher O, et al. Mode of delivery following external cephalic version and induction of labor at term. *Am J Perinatol.* 1995;12(6):404–406.

151. Mashiach R, Hod M, Kaplan B, et al. External cephalic version at term using broad criteria: effect on mode of delivery. *Clin Exp Obstet Gynecol.* 1995;22(4):279–284.

152. Gynecologists ACoOa. ACOG practice patterns: external cephalic version. *Int J Gynaecol Obstet.* 2000;413. Feb.

153. Tiran D. Breech presentation: increasing maternal choice. *Complement Ther Nursing Midwifery.* 2004;10(4):233–238.

154. Brocks V, Philipsen T, Secher NJ. A randomized trial of external cephalic version with tocolysis in late pregnancy. *Br J Obstet Gynaecol.* 1984;91(7):653–656.

155. Fernandez CO, Bloom SL, Smulian JC, et al. A randomized placebo-controlled evaluation of terbutaline for external cephalic version. *Obstet Gynecol.* 1997;90(5):775–779.

156. Neri I, Airola G, Contu G, et al. Acupuncture plus moxibustion to resolve breech presentation: a randomized controlled study. *J Maternal-Fetal Neonat Med.* 2004;15(4):247–252.

157. Ewies A, Olah K. Moxibustion in breech version—a descriptive review. *Acupunct Med.* 2002;20(1):26–29.

158. Coyle ME, Smith CA, Peat B. Cephalic version by moxibustion for breech presentation. *Cochrane Database Syst Rev.* 2005;(2):D003928.

159. Hofmeyr GJ, Kulier R. Cephalic version by postural management for breech presentation. [update of Cochrane Database Syst Rev. 2000(2):D000051; PMID: 10796105]. *Cochrane Database Syst Rev.* 2000;(3):D000051.

CHAPTER 20

1. Wing D. Induction of labor: indications, techniques, and complications; 2006. Up to Date.

2. Martin J, Hamilton B, Sutton P, et al. Births: final data for 2002. *Natl Vital Stat Rep.* 2003;52(10):1–113.

3. Zhang J, Yancey M, Henderson C. U.S. national trends in labor induction. *1989-1998, J Reprod Med.* 2002;47(2):120–124.

4. Rayburn W, Zhang J. Rising rates of labor induction: present concerns and future strategies. *Obstet Gynecol.* 2002;100(1):164–167.

5. Cammu H, Martens G, Ruyssinck G, Amy J. Outcome after elective labor induction in nulliparous women: a matched cohort study. *Am J Obstet Gynecol.* 2002;186(2):240–244.

6. Gülmezoglu A, Crowther C, Middleton P. Induction of labour for improving birth outcomes for women at or beyond term. *Cochrane Database Syst Rev.* 2006;4. http://dx.doi.org/10.1002/14651858.CD004945.pub2. Art. No.: CD004945.

7. Vahratian A, Zhang J, Troendle J, et al. Labor progression and risk of cesarean delivery in electively induced nulliparas. *Obstet Gynecol.* 2005;105(4):698–704.

8. Vrouenraets F, Roumen F, Dehing C, et al. Bishop score and risk of cesarean delivery after induction of labor in nulliparous women. *Obstet Gynecol.* 2005;105(4):690–697.

9. Luthy D, Malmgren J, Zingheim R. Cesarean delivery after elective induction in nulliparous women: the physician effect. *Am J Obstet Gynecol.* 2004;191(5):1511–1515.

10. Seyb S, Berka R, Socol M, Dooley S. Risk of cesarean delivery with elective induction of labor at term in nulliparous women. *Obstet Gynecol.* 1999;94(4):600–607.

11. Kelly A, Tan B. Intravenous oxytocin alone for cervical ripening and induction of labour. *Cochrane Database Syst Rev.* 2001;(3). http://dx.doi.org/10.1002/14651858.CD003246. Art. No.: CD003246.

12. Enkin M. *A Guide to Effective Care in Pregnancy and Childbirth.* Oxford: Oxford University Press; 1995.

13. Boulvain M, Stan C, Irion O. Membrane sweeping for induction of labour. *Cochrane Database Syst Rev.* 2005;(1). http://dx.doi.org/10.1002/14651858.CD000451.pub2. Art. No.: CD000451.

14. Howarth G, Botha D. Amniotomy plus intravenous oxytocin for induction of labour. *Cochrane Database Syst Rev.* 2001:(CD003250).

15. Khan K. Amniotomy to shorten spontaneous labour: RHL commentary. *WHO Reproductive Health Library.* 2006;9.

16. Kelly A, Kavanagh J, Thomas J. Vaginal prostaglandin (PGE2 and PGF2a) for induction of labour at term. *Cochrane Database Syst Rev.* 2003;(4). http://dx.doi.org/10.1002/14651858.CD003101. Art. No.: CD003101.

17. Sanchez-Ramos L, Kaunitz A, Wears R. Misoprostol for cervical ripening and labor induction: a meta-analysis. *Obstet Gynecol.* 1997;89:633–642.

18. Wing D. Labor induction with misoprostol. *Am J Obstet Gynecol.* 1999;181:339–345.

19. Alfirevic Z, Weeks A. Oral misoprostol for induction of labour. *Cochrane Database Syst Rev.* 2006;(2). http://dx.doi.org/10.1002/14651858.CD001338.pub2. Art. No.: CD001338.

20. Hofmeyr G, Gülmezoglu A. Vaginal misoprostol for cervical ripening and induction of labour. *Cochrane Database Syst Rev.* 2003;(1). http://dx.doi.org/10.1002/14651858.CD000941. Art. No.: CD000941.

21. Kelly A, Kavanagh J, Thomas J. Castor oil, bath and/or enema for cervical priming and induction of labour. *Cochrane Database Syst Rev.* 2001;(2). http://dx.doi.org/10.1002/14651858.CD003099. Art. No.: CD003099.

22. Moerman D. *Native American Ethnobotany.* 3rd ed. Portland, OR: Timber Press; 2000.

23. Felter H, Lloyd J. *King's American Dispensatory*. Cincinnati: reprinted by Eclectic Medical Publications., 1898; 1983.

24. Low Dog T. *Women's Health in Complementary and Integrative Medicine: A Clinical Guide*. St. Louis: Elsevier; 2004.

25. McFarlin B, Gibson M, O'Rear J, Harman P. A national survey of herbal preparation use by nurse-midwives for labor stimulation. Review of the literature and recommendations for practice. *J Nurse Midwifery*. 1999;44:205–216.

26. BHMA. *British Herbal Pharmacopoeia*. Keighley, UK: British Herbal Medicine Association; 1983.

27. Mills S, Bone K. *The Essential Guide to Herbal Safety*. St. Louis: Elsevier Churchill Livingstone; 2005.

28. Trickey R. *Women, Hormones, and the Menstrual Cycle*. St. Leonards: Australia: Allen and Unwin; 1998.

29. Finkel R, Zarlengo K. Blue cohosh and perinatal stroke [correspondence]. *NEJM*. 2004;351(3):302–303.

30. Jones T, Lawson B. Profound neonatal congestive failure caused by maternal consumption of blue cohosh herbal medication. *J Pediatr*. 1998;132:550–552.

31. Wright I. Neonatal effects of maternal consumption of blue cohosh. *J Pediatr*. 1999;134(3):384–385.

32. Gunn T, Wright I. The use of black and blue cohosh in labour. *NZ Med J*. 1996;109(1032):410–411.

33. Rao R, Hoffman R. Nicotinic toxicity from tincture of blue cohosh (*Caulophyllum thalictroides*) used as an abortifacient. *Vet Hum Toxicol*. 2002;44(4):221–222.

34. Kennelly E, Flynn T, Mazzola E, Roach J, McCloud T, Danford D, et al. Detecting potential teratogenic alkaloids from blue cohosh rhizomes using an in vitro rat embryo culture. *J Nat Prod*. 1999;62(10):1385–1389.

35. McGuffin M, Hobbs C, Upton R, Goldberg A. Boca Raton: CRC Press; 1997.

36. Belew C. Herbs and the childbearing woman. *J Nurse Midwifery*. 1999;44(3):231–252.

37. Westfall E. Herbal medicine in pregnancy and childbirth. *Adv Ther*. 2001;18(1):47–55.

38. Allaire AD. Complementary and alternative medicine in the labor and delivery suite. *Clin Obstet Gynecol*. 2001;44(4):681–691.

39. Zick S, Raisler J, Warber S. Pregnancy. *Clin Fam Pract*. 2002;4(4):1005–1028.

40. Westfall R, Benoit C. The rhetoric of "natural" in natural childbirth: childbearing women's perspectives on prolonged pregnancy and induction of labour. *Soc Sci Med*. 2004;59:1397–1408.

41. Ellingwood F. Cincinnati: Eclectic Medical Publications; 1919.

42. Evans W. *Trease and Evans' Pharmacognosy*. 14th ed. London: WB Saunders; 1998.

43. AltMedDex. *AltMedDex(TM) Protocols, Gossypol*. Montvale, NJ: Thomson; 2003.

44. Simpson M, Parsons M, Greenwood J, Wade K. Raspberry leaf in pregnancy: its safety and efficacy in labor. *J Midwif Women's Health*. 2001;46:51–59.

45. Parsons M, Simpson M, Ponton T. Raspberry leaf and its effect on labor: safety and efficacy. *Aust Coll Midwives J*. 1999;12(20-25).

46. Dove D, Johnson P. Oral evening primrose oil: its effect on length of pregnancy and selected intrapartum outcomes in low-risk nulliparous women. *J Nurse-Midwif*. 1999;44(3):320–324.

47. Rakel D. *Integrative Medicine*. Philadelphia: Saunders; 2003.

48. Uterine remedies. The Eclectic Medical Journals—The John M. Scudder Organ Remedies—1892-1898. *reprinted in Eclectic Med J*. 1996;2:73–75.

49. The influence of Cimicifuga racemosa on parturition. *NY Med J*. 1885:267. reprinted in Eclectic Med J 1995.

50. Jarry H. Untersuchungen zur endokrinen wirksamdeit von inhaltssoffen aus cimicifuga racemosa. *Planta Medica*. 1984;4:46–49.

51. AltMedDex. *AltMedDex(TM) Protocols: Dysmenorrhea*. Montvale, NJ: Thomson; 2004.

52. Blumenthal M. *The Complete German Commission E Monographs: Therapeutic Guide to Herbal Medicine*. Boston: American Botanical Council; 1998.

53. Wichtl M. *Herbal Drugs and Phytopharmaceuticals: A Handbook for Practice on a Scientific Basi*. 4th ed. Stuttgart: Medpharm; 2004.

54. Sakurai N, Nagai M. Chemical constituents of original plants of *Cimicifuga rhizoma* in Chinese medicine. *Yakugaku Zasshi*. 1996;116:850–865.

55. Bone K. *A Clinical Guide to Blending Liquid Herbs: Herbal Formulations for the Individual Patient*. St. Louis: Churchill Livingstone; 2003.

56. Felter H. *The Eclectic Materia Medica, Pharmacology and Therapeutics*. Cincinnati: Eclectic Materia Medica; 2002: 1922.

57. Kavanagh J, Kelly A, Thomas J. Breast stimulation for cervical ripening and induction of labour. *Cochrane Database Syst Rev*. 2005;(3). http://dx.doi.org/10.1002/14651858.CD003392.pub2. Art. No.: CD003392.

58. Chayen B, Kim Y. Results of 317 contraction stress tests with controlled nipple stimulation using an electric breast pump. *J Reprod Med*. 1988;33(2):214–216.

59. Stein JL, Bardeguez AD, Verma UL, Tegani N. Nipple stimulation for labor augmentation. *J Reprod Med*. 1990;35(7):710–714.

60. Kavanagh J, Kelly A, Thomas J. Sexual intercourse for cervical ripening and induction of labour. *Cochrane Database Syst Rev*. 2001;(2). http://dx.doi.org/10.1002/14651858.CD003093. Art. No.: CD003093.

61. Yip S, Pang, Sung M. Induction of labor by acupuncture electro-stimulation. *Am J Chin Med*. 1976;04(03):257–265.

62. Smith C, Crowther C. Acupuncture for induction of labour. *Cochrane Database Syst Rev*. 2004;(1). http://dx.doi.org/10.1002/14651858.CD002962.pub2. Art. No.: CD002962.

63. Priestman KG. A few useful remedies in pregnancy, labour, and the first few days of the babies' life. *Br Homeo J*. 1988;77(3):172–173.

64. Beer A, Heiliger F. Randomized, double blind trial of Caulophyllum D4 for induction of labour after premature rupture of membranes at term. *Gerburtshilfe und Frauenheilkunde [German]*. 1999;59:431–435.

65. Dorfman P, Lasserre M, Tetau M. Homoeopathic preparation for labour: two fold experiment comparing a less widely known therapy with a placebo. *Cahiers de Biotherapie*. 1987;94:77–81.

66. Smith C. Homoeopathy for induction of labour. *Cochrane Database Syst Rev*. 2003;(4):CD003399. http://dx.doi.org/10.1002/14651858.CD003399. 2003;(4):CD003399. http://dx.doi.org/10.1002/14651858.CD003399).

67. Carlson JM, Diehl JA, Sachtleben-Murray M, McRae M, Fenwick L, Friedman EA. Maternal position during parturition in normal labor. *Obstet Gynecol*. 1986;68(4):443–447.

68. Gupta J, Nikodem V. Position for women during second stage of labour (Cochrane Review). *The Cochrane Library.* 2002;2.

69. Andrews C, Chrzanowski M. Maternal position, labour and comfort. *Appl Nursing Res.* 1990;3(1):7–13.

70. Lewis L, Webster J, Carter A, McVeigh C, Devenish-Meares P. Maternal positions and mobility during first stage labour. *(Protocol) Cochrane Database Syst Rev.* 2002;(4). http://dx.doi.org/10.1002/14651858.CD003934. Art. No.: CD003934.

71. Adachi K, Shimada M, Usui A. The relationship between the parturient's positions and perceptions of labor pain intensity. *Nurs Res.* 2003;52(1):47–51.

72. Nikolov A, Dimitrov A, Kovachev I. [Influence of maternal position during delivery of fetal oxygen saturation]. *Akusherstvo i Ginekologiia.* 2001;40(3):8–10.

73. Shachar IB, Weinstein D, Elchalal U. Maternal position and fetal pulse oximetry. *Int J Gynaecol Obstet.* 1998;60(1):67–68.

74. Carbonne B, Benachi A, Leveque ML, Cabrol D, Papiernik E. Maternal position during labor: effects on fetal oxygen saturation measured by pulse oximetry. *Obstet Gynecol.* 1996;88(5):797–800.

75. Hofmeyr G, Kulier R. Hands and knees posture in late pregnancy or labour for fetal malposition (lateral or posterior). *Cochrane Database Syst Rev.* 2005;(2). http://dx.doi.org/10.1002/14651858.CD001063.pub2. Art. No.: CD001063.

76. Stremler R, Hodnett E, Petryshen P, Stevens B, Weston J, Willan AR. Randomized controlled trial of hands-and-knees positioning for occipitoposterior position in labor [see comment]. *Birth.* 2005;329(4):243–251.

77. Sakala C. Content of care by independent midwives: assistance with pain in labor and birth. *Soc Sci Med.* 1988;26(11):1141–1158.

78. Declercq E, Sakala C, Corry M, Applebaum S, Risher P. *Listening to mothers: report of the first national U.S. survey of women's childbearing experiences.* New York: Maternity Center Association; 2002.

79. Leeman L, Fontaine P, King V, Klein M, Ratcliffe S. Management of Labor Pain: Promoting Patient Choice. *Am Fam Physician.* 2003;68(6):1023.

80. Chaillet N, Belaid L, Crochetière C, et al. Nonpharmacologic approaches for pain management during labor compared with usual care: a meta-analysis. *Birth.* 2014;41(2):122–137. United States.

81. Steel A, Adams J, Sibbritt D, Broom A, Frawley J, Gallois C. The influence of complementary and alternative medicine use in pregnancy on labor pain management choices: results from a nationally representative sample of 1,835 women. *J Altern Complement Med.* 2014;20(2):87–97. United States.

82. Simkin P, Bolding A. Update on nonpharmacologic approaches to relieve labor pain and prevent suffering. *J Midwif Women's Health.* 2004;49(6):489–504.

83. Romm A. *The Natural Pregnancy Book.* San Francisco: Celestial Arts; 2003.

84. Romm A. *Pocket Guide to Midwifery Care.* Berkeley, CA: Crossing Press; 1998.

85. Moore M. Adopting birth philosophies to guide successful birth practices and outcomes. *J Perinat Educ.* 2001;10(2):43–45.

86. Kennell J, Klaus M, McGrath S, Robertson S, Hinkley C. Continuous emotional support during labor in a US hospital. A randomized controlled trial [see comment]. *JAMA.* 1991;265(17):2197–2201.

87. Hodnett E, Gates S, Hofmeyr G, Sakala C. Continuous support for women during childbirth. *Cochrane Database Syst Rev.* 2007;(3).

88. Saisto T, Kaaja R, Ylikorkala O, Halmesmaki E. Reduced pain tolerance during and after pregnancy in women suffering from fear of labor. *Pain.* 2001;93(2):123–127.

89. Chang M-Y, Chen C-H, Huang K-F. A comparison of massage effects on labor pain using the McGill Pain Questionnaire. *J Nursing Res.* 2006;14(3):190–197.

90. Capogna G, Alahuhta S, Celleno D, et al. Maternal expectations and experiences of labour pain and analgesia: a multi-centre study of nulliparous women. *Int J Obstet Anaesth.* 1996;5:229–235.

91. Nabb MTM, Kimber L, Haines A, McCourt C. Does regular massage from late pregnancy to birth decrease maternal pain perception during labour and birth? A feasibility study to investigate a programme of massage, controlled breathing and visualization, from 36 weeks of pregnancy until birth. *Complement Ther Clin Pract.* 2006;12(3):222–231.

92. Lund I, Yu C, Uvnas-Moberg K, Wang J, Kurosawa M. Repeated massage-like stimulation induces long-term effects on nociception: contribution of oxytocinergic mechanisms. *Eur J Neurosci.* 2002;16:330–338.

93. Field T, Hernandez-Reif M, Taylor S, Quintino O, Burman I. Labor pain is reduced by massage therapy. *J Psychosom Obstet Gynaecol.* 1997;18(4):286–291.

94. Mortazavi SH, Khaki S, Moradi R, Heidari K, Vasegh Rahimparvar SF. Effects of massage therapy and presence of attendant on pain, anxiety and satisfaction during labor. *Arch Gynecol Obstet.* 2012;286(1):19–23. Germany.

95. Taghinejad H, Delpisheh A, Suhrabi Z. Comparison between massage and music therapies to relieve the severity of labor pain. *Womens Health (Lond Engl).* 2010;6(3):377–381. England.

96. Chang MY, Chen CH, Huang KF. A comparison of massage effects on labor pain using the McGill Pain Questionnaire. *J Nurs Res.* 2006;14(3):190–197. China (Republic : 1949-).

97. Kamalifard M, Shahnazi M, Sayyah Melli M, Allahverdizadeh S, Toraby S, Ghahvechi A. The efficacy of massage therapy and breathing techniques on pain intensity and physiological responses to labor pain. *J Caring Sci.* 2012;1(2):73–78. Iran.

98. Dolatian M, Hasanpour A, Montazeri S, Heshmat R, Alavi Majd H. The Effect of Reflexology on Pain Intensity and Duration of Labor on Primiparas. *Iran Red Crescent Med J.* 2011;13(7):475–479.

99. Valiani M, Shiran E, Kianpour M, Hasanpour M. Reviewing the effect of reflexology on the pain and certain features and outcomes of the labor on the primiparous women. *Iran J Nurs Midwifery Res.* 2010;15(suppl 1):302–310. India.

100. Benfield RD, Herman J, Katz VL, Wilson SP, Davis JM. Hydrotherapy in labor. *Res Nursing Health.* 2001;24(1):57–67.

101. Lee SL, Liu CY, Lu YY, Gau ML. Efficacy of warm showers on labor pain and birth experiences during the first labor stage. *J Obstet Gynecol Neonatal Nurs.* 2013;42(1):19–28. United States.

102. Benfield RD, Hortobágyi T, Tanner CJ, Swanson M, Heitkemper MM, Newton ER. The effects of hydrotherapy on anxiety, pain, neuroendocrine responses, and contraction dynamics during labor. *Biol Res Nurs.* 2010;12(1):28–36. United States.

103. Benfield RD. Hydrotherapy in labor. *J Nursing Schol.* 2002;344(4):347–352.

104. Mackey M. Use of water in labor and birth. *Clin Obstet Gynecol.* 2001;44(4):733–749.

105. Namazi M, Amir Ali Akbari S, Mojab F, Talebi A, Alavi Majd H, Jannesari S. Effects of citrus aurantium (bitter orange) on the severity of first-stage labor pain. *Iran J Pharm Res.* 2014a;13(3):1011–1018. Iran.

106. Namazi M, Amir Ali Akbari S, Mojab F, Talebi A, Alavi Majd H, Jannesari S. Aromatherapy with citrus aurantium oil and anxiety during the first stage of labor. *Iran Red Crescent Med J.* 2014b;16(6):e18371. United Arab Emirates.

107. Freeman R, Macaulay A, Eve L, Chamberlain G. Randomised trial of self hypnosis for analgesia in labor. *BMJ.* 1986;8(657-658).

108. Burns E, Blamey C, Ersser SJ, Lloyd AJ, Barnetson L. The use of aromatherapy in intrapartum midwifery practice an observational study. *Comp Ther Nursing Midwifery.* 2000;6(1):33–34.

109. Labrecque M, Nouwen A, Bergeron M, Rancourt JF. A randomized controlled trial of nonpharmacologic approaches for relief of low back pain during labor. *J Fam Practice.* 1999;48(4):259–263.

110. Ader L, Hansson B, Wallin G. Parturition pain treated by intracutaneous injections of sterile water [see comment]. *Pain.* 1990;41(2):133–138.

111. Huntley AL, Coon JT, Ernst E. Complementary and alternative medicine for labor pain: a systematic review. *Am Obstet Gynecol.* 2004;191(1):36–44.

112. Sehhatie-Shafaie F, Kazemzadeh R, Amani F, Heshmat R. The effect of acupressure on sanyinjiao and hugo points on labor pain in nulliparous women: a randomized clinical trial. *J Caring Sci.* 2013;2(2):123–129. Iran.

113. Nesheim B-I, Kinge R. Performance of acupuncture as labor analgesia in the clinical setting. *Acta Obstet Gynecol Scand.* 2006;85(4):441–443.

114. Lee H, Ernst E. Acupuncture for labor pain management: a systematic review. *Am J Obstet Gynecol.* 2004;191(5):573–1579.

115. Hamidzadeh A, Shahpourian F, Orak RJ, Montazeri AS, Khosravi A. Effects of LI4 acupressure on labor pain in the first stage of labor. *J Midwifery Womens Health.* 2012;57(2):133–138. United States.

116. Hjelmstedt A, Shenoy ST, Stener-Victorin E, et al. Acupressure to reduce labor pain: a randomized controlled trial. *Acta Obstet Gynecol Scand.* 2010;89(11):1453–1459. England.

117. Madden K, Middleton P, Cyna AM, Matthewson M, Jones L. Hypnosis for pain management during labour and childbirth. *Cochrane Database Syst Rev.* 2012;11:CD009356. England.

118. Chuntharapat S, Petpichetchian W, Hatthakit U. Yoga during pregnancy: effects on maternal comfort, labor pain and birth outcomes. *Complement Ther Clin Pract.* 2008;14(2):105–115. England.

119. Abdolahian S, Ghavi F, Abdollahifard S, Sheikhan F. Effect of dance labor on the management of active phase labor pain & clients' satisfaction: a randomized controlled trial study. *Glob J Health Sci.* 2014;6(3):219–226. Canada.

CHAPTER 21

1. Romm A. *Natural Health After Birth: The Complete Guide to Postpartum Wellness.* Rochester, VT: Healing Arts Press; 2002.

2. MacArthur C, Lewis M, Knox E. Health after childbirth. *Br J Obstet Gynaecol.* 1991;98:1193–1195.

3. Bick D, MacArthur C. Attendance, content and relevance of the sex week postnatal examination. *Midwifery.* 1995;11(2):69–73.

4. Ball J. *Reactions to Motherhood.* St. Louis: Elsevier; 1994.

5. Buchart WA, et al. Listening to women: focus group discussions of what women want from postnatal care. *Curationis.* 1999;22:4–8.

6. Pinn G. Herbs used in obstetrics and gynecology. *Aust Fam Physician.* 2001;30(4):351–356.

7. Hardy M. Herbs of special interest to women. *J Am Pharm Assoc.* 2000;40(2):234–239.

8. Molina J. Traditional Native American practices in obstetrics. *Clin Obstet Gynecol.* 2001;44(4):661–669.

9. Pinn G, Pallett L. Herbal medicine in pregnancy. *Comp Ther Nurs Midwif.* 2002;8:77–80.

10. Chez RA, Jonas WB. Complementary and alternative medicine. Part I: Clinical studies in obstetrics. *Obstet Gynecol Surv.* 1997;52(11):704–708.

11. Dunham C. *Mamatoto: A Celebration of Birth.* New York: Penguin; 1992.

12. Placksin S. *Mothering the New Mother.* New York: New Market Press; 2000.

13. Upton R. *American Herbal Pharmacopoeia and Therapeutic Monographs: Black Haw.* Santa Cruz: American Herbal Pharmacopoeia; 2000.

14. Upton R. *American Herbal Pharmacopoeia and Therapeutic Monographs: Cramp Bark.* Santa Cruz: American Herbal Pharmacopoeia; 2000.

15. Romm A. *The Natural Pregnancy Book.* San Francisco: Celestial Arts; 2003.

16. Beck CT. Postpartum depression: it isn't just the blues. *Am J Nurs.* 2006;106(5):40–50. quiz 50–51.

17. Berggren-Clive K. Out of the darkness and into the light: women's experience with depression after childbirth. *Can J Commun Mental Health.* 1998;17:103–120.

18. Tcheremissine OV, Lieving LM. Pharmacotherapy of postpartum depression: current practice and future directions. *Expert Opin Pharmacother.* 2005;6(12):1999–2005.

19. Logsdon MC, Wisner K, Billings DM, Shanahan B. Raising the awareness of primary care providers about postpartum depression. *Issues Mental Health Nurs.* 2006;27(1):69–73.

20. Small R. Depression after childbirth: the views of medical students and women compared. *Birth.* 1997;24(2):109–115.

21. Beck CT, Indman P. The many faces of postpartum depression. *JOGNN.* 2005;34:569–576.

22. Chen TH, Lan TH, Yang CY, Juang KD. Postpartum mood disorders may be related to a decreased insulin level after delivery. *Med Hypoth.* 2006;66(4):820–823.

23. McCoy SJ, Beal JM, Shipman SB, et al. Risk factors for postpartum depression: a retrospective investigation at 4-weeks postnatal and a review of the literature [see comment]. *J Am Osteopath Assoc.* 2006;106(4):193–198.

24. Eilat-Tsanani S, Merom A, Romano S, Reshef A, Lavi I, Tabenkin H. The effect of postpartum depression on women's consultations with physicians. *Israel Med Assoc J.* 2006;8(6):406–410.

25. Bloch M, Rotenberg N, Koren D, Klein E. Risk factors for early postpartum depressive symptoms [see comment]. *Gen Hosp Psychiatr.* 2006;28:1–8.

26. Abou-Saleh M. Hormonal aspects of postpartum. *Psychneuroendocrinology.* 1998;23(5):465–475.

27. Groer M, Davis M, Hemphill J. Postpartum stress: current concepts and the possible protective role of breastfeeding. *JOGNN.* 2002;31:411–417.

28. Beck CT. Revision of the Postpartum Depression Predictors. *J Obstet Gynecol Neonat Nurs*. 2002;31(4):394–402.

29. Bernazzani O. Psychosocial predictors of depressive symptomatology level in postpartum Women. *J Affect Dis*. 1997;46(1):39–49.

30. Nielsen F. Postpartum depression: identification of women at risk. *Br J Obstet Gynecol*. 2000;107(10):1210–1217.

31. Gjerdingen D. The effects of social support on women's health during pregnancy, labor and delivery, and the postpartum period. *Fam Med*. 1991;23(5):370–375.

32. Ellis D, Hewat R. Mothers' postpartum perceptions of spousal relationships. *J Obstet Gynecol Neonat Nurs*. 1985;14(2):140–146.

33. Misri S. The impact of partner support in the treatment of postpartum depression. *Can J Psychiatr*. 2000;45(6):554–558.

34. Driscoll JW. Postpartum depression: the state of the science. *J Perinat Neonat Nurs*. 2006;20(1):40–42.

35. Corwin E, Brownstead J, Barton N, Heckard S, Morin K. The impact of fatigue on the development of postpartum depression. *JOGNN*. 2005;34(5):577–584.

36. Dankner R. Cultural elements of postpartum depression. *J Reprod Med*. 2000;45(2):97–104.

37. Small R. Depression after childbirth. Does social context matter? *Med J Aust*. 1994;161(8):473–477.

38. O'Hara M. Effect of interpersonal psychotherapy for postpartum depression. *Arch Gen Psychiatry*. 2000;57(11):1039–1045.

39. Righetti-Veltema M. Risk factors and predictive signs of postpartum depression. *J Affect Disord*. 1998;49(3):167–180.

40. Astbury J. Birth events, birth experiences and social differences in postnatal depression. *Austr J Pub Health*. 1994;18(2):176–184.

41. Gjerdingen D. A causal model describing the relationship of women's postpartum health to social support, length of leave, and complications of childbirth. *Women's Health*. 1990;2:81–87.

42. Edwards D. A pilot study of postnatal depression following cesarean section using two retrospective self-rating instruments. *J Psychosom Res*. 1994;38:111–117.

43. Astbury J. Birth events, birth experiences and social differences in postnatal depression. *Austr J Pub Health*. 1994;18(2):176–184.

44. Shields N. Impact of midwife-managed care in the postnatal period: an exploration of psychosocial outcomes. *J Reprod Infant Psychol*. 1997;15:91–108.

45. Youngkin E, Davis M. *Women's Health: A Primary Care Clinical Guide*. Stamford: Appleton and Lange; 1998.

46. Burt V, Suri R, Altshuler L, Stowe Z, Hendrick V, Muntean E. Use of psychotropic medications during breastfeeding. *Am J Psychiatry*. 2001;158:1001–1009.

47. Hale TW. Maternal medications during breastfeeding. *Clin Obstet Gynecol*. 2004;47(3):696–711.

48. Chambers C, Hernandez-Diaz S, Van Marter L. Selective serotonin-reuptake inhibitors and risk of persistent pulmonary hypertension of the newborn. *NEJM*. 2006;354(6):579–587.

49. Campagne DM. Comment on "the effectiveness of various postpartum depression treatments and the impact of antidepressant drugs on nursing infants" [comment]. *Medgenmed [Computer File]: Medscape Gen Med*. 2004;6(1):43.

50. Weier KM, Beal MW. Complementary therapies as adjuncts in the treatment of postpartum depression. *J Midwif Wom Health*. 2004;49(2):96–104.

51. Muzik M, Hamilton SE, Rosenblum KL, et al. Mindfulness yoga during pregnancy for psychiatrically at-risk women: preliminary results from a pilot feasibility study. *Complement Ther Clin Pract*. 2012;18:235–240.

52. Schulz V, Hansel R, Blumenthal M, Tyler V. *Rational Phytotherapy: A Reference Guide for Physicians and Pharmacists*. 5th ed. Berlin: Springer-Verlag; 2004.

53. Blumenthal M, ed. *The complete German Commission E monographs: Therapeutic guide to herbal medicines*. Austin: American Botanical Council; 1998.

54. Upton R. *American Herbal Pharmacopoeia and Therapeutic Monographs: Ashwagandha Root*. Santa Cruz: American Herbal Pharmacopoeia; 2000.

55. Upton R. *American Herbal Pharmacopoeia and Therapeutic Compendium: Schisandra berry*. Santa Cruz: American Herbal Pharmacopoeia; 1999.

56. Linde K, Berner MM, Kriston L. St John's wort for major depression. *Cochrane Database Syst Rev*. 2008;(4):CD000448.

57. Low Dog T. *Women's Health in Complementary and Integrative Medicine: A Clinical Guide*. St. Louis: Elsevier; 2004.

58. Klier C, Schafer M, Schmid-Siegal B, et al. St. John's Wort (*Hypericum perforatum*): is it safe during breastfeeding? *Pharmacopsychiatry*. 2002;35:29–30.

59. Klier CM, Schmid-Siegel B, Schäfer MR, et al. St. John's wort (Hypericum perforatum) and breastfeeding: plasma and breast milk concentrations of hyperforin for 5 mothers and 2 infants. *J Clin Psychiatry*. 2006, Feb;67(2):305–309.

60. McIntyre M. A review of the benefits, adverse effects, drug interactions and safety of St. John's wort: the implications with regard to the regulation of herbal medicines. *J Alt Comp Med*. 2000;6:115–124.

61. McKenna D, Jones K, Hughes K, Humphrey S. *Botanical Medicines: The Desk Reference for Major Herbal Supplements*. New York: Haworth Press; 2002.

62. Cott J. Dietary supplements and natural products as psychotherapeutic agents. *Psychosom Med*. 1999;61:712–728.

63. Sarris J, Kavanagh DJ, Byrne G, Bone KM, Adams J, Deed G. The Kava Anxiety Depression Spectrum Study (KADSS): a randomized, placebo-controlled crossover trial using an aqueous extract of Piper methysticum. *Psychopharmacology (Berl)*. 2009, Aug;205(3):399–407.

64. Kinzler E, Kromer J, Lehmann E. Effect of a special kava extract in patients with anxiety, tension, and excitation states of non-psychotic genesis. *Arzneimittel-Forschung*. 1991;41:585–588.

65. Pittler M, Ernst E. Efficacy of kava extract for treating anxiety: systematic review and meta-analysis. *J Clin Psychopharmacol*. 2000;20:84–90.

66. Malsch U, Keiser M. Efficacy of kava-kava in the treatment of non-psychotic anxiety, following pretreatment with benzodiazepines. *Psychopharmacology*. 2001;157:277–283.

67. Wichtl M. *Herbal Drugs and Phytopharmaceutical: A Handbook for Practice on a Scientific Basis*. 4th ed. Stuttgart: Medpharm; 2004.

68. Bone K. *A Clinical Guide to Blending Liquid Herbs: Herbal Formulations for the Individual Patient*. St. Louis: Churchill Livingstone; 2003.

69. ESCOP. *ESCOP Monographs: The Scientific Foundation for Herbal Medicinal Products*. Stuttgart: Thieme; 2003.

70. Brock C, Whitehouse J, Tewfik I, Towell T. American Skullcap (Scutellaria lateriflora): a randomised, double-blind placebo-controlled crossover study of its effects on mood in healthy volunteers. *Phytother Res*. 2014;28(5):692–698. England.

71. Wolfson P, Hoffmann DL. An investigation into the efficacy of *Scutellaria lateriflora* in healthy volunteers. *Alt Ther Health Med*. 2003;9(2):74–78.

72. Marszalek JR, Lodish HF. Docosahexaenoic acid, fatty acid-interacting proteins, and neuronal function: breastmilk and fish are good for you. *Annu Rev Cell Dev Biol*. 2005;21:633–657.

73. Naliwaiko K, Araujo RL, da Fonseca RV, et al. Effects of fish oil on the central nervous system: a new potential antidepressant? *Nutr Neurosci*. 2004;7(2):91–99.

74. Otto SJ, de Groot RH, Hornstra G. Increased risk of postpartum depressive symptoms is associated with slower normalization after pregnancy of the functional docosahexaenoic acid status. *Prostagland Leukotrienes Essent Fatty Acids*. 2003;69(4):237–243.

75. Hibbeln JR. Seafood consumption, the DHA content of mothers' milk and prevalence rates of postpartum depression: a cross-national ecological analysis. *J Affect Disord*. 2002;69(1-3):25–29.

76. Sontrop J, Campbell MK. Omega-3 polyunsaturated fatty acids and depression: a review of the evidence and a methodological critique. *Prev Med*. 2006;42(1):4–13.

77. Mozurkewich EL, Clinton CM, Chilimigras JL, et al. The Mothers, Omega-3, and Mental Health Study: a double-blind, randomized controlled trial. *Am J Obstet Gynecol*. 2013;208(4):313.e1–313.e9. United States.

78. Wojcicki JM, Heyman MB. Maternal omega-3 fatty acid supplementation and risk for perinatal maternal depression. *J Matern Fetal Neonatal Med*. 2011;24(5):680–686. England.

79. Makrides M, Gibson RA, McPhee AJ, Yelland L, Quinlivan J, Ryan P. DOMInO Investigative Team. Effect of DHA supplementation during pregnancy on maternal depression and neurodevelopment of young children: a randomized controlled trial. *JAMA*. 2010;304(15):1675–1683. United States.

80. Peet M, Stokes C. Omega-3 fatty acids in the treatment of psychiatric disorders. *Drugs*. 2005;65(8):1051–1059.

81. Parker G, Gibson NA, Brotchie H, Heruc G, Rees AM, Hadzi-Pavlovic D. Omega-3 fatty acids and mood disorders. *Am J Psychiatr*. 2006;163(6):969–978.

82. Arteca RN, Schlagnhaufer CD, Arteca JM. Root applications of gibberellic acid enhance growth of seven *Pelargonium* cultivars. *Hortscience*. 1991;26(5):555–556.

83. Field T, Grizzle N, Scafidi F, Schanberg S. Massage and relaxation therapies' effects on depressed adolescent mothers. *Adolescence*. 1996;31:903–1002.

84. Onozawa K, Glover V, Adams D, Modi N, Kumar R. Infant massage improves mother-infant interaction for mothers with postnatal depression. *J Affect Disord*. 2001;63:201–207.

85. Conrad P, Adams C. The effects of clinical aromatherapy for anxiety and depression in the high risk postpartum woman - a pilot study. *Complement Ther Clin Pract*. 2012;18(3):164–168. England.

86. Imura M, Misao H, Ushijima H. The psychological effects of aromatherapy-massage in healthy postpartum mothers. *J Midwifery Womens Health*. 2006;51(2):e21–e27. United States.

87. American College of O-G. ACOG Practice Bulletin. Episiotomy. Clinical management guidelines for obstetrician-gynecologists. *Obstet Gynecol*. 2006;107(4):957–962.

88. Albers LL, Sedler KD, Bedrick EJ, Teaf D, Peralta P. Midwifery care measures in the second stage of labor and reduction of genital tract trauma at birth: a randomized trial. *J Midwif Women's Health*. 2005;50(5):365–372.

89. Hartmann K, Viswanathan M, Palmieri R, Gartlehner G, Thorp J, Lohr K. Outcomes of routine episiotomy: a systematic review. *JAMA*. 2005;293:2141–2148. (Level III).

90. Nager C, Helliwell J. Episiotomy increases perineal laceration length in primiparous women. *Am J Obstet Gynecol*. 2001;185(29):444–450.

91. Myles T, Santolaya J. Maternal and neonatal outcomes in patients with prolonged second stage of labor. *Obstet Gynecol*. 2003;102:52–58.

92. Bodner-Adler B, Bodner K, Kimberger O, Wagenbichler P, Mayerhofer K. Management of the perineum during forceps delivery. Association of episiotomy with the frequency and severity of perineal trauma in women undergoing forceps delivery. *J Reprod Med*. 2003;48:239–242.

93. Premkumar G. Perineal trauma: reducing associated postnatal maternal morbidity. *RCM Midwives*. 2005;8(1):30–32.

94. Renfrew MJ, Hannah W, Albers L, Floyd E. Practices that minimize trauma to the genital tract in childbirth: a systematic review of the literature. *Birth*. 1998;25(3):143–160.

95. Shorten A, Donsante J, Shorten B. Birth position, accoucheur, and perineal outcomes: informing women about choices for vaginal birth. *Birth*. 2002;29(1):18–27.

96. Aikins Murphy P, Feinland JB. Perineal outcomes in a home birth setting. *Birth*. 1998;25(4):226–234.

97. Signorello L, Harlow B, Chekos A, Repke J. Postpartum sexual functioning and its relationship to perineal trauma: a retrospective cohort study of primiparous women. *Am J Obstet Gynecol*. 2001;184(5):881–888.

98. Beckmann MM, Garrett AJ. Antenatal perineal massage for reducing perineal trauma. *Cochrane Database of Systematic Reviews*. 2006:1D005123.

99. Davidson K, Jacoby S, Brown MS. Prenatal perineal massage: preventing lacerations during delivery. *JOGNN*. 2000;29(5):474–479.

100. Labrecque M, Eason E, Marcoux S. Women's views on the practice of prenatal perineal massage. *BJOG*. 2001;108(5):499–504.

101. Faruel-Fosse H, Vendittelli F. [Can we reduce the episiotomy rate?] *J Gynecol Obstet Biol Reprod*. 2006;35(suppl 1):1S68–61S76.

102. Lehrer L. Easing the baby out. *Midwif Today Int Midwife*. 2003;(65):8.

103. Cornwell S, Dale A. Lavender oil and perineal repair. *Modern Midwife*. 1995;5(3):31–33.

104. Sheikhan F, Jahdi F, Khoei EM, Shamsalizadeh N, Sheikhan M, Haghani H. Episiotomy pain relief: use of Lavender oil essence in primiparous Iranian women. *Complement Ther Clin Pract*. 2012;18(1):66–70. England.

105. Vakilian K, Atarha M, Bekhradi R, Chaman R. Healing advantages of lavender essential oil during episiotomy recovery: a clinical trial. *Complement Ther Clin Pract*. 2011;17(1):50–53. England.

CHAPTER 22

1. American Academy of Pediatrics Work Group on Breastfeeding. Breastfeeding and the use of human milk. *Pediatrics*. 1999;100(6):1035–1039.

2. Protecting, promoting and supporting breastfeeding. The special role of maternity services. A joint WHO/UNICEF statement. *Int J Gynaecol Obstet*. 1990;31(suppl 1):171–183.

3. Blumenthal M, Gruenwald J, Hall T, et al. *The Complete German Commission E Monographs: Therapeutic Guide to Herbal Medicines.* Austin: American Botanical Council; 1998.

4. Tyler VE. *The Honest Herbal: A sensible guide to the use of herbs and related remedies.* New York: Pharmaceutical Product Press (Haworth Press); 1993.

5. Brinker F. *Herb Contraindications and Drug Interactions.* 2nd ed. Sandy, OR: Eclectic Medical Publications; 1998.

6. Newall CA, Anderson LA, Phillipson JD. *Herbal Medicines: A guide for health-care professionals.* London: Pharmaceutical Press; 1996.

7. McKenna D, Jones K, Hughes K, et al. *Botanical Medicines: The Desk Reference for Major Herbal Supplements.* 2nd ed. Binghamton, NY: Haworth Press; 2002.

8. Mills S, Bone K. *The Complete Guide to Botanical Medicine Safety.* St. Louis: Churchill Livingstone; 2005.

9. Feltrow CW, Avila JR. *Professional's Handbook of Complementary & Alternative Medicines.* Springhouse, PA: Springhouse Corporation; 1999.

10. McGuffin M, Hobbs C, Upton R, et al. *Botanical Safety Handbook: Guidelines for the safe use and labelling for herbs in commerce.* Boca Raton: CRC Press; 1997.

11. American Academy of Pediatrics Committee on Drugs. The transfer of drugs and other chemicals into human milk. *Pediatrics.* 2001;108(3):776–789.

12. Hale T. *Medications and Mother's Milk.* 10th ed. Amarillo, TX: Pharmasoft Medical Publishing; 2002.

13. Lawrence R. A review of the medical benefits and contraindications to breastfeeding in the United States. *Maternal & Child Health Technical Information Bulletin.* US Department of Health & Human Resources Public Health Service; October 1997.

14. Newman J, Pitman T. *Dr. Jack Newman's Guide to Breastfeeding.* Toronto: HarperCollins Publishers; 2000.

15. Lawrence R, Lawrence R. *Breastfeeding: A Guide to the Medical Profession.* 4th ed. St. Louis: Mosby; 1999.

16. Farnsworth NR. Relative Safety of Herbal Medicines. *Herbalgram.* 1993;29. 36A-36H.

17. Ernst E. Herbal medicinal products: an overview of systematic reviews and meta-analyses. *Perfusion.* 2001;14:398–404.

18. De Smet PAGM, Brouwers JRBJ. Pharmacokinetic evaluation of herbal remedies. Basic introduction, applicability, current status and regulatory needs. *Clin Pharmacokinet.* 1997;32(6):427–436.

19. Stock S, Holzl J. Pharmacokinetic tests of [14C]-labeled hypericin and pseudohypericin from Hypericum perforatum and serum kinetics of hypericin in man. *Planta Medica.* 1991;57(suppl 2):A61.

20. Franke AA, Custer LJ, Tanaka Y. Isoflavones in human breast milk and other biological fluids. *Am J Clin Nutr.* 1998;68(suppl): 1466S–1473S.

21. Divi RL, Chang HC, Doerge DR. Anti-thyroid isoflavones from soybean: isolation, characterization, and mechanisms of action. *Biochem Pharmacol.* 1997;54(1):10087–10096.

22. Faber P, Strenge-Hesse A. Relevance of rhein excretion into breast milk. *Pharmacology.* 1988;36(suppl 1, 7258):212–220.

23. Farnsworth NR, Bingel AS, Cordell GA, et al. Potential value of plants as sources of new antifertility agents Part I. *J Pharmaceut Sci.* 1975;64(5):535–598.

24. Farnsworth NR, Bingel AS, Cordell GA, et al. Potential value of plants as sources of new antifertility agents Part II. *J Pharmaceut Sci.* 1975;64(5):717–754.

25. Bingel AS, Farnsworth NR. *Higher plants as potential sources of galactagogues.* New York: Academic Press; 1994:1–54.

26. Daly S, Hartmann P. Infant demand and supply. Part 2: The short-term control of milk synthesis in lactating women. *J Hum Lact.* 1995;11(1):27–31.

27. Lust KD, Brown JE, Thomas W. Maternal intake of cruciferous vegetables and other foods and colic symptoms in exclusively breast-fed infants. *J Am Diet Assoc.* 1996;96(1):46–48.

28. Mennella JA, Beauchamp GK. The effects of repeated exposure to garlic-flavored milk on the nursling's behavior. *Pediatr Res.* 1993;34:805–808.

29. He M, Ma J, Chen Q, et al. Growth and feeding practices of 4 and 8 months infants in Southern China. *Nutr Res.* 2001;21:103–120.

30. Mohrbacher N, Stock J. *The Breastfeeding Answer Book.* Schaumburg, IL: La Leche League International Publications; 2003.

31. Riordan J, Auerbach KG, eds. *Breastfeeding and Human Lactation.* London: Jones & Bartlett; 1993.

32. Awang DVC. Maternal use of ginseng and neonatal androgenization (letter). *JAMA.* 1991;265:1828.

33. Waller DP, Martin AM, Farnsworth NR, et al. Lack of androgenicity of Siberian ginseng (letter). *JAMA.* 1992;267:2329.

34. Rosti L, Nardini A, Bettinelli ME, et al. Toxic effects of a herbal tea mixture in two newborns (letter). *Acta Paediatr.* 1994;83(6):83.

35. Nambiar S, Schwartz RH, Constantino A. Hypertension in mother and baby linked to ingestion of Chinese herbal medicine (letter). *West J Med.* 1999;99(171):152.

36. Roberge RJ, Leckey R, Spence R, et al. Garlic burns of the breast (letter). *Am J Emerg Med.* 1997;15:548.

37. McGeorge BCL, Steele MC. Allergic contact dermatitis of the nipple from Roman chamomile ointment. *Contact Dermat.* 1991;24:139–140.

38. Huggins K. Fenugreek: one remedy for low milk production. *Medela Rental Round-up Winter.* 1998;15(1):16–17.

39. Werbach MR, Murray MT. *Botanical Influences on Illness, a sourcebook of clinical research.* Tarzana, CA: Third Line Press; 1994.

40. Swafford S, Berns B. Effect of fenugreek on breast milk volume, Annual Meeting Abstracts. *ABM News and Views.* 2000;6(3).

41. Mohr H. Clinical investigations of means to increase lactation. *Dtsch med Wschr.* 1954;79(41):1513–1516.

42. Winterhoff H, Munster CG, Behr B. Die Hemmung der Laktation bei Ratten als indirekter Beweis fur die Senkung von Prolaktin durch Agnus Castus [Reduced lactation in rats followed Vitex extract application]. *Zeitschrift fur Phytotherapie.* 1991;12:175–179.

43. Sliutz G, Speiser P, Schultz AM, et al. Agnus castus extracts inhibit prolactin secretion of rat pituitary cells. *Horm Metab Res.* 1993;25:253–255.

44. Jarry H, Leonhardt S, Gorkow C, et al. In vitro prolactin but not LH and FSH release is inhibited by compounds in extracts of Agnus Castus: direct evidence for a dopaminergic principle by the dopamine receptor assay. *Exp Clin Endocrinol.* 1994;102:448–454.

45. Merz PG, Gorkow C, Schrodter A, et al. The effects of a special Agnus castus extract (BP1095E1) on prolactin secretion in healthy male subjects. *Exp Clin Endocrinol Diabetes.* 1996;104(6):447–453.

46. Sourgens H, Winterhoff H, et al. Antihormonal effects of plant extracts: TSH- and prolactin-suppressing properties of Lithospermum officinale and other plants. *Planta Med.* 1982;45:78–86.

47. Cott J. Therapeutics section In American Herbal Pharmacopoeia and Therapeutic Compendium. *St. John's Wort: quality control, analytical and therapeutic monograph, as published in Herbalgram 40, special section (32 pages).* 1997.

48. Franklin M, Cowen PJ. Researching the antidepressant actions of Hypericum perforatum (St John's wort) in animals and man. *Pharmacopsychiatry.* 2001;34(1):S29–S37.

49. Briggs GG, Freeman RK, Jaffe SJ. *Drugs in Pregnancy and Lactation: A Reference Guide to Fetal and Neonatal Risk.* 5th ed. New York: Lippincott Williams & Wilkins; 1998.

50. O'Dowd M. *The History of Medications for Women: Materia medica woman.* New York: Parthenon Publishing Group; 2001.

51. Marx C, Izquierdo A, Driscoll J, Murray M. Vitamin E concentrations in serum of newborn infants after topical use of vitamin E by nursing mothers. *Am J Obstet Gynecol.* 1985;(152):668.

52. ESCOP Monographs. *The Scientific Foundation for Herbal Medicinal Products.* Stuttgart: Thieme; 2003.

53. Schulz V, Hansel R, Blumenthal M, Tyler V. *Rational Phytotherapy: A Reference Guide for Physicians and Pharmacists.* 5th ed. Berlin: Springer-Verlag; 2004.

54. Blumenthal M. *The ABC Clinical Guide to Herbs.* Austin: American Botanical Council; 2003.

55. Lavergne N. Does application of tea bags to sore nipples while breastfeeding provide effective relief? *J Obstet Gynecol Neonat Nursing.* 1997;26(26):53–58.

56. Low Dog T. *Women's Health in Complementary and Integrative Medicine: A Clinical Guide.* St. Louis: Elsevier; 2004.

57. Wichtl M. *Herbal Drugs and Phytopharmaceuticals: A Handbook for Practice on a Scientific Basis.* 4th ed. Stuttgart: Medpharm; 2004.

58. Schilcher H. *Phytotherapy in paediatrics: handbook for physicians and pharmacists.* 2nd ed. Stuttgart: Medpharm Scientific Publishers; 1997.

59. Carson CF, Hammer KA, Riley TV. Melaleuca alternifolia (tea tree) oil: a review of antimicrobial and other medicinal properties. *Clin Microbiol Rev.* 2006;19(1):50–62.

60. Cox SD, Mann CM, Markham JL, et al. The mode of antimicrobial action of the essential oil of Melaleuca alternifolia (tea tree oil). *J Appl Microbiol.* 2000;88(1):170–175.

61. Cox SD, Gustafson JE, Mann CM, et al. Tea tree oil causes K+ leakage and inhibits respiration in Escherichia coli. *Letta Appl Microbiol.* 1998;26(5):355–358.

62. Hada T, Inoue Y, Shiraishi A, Hamashima H. Leakage of K+ ions from Staphylococcus aureus in response to tea tree oil. *J Microbiol Meth.* 2003;53(3):309–312.

63. Carson CF, Mee BJ, Riley TV. Mechanism of action of Melaleuca alternifolia (tea tree) oil on Staphylococcus aureus determined by time-kill, lysis, leakage, and salt tolerance assays and electron microscopy. *Antimicrob Agents Chemother.* 2002;46(6):1914–1920.

64. Nelson RR. Selection of resistance to the essential oil of Melaleuca alternifolia in Staphylococcus aureus. *J Antimicrob Chemother.* 2000;45(4):449–550.

65. Gustafson JE, Liew YC, Chew S, et al. Effects of tea tree oil on Escherichia coli. *Letts Appl Microbiol.* 1998;26(3):194–198.

66. Snowden H, Renfrew M, Woolridge M. Treatments for breast engorgement during lactation. *Cochrane Database Syst Rev.* 2001;(2):D000046.

67. Roberts K, Reiter M, Schuster D. The effectiveness of cabbage leaf extract was compared with that of a placebo in treating breast engorgement in lactating women. In a double-blind experiment with a pretest/posttest design. Effects of cabbage leaf extract on breast engorgement. *J Hum Lact.* 1998;14(3):231–236.

68. Pediatrics AAO. Transfer of drugs and other chemicals into human milk. *Pediatrics.* 2001;108(3):776–789.

69. Kee W, Tan S, Lee V, Salmon Y. The treatment of breast engorgement with Serrapeptase (Danzen): a randomized double-blind controlled trial. *Singapore Med J.* 1989;30(1):48–54.

70. Foxman B, D'Arcy H, Gillespie B. Lactation mastitis: occurrence and medical management among 946 breastfeeding women in the United States. *Am J Epidemiol.* 2002;155:103.

71. Berens P. Prenatal, intrapartum, and postpartum support of the lactating mother. *Pediatr Clin North Am.* 2001;48:365.

72. Mastitis. *Causes and Management.* Geneva: World Health Organization Department of Child and Adolescent Health and Development; 2000.

73. Dener C, Inan A. Breast abscesses in lactating women. *World J Surg.* 2003;27:130.

74. Vaidya K, Sharma A, Dhungel S. Effect of early mother-baby close contact over the duration of exclusive breastfeeding. *NMCJ.* 2005;7(2):138–140.

75. Mikiel-Kostyra K, Mazur J, Boltruszko I. Effect of early skin-to-skin contact after delivery on duration of breastfeeding: a prospective cohort study [see comment]. *Acta Paediatr.* 2002;91(12):1301–1306.

76. Humphrey S. *The Nursing Mother's Herbal.* Minneapolis: Fairview Press; 2003.

77. Gabay M. Galactagogues: medications that induce lactation. *J Hum Lact.* 2002;18:274–279.

78. Malini T, Vanithakumari G, Megala N, Anusya S, Devi K, Elango V. Effect of Foeniculum vulgare Mill. seed extract on the genital organs of male and female rats. *Indian J Physiol Pharmacol.* 1985;29(31):21–26.

79. Jarry H, Spengler B, Wuttke W, Christoffel V. Phytotherapy in gynecology: pharmacological rationale for the use of dopaminergic principles. *Phytomedicine.* 2000;7(suppl 2).

80. Jarry H, Leonhardt S, Gorkow C, Wuttke W. In vitro prolactin but not LH and FSH release is inhibited by compounds in extracts of Agnus castus: direct evidence for a dopaminergic principle by the dopamine receptor assay. *Exp Clin Endocrinol.* 1994;102(6):448–454.

81. Sliutz G, Speiser P, Schultz AM, Spona J, Zeillinger R. Agnus castus extracts inhibit prolactin secretion of rat pituitary cells. *Horm Metab Res.* 1993;25(5):253–255.

82. Wuttke W, Jarry H, Christoffel V, Spengler B, Seidlova-Wuttke D. Chaste tree (Vitex agnus-castus): pharmacology and clinical indications. *Phytomedicine.* 2003;10(4):348–357.

83. Winterhoff H. Vitex agnus-castus (chaste tree): pharmacological and clinical data. *Abstr Am Chem Soc.* 1996;212(1-2).

84. Barrett M. Binghamton, NY: Haworth Press; 2004.

85. Betzold C. Galactagogues. *J Midwif Women's Health.* 2004;49(2):151–154.

86. Mills E, Duguoa J, Perri D, Koren G. *Herbal Medicines in Pregnancy and Lactation: An Evidence-Based Approach.* Boca Raton, FL: Taylor and Francis; 2006.

87. Turkyılmaz C, Onal E, Hirfanoglu IM, et al. The effect of galactagogue herbal tea on breast milk production and short-term catch-up of birth weight in the first week of life. *J Altern Complement Med.* 2011;17(2):139–142. United States.

88. Remington J, Wood H. *The Dispensatory of the United States of America*; 1918.

89. Rosti L, Nardini A, Bettinelli ME, Rosti D. Toxic effects of a herbal tea mixture in two newborns. *Acta Paediatr.* 1994;83(6):683.

CHAPTER 23

1. Grizzard T, Barbieri R. *Cross-cultural considerations in menopausal women*; 2007. Up-to-Date.

2. Beyenne Y. *Menarche to menopause: reproductive lives of peasant women in two cultures.* New York: University of New York Press; 1989.

3. Beyenne Y. Cultural significance and physiological manifestations of menopause. A biocultural analysis. *Cult Med Psychiatry.* 1986;10(1):47–71.

4. Flint M, Samil RS. Cultural and subcultural meanings of the menopause. *Ann NY Acad Sci.* 1990;592:134–148. 185-192.

5. Rasmussen SJ. From childbearers to culture-bearers: transition to post childbearing among Tuareg women. *Med Anthropol.* 2000;19(1):111–116.

6. Steinem G. *Revolution from within.* Boston: Little Brown; 1993.

7. World Health Organization. Research on the menopause. *Prog Reprod Health.* 1996;40(Part 1):1–8.

8. Woods NF, Mitchell ES. Symptoms during the perimenopause: prevalence, severity, trajectory, and significance in women's lives. *Am J Med.* 2005;118(12):14–24.

9. Woods NF, Mitchell ES. Pathways to depressed mood for midlife women: observations from the Seattle Midlife Women's Health Study. *Res Nurs Health.* 1997;20(2):119.

10. Bosworth HB, Bastian LA, Kuchibhatla MN, et al. Depressive symptoms, menopausal status, and climacteric symptoms in women at midlife. *Psychosom.* 2001;63(4):607.

11. Pearlstein TB. Hormones and depression: what are the facts about premenstrual syndrome, menopause, and hormone replacement therapy? *Am J Obstet Gynecol.* 1995;173(2):650.

12. Woods NF, Mariella A, Mitchell ES. Patterns of depressed mood across the menopausal transition: approaches to studying patterns in longitudinal data. *Acta Obstet Gynecol Scand.* 2002;81(7):630.

13. Coleman PM. Depression during the female climacteric period. *J Adv Nurs.* 1993;18(10):1541.

14. Kaufert PA, Gilbert P. The context of menopause: psychotropic drug use and menopausal status. *Soc Sci Med.* 1986;23(8):753.

15. Kaufert PA, Gilbert P, Tate R. The Manitoba Project: a re-examination of the link between menopause and depression. *Maturitas.* 1992;14(2):153.

16. Whooley MA, Grady D, Cauley JA. Postmenopausal estrogen therapy and depressive symptoms in older women. *J Gen Intern Med.* 2000;15(8):539.

17. Avis NE, Brambilla D, McKinlay SM, et al. A longitudinal analysis of the association between menopause and depression. Results from the Massachusetts Women's Health Study. *Ann Epidemiol.* 1994;4(3):214–220.

18. Kenton L. *Passage to Power.* London: Ebury Press; 1995.

19. Mucclough M. *Hope or hype? Philadelphia Enquirer*; May 13, 1996.

20. Love S, Dr. *Susan Love's Hormone Book.* New York: Random House; 1997.

21. Northrup C. *The Wisdom of Menopause.* New York: Bantam; 2001.

22. Collaborative Group on Hormonal Factors in Breast Cancer. Breast cancer and hormone replacement therapy: collaborative reanalysis of data from 51 epidemiological studies of 52,705 women with breast cancer and 108,411 women without breast cancer. *Lancet.* 1997;350(9084):1047–1059.

23. Grodstein F. Postmenopausal hormone therapy and mortality. *NEJM.* 1997;336:1769–1775.

24. Ettinger B. Reduced mortality associated with long-term postmenopausal estrogen therapy. *Obst Gynecol.* 1996;87:6–12.

25. Schairer C, Lubin J, Troisi R, et al. Menopausal estrogen and estrogen-progestin replacement therapy and breast cancer risk. *JAMA.* 2000;283(4):485–491.

26. Chen CL. Hormone replacement therapy in relation to breast cancer. *JAMA.* 2002;287:734–741.

27. Doshani AG. Getting to the HeaRT of hormone replacement therapy, Abstract from Twelfth Annual Meeting of NAMS. *J NAMS.* 2001;8(6):480.

28. Begley S. A clear signal on estrogen. *Newsweek.* June 30, 1997.

29. Angier N. Is menopause a key to survival? The grandmother hypothesis. *New York Times.* August 18, 1997.

30. Greenwood S. *Menopause naturally.* San Francisco: Volcano; 1984.

31. Schoenbeck L. *Menopause, bridging the gap between natural and conventional medicine, Menopause Across Cultures.* New York: Kensington; 2002.

32. Taylor Sumrall. *Women of the 14th Moon.* Vermont: Crossing Press; 1991.

33. Data from Finnish National Institute of Public Health. *as reported in Health*; 1996. 1996.

34. Int J. *Cancer as reported in Health.* 2002;1-2:144.

35. Fallon S. *Nourishing traditions.* San Diego: ProMotion; 1995.

36. Wolk A, Bergström R, Hunter D, et al. A prospective study of association of monounsaturated fat and other types of fat with risk of breast cancer. *Arch Intern Med.* 1998;158(1):41–45.

37. Carper J. *Food Pharmacy Guide to Good Eating.* New York: Bantam; 1991.

38. Trichopoulou A. Consumption of olive oil and specific food groups in relation to breast cancer risk in Greece. *J Natl Cancer Inst.* 1995;87:110–116.

39. Pedersen M. *Nutritional Herbology.* Bountiful, UT: Pedersen Publishing; 1987.

40. Bergner P. *The Healing Power of Minerals.* Rocklin, CA: Prima; 1997.

41. *United States Department of Agriculture, Handbook of the Nutritional Value of Foods in Common Units.* New York: Dover; 1975.

42. Feskanich D, Willett WC, Stampfer MJ, et al. Milk, dietary calcium, and bone fractures in women: a 12-year prospective study. *Am J Pub Health.* 1997;87:992–997.

43. Hu JF, Zhao XH, Jia JB, et al. Dietary calcium and bone density among middle-aged and elderly women in China. *Am J Clin Nutr.* 1993;58:219–227.

44. Cumming RG, Cummings SR, Nevitt MC, et al. Calcium intake and fracture risk: results from the study of osteoporotic fractures. *Am J Epidemiol.* 1997;145:926–934.

45. Burgess I. *Results of studies done by the New Zealand Agricultural Commission on the mineral content of herbal infusions*; 1995-1998. unpublished.

46. Carlson KJ.

47. Roth D. *No, It's Not Hot in Here*. Georgetown, MA: Ant Hill Press; 1999.

48. Wolfe HL. Second Spring. *A Guide to Healthy Menopause through Traditional Chinese Medicine*. Boulder, CO: Blue Poppy; 1990.

49. Hudson T. *Women's Encyclopedia of Natural Medicine*. Lincolnwood, IL: Keats; 1999.

50. Weirauch JL. Sterol content of foods of plant origin. *J Am Diet Assoc*. 73:39–47.

51. Raloff J. Plant estrogens may ward off breast cancer. *Science News*. Oct 11, 1997;152.

52. Clarke R, Hilakivi-Clarke L, Cho E. Estrogens, Phytoestrogens and breast cancer. *Adv Experiment Med Biol*. 1996;401:63–85.

53. Ingram D. Case control study of phytoestrogens and breast cancer. *Lancet*. 1997;350:990–994.

54. Duncan AM. Soy isoflavones exert modest effects in premenopausal women. *J Clin Endocrinol Metab*. 1999;84(1):92–97.

55. Aldercreutz H, Mazur W. Phytoestrogens and western diseases. *Annals Med*. 1997;29:95–120.

56. Miksicek RJ. Interaction of naturally occurring nonsteroidal estrogens with expressed recombinant human estrogen receptor. *J Steroid Biochem Mol Bio*. 1994;49:153–160.

57. Facklemann K. Medicine for menopause, researchers study herbal remedies for hot flashes. *Sci News*. 1998;153:392–393.

58. Ballard JE, McKeown BC, Graham HM, et al. Effect of high level physical activity and estrogen replacement therapy upon bone mass in postmenopausal women. *Lancet*. 1990;335:265–269.

59. Doress-Worters P, Siegal D. *The New Ourselves, Growing Older: Women Aging with Knowledge and Power*. New York: Simon & Schuster; 1994.

60. Pearlstein T, Rosen K, Stone AB. Mood disorders and menopause. *Endocrinol Metab Clin North Am*. 1997;26(2):279.

61. Amato P, Christophe S, Mellon PL. Estrogenic activity of herbs commonly used as remedies for menopausal symptoms. *Menopause*. 2002;9(2):145–150.

62. Coope J. Hormonal and nonhormonal interventions for menopausal symptoms. *Maturitas*. 1996;23(2):160.

63. Soares CN, Almeida OP, Joffe H, Cohen LS. Efficacy of estradiol for the treatment of depressive disorders in perimenopausal women: a double-blind, randomized, placebo-controlled trial. *Arch Gen Psychiatry*. 2001;58(6):529–534.

64. Zweifel JE, O'Brien WH. A meta-analysis of the effect of hormone replacement therapy upon depressed mood. *Psychoneuroendocrinology*. 1997;22(3):189–212.

65. Stewart DE, Boydell K, Derzko C, et al. Psychologic distress during the menopausal years in women attending a menopause clinic. *Int J Psychiatry Med*. 1992;22(3):213.

66. Stephens C, Ross N. The relationship between hormone replacement therapy use and psychological symptoms: no effects found in a New Zealand sample. *Health Care Women Int*. 2002;23(4):408–414.

67. Pearce J, Hawton K, Blake F. Psychological and sexual symptoms associated with the menopause and the effects of hormone replacement therapy. *Br J Psychiatry*. 1995;167(2):163–173.

68. Iatrakis G, Haronis N, Sakellaropoulos G, et al. Psychosomatic symptoms of postmenopausal women with or without hormonal treatment. *Psychother Psychosom*. 1986;46(3):116–121.

69. Palinkas LA, Barrett-Connor E. Estrogen use and depressive symptoms in postmenopausal women. *Obstet Gynecol*. 1992;80(1):35.

70. Dennerstein L, Dudley E, Guthrie J, Barrett-Connor E. Life satisfaction, symptoms, and the menopausal transition. *Medscape Women's Health*. 2000;5(4):E4.

71. Dennerstein L, Lehert P, Dudley E, et al. Factors contributing to positive mood during the menopausal transition. *J Nerv Ment Dis*. 2001;189(2):84–89.

72. Santen R. *Treatment of menopausal symptoms in women not taking estrogen*; 2002 Aug:8. UpToDateOnline10.3.

73. Goroll A, May L, Mulley A. *Primary Care Medicine: Office Evaluation and Management of the Adult Patient*. 4th ed. Philadelphia: Lippincott; 2000.

74. Edington R, Chagnon J, Steinberg W. Clonidine (Dixarit) for menopausal flushing. *Can Med Assoc J*. 1980;123:25.

75. Chlebowski R, Hendrix S, Langer R, et al. Influence of Estrogen Plus Progestin on Breast Cancer and Mammography in Healthy Postmenopausal Women: the Women's Health Initiative Randomized Trial. *JAMA*. 2003;289(24):3243–3253.

76. Li C, Malone K, Porter P, et al. Relationship between long durations and different regimens of hormone therapy and risk of breast cancer. *JAMA*. 2003;289(24):3254–3263.

77. Herrington D, Howard T. From presumed benefit to potential harm—hormone therapy and heart disease. *NEJM*. 2003;349(6):519–521.

78. Manson J, Hsia J, Johnson K, et al. Estrogen plus progestin and the risk of coronary heart disease. *NEJM*. 2003;349(6):523–534.

79. Baker V. Alternatives to oral estrogen replacement. *Obstet Gynecol Clin North Am*. 1994;21(2):273.

80. Birkhauser M. Depression, menopause and estrogens: is there a correlation? *Maturitas*. 2002;41(suppl 1):S3.

81. Choby B. *Midlife care in women*. Monograph 278: Am Acad Fam Physicians; 2002.

82. Keating NL, Cleary PD, Rossi AS, et al. Use of hormone replacement therapy by postmenopausal women in the United States. *Ann Intern Med*. 1999;130:545–553.

83. Fletcher SW, Colditz G. Failure of oestrogen plus progestin therapy for prevention. *JAMA*. 2002;288:366–368.

84. Johnson SR. Menopause and hormone replacement therapy. *Med Clin North Am*. 1998;82:297–320.

85. Speroff L, Gass RH, Kase NG. *Clinical Gynecologic Endocrinology and Infertility*. 6th ed. Baltimore: Lippincott Williams & Wilkins; 1999.

86. Cutson TM. Managing Menopause. *Am Fam Physician*. 2000;61:1391–1400. 1405-1406.

87. AltMedDex: Menopause protocol, MICROMEDEX(R) Healthcare Series, 116 6/2003.

88. Rymer J, Morris EP. Extracts from clinical evidence: menopausal symptoms. *BMJ*. 2002;321:1516–1519.

89. Fantl JA, Bump RC, Robinson D, et al. Efficacy of estrogen supplementation in the treatment of urinary incontinence. The Continence Program for Women Research Group. *Obstet Gynecol*. 1996;88:745–749.

90. Rymer J, Wilson R, Ballard K. Making decisions about hormone replacement therapy. *BMJ*. 2003;326:322–326.

91. https://www.iofbonehealth.org/facts-statistics#category-14

92. Prestwood KM, Kenny AM. Osteoporosis: pathogenesis, diagnosis, and treatment in older adults. *Clin Geriatr Med.* 1998;14:577–599.

93. Christiansen C, Christensen MS, Transbol I. Bone mass in postmenopausal women after withdrawal of oestrogen/gestagen replacement therapy. *Lancet.* 1981;1:459–461.

94. Torgerson DJ, Bell-Syer SE. Hormone replacement therapy and prevention of nonvertebral fractures: a meta-analysis of randomized trials. *JAMA.* 2001;285(22):2891–2897.

95. Writing Group for the 18 Investigators. Risks and benefits of estrogen plus progestin in healthy post-menopausal women: principal results from the Women's Health Initiative randomized controlled trial. *JAMA.* 2002;288(3):321–333.

96. Gruenwald J. *Physicians Desk Reference for Herbal Medicines.* 1st ed. Montvale, NJ: Medical Economics; 1999.

97. Lieberman UA, Weiss SR, Broll J, et al. Effect of oral alendronate on bone mineral density and the incidence of fractures in postmenopausal osteoporosis. The Alendronate Phase III Osteoporosis Treatment Study Group. *NEJM.* 1995;333:1437–1443.

98. Hulley S, Grady D, Bush T, et al. Randomized trial of estrogen plus progestin for secondary prevention of coronary heart disease in postmenopausal women. Heart and Estrogen/Progestin Replacement Study (HERS) Research Group. *JAMA.* 1998;280:605–613.

99. Grady D, Wenger NK, Herrington D, et al. Postmenopausal hormone replacement therapy increases risk for venous thromboembolism disease: the heart and estrogen/progestin replacement study. *Ann Intern Med.* 2000;132:689–696.

100. Daly E, Vessey MP, Hawkins MM, et al. Risk of venous thromboembolism in users of HRT. *Lancet.* 1996;348:977–980.

101. Faulkner DL, Young C, Hutchins D, McCollam JS. Patient noncompliance with hormone replacement therapy: a nationwide estimate using a large prescription claims database. *Menopause.* 1998;5:226–229.

102. Berman RS. Patient compliance of women taking estrogen replacement therapy. *Drug Information J.* 1997;31:71–83.

103. Newton KM, LaCroix AZ, Leveille SG, et al. Women's beliefs and decisions about hormone replacement therapy. *J Women's Health.* 1997;6:459–465.

104. Ettinger B, Li D, Klein R. Unexpected vaginal bleeding and associated gynecologic care in postmenopausal women using hormone replacement therapy. *Fertil Steril.* 1998;69:865–869.

105. Hunter MS, O'Dea I, Britten N. Decision making and hormone replacement: a qualitative analysis. *Soc Sci Med.* 1997;45:1541–1548.

106. Ravnikar VA. Compliance with hormone therapy. *Am J Obstet Gynecol.* 1998;156:1332–1334.

107. Cox D. Should a doctor prescribe hormone replacement therapy which has been manufactured from mare's urine? *J Med Ethics.* 1996;22:199.

108. Thiedke C, Menopause. *Clin Fam Pract.* 2002;4(4):985.

109. Wright JV, Morgenthaler J. *Natural Hormone Replacement.* Petaluma, CA: Smart Publications; 1997.

110. Schiff I, Tulchinsky D, Cramer D, et al. Oral medroxyprogesterone in the treatment of postmenopausal symptoms. *JAMA.* 1980;244:1443–1445.

111. Morrison JC, Martin DC, Blair RA, et al. The use of medroxyprogesterone acetate for relief of climacteric symptoms. *Am J Obstet Gynecol.* 1980;138:99–104.

112. Apgar BS. Using progestins in clinical practice. *Am Fam Physician.* 2002;62(8):1839–1846. 1849-1850.

113. Ottosson UB, Johansson BG, von Schoultz B. Subfractions of high-density lipoprotein cholesterol during estrogen replacement therapy. *Am J Obstet Gynecol.* 1985;151:746–750.

114. Writing Group for the PEPI Trial. Effects of estrogen or estrogen/progestin regimens on heart disease risk factors in postmenopausal women. The Postmenopausal Estrogen/Progestin Interventions (PEPI) Trial. *JAMA.* 1995;273:199–208. [erratum appears in JAMA 274:1676, 1995].

115. Taylor M. Alternatives to conventional hormone replacement therapy. *Comp Ther.* 1997;23:514–532.

116. Cooper A, Spencer C, Whitehead MI, et al. Systemic absorption of progesterone from Pro-Gest cream in postmenopausal women. *Lancet.* 1998;351:1255–1256.

117. Leonetti HB, Longo S, Anasti JN. Transdermal progesterone cream for vasomotor symptoms and postmenopausal bone loss. *Obstet Gynecol.* 1999;94(2):225–228.

118. Porter M, Penney GC, Russell D, et al. A population based survey of women's experience of the menopause. *Br J Obstet Gynaecol.* 1996:1025–1028.

119. Liu J, Burdette JE, Xu H, et al. Evaluation of estrogenic activity of plant extracts for the potential treatment of menopausal symptoms. *J Agric Food Chem.* 2001;49(5):2472–2479.

120. Zava DT, Dollbaum CM, Blen M. Estrogen and progestin bioactivity of foods, herbs, and spices. *Proc Soc Exp Biol Med.* 1998;217(3):369–378.

121. Hale GE, Hughes CL, et al. A double-blind randomized study on the effects of red clover isoflavones on the endometrium. *Menopause.* 2001;8(5):338–346.

122. Rosenberg Zand RS, Jenkins DJ, Diamandis EP. Effects of natural products and nutraceuticals on steroid hormone-regulated gene expression. *Clin Chim Acta.* 2001:213–219.

123. Baker RJ, Templeman CMT, et al. Randomized placebo-controlled trial of an isoflavone supplement and menopausal symptoms in women. *Climacteric.* 1999:85–92.

124. Knight DC, Howes JB, Eden JA. The effect of Promensil, an isoflavone extract, on menopausal symptoms. *Climacteric.* 1999;2(2):79–84.

125. Nestel PJ, Pomeroy S, Kay S, et al. Isoflavones from red clover improve systemic arterial compliance but not plasma lipids in menopausal women. *J Clin Endocrinol Metab.* 1999;84:898.

126. Hidalgo LA, Chedraui PA, Morocho N, et al. The effect of red clover isoflavones on menopausal symptoms, lipids and vaginal cytology in menopausal women: a randomized, double-blind placebo-controlled study. *Gynecol Endocrinol.* 2005;21(5):257–264.

127. Low Dog T. Menopause: a review of botanical dietary supplements. *Am J Med.* 2005;118(12 suppl 2):98–108.

128. Nelson HD, Vesco KK, Haney E, et al. Nonhormonal therapies for menopausal hot flashes: systematic review and meta-analysis. *JAMA.* 2006;295(17):2057–2071.

129. Fetrow CW, Avila JR. *Professional's Handbook of Complementary and Alternative Medicines.* Springhouse, PA: Springhouse; 1999.

130. Newall C, Anderson LA, Phillipson JD. *Herbal Medicines: A Guide for Health Care Professionals.* London: The Pharmaceutical Press; 1996.

131. Hirata JD, Swiersz LM, Zell B, et al. Does dong quai have estrogenic effects in postmenopausal women? A double-blind placebo-controlled trial. *Fertil Steril.* 1997;68:981–986.

132. Murray M. Cimicifuga extract Black Cohosh: a natural alternative to estrogen for menopause. *Health Counselor* 8:36–37.

133. Blumenthal M. *The complete German Commission E monographs; therapeutic guide to herbal medicines.* Austin: American Botanical Council; 1998.

134. Liske E. Therapeutic efficacy and safety of Cimicifuga racemosa for gynecologic disorders. *Adv Ther.* 1998;15:45–53.

135. Zierau O, Bodinet C, Kolba S, et al. Antiestrogenic activities of Cimicifuga racemosa extracts. *J Steroid Biochem Mol Biol.* 2002;80(1):25–30.

136. Bodinet C, Freudenstein J. Influence of Cimicifuga racemosa on the proliferation of estrogen receptor-positive human breast cancer cells. *Breast Cancer Research Treatment.* 2002;76(1):1–10.

137. Hernandez Munoz G, Pluchino S. Cimicifuga racemosa for the treatment of hot flashes in women surviving breast cancer. *Maturitas.* 2003;44(suppl 1):S59–S65.

138. Davis VL, et al. *American Association for Cancer Research annual meeting.* July 11-14, 2003. Washington, D.C., abstract #R910.

139. Pockaj BA, Loprinzi CL, Sloan JA, et al. Pilot evaluation of black cohosh for the treatment of hot flashes in women. *Cancer Invest.* 2004;22(4):215–521.

140. Foster S. Black cohosh, Cimicifuga racemosa, a literature review. *Herbalgram.* 1999:35–49.

141. Gruenwald J: Standardized black cohosh extract clinical monograph, *Quart Rev Nat Med.* 98:117–125.

142. Stolze H. The other way to treat symptoms of menopause. *Gynecology.* 1982;1.

143. Cmiicifuga and Hypericum for Menopause. *Br J Phytotherapy.* 1995;4:96.

144. Vorberg G. Treatment of menopause symptoms. *ZFA.* 1984;60:626.

145. Warnecke G. Using phyto-treatment to influence menopause symptoms. *Med Welt.* 1985;36.

146. Stoll W. Phytotherapy influences atrophic vaginal epithelium. *Therapeutikon.* 1987;1.

147. Liske E, et al. Therapy of climacteric complaints with Cimicifuga racemosa: herbal medicine with clinically proven evidence. *Menopause.* 1998;4:250.

148. Lehmann-Willenbrock E, Riedel HH. Clinical and endocrinologic studies of the treatment of ovarian insufficiency manifestations following hysterectomy with intact adnexa. *Zentralbl Gynakol.* 1998;110:611–618.

149. Wuttke W, Seidlova-Wuttke D, Gorkow C. The Cimicifuga preparation BNO 1055 vs. conjugated estrogens in a double-blind placebo-controlled study: effects on menopause symptoms and bone markers. *Maturitas.* 2003;44(suppl 1):S67–S77.

150. Vermes G, Banhidy F, Acs N. The effects of Remifemin on subjective symptoms of menopause. *Adv Ther.* 2005;22(2):148–154.

151. Osmers R, Friede M, Liske E, et al. Efficacy and safety of isopropanolic black cohosh extract for climacteric symptoms. *Obstet Gynecol.* 2005;105(5 pt 1):1074–1083.

152. Geller SE, Studee L. Botanical and dietary supplements for menopausal symptoms: what works, what does not. *J Health (Larchmt).* 2005;14(7):634–649.

153. Mahady GB. Black cohosh (Actaea/Cimicifuga racemosa): review of the clinical data for safety and efficacy in menopausal symptoms. *Treat Endocrinol.* 2005;4(3):177–184.

154. Low Dog T. *Herbal Medicine: Women's Health, Dermatology and Cardiology.* Holyoke: Lecture; March 28, 2003.

155. Huntley A. The safety of black cohosh (Actaea racemosa, Cimicifuga racemosa). *Expert Opin Drug Saf.* 2004;3(6):615–623.

156. Schaper, Brummer GmbH, Co KG. *Remifemin scientific brochure.* Salzgitter: Schaper & Brummer; 1997.

157. Levitsky J, Alli TA, Wisecarver J, et al. Fulminant liver failure associated with the use of black cohosh. *Dig Dis Sci.* 2005;50(3):538–539.

158. Minciullo PL, Saija A, Patafi M, et al. Muscle damage induced by black cohosh (Cimicifuga racemosa). *Phytomedicine.* 2006;13(1-2):115–118.

159. Chenoy R, Hussain S, Tayob Y, et al. Effect of oral gamolenic acid from evening primrose oil on menopausal flashing. *BMJ.* 1994;308:501–503.

160. Kuppurajen K, Srinivasan K, Janak K. A double-blind study of the effect of Mandukapami on the general mental ability of normal children. *J Res Ind Med Yog Homeopath.* 1978;13:37–41.

161. Lindgren R, Mattsson L-A, Meier W, et al. *Has Ginsana G 115 estrogenic effects when measured by maturity index, plasma FSH and estradiol?* Boston, MA: North American Menopause Society 8th Annual Meeting; Sept 4–6, 1997. Abstract S7.

162. Wiklund IK, Mattsson LA, Lindgren R, et al. Effects of a standardized ginseng extract on quality of life and physiological parameters in symptomatic postmenopausal women: a double-blind placebo-controlled trial, Swedish Alternative Medicine Group. *Int J Clin Pharmacol Res.* 1999;19(3):89–99.

163. AltMedDex, Panax Ginseng, MICROMEDEX(R) Healthcare Series, Vol. 116 6/2003.

164. Greenspan EM. Ginseng and vaginal bleeding. *JAMA.* 1983;249:2018.

165. Punnonen R, Lukola A. Oestrogen-like effect of ginseng. *BMJ.* 1980;281:1110.

166. Hopkins MP, Androff L, Benninghoff AS. Ginseng face cream and unexplained vaginal bleeding. *Am J Obstet Gynecol.* 1988;159:1121–1122.

167. Knight DC, Eden JA. A review of the clinical effects of phytoestrogens. *Obstet Gynecol.* 1996;87:897–904.

168. Murkies AL, Lombard C, Strauss BJ, et al. Dietary flour supplementation decreases post-menopausal hot flashes: effect of soy and wheat. *Maturitas.* 1995;21:189–195.

169. Scambia G, Mango D, Signorile PG, et al. Clinical effects of a standardized soy extract in postmenopausal women: a pilot study. *Menopause.* 2000;7:105–111.

170. Albertazzi P, Pansini F, Bonaccorsi G, et al. The effect of dietary soy supplementation on hot flashes. *Obstet Gynecol.* 1998;91:6–11.

171. Han KK, Soares JM, Haidar MA, et al. Benefits of soy isoflavone therapeutic regimen on menopausal symptoms. *Obstet Gynecol.* 2002;99:389–394.

172. Baird DD, Umbach DM, Lansdell L, et al. Dietary intervention study to assess estrogenicity of dietary soy among postmenopausal women. *J Clin Endocrinol Metab.* 1995;80:1685–1690.

173. Krebs EE, Ensrud KE, MacDonald R, et al. Phytoestrogens for treatment of menopausal symptoms: a systematic review. *Obstet Gynecol.* 2004;104(4):824–836.

174. Huntley AL, Ernst E. Soy for the treatment of perimenopausal symptoms—a systematic review. *Maturitas.* 2004;47(1):1–9.

175. Collins A, Landren BM. Experience of symptoms during transition to menopause: a population-based longitudinal study. In: *The modern management of menopause, a perspective for the 21(st) century: Proceedings of the VII International Congress on Menopause, Stockholm.* New York: Parthenon Books; 1993:1994.

176. Ivarsson T, Spetz AC, Hammar M. Physical exercise and vasomotor symptoms in postmenopausal women. *Maturitas.* 1998;29:139–146.

177. Freedman RR, Woodward S. Behavioral treatment of menopausal hot flashes: evaluated by ambulatory monitoring. *Am J Obstet Gynecol.* 1992;167:4346–4349.

178. Dawson-Hughes B, Dallal G, Krall L, et al. Effect of vitamin D supplementation on wintertime and overall bone loss in healthy postmenopausal women. *Ann Int Med.* 1991;115:505.

179. Reid IR. The role of calcium and vitamin D in the prevention of osteoporosis. *Endocrinol Metab Clin North Am.* 1998;27:389–398.

180. Tucker K, Hannan M, Chen H, et al. Potassium, magnesium, and fruit and vegetable intakes are associated with greater bone mineral density in elderly men and women. *Am J Clin Nutr.* 1999;69:727–736.

Note: Pages followed by "*b*", "*t*", and "*f*" refer to boxes, tables, and figures respectively.

623